Management of Acute Kidney Problems

Achim Jörres
Claudio Ronco
John A. Kellum (Eds.)

Management of Acute Kidney Problems

Springer

Achim Jörres, MD
Professor of Medicine
Deputy Director
Chief, Department of Nephrology and
Medical Intensive Care
Charité University Hospital
Campus Virchow-Klinikum
Augustenburger Platz 1
13353 Berlin
Germany
achim.joerres@charite.de

Claudio Ronco, MD
St. Bortolo Hospital
Director, Department of Nephrology
Dialysis and Transplantation
Viale Rodolfi, 16
36100 Vicenza
Italy
claudioronco@ulssvicenza.it

John A. Kellum Jr., MD, FACP, FCCM
Professor of Critical Care Medicine,
University of Pittsburgh
School of Medicine
Department Critical Care Medicine
3550 Terrace Street, 606 Scaife Hall
Pittsburgh, PA 15261
USA
kellumja@ccm.upmc.edu

ISBN: 978-3-662-50155-9 ISBN: 978-3-540-69441-0 (eBook)

DOI: 10.1007/978-3-540-69441-0

Springer Heidelberg Dordrecht London New York

Cover design: Frido Steinen-Broo, eStudio Calamar, Figueres/Berlin

Printed on acid-free paper

Springer is part of Springer Science+Business Media (www.springer.com)

To Dinah, Marc, and Ann-Kristin; you are always at the center of my heart and my thoughts.

Achim

To my wife, Paola, who gives true meaning to all my efforts.

Claudio

To my sister, Janine, whose tireless care at the bedside of critically ill patients has made a world of difference and reminds me that all intensive care nurses are our great unsung heroes.

John

Preface

Acute kidney disease (from injury to failure) is an important clinical area particularly in the intensive care unit setting. As many as two thirds of critically ill patients experience an episode of acute kidney injury during the course of their illness, and about 5% of patients admitted to an intensive care unit will eventually require renal replacement therapy. In these patients, in-hospital mortality is extremely high, exceeding 50%, with acute kidney failure constituting a significant independent risk factor for death.

As intensive care practitioners are often the initial or even sole providers of care to seriously ill patients at risk for acute kidney injury, it is their responsibility to ensure that adequate measures to prevent its occurrence are taken. Moreover, it is their task to diagnose and evaluate incipient acute kidney disease, to initiate optimal supportive care, and where possible, definitive treatment of this disorder.

It is the editors' hope that this book will provide a reference for clinicians practicing in the intensive care unit, to help guide their care of patients with acute kidney disease. In addition, we would like to address clinicians from many other fields who are regularly involved in the care of patients at risk for acute kidney injury. To that end we have brought together a group of international authors to cover the most recent information on definition, epidemiology, pathophysiology, and clinical causes of acute kidney injury and failure. Their understanding is a fundamental prerequisite for the prevention of this disorder. Moreover, the earlier parts of this book present differential diagnostic approaches for patients with acute kidney disease and a detailed outline of important measures for its clinical management and the prevention of complications. The subsequent parts are dedicated to the diagnosis and management of acute kidney disease in specific patient groups and in particular disorders. Finally, the various key aspects related to the adequate delivery of acute renal replacement therapy are detailed in the final parts of the book.

The chapters included in this book are derived from clinical experience and report the evidence for current clinical practice extracted from consensus statements or systematic analyses of the literature. We are truly indebted to the authors for their timely and expert contributions. We very much hope that the present book will be a tool for clinicians and a reference for investigators, students, and fellows.

The enormous effort of putting together such compilation of information and references should stimulate all colleagues to use this book as a starting point for good clinical practice that will certainly be enriched day by day in the coming months and years, by the expanding body of literature that the field of acute kidney disease requires and also as a resource for continuous progress toward better care for our patients.

Berlin, Germany — Achim Jörres
Vicenza, Italy — Claudio Ronco
Pittsburgh, Pennsylvania, USA — John A. Kellum

Contents

Part VI Diagnosis and Management of Specific Disorders

Contributors

Tariq Ali Kent and Canterbury Hospital, Ethelbert Road, Canterbury, Kent CT1 3NG, UK
tariq.ali@nhs.net

Robert J. Anderson Department of Medicine, University of Colorado, Health Science Center, 4200 East 9th Avenue., Denver, CO 80262, USA
robert.anderson@uchsc.edu

Sean M. Bagshaw Division of Critical Care Medicine, University of Alberta Hospital, University of Alberta, 3C1.12 Walter C. Mackenzie Centre, 8440–112 Street, Edmonton, Alberta T6G 2B7, Canada
bagshaw@ualberta.ca

Shweta Bansal University of Colorado, School of Medicine, 4200 East 9th Avenue C281, Denver, CO 80262, USA
shweta.bansal@uchsc.edu

Richard J. Baker Department of Renal Medicine, St James's University Hospital, Beckett Street, Leeds, LS9 7TF, UK
richard.baker@leedsth.nhs.uk

Rashad S. Barsoum Cairo University, Cairo Kidney Center, 3 Hussein El-Memar Street, Antique Khana, P.O. Box 91, Bab El-Louk, Cairo 11513, Egypt
rashad.barsoum@gmail.com

Rinaldo Bellomo Department of Intensive Care, Austin Hospital, Studley Rd, Heidelberg, Victoria 3084, Australia
rinaldo.bellomo@austin.org.au

Mourad Benyamina Burn ICU, Department of Emergency Medicine and ICU, Cochin Hospital, Assistance Publique – Hôpitaux de Paris, Paris Descartes University, Paris, France

Thomas Berg Hepatology & Gastroenterology, Charité-Universitätsmedizin Berlin, Campus Virchow-Klinikum, Augustenburger Platz 1, 13353, Berlin, Germany
thomas.berg@charite.de

Daniela Bergamo Department of Internal Medicine, Division of Nephrology and Dialysis, CTO Hospital, Turin, Italy

Annette Beyea Departments of Medicine and Anesthesiology, Dartmouth-Hitchcock Medical Center, One Medical Center Drive, Lebanon, NH 03756, USA

Joseph V. Bonventre Brigham and Women's Hospital, Renal Division, 75 Francis Street, Boston, MA 02115, USA
jbonventre@partners.org

David J. Border Department of Renal Medicine, York Hospital, Wigginton Road, York YO31 8HE, England,
david.border@york.nhs.uk

Marie L. Borum Division of Gastroenterology and Liver Diseases, George Washington University, 2150 Pennsylvania Avenue, NW, Suite 3-408, Washington, DC 20037, USA
mborum@mfa.gwu.edu

Josée Bouchard Department of Medicine, Division of Nephrology, University of California, San Diego, CA 92103, USA
joseebouchard123@yahoo.ca

Raf Brouns Memory Clinic, Department of Neurology, Middelheim General Hospital, Antwerp, Belgium and Laboratory of Neurochemistry and Behaviour, Institute Born-Bunge, University of Antwerp, Belgium

David F. M. Brown Department of Emergency Medicine, Massachusetts General Hospital, 55 Fruit St., Boston, MA 02114-2696, USA
dbrown2@partners.org

Bernard Canaud Nephrology, Dialysis & Intensive Care Unit, Renal Research and Training Institute, Lapeyronie University Hospital, CHU Montpellier, 34295 Montpellier, France
b-canaud@chu-montpellier.fr

Barbara Ceradini Department of Intensive Care, Erasme Hospital, Université libre de Bruxelles, 808, route de Lennik, 1070-Brussels, Belgium

Leila Chenine Nephrology, Dialysis & Intensive Care, Lapeyronie Hospital, Montpellier Cedex, France

Howard L. Corwin Departments of Medicine and Anesthesiology, Dartmouth-Hitchcock Medical Center, One Medical Center Drive, Lebanon, NH 03756, USA
howard.l.corwin@hitchcock.org

Angela D'Angelo Università di Padova, CNR, Via Giustiniani, 2 35128 Padova, Italy
angela.dangelo@unipd.it

Joseph F. Dasta The Ohio State University, College of Pharmacy, University of Texas, College of Pharmacy, P.O. Box 967, Hutto, TX 78634-0967, USA
dasta@mail.utexas.edu

Andrew Davenport Royal Free Hospital, Pond Street, London NW3 2QG , UK
andrew.davenport@royalfree.nhs.uk

Peter Paul De Deyn Department of Neurology and Memory Clinic, Middelheim General Hospital, Lindenreef 1, 2020 Antwerp, Belgium
peter.dedeyn@ua.ac.be

An S. De Vriese The Renal Unit, AZ Sint-Jan AV, Ruddershove, 10, 8000 Brugge, Belgium
an.devriese@azbrugge.be

Dorella Del Prete Universitá di Padova, CNR, Via Giustiniani 2, 35128 Padova, Italy

Wilfred Druml Department of Medicine III, Division of Nephrology, Vienna General Hospital, Währinger Gürtel 18–20, 1090 Vienna, Austria
wilfred.druml@meduniwien.ac.at

Duska Dragun Department of Nephrology and Intensive Care Medicine, Charité Campus Virchow-Klinikum, 13343 Berlin, Germany

Pieter Evenepoel Department of Nephrology, University Hospital Gasthuisberg, Herestraat 49, 3000 Leuven, Belgium
Pieter.evenepoel@uz.kuleuven.ac.be

Ken Farrington Renal Unit, Lister Hospital, Corey Mill Lane, Stevenage, SG 14AB, UK
ken.farrington@nbs.net

Donald A. Feinfeld Division of Nephrology & Hypertension, Department of Medicine, Beth Israel Medical Center, 350 17th Street, 18BH20, New York, NY 10003, USA

Danilo Fliser Division of Renal and Hypertensive Disease, Department of Internal Medicine, Saarland University Centre, Kirrberger Strasse, 66421 Homburg/Saar, Germany
indfli@uks.eu

Miriam Galbusera Clinical Research Center for Rare Diseases "Aldo e Cele Daccò", Mario Negri Institute for Pharmacological Research, 24125 Bergamo, Italy

Ezio Nicola Gangemi Department of Plastic Surgery, Burns Unit, CTO Hospital, Turin, Italy
indfli@uks.eu

Herwig Gerlach Department of Anesthesia, Intensive Care Medicine, and Pain Management, Vivantes–Klinikum Neukölln, Klinik fuer Anaesthesie, Operative Intensivmedizin und Schmerztherapie, Rudower Strasse 48, 12313 Berlin, Germany
herwig.gerlach@vivantes.de

Griet Glorieux Nephrology Unit, Department of Internal Medicine, University Hospital, Gent University, De pintelaan 185, 9000 Gent, Belgium

Stuart L. Goldstein Baylor College of Medicine, Medical Director, Renal Dialysis Unit and Pheresis Service, Texas Children's Hospital, 6621 Fannin Street, MC 3-2482, Houston, Texas 77054, USA
stuartg@bcm.tmc.edu

Jan Gunst Department of Intensive Care Medicine, University Hospitals, University of Leuven, Herestraat 49, 3000 Leuven, Belgium
jan_gunst@hotmail.com

Michael Haase Department of Nephrology and Intensive Care Medicine, Charité Campus Virchow-Klinikum, 13343 Berlin, Germany
michael.haase@charite.de

Anja Haase-Fielitz Department of Nephrology and Intensive Care Medicine, Charité University Medicine, Humboldt University Berlin, Berlin, Germany

Nikolas B. Harbord Albert Einstein College of Medicine, Bronx, New York, USA

Dietrich Hasper Nephrology & Medical Intensive Care, Charité-Universitätsmedizin Berlin, Campus Virchow-Klinikum, 13353, Berlin, Germany
dietrich.hasper@charite.de

Delphine Henriet Nephrology, Dialysis & Intensive Care Unit, Renal Research and Training Institute, Lapeyronie University Hospital, CHU Montpellier, 34295 Montpellier, France

Zsuzsanna Hollo Department of Area of Medicine, Division of Nephrology and Dialysis, CTO Hospital, Turin, Italy

Eric A. J. Hoste Department of Intensive Care Medicine, 2K12-C, Gent University Hospital, De pintelaan 185, 9000 Gent, Belgium
eric.hoste@ugent.be

Todd S. Ing Department of Nephrology, Loyola University Medical Center, 2160 First Avenue, Maywood, IL 60153, USA
todding@att.net

Hassane Izzedine Department of Nephrology, La Pitié-Salpêtrière Hospital, 47-80 Boulevard de l'Hôpital, Assistance Publique-Hopitaux de Paris, Pierre et Marie Curie University, 75013 Paris, France
hassan.izzedine@psl.aphp.fr

Michael Joannidis Medical Intensive Care Unit, Department of General Internal Medicine, Medical University Innsbruck, Anichstrasse 35, 6020 Innsbruck, Austria

Achim Jörres Department of Nephrology and Medical Intensive Care, Charite University Hospital Campus Virchow-Klinikum, Augustenburger Platz 1, 13353 Berlin, Germany
achim.joerres@charite.de

Dinah Jörres Department of Anaesthesiology and Intensive Care Medicine, Charité University Campus Virchow-Klinikum, Augustenburger Platz 1, 13353 Berlin, Germany
dinah.joerres@charite.de

Sandra L. Kane-Gill University of Pittsburgh School of Pharmacy, 918 Salk Hall, 3501 Terrace St., Pittsburgh, PA 15261, USA
slk54@pitt.edu

Vijay Karajala CRISMA Laboratory, Department of Ciritical Care Medicine, University of Pittsburgh, 3550 Terrace Street, Pittsburgh, PA 15261, USA
karajalavs@upmc.edu

John A. Kellum Department of Critical Care Medicine, University of Pittsburgh, 608 Scaife Hall, 3550 Terrace Street, Pittsburgh, PA 15261, USA
kellumja@ccm.upmc.edu

Jan T. Kielstein Division of Nephrology and Hypertension, Department of Internal Medicine, Medical School Hannover, Carl-Neuberg-Straße 1, 30625 Hannover, Germany
kielstein@yahoo.com

Detlef H. Krieter University Hospital Würzburg, Department of Medicine, Division of Nephrology, Josef-Schneider-Strasse 2, 97080 Würzburg, Germany
krieter_d@medizin.uni-wuerzburg.de

Norbert Lameire Nephrology Unit, Department of Internal Medicine, University Hospital, Gent University, 4K4, NDT-COMGAN Office, De pintelaan 185, 9000 Gent, Belgium
norbert.lameire@ugent.be

Martine Leblanc University of Montreal, Nephrology and Critical Care, Maisonneuve-Rosemont Hospital, 5415 boulevard de l'Assomption, Montreal, QC H1T 2M4, Canada
martine.leblanc@sympatico.ca

Hélène Leray-Moragués Nephrology, Dialysis & Intensive Care Unit, Renal Research and Training Institute, Lapeyronie University Hospital, CHU Montpellier, 34295 Montpellier, France

Susie Q. Lew Division of Renal Diseases and Hypertension, George Washington University, 2150 Pennsylvania Avenue, NW, Suite 1-200, Washington, DC 20037, USA
sqlew@gwu.edu

Andrew Liteplo Department of Emergency Medicine, Zero Emerson #3B, Massachusetts General Hospital, 55 Fruit St., Boston, MA 02114, USA

Wai-Kei Lo Department of Medicine, Tung Wah Hospital, 12 Po Yan Street, Hong Kong
wkloc@hkucc.hku.hk

Sing-Leung Lui Department of Medicine, Tung Wah Hospital, 12 Po Yan Street, Hong Kong
sllui@hkucc.hku.hk

Filippo Mariano Department of Internal Medicine, Division of Nephrology and Dialysis, CTO Hospital, Via G. Zurreti 29, 10126 Turin, Italy
filippo.mariano@cto.to.it

Roy Mathew Division of Nephrology, Department of Medicine, University of California, San Diego, CA 92103, USA
roy.rom75@gmail.com

Peter A. McCullough Division of Nutrition and Preventive Medicine, William Beaumont Hospital, 4949 Coolidge Highway, Royal Oak, MI 48073, USA
pmc975@yahoo.com

Ravindra L. Mehta Division of Nephrology, Department of Medicine, University of California, San Diego, CA 92103, USA
rmehta@ucsd.edu

Philipp G.H. Metnitz Department of Anesthesiology and General Intensive Care, University Hospital of Vienna, Währinger Gürtel 18-20, 1090 Vienna, Austria
philipp@metnitz.biz

Bruce A. Mueller Department of Clinical, Social and Administrative Sciences, College of Pharmacy, University of Michigan, 428 Church Street, Ann Arbor, MI 48109–1065, USA
muellerb@umich.edu

Nathalie Neirynck The Renal Unit, University Hospital Gent, Gent, Belgium

Vicki E. Noble Department of Emergency Medicine, Zero Emerson #3B, Massachusetts General Hospital, 55 Fruit St., Boston, MA 02114, USA
vnoble@partners.org

Marina Noris Clinical Research Center for Rare Diseases "Aldo e Cele Daccò", Mario Negri Institute for Pharmacological Research, 24125 Bergamo, Italy

Michael Oppert Nephrology & Medical Intensive Care, Charité Campus Virchow-Klinikum, 13343 Berlin, Germany
oppert@charite.de

Michael R. Pinsky Department of Critical Care Medicine, University of Pittsburgh, 606 Scaife Hall, 3550 Terrace Street, Pittsburgh, PA 15261, USA
pinskymr@upmc.edu

Isabelle Plamondon University of Montreal, Nephrology and Critical Care, Maisonneuve-Rosemont Hospital, Montreal, P.Q., Canada

Gesine Pless Klinik für Allgemein-, Visceral- und Transplantationschirurgie, Experimentelle Chirurgie und Regenerative Medizin, Charité – Campus Virchow, Universitätsmedizin Berlin, Augustenburger Platz 1, 13353 Berlin, Germany

Jai Prakash Department of Nephrology, Institute of Medical Sciences, Banaras Hindu University, Varanasi-221005, India
jpojha555@hotmail.com; jprakash53@gmail.com

John R. Prowle Department of Intensive Care, Austin Hospital, Melbourne, Victoria 3084, Australia

Ana Reiter Department of Anesthesiology and General Intensive Care, University Hospital of Vienna, Vienna, Austria

Giuseppe Remuzzi Clinical Research Center for Rare Diseases "Aldo e Cele Daccò", Mario Negri Institute for Pharmacological Research, Bergamo, Via Gavazzeni, 11, 24125 Bergamo, Italy
gremuzzi@marionegri.it

Zaccaria Ricci Department of Pediatric Cardiosurgery, Bambino Gesù Hospital, Piazza S. Onofrio 4, 00100 Rome, Italy
zaccaria.ricci@fastwebnet.it

Paul Roderick Public Health Sciences and Medical Statistics, C Floor, South Academic Block, Southampton General Hospital, Southampton SO166YD, UK
pjr@soton.ac.uk

Claudio Ronco Department of Nephrology, Dialysis and Transplantation, S. Bortolo Hospital, Viale Rodolfi 37, 36100 Vicenza, Italy
claudio.ronco@vlssvicenza.it

Herman Rosen Division of Nephrology and Hypertension, Beth Israel Medical Center, New York, NY 10003, USA

Alan D. Salama Renal Section, Division of Medicine, Imperial College London, Hammersmith Hospital, Du Cane Road, London W12 0NN, UK
a.salama@imperial.ac.uk

Igor Maximilian Sauer Department of Surgery, Charité Campus Virchow, Augustenburger Platz 1, 13353 Berlin, Germany
igor.sauer@charite.de

Jörg Christian Schefold Department of Nephrology and Medical Intensive Care, Charité-Universitätsmedizin Berlin, Campus Virchow-Klinikum, 13343 Berlin, Germany
joerg.schefold@charite.de

Miet Schetz Department of Intensive Care Medicine, University Hospitals, University of Leuven, Herestraat 49, 3000 Leuven, Belgium
marie.schetz@uz.kuleuven.be

Ralf Schindler Department of Nephrology and Intensive Care Medicine, Charité, Campus Virchow-Klinikum, Augustenburger Platz 1, 13353 Berlin, Germany
ralf.schindler@charite.de

Robert W. Schrier University of Colorado School of Medicine, 4200 East Ninth Avenue, B173, Biomedical Research Building, Room 723, Denver, CO 80262, USA
robert.schrier@uchsc.edu

Maurizio Stella Department of Plastic Surgery, Burns Unit, CTO Hospital, Turin, Italy

Mathavakkannan Suresh Renal Unit, Lister Hospital, Corey Mill Lane, Stevenage, SG 14AB, UK

Mehmet Sükrü Sever Department of Internal Medicine/Nephrology, Istanbul School of Medicine, Millet caddesi, Çapa Topkapi TR 34390, Istanbul, Turkey
severm@hotmail.com

Jordan M. Symons Division of Nephrology, Children's Hospital and Regional Medical Center, Department of Pediatrics, University of Washington School of Medicine, 4800 Sand Point Way NE, Seattle, WA 98105–0371, USA
jordan.symons@seattlechildrens.org

Susanne Toussaint Department of Anesthesia, Intensive Care Medicine, and Pain Management, Vivantes – Klinikum Neukölln, Klinik fuer Anaesthesie, Operative Intensivmedizin und Schmerztherapie, Rudower Strasse 48, 12313 Berlin, Germany
susanne.toussaint@vivantes.de

Giorgio Triolo Department of Internal of Medicine, Division of Nephrology and Dialysis, CTO Hospital, Turin, Italy

Pallavi Tyagi Private Practice, Singapore

Shigehiko Uchino Intensive Care Unit, Department of Anesthesiology, Jikei University School of Medicine, 3-19-18, Nishi-Shinbashi, Minato-ku, Tokyo 105–8471, Japan
s.uchino@jikei.ac.jp

Wim Van Biesen Renal Division, Department of Internal Medicine, University Hospital Gent, ICU De pintelaan 185, 9000 Gent, Belgium
wim.vanbiesen@ugent.be

Greet Van den Berghe Department of Intensive Care Medicine, University Hospitals, University of Leuven, Herestraat 49, 30000 Leuven, Belgium
greet.vandenberghe@med.kuleuven.be

Bert-Jan H. Van den Born Department of Internal and Vascular Medicine, Academic Medical Centre, Meibergdreef 9, 1105 AZ Amsterdam, The Netherlands
b.j.vandenborn@amc.uva.nl

Gert A. van Montfrans Department of Internal and Vascular Medicine, Academic Medical Centre, Meibergdreef 9, 1105 AZ Amsterdam, The Netherlands

Raymond Vanholder Renal Division, Department of Internal Medicine, University Hospital Gent, De pintelaan 185, 9000 Gent, Belgium
raymond.vanholder@ugent.be

Ilse Vanhorebeek Department of Intensive Care Medicine, University Hospitals, University of Leuven, Herestraat 49, 3000 Leuven, Belgium
ilse.vanhorebeek@med.kuleuven.be

A. Mary Vilay Critical Care Nephrology Research Fellow and Clinical Instructor, Department of Clinical, Social and Administrative Sciences, College of Pharmacy, University of Michigan, 428 Church Street, Ann Arbor, MI 48109–1065, USA
amvilay@umich.edu

Jean-Louis Vincent Department of Intensive Care, Erasme Hospital, Université libre de Bruxelles, 808, route de Lennik, 1070-Brussels, Belgium
jlvincent@ulb.ac.be

Christophe Vinsonneau Department of Intensive Care, Cochin Port-Royal University Hospital, René Descartes University, 75014 Paris, France
christophe.vinsonneau@cch.aphp.fr

Non Wajanaponsan Department of Critical Care Medicine, University of Pittsburgh, 606 Scaife Hall, 3550 Terrace Street, Pittsburgh, PA 15261, USA

Wei Wang University of Colorado, School of Medicine, 4200 East Ninth Avenue C281, Denver, CO 80262, USA

Christoph Wanner University Hospital Würzburg, Department of Medicine, Division of Nephrology, Josef-Schneider-Strasse 2, 97080 Würzburg, Germany
wanner_c@medizin.uni-wuerzburg.de

James F. Winchester Division of Nephrology & Hypertension, Department of Medicine, Beth Israel Medical Center, 350 East 17th Street, 18BH20, New York, NY 10003, USA
jwinches@bethisraelny.org

Terence Pok-Siu Yip Department of Medicine, Tung Wah Hospital, 12 Po Yan Street, Hong Kong
yipterence@gmail.com

Michael Zappitelli McGill University Health Center, Montreal Children's Hospital, 2300 Tupper, Room E-222, Montreal, Quebec, H3J 2S6 Canada
mzaprdr@yahoo.ca

Part I

Definition and Classification of Acute Kidney Failure

Definition and Classification of Acute Kidney Injury

1.1

Vijay Karajala and John A. Kellum

Core Messages

- Appreciation for the clinical meaning of even small changes in kidney function has radically changed the way patients are being cared for. Analogous to chronic kidney *disease* (CKD) in the outpatient arena, acute kidney injury (AKI) is associated with both short- and long-term adverse outcomes in hospitalized patients.
- The RIFLE classification has been validated in multiple studies and may be utilized as a prognostic tool.
- Evaluation of the epidemiology of AKI has been hampered by the lack of a standard definition and classification system. New studies involving multiple, different populations are clarifying the incidence and prevalence of this syndrome. However, the condition appears to be common (approximately 30–50% of critically ill patients) and is associated with a large increase in the risk of death (3–5-fold increase).
- As new treatments for AKI emerge, RIFLE classifications will undoubtedly be used to reference recommendations for prevention and treatment.

J. A. Kellum (✉)
Department of Critical Care Medicine, University of Pittsburgh, 608 Scaife Hall, 3550 Terrace Street, Pittsburgh, PA 15261, USA
e-mail: kellumja@ccm.upmc.edu

1.1.1 Introduction

Acute kidney injury (AKI) is a common condition in hospitalized patients. A standardized definition of AKI is critical to enable clinicians to consistently identify the disorder. Until recently, no consensus definition existed. This chapter describes the new nomenclature of AKI as well as the validated consensus-based RIFLE criteria.

To illustrate the difficulty associated with a lack of standardization in the definition of renal dysfunction, most chapters and review articles on "acute renal failure" begin with words such as "Depending on the definition used and population studied, incidence in critically ill patients is approximately 1–25%." Indeed, there have been more than 35 definitions of acute renal failure in the literature [1–5], and the lack of a standard consensus definition has also been a major impediment to the progress of clinical and basic research in this field [6].

1.1.2 What Is Acute Kidney Injury? Current Controversies

The term "acute renal failure" was introduced by Homer W. Smith [7] in the chapter "Acute Renal Failure Related to Traumatic Injuries" in his textbook "*The Kidney: Structure and Function in Health and Disease*" (1951). Since then the term acute renal failure has been widely used in the medical literature. The excretion of water-soluble solutes and urine production are the result of glomerular filtration, and clinicians have generally equated these functions of the kidney to the glomerular filtration rate (GFR). As a result, most definitions of renal acute failure use indirect estimates

A. Jörres et al. (eds.), *Management of Acute Kidney Problems*,
DOI: 10.1007/978-3-540-69441-0_1.1, © Springer-Verlag Berlin Heidelberg 2010

of GFR (serum creatinine [SCr]), solute clearance (blood urea nitrogen [BUN]), and/or urine output over time. However, this paradigm has serious limitations.

1.1.3 Renal "Failure" or Renal "Success"

Fluid and electrolytes problems are commonly faced in the intensive care unit (ICU) setting. Urine output is an important physiological sign, and fluid imbalance is common in the critically ill due to their inability to drink fluids, excess volume losses, obligatory volume losses, and not least, renal dysfunction. Measurement of BUN and SCr are routinely performed in ICUs to assess renal function. An increase in BUN and SCr is known as azotemia (from "azote" – an old name for nitrogen). Azotemia and oliguria (i.e., decreased urine output) or anuria (i.e., no urine output) together form the cardinal features of renal failure.

Before examining the pathological state of this condition, it will be useful to review the normal renal physiology. The normal kidney functions to remove nitrogenous waste and other solutes, as well as regulate fluid, electrolyte, and acid–base balance. Although it does each of these with remarkable efficiency, there are limits to what the kidney can do when stressed. For example, in the face of severe extracellular fluid depletion, GFR is reduced. This reduction is sometimes called "single-nephron" GFR to distinguish it from the loss of nephrons that occurs with renal disease (e.g., diabetic nephropathy), but it actually refers to all nephrons. The reduced GFR means that a greater fraction of salt and water can be absorbed, and thus, less will enter the tubules. Of course, less tubular filtrate means less urine and less nitrogen excretion. This physiology has also given rise to the observation that some cases of azotemia and oliguria actually represent a perfectly normal response (not failure) and thus "acute renal success" [8].

1.1.4 Oliguria and Anuria

Urine output when severely decreased can be both a reasonably sensitive and functional index for the kidney as well as a biomarker of tubular function or injury; however, this relationship between urine output and renal function/injury is complex. For example, oliguria may be more profound when tubular function is intact. Volume depletion and hypotension are profound stimuli for vasopressin secretion. As a consequence, the distal tubules and collecting ducts become fully permeable to water. Concentrating mechanisms in the inner medulla are also aided by low flow through the loops of Henle, and thus urine volume is minimized and urine concentration maximized (> 500 mOsm/kg). Conversely, when the tubules are injured, maximal concentrating ability is impaired and urine volume may even be normal (i.e., non-oliguric renal failure). Also, in critically ill patients, large doses of diuretics are commonly used, and urine output which would otherwise be used to categorize renal failure loses its diagnostic value in these patients (i.e., poor negative predictive value). Thus, urine output may be adequate in the presence of renal failure and does not necessarily correlate with the severity of renal injury. Furthermore, changes in urine output or GFR are neither essential nor adequate for the accurate diagnosis of renal pathology.

1.1.5 Prerenal Azotemia and Acute Tubular Necrosis

Conventionally, acute renal failure is categorized in terms of physiology into prerenal or postrenal (effecting kidney function secondary to conditions "outside" the kidney, otherwise called "functional" renal failure) and renal (directly injuring the kidney, so-called structural renal failure or acute tubular necrosis [ATN]). This classification was proposed to enhance understanding of the pathophysiology. In reality, however, the mechanisms are not clearly understood, and these mechanisms often overlap and have limited relevance to clinical practice.

The entity "prerenal" is considered as any "before the kidney" process affecting kidney function: for example, acute myocardial infarction and low cardiac output syndrome causing low perfusion states or a patient with major volume loss. This prerenal concept assumes that there is no intrinsic structural kidney injury. However, several logical questions have been posed. It is very difficult to know when functional renal failure becomes structural renal failure. It is also unclear from this definition how much structural injury is necessary to consider it "intrarenal". Although in clinical practice we utilize urine studies (urine creatinine, urine electrolytes, fractional excretion of sodium, tubular casts, etc.) to classify patients as either with prerenal or renal conditions, this urinalysis-based approach has limited validation [9]. Intact tubular function, particularly early on, may be seen with various forms of renal disease. A high volume osmolality coupled with low urine Na^+ in the face of oliguria and azotemia is strong evidence of intact tubular function. Sepsis, the most common condition associated with renal failure in the ICU [10], may alter function without characteristic changes in urine indices. In early post mortem studies of patients who died in ICU with acute renal failure (ARF) and sepsis, the histopathology of the kidney was often normal in ARF. In a recent systematic review of six histopathological studies of septic renal failure, only 22% of patients showed evidence of ATN [11].

Finally, it may be quite tempting to extrapolate the prerenal/renal paradigm to a benign and malignant azotemia, but as we and others have argued elsewhere [9, 12, 13], pure prerenal physiology is unusual in hospitalized patients and its effects are not necessarily benign. So classification of a case as benign "prerenal" azotemia will lead to incorrect management decisions.

1.1.6 Limitations of Biomarkers

GFR has traditionally been used as the performance index for renal function. However, without knowing what the maximal GFR (renal reserve) would be in a given patient, measurements of GFR will not yield an accurate estimate of the global renal function. A noninvasive method of measuring real-time GFR has yet to be developed, and we still continue to rely on SCr and BUN as surrogate markers of GFR. However, there are significant limitations when these markers are used. BUN can vary independently of renal function for a variety of reasons, including gastrointestinal bleeding, steroid use, and nutritional status. Thus, changes in BUN do not reliably convey the degree of uremia in any given patient.

Similarly, SCr is a marker of late-stage disease. In some cases, SCr levels might not increase until a substantial amount of functioning renal mass (up to 50%) has been lost. There are many renal and nonrenal factors that can markedly affect the SCr concentration independent of GFR, including age, sex, muscle mass, metabolism, drugs, and volume status [14, 15]. Furthermore, as GFR decreases, tubular secretion of creatinine increases. Thus, SCr can underestimate the degree of GFR decline during the evolution of ARF. Finally, changes in SCr reflect changes in the GFR only in a steady state, and no single creatinine value correlates to a given GFR across all patients. By definition, AKI is not a steady state, and the SCr may lead to falsely high or low GFR estimates [15].

1.1.7 Renal Failure Defined by RIFLE Criteria

Over the last few years the case for a consensus definition and a classification system for ARF has repeatedly been made [16, 17]. The major aim of such a system would be to bring one of the major intensive care syndromes to a standard of definition and a level of classification similar to that achieved by two other common ICU syndromes (i.e., sepsis and acute respiratory distress syndrome). Furthermore, the need to classify the severity of the syndrome rather than only consider the most severe form was emphasized. Following such advocacy and through the persistent work of the Acute Dialysis Quality Initiative (ADQI) group, such a system was developed through a broad consensus of experts [1]. The characteristics of this system are summarized in Figure 1.1.1. The acronym RIFLE stands for the increasing severity classes Risk, Injury, and Failure, and the two outcome classes Loss and End Stage Kidney Disease. The three severity grades are defined on the basis of the changes in SCr or urine output where the worst of each criterion is used. The two outcome criteria, Loss and End-Stage Kidney Disease, are defined by the duration of loss of kidney function. Since its publication, the RIFLE classification system has received much attention, with more than 100,000 electronic hits for its publication site and more than 80 citations in 2 years. It has also spawned several investigations of its predictive ability, internal validity, robustness, and clinical relevance in a variety of settings.

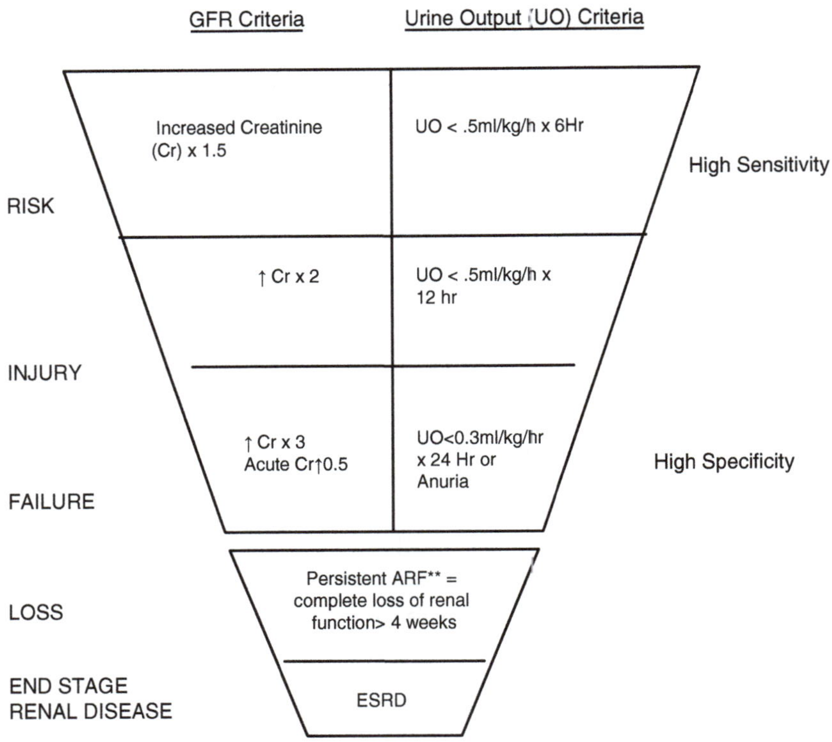

Fig. 1.1.1 RIFLE criteria

1.1.8 The Concept of Acute Kidney Injury: A Paradigm Shift

The concept of AKI, as defined by RIFLE creates a new paradigm [19]. It is not acute renal failure. Instead, it encompasses both severe and less severe alterations in renal function. Rather than focusing exclusively on patients with renal failure or those who receive dialysis, we find that the strong association with hospital mortality demands that we change the way we think about this disorder. In a study by Hoste et al. [20], only 14% of patients reaching RIFLE class F received renal replacement therapy, yet these patients experienced hospital mortality more than five times that of the same ICU population without AKI. Is renal support underutilized or delayed? Are there any supportive measures that should be employed for these patients? Sustained AKI leads to profound alterations in fluid, electrolyte, acid–base, and hormonal regulation. AKI results in abnormalities in the central nervous system, immune system, and coagulation system. Many patients with AKI already have multiple organ failure. What is the incremental influence of AKI on remote organ function, and how does it affect outcome?

A recent study by Levy et al. [21] examined outcomes for over 1,000 patients enrolled in the control arm of two large sepsis trials. The early improvement (within 24 h) in cardiovascular ($p = 0.001$), renal ($p < 0.0001$), or respiratory ($p = 0.046$) function was significantly related to survival. This study suggests that outcomes for patients with severe sepsis in the ICU are closely related to early resolution of AKI. While rapid resolution of AKI may simply be a marker of good prognosis, it may also indicate a window of therapeutic opportunity to improve outcome in such patients. AKIN has also put forth a conceptual framework for AKI that may aid in future studies (Figure 1.1.2).

1.1.9 Validation Studies Using RIFLE

Over 76,000 patients have been enrolled in studies to validate the RIFLE criteria as a means of classifying patients with AKI. One of the earliest studies by Abosaif et al. [22] studied 247 patients admitted to ICU with a SCr > 150 μmol/l. These investigators found that the ICU mortality was greatest among patients classified as RIFLE class F, with 74.5% mortality, compared with

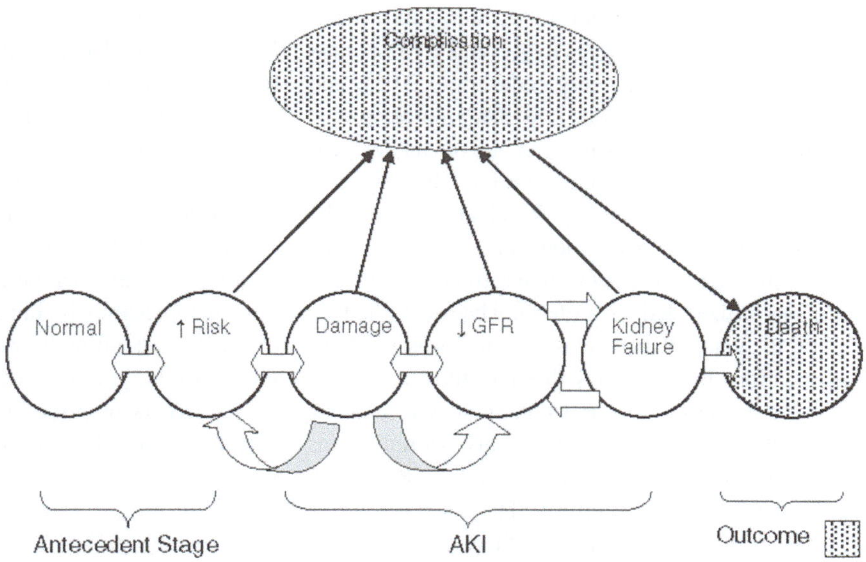

Fig. 1.1.2 Conceptual model of acute kidney injury (AKI) (Adapted from www.AKINet.org)

50% among those who were class I, 38.3% in those who were class R. In a significantly larger single-center multi-ICU study, Hoste and colleagues [20] evaluated RIFLE as an epidemiological and predictive tool in 5,383 critically ill patients. They found that AKI occurred in a staggering 67% of patients, with 12% achieving a maximum class of R, 27% class I, and 28% class F. Of the 1,510 patients who reached class R, 56% progressed to either I or F. Patients with a maximum score of class R had a mortality rate of 5.5%. Furthermore, RIFLE class I (hazard ratio of 1.4) and class F (hazard ratio of 2.7) were independent predictors of mortality after controlling for other variables known to predict outcome in critically ill patients.

Uchino and colleagues [2] focused on the predictive ability of RIFLE classification in a cohort of 20,126 patients admitted to a teaching hospital for > 24 h over a 3-year period. The authors used the electronic laboratory database to classify patients into RIFLE class R, I, and F, and followed then to hospital discharge or death. Nearly 10% of patients achieved a maximum RIFLE class R, 5% class I, and 3.5% class F. There was a nearly linear increase in hospital mortality with increasing RIFLE class with patients who were class R having more than three times the mortality rate of patients without AKI. Patients who were class I had close to twice the mortality of those who were class R, and patients who were class F had ten times the mortality rate of hospitalized patients without AKI. The investigators performed multivariate logistic regression analyses to test whether RIFLE classification was an independent predictor of hospital mortality. They found that class R carried an odds ratio for hospital mortality of 2.5, class I of 5.4, and class F of 10.1.

Ali and coworkers [6] studied the incidence of AKI in northern Scotland, a geographical population base of 523,390. The annual incidence of AKI was 2,147 per million population. Sepsis was a precipitating factor in 47% of patients. RIFLE classification was useful for predicting recovery of renal function ($p < 0.001$), requirement for renal replacement therapy ($p < 0.001$), length of hospital stay for survivors ($p < 0.001$), and in-hospital mortality ($p = 0.035$). Although subjects with AKI no longer had statistically significantly higher mortality at 3 and 6 months.

Another study by Ostermann and Chang [23] analyzed 41,972 patients admitted to 22 ICUs in the United Kingdom and Germany between 1989 and 1999 as part of the Riyadh Intensive Care Program database. AKI defined by RIFLE occurred in 15,019 patients (35.8%): 7,207 (17.2%) who were class R, 4,613 (11%) class I, and 3,199 (7.6%) class F. Hospital mortality rates were RIFLE class R 20.9%, class I 45.6%, and class F 56.8%, compared with 8.4% among patients without AKI. Independent risk factors for hospital mortality were age (odds ratio 1.02); APACHE II score on admission to ICU (odds ratio 1.10); presence of preexisting end-stage disease (odds ratio 1.17); mechanical ventilation (odds ratio 1.52); RIFLE class R (odds ratio 1.40), class I (odds ratio 1.96), and class F (odds ratio 1.59); maximum number of failed organs (odds ratio 2.13); admission after emergency surgery (odds ratio 3.08); and nonsurgical admission (odds ratio 3.92). Interestingly, renal replacement therapy for AKI was not an independent risk factor for hospital mortality. Finally, in a recent systematic review by Ricci et al. [18], the authors analyzed data for more than 71,000 patients from published reports from August 2004 to June 2007 that have utilized RIFLE criteria. They identified 24 studies in which RIFLE classification was used for classification. In 13 studies that had mortality as an outcome, mortality was 6.9% in non-AKI patients compared with 31.2% in AKI patients. Mortality was 18.9%, 36.1%, and 46.5% in RIFLE class R, class I, and class F groups, respectively. They also noted that with respect to non-AKI patients, there appeared to be a stepwise increase in relative risk (RR) for death going from class R to F: 2.40, 4.15, and 6.15, respectively. The mortality with AKI seemed more pronounced among cardiovascular patients with class F versus non-AKI (RR = 13.85, $p = 0.01$); however, the 95% confidence interval (95% CI) in this group was quite large (95% CI, 1.8–106.7).

1.1.10 Conceptual Development and Future Directions

The goal of a standard definition and classification of renal failure is now close to being realized. Further refinement of RIFLE definitions and classifications is ongoing. Recently, AKIN proposed to include an increase in $SCr \geq 0.3$ mg/dl within 48 h under the RIFLE R classification even if that increase failed to reach the 50% cutoff. In a recent study, Bagshaw et al. [24] compared this modification to the original RIFLE criteria. This study included 120,123 patients enrolled from January 2000 to December 2005 from 57 ICUs from the Australian New Zealand Intensive Care Society (ANZICS) Adult Patient Database (APD). This study found that compared with RIFLE criteria, the AKIN modification slightly increased the number of patients with AKI, by a modest 2%; furthermore, the modification did not significantly increase the predictive ability of RIFLE for mortality.

The use of functional markers (urine output and SCr) will be replaced or augmented in the near future by injury markers. Several potential urine and plasma markers have been identified, but no single biochemical marker so far provides the levels of sensitivity and specificity necessary to be clinically useful across the full spectrum of ARF, and these markers are reviewed elsewhere [14, 25]. In the future, biomarkers will likely identify this disorder before functional decline, and new therapies may be introduced earlier in the course of the disease, possibly mitigating and/or potentiating the recovery of this disorder. Until, then, the "tried and true" markers of urine output and serum creatinine, categorized by RIFLE criteria, will be the best we can provide.

1.1.11 Conclusions

Even small changes in kidney function in hospitalized patients are associated with both short- and long-term adverse outcomes. The RIFLE classification provides a uniform definition for the whole range of AKI. It has been validated in multiple studies and may be utilized as a prognostic tool. The RIFLE classification for AKI is quite analogous to the Kidney Disease Outcomes Quality Initiative for chronic kidney disease (CKD) staging, which is well known to correlate disease severity with cardiovascular complications and other morbidities. CKD stages have also been linked to specific treatment recommendations, which have proven extremely useful in managing this disease. As the epidemiology of AKI becomes clearer and as new treatments emerge (both made all the more possible by standards for diagnosis and classification), RIFLE classifications will undoubtedly be used to reference recommendations for prevention and treatment. Indeed this was the ultimate purpose that RIFLE criteria was intended to serve.

References

1. Bellomo, R. et al., *Acute renal failure – definition, outcome measures, animal models, fluid therapy and information technology needs: the Second International Consensus*

Conference of the Acute Dialysis Quality Initiative (ADQI) Group. Crit Care, 2004. 8(4): p. R204–12.
2. Uchino, S., *The epidemiology of acute renal failure in the world.* Curr Opin Crit Care, 2006. 12(6): p. 538–43.
3. Bellomo, R., J.A. Kellum, and C. Ronco, *Defining and classifying acute renal failure: from advocacy to consensus and validation of the RIFLE criteria*. Intensive Care Med, 2007. 33(3): p. 409–13.
4. Hoste, E.A. and J.A. Kellum, *Incidence, classification, and outcomes of acute kidney injury*. Contrib Nephrol, 2007. 156: p. 32–8.
5. Kellum, J.A. et al., *Developing a consensus classification system for acute renal failure*. Curr Opin Crit Care, 2002. 8(6): p. 509–14.
6. Venkataraman, R. and J.A. Kellum, *Defining acute renal failure: the RIFLE criteria*. J Intensive Care Med, 2007. 22(4): p. 187–93.
7. Smith, H.W., *Acute renal failure related to traumatic injuries;* in *The Kidney: Structure and Function in Health and Disease*. 1951, Oxford University Press, Cary.
8. Thurau, K. and J.W. Boylan, *Acute renal success. The unexpected logic of oliguria in acute renal failure*. Am J Med, 1976. 61(3): p. 308–15.
9. Bagshaw, S.M., C. Langenberg, and R. Bellomo, *Urinary biochemistry and microscopy in septic acute renal failure: a systematic review*. Am J Kidney Dis, 2006. 48(5): p. 695–705.
10. Uchino, S. et al., *Acute renal failure in critically ill patients: a multinational, multicenter study*. JAMA, 2005. 294(7): p. 813–8.
11. Langenberg, C. et al., *The histopathology of septic acute kidney injury: a systematic review*. Crit Care, 2008. 12(2): p. R38.
12. Kellum, J.A., *Prerenal azotemia: still a useful concept?* Crit Care Med, 2007. 35(6): p. 1630–1.
13. Bagshaw, S.M. et al., *A systematic review of urinary findings in experimental septic acute renal failure*. Crit Care Med, 2007. 35(6): p. 1592–8.
14. Bonventre, J.V., *Diagnosis of acute kidney injury: from classic parameters to new biomarkers*. Contrib Nephrol, 2007. 156: p. 213–9.
15. Dennen, P. and C.R. Parikh, *Biomarkers of acute kidney injury: can we replace serum creatinine?* Clin Nephrol, 2007. 68(5): p. 269–78.
16. Bellomo, R., J. Kellum, and C. Ronco, *Acute renal failure: time for consensus*. Intensive Care Med, 2001. 27(11): p. 1685–8.
17. Kellum, J.A., R.L. Mehta, and C. Ronco, *Acute dialysis quality initiative (ADQI)*. Contrib Nephrol, 2001 132: p. 258–65.
18. Ricci, Z., D. Cruz, and C. Ronco, *The RIFLE criteria and mortality in acute kidney injury: a systematic review*. Kidney Int, 2008. 73(5): p. 538–46.
19. Mehta, R.L. et al., *Acute Kidney Injury Network: report of an initiative to improve outcomes in acute kidney injury*. Crit Care, 2007. 11(2): p. R31.
20. Hoste, E.A. et al., *RIFLE criteria for acute kidney injury are associated with hospital mortality in critically ill patients: a cohort analysis*. Crit Care, 2006. 10(3): p. R73.
21. Levy, M.M. et al., *Early changes in organ function predict eventual survival in severe sepsis*. Crit Care Med, 2005. 33(10): p. 2194–201.
22. Abosaif, N.Y. et al., *The outcome of acute renal failure in the intensive care unit according to RIFLE: model application, sensitivity, and predictability*. Am J Kidney Dis, 2005. 46(6): p. 1038–48.
23. Ostermann, M. and R.W. Chang, *Acute kidney injury in the intensive care unit according to RIFLE*. Crit Care Med, 2007. 35(8): p. 1837–43; quiz 1852.
24. Bagshaw, S.M., C. George, and R. Bellomo, *A comparison of the RIFLE and AKIN criteria for acute kidney injury in critically ill patients*. Nephrol Dial Transplant, 2008. 23(5): p. 1569–74.
25. Nickolas, T.L., J. Barasch, and P. Devarajan, *Biomarkers in acute and chronic kidney disease*. Curr Opin Nephrol Hypertens, 2008. 17(2): p. 127–132.

Part II

Overview of Pathophysiology, Etiology and Epidemiology

II

Mechanisms of Acute Kidney Injury and Repair

2.1

Joseph V. Bonventre

Core Messages

- The pathogenesis of acute kidney injury (AKI) is complex and varies to some extent based on the particular cause.
- Inflammation contributes to this pathophysiology in a variety of contexts. Inflammation can result in reduction in local blood flow to the outer medulla, with adverse consequences on tubule function and viability. Both the innate and adaptive immune responses are important contributors to inflammation.
- With ischemia/reperfusion, endothelial cells express a number of adhesion molecules which have counterreceptors on leukocytes. A number of vasoactive mediators that are released with injury, such as nitric oxide, may also affect leukocyte–endothelial interactions.
- There is obstruction of the microvasculature as well as enhanced vasoconstriction. Tubule epithelial cells generate proinflammatory and chemotactic cytokines. In response to bilateral ischemia/reperfusion injury, mouse kidneys produce D series resolvins and protectins which reduce intrarenal inflammation and limit injury.
- Injection of mesenchymal stem (stromal) cells is protective against renal injury as assessed by serum creatinine measured 24 h after ischemia. The mechanism of such protection may be through intrarenal paracrine effects to decrease inflammation or by systemic immune modulation.
- The epithelial cells that replace the lost cells derive from surviving tubular epithelial cells.

2.1.1 Introduction

The mechanisms involved in kidney injury and repair are complex. In this chapter, I will briefly summarize various components of this complexity. There are many potential causes of acute kidney injury (AKI), and each has its own characteristics, but I will focus on overriding themes, recognizing that the importance of some mechanisms may be dependent on the factors leading to the development of acute kidney dysfunction. The kidney is particularly susceptible to ischemia and toxins with resultant vasoconstriction, endothelial damage, and activation of inflammatory processes. This susceptibility derives in part from the vascular–tubular structural associations in the outer medulla of the kidney which lead to enhanced susceptibility to compromise of blood flow to critical nephron structures that are present there. In addition, because the nephron concentrates many substances as glomerular filtrate is reabsorbed from the tubular lumen, the concentrations of these substances may reach thresholds of toxicity to the surrounding epithelial cells. It is increasingly recognized that AKI is frequently superimposed on chronic renal disease and may be an important precipitant for progression to end-stage

J. V. Bonventre
Brigham and Women's Hospital, Renal Division, 75 Francis Street, Boston, MA 02115, USA
e-mail: jbonventre@partners.org

A. Jörres et al. (eds.), *Management of Acute Kidney Problems*,
DOI: 10.1007/978-3-540-69441-0_2.1, © Springer-Verlag Berlin Heidelberg 2010

renal disease. The interplay between chronic and acute kidney disease contributes to additional complexity in understanding the mechanisms. The kidney is robust in its ability to repair itself, but often this ability is not manifest in our patients. To better understand how to facilitate recovery from AKI, it is important to understand the processes of repair under circumstances where repair is effective. This has led to a great deal of excitement in the area of stem cell biology as it relates to the kidney. We will discuss injury in the first part of this chapter and repair in the second.

2.1.2 Injury

In response to a variety of insults, including ischemia and many toxins, there are many common features of the epithelial cell response. The processes of injury and repair to the kidney epithelium are depicted schematically in Fig. 2.1.1. Injury results in rapid loss of cytoskeletal integrity and cell polarity. There is shedding of the proximal tubule brush border, loss of polarity with mislocalization of adhesion molecules and other membrane proteins such as Na^+,K^+-ATPase and β-integrins [50]. Cells die by apoptosis and necrosis [42]. With severe injury, viable and nonviable cells are desquamated leaving regions where the basement membrane remains as the only barrier between the filtrate and the peritubular interstitium. This allows for backleak of the filtrate, especially under circumstances where the pressure in the tubule is increased due to intratubular obstruction resulting from cellular debris in the lumen interacting with proteins such as fibronectin which enter the lumen [51]. Many cellular factors are involved with injury of the epithelial cell. Some of

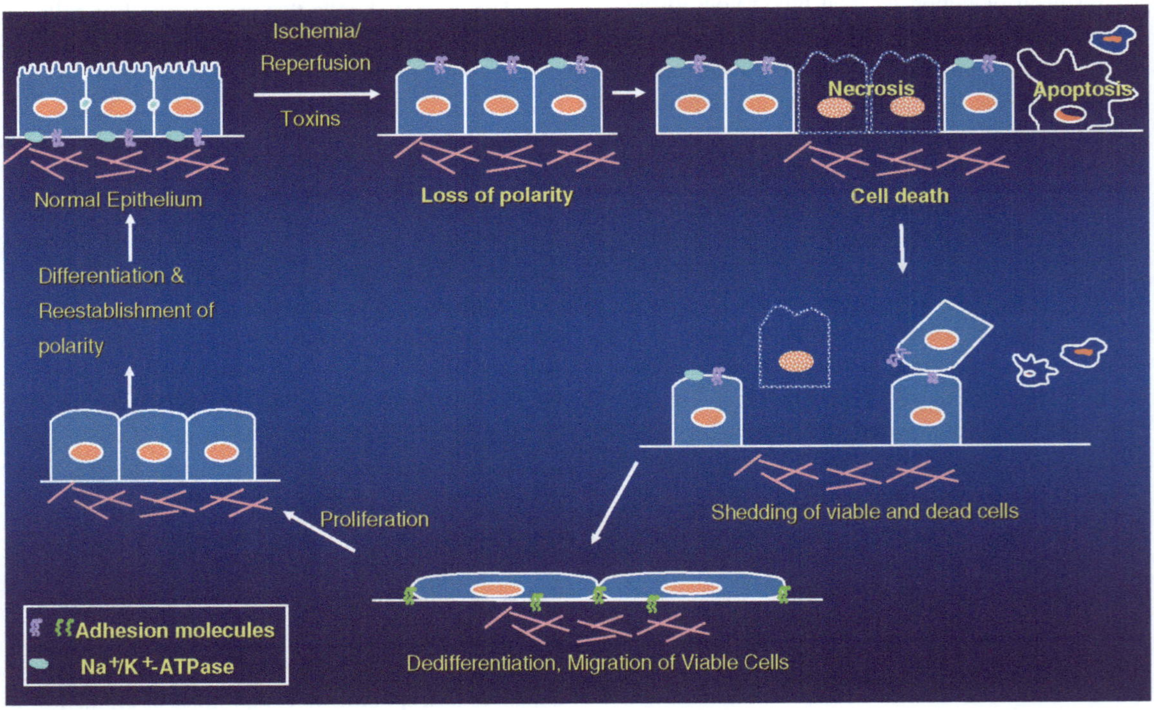

Fig. 2.1.1 Injury and repair to the epithelial cell of the kidney with ischemia/reperfusion. One of the first things to happen to the proximal epithelial cell after injury to the kidney is loss of the brush border and loss of the polarity of the epithelial cell with mislocation of adhesion molecules and Na^+,K^+-ATPase and other proteins. If the insult is severe, there is cell death by either necrosis or apoptosis. In addition, because of the mislocation of adhesion molecules, viable epithelial cells lift off the basement membrane and are found in the urine. The desquamated cells and cellular debris can interact with luminal proteins to physically obstruct the tubule lumen. If provided with the proper nutrients and oxygen supply, the kidney can then initiate a repair process. Viable epithelial cells dedifferentiate and migrate over the basement membrane. The source of these cells appears to be the kidney itself and not the bone marrow. Cells replacing the epithelium may derive from differentiated epithelial cells or from a subpopulation of progenitor cells within the tubule. The cells then differentiate and reestablish the normal polarity of the epithelium

Table 2.1.1 Proximate cellular causes of injury

- ATP depletion
- Increased intracellular free Ca2± concentration
- Phospholipase activation
- Protease activation including caspases
- Endonuclease activation
- Mitochondrial injury with cytochrome C leakage
- Reactive oxygen species
- Increased mitochondrial and plasma membrane permeability
- Decreased protein synthesis
- Endoplasmic reticulum swelling
- Clumping of nuclear chromatin

these are summarized in Table 2.1.1. The endothelium likely also plays an important role in the injury, since blood flow and hence oxygen and nutrient delivery to the epithelial cell, as well as waste product removal, depends critically on the integrity of the vasculature. In turn, the integrity of the vasculature depends critically on a normal functioning endothelium. Damage to endothelial cells and subsequent distortion of peritubular capillary blood flow are characteristics of ischemic injury [2]. The damage to the endothelium may then result in impaired blood flow and lead to epithelial cell injury. Diminished blood flow may be particularly problematic in the outer medulla where endothelial edema may be particularly prone to result in stasis, given the confined space. Furthermore, in this region of the kidney, the oxygen tension is low at baseline due to countercurrent exchange in the vasa recta [8]; hence, impaired flow is particularly likely to lead to proximal tubule cell death.

The epithelium is likely not to just be an innocent bystander in the process of kidney injury. Activation and damage to the epithelium results in the generation of inflammatory and vasoactive mediators, which can feed back on the vasculature to worsen the vasoconstriction and inflammation. Furthermore, there is activation of innate immunity which may play a critical role in the acute and chronic sequelae of initiation of injury. Inflammation contributes in a critical way to injury in AKI [7].

2.1.3 Inflammation

The innate immune response. Both the innate and adaptive immune responses are important contributors to the pathobiology of ischemic injury. The innate component is responsible for the early response to infection or injury and is foreign-antigen independent. Toll-like receptors (TLRs), which are important for the detection of exogenous microbial products [1] and development of antigen-dependent adaptive immunity [22], also recognize host material released during injury [21]. TLRs are present in epithelial cells and up-regulated in response to endogenous ligands which are released by damaged tissue. TLRs can mediate a strong proinflammatory response, which, in many organs, includes activation and maturation of dendritic cells, the most potent antigen-presenting cells of the immune system [39]. Dendritic cells then activate naïve T cells to be antigen-specific, hence triggering the adaptive immune response. With ischemia/reperfusion in rats there was an increase in the number of dendritic cells that differentiated from peripheral blood monocytes, as well as a higher production of interleukin-12 (IL-12), greater expression of major histocompatibility complex (MHC) class II, and greater production of interferon-γ (IFN-γ) by T cells stimulated by dendritic cells [48]. Furthermore, it has been demonstrated that hypoxia in vitro and ischemia/reperfusion in vivo result in differentiation of dendritic cells that is comparable to allogeneic stimulation [36].

The role of TLRs was evaluated using an ischemia/reperfusion model in $TLR2^{-/-}$ and $TLR2^{+/+}$ mice [27]. Significantly fewer granulocytes were present in the interstitium of the kidney 1 day post ischemia/reperfusion in the $TLR2^{-/-}$ mice, and fewer macrophages were present 1–5 days after ischemia/reperfusion. Kidney homogenate cytokines KC, MCP-1, IL-1b, and IL-6 were also significantly lower in the $TLR2^{-/-}$ animals as compared with the $TLR^{+/+}$ mice. Hence the absence of TLR2 clearly had an antiinflammatory effect on the response to ischemia/reperfusion. This antiinflammatory effect was associated with a functional protection as measured by serum creatinine at 1 day post ischemia/reperfusion and blood urea nitrogen and tubular injury score 1 and 5 days post ischemia/reperfusion. In a study of the role of TLR4 in ischemia/reperfusion injury of the kidney, Wu et al. [49] found that TLR4 expression by tubular epithelial cells is up-regulated by ischemia in vivo or in vitro. $TLR4^{-/-}$ animals were protected against ischemic injury, and injury was not significantly enhanced by a bone marrow transplant with marrow from $TLR4^{+/+}$ mice, indicating that the protection afforded the $TLR4^{-/-}$ animals was due to prevention of TLR4 signaling in intrinsic kidney cells.

Additional tubule contributions to inflammatory injury. Both the S3 segment of the proximal tubule and the medullary thick ascending limb (MTAL) are located in the outer stripe of the outer medulla. This region of the kidney is marginally oxygenated under normal conditions, and after an ischemic insult, oxygenation is further compromised because the return in blood flow is delayed. Both segments of the nephron contribute to the inflammatory response in AKI [5]. The distal tubule is physically closely associated with the proximal tubule and the vasa recta in the outer medulla. The distal cells are more adapted to the hypoxic environment of the medulla. Hence, with the increasing hypoxia associated with AKI, these cells are able to survive the insult more effectively than the S3 segment cells of the proximal tubule. This does not mean, however, that the distal cells are not involved in an important way in the overall response to ischemia including the modulation of inflammatory pathways. The distal tubule cells adaptively increase the production of survival factors, including growth factors, which may enhance the survival of the adjacent proximal tubule cells [17].

The tubule epithelial cells are known to generate proinflammatory and chemotactic cytokines such as TNF-α, MCP-1, IL-8, IL-6, IL-1β, and TGF-β, MCP-1, IL-8, RANTES, and ENA-78 [7]. Proximal tubular epithelia may respond to T lymphocyte activity through activation of receptors for T cell ligands [28]. When CD40 on the proximal tubule cell is ligated in response to interaction with CD154, MCP-1 and IL-8 production is enhanced, as is TRAF6 recruitment and MAPK activation [28]. CD40 also induces RANTES production by human renal tubular epithelia, an effect which is amplified by production of IL-4 and IL-13 by T helper 2 (Th2) cells, a subpopulation of T cells [11]. B7-1 and B7-2 can be induced on proximal tubule epithelial cells in vivo and in vitro. After B7-1 and B7-2 induction, proximal tubule epithelial cells costimulate CD28 on T lymphocytes resulting in cytokine production [34].

Leukocyte–endothelial interactions. With ischemia/reperfusion, endothelial cells up-regulate integrins, selectins, and members of the immunoglobulin superfamily, including intercellular adhesion molecule-1 (ICAM-1) [24] and vascular cell adhesion molecule (VCAM). Interrupting the production of ICAM-1 either with antibodies or by genetic changes, results in protection of the mouse against ischemic injury [23, 24]. We proposed that this up-regulation of ICAM-1 was related to the up-regulation of the proinflammatory cytokines TNF-α and IL-1β, which we measured to be increased by ischemia/reperfusion.

A number of vasoactive compounds may also affect leukocyte–endothelial interactions. Vasodilators, such as nitric oxide (NO), also can have effects that decrease inflammation. NO inhibits adhesion of neutrophils to TNF-α-activated endothelial cells [30]. A normal endothelium appropriately regulates vascular tone and vascular permeability, limits adhesion and transmigration of inflammatory cells, and minimizes activation of the pro-coagulation pathways. With injury to the endothelium that characterizes many forms of kidney disease including AKI, there is enhanced leukocyte–endothelial cell adhesion, and activation of platelets and the local coagulation pathway. There is increasing vascular permeability and interstitial edema [41]. Activated platelets bind avidly to leukocytes, forming platelet–leukocyte complexes which roll on the endothelium and produce cytokines which further enhance the inflammatory response [46]. Inhibition of platelet-activating factor protects against ischemia/reperfusion injury in the rat [23].

It has been known for quite some time now that there is less flow to the outer medulla in the postischemic kidney [45]. Enhanced platelet–leukocyte–endothelial interactions can physically impede blood flow especially in the setting of tissue edema [6]. Furthermore, these interactions will additionally activate both leukocytes and endothelial cells and contribute to the generation of local factors that promote vasoconstriction especially in the presence of other vasoactive mediators, resulting in compromised local blood flow and impaired tubule cell metabolism [38]. Due to the anatomical relationships of vessels and tubules in the outer medulla these leukocyte–endothelial interactions impact the outer medulla to a greater extent than in the cortex.

Neutrophils, Lymphocytes, and Macrophages. There has been some controversy about the relative importance of various subgroups of leukocytes to AKI. We found a robust influx of neutrophils early after reperfusion in the mouse. To evaluate whether prevention of neutrophil infiltration could be responsible for the protection observed in the ICAM$^{-/-}$mice, we treated normal mice with antineutrophil serum to reduce absolute neutrophil counts to <100 cells/mm^3. These neutrophil-depleted animals were protected against ischemic renal failure [25]. Early involvement of neutrophils may be important for blockage of the small vessels in the kidney, and because they do not transmigrate into the interstitium, their early involvement may be underappreciated.

There are data from a number of groups indicating that T cells participate in an important way in the injury associated with ischemia/reperfusion [15]. In a recent study Li et al. found that within 30 min after reperfusion there was an increase in kidney tissue $CD4^+$ T cells. At 3 h after reperfusion there was a large number of IFN-γ producing GR-1^+CD11b^+ neutrophils [29]. These investigators found that IFN-γ–producing $CD4^+$ T cells and/or natural killer T cells (NKT) were very important in inducing neutrophil infiltration and kidney injury after ischemia. Depletion of NKT cells attenuated ischemia/reperfusion injury.

Macrophage infiltration is a prominent feature of ischemia/reperfusion injury. While it has generally been considered that macrophages contribute to the injury, it is increasingly recognized that macrophage biology is marked by different subclasses of macrophages, some of which are proinflammatory and some antiinflammatory [32]. Macrophages can be broadly classified into two main groups: M1, whose prototypical activating stimuli are the Th1 cytokine IFN-γ and lipopolysaccharide (LPS); and M2, further subdivided into M2a (activated by IL-4 or IL-13), M2b (activated by immune complexes in combination with IL-1β or LPS) and M2c (activated by IL-10, TGF-β, or glucocorticoids). M2a cells produce cytokines, which recruit eosinophils, basophils, and Th2 cells and are involved in proangiogenic pathways. M2b cells produce high levels of IL-10, an important antiinflammatory cytokine believed to play a critical role in down-regulation of the immune response. M2b cells, however, also produce some proinflammatory cytokines including TNFα, IL-1β, and IL-6. M2c cells are generally considered deactivated macrophages that are involved in down-regulation of the immune response. Hence macrophage activation can be either proinflammatory or antiinflammatory. It is therefore reasonable to suspect that the involvement of macrophages in ischemic injury is complex and may be different depending on the stage of injury/repair.

2.1.4 Paracrine Effects of Bone Marrow–Derived Stem Cells

There is a potential role for bone marrow–derived cells in the production of protective paracrine factors that may facilitate repair of the epithelium. We and others have found that intrava injection of mesenchymal stem (stromal) cells (MSCs) is protective against renal injury as assessed by serum creatinine measured 24 h after ischemia, despite the fact that there is no transdifferentiation of MSCs into tubular cells [13]. Other groups have also found that MSCs protect against ischemic renal injury by a differentiation-independent mechanism [43]. In the adriamycin nephropathy model, injection of the side-population of cells derived from the kidney (possibly progenitor cells) was also found to be protective in the absence of tubular integration [10]. The mechanism of such protection may be through intrarenal paracrine effects to decrease inflammation or by systemic immune modulation, since injected cells may be rapidly ingested by immune cells in the spleen, liver, and lungs. Togel et al. have found that MSC-conditioned media contains VEGF, HGF, and IGF-1 and augments aortic endothelial cell survival and growth [44]. They concluded that areas of the kidney characterized by significant numbers of injected MSCs had fewer apoptotic kidney cells compared with those areas not containing MSCs. Recently it has been reported that homing to the kidney is not necessary for the beneficial effect of MSC-based therapy. Bi et al. [3] reported protective effects of intravenous or intraperitoneally administered bone marrow–derived stromal cells even though there were very few cells found in the kidney. It has been increasingly recognized that MSCs can modulate innate immunity by generating a large number of agents that modify this response [40].

2.1.5 Other Mechanisms to Limit or Stop Inflammation

We have already discussed some mechanisms brought to bear to limit the inflammatory process. As indicated above, NO and subclasses of macrophages may fulfill this role. In addition, infiltrating cells, some of which may come from the bone marrow, appear to have paracrine effects to limit inflammation and the injury process. There is evidence that some growth factors, such as hepatocyte growth factor (HGF), can have an antiinflammatory action. HGF has been reported to inhibit renal inflammation by attenuating tubular cell apoptosis, inhibiting endothelial injury and neutrophil extravasation via processes that involve disrupting NF-kB signaling [16, 33].

We have worked on another class of molecules, the resolvins (Rv) and protectins (PD). These are two families of naturally occurring omega-3 fatty acid docosahexaenoic acid metabolites. These compounds were initially identified by Serhan and colleagues [37], and have been found to be important for resolution of inflammation in a number of organ systems. In collaboration with the Serhan laboratory, we found that bilateral ischemia/reperfusion injury resulted in increased D series resolvins (RvDs) and PD1 production in mouse kidney [14]. Administration of RvDs or PD1 to mice prior to, and subsequent to, ischemia resulted in a reduction in functional and morphological kidney injury. Administration of RvD1 10 min after reperfusion also protected the kidneys, as was reflected histologically with reduced injury and reduced inflammatory cell infiltrate. Interstitial fibrosis after ischemia/reperfusion was reduced in mice treated with RvDs.

Thus, there are a number of factors which may represent adaptive responses to ischemia, which are developed by the body to limit the inflammatory response. In many cases this may be sufficient to prevent organ failure. In other cases, however, either because these processes are not activated or because they are overwhelmed, the organ fails and the consequences to the patient are often cataclysmic.

2.1.6 Repair

In contrast to the heart or brain, the kidney can recover from an ischemic or toxic insult that results in cell death [47], although it is becoming increasingly recognized that there are longer term detrimental effects of even brief periods of ischemia [35]. The source of the cells responsible for replacement of the epithelial cells that have been lost has been a topic of great interest especially given all the enthusiasm about the possibility of using adult stem cells therapeutically. We had proposed that surviving cells that remain adherent are responsible for replacement of the lost epithelial cells during repair with the potential to recover normal renal function. The viable cells spread, dedifferentiate, and migrate to cover the exposed areas of the basement membrane, and then proliferate to restore cell number (Fig. 2.1.1). Finally differentiation of the cell restores the functional integrity of the nephron [4]. As described above, we and others have concluded that the bone marrow does not contribute directly to the replacement of cells but bone marrow–derived cells may have paracrine effects that may facilitate repair potentially by reducing inflammation [19]. Putative adult kidney stem cells have been isolated, and some researchers have found that these cells can facilitate functional recovery after injury [9, 12, 18, 26, 31]. Using genetic fate–mapping techniques we generated transgenic mice in which 94–95% of tubular epithelial cells, but no interstitial cells, were labeled with either beta-galactosidase (LacZ) or red fluorescent protein [20]. After ischemia, despite extensive cell proliferation, no dilution of either cell fate marker was observed. These results indicate that regeneration by surviving tubular epithelial cells is the predominant mechanism of repair after ischemic tubular injury in the adult mammalian kidney.

2.1.7 Conclusions

The pathophysiology of AKI is complex and is further complicated by the fact that AKI often exists in the context of multiple organ failure. Hemodynamic and tubular factors contribute to the dysfunction of the kidney. Inflammation plays an important role, but we remain frustrated by not being able to interrupt this inflammatory process in ways that are effective in humans to prevent the devastating consequences of AKI. It is increasingly recognized that there are endogenous mechanisms that the organism brings to bear to control the inflammation. Understanding how these antiinflammatory processes are regulated may provide insights into how we might intervene to facilitate and enhance them to prevent or mitigate the devastating consequences of AKI. Repair of the kidney can be very robust. Infiltrating cells may play a role in this repair by producing factors which promote the growth of the epithelium and/or limit the inflammation. The ability of the surviving cells to proliferate and replace the lost cells is very impressive. The role of infiltrating cells or interstitial "stem" or "progenitor" cells to become epithelial cells either does not occur or occurs in so small a percentage of cases as to not be of physiological importance.

Acknowledgments This work was supported by the US National Institutes of Health (grants DK 39773, DK54741, DK72381).

References

1. Aderem, A and RJ Ulevitch (2000). "Toll-like receptors in the induction of the innate immune response." *Nature* 406(6797): 782–787.
2. Basile, DP (2007). "The endothelial cell in ischemic acute kidney injury: implications for acute and chronic function." *Kidney Int* 72(2): 151–156.
3. Bi, B, R Schmitt, M Israilova, et al. (2007). "Stromal cells protect against acute tubular injury via an endocrine effect." *J Am Soc Nephrol* 18(9): 2486–2496.
4. Bonventre, JV (2003). "Dedifferentiation and proliferation of surviving epithelial cells in acute renal failure." *J Am Soc Nephrol* 14(Suppl 1): S55–61.
5. Bonventre, JV, M Brezis, N Siegel, et al. (1998). "Acute renal failure. I. Relative importance of proximal vs. distal tubular injury." *Am J Physiol* 275: F623–F631.
6. Bonventre, JV and JM Weinberg (2003). "Recent advances in the pathophysiology of ischemic acute renal failure." *J Am Soc Nephrol* 14(8): 2199–2210.
7. Bonventre, JV and A Zuk (2004). "Ischemic acute renal failure: an inflammatory disease?" *Kidney Int* 66(2): 480–485.
8. Brezis, M and FH Epstein (1993). "Cellular mechanisms of acute ischemic injury in the kidney." *Annu Rev Med* 44: 27–37.
9. Bussolati, B, S Bruno, C Grange, et al. (2005). "Isolation of renal progenitor cells from adult human kidney." *Am J Pathol* 166(2): 545–555.
10. Challen, GA, I Bertoncello, JA Deane, et al. (2006). "Kidney side population reveals multilineage potential and renal functional capacity but also cellular heterogeneity." *J Am Soc Nephrol* 17(7): 1896–1912.
11. Deckers, JG, S De Haij, FJ van der Woude, et al. (1998). "IL-4 and IL-13 augment cytokine- and CD40-induced RANTES production by human renal tubular epithelial cells in vitro." *J Am Soc Nephrol* 9(7): 1187–1193.
12. Dekel, B, L Zangi, E Shezen, et al. (2006). "Isolation and characterization of nontubular sca-1+lin- multipotent stem/progenitor cells from adult mouse kidney." *J Am Soc Nephrol* 17(12): 3300–3314.
13. Duffield, JS and JV Bonventre (2005). "Kidney tubular epithelium is restored without replacement with bone marrow-derived cells during repair after ischemic injury." *Kidney Int* 68(5): 1956–1961.
14. Duffield, JS, S Hong, VS Vaidya, et al. (2006). "Resolvin d series and protectin d1 mitigate acute kidney injury." *J Immunol* 177(9): 5902–5911.
15. Friedewald, JJ and H Rabb (2004). "Inflammatory cells in ischemic acute renal failure." *Kidney Int* 66(2): 486–491.
16. Giannopoulou, M, C Dai, X Tan, et al. (2008). "Hepatocyte growth factor exerts its anti-inflammatory action by disrupting nuclear factor-kappaB signaling." *Am J Pathol* 173(1): 30–41.
17. Gobe, GC and DW Johnson (2007). "Distal tubular epithelial cells of the kidney: potential support for proximal tubular cell survival after renal injury." *Int J Biochem Cell Biol* 39(9): 1551–1561.
18. Gupta, S, C Verfaillie, D Chmielewski, et al. (2006). "Isolation and characterization of kidney-derived stem cells." *J Am Soc Nephrol* 17(11): 3028–3040.
19. Humphreys, BD, JD Duffield, and JV Bonventre (2006). "Renal stem cells in recovery from acute kidney injury." *Minerva Urol Nefrol* 58(1): 13–21.
20. Humphreys, BD, MT Valerius, A Kobayashi, et al. (2008). "Intrinsic epithelial cells repair the kidney after injury." *Cell Stem Cell* 2(3): 284–291.
21. Johnson, GB, GJ Brunn, and JL Platt (2003). "Activation of mammalian Toll-like receptors by endogenous agonists." *Crit Rev Immunol* 23(1–2): 15–44.
22. Kaisho, T and S Akira (2006). "Toll-like receptor function and signaling." *J Allergy Clin Immunol* 117(5): 979–987; quiz 988.
23. Kelly, KJ, NE Tolkoff-Rubin, RH Rubin, et al. (Eds.) (1996). An oral platelet activating factor antagonist, Ro 24-4736, protects the rat kidney from ischemic injury. *Am J Physiol* 271: F1061–F1067.
24. Kelly, KJ, WW Williams, RB Colvin, et al. (1994). "Antibody to intercellular adhesion molecule-1 protects the kidney against ischemic injury." *Proc Natl Acad Sci USA* 91: 812–816.
25. Kelly, KJ, WW Williams, RB Colvin, et al. (1996). "Intercellular adhesion molecule-1 deficient mice are protected against renal ischemia." *J Clin Invest* 97: 1056–1063.
26. Kitamura, S, Y Yamasaki, M Kinomura, et al. (2005). "Establishment and characterization of renal progenitor like cells from S3 segment of nephron in rat adult kidney." *FASEB J* 19(13): 1789–1797.
27. Leemans, JC, G Stokman, N Claessen, et al. (2005). "Renal-associated TLR2 mediates ischemia/reperfusion injury in the kidney." *J Clin Invest* 115(10): 2894–2903.
28. Li, H and EP Nord (2002). "CD40 ligation stimulates MCP-1 and IL-8 production, TRAF6 recruitment, and MAPK activation in proximal tubule cells." *Am J Physiol Renal Physiol* 282(6): F1020–1033.
29. Li, L, L Huang, SS Sung, et al. (2007). "NKT cell activation mediates neutrophil IFN-gamma production and renal ischemia-reperfusion injury." *J Immunol* 178(9): 5899–5911.
30. Linas, S, D Whittenburg, and JE Repine (1997). "Nitric oxide prevents neutrophil-mediated acute renal failure." *Am J Physiol* 272(1 Pt 2): F48–54.
31. Maeshima, A, H Sakurai, and SK Nigam (2006). "Adult kidney tubular cell population showing phenotypic plasticity, tubulogenic capacity, and integration capability into developing kidney." *J Am Soc Nephrol* 17(1): 188–198.
32. Martinez, FO, A Sica, A Mantovani, et al. (2008). "Macrophage activation and polarization." *Front Biosci* 13: 453–461.
33. Mizuno, S and T Nakamura (2005). "Prevention of neutrophil extravasation by hepatocyte growth factor leads to attenuations of tubular apoptosis and renal dysfunction in mouse ischemic kidneys." *Am J Pathol* 166(6): 1895–1905.
34. Niemann-Masanek, U, A Mueller, BA Yard, et al. (2002). "B7-1 (CD80) and B7-2 (CD 86) expression in human tubular epithelial cells in vivo and in vitro." *Nephron* 92(3): 542–556.
35. Park, KM, JY Byun, C Kramers, et al. (2003). "Inducible nitric oxide synthase is an important contributor to prolonged protective effects of ischemic preconditioning in the mouse kidney." *J Biol Chem* 278(29): 27256–27266.

36. Rama, I, B Bruene, J Torras, et al. (2008). "Hypoxia stimulus: an adaptive immune response during dendritic cell maturation." *Kidney Int* 73(7): 816–825.
37. Serhan, C, S Hong, K Gronert, et al. (2002). "Resolvins: a family of bioactive products of omega-3 fatty acid transformation circuits initiated by aspirin treatment that counter proinflammation signals." *J Exp Med* 196: 1025–1037.
38. Sheridan, AM and JV Bonventre (2000). "Cell biology and molecular mechanisms of injury in ischemic acute renal failure." *Curr Opin Nephrol Hypertens* 9(4): 427–434.
39. Shirali, AC and DR Goldstein (2008). "Tracking the toll of kidney disease." *J Am Soc Nephrol* 19:1444–1450.
40. Stagg, J (2007). "Immune regulation by mesenchymal stem cells: two sides to the coin." *Tissue Antigens* 69(1): 1–9.
41. Sutton, TA, CJ Fisher, and BA Molitoris (2002). "Microvascular endothelial injury and dysfunction during ischemic acute renal failure." *Kidney Int* 62(5): 1539–1549.
42. Thadhani, R, M Pascual, and JV Bonventre (1996). "Acute renal failure." *New Engl J Med* 334: 1448–1460.
43. Togel, F, Z Hu, K Weiss, et al. (2005). "Administered mesenchymal stem cells protect against ischemic acute renal failure through differentiation-independent mechanisms." *Am J Physiol Renal Physiol* 289(1): F31–42.
44. Togel, F, K Weiss, Y Yang, et al. (2007). "Vasculotropic, paracrine actions of infused mesenchymal stem cells are important to the recovery from acute kidney injury." *Am J Physiol Renal Physiol* 292(5): F1626–1635.
45. Vetterlein, F, A Pethö, and G Schmidt (1986). "Distribution of capillary blood flow in rat kidney during postischemic renal failure." *Am J Physiol* 251: H510–H519.
46. Wagner, DD and PS Frenette (2008). "The vessel wall and its interactions." *Blood* 111(11): 5271–5281.
47. Witzgall, R, D Brown, C Schwarz, et al. (1994). "Localization of proliferating cell nuclear antigen, vimentin, c-Fos, and clusterin in the postischemic kidney. Evidence for a heterogenous genetic response among nephron segments, and a large pool of mitotically active and dedifferentiated cells." *J Clin Invest* 93(5): 2175–2188.
48. Wu, CJ, JR Sheu, HH Chen, et al. (2006). "Modulation of monocyte-derived dendritic cell differentiation is associated with ischemic acute renal failure." *J Surg Res* 132(1): 104–111.
49. Wu, H, G Chen, KR Wyburn, et al. (2007). "TLR4 activation mediates kidney ischemia/reperfusion injury." *J Clin Invest* 117(10): 2847–2859.
50. Zuk, A, JV Bonventre, D Brown, et al. (1998). "Polarity, integrin, and extracellular matrix dynamics in the postischemic rat kidney." *Am J Physiol* 275(3 Pt 1): C711–731.
51. Zuk, A, JV Bonventre, and KS Matlin (2001). "Expression of fibronectin splice variants in the postischemic rat kidney." *Am J Physiol Renal Physiol* 280(6): F1037–1053.

Uremic Toxins

2.2

Griet Glorieux, Wim Van Biesen, Norbert Lameire, and Raymond Vanholder

Core Messages

- In acute kidney injury (AKI), the specific metabolic conditions induced by renal failure are obscured by many interfering factors (e.g., sepsis, pulmonary dysfunction, and hemodynamic instability).
- Many low-molecular-weight uremic retention solutes contribute to the uremic syndrome, but also the middle-molecular-weight molecules are an important group of biologically active uremic retention solutes.
- Some uremic compounds are difficult to remove by standard dialysis strategies. Increasing pore size, adding convection, and/or increasing dialysis time and frequency improve their removal.
- Optimal toxin removal should be one of the primary aims in the treatment of AKI.

2.2.1 Introduction

The uremic syndrome is characterized by a progressive deterioration of biochemical and physiologic functions, and a quantitative and qualitative deterioration of performance, in parallel with the progression of renal failure. This is largely attributed to the retention of a myriad of compounds that under normal conditions are excreted by the healthy kidneys. The clinical characteristics are aspecific, in a way mimicking the picture of poisoning by drug overdosage. The most pronounced changes are found in the cardiovascular, neurologic, hematologic, and immunologic systems (Table 2.2.1).

The basic pathophysiologic mechanisms are related to the dysfunction of several hormonal, homeostatic, and metabolic systems. Although extensive information is available about the basic functional disturbances in uremia, most studies regarding this issue have been focusing on chronic kidney disease (CKD); one of the reasons for this preference may be the relatively stable clinical condition of CKD patients, whereby clinical, biochemical, and functional investigations can be planned. The acute kidney injury (AKI) patient is in an unstable condition, and in addition, many interfering factors (e.g., sepsis, pulmonary dysfunction, and hemodynamic instability) will obscure the picture. Therefore, most of the accumulated experience on the pathophysiology of uremic toxicity has been obtained in CKD patients. It is, however, conceivable that much can be extrapolated to AKI, in as far as both conditions emanate in uremic toxin accumulation and/or changes in the specific metabolic conditions induced by renal failure.

2.2.2 Interfering Factors Due to Renal Replacement Therapy

Renal replacement therapy, in spite of its beneficial effect on uremic retention, may cause a number of adverse effects or trade-off effects mimicking uremic toxicity.

Dialysis with dialyzers containing complement and leukocyte-activating membranes may affect the immunologic, metabolic, and hematologic status of

R. Vanholder (✉)
Renal Division, Department of Internal Medicine, University Hospital Gent, De pintelaan 185, 9000 Gent, Belgium
e-mail: raymond.vanholder@ugent.be

A. Jörres et al. (eds.), *Management of Acute Kidney Problems*,
DOI: 10.1007/978-3-540-69441-0_2.2, © Springer-Verlag Berlin Heidelberg 2010

Table 2.2.1 Affected organ systems

Affected system	Effect
Cardiovascular system	– Severe inflammation, with the potential to modify the vascular status – Cardiac hypertrophy and dilated cardiomyopathy due to fluid overload and hypoproteinemia
Neurologic system	– Functional and morphologic nervous damage leading to neuropathy (e.g., complex reflex pathways such as F-waves and H-reflexes)
Hematology	– Repeated blood losses or samplings, overt inflammation, and malnutrition might aggravate anemia
Coagulation	– Presence of inflammation should result in a pro-coagulatory effect
Immune status	– Extra morbidity and mortality due to an enhanced susceptibility to infection – The presence of a number of uremic retention solutes (guanidines, AGEs, p-cresylsulphate, cytokines) have the potential to modify immune response
Endocrinology	*Carbohydrate metabolism*: Inadequate response to insulin will result in inadequate cellular uptake of glucose and inadequate calorie utilization *Thyroid hormone*: Thyroid-stimulating hormone release in response to thyroid-releasing hormone is suppressed *Growth hormone*: Administration of growth hormone to ICU patients was shown to have a negative impact on outcome; nevertheless, it appeared to have a positive metabolic effect on critically ill patients with acute renal failure

the patient, irrespective of general toxicity [1]. The insertion of central vein catheters for acute hemodialysis, as well as the use of peritoneal dialysis catheters, may enhance the risk of infection. Both fresh and spent peritoneal dialysis fluid affects leukocyte functional capacity, but in spent dialysate, part of the functional depression may be the consequence of the presence of toxic solutes in the fluid.

Hemodialysis fluid may also have proinflammatory activity, if it contains microbiological contaminants [2, 3]. Although the problem of water purity has been solved in many chronic maintenance dialysis units, appropriate water purification systems are more frequently missing in intensive care units (ICUs). Batch hemodialysis with the Genius system, which makes ultrapure dialysis water available at the bedside, may solve this problem [4].

Arteriovenous fistulae may cause cardiac decompensation. The use of immunosuppressive agents after renal transplants and in autoimmune diseases enhances the risk of infection and cancer. All of these factors may cause problems that at first glance could be related to uremia, as much in CKD as in AKI.

2.2.3 Biochemical Alterations

The uremic syndrome is characterized by a virtually ubiquitous disturbance of biochemical functions. These are at the basis of the clinical epiphenomena. In as far as toxin accumulation is similar in AKI and CKD, these functional disturbances can, by extrapolation, be expected to be similar.

2.2.3.1 *Enzymatic Processes*

In the course of renal failure and uremic retention, a host of enzymatic and metabolic functions are depressed [5]: gluconeogenesis, lactate dehydrogenase, mitochondrial storage of calcium, mitochondrial oxygen consumption, alkaline phosphatase isoenzyme activity, insulin degradation, etc.

Due to a host of enzymatic and functional disturbances, resting cellular and cytosolic Ca^{++} contents are increased, which results in the impairment of various metabolic processes, e.g., pancreatic glucose-dependent insulin secretion [6]. Increased intracellular or cytosolic Ca^{++} has been related to increased peripheral vascular resistance and hence hypertension [7], as well as to a blunted phagocytic response [8]. According to Gafter et al., uremic high red blood cell (RBC) calcium can at least in part be attributed to deficient extrusion after deactivation of Ca^{++}-ATPase [9]. Lindner et al. demonstrated the presence of a circulating inhibitor of the RBC membrane calcium pump in uremic plasma ultrafiltrate [10]. The responsible factor was partially identified and characterized as of low molecular weight, dialyzable, and heat stable.

Both production and metabolic clearance of calcitriol were demonstrated to be disturbed in AKI as well as in CKD [11–13]. In further studies, it was demonstrated that uremic ultrafiltrate contained factors inhibiting both production and metabolization of calcitriol [14]. Some of these factors showed an elution pattern on high-performance liquid chromatography (HPLC), consistent with purines, such as uric acid, or xanthine. Administration of purines induced alterations similar to uremic ultrafiltrate [15]. Infusion of uremic ultrafiltrate to normal rats further reduced the intestinal calcitriol receptor concentration as well as the receptor interaction with DNA in vitro, hence pointing to a reduction of the biological action of calcitriol in renal failure.

From these data it becomes clear that a host of biological processes are depressed or altered in uremia, and that the causative factors are variable and remain to a large part unidentified.

2.2.3.2 Drug Protein Binding

As reviewed previously [16, 17], two binding defects are possible: in one group of essentially acidic drugs, binding is decreased, which means an increase in the free, active fraction; because for most drugs, total (bound plus unbound) concentrations are monitored, lower than normal total concentrations should be aimed at in this situation. At "normal" total levels, toxic adverse effects are to be expected. Current examples are theophylline, phenytoin, methotrexate, diazepam, digoxin, and salicylate [18, 19]. Basic drugs – e.g., propranolol, cimetidine, clonidine, or imipramine – show an increased protein binding. This causes a decrease in available free concentration, diminishing the therapeutic effect. For these drugs, higher total concentrations should be pursued.

Attempts to identify the ligands responsible for decreased protein binding have been scant. Several studies suggest that hippuric acid is one of the main contributing compounds [19–21], but its relative importance remains undefined. Other potential competitors are indoxyl sulphate [21], derivatives of furanpropanoic acid [22, 23], and other furancarboxylic acids [24], β-(*m*-hydroxyphenyl)-hydracrylate and *p*-hydroxyphenylacetate [20].

The rise in binding site number for basic drugs is related to a rise in α1-acid glycoprotein concentration [25], due to its decreased removal by the kidneys.

The altering relations between bound and unbound drug fractions emphasize the importance of monitoring free rather than total drug concentrations in uremic patients.

It should be stressed that changes in drug protein binding are not the only adverse effect of uremia related to pharmacology. Decreased renal clearance and/or metabolism, and changes in distribution volume may also enhance drug toxicity. Increments in active concentration may be compensated for by alternative pathways of metabolization, e.g., hepatic or intestinal. In addition, accumulation of active drug metabolites may add to the toxicity of the accumulation of the genuine drug per se, as is the case for theophylline [26].

Protein binding is not only related to efficacy and toxicity of drugs. In addition, uremic solute protein binding also may alter toxicity, as conceivably only free, nonbound compounds may exert toxicity. Many potential toxins are protein bound (e.g., indoxyl sulphate, the hippuric and propionic acids, phenols, and indoles). Guanidino compounds provoke structural alterations in albumin, decreasing its binding capacity for homocysteine, hence generating more free homocysteine with the potential to enhance the toxic impact of this compound [27]. Peritoneal dialysis may induce a more efficient removal of protein-bound compounds than hemodialysis [28]. Also, albumin-leaking hemodialysis membranes have the capacity to enhance removal of protein-bound molecules [29].

Changes in protein binding of drugs may be an extra source of pathophysiology in AKI because of the multiplicity of drugs that are most often administered to these patients. In addition, patients with AKI often have low plasma protein levels due to inflammation, malnutrition, and protein losses through capillary leaks. All of these conditions, together with uremic toxin accumulation, tend to liberate drugs from binding sites, thus increasing their potential toxicity.

2.2.4 Factors Responsible for the Uremic Syndrome

Our knowledge about the factors responsible for the uremic syndrome remains inconsistent and incomplete. The concept that one single uremic toxin is responsible for the uremic syndrome is likely to be abandoned. In a review, approximately 90 uremic retention solutes were identified as reported in the literature [30]. It is likely, however, that a much larger number of solutes with a toxic potential remain unidentified [31]. Also, the extrapolation of in vitro data to the clinical situation has sometimes resulted in incorrect conclusions, as trivial factors with a potential to introduce bias in the results, such as use of incorrect concentrations [30] or determination errors due to analytical mistakes [32], have often been overlooked.

The uremic syndrome results from the retention of compounds that are cleared by the healthy kidneys; the intake of precursors, mainly via nutrition, also plays a role. This concept is underscored by the success of dialysis in stage 5 CKD and the symptomatic improvement following decreases in dietary protein intake. The uremic syndrome is, however, not only the result of retention of compounds but also of deranged hormonal and enzymatic homeostasis.

Several secondary factors contribute to the uremic syndrome, such as the speed of progression of renal failure and fluctuations in toxin concentration. Analogous to what happens with drugs, peak levels may be more important than trough levels.

Historically, uremic toxicity was at first attributed to low-molecular-weight compounds (molecular weight [MW] < 500 Da). This could not explain the favorable results with continuous ambulatory peritoneal dialysis, however, and as a consequence, the concept of middle molecules was developed. Middle molecules are hypothetical uremic toxins with a molecular weight roughly between 500 and 12,000 Da [33]. The problem when the middle molecule hypothesis was formulated was that no compounds with their characteristics and a definite biological impact were known at that time. Therefore, attention was focused again in the direction of low-molecular-weight solutes, and urea was identified as a useful marker for the biochemical follow-up of maintenance dialysis patients; urea kinetics during and in between dialyses were applied for the calculation of parameters related to dialysis adequacy (Kt/V) and nutritional and metabolic status (protein catabolic rate – PCR). One drawback of urea, however, was that reports on its toxic capacity remained scanty. For that reason, the most recent research has again focused on the characterization of other responsible toxins, which might be characterized by a different kinetic behavior from that of urea.

With improved analytic techniques, it became evident that presumed middle molecular fractions are in fact heterogeneous mixtures containing many lower-molecular-weight compounds [34]. The reason may be that molecular weight is only one factor influencing solute behavior in uremia. Factors which play an additional role include electrostatic charge, hydrophobicity, steric configuration, protein binding, compartmental behavior, and resistance of cell membranes towards gradient-dependent solute transfer. Each of these factors may slow down intradialytic solute movement, either from the plasma to the dialysate compartment or from the intracellular compartment to the plasma. Thus the definition of middle molecules may be extended to much smaller molecules with protein binding and/or multicompartmental distribution.

2.2.5 Major Low-Molecular-Weight Uremic Retention Products

The definition of uremic retention in acute renal failure, as compared with chronic renal failure remains a matter of debate. Most studies on uremic toxicity have at present been undertaken in CKD, which can be attributed to the more stable condition of these chronic renal failure patients. Nevertheless, because in both conditions glomerular filtration decreases substantially, it is conceivable that similar compounds will be retained to a fairly similar extent. However, enhanced tissue breakdown, deficient nutritional status, inflammatory condition, and/or altered bacterial production in the intestines may provoke substantial differences in generation, in spite of similar disturbances of excretion. Whether this results in differences in retention pattern remains largely unknown.

2.2.5.1 Advanced Glycosylation End Products

Advanced glycosylation end products (AGEs) are generated and retained at increasing concentrations during the aging process, but also during diabetes mellitus and uremia [35]. They intrinsically result from nonenzymatic glycosylation, and their presence in diabetes is related to cumulative glucose concentrations resulting in the production of ligands that are linked in a progressive way to other compounds, mainly proteins [36]. In uremia, AGEs are rather generated by oxidative processes. The production process takes a substantial period of time (several weeks). At the end of this period, the resulting modified proteins have not only changed structurally but also functionally. The molecules at the basis of these modifications have a low molecular weight [36]; due to the linkage to amino acids which are part of (poly)peptides, the end products are larger, and often in the middle molecular range. As the development of these compounds takes several weeks, their pathophysiologic importance in AKI, with its relatively short course, may be less prominent, although less stable precursors such as Schiff bases and Amadori products develop in the range of hours to days and may also exert toxicity.

There is not much debate over whether AGEs are retained in uremia [37] and whether they interfere with biological function. Among their influences, a proinflammatory effect has been found quite consistently [38]. Most data in that direction have been obtained with artificially prepared AGEs, however, which do not necessarily conform with the structures retained in uremia. A more recent study showed similar immune-stimulating effects for AGEs definitely retained in uremic patients, albeit not for all compounds submitted to evaluation [39]. Dialytic removal of AGEs is difficult, and only highly efficient strategies, applying very open membranes and convection, seem to affect positively AGE removal [40].

To the best of our knowledge, no information is available about AGE retention in AKI; the long-lasting generation process, covering several weeks, suggests a lower generation than in CKD, unless the general condition of the patient has already stimulated AGE production (e.g., in diabetes mellitus or the aged).

2.2.5.2 Creatinine

The rise in serum creatinine during kidney failure is not linearly related to the decrease in glomerular filtration rate (GFR), which may decrease by 50% or more without marked changes in serum creatinine. Changes become more prominent in the lower range of filtration. There are virtually no convincing arguments in favor of a toxic effect of creatinine, although it may be a precursor of the toxic compound methylguanidine [41].

Serum creatinine concentration is not only affected by kidney failure, but also by muscular status. In AKD, creatinine levels may be at the root of an overestimation of GFR and a false feeling of safety in the case of patients with muscular wasting, which is common after a prolonged stay in the ICU in an inflammatory state [42]. It has been suggested that serum creatinine may be more elevated than can be expected from renal function, in the presence of acute massive muscle necrosis in rhabdomyolysis, but this supposition could not be corroborated clinically. Already small increases in serum creatinine in AKI are related to important increases in mortality [43].

2.2.5.3 Dimethylarginine

Asymmetric dimethylarginine (N,N-dimethylarginine [ADMA]) is an endogenous structure analog of L-arginine, the latter compound being a precursor of nitric oxide (NO) synthesis. NO synthesis which contributes to endothelial protection, is blocked by excess ADMA accumulation in the blood, as is the case in renal failure [44]. In CKD, ADMA concentrations are related to indices of vascular damage [45], although concentration in many studies is below the one inducing NO synthase blockade. Convective strategies enhance ADMA removal in AKI [46].

2.2.5.4 Guanidines

Several guanidines have been related to neurotoxic effects [47, 48]. More recently, it was demonstrated that guanidines interfered with immune function, either in an immune-inhibiting or an immune-enhancing way [49]; guanidine compounds were shown to suppress the natural killer cell response to interleukin 2 [50].

Although guanidine compounds are small and water soluble, most of them distribute over a much larger volume than urea, resulting in a substantial post-dialytic rebound [51]. From this it can be supposed that long, slow dialysis strategies, as are often applied in AKI, may benefit their removal.

2.2.5.5 Hippuric Acid

Indirect data reported by MacNamara et al. [21] and by Gulyassy et al. [20] and more direct studies on ultrafiltrate collected in dialyzed patients [19] demonstrated an interference of hippuric acid with the protein binding of drugs such as phenytoin and theophylline. It also interferes with tubular transport of organic acids. Hippuric acid (MW 179 Da) behaves like larger molecules, due to its protein binding, which even tends to increase during dialysis [52].

The role of hippuric acid in AKI might be substantial due to its interference with drug protein binding and tubular organic acid excretion. Since most patients with AKI receive many drugs, hippuric acid retention results in the liberation of protein-bound drugs from their binding sites and in an enhanced risk for drug toxicity, which is often difficult to quantify. Most drug concentrations are actually monitored as total and in that case pursuing a maximal "acceptable" total drug concentration will lead to a free, active concentration that is too high. The problem of drug protein binding in AKI has to our knowledge, however, not been subjected to in-depth evaluation.

2.2.5.6 Homocysteine

Homocysteine concentration increases in inverse relation to the evolution of renal function [53]. Hyperhomocysteinemia has been limited to premature arterial occlusion in the general population, but it has been more difficult to demonstrate such a relationship in CKD [54]. One might wonder whether exposure to homocysteine in AKI is sufficiently long to induce vascular damage. Dialytic removal of homocysteine is difficult but more efficacious with the use of larger pore sizes [29].

2.2.5.7 Indoxyl Sulphate

Indoxyl sulphate, an indole derivative, is found at high concentrations in uremic serum. It is to a large extent bound to protein. Indoxyl sulphate has been associated with decreases in drug protein binding [21] and with defects of cellular organic acid transport [55]. It has been shown in vitro to interfere with endothelial function and repair [56, 57], an aspect which might play an important role in AKI as well.

Due to its substantial protein binding (about 100% in normals and 90% in uremics), indoxyl sulphate has an intradialytic behavior which is not typical of other low-molecular-weight compounds such as creatinine.

2.2.5.8 Phosphate

Phosphate levels are related to itching, and stimulate parathyroid activity, resulting in hyperparathyroidism. More recently, phosphate has been linked to vascular damage, by deposition of calcium–phosphorus complexes in the vessel wall [58]. Since phosphate accumulates in AKI as well, and since calcium–phosphorus complexes are generated readily once the product exceeds a certain threshold, phosphate retention might be deleterious in AKI as well, but is not necessarily taken into account clinically. Intradialytic kinetics are not straightforward and are not comparable to those of urea, creatinine, or uric acid [59]. Dialytic phosphate removal is followed by a marked rebound [60], suggesting multicompartmental behavior and does not correlate with urea elimination. Standard dialysis, as applied in CKD (alternate days 4 h); might be insufficient for phosphate removal in AKI.

2.2.5.9 Purines

Several purine analogs are retained in uremia: uric acid, xanthine, and hypoxanthine. It has been demonstrated that purines were involved in disturbances of calcitriol production and metabolization. Uric acid, xanthine, and hypoxanthine also inhibit the monocytic response to the cytokine effect of calcitriol [61].

2.2.5.10 Urea

It is accepted that in general urea may only be toxic at higher concentrations than those currently encountered in uremia.

In AKI, urea has been used as a marker for making the decision to start dialysis or not, whereby the molecule is considered both as an indicator of protein catabolism and of uremic retention.

2.2.6 Middle Molecules

For the time being, a substantial number of uremic retention solutes with a molecular weight in excess of 500 Da (so-called middle molecules) have been identified [40, 62–92] (Table 2.2.2). Most of them exert biological actions and interfere especially with immune function and cardiovascular response.

Among these middle molecules, the **peptides** constitute a heterogeneous group of molecules. **Granulocyte-inhibiting protein I (GIP I**; MW 28 kDa), recovered from uremic sera or ultrafiltrate, suppresses the killing of invading bacteria by polymorphonuclear cells [80]. The compound has structural analogy with the variable part of kappa light chains. Another peptide with granulocyte inhibitory effect (**GIP II**; MW 9.5 kDa) is partially homologous with β2-*microglobulin,* and inhibits granulocyte glucose uptake and respiratory burst activity [74]. A **degranulation-inhibiting protein** (DIP; MW: 24 kDa), identical to *angiogenin*, was isolated from plasma ultrafiltrate of uremic patients [91]. The structure responsible for the inhibition of degranulation is different from the sites that are responsible for the angiogenic activity of angiogenin. A structural variant of *ubiquitin* inhibits polymorphonuclear chemotaxis (**chemotaxis-inhibiting protein** [CIP]; MW 8.5 kDa) [65]. The presence of these granulocyte inhibitory proteins might hamper immune defenses, which might be deleterious in AKI patients who suffer often from infection. Also **kappa and lambda light chains** have a negative impact on immune activity [64].

Leptin is a 16-kDa compound, which in addition is protein bound and thus difficult to remove by dialysis. Its pathophysiologic role has been linked to malnutrition, again a current problem in AKI [93].

Parathyroid hormone is secreted in a compensatory reaction to hypocalcemia, hyperphosphatemia, and a shortage of active vitamin D analogs, which are all induced by kidney failure [94]. Also in AKI, parathyroid levels start to rise soon after its development [95]. The toxic role of parathyroid hormone is essentially linked to its capacity to enhance calcium uptake into the cell, with the subsequent modification of several essential functions [96].

Table 2.2.2 Middle molecules ($N = 32$)

Middle molecule	Molecular weight (kDa)	Reference
Adiponectin	30.0	[89]
Adrenomedullin	5.7	[81]
Atrial natriuretic peptide	3.1	[69]
β_2-Microglobulin	11.8	[40, 82]
β-Endorphin	3.5	[75]
Basic fibroblast growth factor (bFGF)	18–24.0	[90]
Calcitonin gene-related peptide (CGRP)	3.8	[85]
Cholecystokinin	3.9	[62]
Chemotaxis-inhibiting protein	8.5	[65]
Clara cell protein	15.8	[82]
Complement factor D	23.7	[86]
Cystatin C	13.3	[82]
Degranulation-inhibiting protein	14.1	[88]
Delta-sleep-inducing peptide	0.8	[77]
Endothelin	4.3	[69]
Guanylin	1.5	[84]
Granulocyte-inhibiting protein (GIP I;GIP II)	28; 9.5	[74, 80, 91]
Hyaluronic acid	25.0	[68]
Interleukin-1β	32.0	[87]
Interleukin-6	24.5	[83]
Interleukin-18	20.0	[73]
kappa-Ig light chain	25.0	[64, 66]
lambda-Ig light chain	25.0	[64, 66]
Leptin	16.0	[67, 79]
Methionine-enkephalin	0.5	[75]
Motiline	2.7	[78]
Neuropeptide Y	4.3	[62]
Parathyroid hormone	9.2	[92]
Retinol-binding protein	21.2	[82]
Substance P	1.3	[76]
Tumor necrosis factor-a	26.0	[70, 83]
Uroguanylin	1.7	[72]
Vasopressin	1.1	[63]
Vasoactive intestinal peptide (VIP)	3.3	[71]

β_2–Microglobulin is a 11.8-kDa molecule, which has most essentially been related to renal failure and dialysis-related amyloidosis [97]. The latter is a slowly developing complication which takes many years of dialysis in proinflammatory conditions, and the course of AKI is probably too short in most cases to induce this disease. The further role of β_2-microglobulin is related to its frequent use as a marker of large-molecule removal by dialysis.

Perhaps the pathophysiologically most relevant middle molecules in AKI are the **cytokines**, which are retained in renal failure and generated in infection. Since many patients with AKI are septic, they may often develop overwhelmingly high cytokine concentrations in their blood. These cytokines are essential for the immune response, but may become toxic by themselves by inducing inflammatory damage (multiorgan failure).

2.2.7 Factors Influencing Plasma Concentration of Uremic Solutes

It is difficult to define per individual patient which concentration is useful and which is deleterious, and this weighs on the decision-making regarding whether or not to remove these molecules. All middle molecules are hardly if at all removed by standard dialysis strategies. Removal becomes only possible by increasing pore size, adding convection, and/or increasing dialysis length and frequency [98, 99]. When doing this in a setting of continuous renal replacement therapy (CRRT), blood and dialysate flows are generally low, so that removal is restricted, unless extreme quantities of ultrafiltration and substitution fluid are imposed [100]. Alternatively, intermittent dialysis may be applied with larger-pore, high-flux membranes. In general, however, intermittent dialysis for AKI is conducted with low-flux membranes, essentially because guarantees of water purity are insufficient in ICUs. In this setting, middle molecule removal is nil. For that reason, dialysis strategies with large-pore membranes and ultrapure water, if possible prolonged, daily, and at intermediate blood and dialysate flow rates, should be preferred.

It has been claimed that membranes for CRRT provoke substantial removal by adsorption of middle molecules, especially cytokines. Careful kinetic studies, however, have shown that adsorptive and global removal by these devices is relatively small and rapidly overwhelmed by massive generation, and even more importantly, that removal of both proinflammatory and antiinflammatory cytokines is similar, resulting in a neutral net effect on the immune system [101].

2.2.8 Conclusions and Therapeutic Implications

The uremic syndrome is related to a complex set of biochemical and pathophysiologic alterations, which result in a state of malaise and generalized dysfunction. The basic process at the origin of this malfunction is the retention of toxic solutes due to the decrease of GFR, in CKD as well as AKI. This condition should be corrected by the removal of these toxins, although many of the retention compounds are difficult to remove by standard dialysis strategies: e.g., protein-bound and/or larger "middle" molecules. It has been demonstrated that several of these compounds exert biological and biochemical action, and hence may induce complications and affect clinical condition. Remarkably enough, solute retention and removal are estimated essentially by studying the behavior of small water soluble compounds, such as urea and creatinine, which, however, are biochemically inert.

In AKI, functional disturbances attributable to toxins may be induced to an equal extent as in CKD but may be paralleled or even overwhelmed by other pathophysiologic events, such as sepsis, fluid overload, inflammation, blood losses, malnutrition, and vitamin deficiency. For that reason, it is not always possible to induce functional improvement by specifically removing uremic solutes alone; this aim should rather be pursued by applying a whole set of therapies. Optimal toxin removal should, however, be one of these primary aims.

Analogous to CKD, it might also be reasonable in AKI to enhance removal of the difficult-to-remove molecules, by increasing membrane pore size, convection, dialysis frequency, and dialysis length. One drawback in this setting might be the relative impurity of dialysis water at many ICUs. Therefore, dialysis water purity should be another aim to be pursued.

References

1. Vanholder R, Ringoir S, Dhondt A, et al (1991) Phagocytosis in uremic and hemodialysis patients: a prospective and cross sectional study. Kidney Int 39: 320–327.
2. Lonnemann G (2000) Chronic inflammation in hemodialysis: the role of contaminated dialysate. Blood Purif 18: 214–223.
3. Lonnemann GR (2000) The quality of dialysate: an integrated approach. Kidney Int 58: S112–S119.

4. Lonnemann G (2000) Should ultra-pure dialysate be mandatory? Nephrol Dial Transplant 15: 55–59.
5. Ringoir S, Schoots A, and Vanholder R (1988) Uremic toxins. Kidney Int Suppl 24: S4–S9.
6. Fadda GZ, Hajjar SM, Perna AF, et al (1991) On the mechanism of impaired insulin secretion in chronic renal failure. J Clin Invest 87: 255–261.
7. Raine AE, Bedford L, Simpson AW, et al (1993) Hyperparathyroidism, platelet intracellular free calcium and hypertension in chronic renal failure. Kidney Int 43: 700–705.
8. Alexiewicz JM, Smogorzewski M, Fadda GZ, et al (1991) Impaired phagocytosis in dialysis patients: studies on mechanisms. Am J Nephrol 11: 102–111.
9. Gafter U, Malachi T, Barak H, et al (1990) Red blood cell calcium level in chronic renal failure: effect of continuous ambulatory peritoneal dialysis. J Lab Clin Med 116: 386–392.
10. Lindner A, Gagne ER, Zingraff J, et al (1992) A circulating inhibitor of the RBC membrane calcium pump in chronic renal failure. Kidney Int 42: 1328–1335.
11. Hsu CH, Patel S, Young EW, et al (1987) Production and degradation of calcitriol in renal-failure rats. Am J Physiol 253: F1015–F1019.
12. Hsu CH, Patel S, Young EW, et al (1988) Production and metabolic-clearance of calcitriol in acute renal-failure. Kidney Int 33: 530–535.
13. Hsu CH and Patel S (1990) Factors influencing calcitriol metabolism in renal failure. Kidney Int 37: 44–50.
14. Hsu CH, Vanholder R, Patel S, et al (1991) Subfractions in uremic plasma ultrafiltrate inhibit calcitriol metabolism. Kidney Int 40: 868–873.
15. Hsu CH, Patel SR, Young EW, et al (1991) Effects of purine derivatives on calcitriol metabolism in rats. Am J Physiol 260: F596–F601.
16. Piafsky KM (1980) Disease-induced changes in the plasma binding of basic drugs. Clin Pharmacokinet 5: 246–262.
17. Lindup WE, Bishop KA, and Collier R (1986) Drug binding defect of uremic plasma: contribution of endogenous binding inhibitors. In: Tillement JP and Lindenlaub E (eds) Protein binding and drug transport, pp 397–414. Schattauer Verlag, Stuttgart.
18. Roman S, Gulyassy PF, and Depner TA (1984) Inhibition of salicylate binding to normal plasma by extracts of uremic fluids. Am J Kidney Dis 4: 153–161.
19. Vanholder R, Van Landschoot N, de Smet R, et al (1988) Drug protein binding in chronic renal failure: evaluation of nine drugs. Kidney Int 33: 996–1004.
20. Gulyassy PF, Bottini AT, Stanfel LA, et al (1986) Isolation and chemical identification of inhibitors of plasma ligand binding. Kidney Int 30: 391–398.
21. McNamara PJ, Lalka D, and Gibaldi M (1981) Endogenous accumulation products and serum protein binding in uremia. J Lab Clin Med 98: 730–740.
22. Mabuchi H and Nakahashi H (1986) Isolation and characterization of an endogenous drug-binding inhibitor present in uremic serum. Nephron 44: 277–281.
23. Mabuchi H and Nakahashi H (1986) Profiling of endogenous ligand solutes that bind to serum proteins in sera of patients with uremia. Nephron 43: 110–116.
24. Niwa T, Takeda N, Maeda K, et al (1988) Accumulation of furancarboxylic acids in uremic serum as inhibitors of drug binding. Clin Chim Acta 173: 127–138.
25. Paxton JW (1983) Alpha 1-acid glycoprotein and binding of basic drugs. Methods Find Exp Clin Pharmacol 5: 635–648.
26. Nicot G, Charmes JP, Lachatre G, et al (1989) Theophylline toxicity risks and chronic renal failure. Int J Clin Pharmacol Ther Toxicol 27: 398–401.
27. Perna AF, Ingrosso D, Satta E, et al (2004) Plasma protein aspartyl damage is increased in hemodialysis patients: studies on causes and consequences. J Am Soc Nephrol 15: 2747–+.
28. Gulyassy PF (1994) Can dialysis remove protein bound toxins that accumulate because of renal secretory failure? ASAIO J 40: 92–94.
29. Galli F, Benedetti S, Buoncristiani U, et al (2003) The effect of PMMA-based protein-leaking dialyzers on plasma homocysteine levels. Kidney Int 64: 748–755.
30. Vanholder R, de Smet R, Glorieux G, et al (2003) Review on uremic toxins: classification, concentration, and interindividual variability. Kidney Int 63: 1934–1943.
31. Weissinger EM, Kaiser T, Meert N, et al (2004) Proteomics: a novel tool to unravel the patho-physiology of uraemia. Nephrol Dial Transplant 19: 3068–3077.
32. Martinez AW, Recht NS, Hostetter TH, et al (2005) Removal of p-cresol sulphate by hemodialysis. J Am Soc Nephrol 16: 3430–3436.
33. Schoots A, Mikkers F, Cramers C, et al (1984) Uremic toxins and the elusive middle molecules. Nephron 38: 1–8.
34. Schoots AC, Mikkers FE, Claessens HA, et al (1982) Characterization of uremic "middle molecular" fractions by gas chromatography, mass spectrometry, isotachophoresis, and liquid chromatography. Clin Chem 28: 45–49.
35. Ritz E, Deppisch R, and Nawroth P (1994) Toxicity of uremia – does it come of age. Nephrol Dial Transplant 9: 1–2.
36. Bucala R, Tracey KJ, and Cerami A (1991) Advanced glycosylation products quench nitric oxide and mediate defective endothelium-dependent vasodilatation in experimental diabetes. J Clin Invest 87: 432–438.
37. Dolhoferbliesener R, Lechner B, Deppisch R, et al (1995) Immunological determination of advanced glycosylation end-products in human blood and urine. Nephrol Dial Transplant 10: 657–664.
38. Witko-Sarsat V, Friedlander M, Nguyen KT, et al (1998) Advanced oxidation protein products as novel mediators of inflammation and monocyte activation in chronic renal failure. J Immunol 161: 2524–2532.
39. Glorieux G, Helling R, Henle T, et al (2004) In vitro evidence for immune activating effect of specific AGE structures retained in uremia. Kidney Int 66: 1873–1880.
40. Stein G, Franke S, Mahiout A, et al (2001) Influence of dialysis modalities on serum AGE levels in end-stage renal disease patients. Nephrol Dial Transplant 16: 999–1008.
41. Yokozawa T, Fujitsuka N, and Oura H (1991) Studies on the precursor of methylguanidine in rats with renal-failure. Nephron 58: 90–94.
42. Hoste EA, Lameire NH, Vanholder RC, et al (2003) Acute renal failure in patients with sepsis in a surgical

ICU: predictive factors, incidence, comorbidity, and outcome. J Am Soc Nephrol 14: 1022–1030.
43. Hoste EA and Kellum JA (2006) RIFLE criteria provide robust assessment of kidney dysfunction and correlate with hospital mortality. Crit Care Med 34: 2016–2017.
44. Vallance P, Leone A, Calver A, et al (1992) Accumulation of an endogenous inhibitor of nitric oxide synthesis in chronic renal failure. Lancet 339: 572–575.
45. Zoccali C, Benedetto FA, Maas R, et al (2002) Asymmetric dimethylarginine, C-reactive protein, and carotid intima-media thickness in end-stage renal disease. J Am Soc Nephrol 13: 490–496.
46. Kielstein JT, Boger RH, Bode-Boger SM, et al (2004) Low dialysance of asymmetric dimethylarginine (ADMA) – in vivo and in vitro evidence of significant protein binding. Clin Nephrol 62: 295–300.
47. D'Hooge R, Pei YQ, Manil J, et al (1992) The uremic guanidino compound guanidinosuccinic acid induces behavioral convulsions and concomitant epileptiform electrocorticographic discharges in mice. Brain Res 598: 316–320.
48. Giovannetti S, Balestri PL, and Barsotti G (1973) Methylguanidine in uremia. Arch Intern Med 131: 709–713.
49. Glorieux GL, Dhondt AW, Jacobs P, et al (2004) In vitro study of the potential role of guanidines in leukocyte functions related to atherogenesis and infection. Kidney Int 65: 2184–2192.
50. Asaka M, Iida H, Izumino K, et al (1988) Depressed natural killer cell activity in uremia. Evidence for immunosuppressive factor in uremic sera. Nephron 49: 291–295.
51. Eloot S, Torremans A, de Smet R, et al (2005) Kinetic behavior of urea is different from that of other water-soluble compounds: the case of the guanidino compounds. Kidney Int 67: 1566–1575.
52. Farrell PC, Gotch FA, Peters JH, et al (1978) Binding of hippurate in normal plasma and in uremic plasma pre- and postdialysis. Nephron 20: 40–46.
53. Chauveau P, Chadefaux B, Coude M, et al (1993) Hyperhomocysteinemia, a risk factor for atherosclerosis in chronic uremic patients. Kidney Int 43: S72–S77.
54. Suliman ME, Qureshi AR, Barany P, et al (2000) Hyperhomocysteinemia, nutritional status, and cardiovascular disease in hemodialysis patients. Kidney Int 57: 1727–1735.
55. Boumendil-Podevin EF, Podevin RA, et al (1975) Uricosuric agents in uremic sera. Identification of indoxyl sulphate and hippuric acid. J Clin Invest 55: 1142–1152.
56. Dou L, Bertrand E, Cerini C, et al (2004) The uremic solutes p-cresol and indoxyl sulphate inhibit endothelial proliferation and wound repair. Kidney Int 65: 442–451.
57. Dou L, Jourde-Chiche N, Faure V, et al (2007) The uremic solute indoxyl sulphate induces oxidative stress in endothelial cells. J Thromb Haemost 5: 1302–1308.
58. Block GA and Port FK (2000) Re-evaluation of risks associated with hyperphosphatemia and hyperparathyroidism in dialysis patients: recommendations for a change in management. Am J Kidney Dis 35: 1226–1237.
59. Sugisaki H, Onohara M, and Kunitomo T (1982) Dynamic behavior of plasma phosphate in chronic dialysis patients. Trans Am Soc Artif Intern Organs 28: 302–311.
60. Haas T, Hillion D and Dongradi G (1991) Phosphate kinetics in dialysis patients. Nephrol Dial Transplant 6 (Suppl 2): 108–113.
61. Glorieux G, Hsu CH, de Smet R, et al (1998) Inhibition of calcitriol-induced monocyte CD14 expression by uremic toxins: role of purines. J Am Soc Nephrol 9: 1826–1831.
62. Aguilera A, Codoceo R, Selgas R, et al (1998) Anorexigen (TNF-alpha, cholecystokinin) and orexigen (neuropeptide Y) plasma levels in peritoneal dialysis (PD) patients: their relationship with nutritional parameters. Nephrol Dial Transplant 13: 1476–1483.
63. Andersson U, Sylven C, Lindvall K, et al (1988) Cardiac function and cardiovascular hormone balance during hemodialysis with special reference to atrial natriuretic peptide. Clin Nephrol 30: 303–307.
64. Cohen G, Mai B, Haagweber M, et al (1995) Effect of immunoglobulin light-chains on Pmn functions. Kidney Int 47: 969.
65. Cohen G, Rudnicki M, and Horl WH (1998) Isolation of modified ubiquitin as a neutrophil chemotaxis inhibitor from uremic patients. J Am Soc Nephrol 9: 451–456.
66. Cohen G, Rudnicki M, Schmaldienst S, et al (2002) Effect of dialysis on serum/plasma levels of free immunoglobulin light chains in end-stage renal disease patients. Nephrol Dial Transplant 17: 879–883.
67. Dagogo-Jack S, Ovalle F, Landt M, et al (1998) Hyperleptinemia in patients with end-stage renal disease undergoing continuous ambulatory peritoneal dialysis. Perit Dial Int 18: 34–40.
68. de Medina M, Ashby M, Diego J, et al (1999) Factors that influence serum hyaluronan levels in hemodialysis patients. ASAIO J 45: 428–430.
69. Deray G, Carayon A, Maistre G, et al (1992) Endothelin in chronic renal failure. Nephrol Dial Transplant 7: 300–305.
70. Descamps-Latscha B, Herbelin A, Nguyen AT, et al (1995) Balance between IL-1 beta, TNF-alpha, and their specific inhibitors in chronic renal failure and maintenance dialysis. Relationships with activation markers of T cells, B cells, and monocytes. J Immunol 154: 882–892.
71. Doherty CC, Buchanan KD, Ardill J, et al (1978) Elevations of gastrointestinal hormones in chronic renal failure. Proc Eur Dial Transplant Assoc 15: 456–465.
72. Fukae H, Kinoshita H, Fujimoto S, et al (2000) Plasma concentration of uroguanylin in patients on maintenance dialysis therapy. Nephron 84: 206–210.
73. Gangemi S, Mallamace A, Minciullo PL, et al (2002) Involvement of interleukin-18 in patients on maintenance haemodialysis. Am J Nephrol 22: 417–421.
74. Haag-Weber M, Mai B, and Horl WH (1994) Isolation of a granulocyte inhibitory protein from uraemic patients with homology of beta 2-microglobulin. Nephrol Dial Transplant 9: 382–388.
75. Hegbrant J, Thysell H, and Ekman R (1991) Elevated plasma levels of opioid peptides and delta sleep-inducing peptide but not of corticotropin-releasing hormone in patients receiving chronic hemodialysis. Blood Purif 9: 188–194.
76. Hegbrant J, Thysell H, and Ekman R (1991) Plasma levels of gastrointestinal regulatory peptides in patients receiving maintenance hemodialysis. Scand J Gastroenterol 26: 599–604.

77. Hegbrant J, Thysell H, and Ekman R (1992) Erythropoietin treatment and plasma levels of corticotropin-releasing hormone, delta sleep-inducing peptide and opioid peptides in hemodialysis patients. Scand J Urol Nephrol 26: 393–396.
78. Hegbrant J, Thysell H, Martensson L, et al (1993) Changes in plasma levels of vasoactive peptides during standard bicarbonate hemodialysis. Nephron 63: 303–308.
79. Heimburger O, Lonnqvist F, Danielsson A, et al (1997) Serum immunoreactive leptin concentration and its relation to the body fat content in chronic renal failure. J Am Soc Nephrol 8: 1423–1430.
80. Horl WH, Haag-Weber M, Georgopoulos A, et al (1990) Physicochemical characterization of a polypeptide present in uremic serum that inhibits the biological activity of polymorphonuclear cells. Proc Natl Acad Sci USA 87: 6353–6357.
81. Ishimitsu T, Nishikimi T, Saito Y, et al (1994) Plasma levels of adrenomedullin, a newly identified hypotensive peptide, in patients with hypertension and renal failure. J Clin Invest 94: 2158–2161.
82. Kabanda A, Jadoul M, Pochet JM, et al (1994) Determinants of the serum concentrations of low molecular weight proteins in patients on maintenance hemodialysis. Kidney Int 45: 1689–1696.
83. Kimmel PL, Phillips TM, Simmens SJ, et al (1998) Immunologic function and survival in hemodialysis patients. Kidney Int 54: 236–244.
84. Kinoshita H, Nakazato M, Yamaguchi H, et al (1997) Increased plasma guanylin levels in patients with impaired renal function. Clin Nephrol 47: 28–32.
85. Odar-Cederlof I, Theodorsson E, Eriksson CG, et al (1993) Vasoactive agents and blood pressure regulation in sequential ultrafiltration and hemodialysis. Int J Artif Organs 16: 662–669.
86. Pascual M, Steiger G, Estreicher J, et al (1988) Metabolism of complement factor D in renal failure. Kidney Int 34: 529–536.
87. Pereira BJ, Shapiro L, King AJ, et al (1994) Plasma levels of IL-1 beta, TNF alpha and their specific inhibitors in undialyzed chronic renal failure, CAPD and hemodialysis patients. Kidney Int 45: 890–896.
88. Shimoyama S, Yamasaki K, Kawahara M, et al (1999) Increased serum angiogenin concentration in colorectal cancer is correlated with cancer progression. Clin Cancer Res 5: 1125–1130.
89. Stenvinkel P, Marchlewska A, Pecoits-Filho R, et al (2004) Adiponectin in renal disease: relationship to phenotype and genetic variation in the gene encoding adiponectin. Kidney Int 65: 274–281.
90. Stompor T, Rajzer M, Sulowicz W, et al (2003) An association between aortic pulse wave velocity, blood pressure and chronic inflammation in ESRD patients on peritoneal dialysis. Int J Artif Organs 26: 188–195.
91. Tschesche H, Kopp C, Horl WH, et al (1994) Inhibition of degranulation of polymorphonuclear leukocytes by angiogenin and its tryptic fragment. J Biol Chem 269: 30274–30280.
92. Tsukamoto Y, Hanaoka M, Matsuo T, et al (2000) Effect of 22-oxacalcitriol on bone histology of hemodialyzed patients with severe secondary hyperparathyroidism. Am J Kidney Dis 35: 458–464.
93. Stenvinkel P, Pecoits R, and Lindholm B (2003) Leptin, ghrelin, and proinflammatory cytokines: compounds with nutritional impact in chronic kidney disease?. Adv Renal Repl Ther 10: 332–345.
94. Felsenfeld AJ and Rodriguez M (1996) Parathyroid gland function in the hemodialysis patient. Semin Dial 9: 303–309.
95. Druml W, Schwarzenhofer M, Apsner R, et al (1998) Fat-soluble vitamins in patients with acute renal failure. Miner Electrolyte Metab 24: 220–226.
96. Massry SG and Smogorzewski M (1994) Mechanisms through which parathyroid hormone mediates its deleterious effects on organ function in uremia. Semin Nephrol 14: 219–231.
97. Gejyo F, Yamada T, Odani S, et al (1985) A new form of amyloid protein associated with chronic hemodialysis was identified as beta 2-microglobulin. Biochem Biophys Res Commun 129: 701–706.
98. Locatelli F, Mastrangelo F, Redaelli B, et al (1996) Effects of different membranes and dialysis technologies on patient treatment tolerance and nutritional parameters. The Italian Cooperative Dialysis Study Group. Kidney Int 50: 1293–1302.
99. Raj DS, Ouwendyk M, Francoeur R, et al (2000) beta(2)-microglobulin kinetics in nocturnal haemodialysis. Nephrol Dial Transplant 15: 58–64.
100. Ronco C, Bellomo R, Homel P, et al (2000) Effects of different doses in continuous veno-venous haemofiltration on outcomes of acute renal failure: a prospective randomised trial. Lancet 356: 26–30.
101. De Vriese AS, Colardyn FA, Philippe JJ, et al (1999) Cytokine removal during continuous hemofiltration in septic patients. J Am Soc Nephrol 10: 846–853.

Prerenal Acute Kidney Failure

2.3

Eric A. J. Hoste

Core Messages

- Prerenal acute kidney failure is a form of acute kidney injury (AKI) that is rapidly reversible. It can be differentiated from intrinsic acute kidney failure, a condition that is not rapidly reversible, and often needs treatment with renal replacement therapy, by a series of biochemical and urine variables.
- Prerenal acute kidney failure is a heterogeneous group of conditions, with different pathogeneses. While some forms are caused by hypoperfusion of the kidneys, others are probably caused by inflammation and microcirculatory abnormalities of the kidneys.
- Prerenal acute kidney failure is a frequently occurring condition in hospitalized and intensive care unit (ICU) patients. When AKI is classified according to the most severe form during hospitalization, pre-renal acute kidney failure accounts for almost half of the cases of AKI, and is associated with a better prognosis than intrinsic acute kidney failure.

2.3.1 Introduction

Prerenal acute kidney failure is commonly used term for a well-established form of acute kidney injury (AKI), referred to in textbooks and the medical literature [10, 22, 31]. However, there is actually not a uniform definition for this condition. Prerenal acute kidney failure is characterized by a reversible decrease of kidney function or glomerular filtration rate caused by decreased kidney perfusion. There are no structural abnormalities of the kidneys, although this paradigm is not supported by hard data. Restoration of kidney perfusion results in rapid normalization of kidney function. In many patients the therapy for restoration of kidney perfusion consists of administration of fluids. Therefore, an alternative, much-used terminology for prerenal acute kidney failure is volume-responsive acute kidney injury. However, not all causes of kidney hypoperfusion can be treated with volume; for instance, patients with congestive heart failure may need inotropic support for restoration of blood flow.

The generally accepted paradigm for prerenal acute kidney failure states that when prerenal acute kidney failure persists for a longer period, hypoperfusion of the kidneys will lead to ischemia and acute tubular necrosis, or intrinsic acute kidney failure [10, 22, 31], a condition in which the kidney is affected, and which is not rapidly reversible. Especially, the outer medullary region is at risk for this, because as a consequence of the particular renal vasculature, oxygen supply in this region of the kidney is limited, while energy demands are high [31]. It is less clear when exactly a patient progresses from prerenal to intrinsic acute kidney failure, and how to detect this progression. Especially as histological data that may support this are scarce or nonexistent [24]. In fact, biopsy studies in patients with the clinical syndrome of acute tubular necrosis were normal in many patients. The ischemia and necrosis paradigm for progression of prerenal to intrinsic acute kidney failure is supported by several observations in animal models [7–9]. However, alternative mechanisms may underlie the pathogenesis of

E. A. J. Hoste
Department of Intensive Care Medicine, 2K12-C, Gent University Hospital, De pintelaan 185, 9000 Gent, Belgium
e-mail: eric.hoste@ugent.be

A. Jörres et al. (eds.), *Management of Acute Kidney Problems,*
DOI: 10.1007/978-3-540-69441-0_2.3, © Springer-Verlag Berlin Heidelberg 2010

prerenal acute kidney failure. There are an increasing number of observations in patients and in animal models of sepsis, one of the conditions that may cause prerenal acute kidney failure, that demonstrate that kidney perfusion, including blood flow in the outer medullary region, is not decreased in sepsis [6, 14, 16, 17, 23]. In addition, it was anticipated that vasoconstrictor agents such as norepinephrine would decrease renal blood flow; however, the opposite is true. Norepinephrine leads to improvement of renal blood flow, medullary blood flow, and creatinine clearance [1, 15, 16]. The current evidence for the pathogenesis of prerenal acute kidney injury in sepsis points therefore to a deficient microcirculation in the kidneys secondary to inflammation.

2.3.2 Pathophysiology

Prerenal acute kidney failure is a heterogeneous group of conditions, and multiple pathways may lead to the clinical condition of prerenal acute kidney failure.

(a) *Hypoperfusion*

Hypoperfusion of the kidneys will lead to activation and a complex interplay of several neurohormonal processes that act to correct for hypoperfusion of the kidneys [4]. Activation of the sympatic nervous system, the renin-angiotensin-aldosterone system, vasopressin, and endothelin, will lead to vasoconstriction, increase of blood pressure, and sodium and water retention. These actions are counterbalanced by the actions of prostaglandins, nitric oxide, natriuretic peptides, and bradykinin. Also, right-sided heart failure with venous congestion will contribute to a decreased glomerular perfusion [25, 34].

(b) *Inflammation*

Inflammation plays an important role in the pathophysiology in certain conditions of prerenal acute kidney injury where kidney perfusion is not decreased, e.g., sepsis. Infection leads to release of tumor necrosis factor, interleukin-1 (IL-1), and IL-6, and platelet-activating factor, and this sets off a whole cascade of proinflammatory and antiinflammatory cytokines. The resultant localized and systemic inflammatory response induces vasoconstriction, neutrophil aggregation, production of reactive oxygen species, induction of tissue factor, and thrombosis [20, 33]. Kidneys are especially vulnerable to cytokine-mediated injury. The intrarenal microcirculation is affected by several inflammatory mediators, inducible nitric oxide synthase (iNOS), a vasodilator, and endothelins, which are potent vasoconstrictors. Deficient microcirculation in the kidney is probably an important factor for development of certain forms of prerenal acute kidney failure as in sepsis and severe inflammation.

(c) *Low levels of activated protein C*

Activated protein C (aPC) concentrations are decreased in patients with sepsis, and it has been shown that administration of aPC leads to improved survival [3]. It has also been demonstrated in an animal model of sepsis that treatment with aPC results in improved microcirculatory blood flow in the kidney, and reduced leukocyte rolling and adherence [18, 19]. In addition, substitution with aPC, decreased iNOS, reduced activation of the renin-angiotensin system and caspase-3 activity, and led to an improvement of kidney function [18, 19].

(d) *Drug nephrotoxicity*

Certain drugs, such as calcineurin inhibitors [5], can cause renal vasoconstriction and a prerenal form of acute kidney failure.

2.3.3 Causes of Prerenal Acute Kidney Failure

A wide variety of conditions may lead to prerenal acute kidney failure. These can be categorized into conditions leading to low effective arterial blood volume, low cardiac output, or decreased perfusion as a consequence of vascular problems (Table 2.3.1).

Low effective arterial blood volume can be present in patients who are volume depleted, such as in hemorrhagic shock, or after dehydration by, e.g., diarrhea, fever, or as a result of excessive perspiration or transpiration. But also sepsis patients who are fluid overloaded and present with massive edema can develop low effective arterial blood volume by redistribution of volume from the arterial compartment to the venous and interstitial compartments.

Table 2.3.1 Major causes of prerenal acute kidney failure

A. ***Low effective arterial blood volume***
• Absolute volume depletion:
– Hemorrhagic shock
– Diarrhea
– Fever
• Relative volume depletion:
– Sepsis
– Hepatorenal syndrome
B. ***Low cardiac output***
• Cardiogenic shock
• Pulmonary embolism
• Mechanical ventilation
C. ***Vascular problems***
• Renal artery stenosis
• Decreased perfusion of single nephron by NSAIDs,ACEIs, ARBs

NSAID = nonsteroidal antiinflammatory drug; ACEI = angiotensin-converting enzyme inhibitor; ARB = angiotensin II receptor blocker.

Table 2.3.2 Biochemical indices for the differential diagnosis of prerenal and renal acute kidney failure (AKF)

	Prerenal AKF	Renal AKF
Urine analysis	Hyaline casts	abnormal
Specific gravidity urine	>1.020	<1.010
U_{Osm} (mOsm/kg H_2O)	>500	<300–500
U_{Osm}/S_{Osm}	>1.5	<1.1
U_{Na} (mmol/L)	<20	>40
FE_{Na} (%)	<1	>2
FE_{urea} (%)	<0.35	>0.35
$FE_{uric\ acid}$ (%)	<7	>15
Renal failure index	<1	>1
$U_{creatinine}/S_{creatinine}$	>40	<20
$S_{urea}/S_{creatinine}$	>40	<20–30

U_{Osm} = urine osmolality; U_{Na} = urine sodium concentration; FE = fractional excretion; S_{Osm} = serum osmolality

Low cardiac output can be caused by a wide variety of acute or chronic cardiac diseases, e.g., acute myocardial infarction, aortic valve stenosis, congestive heart failure, or pericardial tamponade. But also mechanical ventilation may lead to a decreased cardiac output, decreased renal perfusion, and prerenal acute kidney failure [21, 32]. Mechanical ventilation leads to increased thoracic pressure, which will decrease cardiac preload, and increase cardiac afterload, and as a result of this may lead to decreased cardiac output. In addition, permissive hypoxemia and hypercapnia may alter renal hemodynamics. Also, mechanical ventilation may cause biotrauma, leading to an inflammatory response in the lung, which in turn may affect kidney function [13]. This also illustrates that the traditional paradigm that prerenal acute kidney failure is not associated with structural abnormalities of the kidney is probably a simplification of the complex mechanisms underlying it.

2.3.4 Diagnosis of Prerenal Acute Kidney Injury

Prerenal acute kidney injury is essentially an oliguric form of acute kidney failure, although nonoliguric prerenal acute kidney injury has also been described [29].

Urine analysis is a central element in the diagnosis of prerenal acute kidney failure and the differentiation with intrinsic acute kidney failure (Table 2.3.2). The kidney is not affected in prerenal acute kidney failure, therefore the tubules function normally, and a series of biochemical indices may indicate whether there is hypoperfusion of the kidney or prerenal acute kidney injury. Although the various variables listed in Table 2.3.2 have been used in clinical practice for years, and are widely cited in literature, the level of evidence supporting their use is limited [2].

2.3.5 Epidemiology of Prerenal Acute Kidney Failure

The annual incidence of prerenal acute kidney failure has been reported in a range between 7% and 48%, depending on the characteristics of the population studied. In the early 1990s, Liaño et al. found that 24.5% of hospitalized patients with a serum creatinine equal or greater than 2.0 mg/dl, had a prerenal type of AKI [26]. Brivet et al. found in the same period in a cohort of patients with serum creatine ≥3.5 mg/dl, an incidence of 7% [11]. In other words, more severe AKI, defined by a higher serum creatinine, has a lower incidence of prerenal acute kidney failure. Also, severity of illness has an impact on the incidence of prerenal acute kidney failure. Liaño et al. found that hospitalized non-ICU patients with acute kidney failure had a lower incidence of prerenal acute kidney failure compared with ICU patients (17.8% vs 28.1%) [27].

Finally, the incidence of prerenal acute kidney failure seems to be higher in recent years compared with that observed in the early 1990s. In a prospective multicenter study in Belgium, 48.1% of ICU patients had prerenal acute kidney failure when serum creatinine was equal or greater than 2 mg/dl [28]. Nash et al. found an incidence of 39% in hospitalized patients [30], and recently, Cruz et al. recorded in Italy an incidence of 38.9% in ICU patients [12]. However, these numbers most probably underestimate the true incidence of this condition. The majority of ICU patients with intrinsic acute kidney failure will progress through a phase of prerenal acute kidney failure. Therefore, probably the majority of ICU patients with AKI either have prerenal acute kidney failure or had an evolutionary form, progressing through acute intrinsic failure.

Prerenal acute kidney failure is a less severe form of AKI, therefore, it is not surprising that in most studies, in-hospital mortality was almost half in prerenal acute kidney failure compared with intrinsic acute kidney failure (48–65% vs 29–39%) [26–28]. Although not all authors could demonstrate this [12].

References

1. Albanese J, Leone M, Garnier F, Bourgoin A, Antonini F, Martin C, (2004) Renal effects of norepinephrine in septic and nonseptic patients. Chest 126: 534–539
2. Bagshaw SM, Langenberg C, Bellomo R, (2006) Urinary biochemistry and microscopy in septic acute renal failure: a systematic review. Am J Kidney Dis 48: 695–705
3. Bernard GR, Vincent JL, Laterre PF, LaRosa SP, Dhainaut JF, Lopez-Rodriguez A, Steingrub JS, Garber GE, Helterbrand JD, Ely EW, (2001) Efficacy and safety of recombinant human activated protein C for severe sepsis. N Engl J Med 344: 699–709
4. Blantz RC, (1998) Pathophysiology of pre-renal azotemia. Kidney Int 53: 512–523
5. Bobadilla NA, Gamba G, (2007) New insights into the pathophysiology of cyclosporine nephrotoxicity: a role of aldosterone. Am J Physiol Renal Physiol 293: F2–9
6. Brenner M, Schaer GL, Mallory DL, Suffredini AF, Parrillo JE, (1990) Detection of renal blood flow abnormalities in septic and critically ill patients using a newly designed indwelling thermodilution renal vein catheter. Chest 98: 170–179
7. Brezis M, Rosen S, Silva P, Epstein FH, (1984) Selective vulnerability of the medullary thick ascending limb to anoxia in the isolated perfused rat kidney. J Clin Invest 73: 182–190
8. Brezis M, Rosen S, Silva P, Epstein FH, (1984) Renal ischemia: a new perspective. Kidney Int 26: 375–383
9. Brezis M, Heyman SN, Epstein FH, (1994) Determinants of intrarenal oxygenation. II. Hemodynamic effects. Am J Physiol Renal Physiol 267: F1063–1068
10. Brezis M, Rosen S, (1995) Hypoxia of the renal medulla – its implications for disease. N Engl J Med 332: 647–655
11. Brivet F, Kleinknecht D, Loirat P, Landais P, The French Study Group on Acute Renal Failure, (1996) Acute renal failure in intensive care units-causes, outcome, and prognostic factors on hospital mortality; a prospective, multicenter study. Crit Care Med 24: 192–198
12. Cruz DN, Bolgan I, Perazella MA, Bonello M, de Cal M, Corradi V, Polanco N, Ocampo C, Nalesso F, Piccinni P, Ronco C, for the North East Italian Prospective Hospital Renal Outcome Survey on Acute Kidney Injury I, (2007) North East Italian Prospective Hospital Renal Outcome Survey on Acute Kidney Injury (NEiPHROS-AKI): Targeting the Problem with the RIFLE Criteria. Clin J Am Soc Nephrol 2: 418–425
13. Dhanireddy S, Altemeier WA, Matute-Bello G, O'Mahony DS, Glenny RW, Martin TR, Liles WC, (2006) Mechanical ventilation induces inflammation, lung injury, and extra-pulmonary organ dysfunction in experimental pneumonia. Lab Invest 86: 790–799
14. Di Giantomasso D, May CN, Bellomo R, (2003) Vital organ blood flow during hyperdynamic sepsis. Chest 124: 1053–1059
15. Di Giantomasso D, May CN, Bellomo R, (2003) Norepinephrine and vital organ blood flow during experimental hyperdynamic sepsis. Intensive Care Med 29: 1774–1781
16. Di Giantomasso D, Morimatsu H, May CN, Bellomo R, (2003) Intrarenal blood flow distribution in hyperdynamic septic shock: Effect of norepinephrine. Crit Care Med 31: 2509–2513
17. Di Giantomasso D, Bellomo R, May CN, (2005) The haemodynamic and metabolic effects of epinephrine in experimental hyperdynamic septic shock. Intensive Care Med 31: 454–462
18. Gupta A, Berg DT, Gerlitz B, Sharma GR, Syed S, Richardson MA, Sandusky G, Heuer JG, Galbreath EJ, Grinnell BW, (2007) Role of protein C in renal dysfunction after polymicrobial sepsis. J Am Soc Nephrol 18: 860–867
19. Gupta A, Rhodes GJ, Berg DT, Gerlitz B, Molitoris BA, Grinnell BW, (2007) Activated protein C ameliorates LPS-induced acute kidney injury and downregulates renal INOS and angiotensin 2. Am J Physiol Renal Physiol 293: F245–254
20. Knotek M, Rogachev B, Wang W, Ecder T, Melnikov V, Gengaro PE, Esson M, Edelstein CL, Dinarello CA, Schrier RW, (2001) Endotoxemic renal failure in mice: Role of tumor necrosis factor independent of inducible nitric oxide synthase. Kidney Int 59: 2243–2249
21. Kuiper JW, Groeneveld AB, Slutsky AS, Plotz FB, (2005) Mechanical ventilation and acute renal failure. Crit Care Med 33: 1408–1415
22. Lameire N, Van Biesen W, Vanholder R, (2005) Acute renal failure. Lancet 365: 417–430
23. Langenberg C, Wan L, Egi M, May CN, Bellomo R, (2006) Renal blood flow in experimental septic acute renal failure. Kidney Int 69: 1996–2002

24. Langenberg C, Bagshaw SM, May CN, Bellomo R, (2008) The histopathology of septic acute kidney injury: a systematic review. Critical care (London, England) 12: R38
25. Liang KV, Williams AW, Greene EL, Redfield MM, (2008) Acute decompensated heart failure and the cardiorenal syndrome. Crit Care Med 36: S75–88
26. Liaño F, Pascual J, the Madrid Acute Renal Failure Study Group, (1996) Epidemiology of acute renal failure: A prospective, multicenter, community-based study. Kidney Int 50: 811–818
27. Liaño F, Junco E, Pascual J, Madero R, Verde E, the Madrid Acute Renal Failure Study Group, (1998) The spectrum of acute renal failure in the intensive care unit compared to that seen in other settings. Kidney Int 53, Suppl. 66: S16–S24
28. Lins RL, Elseviers MM, Daelemans R, Arnouts P, Billiouw JM, Couttenye M, Gheuens E, Rogiers P, Rutsaert R, Van Der Niepen P, De Broe ME, (2004) Re-evaluation and modification of the Stuivenberg Hospital Acute Renal Failure (SHARF) scoring system for the prognosis of acute renal failure: an independent multicentre, prospective study. Nephrol Dial Transplant 19: 2282–2288
29. Miller PD, Krebs RA, Neal BJ, McIntyre DO, (1980) Polyuric prerenal failure. Arch Internal Med 140: 907–909
30. Nash K, Hafeez A, Hou S, (2002) Hospital-acquired renal insufficiency. Am J Kidney Dis 39: 930–936
31. Schrier RW, Wang W, (2004) Acute renal failure and sepsis. N Engl J Med 351: 159–169
32. The Acute Respiratory Distress Syndrome Network, (2000) Ventilation with lower tidal volumes as compared with traditional tidal volumes for acute lung injury and the acute respiratory distress syndrome. N Engl J Med 342: 1301–1308.
33. Thijs A, Thijs LG, (1998) Pathogenesis of renal failure in sepsis. Kidney Int 66: S34–37
34. Wencker D, (2007) Acute cardio-renal syndrome: progression from congestive heart failure to congestive kidney failure. Curr Heart Fail Rep 4: 134–138

Intrinsic Acute Kidney Injury

2.4

Norbert Lameire

Core Messages

- Acute kidney injury (AKI) in the intensive care unit (ICU) can be the result of a wide range of disease processes, so that it is likely to be encountered by physicians from all specialties.
- The increasing recognition of the overlap between critical care medicine and nephrology has resulted in what nowadays is called critical care nephrology. Nephrologists should be familiar with the rapid advances in the field of intensive care medicine and the impact these advances may have on the occurrence of AKI in these patients. At the same time, the intensivist should also consider the kidney in the management of critically ill patients.
- The nondialytic therapy of practically all patients with AKI includes optimising renal perfusion with volume expansion, use of inotropes and vasopressors, and eventually trials with loop diuretics.
- The moment of initiation of renal replacement therapy (RRT), the selection of the RRT modality, and the dose and frequency of dialysis should be decided in daily consultations between nephrologist and intensivist. Flex-ibility and willingness to listen and to take the advice of both teams is a great asset which can only be to the advantage of the critically ill patient. The slow but steady improvement of the, at least short-term, prognosis of the patient with AKI is testimony to this growing cooperation between the two disciplines. In recent years, it has been recognised that the term acute renal failure (ARF) fails to adequately describe what is a dynamic process extending across initiation, maintenance and recovery phases, each of which may be of variable duration and severity [1].The term acute renal *failure* suggests that the syndrome is dichotomous and places an undue emphasis on whether or not renal function has overtly failed. This belies the now well-established fact that even mild decrements in glomerular filtration may be associated with adverse clinical outcomes. The alternative proposed term acute kidney injury (AKI) better captures the diverse nature of this syndrome, and has entered into widespread clinical use

The terminology of acute kidney injury (AKI) acknowledges that, although there are different causative factors, in most instances, an acute decline in kidney function is secondary to an injury that leads to a functional or structural change in the kidney. In addition, the word 'failure' reflects only one end of the spectrum of clinical conditions that are seen in this disease. It is therefore recommended that the term acute renal failure (ARF) should be used only for those cases of AKI in need of renal replacement therapy (RRT).

The clinical studies of AKI in different settings, including the intensive care unit (ICU), and described in the literature have used multiple operational definitions, making it difficult to compare epidemiologic studies and to evaluate interventions for its prevention and treatment.

N. Lameire
Nephrology Unit, Department of Internal Medicine, University Hospital, Gent University, 4K4, NDT-COMGAN Office, De pintelaan 185, 9000 Gent, Belgium
e-mail: norbert.lameire@ugent.be

A. Jörres et al. (eds.), *Management of Acute Kidney Problems,*
DOI: 10.1007/978-3-540-69441-0_2.4, © Springer-Verlag Berlin Heidelberg 2010

Between 5% and 20% of critically ill patients experience an episode of AKI, often accompanied by a multiorgan dysfunction syndrome [2, 3].

Historically, AKI has been described as prerenal, intrinsic renal or postrenal [4]. Pre-renal and intrinsic renal failure due to ischaemia and nephrotoxins are responsible for most episodes of AKI. AKI due to primary intrarenal disease is called intrinsic renal failure and accounts for 35–40% of all patients with acute renal dysfunction. Intrinsic ARF can be categorised anatomically by the area of the kidney parenchyma involved: vascular, glomerular, tubular or interstitial areas. Ischaemic or toxic acute tubular necrosis (ATN) accounts for 80–90% of acute intrinsic ARF in most series of AKI observed in the critically ill patient. The remaining 10–20% of intrinsic ARF are caused by acute glomerulonephritis, acute interstitial nephritis or renal vasculitis.

The purpose of this chapter is to provide a general overview of the different causes of AKI in the ICU and to focus mainly on the general diagnostic approach for these patients. The individual diseases will be described in separate chapters of this book.

2.4.1 Epidemiology of AKI in the ICU Focusing on Non-ATN Etiologies

A study of the epidemiology of AKI in the ICU, identified 254 cases of ARF over a 10-month period, 57 cases of end-stage renal disease (ESRD) and 1,219 cases of no renal failure; this corresponded with an incidence of ARF of 17%. Unfortunately, this study did not differentiate among the different etiologies [5].

In Scotland (total population 5,054,800), 809 patients with ARF (group A) or acute on chronic kidney disease (ACKD; group B) started RRT over a 36-week interval. This equates to an overall age-standardised incidence of 286 per million of the adult population (pmp) per year (95% confidence interval [95% CI], 269–302). The incidence was 212 pmp (95% CI, 195–230) for group A and 74 pmp (95% CI, 64–85) for group B; 51% of these patients were treated in an ICU, and only 18 of a total of 809 (or 3%) suffered from acute glomerulonephritis; in these last cases, five cases of acute vasculitis were presumably included [6].

The largest prospective observational study of ICU patients with AKI who either were treated with RRT or fulfilled at least one of the predefined criteria for ARF from September 2000 to December 2001 at 54 hospitals in 23 countries was described by Uchino et al. [7]. Of 29,269 critically ill patients admitted during the study period, 1,738 patients (5.7%) had ARF during their ICU stay, including 1,260 who were treated with RRT. The most common contributing factor to ARF was septic shock (47.5%). Approximately 30% of patients had preadmission renal dysfunction. Unfortunately, also in this study, no detailed information of the number of different etiologies is given.

The most comprehensive study on the etiology of AKI in ICU compared with non-ICU patients is the study by Liano et al. in Madrid hospitals [8].

Figure 2.4.1 summarizes the percentage distribution of these etiologies in the two different populations. Whereas in both groups, acute prerenal and ATN were

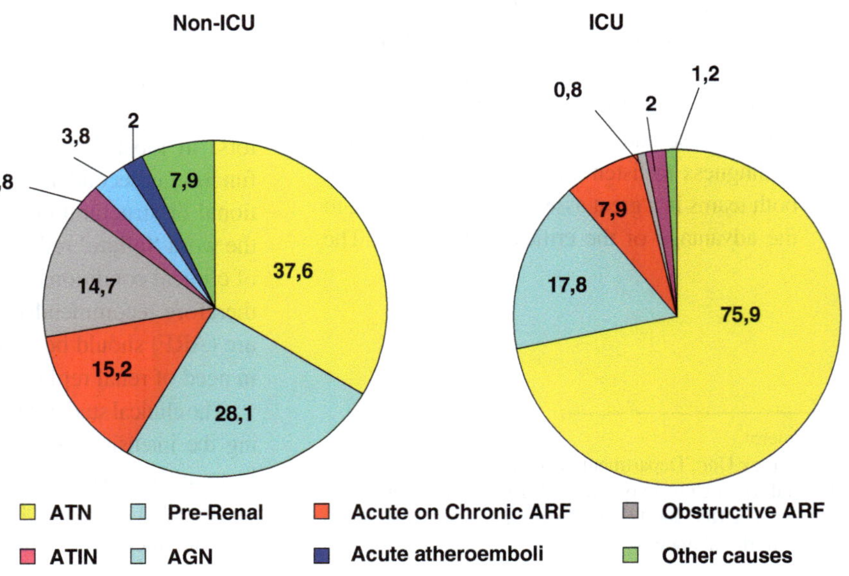

Fig. 2.4.1 Percentual distribution of causes of ARF in the ICU and non-ICU setting. (Modified from [8])

the most common causes of AKI, acute glomerular diseases accounted for only 2% and 3.8%, respectively, while acute tubulointerstitial diseases were only present in 2% of the non-ICU patients. It is important to draw attention to the relatively high incidence of acute on chronic renal failure in both populations (7.9% and 15.2% in the ICU and non-ICU populations, respectively).

Based on these data it is suggested that non-ATN causes of AKI are relatively rare in an ICU population, at least in the developed world.

Conversely, in tropical countries, medical causes of AKI predominate, accounting for 60–67% of cases of AKI. Specific infections have an important role; severe malaria is particularly predominant. Based on the recent review by Cerda et al. [9], acute glomerulonephritis remains an important cause of AKI in the developing world. In areas such as southeast Anatolia in Turkey, acute glomerulonephritis causes more than 60% of cases of AKI. In Egypt and Morocco, poststreptococcal acute glomerulonephritis develops in response to cutaneous infections for which flies or scabies are vectors; similar mechanisms of dissemination operate in Dunbar, South Africa. Conversely, acute glomerulonephritis in Libya is secondary to pharyngeal streptococcal infection; vectors have a less prominent role, presumably because of the more temperate climate. Recently, a form of acute eosinophilic glomerulonephritis has been described in children of south-western Uganda, presumably related to malarial or other infections.

Most cases of AKI in developing countries are, however, either unrecognised or treated in rural hospitals and only occasionally in ICUs.

Based on the rather scarce data on the epidemiology of non-ATN intrinsic AKI in the ICU, it can be reasonably estimated that the occurrence of this type of AKI is rather low (between 5% and 10% of all ICU admissions), but nevertheless these etiologies should be taken into account in the work-up of any case of AKI.

2.4.2 Clinical Evaluation of the Critically Ill Patient with AKI

The clinical evaluation of AKI should aim to answer the following five questions:

1. Is the renal failure acute, acute-on-chronic or chronic?
2. Is there evidence of true hypovolaemia or reduced effective arterial blood volume, i.e. 'prerenal' AKI?
3. Has there been a major vascular occlusion?
4. Is there evidence of parenchymal renal disease other than ATN?
5. Is there renal tract obstruction, i.e. 'postrenal' AKI?

An algorithm summarising the approach to a patient with presumed AKI is provided in Fig. 2.4.2. This approach will reveal the likely cause of AKI in most patients. This enables the clinician to develop a rational therapeutic plan that will facilitate the rapid restoration of renal function in patients with prerenal or postrenal AKI and will provide a logical basis for the treatment of patients with intrinsic parenchymal renal diseases [10].

2.4.2.1 Acute Prerenal Kidney Injury

Prerenal factors range from obvious renal hypoperfusion in patients with hypotension or haemorrhage to more subtle renal hypoperfusion, such as that seen in patients with heart failure or cirrhosis. A high ratio of urea nitrogen to creatinine, a low urinary output and a fractional excretion of urinary sodium of less than 1% are suggestive, but not confirmatory, of a prerenal cause.

Hypovolaemia leading to renal hypoperfusion is the most common prerenal cause of decreased glomerular filtration, which may be exacerbated by vasoconstriction via prostanoids, cytokines and activation of the renin–angiotensin–aldosterone axis in the setting of sepsis, or by vasoconstrictors such as vasopressors and aminoglycoside antibiotics.

ATN is the most common intrinsic mechanism of AKI and is generally caused by a toxic or ischaemic insult to the kidney. Most toxins such as antibiotics, intravascular contrast media and nonsteroidal antiinflammatory drugs lead to ATN-mediated AKI, whereas sepsis and cardiopulmonary bypass may cause both prerenal and intrinsic AKI. Only a small proportion of ICU-associated ATN occurs in the absence of failure of another organ.

Obstructions distal to the collecting system, such as nephrolithiasis, prostatic hypertrophy or operative injury, represent the most common causes of postrenal AKI.

Once a diagnosis of AKI is established, the patient's history, physical findings, laboratory tests and imaging procedures usually answer the remainder of the above questions and identify a specific etiology of AKI.

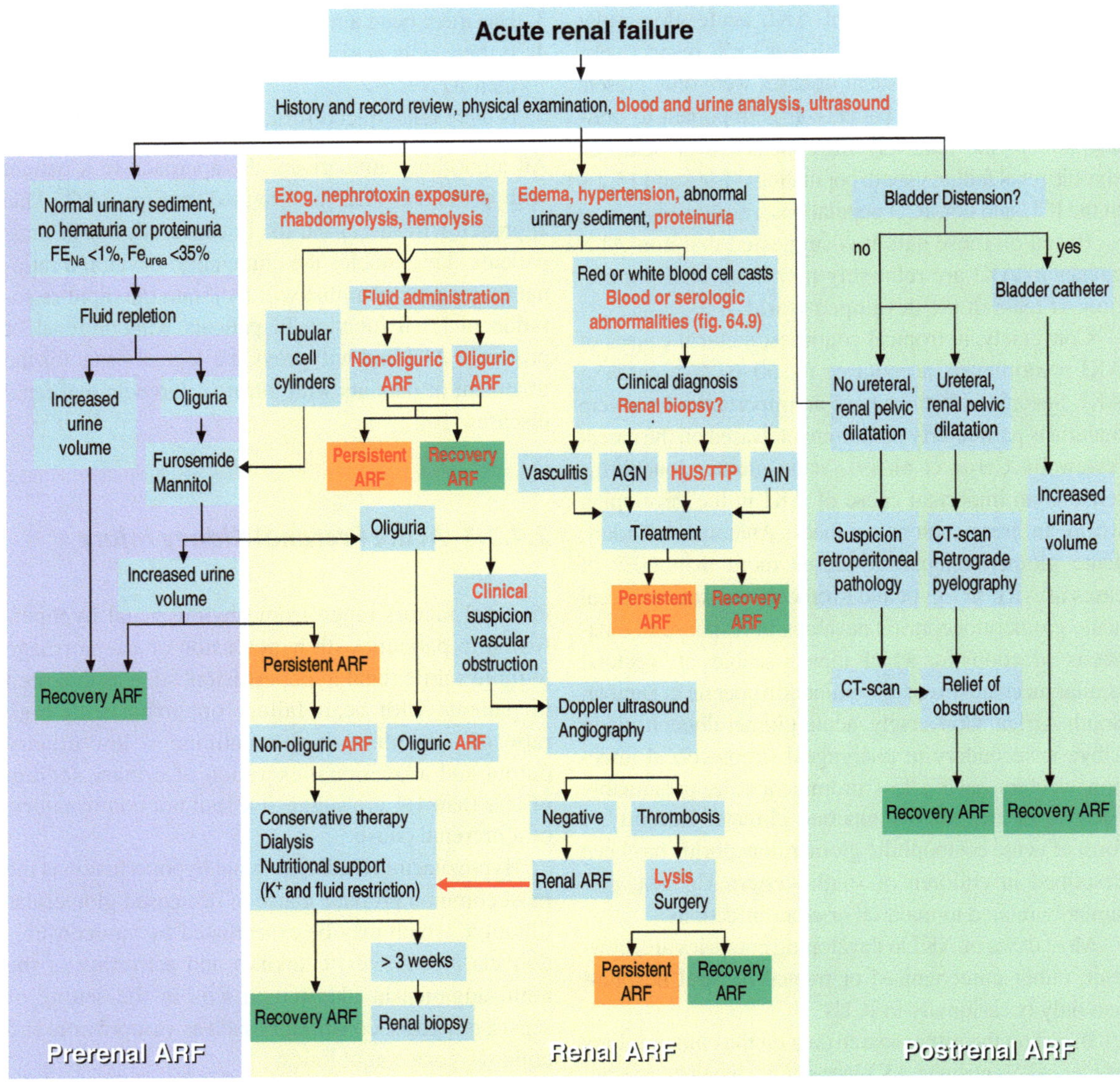

Fig. 2.4.2 Algorithm for the diagnostic approach to a patient with suspected AKI. Abbreviations: abno – abnormal; AGN – acute glomerulonephritis; AIN – acute interstitial nephritis; RF – renal failure; UV – urine volume

2.4.2.2 Intrinsic Intrarenal Acute Failure

Differences in the clinical setting and presentation, particularly in the history, physical examination and urinalysis, will distinguish between these types of ARF. Determining if a patient has ATN, acute interstitial nephritis or acute glomerulonephritis and/or acute vasculitis as the cause of ARF is necessary because the treatment and prognosis of each may differ. Unlike prerenal and postrenal ARF, the decrement in glomerular filtration rate (GFR) in intrinsic AKI is directly linked to kidney damage and not the result of reduced renal perfusion or elevated pressures in the renal conduits. Since urea reabsorption is not preferentially increased, urea and creatinine concentrations rise in parallel and the blood urea nitrogen to creatinine ratio is usually preserved (10–20:1). Similarly, because the impaired kidney function results from direct kidney injury, the urinalysis is usually abnormal. Specific findings on dipstick and microscopic examination of the urine provide important clues to the location of the parenchymal injury responsible for the kidney dysfunction. In some cases, despite a careful history, physical exam, urinalysis and additional specific tests, the type of the kidney disorder (tubular, vascular, glomerular or interstitial) remains undefined, and a percutaneous kidney biopsy will be needed to determine the cause.

2.4.2.2.1 History and Record Review

The past medical history should include previous urea, creatinine and electrolyte results; previous health checks; systemic conditions (e.g. diabetes, hypertension, ischaemic heart or peripheral artery disease and jaundice); previous urinary symptoms (pyelonephritis or urinary tract infection); recent procedures (surgery, angiography and other radiologic procedures); known infections (e.g. HIV and hepatitis) and known immunosuppressive therapy (transplant patients and patients with malignancies). Drug history should include over-the-counter formulations and herbal remedies or recreational drugs. The social history should include foreign travel (malaria and schistosomiasis), exposure to waterways or sewage systems (leptospirosis) and exposure to rodents (Hantavirus).

In contrast with community-acquired AKI where it can usually be attributed to a single cause, AKI acquired on a hospital ward or acquired in the ICU mostly occurs in the setting of comorbidity and is multifactorial, often associated with sepsis and multiorgan failure. Unique causes of AKI can be seen in the setting of malignancy, HIV infection, pregnancy and the postoperative state. Patients with liver disease are susceptible to prerenal and renal AKI as well as to hepatorenal syndrome.

The clinical history with regard to events associated with intravascular volume loss or volume sequestration and impaired cardiac function is important in determining the cause of AKI. A history of thirst, orthostatic lightheadedness or hypotension and symptoms of congestive heart failure support a prerenal etiology of AKI.

A history of factors that predispose to vascular disease or preexistent cardiovascular morbidity, arterial catheterisation involving the aorta and atrial fibrillation are compatible with vascular embolic events leading to AKI. A history of systemic infection or the presence of systemic symptoms may support a glomerular cause of AKI. Medication exposure or a history of acute pyelonephritis may point to acute interstitial nephritis as the cause of AKI. The presence of disorders associated with either rhabdomyolysis or intravascular haemolysis suggests the possibility of haem pigment nephropathy.

Postrenal causes of AKI are common at the extremes of age, with a history of changes in the size and force of urine stream; the presence of bladder, prostate or pelvic cancer; the use of anticholinergic and alpha-adrenergic medications; the presence of anuria, suprapubic pain or urolithiasis; or exposure to medications known to cause hyperuricaemia or crystalluria. Patients with either a single kidney or a significant baseline decrease in the function of one kidney should make the clinician even more concerned about the possibility of postrenal AKI because a single lesion may obstruct the normal kidney. In this case, anuria is frequent.

2.4.2.2.2 Physical Examination

Assessing the volume status of patients with AKI is critical but sometimes difficult. Orthostatic tachycardia and hypotension have diagnostic value in detecting hypovolaemia. Decreased skin turgor or impaired capillary refill time have limited sensitivity and specificity. Assessment of the jugular venous pressure (JVP) with the patient reclining at 45° is mandatory. The normal JVP is between 0 and 3 cm above the sternal angle, which corresponds to a right atrial pressure of approximately 8 cm of water. If the JVP is difficult to visualise, gentle pressure over the liver to increase venous return can be helpful (the hepatojugular reflux). Recording the patient's daily body weight in conjunction with fluid balance charts and clinical examination can aid in estimating the evolution of the fluid balance. Although clinical assessment provides a satisfactory index of cardiac output and tissue perfusion in most patients, invasive haemodynamic monitoring (central venous and/or Swan-Ganz catheterisation) is often necessary in critically ill patients. The role of less invasive serial transesophageal Doppler monitoring in the following up and guidance of the volume status in the ICU patient is promising [11].

Ophthalmic examination may reveal plaques suggestive of atheroemboli (Hollenhorst plaques, i.e. intraluminal retinal cholesterol/fibrin deposits) or findings compatible with bacterial endocarditis, vasculitis or malignant hypertension. Neck examination for JVP and carotid pulses and sounds may be helpful in detecting heart failure, aortic valve disease or vascular disease. Cardiovascular examination for rate, rhythm, murmurs, gallops and rubs may be helpful in detecting the presence of heart failure and possible sources of emboli.

Lung examination can assist in determining the presence of either heart failure or a pulmonary-renal syndrome associated with AKI. Abdominal examination can reveal findings compatible with vascular disease (e.g. bruits and palpable abdominal aortic aneurysm), masses that could be malignant, a distended bladder, possible sources of bacteremia or evidence of liver disease. Examination of the extremities for symmetry and strength of pulses and edema can be helpful. Skin examination may reveal palpable purpura (vasculitis), a fine maculopapular rash (drug-induced interstitial nephritis), livedo reticularis, purple toes and other embolic stigmata (atheroemboli). If neurologic signs are present, systemic disorders such as vasculitis, thrombotic microangiopathy, subacute bacterial endocarditis and malignant hypertension warrant consideration. Peripheral neuropathy in the presence of AKI raises the possibility of nerve compression caused by rhabdomyolysis, heavy metal intoxication or plasma cell dyscrasia. Pelvic examination in females and rectal examination in both females and males may detect an obstructive cause of AKI.

Monitoring of Intra-abdominal Pressure

Markedly raised intra-abdominal pressures (>20 mm Hg) may occur after trauma, abdominal surgery or secondary to massive fluid resuscitation resulting in AKI [12–14]. The mechanism remains unclear but may be due to increased renal venous pressure and vascular resistance. It is difficult to find a good gold standard for intra-abdominal pressure measurement. Bladder pressure can be used as an intra-abdominal pressure estimate provided it is measured in a reproducible way. Automated continuous intra-abdominal pressure monitoring has recently be-come available.

This measurement may be particularly useful in the sometimes abrupt decline in GFR in the patients with severe heart failure; this form of haemodynamically mediated AKI is often called the cardiorenal syndrome [15].

Since the kidneys are intricately involved in fluid and electrolyte homeostasis, they are critical to the body's compensatory mechanisms responsible for the pathophysiologic changes in heart failure. In advanced heart failure, however, the kidney may be unable to compensate properly, and in fact several of the compensatory mechanisms which are active can be counterproductive and ultimately worsen both the heart failure and the renal dysfunction, leading to cardiorenal syndrome, present in 20–30% of patients admitted to the hospital for acute decompensated heart failure [16]

Relation with high intra-abdominal pressure [17] or increased renal vein pressure [16] have been thought to play a role in the decreased renal perfusion in severe heart failure.

2.4.2.2.3 Laboratory Tests

Urine Volume

Urine volume in AKI can vary from oliguria (i.e. <500 mL/24 h or <20 mL/h) to anuria (i.e. <100 mL/24 h) to extreme polyuria. In most patients with AKI in the ICU, an indwelling urinary catheter allows accurate measurement of hourly urine output, a parameter useful in monitoring the initial response to fluid resuscitation until the intravascular fluid volume of the patient is adequately restored. Once this state is reached, hourly urine volumes are less useful in guiding management, and increased urine flow should not be regarded as a primary treatment goal. Once patients are established to be oligo-anuric, the urinary catheter should be removed to reduce the risk of infection. Severe AKI can exist despite normal urine output (i.e. non-oliguria), but changes in urine output can occur long before biochemical changes are apparent. Non-oliguric AKI is nowadays more common than oliguric AKI, particularly in ICU patients, because of the more frequent monitoring via daily serum creatinine changes and/or earlier intervention with fluid loading and diuretics. The 'spontaneous' non-oliguric forms usually have a better prognosis compared with the oliguric forms. This may well relate to a less severe renal insult or a higher incidence of nephrotoxin-induced AKI in the non-oliguric group.

Anuria is seen with cessation of glomerular filtration (e.g. rapidly progressive glomerulonephritis, acute cortical necrosis or total renal arterial or venous occlusion) or complete urinary tract obstruction. Brief (<24–48 h) episodes of oligo-anuria occur in some cases of ATN. Prerenal forms of AKI nearly always present with oliguria, although non-oliguric forms have been reported. Postrenal and renal forms of AKI can present with any pattern of urine flow. The presence of alternating anuria and polyuria is an uncommon but classic manifestation of urinary tract obstruction, e.g., due to a stone that changes its position. In rare cases, unilateral obstruction can lead to anuria and AKI; vascular or ureteral spasm, mediated by autonomic activation, is thought to be responsible for the loss of function in the non-obstructed kidney.

Urine Dipstick and Microscopic Examination

Routine dipstick and microscopic analysis of urine are often helpful in determining the cause of AKI. Generally, a normal urine analysis in the setting of AKI suggests a prerenal or postrenal cause and an abnormal urinalysis a 'renal' cause. However, patients with prerenal AKI can have a significant number of casts (due to the precipitation of Tamm Horsfall protein in concentrated, acidic urine) and cellular elements in their urine in addition to small urine volumes, high specific gravity and acidic urine.

Urinary protein measurement by dipstick is specific for albumin. Small amounts of protein found by dipstick, with larger amounts found by laboratory urinary protein tests (such as sulfosalicylic acid) suggest the presence of light chains. If the dipstick reaction for protein is moderately or strongly positive in the setting of AKI, quantification is indicated. The presence of more than 1–2 g/day of urine protein suggests a glomerular cause of AKI.

Examination of the urine sediment is of great value in AKI. Gross or microscopic haematuria suggests a glomerular, vascular, interstitial or other structural renal cause (e.g. stone, tumour, infection or trauma) of AKI and is rarely seen with ATN. Red blood cell casts in the urine sediment strongly suggest a glomerular or vascular cause of AKI but have also been observed with acute interstitial nephritis. Studies of the urinary red cell morphology in AKI of different causes are lacking. Lack of urinary red cells despite a positive dipstick reaction for blood is typical of AKI induced by myoglobinuria or haemoglobinuria.

A recent systematic review investigated the value of urinary microscopy in patients with septic ARF [18]. Because of substantial heterogeneity, no formal quantitative analysis could be performed; urinary microscopy was described in only seven articles (26%). The majority were small single-centre reports and had serious limitations. For example, only 52% of patients were septic, only 54% of patients had ARF, many studies failed to include a control group, time from diagnosis of sepsis or ARF to measure of urinary tests was variable, and there were numerous potential confounders. A few reports of urinary microscopy described muddy brown epithelial cell casts and renal tubular cells in patients with septic ARF, whereas others described a normal urinary sediment. This systematic review concluded that the scientific basis for the use of urinary biochemistry indices and urinary microscopy in patients at least with septic ARF is weak. On the other hand, a careful examination of the urinary sediment may be very helpful in directing the diagnosis to a non-ATN etiology of intrinsic renal AKI.

Large numbers of white blood cells (WBCs) and in particular of leukocyte casts on urinalysis suggest either pyelonephritis or interstitial nephritis. Eosinophiluria (>1% urine WBCs) is nonspecific. However, this finding is diagnostically valuable when AKI occurs in a setting compatible with either allergic interstitial nephritis (drug exposure, fever, rash or peripheral eosinophiluria) or cholesterol embolism.

Collecting duct cells and total casts in urine detected by cytodiagnostic quantitative assessment are increased in AKI but, as illustrated by the above-mentioned systematic review [18], lack sufficient sensitivity, specificity and predictive power for routine clinical use.

Crystals in the urine sediment should be assessed using fresh warm urine, by polarising microscopy, with a knowledge of urine pH and by an experienced microscopist. A large number of uric acid crystals suggest acute uric acid nephropathy, tumour lysis syndrome or catabolic AKI. Oxalate crystals are compatible with ethylene glycol intoxication, jejunoileal bypass or massive doses of vitamin C underlying AKI. Drug-induced crystals can result from sulphonamides, indinavir and triamterene.

Urinary Indices

In prerenal AKI, tubular function is intact and renal vasoconstriction is associated with enhanced tubular sodium reabsorption. Thus, when creatinine accumulates in the blood due to a fall in GFR secondary to renal vasoconstriction with intact tubular function, the fractional excretion (FE) of filtered sodium (FE_{Na} = [(urine sodium × plasma creatinine)/(plasma sodium × urine creatinine)]) is less than 1%. A paradoxically high FE_{Na} despite the presence of prerenal azotemia occurs during diuretic treatment, including mannitol, within the preceding 24 h, or glycosuria or excretion of an alkaline urine. In the last case, the obligatory excretion of bicarbonate requires the excretion of sodium. In the presence

Table 2.4.1 Diagnostic urinary indices in ARF

Indices	Prerenal	Renal
Urine sediment	Hyaline casts	Abnormal
Specific gravity	>1.020	~1.010
Urine osmolality (mOsm/kg H_2O)	>500	<350
U_{Na} (mmol/L)	<20	>40
Fractional excretion		
Sodium (%)	<1	>2
Urea (%)	<35	>35
Uric acid (%)	<7	>15
Lithium (%)	<7	> 20
Low-molecular-weight proteins	Low	High
Brush border enzymes	Low	High

of alkalosis and suspicion of prerenal failure, calculation of the FE of chloride may therefore be more appropriate than the FE of sodium. Finally, renal vasoconstriction in a patient with advanced chronic renal failure may not be expected to be associated with an FE_{Na} of less than 1%, because of chronic adaptation to an increased single-nephron GFR (Table 2.4.1) [10].

A reduced effective circulating volume also stimulates antidiuretic hormone (ADH) release. ADH results in increased distal water and urea reabsorption. Thus, a low FE of urea (FE_{urea}) (<35%) is more sensitive and specific than FE_{Na} in differentiating between prerenal and renal causes of AKI, especially when diuretics have been administered. In a recent prospective study in patients with AKI [19], the diagnostic accuracy of this combination of FE_{Na} and FE_{urea} was described. The performance of the tests was investigated in 99 patients hospitalised at a tertiary-care centre who developed AKI (defined as a 30% increase in serum creatinine level from baseline within 1 week). Patients were classified as having transient or persistent AKI according to the clinical context and whether serum creatinine level returned to baseline within 7 days. Each group was also subdivided according to exposure to diuretics. FE_{urea} of 35% or less and FE_{Na} of 1% or less were used to define transient AKI. Sensitivity, specificity and receiver operating characteristic curves were generated for each index test. Sensitivity and specificity of FE_{urea} were 48% and 75%, respectively, in patients not administered diuretics and 79% and 33% in patients administered diuretics. Sensitivity and specificity of FE_{Na} were 78% and 75% in patients not administered diuretics and 58% and 81% in those administered diuretics. Receiver operating characteristic curves did not identify a better diagnostic cutoff value for FE_{urea} or FE_{Na}.

It was concluded from this study that in patients without diuretic use, FE_{Na} is better able to distinguish transient from persistent AKI. In patients administered diuretics, this distinction cannot be made accurately by means of FE_{Na}. FE_{urea} cannot be used as an alternative tool because it lacks specificity. Further investigations of the concomitant use of both urinary parameters are thus warranted.

Another caveat is that a low FE_{Na} does not always indicate prerenal azotemia and can be observed in the early stages of obstruction, acute glomerulonephritis, pigment nephropathy and intrinsic AKI, induced by radiographic contrast agents. This may be related to the early presence of severe renal vasoconstriction and intact distal tubule function, which can occur in the presence of proximal tubule injury. FE_{Na} has only approximately 80% diagnostic sensitivity in distinguishing azotemia associated with renal vasoconstriction and intact tubular function from established AKI with tubular dysfunction. This may result from the limited sensitivity of this parameter, or perhaps more likely, the patient may actually be progressing from a prerenal azotemic state to established AKI.

The above-mentioned systematic review [18] also explored the diagnostic accuracy of the traditional urinary parameters in septic patients. Urinary biochemistry or derived indices were reported in 24 articles (89%). Urinary sodium, FE_{Na}, urinary to plasma creatinine ratio, urinary osmolality, urinary to plasma osmolality ratio and serum urea to creatinine ratio showed variable and inconsistent results.

In general it can thus be concluded that, although useful as a first approach, the 'classical' urinary parameters are not always reliable to make a clear distinction between the different forms of AKI.

Serum Creatinine

AKI is very frequently monitored by following the daily variations in serum creatinine. A direct relationship exists between the magnitude of serum creatinine increase and mortality from AKI, and even minimal changes in serum creatinine are already related to mortality [20, 21].

In the complete absence of glomerular filtration, serum creatinine will rise by 1.0–1.5 mg/dL (88–132 µmol/L) per day. A disproportionate rise of creatinine occurs in rhabdomyolysis or when medications that interfere with creatinine excretion (e.g. cimetidine, trimethoprim and pyrimethamine) or its measurement (e.g. cefoxitin, ascorbic acid, methyldopa, flucytosine and barbiturates) are taken.

Important limitations of using serum creatinine as a GFR marker in patients with AKI include tubular backleak of creatinine into the blood, and altered tubular secretion of creatinine. Critically ill patients may have abnormal liver function that alters creatinine metabolism significantly. Increased release of creatinine into the blood may occur with muscle trauma, fever and immobilisation, whereas low muscle mass, such as that observed with liver disease and ageing, will result in lower basal creatinine levels. Marked increases in extracellular fluid, which are common in critically ill patients, may increase the volume of distribution and thereby dilute down the serum creatinine. There is currently no information on extrarenal creatinine clearance in AKI, and a steady-state condition seldom exists. It is important to keep in mind that during the development of AKI, serum creatinine levels will underestimate the degree of renal dysfunction, whereas the opposite will be true as renal function recovers.

After an acute nephrotoxic insult, the number of days that the serum creatinine continues to increase has prognostic value. A progressive increase of serum creatinine over more than 5 days is characteristic of AKI during which recovery has not yet started or at least is still grossly insufficient. When an abrupt and complete interruption of the GFR is followed by a progressive recovery, the serum creatinine will continue to increase with peak values on days 3 to 5. Even when the recovery is slower, this will not affect the time of creatinine increase; the peak creatinine value in that case will usually be observed at day 4 but at a higher level.

Serum Cystatin C

Cystatin C is more sensitive and accurate than serum creatinine in several settings and was an early and reliable marker of AKI in ICU patients [22]. Usually cystatin C levels rise 1–2 days earlier than the serum creatinine in incipient AKI. However, cystatin C levels are also influenced by nonrenal factors, and more data are needed before recommending its routine use in AKI patients.

By contrast, to rapidly evaluate the basal renal function in the newly admitted critically ill patient, cystatin C may be a more reliable parameter for GFR than creatinine [23].

Biomarkers

Traditional urinary biomarkers, including low- and high-molecular-weight proteins, brush border antigens, urinary enzymes and Tamm Horsfall protein have not entered clinical routine in AKI patients due to the lack of sufficient validation, lack of standardised assays and changes in the specificity of patterns of urinary marker excretion with advancing renal dysfunction [24].

The last few years have seen an explosion of papers describing the basic molecular biological research and the beginning of the clinical application of a great number of biomarkers in the field of AKI. It seems, however, that based on the initial clinical trials that likely a combination of these markers will be the most useful approach since some of them appear early, and others later, in the evolution of AKI [24].

A recent paper [25] concluded that a combination of three biomarkers achieved a perfect score diagnosing acute kidney injury. In the case-control study, KIM-1 was better than NAG at all time points, but combining both was no better than KIM-1 alone.

Urinary MMP-9 was not a sensitive marker in the case-control study. This study suggests that urinary biomarkers allow diagnosis of acute kidney injury earlier than a rise in serum creatinine.

Another recent paper showed that urinary levels of liver fatty acid binding protein (L-FABP) represent a sensitive and predictive early biomarker of AKI after cardiac surgery [26].

Endre and Westhuyzen [27] summarised the most important biomarkers that have recently been proposed for the early diagnosis of AKI. All of them, however, still have to go through more clinical validation before they can be recommended in clinical practice.

2.4.2.2.4 Other Laboratory Tests to Establish the Cause of AKI

Various findings in the complete blood count, coagulation assays, changes in serum electrolytes and other parameters and immunologic investigations can suggest specific causes of AKI. These laboratory tests are summarised in Table 2.4.2.

Table 2.4.2 Blood and serum findings pointing to specific causes of acute renal failure (ARF)

Laboratory finding	Observed in AKI due to
Anaemia	Preexistent chronic renal failure, haemorrhage, haemolysis
Anaemia with rouleaux formation	Plasma cell dyscrasia
Eosinophilia	Atheroemboli, acute interstitial nephritis or polyarteritis nodosa
Leukopenia	SLE
Thrombocytopenia	SLE, Hantavirus infection, DIC, rhabdomyolysis, advanced liver disease with hypersplenism, 'white clot syndrome' due to heparin administration
Thrombocytopenia, reticulocytosis, elevated LDH, schistocytes on peripheral smear, low ADAMTS13 levels	Thrombotic microangiopathy
Coagulopathy	Liver disease, DIC, antiphosholipid antibody syndrome
Hypercalaemia < 5.5 mEq/L Marked hypercalaemia	Various causes Tumor lysis syndrome, haemolysis, use of NSAIDs, ACEi or ARB
Marked hypercalaemia, hyperphosphataemia, hypocalcaemia, elevated serum uric acid and CK, AST and LDH	Rhabdomyolysis
Marked hypercalaemia, hyperphosphataemia, hypocalcaemia, very high serum uric acid, normal or marginally elevated CK	Acute uric acid nephropathy, tumour lysis syndrome, heat stroke
Hypercalcaemia	Malignancy, sarcoidosis, vitamin D intoxication, etc.
Widening of serum anion and osmolal gap*	Ethylene glycol or methanol intoxication
Marked acidosis, anion gap >5–10 mEq/L	ethylene glycol poisoning, rhabdomyolysis, lactic acidosis from sepsis
Hypergammaglobulinaemia	SLE, bacterial endocarditis and other chronic infections
Paraprotein (M-gradient), hypergammaglobulinaemia	Myeloma
Urine electrophoresis showing free light chains	Myeloma, low-grade plasma cell dyscrasias (even in the absence of serum abnormalities)
Elevated serum IgA	IgA nephropathy
Elevated antinuclear antibodies	Autoimmune diseases including SLE, scleroderma, mixed connective tissue disease, Sjögren's syndrome, etc.
Elevated anti-double stranded DNA antibodies	SLE
Elevated anti-C1q antibodies	SLE, MPGN, some cases of IgA nephropathy
Elevated ANCA titer	Wegener's granulomatosis, microscopic polyangiitis
Antiglomerular basement membrane antibodies	Anti-GBM nephritis, Goodpasture syndrome
Cryoglobulins	Hepatitis C, lymphoproliferative disorders

DIC – disseminated intravascular coagulation; LDH – lactate dehydrogenase; CK – creatinine kinase; AST – asparagine aminotransferase; SLE – systemic lupus erythematosus; NSAID – non-steroidal antiinflammatory drug; ACEI – angiotensin-converting enzyme inhibitor; MPGN – membranoproliferative glomerulonephritis; ADAMTS13: a disintegrin and metalloprotease with thrombospondin-1–like domains.

*Mild metabolic acidosis occurs frequently as a consequence of AKI and is often associated with a modest (5–10 mEq/L) increase in the anion gap.

2.4.2.2 *Imaging Procedures in the Patient with AKI*

2.4.2.2.1 Ultrasound

Ultrasonography exhibits high sensitivity (90–98%) but a lower specificity (65–84%) for the detection of obstructive nephropathy. However, it is not a reliable method for identifying the anatomic site of obstruction. Sensitive ultrasonographic findings to rule out postrenal azotemia are a post-void residual bladder urine below 50 mL and absence of pelvicalyceal dilatation. Patients with highly distensible collecting systems or with pyelocaliectasis may be misdiagnosed as having hydronephrosis. False-negative findings have been reported in patients with very early (<8 h) obstruction. In many other false-negative cases, the patients were of an older age, and the obstructing process, usually prostatic carcinoma or retroperitoneal fibrosis, encased the retroperitoneal ureters and renal pelvis, preventing their dilatation. In the elderly, partial obstruction may be obscured by volume depletion. When there is a strong suspicion of obstruction, the ultrasonographic examination should be repeated after volume repletion.

Increased ultrasonographic renal size without hydronephrosis may occur with acute glomerulonephritis, with infiltration by amyloid or malignancy, in diabetes and in renal vein thrombosis. The finding of reduced renal size and increased echogenicity points to chronic renal failure. Even if the kidneys are reduced in size, the possibility of prerenal AKI or acute-on-chronic renal failure must always be considered.

Ultrasound contrast media can improve the diagnostic capabilities in AKI by allowing the visualisation of altered renal blood flow and of renal perfusion defects.

2.4.2.2.2 Renal Doppler Ultrasonography

Doppler studies have been suggested to differentiate prerenal cause from renal AKI. Partly as a result of intrarenal vasoconstriction, ATN usually produces a reduction in renal blood flow. Increases of the resistance index (RI) to >0.75 have been described in 91% of kidneys with ATN, compared with less than 0.75 in kidneys with acute prerenal failure. However the RI results overlap between these two major causes, and high RIs are also observed in acute obstruction, which markedly reduces its usefulness to obtain a specific diagnosis.

2.4.2.2.3 Other Radiologic Investigations

Intravenous urography nowadays is largely abandoned in patients with AKI, in particular given the need for potentially nephrotoxic radiocontrast agents.

A plain radiograph of the abdomen (sometimes called KUB – 'kidney, ureter and bladder') is a mandatory investigation in any patient in whom an obstructive cause of AKI is suspected, since it can detect even small radio-opaque stones and ureteral stones not found by ultrasound.

The presence and site of obstruction is accurately diagnosed by antegrade or retrograde pyelography. If obstruction is present, a ureteral stent or percutaneous nephrostomy can be placed in the same session.

A computed tomography (CT) scan performed without contrast is of comparable diagnostic value to the renal ultrasound but more costly and less convenient. However, CT is superior in the evaluation of ureteral obstruction, because it can delineate the level of obstruction and define retroperitoneal inflammatory tissue (in retroperitoneal fibrosis) or a retroperitoneal malignant mass.

Magnetic resonance imaging (MRI) is not usually used for evaluation of AKI, but if imaging is necessary, it should be preferred to contrast-enhanced CT and other radiocontrast-requiring radiographic techniques. An altered corticomedullary relationship is frequently recognised in patients with AKI but also in other acute renal diseases on T-weighed images. When postrenal AKI is suspected, MRI is valuable in assessing hydronephrosis and detecting the cause and site of obstruction. MR angiography can be useful for detecting abnormalities in the renal artery and vein. Particularly the diagnosis of acute renal cortical necrosis becomes more reliable with gadolinium-enhanced MRI. The 'rim sign' is characteristic for this infrequent cause of AKI.

In view of the increasingly reported incidence of the syndrome of nephrogenic systemic fibrosis in patients who have been exposed to gadolinium-containing contrast media – and such cases have also been described in patients with ARF – it is actually not recommended to use certain types of gadolinium-containing molecules, such as gadodiamide-Omniscan unless absolutely indicated, in patients with a GFR <30–40 mL/min [28, 29].

Renal angiography can be indicated when renal artery occlusion (by embolisation, thrombosis or a dissecting aneurysm) is suspected based on the clinical history (e.g. in patients with atrial fibrillation and acute flank pain) or on duplex scanning, to confirm the exact anatomy of the occlusion and to assess the potential for intervention. However, in this setting, MR angiography or spiral CT is superior. Hepatic or renal angiography may also be useful in diagnosing classical polyarteritis nodosa.

Although Doppler ultrasound, MRI, MR angiography and CT are used more frequently in the evaluation of thromboembolic disease and acute cortical necrosis, renal venography may be indicated to confirm a clinical or duplex ultrasound suspicion of renal vein thrombosis. When a diagnosis of acute renal artery occlusion is considered, renal angiography should be obtained urgently, as early surgical or thrombolytic therapy may be necessary to salvage the kidney. However, where the complete occlusion occurs in a background of chronic occlusive disease, sufficient collateral blood supply may be provided, and even delayed intervention can result in recovery of renal function.

2.4.2.2.4 Renal Biopsy

Renal biopsy is reserved for patients in whom prerenal and postrenal failure have been excluded and the cause of intrinsic renal AKI is unclear. Renal biopsy is particularly useful when clinical assessment, urinalysis and laboratory investigation suggest diagnoses other than ischaemic or nephrotoxic injury that may respond to specific therapy – for example, rapidly progressive glomerulonephritis and allergic interstitial nephritis. Renal biopsy should also be considered in AKI when there are symptoms or signs of a systemic illness, such as persistent fever or unexplained anaemia. Unexpected causes of AKI, such as myeloma, interstitial nephritis, endocarditis or cryoglobulinaemia, or cholesterol emboli may be revealed by renal biopsy in these situations. In studies of patients with biopsy-proven atheroembolic kidney disease, anticoagulation was thought to be a precipitating factor in 33–55% of cases. Anticoagulant agents are thought to destabilise atherosclerotic plaques by allowing cholesterol crystals that were previously covered by clot to be exposed to the circulation. The prognosis for patients with atheroembolic kidney disease is poor; in up to 25%, the condition progresses to ESRD, and in a recent prospective study, 38% died within 5 years [30].

In patients diagnosed with ATN and normal-sized kidneys, who do not recover renal function after 3–4 weeks, a renal biopsy may be indicated to confirm the cause of AKI, exclude other treatable causes and determine the prognosis. Finally, renal biopsy is a routine diagnostic procedure in patients with AKI after transplant, when it is often essential for distinguishing between ischaemic ATN, acute rejection and calcineurin inhibitor toxicity.

2.4.3 Summary of General Therapeutic Principles of AKI in the ICU

From this chapter, it is hopefully clear that AKI in the ICU can be the result of a wide range of disease processes so that it is likely to be encountered by physicians from all specialties. In particular the increasing recognition of the overlap between critical care medicine and nephrology has resulted in what nowadays is called critical care nephrology. In this specialty, nephrologists should be familiar with the rapid advances in the field of general intensive care medicine (euglycaemic control with continuous insulin, low doses of corticosteroids in septic shock, administration of activated protein C, general infection control, advances in nutrition for the critically ill, etc.), and the impact these advances may have on the occurrence of AKI in these patients. At the same time, the intensivist, while still keeping the overall responsibility and coordination of the management of these often complex patients, should involve the nephrologist in the critical care unit, not only for determining the initiation, selection and practical supervision of the applied RRT modalities, but also in the management of fluid and electrolyte disturbances, acid–bases disorders, management of cardiac and liver failure, control of hypertension, management of intoxications, giving advice on dose adaptations according to the changed renal pharmacokinetics of many drugs and the specific drug interventions in many non-ATN cases of AKI. The discussion of the many diverse medical treatments of the different intrinsic renal causes of AKI is beyond the scope of this chapter and will be described in other chapters devoted to these individual diseases.

The nondialytic therapy of practically all patients with AKI includes optimising renal perfusion with volume expansion, use of inotropes and vasopressors, eventual trials with renal vasodilators and loop diuretics and/or mannitol, and modulation of renal metabolism and avoidance of tubular obstruction. A very important aspect of this nondialytic therapy is nephrological advice related to the prevention of AKI in at-risk patients and the role of the nephrologists in the prevention of the many complications associated with AKI. An example of the cooperation between nephrology and intensive care is the willingness of the nephrologist to intervene at any moment with dialysis and ultrafiltration in the 'spontaneously' or 'therapeutically-induced' volume-overloaded patient.

The moment of initiation of RRT, the selection of the RRT modality and the dose and frequency of dialysis should be decided in daily consultations between nephrologist and intensivist. Flexibility and willingness to listen and to take the advice of both teams is a great asset which can only be to the advantage of the critically ill patient. The slow but steady improvement of the, at least short-term, prognosis of the patient with AKI is testimony to this growing cooperation between the two disciplines [31].

References

1. Mehta RL, Kellum JA, Shah SV et al. Acute Kidney Injury Network: report of an initiative to improve outcomes in acute kidney injury. *Crit Care* 2007; 11: R31
2. Joannidis M, Metnitz PG. Epidemiology and natural history of acute renal failure in the ICU. *Crit Care Clin* 2005; 21: 239–249
3. Lameire N, Van Biesen W, Vanholder R. The changing epidemiology of acute renal failure. *Nature Clin Pract Nephrol* 2006; 2: 364–377
4. Lameire N, Van Biesen W, Vanholder R. Acute renal failure. *Lancet* 2005; 365: 417–430
5. Clermont G, Acker CG, Angus DC, Sirio CA, Pinsky MR, Johnson JP. Renal failure in the ICU: comparison of the impact of acute renal failure and end-stage renal disease on ICU outcomes. *Kidney Int* 2002; 62: 986–996
6. Prescott GJ, Metcalfe W, Baharani J et al. A prospective national study of acute renal failure treated with RRT: incidence, aetiology and outcomes. *Nephrol Dial Transplant* 2007; 22: 2513–2519
7. Uchino S, Kellum JA, Bellomo R et al. Acute renal failure in critically ill patients: a multinational, multicenter study. *JAMA* 2005; 294: 813–818
8. Liano F, Junco E, Pascual J, Madero R, Verde E. The spectrum of acute renal failure in the intensive care unit compared with that seen in other settings. The Madrid Acute Renal Failure Study Group. *Kidney Int Suppl* 1998; 66: S16-S24
9. Cerda J, Bagga A, Kher V, Chakravarthi RM. The contrasting characteristics of acute kidney injury in developed and developing countries. *Nat Clin Pract Nephrol* 2008; 4: 138–153
10. Lameire N, Van Biesen W, Vanholder R. Epidemiology, clinical evaluation, and prevention of acute renal failure. In: Feehally J, Floege J, Johnson RJ, eds. *Comprehensive Clinical Nephrology*. Mosby-Elsevier, Philadelphia: 2007; 771–785
11. Abbas SM, Hill AG. Systematic review of the literature for the use of oesophageal Doppler monitor for fluid replacement in major abdominal surgery. *Anaesthesia* 2008; 63: 44–51
12. De Waele JJ, De L, I. Intra-abdominal hypertension and the effect on renal function. *Acta Clin Belg Suppl* 2007; 371–374
13. Malbrain ML. Is it wise not to think about intraabdominal hypertension in the ICU? *Curr Opin Crit Care* 2004; 10: 132–145
14. Sugrue M. Abdominal compartment syndrome. *Curr Opin Crit Care* 2005; 11: 333–338
15. Rea ME, Dunlap ME. Renal hemodynamics in heart failure: implications for treatment. *Curr Opin Nephrol Hypertens* 2008; 17: 87–92
16. Wencker D. Acute cardio-renal syndrome: progression from congestive heart failure to congestive kidney failure. *Curr Heart Fail Rep* 2007; 4: 134–138
17. Mullens W, Abrahams Z, Skouri HN et al. Elevated intra-abdominal pressure in acute decompensated heart failure: a potential contributor to worsening renal function? *J Am Coll Cardiol* 2008; 51: 300–306
18. Bagshaw SM, Langenberg C, Bellomo R. Urinary biochemistry and microscopy in septic acute renal failure: a systematic review. *Am J Kidney Dis* 2006; 48: 695–705
19. Pepin MN, Bouchard J, Legault L, Ethier J. Diagnostic performance of fractional excretion of urea and fractional excretion of sodium in the evaluations of patients with acute kidney injury with or without diuretic treatment. *Am J Kidney Dis* 2007; 50: 566–573
20. Lassnigg A, Schmidlin D, Mouhieddine M et al. Minimal changes of serum creatinine predict prognosis in patients after cardiothoracic surgery: a prospective cohort study. *J Am Soc Nephrol* 2004; 15: 1597–1605
21. Weisbord SD, Chen H, Stone RA et al. Associations of increases in serum creatinine with mortality and length of hospital stay after coronary angiography. *J Am Soc Nephrol* 2006; 17: 2871–2877
22. Herget-Rosenthal S, Marggraf G, Husing J, et al. Early detection of acute renal failure by serum cystatin C. *Kidney Int* 2004; 66: 1115–1122
23. Villa P, Jimenez M, Soriano MC, Manzanares J, Casasnovas P. Serum cystatin C concentration as a marker of acute renal dysfunction in critically ill patients. *Crit Care* 2005; 9: R139–R143
24. Thurman JM, Parikh CR. Peeking into the black box: new biomarkers for acute kidney injury. *Kidney Int* 2008; 73: 379–381
25. Han WK, Waikar SS, Johnson A, et al. Urinary biomarkers in the early diagnosis of acute kidney injury. *Kidney Int* 2008; 73: 863–869
26. Portilla D, Dent C, Sugaya T, et al. Liver fatty acid-binding protein as a biomarker of acute kidney injury after cardiac surgery. *Kidney Int* 2008; 73: 465–472
27. Endre ZH, Westhuyzen J. Early detection of acute kidney injury: emerging new biomarkers (Review Article). *Nephrology (Carlton)* 2008; 13: 91–98
28. Nortier JL, del Marmol V. Nephrogenic systemic fibrosis – the need for a multidisciplinary approach. *Nephrol Dial Transplant* 2007; 22: 3097–3101
29. Swaminathan S, Shah SV. New insights into nephrogenic systemic fibrosis. *J Am Soc Nephrol* 2007; 18: 2636–2643
30. Scolari F, Ravani P, Pola A, et al. Predictors of renal and patient outcomes in atheroembolic renal disease: a prospective study. *J Am Soc Nephrol* 2003; 14: 1584–1590
31. Waikar SS, Curhan GC, Wald R, McCarthy EP, Chertow GM. Declining mortality in patients with acute renal failure, 1988 to 2002. *J Am Soc Nephrol* 2006; 17: 1143–1150

Urinary Tract Obstruction

2.5

Angela D'Angelo and Dorella Del Prete

Core Messages

- Urinary tract obstruction is a common major cause of acute and chronic renal insufficiency.
- Obstructive uropathy is a condition common to all age groups, even very early and late in life.
- Regardless of the age of obstruction, the renal response involves progressive tubular dilation, tubular atrophy, and interstitial fibrosis.
- Although urinary tract obstructions can develop entirely asymptomatically, it is more common, especially in chronic cases and in pediatric ages, for an obstruction to cause more or less evident signs and symptoms, particularly because most cases of obstructive uropathy that become clinically manifest are caused by a partial rather than a total obstruction of the urinary tract.
- In patients presenting with acute or chronic renal problems, it is always important to confirm or exclude an obstructive uropathy, given the frequency of this condition and because it is the most common cause of reversible renal insufficiency.
- It is always important to remove an obstruction in order to preserve renal function and prevent complications, one of the most important of which is infection.

2.5.1 Introduction

Urinary tract obstruction is a common major cause of acute and chronic renal insufficiency. It is the postrenal cause of acute renal insufficiency, and the potentially suitable treatment measures should always prompt this syndrome to be suspected. It can give rise to three different clinical pictures:

- Hydronephrosis, or distension of the renal pelvis and calyces
- Obstructive uropathy, or functional and partly structural changes after the urinary tract obstruction between the renal pelvis and urethra, obstruction that alters the normal urine flow, demanding a greater pressure upstream in the attempt to overcome the obstacle
- Obstructive nephropathy, or functional and structural changes affecting the renal parenchyma as a consequence of a protracted obstruction

In general, any obstacle to urine outflow induces a series of functional modifications in the urinary tract that come under the term of obstructive uropathy. If this condition is not treated, it leads to progressive renal damage or obstructive nephropathy.

The obstruction may be congenital or acquired; partial (low grade) or complete (high grade); unilateral or bilateral; occurring in the upper (above the ureterovesical junction) or lower urinary tract; and intraluminal, intramural (intrinsic), or extramural (extrinsic).

In the past, this condition went largely underdiagnosed, especially when it was accompanied by chronic renal insufficiency. It was with the advent of ultrasound that its diagnosis became easier, and physicians have consequently become more aware that this condition is important, frequent, and in several cases treatable. In fact, recognizing an obstructive uropathy is important

A. D'Angelo (✉)
Università di Padova, CNR , Via Giustiniani, 2 35128 Padova, Italy
e-mail: angela.dangelo@unipd.it

A. Jörres et al. (eds.), *Management of Acute Kidney Problems*,
DOI: 10.1007/978-3-540-69441-0_2.5, © Springer-Verlag Berlin Heidelberg 2010

not only because the condition is rather common (lifelong incidence of approximately 1/1,000), but also because, given a timely diagnosis, it can be treated in the majority of cases, and the related renal functional alterations are often reversible. Conversely, if an obstruction goes undiagnosed and consequently without treatment for some time, then chronic obstructive nephropathy sets in, the most severe final outcome of which is interstitial fibrosis, as in all chronic forms of renal disease.

At present, surgical relief of obstruction is the primary treatment at least for congenital urinary tract obstruction. An additional concern is the long-term outcome of patients with obstructive uropathy – that is, the impact of tubulointerstitial disease and nephron loss on renal function and blood pressure. The cellular and molecular approach to the study of this disease should lead to new therapies that will attenuate the early injurious renal responses to urinary tract obstruction, and also the factors that lead to progressive renal deterioration [1].

2.5.2 Causes of Obstruction

Obstructive uropathy is a condition common to all age groups, even very early and late in life.

In early infancy and childhood, numerous congenital disorders may be accompanied by obstructions coinciding with anomalies affecting the ureter and bladder (at the ureteropelvic or ureterovesical junction, collector system duplicity with ureterocele), and urethra (posterior urethra valves, urethral stenosis, or atresia).

The most common of these disorders is the obstruction at the ureteropelvic junction, followed by obstruction at the ureterovesical junction and bladder outlet obstruction. The changes from hydronephrosis to renal dysplasia or agenesis suggest that a late or an early obstruction, respectively, has interfered with the kidney development. The obstructed fetal kidney is replaced by expanded mesenchymal stroma and primitive nephrons, indicating decreased mesenchymal-epithelial transformation [2].

In children the obstruction is frequently associated with vesicoureteral reflux, and the progression to chronic renal insufficiency is generally due to a late diagnosis of the obstruction, to surgical complications, or, more frequently, to overlying infections. The consequent obstructive nephropathy can progress toward end-stage renal insufficiency in a variable period of months or years, when a patient is still a child or much later in adult age.

Table 2.5.1 Congenital causes of urinary tract obstruction

Renal pelvis	Ureteropelvic junction anomalies
	Aberrant renal artery
Ureter	Collector system duplicity
	Ectopic ureter
	Ureterocele
	Ureterovesical junction anomalies
Bladder	Neurogenic (spina bifida)
Urethra	Atresia
	Valves
	Stenosis

The main causes of obstruction involved in the congenital forms are listed in Table 2.5.1.

Upper urinary tract obstructions (above the ureterovesical junction) usually are unilateral, whereas lower urinary tract obstructions are, by definition, bilateral. The etiology varies according to patient age and sex. In young and middle-aged men, acute obstruction due to renal stones is common but temporary, whereas pelvic cancer is an important cause of obstructive uropathy in women of this age group. In older age groups, urinary tract obstruction is more common in the men, resulting from prostatic hypertrophy or malignancy [3].

In the elderly in fact, the most frequent type of obstructive nephropathy affects the neck of the bladder, secondary mainly to benign prostate hypertrophy. With adequate surgical treatment, this is rarely accompanied by progression toward renal insufficiency. Cases of prostatic, pelvic, or intra-abdominal cancer always warrant assessment for the risk of urinary tract obstruction.

Of course there are numerous other causes of obstruction in children, adults, and the elderly, including stones, neoplasms, surgical procedures, clots, detached renal papillae, traumas, infections, autonomic neuropathy, genital diseases, and retroperitoneal fibrosis, and different causes naturally carry very different prognoses.

It is important to bear in mind that an obstruction may overlap a prior chronic renal disease, as in the case of papillary necrosis, in which papillae become detached and constitute an obstruction. The patient may have a history of analgesics abuse, as well as renal amyloidosis and acute pyelonephritis, especially in cases associated with diabetes mellitus. Then there is necrotizing papillitis or diabetic neurogenic bladder,

Table 2.5.2 Causes of obstructions developing in existing renal disease

Detachment of papillae	Analgesic-induced nephropathy
	Diabetic necrotizing papillitis
Clots	Polycystic kidney
Neurogenic bladder	Diabetes mellitus
Ureteral and vesical fibrosis	Renal tuberculosis

and other causes of obstruction in polycystic kidney, and in the case of renal tuberculosis. These causes are listed in Table 2.5.2.

Obstructive uropathy varies in severity, depending on the site and degree of the obstruction and its duration. There are numerous causes of acquired obstruction, the majority of them in the renal pelvis, ureter, bladder, and urethra are listed in Table 2.5.3, divided according to their intrinsic or extrinsic nature.

Stones are the most common extrarenal cause of intraluminal obstruction in young male adults, who generally have a family or personal history of renal stones or colic, hematuria, gout, or renal tubular acidosis, and, in females, recurrent infections as a cause or complication, in addition to signs of hyperparathyroidism. The passage of a stone along the ureter does not usually interfere with diuresis and does not necessarily lead to renal insufficiency, since the contralateral kidney usually functions normally.

Table 2.5.3 Main causes of acquired obstruction and related sites

Renal pelvis	Lumen	Stones, clots, neoplasms, urate crystals
	Wall	Ureteropelvic junction obstruction
	Extrinsic	Narrowing due to surgical sequelae
		Neoplasms
Ureter	Lumen	Stones, clots, neoplasms, detached papillae
	Wall	Narrowing induced by trauma, radiation, inflammation
	Extrinsic	Retroperitoneal lesions (fibrosis, neoplastic disease, hemorrhage, sequelae of surgery)
Bladder	Lumen	Stones, clots, neoplasms
	Wall	Interstitial cystitis, tuberculosis
	Extrinsic	Neurogenic bladder (spinal lesions, diabetes mellitus)
		Prostatic or cervical cancer
Urethra	Lumen	Neoplasms, foreign bodies
	Wall	Narrowing (due to trauma, tuberculosis, inflammation)
	Extrinsic	Prostatic hypertrophy or carcinoma

As long as the stone remains at its site of formation, i.e. attached to the renal papilla, it is asymptomatic or may cause sporadic microscopic hematuria. It is only when it becomes detached from the papilla and moves freely in the flow of urine that it may become painful if it acutely obstructs the collector system, and especially if it gets stuck or meets with some difficulty at any point along its course from the ureteropelvic junction to the ureterovesical junction. The resulting pain is due to the increase in pressure and consequent dilation of the renal pelvis and collector system upstream, which is known as renal colic. The pain is usually of sudden onset and, when it reaches its maximum intensity it remains constant and intolerable. If the pain begins on one side and neither irradiates nor shifts in site, then the obstruction is likely to be stuck somewhere along the urinary tract; on the other hand, if the pain moves, shifting downwards and irradiating along the ureter into the lateral and anterior abdomen, this means that the stone is mobile. Stones that become trapped at the ureterovesical junction are often associated not with colic, but with symptoms of infection, dysuria, and pollakiuria (due to inflammation of the vesical triangle), so the pain irradiates to the ipsilateral external genitalia.

Urinary tract stones may also develop without symptoms, however, and be discovered by chance. With the exception of those consisting of uric acid, stones are usually radiopaque: calcium stones because of their calcium content, struvite stones because of their magnesium content, and cystine stones because of their sulfur content.

The obstructed kidney tends to become enlarged and, in the case of urinary tract infections, there may be muscle spasms and pain in the costovertebral angle.

Neoplasms can cause local symptoms, such as pain, a palpable mass, capricious hematuria, or systemic symptoms such as fever and anemia.

Retroperitoneal fibrosis should be suspected in cases with a history of headache and the use of methysergide, or with signs of lymphoma. Invasion to this level from neoplasms originating in the neck of uterus, prostate, bladder, colon, or ovary is also a common finding.

Pelvic surgery can be responsible for obstructions due to accidental ureter ligature, or following radiation for cancer treatment.

Infection or trauma can be responsible for ureteral stenosis.

Other clinical signs and complications of a urinary tract obstruction will vary not only according to cause (congenital or acquired), but also depending on the site of the obstruction, whether it is unilateral or bilateral, how quickly it developed and the degree of obstruction (partial or complete).

Site: If the obstruction is in the neck of the bladder, it is usually accompanied by symptoms of bladder dysfunction (difficulty in starting micturition, intermittent micturition, a sensation of incomplete emptying, pollakiuria, and nycturia), and it is sometimes complicated by urinary tract infections. Obstructions on higher levels are often symptom-free (especially if they are chronic), or they may sometimes be associated with pain and a palpable mass.

Unilateral vs. bilateral: If the obstruction is complete, it causes anuria; if not, the obstruction often goes unnoticed unless the extent of the obstruction is sufficient to cause pain or severe enough to cause hydronephrosis; if the latter is complicated by infection, then bacteremia may develop.

Rate of onset and degree: Pain is common when the obstruction is of sudden onset, but unusual with chronic obstructions; a total obstruction causes anuria, but partial obstructions can also cause anomalies in urine volume that can lead to polyuria; various degrees of partial obstruction can thus give rise to fluctuating urine volumes, which is an important diagnostic sign.

Complications: The most common is infection, which may be spontaneous or after diagnostic tests and urologic procedures; hypertension and polycythemia are less common signs, but may be severe in some cases: uremia or symptomatic renal insufficiency may be due to a prolonged, severe partial obstruction, or to a unresolved total obstruction.

2.5.3 Renal Damage Induced by Urinary Tract Obstructions

Regardless of the age of obstruction, the renal response involves progressive tubular dilation, tubular atrophy, and interstitial fibrosis. An acute obstruction induces a sudden rise in ureteric and intrarenal pressure, causing dilation upstream and increasing the peristaltic activity; the consequent elevation in pressure is transmitted back to the tubular lumen, and is enhanced further by early increments in renal blood flow (RBF) and glomerular filtration rate (GFR). However, this maximal pelvic pressure elevation begins soon to fall with reduction of RBF and GFR because of the increasing dilation of the renal pelvis, and also for the altered pyelolymphatic and pyelovenous backflow. At this point the stretch effect of the continued pooling of urine following obstruction induces the collecting tubules to become resistant to vasopressin, so they cannot produce concentrated urine, and sodium handling (and associated water reabsorption) is progressively impaired both in the distal and proximal tubules [4].

The pressure increase in the renal tubules initially leads to a transient increase in blood flow, then to a more limited renal perfusion due to pre- and post-glomerular capillary vasoconstriction mediated by various vasoactive compounds, such as angiotensin II, thromboxane A2, and vasopressin.

In general, ureteral obstruction results in decreased RBF and GFR in the ipsilateral kidney and increased RBF to the intact opposite kidney. Twenty-four hours after the acute event, renal blood flow will have dropped by about 50%, and the consequent drop in GFR reduces the pressure in the tubules and protects the glomeruli against hypertensive damage. There may be a functional recovery after variable periods of total obstruction, ranging from 1 week even to several months. Partial obstructions that fail to clear and that give rise to hydronephrosis always warrant corrective surgery in adults, whereas in the children they may clear spontaneously with time, without reducing the patient's kidney function.

Conversely, when obstruction persists and becomes chronic, this inevitably entails a slow, progressive, gradual, and irreversible decline in kidney function, because the hemodynamic changes, beginning with renal vasoconstriction mediated by increased activity of the renin-angiotensin system, is followed by an interstitial inflammatory response initially characterized by macrophage infiltration, tubular dilation, and renal tubular cell apoptosis, with consequent tubule atrophy and interstitial fibrosis. Some tubular cells undergo epithelial-mesenchymal transformation and migrate across the damaged tubular basement membrane to the interstitial space, where they can become activated myofibroblasts. The fibroblasts that accumulate in the interstitium are formed via proliferation of resident fibroblasts (49%), and from bone marrow–derived cells (15%), as well as via transformation of epithelial cells (36%) [5].

The renal damage caused by an obstruction is therefore not merely the outcome of a more or less acute mechanical interference with the flow of urine, but it is part of a more complex picture due to the interaction of various vasoactive factors and cytokines responsible for changes in both glomerular hemodynamics and tubule function. [6].

In fact, it has been demonstrated that an obstruction triggers the activation of the infrarenal renin-angiotensin system [7, 8].

Angiotensin II has an important role in the progression of renal damage because it is responsible for an increased production of growth factors, and especially TGF-β, which is a key mediator of renal interstitial fibrosis. It was demonstrated that in the obstructed kidney, the extracellular matrix is synthesized and deposited more rapidly than it is degraded. Oxidative stress, powered partly by angiotensin II, induces tubule cell apoptosis through activation of the NF-κB factor. This factor in fact is prompted by ureteral obstruction, and the administration of angiotensin-converting enzyme (ACE) inhibitors can significantly reduce its levels [9].

Histologic examination of the kidney soon after obstruction shows tubule dilation, confirming the importance of the urine-pooling effect. The transferred pressure gives the epithelial cells lining the nephron a flattened appearance. These initial stressful stimuli in the tubular compartment are known to cause cell injury and death. The affected cells prompt the generation of an inflammatory response. Tubular cell death during unilateral obstruction has been shown to occur principally by way of programmed cell death or apoptosis [10].

2.5.4 Clinical Signs

As mentioned previously, these depend on the causes of the obstruction, whether it involves one or both kidneys, the rate of onset and degree of the obstruction, and any concomitant complications. It is worth emphasizing that urinary tract obstructions can develop entirely asymptomatically, especially in chronic cases and in pediatric ages. It is more common, however, for an obstruction to cause more or less evident signs and symptoms, particularly because most cases of obstructive uropathy that become clinically manifest are caused by a partial rather than a total obstruction of the urinary tract.

Depending on how the obstruction develops, the corresponding clinical syndrome can give rise to the following pictures:

- *Acute renal insufficiency*: If the obstruction is complete or incomplete, unilateral or bilateral; this is accompanied by clearly evident signs and symptoms, pain, dysuria (difficulty in starting micturition, intermittent jet, hesitancy, urgency, pollakiuria, and/or nycturia), hematuria, oligoanuria and fever, and sometimes even urinary sepsis. The patient may be anuric if the obstruction is complete, or intensely polyuric
- *Chronic renal insufficiency*: If the obstruction is partial, bilateral, and severe. It may have been silent or mild enough to go unrecognized for some time
- *Tubule disorders*: If the obstruction is partial and bilateral. These are the effects of a reduced renal concentration and acidification capacity, a metabolic acidosis associated with hypopotassemia.

This clinical syndrome includes postobstructive polyuria (major osmotic diuresis on removal of the obstruction, isosthenuric urine with sodium concentration relatively not very high); nephrogenic diabetes insipidus (diuresis characterized by markedly hyposthenuric urine due to direct renal tubule damage caused by long periods of obstruction severe enough to make the tubule insensitive to the action of antidiuretic hormone and hydrosodic depletion (after the elimination of a bilateral obstruction, the loss of sodium, accompanied by an intense polyuria and concomitant dehydration, is excessive with respect to the nutritional intake and associated with an increased excretion of calcium, phosphorus, and magnesium severe enough to reduce their blood levels, leading to a picture of so-called salt-losing nephritis).

- *Urinary tract infections*: They are a frequent complication of all types of obstruction. They are recurrent infections facilitated by urine stasis and often scarcely amenable to *common* treatments. The increase in ureteral pressure is transmitted upwards to the renal pelvis, causing papillary necrosis, and this predisposes the patient to infections, which alter smooth muscle contractility and may further complicate the situation by making a partial obstruction become complete.
- *Colic-like pain*: If a complete or partial obstruction is unilateral, an intense pain at renal level is caused more by the rapidity of onset than by the severity of the resulting distension of the collector system. In fact, if the obstruction develops slowly and progressively, the related distension may be severe but go clinically

unnoticed, whereas if the obstruction is acute and affects the ureter, the pain to the corresponding side is intense and piercing, radiating to the lower abdomen and to the inguinal and suprapubic area or outer genitals, and it is associated with vomiting, hematuria, and tenesmus. If the obstruction lies on the ureterovesical valve, the signs and symptoms may include a reduced caliber and urine flow rate, difficulty in starting micturition, intermittency of the jet, pollakiuria, and nycturia, all symptoms usually accompanied by either oligoanuresis or severe polyuria.

- *Polycythemia*: It is fairly rare, but it seems that ischemia of a partially obstructed kidney can induce an increase in erythropoietin production.
- *Hypertension*: Coinciding with or *caused* by acute or chronic, unilateral or bilateral hydronephrosis, hypertension is generally due to an increased sodium and water retention. In fact, this symptom is solved by urine drainage through a catheter and consequent osmotic diuresis with a negative hydric balance, which confirms that hypertension was volume-dependent. If the obstruction is unilateral and acute, hypertension is generally correlated with an increase in renin levels, which in fact disappears once the obstruction has been removed. When the obstruction persists and the hydronephrosis becomes chronic, it no longer seems to stimulate an increase in renin secretion, whereas volume changes seem to occur, or the inability to release antihypertensive or vasodepressor substances.

2.5.5 Diagnostic Approach

This is based on recording the patient's clinical history, assessing the symptoms, and conducting a physical examination of the abdomen. But fundamental information is obtained by characterizing the patient's urinary excretion modalities and variables, and essentially by means of urine tests.

Any hematuria is suggestive of an obstructive lesion due to a stone, papillary necrosis, or tumor. If the hematuria is associated with bacteriuria, then a chronic obstruction is likely. If there are associated leukocyturia and cylindruria (leukocytic cylinders), then pyelonephritis is suspected. In cases of acute renal insufficiency, the presence of uric acid crystals suggests an infrarenal obstruction.

It is always essential to assess renal function, blood crasis, electrolytes, and acid–alkaline balance to clarify the condition. If the initial symptoms include pain with no reduction of renal function, the diagnosis directly focuses on establishing the presence or the absence of a stone.

2.5.6 Instrumental Diagnostics

In patients presenting with acute or chronic renal problems, it is always important to confirm or exclude an obstructive uropathy, given the frequency of this condition and because it is the most common cause of reversible renal insufficiency.

Imaging involves using ultrasound, radioisotopic, radiologic, and endoscopic investigations. These are used, in said order, according to their different diagnostic utility, opting for the one that is least invasive, easiest to perform, with the lowest complication rates and costs. The instrumental investigations must nonetheless provide accurate anatomic and functional information to establish not only whether or not there is an obstruction, but also its presumable severity, location and, if possible, its cause. Moreover, these tests must help us to ascertain the feasibility and the methodology of removing the obstruction, in order to achieve the best possible functional recovery.

Ultrasound: This is the first test to use to view the calyceal structures and the upper excretory tract, evaluate their size and shape, and look for any signs of stones. Ultrasound is noninvasive and easy to perform, so it is the screening method of choice for seeking dilations of the urinary tract in adults and children. It is readily repeatable, enabling any hydronephrosis documented to be followed up. It is indispensable for ruling out or confirming an obstruction, especially in the case of renal insufficiency, distinguishing an absent or atrophic kidney from one that is obstructed or hydronephrotic. It can be used in acute renal insufficiency to rule out a causal obstruction. It is unable instead to explore the ureter adequately. It is indispensable for the prenatal diagnosis of congenital obstructive uropathy.

The echo color Doppler extends its use to the study of urodynamics.

3-D ultrasound: In the case of obstructive uropathy, this noninvasive method is very useful because it considerably increases the diagnostic potential of two-dimensional ultrasound, representing a technological development capable of improving the detail of the ultrasound image. Applied to the ureter, it succeeds in providing important information on the shape of a stone, exactly defining its location inside the ureteral lumen. It is also particularly effective in diagnosing an obstruction due not to a stone, but to inflammation or neoplastic disease [11].

Radioisotopic investigations: Sequential renal scintigraphy is particularly important in providing functional, rather than etiologic information on an obstruction causing hydronephrosis, particularly in pediatric patients. In addition to evaluating the functionality of a dilated kidney, it particularly enables a distinction between hydronephrosis due to an obstruction from a simple dilation. The isotopes most often used can be divided according to whether they are eliminated by glomerular filtration or tubular secretion, or, by binding to the proximal tubular cells, they are slowly excreted with the urine, affording more accurate and detailed images with no signal overlap, even in the case of renal insufficiency (providing it is only mild or moderate). This test can be repeated and it enables variations in the dilated kidney's functionality to be monitored over time, in addition to the degree and extent of the dilation concerned. Performing the test with a diuretic completes and further improves the diagnostic work-up because furosemide induces a rapid emptying of the excretory tract in the event of simple stasis (though it has the drawback that response to the diuretic also depends on renal function).

2.5.7 Radiologic Investigations

Excretory urography or descending pyelography, is a radiologic method using contrast enhancement that for many years was irreplaceable as a means for diagnosing and establishing the site and nature of an obstruction, and it is still recommended today when it is important to obtain a detailed assessment of the renal excretory pathways at precalyceal level too, e.g., when sponge kidney is suspected. It is also indicated for calyceal lesions induced by parenchymal conditions, e.g., papillary necrosis. It can be conducted only if renal function is still normal or only moderately reduced, however, and providing the patient has no allergic diathesis or other contraindications. It is preceded by a routine uncontrasted abdominal X-ray, which enables a preliminary assessment of the kidneys' shape and size, and any signs of stones, if radiopaque, along the urinary tract. Using a suitably high dose of iodized water-soluble contrast medium (100 ml of 50–60% solution) and concomitant tomography, it succeeds in providing accurate information on the dimensions, shape, and status not only of the excretory calyceal structures, but also of the ureters (calyceal pyelographic phase) and bladder (cystographic phase), as well as identifying any radiotransparent stones. In the initial (nephrographic) phase, moreover, it also provides useful details on the corticorenal and medullary parenchyma. Before undergoing this type of test, the patient needs to be well hydrated, and it is important to ensure that the information obtainable is proportional to the renal toxicity risk of the contrast medium used.

Computed tomography: Direct computed tomography (CT) can rule out or confirm an obstruction in patients at high risk of contrast medium toxicity, especially in cases of severely reduced renal function. If a kidney is totally obstructed, CT enables an assessment of the site, cause, and extent of the obstruction. Of course, its accuracy cannot always be fully assured; for instance, if the dilated urinary pathways are easy to see, any parapyelic cysts can be interpreted as part of the hydronephrosis. Direct views of the renal parenchyma in the etiologic diagnosis of an obstruction also enable an assessment of the likelihood of a functional recovery after the obstruction has been removed. It has been demonstrated that urography with 3-D CT considerably increases the sensitivity of stone identification at ureteral sites [12].

CT with a contrast medium is particularly suitable for use in the diagnosis of an obstruction involving a dislocation of the urinary pathways due to retroperitoneal fibrosis, para-aortic lymphadenopathies, and ureteral incarceration by cancer.

Magnetic resonance urography: This is particularly indicated in children with hydronephrosis due to an obstruction of the urine flow exceeding the drainage capacity. This is usually a chronic, partial obstruction located between the kidney and the bladder, causing renal functional impairment and a progressive deterioration of the kidney. In very small children, the obstruction may limit the proper development of the kidney. This investigation enables us to ascertain the variable changes in the intensity of the signal within the renal parenchyma after administering a contrast agent, and thus evaluate the changes in the nephrograms produced by perfusion, filtration, and concentration of the contrast medium. The information that we obtain is consequently both anatomic and functional, enabling us to select patients likely to benefit from surgery [13].

Anterograde pyelography: This involves the percutaneous translumbar placement of a needle or catheter, under ultrasound guidance, directly in the calyceal structures of the kidney to obtain their opacification with an iodized contrast medium to view the renal pelvis and corresponding ureter, and thus identify the site and nature of an obstruction. This test is indicated when the anatomy of the upper urinary tract needs to be assessed but excretory urography or retrograde pyelography cannot be used. In addition to diagnosing the site of an obstruction, anterograde pyelography enables us to measure the pressure and thereby distinguish a genuine obstruction from persistent hydronephrosis involving no obstruction. The diagnostic procedure may also prove to be therapeutic, since it enables a catheter to be inserted upstream from the obstruction to drain urine to the outside and reduce the hydronephrosis, while providing information on the feasibility of a functional recovery after any surgical removal of the same obstruction.

Retrograde or ascending pyelography: This enables a definitive assessment of the collector system and ureters. It is useful in characterizing a lesion dealing with an obstruction, and determining whether the dilation observable is due to an obstruction, but it is not used routinely because it facilitates the diffusion of infections. It is conducted under cystoscopic control, positioning the catheter in the ureter. A contrast medium injected directly into the bladder through the catheter identifies the ureter, the renal pelvis, and the calyces, but not the parenchyma. Its use is limited to urologic diagnoses, and particularly to assess the length of an obstruction and the ureter distal to the obstruction.

Cysto-urethrography: This is done as part of a retrograde cystography or excretory urography, to assess the posterior urethral valves in male children, or any narrowing of the posterior and anterior urethra, in both children and adults.

2.5.8 Renal Function After the Removal of an Obstruction

Once an obstruction has been removed, if it has been transient, then the related structural changes can regress and the tubular epithelium is regenerated. The blood flow in the kidney increases immediately, while the glomerular filtrate recovers more slower. If the occlusion was bilateral, a major diuresis and natriuresis follows on the removal of the obstruction, and this may have various causes:

- A physiologic response to the previous sodium and water retention giving rise to an increased sodium pool and expansion of the volumes
- Osmotic diuresis due to the retention of urea and other metabolites
- Loss of the medullary concentration gradient due to back-diffusion of the urea from the interstitial fluid to the vasa recta
- An intrinsic renal tubule cell function defect, which would make the cells incapable of exploiting a normal concentration gradient
- The inability to acidify the urine, with a severe loss of bicarbonate

The renal tubules' failure to respond to vasopressin points to a genuine picture of nephrogenic diabetes insipidus, with hydrosodic depletion and metabolic acidosis. Postobstructive diuresis is more limited after a unilateral ureteral obstruction has been removed. If the obstruction has been short lived, then the drop in glomerular filtrate is rapidly and completely reversible, because the alteration has been merely functional in nature, with no loss of nephrons.

2.5.9 Treatment

It is always important to remove an obstruction in order to preserve renal function and prevent complications, one of the most important of which is infection. The appropriate management for obstructive nephropathy depends on the assessment of the severity of renal damage and the potential recovery of renal function if the obstruction is relieved. In the majority of cases, urinary tract obstructions need surgical treatment, so early urologic consultation is a must.

2.5.9.1 *Surgical and Instrumental Treatment*

Surgery, using the various techniques available, is specific for each type of obstructive disease. It is undeniably important to remove the obstruction and facilitate urine flow as soon as possible.

For the most common forms of obstructive uropathy, extracorporeal shock lithotripsy has practically revolutionized the surgical treatment of renal stones. In the case of acute obstructions due to prostatic hypertrophy, drainage with Foley catheters is usually effective, followed several weeks later by prostatic resection. For ureteral obstructions, cystoscopy and the placement of drainage catheters may suffice to enable the passage of the causes of the obstruction; failing this, surgery may be needed.

Percutaneous nephrostomy consists in the ultrasound-guided positioning of a catheter in the renal pelvis to drain the obstructed kidney. The gauge of the catheter used may vary, and it can be kept in place for more or less long periods of time. It also enables the urine and any drained material to be examined for diagnostic purposes and, if necessary, antibiotics can be injected directly into the infected kidney.

The use of short-term nephrostomy tube drainage with evaluation of creatinine clearance is the best predictor of recovery of renal function after release of the homolateral obstruction.

2.5.9.2 Medical Treatment

Basically, this means antiinflammatory, antibiotic, and pain-killing medication. Postobstructive diuresis replacement therapy is important, first intravenously and then orally, strictly monitoring electrolytes and acid–alkaline balance as well as diuresis, body weight, and blood pressure.

2.5.9.3 Conclusions

Urinary tract obstruction is a common major cause of acute and chronic renal insufficiency. Obstructive uropathy is a condition common to all age groups, even very early and late in life. Regardless of the age of obstruction, the renal response involves progressive tubular dilation, tubular atrophy, and interstitial fibrosis. Although urinary tract obstructions can develop entirely asymptomatically, especially in chronic cases and in pediatric ages, it is more common for an obstruction to cause more or less evident signs and symptoms, particularly because most cases of obstructive uropathy that become clinically manifest are caused by a partial rather than a total obstruction of the urinary tract. In patients presenting with acute or chronic renal problems, it is always important to confirm or exclude an obstructive uropathy, given the frequency of this condition and because it is the most common cause of reversible renal insufficiency. It is always important to remove an obstruction in order to preserve renal function and prevent complications, one of the most important of which is infection.

References

1. R.L. Chevalier: Pathogenesis of renal injury in obstructive uropathy. Curr Opin Pediatr 2006; 18: 153–160
2. H. Liapis: Biology of congenital obstructive nephropathy. Nephron Exp Nephrol 2003; 93: 87–91
3. S. Khlar: Obstructive nephropathy. Internal Med 2000; 39: 355–361.
4. T.S. Pedersen, J.J. Hvistendahl, J.C. Djurhuus, J. Frokiaer: Renal water and sodium handling during gradated unilateral ureter obstruction. Scand J Urol Nephrol 2002; 36: 163–172.
5. R.L. Chevalier: Obstructive nephropathy: towards biomarker discovery and gene therapy. Nature Clin Pract Nephrol 2006; 2: 157–168.
6. J. Frokiaer, T.M. Jorgensen, J.C. Djurhuus: Obstructive nephropathy: an update of the experimental research. Urol Res 1999; 27: 29–39
7. D. Del Prete, F. Anglani, R. Dall'Amico, M. Forino, E. Pagetta, G. Gambaro, G. Zacchello, L. Murer: Intrarenal mRNA expression of angiotensinogen, TGFbeta1 and alfaSMA in different human nephropathies. JASN 1997; 8: 534A
8. S. Klahr, J. Morrissey: Obstructed nephropathy and renal fibrosis. Am J Physiol Renal Physiol 2002; 283: F861–F875
9. S. Klahr: Urinary tract obstruction. Semin Nephrol 2001; 21: 133–145
10. D. Del Prete, A. D'Angelo: Acute obstructive nephropathy. In Critical Care Nephrology Ed. Ronco, Bellomo, Kellum 2008; 65: 358–362
11. S. Elwagdy, S. Ghoneim, S. Moussa, I. Ewis: Three-dimensional ultrasound (3D US) methods in the evaluation of calcular and non-calcular ureteric obstructive uropathy. World J Urol 2008; 26: 263–274
12. J.K. Kim, K.S Cho: CT urography and virtual endoscopy: promising imaging modalities for urinary tract evaluation. Brit J of Radiol 2003; 76: 199–209
13. J.D. Grattan-Smith, S.B. Little, R.A. Jones: MR urography evaluation of obstructive uropathy. Pediatr Radiol 2008; 38(Suppl 1): 49–69

Epidemiology of Acute Kidney Injury

2.6

Tariq Ali and Paul Roderick

Core Messages

- Epidemiologic studies of acute kidney injury (AKI) are bedevilled by differences in definition, which make incidence, prevalence and particularly outcomes difficult to compare.
- The incidence of AKI varies from one study to another, but most studies have shown that incidence is much higher among the elderly.
- The incidence of AKI requiring renal replacement therapy (RRT) has increased over time. Despite advances in medical management, mortality in AKI remains very high even in the milder forms of this condition.
- AKI is associated with prolonged hospital admission resulting in significant burden on health care resources. It is, therefore, important to recognise patients at risk and try to prevent the development of this condition.

2.6.1 History

In the Egyptian medicine, urine was thought to be formed in the bladder [61] but in the Roman period it was established that urine forms in the kidneys [22]. In the seventeenth century the term 'ischuria' was introduced to indicate suppression or retention of urine [22] and in the nineteenth century, this disease was described in more detail; patients presenting with a history of sudden decline in urine output followed by confusion, coma and death. It was named Bright's disease after Richard Bright who later published his work on end-stage kidney disease [22]. In 1916, Frankenthal described traumatic muscle destruction and kidney failure resulting from war injuries [8, 24], and 126 cases were cited in the official German handbook on World War I [15]. This report was neglected and no lessons were learnt from these casualties; none of the British or American surgery books published between 1918 and 1941 mentioned this condition and hence medical authorities were not prepared to deal with this fatal condition at the time of World War II.

In 1941, four cases of crush injury were described; they presented with muscle injuries during the London blitz. They all died within a week due to 'nitrogen retention', and necropsy revealed severe degenerative changes in renal tubules and pigment deposition in the nephrons [16, 17]. These pigments were attributed to the leakage of haemoglobin, myohaemoglobin or bile pigments into the tubular lumen. Similar changes were described following mismatched blood transfusion [5, 14, 26, 71] and in eclampsia [4]. The proposed treatments for this condition were to restore urinary output by means of heat to the loins, by increasing blood volume with serum and hence blood pressure, and by the use of diuretics such as caffeine.

In 1948 Bull et al. classified uraemia into two types: 'non-oliguric uraemia' in which patients would continue to pass urine and 'anuric uraemia' in which there was a little or no urine output [13]. They proposed treatment in the form of nasogastric feeding with a mixture of glucose, peanut oil and acacia, and if the patient vomited, it was filtered and returned to stomach through the tube to ensure the mixture was not lost

T. Ali (✉)
Kent and Canterbury Hospital, Ethelbert Road, Canterbury, Kent CT1 3NG, UK
e-mail: tariq.ali@nhs.net

A. Jörres et al. (eds.), *Management of Acute Kidney Problems*,
DOI: 10.1007/978-3-540-69441-0_2.6, © Springer-Verlag Berlin Heidelberg 2010

with vomit. This regimen was claimed to be effective. In 1951 the term acute renal failure (ARF) was described for the first time, in a publication by Oliver and his associates [55].

In 1960, ARF was further classified into two main types: 'extrinsic renal failure' occurring as a result of prerenal and postrenal causes and 'intrinsic renal failure' due to damage to the renal substance [63]. The terminology of prerenal, renal and postrenal is still used, though not the term extrinsic renal failure.

More recently, the term 'acute-on-chronic renal failure' has been introduced to describe ARF in those with preexisting chronic kidney disease (CKD) [40]. The most recent advance in terminology has been the term 'acute kidney injury' (AKI) which builds on the RIFLE classification and recognises the poorer prognosis of milder degrees of ARF [3, 20, 41]. AKI captures the full range of kidney injury: ARF is used mainly for patients admitted to intensive care units (ICUs) with severe kidney injury needing dialysis, while AKI is used for acute renal failure where dialysis is not required [69]. We shall refer to AKI in the remainder of this chapter for consistency.

In 1914, dialysis was performed on animals [1]. The blood was passed through a system of tubes, anticoagulated with hirudin and subsequently transfused back to animals. In 1924 and 1928 further experiments were carried out and vividialysis was performed in humans [18, 37, 45]. The development of an effective haemodialysis machine was first reported by Kolff et al. in 1943, and the use of an artificial kidney as treatment for AKI was described in an article published in 1944 [37]. This machine was known as a rotating drum kidney. The first patient was dialysed in 1943, and subsequently 15 patients were dialysed in the following year but only one survived [38]. However, with significant technical advances, patients were better dialysed in the 1950s and onwards [38]. Mortality in patients with AKI treated with dialysis was reduced from more than 90% to 50% in 1955 [65].

2.6.2 Incidence

Epidemiologic studies of AKI are bedevilled by differences in definition, which makes incidence, prevalence, and particularly outcomes difficult to compare. There are more than 30 definitions in the literature; hence there is no standard on which incidence can be compared over time or between populations. The definitions may vary by, for example, level of serum creatinine, whether patients are only treated with renal replacement therapy (RRT) or not, and whether patients with acute on chronic renal failure are included. Moreover, studies vary by country, time, method and completeness of ascertainment (e.g. routine biochemistry or diagnosis coding) and whether incidence rates are adjusted for population demographics. Consequently, there is large heterogeneity in incidence and outcomes.

Waikar identified patients by using International Classification of Diseases, 9th Revision, Clinical Modification (ICD-9-CM) codes [70], while Liano included those patients with AKI in whom serum creatinine rose to 177 μmol/l [44]. In a recent retrospective study, the inclusion criterion was serum creatinine of 150 μmol/l in males and 130 μmol/l in female patients [3]. Feest only included those with a serum creatinine of >500 μmol/l [23] and in a Scottish study, the incidence was reported for those patients in whom serum creatinine rose to 300 μmol/l [35]. Some studies have excluded elderly patients [35], while others have included only those who were treated in ICUs [6, 19, 30]. In a prospective population-based study, only those patients were included who required RRT [52], and Liano included only those patients who were admitted to tertiary hospitals [44].

AKI in those with chronic kidney disease poses further problems; some authors would include these patients as having AKI, others would exclude them and some may include them in the category of acute on chronic renal failure [23, 35]. Not surprisingly, using different definitions and including different groups, reported incidence varies from one study to another (Table 2.6.1).

2.6.2.1 Low Threshold Studies

There are very few population-based studies which have reported the incidence of 'early' AKI. A prospective multicentre, community-based study in the Madrid area included all those patients in whom serum creatinine had risen to 177 μmol/l [44]. Of the 788 cases of AKI studied, 665 episodes presented from the Madrid area giving an annual incidence of 209 cases per

Table 2.6.1 Studies of the incidence of acute kidney injury (AKI)

Author	Year	Population (million)	Country	Inclusion	Period	Incidence (pmp[a])
Low threshold studies						
Liano [44]	1996	4.2	Spain	Creatinine >177	9 months	209
Waikar [70]	2006	–	USA	ICD-9-CM codes	15 years	2,880
Ali [3]	2007	0.5	Scotland	Creatinine 150 (male), 130 (female) ACRF[b]	6 months	2,147
High threshold studies						
Feest [23]	1993	0.4	England	Creatinine >500 ACRF[b]	2 years	140
Khan [34]	1997	0.5	Scotland	Creatinine ≥300	12 months	620
Stevens [66]	2001	0.6	England	Creatinine >300 Urea >40	12 months	486
AKI requiring RRT[c]						
Metcalfe [52]	2002	1.1	Scotland	RRT dependence	11 weeks	203
Waikar [70]	2006	–	USA	ICD-9-CM codes	15 years	270
Prescott [58]	2007	5.1	Scotland	RRT dependence ACRF[b]	36 weeks	286

Serum creatinine and blood urea values are in µmol/l
[a]Per million population
[b]Acute-on-chronic renal failure
[c]Renal replacement therapy

million population (pmp). This study, however, included only those patients who were admitted to 13 tertiary-care centres, so it could be an underestimate of the true incidence.

Two recent studies have shown that the incidence of AKI is as high as >2,000 pmp [3, 70]. In the first study, the incidence of AKI was studied in hospitalised patients between 1988 and 2002 using the Nationwide Inpatient Sample (NIS), of those discharged from acute care [70]. The NIS is the largest administrative database of hospitalisation in the United States. Patients were identified by ICD-9-CM codes. Quan et al. found that ICD-9-CM codes for both acute and chronic renal failure were 42% sensitive and 99% specific [59]. They found that percentage of annual discharges with AKI increased from 0.4% in 1988 to 2.1% in 2002. The US population age- and sex-adjusted incidence increased from 610 pmp in 1988 to 2,880 pmp in 2002, with the incidence of AKI requiring dialysis being 270 pmp in 2002. The major limitations in this study were the absence of laboratory and clinical data, and the reliance on ICD codes, which underestimate the frequency of AKI. It was also noted that there was an increase in sensitivity of the ICD codes for AKI between 1994 and 2002 suggesting that coding practice for AKI had increased. Possible reasons for increased AKI coding over time include increasing awareness of mild AKI, reimbursement incentives [31] and increasing number of available fields for diagnoses codes [32]. These may have resulted in increased identification of AKI though there was still underascertainment.

In a population-based study in Grampian Scotland carried out by the author, the incidence of acute and acute on chronic renal failure was also higher [3]. AKI was defined as a rise of serum creatinine to at least 150 µmol/l in male and 130 µmol/l in female patients using RIFLE criteria [3]. AKI developed in 474 patients (annual incidence of 1,811 pmp), and AKI in those with underlying chronic kidney disease was reported in 88 patients (336 pmp). These rates are high because of the low threshold for inclusion and complete ascertainment using a biochemistry laboratory serving a defined population. On the other hand, it is still an underestimate as those patients in whom serum creatinine had not risen to threshold value (150/130 µmol/l) could still have AKI but were not captured. The later two studies confirm that incidence of AKI is indeed very high, if all patients are included. This incidence is still an underestimate, as milder forms of AKI go unnoticed, and many episodes occur in the community.

2.6.2.2 High Threshold Studies

Two population-based UK studies ascertained more severe AKI. Feest et al. found an incidence of 140 pmp for patients whose serum creatinine concentration rose to >500 μmol/l [23]. Khan et al. used a cutoff of 300 μmol/l [36] and found an annual incidence of 620 pmp, in comparison to Feest they found the incidence of severe AKI (rise of serum creatinine > 500 μmol/l) was 102 pmp. Feest showed a strong age-related gradient in AKI. Overall annual incidence was 140 pmp, increasing with age from 17 cases pmp in adults under 50 years of age to 949 cases pmp in the 80–89-year age group. In another prospective UK-based study, Stevens et al found an incidence of 545 pmp in patients whose creatinine rose to 300 μmol/l [66]. They also found that incidence of AKI increased with increasing age, 68% patients were aged 70 or above.

2.6.2.3 AKI Requiring Renal Replacement Therapy

The incidence of AKI (and acute-on-chronic renal failure) requiring RRT is reported to be 203 pmp/year in a population base of over one million [53]. They found that at least one third of these patients had preexisting CKD. Khan et al. has found an annual incidence of AKI requiring RRT of 55 pmp [35]. Waikar et al., 270 pmp [70], and Prescott et al., 268 pmp [58]. Waikar et al. found that the crude incidence of AKI requiring RRT increased from 40 pmp in 1988 to 270 pmp in 2002. Similarly UK-based studies have shown the rise of incidence from 55 pmp in 1993 [35] to 81 pmp in 1997 [66] to >200 pmp in two recent studies [52, 58]. These studies suggest that incidence of AKI requiring RRT has risen over time; whether there is a true rise in the incidence, or whether more patients are being accepted for RRT is not yet clear.

In conclusion, the incidence of mild AKI is high and greater than previously reported, and the number and rate of patients accepted for RRT has gradually risen. It is very difficult to compare the true variation in AKI incidence between different areas or over time because of different definitions, methods of ascertainment and population differences.

2.6.2.4 Age- and Sex-Related Incidence

The population of Western developed countries is ageing due to the increase in life expectancy as a result of improvements in public health and medical and health care advances. In particular, more people are surviving significant illnesses but then live with chronic conditions and associated comorbidity.

In the healthy population, the ageing kidney is associated with important structural and functional changes [57]. In the elderly population, the renal substance is on average reduced by 30% [46, 47, 67], and there is significant reduction in the number of glomeruli [25, 33, 49]. The glomerular filtration rate (GFR) progressively declines with age [27, 48]. Despite all these changes, the ageing kidney is capable of maintaining fluid and electrolyte balance, but its adaptive capacity is restricted during illness, volume changes and in response to exposure to nephrotoxins [57]. CKD is also commoner in the elderly population, and a recent study has shown that the prevalence of CKD was 56% for estimated GFR < 60 [60]. These elderly patients have increased vascular risk and increased comorbidity; they are at greater risk of intercurrent illnesses and are more prone to have various medical or surgical procedures performed. For these reasons, it is not surprising that the incidence of AKI is much higher in the elderly.

The reported median or mean ages of those with AKI vary considerably in the literature, though in most studies mean age is >60 years and males predominate.

The mean age in Liano and Pascual's study [44] was 64; this study included those patients admitted to tertiary-care hospitals in whom serum creatinine rose to at least 177 μmol/l. Liano and Pascual also concluded that 48% of AKI cases occurred in patients over 64 years, whereas these age ranges only represent 16% of the Madrid population. The majority of patients (65%) were male, and mean age was similar in both sexes. It was one of the earlier studies which showed increased frequency in male patients. They did further analysis of their data to see whether hormonal status played a role. Patients were divided into a younger group (up to 45 years of age) and older group (>45 years). The rate of female patients was similar in both groups, and they concluded that hormonal status does not seem to play a role in the development of AKI. It is difficult to be certain, but vascular causes could be related to high frequency in males.

In a UK-based study in which patients were included only if serum creatinine rose to 300 μmol/l, the mean age was 73 years and 64% were male [66]. Two thirds of patients were aged 70 years or over. In an American ICU-based study [68] conducted at 54 ICUs and including 29,269 critically ill patients, 1,738 patients had AKI. The mean age was 67 years and 64% were male.

Another study from the United States reported a median age of 72 years in patients identified between 1988 and 2002 [70], and the median age of patients was relatively constant during this period; 54% patients were male. Another study showed a higher mean age of 76 years [73]; just over 50% patients were male.

In a study of those patients with AKI who required RRT, the median age was reported to be 66 and 75 years in those with AKI and acute-on-chronic renal failure, respectively [53]. The majority of patients (65%) were male. Thus the majority of patients with AKI are elderly, and their incidence is likely to continue to rise in keeping with the projected demographic changes in the Western world. Most of the studies have shown that this condition is more frequent in the male population, perhaps due to increased occurrence of vascular disease, obstructive uropathy and underlying CKD.

2.6.3 Outcomes

2.6.3.1 Mortality

It is difficult to determine true mortality rates from the literature; there are several factors which could potentially introduce bias, including differences in definition, methods used in individual studies, inclusion criteria, severity of AKI, location of management (whether in the critical areas or elsewhere), duration of follow-up, time period of study and whether acute-on-chronic renal failure is included. Before the era of haemodialysis, AKI was universally fatal and mortality was >90% [14, 37]. However, improvement in mortality to 50% was reported in the 1950s with advances in the technical ability to dialyse patients with AKI [38, 65]. Since then, despite further advances in medical techniques, mortality in patients with AKI remains high (Table 2.6.2). Depending on the study characteristics, mortality has been reported anywhere between 20% and 80% for all severities of AKI [39, 44, 50, 52, 54, 62]. In a systematic review of 80 studies, it was concluded that mortality rates seem to have remained unchanged at around 50% [74].

Previously patients died of the complications of AKI, mainly fluid overload and hyperkalemia, but now mortality is due to underlying causes or may be due to AKI itself. Although mortality in AKI has traditionally been attributed to the severity of the underlying condition [10], Levy et al. tried to prove otherwise [42]. They identified 183 patients who developed AKI after radiocontrast procedure and paired them with an equal number of patients who did not develop AKI matched for age and baseline serum creatinine. Mortality in those without AKI was 7% compared with 34% in those with

Table 2.6.2 Mortality in acute kidney injury (AKI)

Author	Settings (year)	AKI definition	No. of patients	Mortality (%)
Feest [23]	Population based (1993)	Creatinine > 500	125	46[a] 58[b]
Brivet [12]	ICU (1996)	Creatinine ≥ 310, BUN ≥ 36	360	58[c]
Bhandari [9]	Consecutive cases of AKI between 1984 and 1995 (1996)	Creatinine ≥ 600	1,095	41[a]
Liano [44]	AKI patients admitted to tertiary units (1996)	Creatinine > 177	748	45[c]
Levy [42]	Contrast-related AKI (1996)	Creatinine > 177	174	34[c]
Stevens [66]	Population based (2001)	Creatinine > 300, BUN > 40	288	44[c] 65[d] 69[b]
Metcalfe [52]	Population based (2002)	RRT requirement	48	74[c]
Bell [6]	Retrospective ICU based (2004)	RRT requirement	207	35[e] 50[c]
Mehta [51]	Multi-centre ICU based (2004)	RRT requirement	618	37[c]
Uchino [68]	Prospective ICU based (2005)	Oliguria, BUN > 30	1,738	60[c]
Ostermann	Retrospective ICU based (2007)	RIFLE criteria	15,019	28[e] 36[c]

Serum creatinine and BUN values are in µmol/l
BUN blood urea nitrogen
[a]90-Day mortality
[b]2-Year mortality
[c]In-hospital mortality
[d]1-Year mortality
[e]ICU mortality

AKI. After adjustment for comorbidity, AKI was associated with an odd ratio risk of dying of 5.5. They concluded that high mortality in AKI was not explained by the underlying condition alone. This is in keeping with the results of some other studies [21, 64].

2.6.3.2 Mortality in All Forms of AKI

Liano et al. found mortality rates of 45% in the Madrid study, corrected mortality attributed to AKI itself was only 26% [44]. They found that the most frequent causes of death were shock, infection, cardiorespiratory diseases and stroke.

The hospital mortality rates of patients with AKI identified by ICD-9-CM codes was 21% in a US-based study [43]. This mortality rate was observed not only in tertiary-care hospitals but throughout the entire spectrum of acute care hospitals in the United States. The data also supported an independent impact of AKI on mortality after adjustment for comorbid conditions.

In a population-based study, Stevens et al. reported mortality of 44% in those patients with AKI whose serum creatinine rose to 300 μmol/l [66]. Survival to discharge was higher in those aged < 70 years (65%) compared with those aged 70 and above. During the follow-up period, overall survival had fallen to 47% at 3 months, 35% at 12 months and 31% at 24 months. This suggested that AKI was not only related to mortality during the in-patient episode, but this effect persisted over the long term. The author did not conclude whether this was purely because of AKI or other factors could have played a role.

In a study of more severe AKI (serum creatinine of > 500 μmol/l) Feest et al. quoted a mortality rate of 46% [23]. They found that survival at 3 months or 2 years was not significantly related to age. This was, however, a small study of only 125 patients with severe AKI.

Chertow et al. linked changes in serum creatinine with in-patient mortality, length of stay (LOS) and costs [20]. They found that modest changes in serum creatinine were significantly associated with mortality; increase in serum creatinine > 0.5 mg/dl was associated with 6.5-fold increase in odds of death. This association remained significant even after adjustment for age, sex, severity of illness, admission ICD coding and underlying CKD. On further analysis, it was found that even a very small increase in serum creatinine (0.3–0.4 mg/dl) was significantly associated with mortality.

In a prospective study of >4,000 patients who underwent cardiac and thoracic aortic surgery, the effect of changes in serum creatinine within 48 h of surgery on 30-day mortality was analysed [41]. The mortality was adjusted for various established demographic risk indicators, intraoperative parameters and postoperative complications. In 200 patients, serum creatinine had risen to >0.5 mg/dl, and among those patients, mortality was 32% in comparison to mortality of 6% in patients in whom serum creatinine remained unchanged or increased to <0.5 mg/dl.

2.6.3.3 Mortality in RRT-Dependent AKI

Mortality in those patients with AKI needing RRT was reported to be 74% in a population-based study [52]; 24% of those patients died within 48 h, and median survival was only 8 days. The mortality of patients was 83% in those who started RRT in an ICU. In another study just over half of the patients with AKI who required RRT survived at 90 days [58]. Prescott et al. found that mortality was associated with increasing age, having first dialysis in ICU and sepsis.

In Liano's study, mortality among dialysed patients was significantly higher than that of nondialysed patients (66% vs. 33%) [44]. Waikar et al. claimed that mortality in AKI declined during 1988 to 2002 [70], and they found mortality of 40% in 1988 and 20% in 2002 across all severities of AKI. They admit that it could be explained in part by changes in coding practice, with less severe cases of AKI being recognised and coded in more recent years. In-hospital mortality was higher (28%) among those patients who required RRT. Other studies have also confirmed that mortality is higher in those patients who require RRT for AKI [11, 51].

2.6.3.4 Mortality of AKI in Intensive Care Units

Several studies have shown higher mortality in AKI patients treated in ICU settings. The argument might be that these patients are usually very ill and have poor prognosis for a variety of reasons including multiorgan failure, shock and severe septicaemia.

The PICARD study included all patients consulted for AKI in the ICU of five academic centres in the United States [51]. Among the 618 patients enrolled, 231 (37%) died during their hospital admission. The 28-day mortality was 22% and ICU mortality was 32%. The mortality was higher among those who required RRT, but there was no relationship between aetiology of AKI and in-hospital mortality. Mortality rates were related to severity of external diseases, exceeding 50% with four or more failed organ systems.

In a prospective muticentre study of 20 French ICUs, 360 patients with AKI were identified (7% of the ICU admissions) [11]. During their hospital stay, 58% patients had died and the majority of deaths occurred in the ICU (50%). Hospital mortality was linked to age, sex (higher mortality in male patients), preadmission health status, sepsis and delayed occurrence of AKI. Mortality was also higher in those who required RRT (64%).

In a prospective study, patients with AKI were enrolled from 23 countries [68]. They were treated in the ICU for various conditions, and AKI was recorded in 6% of the ICU admissions. Overall hospital mortality in patients with AKI was 60%, and 52% deaths occurred in the ICU. Independent risk factors for hospital mortality included use of vasopressors, mechanical ventilation, shock and hepatorenal syndrome.

2.6.3.5 Association of Mortality and RIFLE Classification

The concept of the RIFLE classification was not only to standardise the definition of AKI but a classification which could predict relevant clinical outcomes such as mortality and length of hospital stay [7]. It is probably too early to comment on the RIFLE classification's ability to predict outcomes, but a few studies have used this tool with variable results.

The RIFLE classification was applied to 183 patients with AKI admitted to the ICU of a UK hospital [2]. Patients were assigned to RIFLE categories and compared with a control group who were admitted to the ICU but did not fulfil RIFLE criteria. ICU mortality was 38% in the RIFLE class R (Risk) group, 50% in the class I (Injury) group and 74% in the class F (Failure) group. Similarly, requirement for RRT was highest in the class F group.

Hoste et al. carried out a retrospective study in seven ICUs and found that AKI occurred in 67% of ICU admissions [29]. They found that patients in the R class were at high risk of progression to class I or class F. Patients with RIFLE class I and class F had significantly longer hospital stay and higher mortality compared with those who were in class R or those who never developed AKI. The RIFLE classification was able to predict outcomes even after adjusting for baseline severity of illness, case mix, age and sex.

In a retrospective study carried out by the author, the RIFLE classification was applied to all patients with AKI in a defined population [3]. It was useful for predicting full recovery of renal function, RRT requirement, length of hospital stay and in-hospital mortality. However, the RIFLE classification did not predict mortality at 90 days or 6 months.

One of the biggest studies to evaluate RIFLE classification was carried out by compiling a database of patients admitted to 22 ICUs in the United Kingdom and Germany between 1989 and 1999 [56]. They found that any degree of AKI was associated with a significantly increased mortality compared with not having AKI. Without controlling for any other risk factors, mortality increased with severity of the RIFLE classification. The length of stay was shortest among patients without AKI and increased with increasing severity of the RIFLE classification. However, they also found that in all RIFLE categories, hospital mortality increased as the maximum number of associated failed organ systems increased. They concluded that the RIFLE classification provides useful criteria that correlate with outcomes, but other factors had a greater impact on prognosis than severity of AKI.

In summary, mortality from AKI remains very high, and at present there is no strong evidence to suggest that mortality has decreased in past few decades. Survival is poor across all severities of AKI, and some studies have shown than even a minor change in kidney function is associated with poor outcome. The mortality is particularly higher in patients who require RRT and/or need ICU admission. There is conflicting evidence whether other factors play a role in poor outcomes or whether AKI is independently associated with increased mortality, but evidence suggests that both factors play an important role in survival. The RIFLE classification appears to be a good tool in predicting outcomes but needs further research to confirm its usefulness.

2.6.3.6 Recovery of Renal Function

Recovery of renal function in AKI has not been as extensively studied as mortality. There is no universal definition of renal recovery: in some studies recovery is defined as independence from dialysis, while others have defined it as recovery of renal function to baseline. In the latter studies, serum creatinine is used as a marker of recovery. Again, recovery from AKI can only be evaluated in the context of a specific definition of AKI. The RIFLE group proposed that recovery may be partial or complete. Complete renal recovery is defined as return of renal function to baseline classification within the RIFLE criteria, whereas partial renal recovery occurs if there is a persistent change in RIFLE classification (class R, I or F) but not persistent need for RRT [7].

Feest et al. examined recovery of renal function in patients who survived more than 3 months [23]. Recovery was defined as a fall of serum creatinine value to normal (<110 µmol/l). In 36% of the survivors, serum creatinine had fallen below normal, and in 20% patients serum creatinine did not return to below 300 µmol/l. However, they did not mention baseline renal function, and patients with acute-on-chronic renal failure could have been included.

In a UK-based study, overall survival in 1,095 patients with severe AKI (serum creatinine >600 µmol/l) was 59%. Of these 16% remained on long-term dialysis [9]. Although patients with known CKD were excluded, it is unclear what proportion of those had normal kidney function before this episode and it is possible that some of them actually had acute-on-chronic renal failure.

In the French study, the mortality was 58%, and among the survivors, mean serum creatinine was 233 µmol/l at the time of discharge from ICU [12]. At 6-month follow-up, data were available for only 21% of patients because of deaths and some patients being lost to follow-up. The mean serum creatinine in patients who attended for follow-up was 124 µmol/l, and in the majority (75%), serum creatinine was <150 µmol/l.

In an ICU-based study, the RIFLE classification was used to predict outcomes [2]. At 1-month follow-up, the mean serum creatinine was 159 µmol/l, and mean serum creatinine was still high at 133 µmol/l at the 6-month follow-up. However, persistent renal impairment was similar in all categories of RIFLE classification.

A population-based study of AKI requiring RRT showed that at 90 days some 74% patients had died, only one patient was still on dialysis and the rest had sufficiently recovered to be independent of RRT [52]. In contrast, among those who had acute-on-chronic renal failure, 17% were dialysis dependent at 90 days. In another population-based study, 13% of survivors were dialysis dependent at 90 days [58]. However, 32% of these patients did not have previous creatinine values recorded, so a degree of preexisting CKD could not be excluded. A much higher proportion of patients in the acute-on-chronic renal failure group were still dialysis dependent at 90 days (53%).

Hoste et al. studied the effect of sepsis on the outcomes of AKI in an ICU-based study [28]. They included all patients with AKI who required RRT and found that hospital mortality was around 70%. Among the survivors, 9% without sepsis and 43% with sepsis were still on RRT for more than 30 days, and after 3 months, 0.5% and 8% were receiving RRT, respectively.

In another ICU-based study, Bell et al. identified 207 patients with AKI and applied the RIFLE classification [6]. They found a mortality rate of 50% during the hospital stay, and only 2% of the total 207 patients developed end-stage renal disease.

Long-term data on recovery of renal function is lacking in the literature, but it is evident that the majority of patient who survive recover renal functions sufficiently to be independent of dialysis. Although the general perception is that the majority of patients who survive the acute insult recover normal renal function, there is not sufficient evidence to support this notion. It may be that AKI, some of which could be subclinical or involve patients not admitted to hospital, remains unrecognised. It is possible that repeated episodes of mild AKI lead to eventual poor kidney function in elderly patients.

2.6.3.7 Length of Stay and Costs

AKI has been reported to be present in anywhere between 1% and 25% of hospitalised patients. The effects of AKI on hospital length of stay (LOS) and costs are not very well established [20]. Waikar et al. claimed that median LOS has declined over time in patients with AKI, from 10 days in 1988, to 7 days in 2002 [70]. Among patients who required RRT, median LOS was 14 days in 1988 and 12 days in 2002. However, they admit that there was increased recognition of AKI over time, and more people with mild AKI were coded for this condition in 2002 than in 1988.

This could have resulted in shorter LOS in those with mild AKI. In an ICU-based study of AKI in 23 countries, it was reported that median LOS in the ICU was 10 days and hospital stay was 22 days [68].

Chertow et al. reported on the effect of AKI on mortality, LOS and costs in hospitalised patients [20]. They found that AKI was consistently associated with an independent increase in LOS. Larger increases in serum creatinine were associated with increase in LOS. This effect was more marked when patients who died during hospital stay were excluded. Similarly AKI was associated with a rise in hospital costs: for example, a rise in serum creatinine by 0.3 mg/dl was associated with a mean adjusted increase in total cost of US $4,886, and a rise in serum creatinine by 2 mg/dl was associated with an increase in total cost of US $22,023. They estimated that if 5% of hospitalised patients were to develop AKI and taking into consideration an average cost 20% below those observed in this study, then the estimated annual health care cost of hospital-acquired AKI would exceed US $10 billion.

In another study, presence of discharge diagnosis of AKI was associated with prolonged hospital LOS [43]. This study also demonstrated an association between AKI diagnosis and discharge to short- and long-term facilities. The authors concluded that AKI independently affects recovery of physical function after an acute illness, and consequently AKI may be associated with a substantial cost burden on the health care system that persists even after discharge.

The burden of AKI was studied among nonrenal solid organ recipients [72]. The impact of AKI on LOS and costs was adjusted for age, sex, type of transplant and death. The development of AKI was associated with a significantly increased LOS and higher total costs whether or not RRT was required. LOS was increased by 3 weeks and charges were increased by more than US $115,000 among patients who required RRT.

Although there is limited research done in this area, AKI seems to be associated with a significant burden on health care resources. Some of the studies have shown that the outcomes are directly related to the severity of AKI, and even milder forms of AKI may have an adverse effect on outcomes including mortality, LOS and costs. Usually, AKI requiring RRT is the more obvious factor from a public health perspective, but less severe forms of AKI also pose a significant burden on health resources. This is one of the reasons that prevention of AKI should always be considered in hospitalised patients in terms of fluid management, judicious use of antibiotics and care in using nephrotoxic agents.

2.6.4 Summary

1. The incidence of AKI is very high, and incidence of AKI requiring RRT has increased over time.
2. Although AKI occurs in all ages, the majority of patients who develop this condition are elderly with significant comorbidity.
3. There is increased incidence of AKI in male patients possibly because of vascular disease, obstructive uropathy and underlying CKD.
4. Mortality remains very high despite advances in medical management. The only treatment that improved mortality was introduction of dialysis in the 1940s, and since then there has been hardly any improvement in survival. It is possible that any improvement in mortality is masked by the fact that more people with significant comorbid conditions and severe acute illnesses are now actively managed then in the past.
5. If patients survive acute illness, the majority would have sufficient renal recovery to be independent of dialysis. The long-term effects of a single episode of AKI are unclear, and there is no data on recurrent AKI and its impact on long-term morbidity and mortality.
6. AKI is associated with increased length of hospital stay and poses a significant burden on health care resources.

References

1. Abel JJ, Rowntree LG, and Turner BB (1914) On the removal of diffusible substances from the circulating blood of living animals by dialysis. J Pharmacol Exp Ther 5: 275–316
2. Abosaif NY, Tolba YA, Heap M, et al (2005) The outcome of acute renal failure in the intensive care unit according to RIFLE: model application, sensitivity, and predictability. Am J Kidney Dis 46: 1038–1048
3. Ali T, Khan I, Simpson W, et al (2007) Incidence and outcomes in acute kidney injury: a comprehensive population-based study. J Am Soc Nephrol 18: 1292–1298
4. Baird D and Dunn JS (1933) Renal lesions in eclampsia and nephritis of pregnancy. J Path Bact 37: 291–309

5. Baker SL (1937) Urinary suppression following blood transfusion. Lancet 229: 1390–1395
6. Bell M, Liljestam E, Granath F, et al (2005) Optimal follow-up time after continuous renal replacement therapy in actual renal failure patients stratified with the RIFLE criteria. Nephrol Dial Transplant 20: 354–360
7. Bellomo R, Ronco C, Kellum JA, et al (2004) Acute renal failure – definition, outcome measures, animal models, fluid therapy and information technology needs: the Second International Consensus Conference of the Acute Dialysis Quality Initiative (ADQI) Group. CritCare 8: R204–212
8. Better OS (1997) History of the crush syndrome: from the earthquakes of Messina, Sicily 1909 to Spitak, Armenia 1988. Am J Nephrol 17: 392–394
9. Bhandari S and Turney JH (1996) Survivors of acute renal failure who do not recover renal function. QJM 89: 415–421
10. Boulton-Jones M (1994) Dialysis membranes: clinical effects. Lancet 344: 559
11. Brivet FG, Kleinknecht DJ, Loirat P, et al (1996) Acute renal failure in intensive care units – causes, outcome, and prognostic factors of hospital mortality; a prospective, multicenter study. French Study Group on Acute Renal Failure. Crit Care Med 24: 192–198
12. Brivet FG, Kleinknecht DJ, Loirat P, et al (1996) Acute renal failure in intensive care units – causes, outcome, and prognostic factors of hospital mortality; a prospective, multicenter study. French Study Group on Acute Renal Failure [see comment]. Crit Care Med 24: 192–198
13. Bull GM, Jokes AM, and Lowe KG (1949) Conservative treatment of anuric uraemia. Lancet 2: 229–234
14. Bywaters E and Knochel J (1941) Crush injuries with impairment of renal function. Br Med J 1: 427–432
15. Bywaters EG (1990) 50 years on: the crush syndrome. BMJ 301: 1412–1415
16. Bywaters EG and Beall D (1998) Crush injuries with impairment of renal function. 1941. J Am Soc Nephrol 9: 322–332
17. Bywaters EG, Delory GE, Rimington C, et al (1941) Myohaemoglobin in the urine of air raid casualties with crushing injury. Biochem J 35: 1164–1168
18. Cameron JS (2000) Practical haemodialysis began with cellophane and heparin: the crucial role of William Thalhimer (1884–1961). Nephrol Dial Transplant 15: 1086–1091
19. Carbonell N, Blasco M, Sanjuan R, et al (2004) Acute renal failure in critically ill patients. A prospective epidemiological study. Nefrologia 24: 47–53
20. Chertow GM, Burdick E, Honour M, et al (2005) Acute kidney injury, mortality, length of stay, and costs in hospitalized patients. J Am Soc Nephrol 16: 3365–3370
21. Chertow GM, Levy EM, Hammermeister KE, et al (1998) Independent association between acute renal failure and mortality following cardiac surgery. Am J Med 104: 343–348
22. Eknoyan G (2002) Emergence of the concept of acute renal failure. Am J Nephrol 22: 225–230
23. Feest TG, Round A, and Hamad S (1993) Incidence of severe acute renal failure in adults: results of a community based study. BMJ 306: 481–483
24. Frankenthal L (1916) Uber Verschuttungen. Virchows Arch 222–232
25. Frocht A and Fillit H (1984) Renal disease in the geriatric patient. J Am Geriatr Soc 32: 28–43
26. Goldring W and Graef I (1936) Nephrosis with uremia following transfusion with incompatible blood: report of seven cases with three deaths. Arch Intern Med 58: 825–845
27. Hadj-Aissa A, Dumarest C, Maire P, et al (1990) Renal function in the elderly. Nephron 54: 364–365
28. Hoste EA, Blot SI, Lameire NH, et al (2004) Effect of nosocomial bloodstream infection on the outcome of critically ill patients with acute renal failure treated with renal replacement therapy. J Am Soc Nephrol 15: 454–462
29. Hoste EA, Clermont G, Kersten A, et al (2006) RIFLE criteria for acute kidney injury are associated with hospital mortality in critically ill patients: a cohort analysis. Crit Care 10: R73
30. Hoste EA, Lameire NH, Vanholder RC, et al (2003) Acute renal failure in patients with sepsis in a surgical ICU: predictive factors, incidence, comorbidity, and outcome. J Am Soc Nephrol 14: 1022–1030
31. Hsia DC, Ahern CA, Ritchie BP, et al (1992) Medicare reimbursement accuracy under the prospective payment system, 1985 to 1988. JAMA 268: 896–899
32. Iezzoni LI, Foley SM, Daley J, et al (1992) Comorbidities, complications, and coding bias. Does the number of diagnosis codes matter in predicting in-hospital mortality? JAMA 267: 2197–2203
33. Kaplan C, Pasternack B, Shah H, et al (1975) Age-related incidence of sclerotic glomeruli in human kidneys. Am J Pathol 80: 227–234
34. Khan IH, Catto GR, Edward N, et al (1993) Influence of coexisting disease on survival on renal-replacement therapy. Lancet 341: 415–418
35. Khan IH, Catto GR, Edward N, et al (1997) Acute renal failure: factors influencing nephrology referral and outcome. QJM 90: 781–785
36. Khan IH, Catto GR, Edward N, et al (1997) Acute renal failure: factors influencing nephrology referral and outcome. QJM 90: 781–785
37. Kolff WJ and Berk HTJ (1944) The artificial kidney: a dialyser with a great area. Acta Med Scand 177: 121–134
38. Kolff WJ (1965) First clinical experience with the artificial kidney. Ann Intern Med 62: 608–619
39. Kumar VA, Craig M, Depner TA, et al (2000) Extended daily dialysis: A new approach to renal replacement for acute renal failure in the intensive care unit. Am J Kidney Dis 36: 294–300
40. Lameire N, Van Biesen W, and Vanholder R (2005) Acute renal failure. Lancet 365: 417–430
41. Lassnigg A, Schmidlin D, Mouhieddine M, et al (2004) Minimal changes of serum creatinine predict prognosis in patients after cardiothoracic surgery: a prospective cohort study. J Am Soc Nephrol 15: 1597–1605
42. Levy EM, Viscoli CM, and Horwitz RI (1996) The effect of acute renal failure on mortality. A cohort analysis. JAMA 275: 1489–1494
43. Liangos O, Wald R, O'Bell JW, et al (2006) Epidemiology and outcomes of acute renal failure in hospitalized patients: a national survey. Clin J Am Soc Nephrol 1: 43–51
44. Liano F and Pascual J (1996) Epidemiology of acute renal failure: a prospective, multicenter, community-based study.

Madrid Acute Renal Failure Study Group. Kidney Int 50: 811–818
45. Lim RKS and Necheles H (1927) Recovery of a pancreatic secretory excitant by vividialysis of the circulating blood. Proc Soc Exp Biol Med 64: 28–29
46. Lindeman RD (1990) Overview: renal physiology and pathophysiology of aging. Am J Kidney Dis 16: 275–282
47. Lindeman RD and Goldman R (1986) Anatomic and physiologic age changes in the kidney. Exp Gerontol 21: 379–406
48. Lindeman RD, Tobin J, and Shock NW (1985) Longitudinal studies on the rate of decline in renal function with age. J Am Geriatr Soc 33: 278–285
49. McLachlan MS, Guthrie JC, Anderson CK, et al (1977) Vascular and glomerular changes in the ageing kidney. J Pathol 121: 65–78
50. Mehta RL, McDonald B, Gabbai FB, et al (2001) A randomized clinical trial of continuous versus intermittent dialysis for acute renal failure [see comment]. Kidney Int 60: 1154–1163
51. Mehta RL, Pascual MT, Soroko S, et al (2004) Spectrum of acute renal failure in the intensive care unit: the PICARD experience. Kidney Int 66: 1613–1621
52. Metcalfe W, Simpson M, Khan IH, et al (2002) Acute renal failure requiring renal replacement therapy: incidence and outcome. QJM 95: 579–583
53. Metcalfe W, Simpson M, Khan IH, et al (2002) Acute renal failure requiring renal replacement therapy: incidence and outcome. QJM 95: 579–583
54. Nash K, Hafeez A, and Hou S (2002) Hospital-acquired renal insufficiency. Am J Kidney Dis 39: 930–936
55. Oliver J, MacDowell M, and Tracy A (1951) The pathogenesis of acute renal failure associated with traumatic and toxic injury; renal ischemia, nephrotoxic damage and the ischemic episode. J Clin Invest 30: 1307–1439
56. Ostermann M and Chang RW (2007) Acute kidney injury in the intensive care unit according to RIFLE. Crit Care Med 35: 1837–1843
57. Pascual J, Liano F, and Ortuno J (1995) The elderly patient with acute renal failure. J Am Soc Nephrol 6: 144–153
58. Prescott GJ, Metcalfe W, Baharani J, et al (2007) A prospective national study of acute renal failure treated with RRT: incidence, aetiology and outcomes. Nephrol Dial Transplant 22: 2513–2519
59. Quan H, Parsons GA, and Ghali WA (2002) Validity of information on comorbidity derived rom ICD-9-CCM administrative data. Med Care 40: 675–685
60. Roderick PJ, Atkins RJ, Smeeth L, et al (2008) Detecting chronic kidney disease in older people: what are the implications? Age Ageing 37: 179–186
61. Salem ME and Eknoyan G (1999) The kidney in ancient Egyptian medicine: where does it stand?. Am J Nephrol 19: 140–147
62. Schiffl H, Lang SM, and Fischer R (2002) Daily hemodialysis and the outcome of acute renal failure. N Engl J Med 346: 305–310
63. Shackman R, Milne MD, and Struthers NW (1960) Oliguric renal failure of surgical origin. Br Med J 2: 1473–1482
64. Shusterman N, Strom BL, Murray TG, et al (1987) Risk factors and outcome of hospital-acquired acute renal failure. Clinical epidemiologic study. Am J Med 83: 65–71
65. Smith LH, Jr, Post RS, Teschan PE, et al (1955) Post-traumatic renal insufficiency in military casualties. II. Management, use of an artificial kidney, prognosis. Am J Med 18: 187–198
66. Stevens PE, Tamimi NA, Al-Hasani MK, et al (2001) Non-specialist management of acute renal failure. QJM 94: 533–540
67. Tauchi H, Tsuboi K, and Okutomi J (1971) Age changes in the human kidney of the different races. Gerontologia 17: 87–97
68. Uchino S, Kellum JA, Bellomo R, et al (2005) Acute renal failure in critically ill patients: a multinational, multicenter study. JAMA 294: 813–818
69. Van Biesen W, Vanholder R, and Lameire N (2006) Defining acute renal failure: RIFLE and beyond. Clin J Am Soc Nephrol 1: 1314–1319
70. Waikar SS, Curhan GC, Wald R, et al (2006) Declining mortality in patients with acute renal failure, 1988 to 2002. J Am Soc Nephrol 17: 1143–1150
71. Witts LJ (1929) A note on blood transfusion with an account of a fatal reaction. Lancet 1: 1297–1300
72. Wyatt CM and Arons RR (2004) The burden of acute renal failure in nonrenal solid organ transplantation. Transplantation 78: 1351–1355
73. Xue JL, Daniels F, Star RA, et al (2006) Incidence and mortality of acute renal failure in Medicare beneficiaries, 1992 to 2001. J Am Soc Nephrol 17: 1135–1142
74. Ympa YP, Sakr Y, Reinhart K, et al (2005) Has mortality from acute renal failure decreased? A systematic review of the literature. Am J Med 118: 827–832

Economic Impact of Acute Kidney Failure 2.7

Joseph F. Dasta and Sandra L. Kane-Gill

Core Messages

- Determining the cost of an acute disease is complex.
- Intensive care unit (ICU) stay is a major driver of costs, and averages US $3,500 per day.
- Studies evaluating the costs of acute kidney injury (AKI) used widely different methods.
- Different AKI definitions and patient populations were some of the most notable differences in methods between studies.
- AKI patients generate costs that can be twofold to threefold higher than matched ICU patients not developing AKI.
- Renal replacement therapy and ICU length of stay are important drivers of costs of AKI patients.
- Patients with even small increases in serum creatinine have higher hospital and ICU costs compared with patients with no increases in serum creatinine.
- Therapies that prevent and/or effectively treat AKI can have substantial effects on hospital costs.

J. F. Dasta (✉)
The Ohio State University, College of Pharmacy, University of Texas, College of Pharmacy, P.O. Box 967, Hutto, TX 78634–0967, USA
e-mail: dasta@mail.utexas.edu

2.7.1 Quantifying Costs in the Intensive Care Unit

The government, private insurers, health care providers, pharmaceutical, and device companies, even patients, want to know the costs of patients in the intensive care unit (ICU). The reason for this interest is centered on the finite resources in health care and fixed reimbursement to hospitals. How do ICU patients consume these finite resources? While the question is straightforward, the answer is complex.

It is difficult to obtain an accurate estimate of cost since hospitals often generate a charge for their services. Charge is the price that an institution bills payers. Many studies use the cost-to-charge ratio. This is an estimate of the cost of a given treatment used to care for the patient.

Critical care costs in the United States were approximately US $60 billion in 2000, and it would be reasonable to project a cost of US $90 billion by 2010. These high costs are seen despite ICUs accounting for only 10% of hospital beds [6]. A recent study from a large database revealed a mean ICU cost of US $19,725 ± $31,778 and a mean cost per ICU day of US $3,436 ± $3,550 [7]. Drug costs in the ICU account for 38% of total drug costs, and daily ICU drug costs are three times higher than those for ward patients [12].

2.7.2 Overview of Studies Reporting Costs Associated with Acute Kidney Injury

The available cost studies offer unique insights into different populations acquiring acute kidney injury (AKI). The populations range from uncomplicated

A. Jörres, et al. (eds.), *Management of Acute Kidney Problems,*
DOI: 10.1007/978-3-540-69441-0_2.7, © Springer-Verlag Berlin Heidelberg 2010

Table 2.7.1 Key variables in studies reporting the cost of acute kidney injury (AKI)

Reference	Patient population	Total sample size	Sample with AKI[a]	Mortality (%)	AKI definition
9	Seriously ill patients enrolled in SUPPORT study	9,105	490	73 at 6 months	Hospitalized patients requiring hemodialysis or peritoneal dialysis
10	ICU patients from one hospital	3,447	62	ICU 34, hospital 45, 6 month 55	ICU patients requiring RRT
11	ICU patients from two hospitals	663	261	Hospital 62.5	Require RRT or rapidly rising SCr[i], See text for specifics
4	All patients from one hospital	9,205	2,892 and 352 with the least and most stringent definitions, respectively	8 for SCr change of 0.5–0.9 mg/dl	Multiple definitions used, see text
3	Trauma patients admitted to a SICU[l]	1,033	246	24	SCr > 1.5 mg/dl and/or increase in SCr by 50% and/or increase in SCr of > 0.5 mg/dl
8	Patients with uncomplicated AKI from 23 institutions	4,230	2,252	8	DRG[m] for renal failure
5	CABG[n] developing AKI postoperatively	3,741	258	11.2	RIFLE[o]

AKI in hospitalized patients to varying degrees of AKI in ICU patients, and patients who develop AKI following coronary artery bypass grafting (CABG). The hospital costs of AKI patients range from median values of US $3,300 in uncomplicated AKI to US $48,382 in seriously ill AKI patients requiring renal replacement therapy (RRT) (see Table 2.7.1). The more lenient definition of uncomplicated AKI provides the lowest cost. A more stringent definition, requiring RRT, results in the highest projected 6-month mortality rate and cost. There are many contributing factors to the cost variation, including sample size, patient population, method of cost determination, and starting point for cost calculation, but none are more important than the definition used for AKI. Unfortunately, these study design differences make comparison of costs impossible. Despite the enormous variability in study design, all studies agree that patients developing AKI are costly to the institution. As such, therapies directed at preventing and treating this condition would result in significant cost savings.

When considering costs of AKI using a retrospective approach, it is appropriate to consider if total hospitalization costs accurately reflect the cost attributed to the disease. For example, a trauma patient who develops ventilator-associated pneumonia on ICU day 5, is treated with an aminoglycoside and develops AKI, accrues substantial costs from days 1 to 5. Total hospitalization costs for this individual would therefore overinflate the cost attributable to AKI. We suggest that costs for AKI should be calculated from the time that the AKI is diagnosed. For most patients, this is the time when their serum creatinine (SCr) reaches a predetermined value used in the definition of AKI, or when RRT starts. We further suggest using the RIFLE criteria to define AKI [2].

All AKI studies to date, except one, used retrospective data. A prospective analysis would provide a more accurate cost estimate. For example, a prospective

Method used to determine cost, year determined	Starting point for cost determination	Costs Of AKI[b]	Other costs	Hospital LOS[c] (days)	ICU[d] LOS (days)
Medicare cost-to-charge ratio, transformed to 1994 US dollars	From start of RRT[e]	Median hospital cost $48,382, mean $95,612	Projected cost of long-term dialysis $41,331, cost/QALY[f] $193,909	NP[g]	NP
Based on TISS[h] score, 1992 & 1993	From start of RRT	Mean total hospital cost $56,095	Mean cost per 6 months in survivors $124,671	NP	20 ± 12 from the start of RRT for nonsurvivors, 18 ± 18 for survivors
Hospital costs direct and indirect costs, RRT costs by micro-costing methods, adjusted to 1999 Canadian dollars	After first dialysis	Mean total hospital cost $43,022 for all survivors, $25,341 for dead patients	$2,997 to $4,401 per week for CRRT[j], IHD[k] $1,149 per week	Mean 10.3 from start of RRT	Mean 38.2 from start of RRT
Itemized account of institution's cost	Admission to hospital	Mean $13,400 for SCr change of 0.5–0.9 mg/dl	NP	Mean 3.5 additional days with SCr ≥ 0.5 mg/dl	NP
Hospital cost, details not provided	Admission to hospital	Median, hospital costs, $36,200	Median, hospital costs, $24,100 in controls	Mean 11	NP
Ratio of cost to charges for the hospital center	Admission to hospital	Median direct hospital costs, $3,300	NP	Median 5	NP
Ratio of cost to charges from each departmental cost center	Following CABG	Median postoperative costs $37,674 RIFLE class R $29,697, RIFLE class I $38,924, RIFLE class F $52,618	Median postoperative costs in controls $18,463	Median 11 following CABG	Median 3.2

All costs are listed in US dollars
[a]AKI, acute kidney insufficiency
[b]Costs were transformed to reflect 2008 value using a 3% annual inflation rate
[c]LOS, length of stay
[d]ICU, intensive care unit
[e]RRT, renal replacement therapy
[f]QALY, quality-adjusted life year
[g]NP, not provided
[h]TISS, therapeutic intervention scoring system
[i]SCr, serum creatinine
[j]CRRT, continuous renal replacement therapy
[k]IHD, intermittent hemodialysis
[l]SICU, surgical intensive care unit
[m]DRG, diagnosis-related group
[n]CABG, coronary artery bypass grafting
[o]RIFLE, risk, injury, failure, loss, end-stage renal failure

study design will allow a panel of experts to evaluate if each intervention was related to treating the AKI, and erroneous costs could be eliminated. A prospective analysis would allow micro-costing to be used that also included nursing time. Ideally, the post-AKI cost components from an institutional perspective should contain the following items to assess which additional costs predominate: dialysis, AKI-related consultations, fluids, or pharmacologic management of AKI, room charges for additional length of stay (LOS), physician services for additional LOS, nursing care for additional LOS, pharmacy services for mixing medications for additional LOS, medications received during additional LOS, laboratory testing for additional LOS, and complications associated with additional LOS (e.g., infection, venous thrombosis).

The cost studies for AKI have been performed from an institutional perspective, which is reasonable since this is where most resources are used. However, an evaluation from the societal perspective is needed to fully understand the cost burden associated with AKI. We know AKI is associated with a longer hospital LOS, which can be translated into reduced productivity costs. The number of physician visits for renal-related follow-up subsequent to the hospitalization would also generate additional costs. Costs should be considered for patients that develop chronic renal insufficiency secondary to AKI. Therefore, we suggest the total cost of care for AKI from a societal perspective should be determined.

Researchers should consider an evaluation of quality of life for AKI patients. We know that patients who received RRT have a utility of 0.84, 6 months after their ICU stay [9]. It would be interesting to study the magnitude of this effect in varying degrees of AKI and if these patients require additional treatment for depression or posttraumatic stress disorder.

2.7.3 Clinical Studies of Costs Associated with AKI

The following section summarizes studies that describe costs in AKI patients. We were only able to identify seven articles that describe the costs associated with AKI. These few studies are in contrast to a vast amount of clinical literature on AKI. For example, a PubMed search of the phrase "acute renal failure" yielded 30,000 articles starting in 1946. Table 2.7.1 is a compilation of key outcomes from each study. Since the data were collected from 1991 to 2003, we converted all costs to 2008 US dollars by using an annual inflation rate of 3%.

The first study to quantify costs associated with AKI was published in 1997 [9]. They determined the costs associated with AKI from a large database called Study to Understand Prognoses and Preferences for Outcomes and Risks of Treatments (SUPPORT). This was a clinical outcomes and cost-effectiveness analysis of nearly 500 seriously ill patients requiring RRT, having additional serious illnesses, and an expected 6-month mortality of 50%. They calculated hospital costs from the US Medicare cost-to-charge ratio starting when RRT was initiated. As evidence of the severity of illness in these patients, the median survival from starting RRT was 32 days, and only 27% were alive in 6 months. The mean hospital cost from RRT to either death or hospital discharge was US $63,219. The overall cost-effectiveness, expressed as cost per quality-adjusted life year (QALY), was US $193,909. The projected cost of long-term dialysis per patient was US $41,338. Patients were further stratified by prognosis. In patients with a 10% or less probability of surviving 6 months, the cost/QALY was US $373,751. In contrast, patients with the best survivability (40–60% probability of surviving 6 months), the cost/QALY was US $93,469. The authors conclude that dialysis is not cost-effective in patients with average or worse-than-average prognoses. This is based on a commonly quoted value of US $50,000/QALY or less, for a therapy to be cost-effective. These data are limited to patients who are gravely ill, with multiple organ failure, and who require RRT after admission. This study only assessed costs from the time RRT began and does not account for the time before starting dialysis. Despite these limitations, this is one of the most thorough studies of costs and cost-effectiveness of managing patients with AKI.

One study of patients developing AKI following aortic surgery repair revealed that costs of dialysis patients were 2.6-fold higher than for AKI patients not requiring dialysis. Since neither the definition of AKI nor the sample size was provided, it was not incorporated into Table 2.7.1 [1].

Korkeila and colleagues evaluated AKI costs in 62 patients from one hospital in the Netherlands from the start of RRT to death or discharge [10]. It was also a sick patient population who had a hospital mortality of nearly 50% and an ICU length of stay of 2–3 weeks. Approximately 2% of their ICU admissions developed AKI. They did not perform a cost-effectiveness analysis but reported a mean total hospital cost of US $56,095, which is considerably less than the Hamel study. Their method of calculating costs was very different (Table 2.7.1).

Manns et al. collected data on 261 ICU patients from two hospitals in the Calgary Health Region from 1996 to 1999 [11]. Their AKI definition used either RRT or changes in SCr. It consisted of a rapid rising SCr > 1 mg/dl on two consecutive SCr values more than 24 h apart, or if no history of renal insufficiency, a SCr above 2 mg/dl. They used a micro-costing method for RRT costs only. We converted their Canadian dollar costs to US dollars with an exchange rate of CAN $1 = US $0.66 at the time of their study. Total hospital costs for survivors from the time of RRT were US $43,022 after the first RRT. They do not provide costs of the entire population, hence making it impossible to compare with other studies. They also determined that the cost per week for continuous renal replacement therapy is two to three times higher than intermittent hemodialysis. Hence, they conclude considerable cost savings can occur if intermittent hemodialysis was used more frequently.

Chertow et al. preformed a thorough evaluation of hospital costs associated with increases in SCr by using nine different assessments of changes in SCr [4]. The mean adjusted increase in costs was US $7,499 for patients with an increase in SCr of 0.5 mg/dl. The cost analysis adjusted for age, sex, diagnosis-related group weight, and ICD-9 categories. The marginal cost difference increased as the SCr increased. Four categories of increases in SCr included 0.3–0.4, 0.5–0.9, 1.0–1.9, and ≥2.0 mg/dl. The corresponding average, unadjusted costs, were US $6,700, $13,400, $24,100, and $45,500 per group. It is important to note that AKI was independently associated with an increased length of stay, which provides an explanation for some of these additional costs. They reported that 5% of annualized hospital costs are attributable to AKI. Additionally, annual health care expenditures resulting from hospital-acquired AKI are over US $10 billion.

Approximately, 24% of trauma patients admitted to a surgical ICU developed AKI during a 3-year period. A study by Brandt et al. evaluated the costs of AKI in trauma patients, considering small changes in SCr [3]. Outcomes of interest were a 22.1% increase in mortality, a median three additional days of hospitalization and an average increase in 3.7 days of mechanical ventilation. Every 1 mg/dl increase in SCr was related to a 2.2-day increase in hospital length of stay and a 1.1-day increase in mechanical ventilation time. For any increase in SCr, there was an additional cost of US $3,088 per patient. Twenty-five percent of AKI patients required hemodialysis, which is likely a significant contributor to the cost difference between patients who developed AKI and those who did not. It would have been useful if the authors had preformed an additional analysis comparing the costs of AKI patients with and without hemodialysis. The additional costs per patient would have been influenced by these data.

Fischer et al. performed the largest multicenter evaluation of over 2,200 patients with uncomplicated AKI incorporating data from 23 institutions [8]. The evaluation identified specific hospital charges that were converted to costs using cost-to-charge ratios designated for each hospital center. The costs included room and board, equipment, nursing resources, pharmacy costs, laboratory costs, blood products, and radiology costs. The overall cost for patients with uncomplicated AKI was US $3,300. A delineation of hospital costs based on sex, race, age, income, admission source, hospital type, insurance, and severity of illness was also performed. The most costly uncomplicated AKI was for those with a high degree of illness severity and dialysis being US $4,700 and US $5,400, respectively. For patients with uncomplicated AKI that required dialysis, there was an additional US $2,200 in direct hospital costs, 2 more days of hospitalization and a twofold increase in hospital mortality compared with patients not receiving dialysis. Finally, a cost breakdown was completed for common diagnosis-related groups, with circulatory disorders being the most expensive at US $4,500 and bronchitis/asthma being the least expensive at US $1,800 for patients with uncomplicated AKI.

Interestingly, an analysis was performed of factors associated with direct hospital costs. Factors significantly associated with a decrease in costs included non-white race, male, low severity of illness, and nonacademic institutions. In contrast, high severity of illness and dialysis were factors significantly contributing to higher costs.

A study by Dasta et al. evaluated the costs of AKI following CABG surgery [5]. Their institutional approach to cost determination was conducted using total hospital charges converted to costs using cost-to-charge ratios. As a means to evaluate only the costs attributed to AKI, the focus of this evaluation was postoperative costs because AKI was thought to be result of the CABG surgery. Patients with AKI were matched to controls on age and severity of illness (APACHE III scores). The median hospital cost was US $37,674 and US $18,463 for the AKI group and controls, respectively. The additional 6 days of hospitalization or 1.8 days of ICU length of stay for the patients with AKI compared to non-AKI could explain some of the extra costs.

The analysis also included consideration of the degree of AKI severity using the RIFLE criteria [2]. The RIFLE criteria include categorization by worsening AKI severity as a function of change in SCr from baseline, from renal risk (RIFLE class R) to renal injury (RIFLE class I) and renal failure (RIFLE class F). The total postoperative costs increased with severity of AKI. The difference in median total postoperative costs between groups was US $9,226 (class R to I) and US $22,921 (class R to F). Of note, the ICU costs of RIFLE class F patients accounted for 94% of the total postoperative costs. Even patients with the smallest increase in SCr, namely RIFLE class R patients (peak SCr 1.5 times baseline) had total postoperative costs US $11,234 higher than controls. Costs also increased significantly with worsening AKI severity for each cost center including laboratory, pharmacy, ventilatory, ICU room, and ICU supplies.

This study also evaluated the contributions of RRT to the cost of AKI. The median total postoperative cost for AKI patients who did not require RRT was US $34,953 compared with US $74,040 for those who received RRT. Finally, the cumulative cost generated for CABG patients developing AKI was US $18.3 million over 4 years in this institution.

In summary, AKI is not only a clinically devastating disease, it creates a major economic burden that increases with severity of the renal dysfunction. The main drivers of the increased cost of AKI are prolonged ICU length of stay and use of RRT. These few studies used significantly different study designs and hence, the cost data cannot be compared. Future studies should use the RIFLE classification for acute renal dysfunction, collect data prospectively, quantitate costs using micro-costing methods, calculate attributable costs to AKI, and evaluate quality of life following hospital discharge.

2.7.4 Take Home Pearls

- AKI patients generate significantly higher costs than patients who do not develop AKI
- AKI costs increase with increasing severity of renal dysfunction
- Even small increases in SCr generate significant extra costs
- The small body of evidence on AKI costs cannot be directly compared due to different methods used

References

1. Barry MC, Merriman B, Wiley M, et al. (1997) Ruptured abdominal aortic aneurysm-can treatment costs and outcomes be predicted by using clinical or physiological parameters? Eur J Vasc Endovasc Surg 14:487–491
2. Bellomo R, Ronco C, Kellum JA, et al. (2004) Acute renal failure-definition, outcome measures, animal models, fluid therapy and information technology needs: the second international consensus conference of the acute dialysis quality initiative (ADQI) group. Crit Care 8: R204-R212
3. Brandt M-M, Falvo AJ, Rubinfield IS, et al. (2007) Renal dysfunction in trauma: even a little less costs a lot. J Trauma 62:1362–1364
4. Chertow GM, Burdick E, Honour M, et al. (2005) Acute kidney injury, mortality, length of stay, and costs in hospitalized patients. J Am Soc Nephrol 16:3365–3370
5. Dasta JF, Kane-Gill S, Durtschi, AJ, Pathak D, Kellum J (2008) Costs and outcomes of acute kidney injury following cardiac surgery. Nephrol Dial Transplant 23:1970–4
6. Dasta JF, Durtschi AJ, Kane-Gill SL. Pharmacoeconomics, in critical care. In: Fink MP, Abraham E, Vincent J-L, Kochanek PM (eds) (2005) Textbook of Critical Care. Elsevier, Philadelphia, PA
7. Dasta J, Kim SR, McLaughlin TP, et al. (2005) Incremental daily cost of mechanical ventilation in patients receiving treatment in an intensive care unit. Crit Care Med 33:1266–71
8. Fischer MJ, Brimhall, BB, Lezotte DC, et al. (2005) Uncomplicated acute renal failure and hospital resource utilization: a retrospective multicenter analysis. Am J Kid Dis 46:1049–1057
9. Hamel MB, Phillips RS, Davis RB, et al. (1997) Outcomes and cost-effectiveness of initiating dialysis and continuing aggressive care in seriously ill hospitalized patients. Ann Intern Med 127:195–202
10. Korkeila M, Ruokonen E, Takala J (2000) Costs of care, long-term prognosis and quality of life in patients requiring renal replacement therapy during intensive care. Intensive Care Med 26:1824–1831
11. Manns B, Doig CJ, Lee H, et al. (2003) Cost of acute renal failure requiring dialysis in the intensive care unit: clinical and resource implications of renal recovery. Crit Care Med 31:449–455
12. Weber RJ, Kane SL, Oriolo V, et al. (2003) Impact of intensive care unit drug use on hospital costs: a descriptive analysis, with recommendations for optimizing ICU pharmacotherapy. Crit Care Med 31 (Suppl.):S17–S24

Part III

Diagnostic Evaluation and Procedures

Clinical and Laboratory Evaluation 3.1

Robert J. Anderson

Core Messages

- Early detection of the occurrence of acute kidney injury (AKI) and delineation of the cause(s) of this disorder are important to implement early therapy and perhaps reduce morbidity and mortality.
- The current reliance on measurements of serum creatinine to define and classify severity of AKI (RIFLE criteria) ensures that AKI will be diagnosed relatively late.
- Newer biomarkers offer promise to detect AKI in earlier stages than currently available tests but remain to be fully evaluated.
- A systematic approach to each patient with AKI is necessary to ensure that all causal events are identified and addressed.

Objectives to Understand

- Potential clinical and laboratory manifestations of acute kidney injury (AKI)
- Causes of AKI
- Clinical and laboratory evaluation of AKI

R. J. Anderson
Department of Medicine, University of Colorado, Health Science Center, 4200 East 9th Avenue., Denver, CO 80262, USA
e-mail: robert.anderson@uchsc.edu

3.1.1 Introduction

Acute kidney injury (AKI) occurs with relatively high frequency in contemporary hospital practice and especially in the intensive care unit (ICU) [1–6]. Diverse pathophysiologic events encountered in multiple clinical settings produce an identical clinical picture of AKI [7]. Mild forms of AKI are often reversible, and all degrees and causes of AKI are associated with significant mortality and morbidity [1–12]. Alleviation or attenuation of AKI requires prompt identification and therapy directed at the underlying causal factors. This chapter will review the clinical and laboratory features and various causes of AKI, as well as outline a stepwise approach to timely diagnosis.

3.1.2 Presenting Manifestations of AKI

3.1.2.1 Clinical

The most recently proposed consensus definition and classification of AKI is referred to by the acronym of RIFLE [8, 13]. By this definition, two factors, decreasing urine output and decreasing glomerular filtration rate (GFR) define AKI. The decreasing GFR as defined by RIFLE is usually estimated by increasing serum creatinine concentration and presently forms the primary basis for determining the presence of AKI [8, 13].

The clinical condition that most often leads to a diagnosis of AKI is the presence of either oliguria (<5 ml/kg/day or 0.5 ml/kg/h) or anuria (essentially no urine output). The presence of oligoanuria almost always indicates at least some degree of AKI. However, a significant percentage (perhaps 50% or more) of all cases of AKI

A. Jörres et al. (eds.), *Management of Acute Kidney Problems*,
DOI: 10.1007/978-3-540-69441-0_3.1,

Table 3.1.1 Causes of anuric acute kidney injury (AKI)

1. Complete urinary tract obstruction
2. Renal vascular occlusion
– Renal arterial thrombosis/ligation
– Cortical necrosis (sepsis, obstetric accidents, disseminated intravascular coagulation)
– Rapidly progressive glomerulonephritis and vasculitis
– Renal vein thrombosis
3. Acute kidney injury complicating sepsis, heat stroke, and rhabdomyolysis

are nonoliguric [7, 14]. Moreover, all degrees and processes that result in AKI including decreased renal perfusion (so-called prerenal AKI), obstruction to urine flow (so-called postrenal AKI) and disorders of the kidney vasculature, glomeruli, tubules, and interstitium (so-called renal AKI) can be nonoliguric [7, 14]. Thus, the maintenance of normal urine output does not provide assurance to the clinician that GFR is normal.

The documented complete absence of urine flow (anuria) deserves special mention (Table 3.1.1). A few hours of no urine flow is occasionally seen in selected clinical settings such as septic shock, heat stroke, and severe rhabdomyolysis that result in marked renal hypoperfusion [7]. Sustained anuria however is usually (>90% of cases) due to complete urinary tract obstruction which is almost always amenable to therapy. Less commonly, cessation of renal blood flow via the major or smaller renal blood vessels or severe, rapidly progressive glomerulonephritis result in anuria [7].

On rare occasions, when frequent monitoring of urine output or serum creatinine concentration is not being done, such as in either the ambulatory or hospital ward populations, AKI will initially come to the attention of the clinician by one of the clinical manifestations of loss of kidney function (Table 3.1.2) [7]. Given the central role of the kidney in regulating extracellular fluid volume (ECFV), a volume-overload state should always prompt inquiry into the GFR. Rarely, gastrointestinal symptoms (anorexia, nausea, and vomiting), flank/back pain (due to presumably edematous kidneys or urinary tract obstruction), altered mental status, or seizures will be the presenting manifestation of advanced AKI [7]. The primary role of the kidney in production of erythropoietin and the impact of poor kidney function on diminished platelet adhesion and aggregation can result in anemia and bleeding disorders as an initial manifestation of AKI [7].

Table 3.1.2 Possible clinical manifestations of acute kidney injury (AKI)

1. Oligoanuria
2. Volume overload
– Edema
– Congestive heart failure
– Noncardiac pulmonary edema
– Hypertension
3. Anorexia, nausea, vomiting
4. Encephalopathy
5. Seizures
6. Flank/back pain
7. Gastrointestinal hemorrhage
8. Bleeding disorder
9. Anemia (pallor)

3.1.2.2 Laboratory

Many hospitalized patients have frequent determinations of serum creatinine and blood urea nitrogen (BUN) concentrations. An increase in serum creatinine concentration is the major way in which application of the RIFLE criteria for diagnosing AKI is currently done because the serum creatinine concentration is a better surrogate marker for GFR than the BUN concentration [7]. In the absence of GFR, the serum creatinine and BUN concentrations increase by 1.0–1.5 and 10–15 mg/dl/day, respectively. The BUN to serum creatinine ratio is usually 10–15:1. Based upon the differential effects of diet, medications, and renal function on BUN and creatinine concentrations, some clinicians advocate that the BUN to creatinine ratio can provide diagnostic information (Fig. 3.1.1). To date, clinical validation of this ratio remains to be developed [15].

There are several shortcomings with the use of serum creatinine as a surrogate marker for GFR. First, in individuals with a normal GFR, the relationship between decreasing GFR and rising serum creatinine is logrhythmic rather than linear. For example, in a steady-state setting, a reasonable approximation is that each time the GFR halves, the serum creatinine concentration doubles. Steady-state GFRs of 100, 50, 25, 12.5, and 6.25 ml/min are associated with serum creatinine concentrations of about 1.0, 2.0, 4.0, 8.0, and 16.0 ml/dl, respectively. Thus at higher rates of GFR and lower serum creatinine concentrations, relative large decrements in GFR can be associated with only slight increases in serum creatinine concentration, rendering the test insensitive. Moreover, AKI occurs in a non-steady-state condition in which the three determinants of serum creatinine concentration (production, volume of distribution, and renal elimination) fluctuate [16]. Computerized models derived from

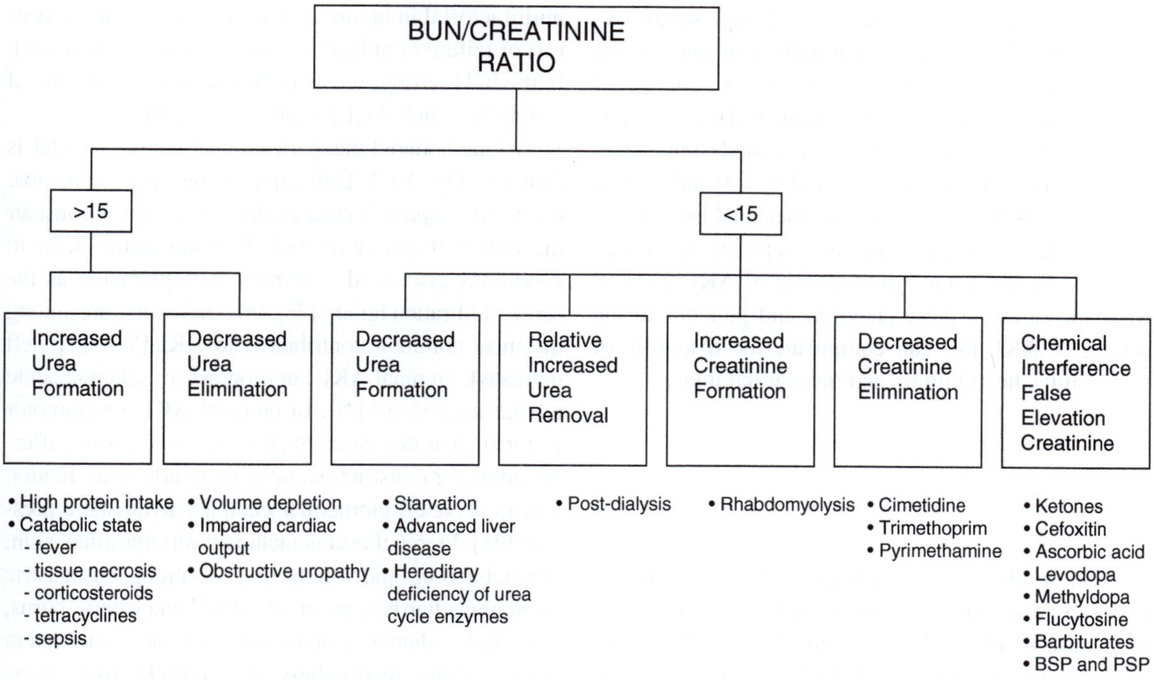

Fig. 3.1.1 Causes of abnormal bun to creatinine ratio

AKI patients demonstrate that several patterns of change in GFR occur during development and recovery from AKI, and often these GFR changes are poorly reflected by daily changes in serum creatinine concentration [16]. Finally, the rise in serum creatinine that occurs with AKI is not a "real-time" occurrence and is usually noted at a time significantly delayed from the onset of AKI. This ensures that the clinician is always significantly delayed in implementation of diagnostic and therapeutic efforts directed toward the AKI. Nevertheless, increases in serum creatinine concentration remain currently as the most practical and well-accepted AKI marker.

As discussed in chapter 3.2, some evidence suggests that increases in cystatin C may be more sensitive than serum creatinine in detecting AKI [17–21]. Cystatin C is a serine protease inhibitor produced in a constant amount by all nucleated cells. The kidney readily filters cystatin C which is then completely catabolized by the renal tubules such that little, if any, appears in the urine. The serum concentration of cystatin C rises in proportion to decreasing GFR. Although accurate nephelometric immunoassays for cystatin C are becoming more widely available, more clinical experience is needed to ascertain if use of cystatin C will lead to earlier determination of the presence of AKI with improved outcomes. Some preliminary information suggests that finding increases in urinary cystatin C may also be an early marker of renal tubular dysfunction and AKI [22].

The kidney is the primary "eliminator" of potassium, phosphorus, uric acid, organic acids, magnesium, and water from the body and activates vitamin D. If serial measurements of serum creatinine, BUN, or cystatin C are not available, then sometimes hyperkalemia, hypocalcemia, hyperphosphatemia, hyperuricemia, hypermagnesemia, metabolic acidosis, or hyponatremia may initially indicate the occurrence of decreased GFR due to AKI (Table 3.1.3). Many experienced clinicians

Table 3.1.3 Possible laboratory manifestations of acute kidney injury (AKI)

1. Elevated serum creatinine, BUN, cystatin C
2. Hyperkalemia
3. Hyponatremia
4. Metabolic acidosis
5. Hypocalcemia
6. Hyperphosphatemia
7. Hyperuricemia
8. Hypermagnesemia
9. Anemia
10. Prolonged bleeding time
11. Increased serum concentration of drugs normally eliminated by the kidneys (e.g., vancomycin)
12. Mild elevation of selected enzymes and biomarkers (creatinine kinase, troponin, brain natriuretic peptide)

have come to realize that unexpectedly high serum levels of selected drugs that are normally eliminated by the kidneys (e.g., vancomycin) are sometimes the initial clue as to the presence of AKI. Decreased GFR is well-known to be associated with slight to modest increases in selected pancreatic (amylase and lipase) and cardiac enzymes (CK-MB, troponin), and selected biomarkers for heart failure (brain natriuretic peptide), and rarely this may be the initial manifestation of AKI [23, 24]. Mild increases of these enzymes and peptides in the setting of AKI also can complicate the diagnosis of pancreatitis, heart failure, and myocardial injury.

3.1.3 Causes of AKI

Diverse conditions and pathophysiologic events can result in an identical pattern of AKI. Identification of the cause(s) of AKI represents the initial step in approaching the patient with AKI. When AKI occurs in the ambulatory or hospital ward setting, a single precipitating factor can often be identified [25, 26]. By contrast, AKI in the ICU setting is almost always multifactorial in nature and usually occurs in the context of failure of at least one other organ system [5–8]. In the ICU setting, sepsis is the most common clinical setting in which AKI develops [5–10, 27].

A time-honored categorization of causes of AKI is shown in Fig. 3.1.2. Utilization of this or a comparable diagnostic approach ensures that the clinician consider the gamut of causes of AKI. Prerenal factors refer to conditions associated with renal hypoperfusion as the cause of filtration failure [28]. Prerenal events are among the most common contributors to AKI [5–10]. If left untreated, prerenal AKI can progress to ischemic acute tubular necrosis (ATN). In prerenal AKI, a vasomotor factor such as decreased renal perfusion pressure, afferent arteriolar constriction, or efferent arteriolar dilation acts to decrease glomerular capillary hydrostatic pressure [28]. Prerenal events include gastrointestinal, skin, or renal loss of fluid volume (e.g., vomiting, nasogastric suctioning, diarrhea, gastrointestinal hemorrhage, burns, heat stroke, diuretics, and glycosuria) or sequestration of extracellular fluid volume (e.g., muscle crush injury, intra-abdominal surgery, pancreatitis, interferon therapy, and early sepsis). Also, impaired cardiac output and hypotension resulting from antihypertensive medications

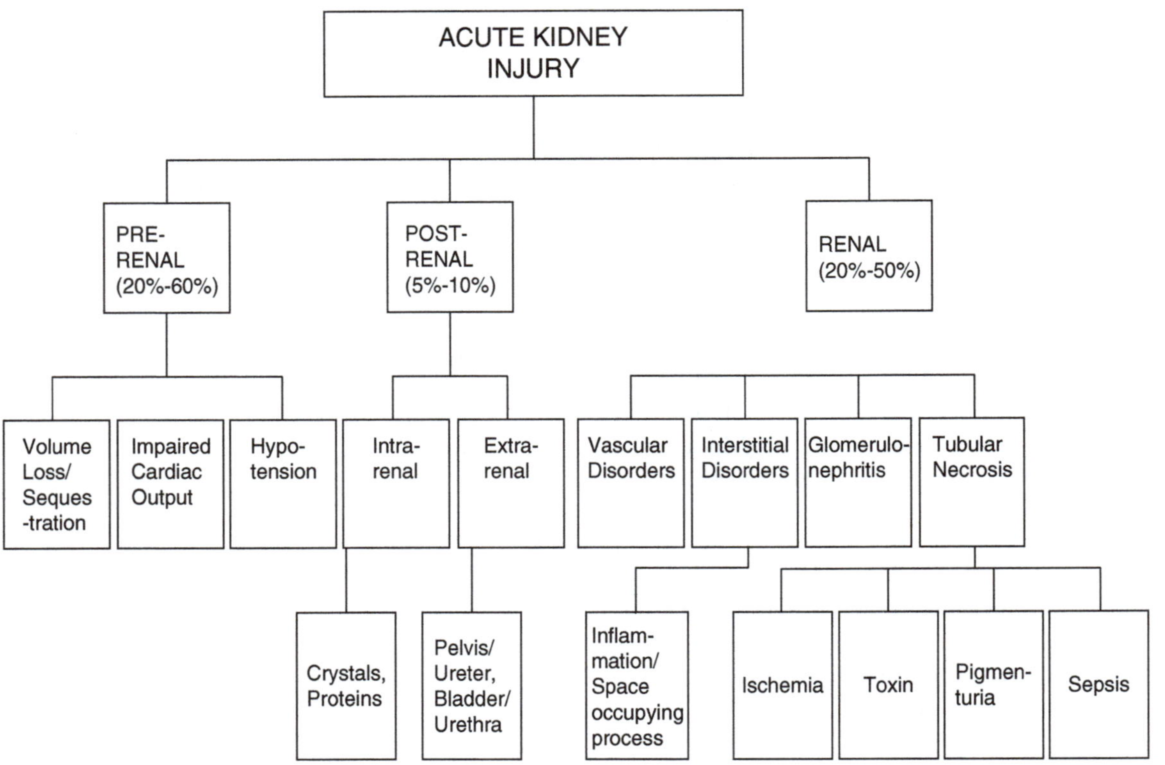

Fig. 3.1.2 Potential causes of acute kidney injury (AKI)

are prerenal factors that can contribute to AKI. Afferent arteriolar constriction caused either by enhanced vasoconstrictor influences (e.g., increased circulating norepinephrine, angiotensin II, endothelin, or enhanced renal adrenergic neural traffic) or by a decrease in vasodilators (e.g., eicosanoids, nitric oxide, and bradykinin) occurs in many cases of prerenal AKI. Such constriction can be due to medications such as nonsteroidal antiinflammatory agents (NSAIDs), cyclosporine, radiocontrast medium, tacrolimus, and amphotericin, and seen in the postoperative state, early sepsis, advanced liver disease, edematous disorders, and volume-depleted states. Efferent arteriolar dilation occurs in the context of angiotensin-converting enzyme inhibitors, angiotensin receptor antagonists, or direct renin inhibitors. These agents diminish the effect of angiotensin II to increase efferent arteriole tone and lower glomerular capillary hydrostatic pressure and GFR.

A relatively unusual "prerenal" form of AKI is that due to a hyperoncotic state. Infusion of either osmotically active substances such as mannitol, dextran, or maltose/sucrose (which is commonly contained in intravenous immunoglobulin preparations) can lead to high oncotic pressure, which exceeds glomerular capillary hydrostatic pressure [7]. This stops glomerular filtration and produces an anuric form of acute renal failure (ARF), which is usually rapidly alleviated by removal of the offending substance [7].

Postrenal causes of AKI are less commonly encountered (2–10% of all cases of AKI), but they are nearly always treatable [7]. Postrenal forms of AKI obstruct flow of either tubular fluid (intrarenal), or formed (extrarenal) urine. Since several proximal tubules drain into a single collecting tubule, intra-collecting tubular precipitation of either relatively insoluble crystals (methotrexate, acyclovir, sulfonamides, indinavir, uric acid, triamterene, and oxalic acid) or protein (plasma cell dyscrasia) can increase intratubular pressure [29]. If sufficiently high, the intratubular pressure opposes glomerular filtration pressure (glomerular hydrostatic pressure minus plasma colloid oncotic pressure) sufficiently to either decrease or stop glomerular filtration. Similarly, obstruction of the extrarenal collecting system at any level (pelvis, ureters, bladder, and urethra), can lead to postrenal AKI. Another cause of form of AKI that is being recognized with increasing frequency in ICU patients is the "intra-abdominal compartment syndrome." In this syndrome, high intra-abdominal pressure leads to diminished renal perfusion and functional ureteric blockade. Relief of intra-abdominal hypertension rapidly reverses AKI in this setting [30, 31].

Once prerenal and postrenal causes have been considered, attention should focus on the kidney itself. It is helpful to consider renal causes of AKI in terms of the anatomic compartments of the kidney. Disorders of the renal vasculature, including the small arteries (e.g., vasculitis, thrombotic thrombocytopenic purpura, hemolytic-uremic syndrome [HUS], malignant hypertension, eclampsia, scleroderma, disseminated intravascular coagulation [DIC]), the large arteries (e.g., thrombosis and emboli), and the renal veins (acute thrombosis) all can result in AKI. All forms of acute glomerulonephritis can, if severe, present as AKI. Acute inflammation and space-occupying processes of the renal interstitium (e.g., drug-induced allergic interstitial nephritis, severe infections such as pyelonephritis, autoimmune disorders, leukemia, or lymphoma, sarcoidosis) can also result in AKI. Collectively, these renal causes are relatively rare. By far the most commonly encountered "renal" form of AKI is presumably due to tubular damage and has been termed ATN. This renal form of AKI usually results from renal ischemia due to prolonged prerenal forms of AKI, nephrotoxins (e.g., radiocontrast medium, aminoglycosides, pentamidine, foscarnet, cisplatin, amphotericin, NSAIDs, heavy metals, and hydrocarbons), and pigmenturia (e.g., from hemoglobinuria due to intravascular hemolysis or from myoglobinuria due to rhabdomyolysis).

Noteworthy is the fact that sepsis, the most common condition associated with ICU-acquired AKI, defies easy classification in the prerenal, postrenal, and renal categorization of AKI and must be strongly considered in every case of AKI [27, 32, 33]. The kidney injury in sepsis and septic shock is likely multifactorial including hypotension, extracellular fluid volume sequestration, vasoconstriction, inflammation of several renal anatomic compartments, intravascular coagulation, and direct renal tubular toxic effects of endotoxin and cytokines [32].

3.1.4 Evaluation of AKI

3.1.4.1 Clinical

A sequential diagnostic approach to AKI is in Fig. 3.1.3. The medical history, record review and physical examination remain the cornerstone for determining the cause(s) of AKI. Table 3.1.4 details some of the key issues of potential relevance. The medical record

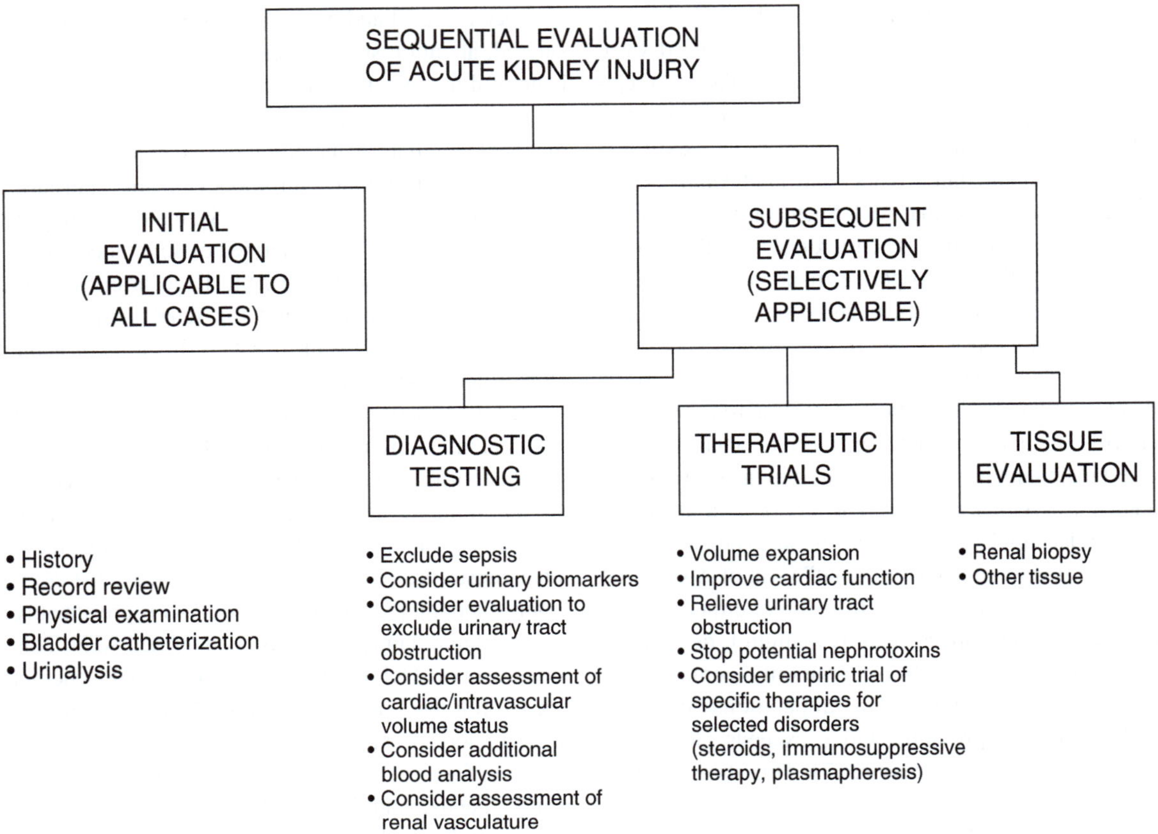

Fig. 3.1.3 Sequential diagnostic approach to acute kidney injury (AKI)

Table 3.1.4 History and physical examination in AKI

AKI predisposing factor	History	Physical exam
Sepsis	Invasive procedures, localized symptoms, fever, chills	Localized findings, SIRS criteria, indwelling catheters and devices
Extracellular fluid volume deficits	GI, renal, skin losses, recent surgery, sepsis, crush injury	Orthostatic hypotension and tachycardia, dry mucus membranes, absence of axillary sweat
Impaired cardiac function	Symptoms of heart failure	Increased jugular venous pressure, cardiac gallops, murmurs, atrial fibrillation, edema, evidence of bacterial endocarditis
Impaired liver function	Increasing abdominal girth, jaundice, edema, alcohol intake, hepatitis B and C infection	Ascites, jaundice, asterixis, edema, spider angiomata
Vascular disease	Diabetes mellitus, hyperlipidemia, hypertension, claudication	Pulses, palpitation of abdominal aorta
Medication/toxin exposure	Medical record and chart review	
Cancer	History of cancer, unexplained weight loss	Masses, adenopathy
Vasculitis	Rash, alopecia, photosensitivity, arthritis/arthralgia, Raynaud's	Palpable purpura
Pigmenturia	Blood transfusion, crush injury, trauma	Swollen/tender muscles
Obstructive uropathy	Voiding difficulties, history of genito-urinary or pelvic cancer	Enlarged bladder/prostate abnormal pelvic exam

review is especially important and should focus on recent clinical events, medication exposures, evidence of hypotension and/or sepsis, serial vital signs, intake/output, and body weights.

3.1.4.2 Laboratory

The laboratory evaluation begins with a routine and careful microscopic urinalysis (Fig. 3.1.4). A review of the hemogram can also be helpful. Significant anemia could point to either recent hemorrhage or intravascular hemolysis as factors contributing to AKI. A microangiopathic state (thrombocytopenia, reticulocytosis, elevated lactic acid dehydrogenase, deformed red blood cells on peripheral smear) with AKI occurs in the setting of thrombotic thrombocytopenic purpura (TTP), HUS, eclampsia of pregnancy, vasculitis, HIV infection, malignant hypertension, and selected medications. Anemia with rouleaux formation in the AKI setting suggests a plasma cell dyscrasia. Acute renal failure with eosinophilia is compatible with renal atheroemboli, acute interstitial nephritis, and polyarteritis nodosa. Leukopenia is common in patients with systemic lupus erythematosus (SLE) and AKI. Thrombocytopenia in the setting of AKI is compatible with TTP, HUS, SLE, DIC, rhabdomyolysis, advanced liver disease with hypersplenism, and "white clot syndrome" resulting from heparin administration as causes of the AKI. The presence of coagulation abnormalities, such as prolongation of the international normalized ratio (INR) and partial thromboplastin time (PTT), suggests underlying liver disease (increased INR), DIC (increased INR and PTT), and antiphospholipid syndrome (increased PTT), all of which can be associated with AKI. Sometimes, especially when the cause of AKI is either unclear or there is evidence of a systemic disorder, additional blood work such as antinuclear antibodies, anti-neutrophilic cytoplasmic antibodies, and anti-glomerular basement membrane antibodies may have diagnostic yield.

Hyperkalemia of modest degree (<5.5 mEq/l) is a common accompaniment of AKI. More marked hyperkalemia suggests the possibility of rhabdomyolysis, tumor lysis syndrome, intravascular hemolysis, or the use of NSAIDs as contributors to AKI. Mild metabolic acidosis occurs frequently as a consequence of AKI and is often associated with a modest (5–10 mEq/l) increase in anion gap. Marked acidosis with large anion gaps

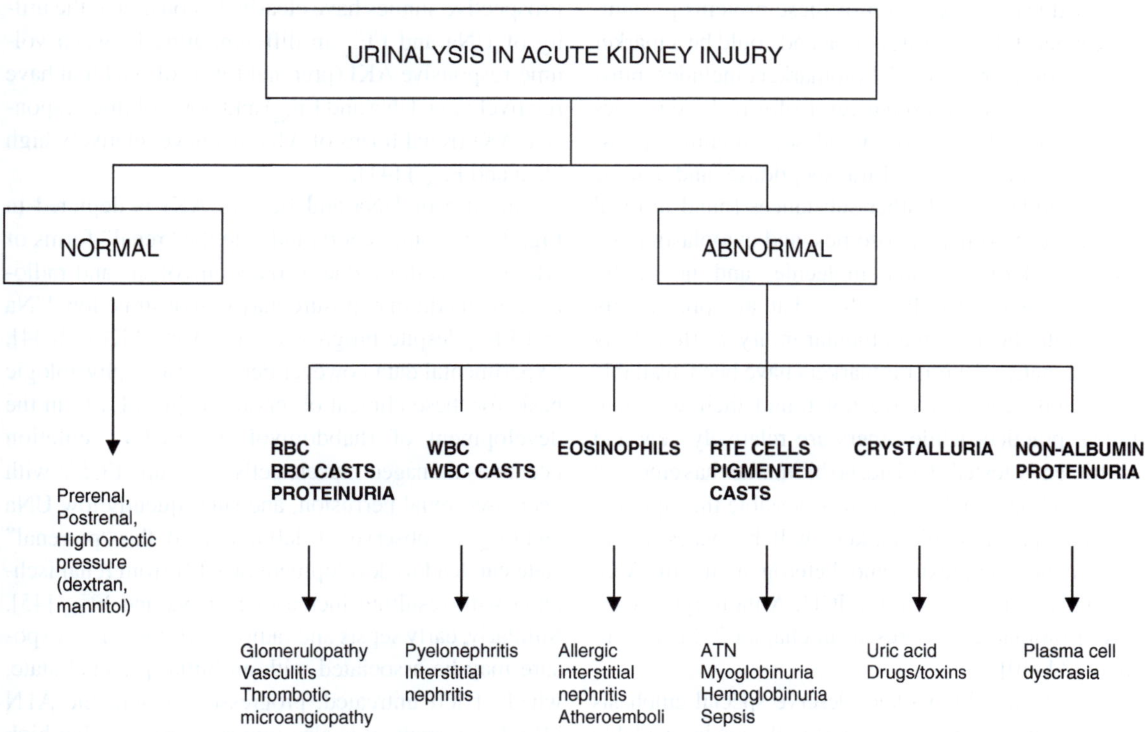

Fig. 3.1.4 Routine urinalysis in acute kidney injury (AKI)

in the setting of ARF should raise the suspicion of ethylene glycol poisoning, marked rhabdomyolysis, and lactic acidosis resulting from sepsis as contributors to AKI. Modest hyperuricemia (<10 mg/dl) usually accompanies AKI. Much higher levels of uric acid occur when tumor lysis syndrome, rhabdomyolysis, and heat stroke are contributors to AKI. Elevations in creatinine kinase, serum glutamic-oxaloacetic transaminase, and lactate dehydrogenase often occur in the setting of tumor lysis- and rhabdomyolysis-associated AKI.

The "Holy Grail" for the early diagnosis of AKI is an excellent biomarker for this disorder. The ideal AKI biomarker would be sensitive, specific, inexpensive, available noninvasively as a point-of-care test and would provide a real-time assessment of kidney function. Other potential uses for a biomarker include detection of predisposition to AKI, determination if the AKI is due to a prerenal, postrenal, or renal cause, localization of the anatomic site of kidney injury, and provision of prognostic information.

Available biomarkers include urinary excretion of small-molecular-weight proteins (e.g., amylase, lysozyme, β2-microglobulin, α1-microglobulin, and retinol-binding protein) that are readily filtered by the glomerulus and reabsorbed by normal tubules. Increased urinary excretion of these proteins presumably reflects tubular dysfunction and could be a marker of AKI. Another set of AKI biomarkers includes transporters (e.g., Na/H exchanger isoform 3), enzymes (e.g., *N*-acetyl-B-glucosaminidase, alkaline phosphatase, gamma-glutamyl transpeptidase, and alanine aminopeptidase), and other substances found in renal tubular brush borders, exosomes, and cytoplasm (e.g., cytokines, kidney injury molecule, and neutrophil gelatinase-associated lipocalin) that are presumably "shed" into the urine with tubular injury. Suffice it say that that many of these biomarkers have been available for several years but have not found their way into clinical practice, while others are relatively new and insufficiently tested. To date, no biomarker has emerged as an ideal marker for AKI. It is possible that application of a panel of biomarkers will be necessary to address the complexity and heterogenicity of AKI, especially as it occurs in the ICU. A thorough review of AKI biomarkers is present in chapter 3.2 and elsewhere [34–40].

Two of these biomarkers deserve special emphasis because either a point-of-care test will soon be available (interleukin-18 [IL-18]), or recent promising studies suggest clinical utility (neutrophil gelatinase-associated lipocalin [NGAL]) [37–39]. Studies indicate that urinary IL-18 increases 6–12 h after onset of renal injury in patients with a renal form of AKI, while prerenal forms of AKI do not demonstrate an increase in urinary IL-18 [37–39]. In patients with adult respiratory distress syndrome, elevated urinary IL-18 preceded clinical evidence of AKI by 24–48 h and predicted mortality [39].

In a study comprising 633 patients including normal controls and patients with a wide spectrum of renal disorders including AKI, urinary NGAL has been recently demonstrated to be 90% sensitive and nearly 100% specific to detect renal forms of AKI [40]. Urinary NGAL excretion had positive and negative likelihood ratios to detect AKI of 182 and 0.1, respectively [40]. In this study, urinary NGAL significantly outperformed urinary excretion of *N*-acetyl-B-D-glucosaminidase, α_1-acid-glycoprotein, α1 microglobulin, and fractional excretion of sodium (FE_{Na}) in determining the presence of AKI [40].

One widely used diagnostic aid in AKI is the measurement of either the sodium concentration (UNa) or the fractional excretion of sodium (FE_{Na} = urine/plasma sodium concentration divided by urine/plasma creatinine times 100) on a "spot" urine sample. Prospective studies have clearly demonstrated the utility of UNa and FE_{Na} in differentiating between volume-responsive AKI (prerenal forms of AKI that have relatively low UNa and FE_{Na}) and non-volume-responsive AKI (renal forms of AKI that have relatively high UNa and FE_{Na}) [41].

One use of UNa and FE_{Na} in AKI is depicted in Fig. 3.1.5. Some reports indicate the "renal" forms of AKI such as those due to rhabdomyolysis and radiocontrast medium exposure may demonstrate low UNa and FE_{Na} despite progression to severe AKI [42–44]. Experimental data however demonstrate a physiologic basis for these clinical observations [45]. Early in the development of rhabdomyolysis, ECFV depletion occurs as damaged muscle cells "take up" ECFV with decreased renal perfusion, and subsequently low UNa and FE_{Na} are observed. If left untreated, this "prerenal" state can lead to development of ATN from renal ischemia with resulting increases in UNa and FE_{Na} [45]. Similarly, early sepsis and radiocontrast medium exposure may be associated with an initial prerenal state, which if left untreated, progresses to ischemic ATN [46]. Conversely, it is also important to note that high

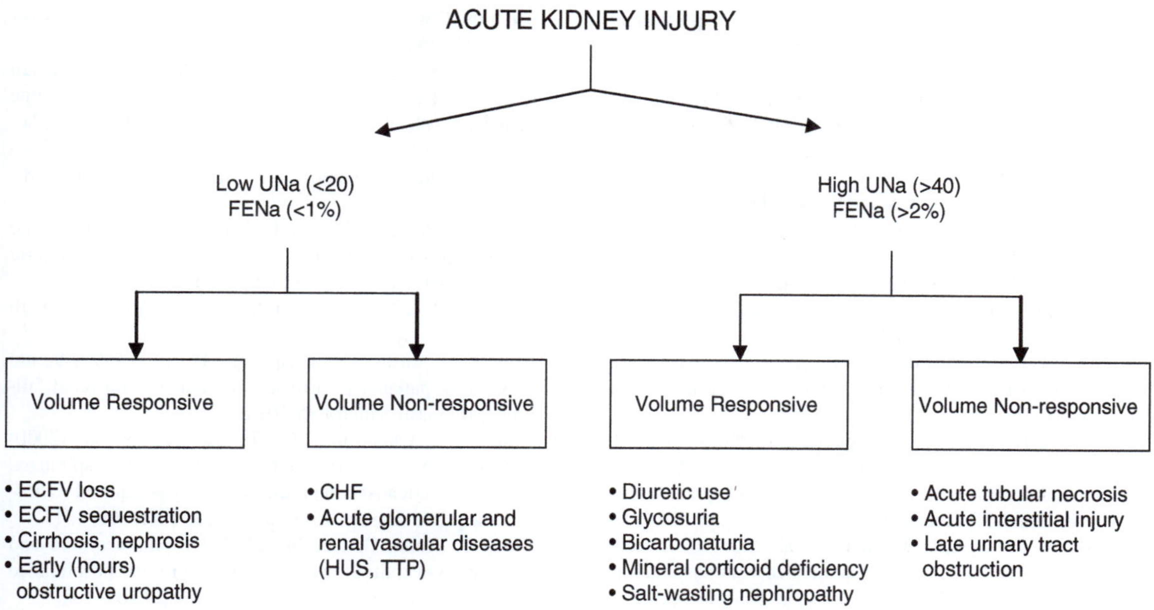

Fig. 3.1.5 Potential utility of fractional excretion of sodium (FE_{Na}) and/or sodium concentration (UNa) done on spot wine samples in the setting of acute kidney injury (AKI)

UNa and FE_{Na} can occur in selected volume-responsive forms of AKI such as those due to ECFV depletion resulting from diuretics, glycosuria, bicarbonaturia, and mineratocorticoid deficiency. In patients who have received diuretics, the fractional excretion of urea nitrogen may be diagnostically helpful in determining if a prerenal form of AKI is present [15].

Sometimes, despite thorough evaluation, the cause of AKI cannot be ascertained with a reasonable degree of certainty. Older observations suggest that the clinical evaluation discussed previously is capable of establishing a diagnosis of the cause of AKI in 75–80% of cases [47]. When doubt exists as to the cause of AKI after careful evaluation, it is appropriate to consider obtaining renal biopsy material. Indications for renal biopsy in the setting of AKI have not been firmly established. Many nephrologists strongly consider a biopsy when prerenal and postrenal factors have been excluded, and the clinical setting and laboratory data do not support a diagnosis of ATN. The presence of extrarenal manifestations that suggest a systemic disorder, heavy proteinuria, and red blood cell casts on urinalysis would also strongly support obtaining renal biopsy material in the AKI setting. Some studies suggest that histologic analysis of renal tissue in cases in which the cause of AKI is not apparent yields at least a 30–50% chance of detection of a treatable form of kidney disease [48–50]. A renal biopsy can be safely done even in ICU patients receiving mechanical ventilation [51].

3.1.5 Summary

Acute kidney injury can be produced through multiple pathophysiologic events in diverse clinical settings. A systematic approach to early detection and delineation of the causes of AKI is a necessary first step to implementing effective therapy. A careful history, medical record review, physical examination, and urinalysis serve as the starting point to detect the cause of AKI. Selected urinary biomarkers offer promise for the early detection of AKI.

References

1. Bagshaw SM, George C, Bellomo R (2007) Changes in the incidence and outcome for early acute kidney injury in a cohort of Australian intensive care units. Crit Care 11(3): R68.

2. Collins AJ, Foley R, Herzog C, et al (2008) Excerpts from the United States Renal Data System 2007 annual data report. Am J Kidney Dis 51(1 Suppl 1):S1–320.
3. Waikar SS, Wald R, Chertow GM, et al (2006) Validity of international classification of diseases, ninth revision, clinical modification codes for acute renal failure. J Am Soc Nephrol 17(6):1688–1694.
4. Xue JL, Daniels F, Star RA, et al (2006) Incidence and mortality of acute renal failure in Medicare beneficiaries, 1992 to 2001. J Am Soc Nephrol 17(4):1135–1142.
5. Mehta RL, Pascual MT, Soroko S, et al (2004) Spectrum of acute renal failure in the intensive care unit: the PICARD experience. Kidney Int 66(4):1613–1621.
6. Uchino S, Kellum JA, Bellomo R, et al (2005) Acute renal failure in critically ill patients: a multinational, multicenter study. JAMA 294(7):813–818.
7. Lee VWS, Harris DCH, Anderson RJ, et al (2007) Chapter 41. Acute renal failure. In: Diseases of the Kidney & Urinary Tract. Schrier RW (ed), vol. 2, 8th edn. Philadelphia: Wolters Kluwer Health/Lippincott Williams & Wilkins, pp 986–1034.
8. Hoste EA, Clermont G, Kersten A, et al (2006) RIFLE criteria for acute kidney injury are associated with hospital mortality in critically ill patients: a cohort analysis. Crit Care 10(3):R73.
9. Uchino S, Bellomo R, Goldsmith D, et al (2006) An assessment of the RIFLE criteria for acute renal failure in hospitalized patients. Crit Care Med 34(7):1913–1917.
10. Ostermann M, Chang RW (2007) Acute kidney injury in the intensive care unit according to RIFLE. Crit Care Med 35(8): 1837–1843; quiz 1852.
11. Lassnigg A, Schmidlin D, Mouhieddine M, et al (2004) Minimal changes of serum creatinine predict prognosis in patients after cardiothoracic surgery: a prospective cohort study. J Am Soc Nephrol 15(6):1597–1605.
12. Coca SG, Peixoto AJ, Garg AX, et al (2007) The prognostic importance of a small acute decrement in kidney function in hospitalized patients: a systematic review and meta-analysis. Am J Kidney Dis 50(5):712–720.
13. Mehta RL, Kellum JA, Shah SV, et al (2007) Acute Kidney Injury Network: report of an initiative to improve outcomes in acute kidney injury. Crit Care 11(2):R31.
14. Anderson RJ, Linas SL, Berns AS, et al (1977) Nonoliguric acute renal failure. New Engl J Med 296:1134.
15. Carvounis CP, Nisar S, Guro-Razuman S (2002) Significance of the fractional excretion of urea in the differential diagnosis of acute renal failure. Kidney Int 62:2223–2229.
16. Moran SM, Myers BD (1985) Course of acute renal failure studied by a model of creatinine kinetics. Kidney Int 27(6): 928–937.
17. Herget-Rosenthal S, Marggraf G, Husing J, et al (2004) Early detection of acute renal failure by serum cystatin C. Kidney Int 66(3):1115–1122.
18. Villa P, Jimenez M, Soriano MC, et al (2005) Serum cystatin C concentration as a marker of acute renal dysfunction in critically ill patients. Crit Care 9(2):R139–143.
19. Delanaye P, Lambermont B, Chapelle JP, et al (2004) Plasmatic cystatin C for the estimation of glomerular filtration rate in intensive care units. Intensive Care Med 30(5): 980–983.
20. Grubb A, Bjork J, Lindstrom V, et al (2005) A cystatin C-based formula without anthropometric variables estimates glomerular filtration rate better than creatinine clearance using the Cockcroft-Gault formula. Scand J Clin Lab Invest 65(2):153–162.
21. Grubb A, Nyman U, Bjork J, et al (2005) Simple cystatin C-based prediction equations for glomerular filtration rate compared with the modification of diet in renal disease prediction equation for adults and the Schwartz and the Counahan-Barraft prediction equations for children. Clin Chem 51(8): 1420–1431.
22. Herget-Rosenthal S, Poppen D, Husing J (2004) Prognostic value of tubular proteinuria and enzymuria in nonoliguric acute tubular necrosis. Clin Chem 50:552–558.
23. Henrich WL (2008) Serum cardiac enzymes in patients with renal failure. UpToDate 16.1.
24. Collen MJ, Ansher AF, Chapman AB, et al (1990) Serum amylase in patients with renal insufficiency and renal failure. Am J Gastroenterol 85(10):1377.
25. Obialo CI, Okonofua EC, Tayade AS, et al (2000) Epidemiology of de novo acute renal failure in hospitalized African Americans: comparing community-acquired vs hospital-acquired disease. Arch Intern Med 160:1309–1313.
26. Wang Y, Zhuan C, Fan M (2007) Hospital-acquired and community-acquired acute renal failure in hospitalized Chinese: a ten-year review. Renal Failure 29:163–168.
27. Bagshaw SM, Uchino S, Bellomo R, et al (2007) Septic acute kidney injury in critically ill patients: clinical characteristics and outcomes. Clin J Am Soc Nephrol 2(3):431–439.
28. Badr KF, Ichikawa I (1988) Prerenal failure: a deleterious shift from renal compensation to decompensation. New Engl J Med 319:623–629.
29. Perazella MA (1999) Crystal-induced acute renal failure. Am J Med 106:459.
30. Daugherty EL, Hongyan L, Taichman D, et al (2007) Abdominal compartment syndrome is common in medical intensive care unit patients receiving large volume fluid resuscitation. J Intensive Care Med 22:294–299.
31. Lui F, Sangosanya A, Kaplan LJ (2007) Abdominal compartment syndrome: clinical aspects and monitoring. Crit Care Clinics 23:415–433.
32. Schrier RW (2006) Urinary indices and microscopy in sepsis-related acute renal failure. Am J Kidney Dis 48:838–841.
33. Bellomo R, Bagshaw S, Langenberg C, et al (2007) Pre-renal azotemia: a flawed paradigm in critically ill septic patients? Contrib Nephrol 156:1–9.
34. Parikh CR, Devarajan P (2008) New Biomarkers of acute kidney injury. Crit Care Med 36(4) Suppl:S159–S165.
35. Bonventre JV (2007) Diagnosis of acute kidney injury: from classic parameters to new biomarkers. Contrib Nephrol 156: 213–219.
36. Dennen P, Parikh CR (2007) Biomarkers of acute kidney injury: can we replace serum creatinine? Clin Nephrol 68: 269–278.
37. Parikh CR, Jani A, Melnikov VY, et al (2004) Urinary interleukin-18 is a marker of human acute tubular necrosis. Am J Kidney Dis 43:405–14.
38. Parikh CR, Mishra J, Thiessen-Philbrook H, et al (2006) Urinary IL-18 is an early predictive biomarker of acute kidney injury after cardiac surgery. Kidney Int 70:199–203.
39. Parikh CR, Abraham E, Ancukiewicz M, et al (2005) Urine IL-18 is an early diagnostic marker for acute kidney injury and predicts mortality in the intensive care unit. J Am Soc Nephrol 16:3046–52.

40. Nickolas TL, O'Roarke MJ, Yong J, et al (2008) Sensitivity and specificity of a single emergency department measurement of urinary neutrophil gelatinase-associated lipocalcin for diagnosing acute kidney injury. Ann Intern Med 148: 810–819.
41. Miller TR, Anderson RJ, Linas SL, et al (1978) Urinary diagnostic indices in acute renal failure: a prospective study. Ann Intern Med 89:47–52.
42. Fang L, Sirota R, Ebert T, et al (1980) Low fractional excretion of sodium with contrast media-induced acute renal failure. Arch Intern Med 140:531–533.
43. Corwin HL, Schreiber MJ, Fang LS (1984) Low fractional excretion of sodium. Occurrence with hemoglobinuric-and myoglobinuric-induced acute renal failure. Arch Intern Med 144:981–2.
44. Vaz AJ (1983) Low fractional excretion of urine sodium in acute renal failure due to sepsis. Arch Intern Med 143:738–9.
45. Reineck HJ, O'Connor GJ, Lifschitz MD, et al (1980) Sequential studies on the pathophysiology of glycerol-induced acute renal failure. J Lab Clin Med 96:356.
46. Kikeri D, Pennell JP, Hwang KH, et al (1986) Endotoxemic acute renal failure in awake rats. Am J Physiol 250:F1098–106.
47. Mustonen J, Pasternak A, Helm H, et al (1984) Renal biopsy in acute renal failure. Am J Nephrol 4:27.
48. Cohen AH, Nast CC, Adler SG, et al (1989) Clinical utility of kidney biopsies in the diagnosis and management of renal disease. Am J Nephrol 9:309.
49. Wilson DM, Turner DR, Cameron JS, et al (1976) Value of renal biopsy in acute intrinsic renal failure. BMJ 2:459.
50. Border WA, Cohen AH (1980) Renal biopsy diagnosis of clinically silent multiple myeloma. Ann Intern Med 93:43.
51. Conlon PJ, Kovalik E, Schwab SJ (1995) Percutaneous renal biopsy of ventilated intensive care unit patients. Clin Nephrol 43:309.

Kidney Function Tests and Urinalysis

3.2

Sean M. Bagshaw

Core Messages

- The most common surrogates of kidney function are serum creatinine, urea, cystatin C; however, these all have limitations, most important of which is that they do not accurately reflecting real-time dynamic changes in glomerular filtration rate (GFR) that occur in acute kidney injury (AKI)
- The Cockcroft-Gault and Modification of Diet in Renal Disease (MDRD) Study Group equations are the most common methods used to estimate GFR; however, they have limited relevance to critically ill patients with AKI.
- Urine output can be a sensitive indicator for changes in renal hemodynamics, but it also has limited sensitivity and specificity
- Several tests of urinary biochemistry, derived indices and microscopy (i.e., FE_{Na}, UNa, FE_{U}) have traditionally been used as aids for the detection and classification of AKI; however, their value in sick patients (i.e., after fluid resuscitation, diuretics, vasopressor infusions, radiocontrast media, and nephrotoxic drugs) remains uncertain
- Novel urinary biomarkers (i.e., NHE3, NGAL, KIM-1, IL-18) have recently been characterized that may provide added diagnostic value and prognostic information for critically ill patients in AKI.

Objectives to Understand

- Overview of kidney function
- Overview of serum markers of kidney function in acute kidney injury
- Overview of urinary tests in acute kidney injury

3.2.1 Introduction

Acute kidney injury (AKI) remains a major therapeutic challenge for the modern clinician. Depending on the criteria used to define its presence, AKI has been described in 5–25% of critically ill patients [1–5]. Recently, a new consensus definition and classification for AKI has been developed and validated [6–8]. This definition, referred to by the acronym RIFLE, divides renal dysfunction into the categories of Risk (class R), Injury (class I), and Failure (class F) [9]. Using this classification, the incidence of at least some degree of renal dysfunction has been shown to be as high as 67% in a recent study of >5,000 critically ill patients [8]. Moreover, the occurrence of renal dysfunction with a maximum RIFLE class F was found in up to 28% of critically ill patients and associated with a several-fold increased risk of hospital death [7, 8]. Thus, despite advances in our understanding of the pathophysiology and application of supportive extracorporeal therapies for AKI, the associated morbidity and mortality remains excessive. Therefore, the timely and accurate diagnosis of AKI is of paramount prognostic and therapeutic importance. In this chapter, the common serum measures of kidney function and urinary tests used in AKI are reviewed. In addition, the potential diagnostic and prognostic role of several novel urinary biomarkers will be discussed.

S. M. Bagshaw
Division of Critical Care Medicine, University of Alberta Hospital, University of Alberta, 3C1.12 Walter C. Mackenzie Centre, 8440–112 Street, Edmonton, Alberta T6G 2B7, Canada
e-mail: bagshaw@ualberta.ca

A. Jörres et al. (eds.), *Management of Acute Kidney Problems*,
DOI: 10.1007/978-3-540-69441-0_3.2, © Springer-Verlag Berlin Heidelberg 2010

3.2.2 Overview of Kidney Function

Before considering the spectrum serum and urinary tests available to evaluate AKI, a logical approach is to begin by understanding the scope of functions performed by the kidney. Moreover, it should be highlighted that many of these functions are either shared with other organs (i.e., acid–base control with the lungs) or involve complex neurohormonal interactions, which in itself also involves other organ systems (i.e., renin–angiotensin–aldosterone axis). In addition, other functions are not routinely measured (i.e., small peptide excretion, tubular metabolism, hormonal production) in the everyday care of the patient with AKI. The kidney contributes several essential functions for maintaining physiologic homeostasis in the body, including:

- Contributing to maintain a constant extracellular milieu through urinary excretion of water, electrolytes, acids, and metabolic waste products (i.e., creatinine, urea, uric acid)
- Regulation of systemic and renal hemodynamics by production of renin, angiotensin II, endothelin, prostaglandins, and nitric oxide
- Secretion of erythropoietin for regulation of red blood cell production
- Secretion of 1,25-dihydroxyvitamin D3 for regulation of calcium, phosphate, and bone metabolism
- Participating in metabolism of small peptides
- Participating in gluconeogenesis during fasting or starvation

Thus, in AKI, some or all of these vital functions may be impaired or absent. The critically ill patient with AKI may have retention of uremic metabolites, decreased capacity for regulation of extracellular volume status, impaired electrolyte and acid–base balance, anemia, and/or accumulation of exogenous toxins.

3.2.3 Assessment of Kidney Function

Generally speaking, the term AKI refers to a syndrome characterized by a rapid (hours to days) decrease in the kidney's ability to eliminate waste products, regulate extracellular volume, and maintain electrolyte and acid–base homeostasis. This loss in excretory function is clinically manifested by an accumulation of end products of metabolism (i.e., creatinine and urea), diminished urine output (i.e., not always present), accumulation of non-volatile acids, and/or an increased serum potassium concentration.

Clinicians at the bedside have relied on these measurable effects to characterize an acute loss in kidney excretory function and for defining and identifying patients with AKI. As a consequence, various serum and urinary tests have been developed and routinely applied in clinical practice.

In view of critically ill patients with AKI having a poor prognosis and increased risk of death, it is clearly desirable to have tests of kidney function that would allow clinicians to diagnose AKI early and that would correlate with true reductions in kidney function associated with acute injury. This would permit the identification of those critically ill patients in whom early and aggressive intervention may be justified.

3.2.3.1 *Glomerular Filtration Rate*

Most tests of kidney function are fashioned to approximate and/or estimate the glomerular filtration rate (GFR). GFR is a global measure of kidney function. The GFR is defined as the sum of the filtration rates for all functioning nephrons in a given patient. GFR is known to vary based on patient age, race, sex, and body mass. In addition, GFR exhibits considerable inter- and intra-patient variation; however, normal values in young health adults are typically in the range of 90 – 120 ml/min/1.73 m² [25]. AKI, therefore, is regarded as an acute decrease in GFR. The main difficulty with GFR is that it cannot be measured directly, but rather can only be estimated by calculating the clearance of a filtered serum marker:

$$\text{GFR (ml/min)} = (U_a \times V)/P_a$$

Where (a) represents an ideal serum marker of GFR, U_a represents the urinary concentration of (a), V represents urine flow rate, and P_a represents the serum concentration of (a), and under ideal circumstances, the filtered load of (a) would equal GFR.

The ideal serum marker to estimate GFR would ideally encompass several characteristics; in particular, such a marker would be endogenous and nontoxic, freely filtered at the glomerulus and excreted unchanged in the urine (i.e., not secreted, metabolized or reabsorbed by renal tubular cells), not influenced by exogenous compounds (i.e., drugs), and be water soluble with minimal protein binding. Moreover, such an ideal marker would be sensitive to both early and small changes in GFR, and would be reliably measured across diverse patient populations and severities of AKI. Finally, an ideal marker should be easy, rapid, and inexpensive to measure. Regrettably, such an ideal serum marker has yet to be discovered. While there are several exogenous serum markers that can be used to estimate GFR (i.e., inulin, iothalamate, EDTA, and iohexol), often their measurement is complex, expensive, and impractical for routine clinical practice in critically ill patients.

3.2.3.2 Serum Markers of Kidney Function in AKI

The most commonly used and practical serum tests to estimate GFR are endogenous markers such as creatinine, urea, and cystatin C. Unfortunately, none are ideal and each has its own limitations. However, one major limitation of all of these endogenous markers is that none reflect real-time dynamic changes in GFR that occur with acute reductions in kidney function. Rather, each endogenous marker requires time to accumulate and before being detected as abnormal, leading to a potential delay in the diagnosis of AKI. In addition, each of these serum markers can potentially be grossly modified by aggressive fluid resuscitation.

3.2.3.3 Serum Creatinine

Creatinine is an amino acid compound derived from the metabolism of creatine in skeletal muscle and from dietary meat intake. Creatinine has a molecular weight of 113 Da, is released into the plasma at a relatively constant rate, is freely filtered by the glomerulus, and is not reabsorbed or metabolized by the kidney. Accordingly, the clearance of creatinine is the most widely used means for estimating GFR [10]. Serum creatinine levels generally have an inverse relationship to GFR. Thus, a rise in serum creatinine is associated with corresponding decrease in GFR and generally implies a reduction in kidney function and vice versa. However, there are limitations with the use of creatinine as a serum marker to estimate GFR.

First, an estimated 10–40% of creatinine clearance occurs by tubular secretion of creatinine into the urine by the organic cation secretory pathways in the proximal renal tubular cells [11]. While this is generally more important for patients with early chronic kidney disease (CKD), where serum creatinine levels appear stable (i.e., generally in range <133 μmol/l) due to compensatory increases in proximal renal tubular secretion. This effect, however, can potentially mask a significant initial decline in GFR. Second, several drugs are known to impair creatinine secretion and thus may cause a transient and reversible increases in serum creatinine (i.e., trimethoprim and cimetidine). Third, the production and release of creatinine into the serum can be highly variable. Differences in dietary intake (i.e., vegetarian or creatine supplements) and/or baseline muscle mass (i.e., neuromuscular disease, malnutrition or amputation) can result in significant variation in baseline serum creatinine. Likewise, certain pathologic states may predispose to variable release of muscle creatinine. For example, in rhabdomyolysis, serum creatinine levels may rise more rapidly due to release of preformed creatinine from damaged muscle and/or peripheral metabolism of creatine phosphate to creatinine in extracellular tissue [12, 13]. Finally, there can be factors that reduce the accuracy of serum creatinine assays and lead to artifactual increases in serum creatinine levels. For example, in diabetic ketoacidosis, increased serum concentration of acetoacetate can cause interference with selected assays (i.e., alkaline picrate method) and present a falsely elevated serum creatinine value [14]. Similarly, some drugs are known to cause similar effects (i.e., cefoxitin and flucytosine).

3.2.3.4 Serum Urea Concentration

Urea is a water-soluble, low-molecular-weight by-product of protein metabolism that is recognized as a useful serum marker of uremic solute retention and elimination. For chronic hemodialysis patients, the degree of urea clearance has clearly shown correlation with clinical outcome and is used to model hemodialysis adequacy over time. Acute and large rises in serum urea concentration are characteristic of development of the uremic syndrome and retention of a large variety of uremic toxins. In addition, the accumulation of urea itself is believe to predispose to adverse metabolic, biochemical, and physiologic effects such as increased oxidative stress, altered function of $Na^+/K^+/Cl^-$ cotransport pathways important in regulation of intracellular potassium and water, and alterations in immune function [15–17].

Similar to serum creatinine, urea exhibits a nonlinear and inverse relationship with GFR. However, the use of urea to estimate GFR is problematic due to the numerous potential extrarenal factors, independent of GFR, that can influence its endogenous production and renal clearance.

First, the rate of urea production is not constant (Table 3.2.1). Urea can increase in response to a high protein intake, critical illness (i.e., sepsis, burns, trauma), gastrointestinal hemorrhage, or drug therapy such as use of corticosteroids or tetracycline [18]. Conversely, patients with chronic liver disease and low protein intake can have lower urea levels without noticeable changes in GFR. In fact, the accurate measurement of kidney function in patients with chronic liver disease can be problematic [19, 20]. For example, cirrhotic patients may have near normal values for urea (i.e., due to decreased production, protein restriction) and serum creatinine (i.e., decreased production due to decreased hepatic creatine synthesis, increased tubular creatinine secretion, and/or loss of skeletal muscle mass) despite severely impaired kidney function.

Table 3.2.1 Reported factors that may influence accuracy of serum measures of kidney function

Serum marker	Factor
Creatinine	Age
	Race
	Sex
	Muscle mass
	Ingestion of meat Amputation
	Chronic illness
	Neuromuscular diseases
	Vegetarian diet
Urea	Liver disease
	Low protein intake
	Trauma
	Burns
	Sepsis
	Gastrointestinal bleeding
	Corticosteroids
	Tetracycline
Cystatin C	Age
	Sex
	Height
	Weight
	Smoking status
	Inflammation
	Thyroid disease
	Corticosteroids

Table 3.2.2 Traditional laboratory tests used to help diagnose "established" acute kidney injury

Test	Prerenal AKI	Established AKI
Urine sediment	Normal	Epithelial casts
Specific gravity	High: > 1.020	Low: < 1.020
Urine sodium (mmol/l)	Low: < 10	High: > 20
Fractional excretion of sodium	< 1%	>1%
Fractional excretion of urea	<35%	>35%
Urine osmolality (mOsm/kg H_2O)	High: > 500	Near serum: <300
U/P creatinine ratio	High: >40	Low: < 10
P urea to creatinine ratio	High	Normal

U = urine; P = plasma

Second, the rate of renal clearance of urea is not constant. An estimated 40–50% of filtered urea is passively reabsorbed by proximal renal tubular cells. Moreover, in states of decreased effective circulating volume (i.e., volume depletion, low cardiac output), there is enhanced reabsorption of sodium and water in the proximal renal tubular cells along with a corresponding increase in urea reabsorption. Consequently, the serum urea concentration may increase out of proportion with changes serum creatinine and be underrepresentative of GFR. The ratio of serum urea to serum creatinine concentration has by tradition been used as an index to discriminate so-called prerenal AKI and more established AKI (i.e., acute tubular necrosis [ATN]) (Table 3.2.2).

3.2.3.5 Serum Cystatin C

Cystatin C is an endogenous cysteine proteinase inhibitor of low molecular weight that holds many ideal features for use as a surrogate marker of kidney function and estimate of GFR. Cystatin C is synthesized at a relatively constant rate and released into plasma by all nucleated cells in the body [21–23]. It is reportedly not affected by patient age, sex, muscle mass, or changes in diet. However, this has recently been challenged (Table 3.2.1). In a large cross-sectional study of 8,058 patients, several factors were found associated with elevated cystatin C levels including: older age, male sex, greater height, greater weight, current smoking status, and elevated C-reactive protein levels [24]. Cystatin C levels have also been found to be influenced by abnormal thyroid function, use of immunosuppressive therapy (i.e., corticosteroids) or the presence of systemic inflammation [24–27].

Nonetheless, the main catabolic site of cystatin C is the kidney with more than 99% freely filtered by the glomerulus. Cystatin C is not notably secreted or reabsorbed. However, it is nearly completely metabolized by proximal renal tubular cells. As a consequence, there is little to no detectable cystatin C in present in the urine. Thus, while a reduction in GFR correlates well with a rise in serum cystatin C level, true clearance of cystatin C cannot be determined. However, serum cystatin C concentrations have demonstrated good inverse correlations with radionuclide-derived measurements of GFR [22, 28].

The diagnostic value of cystatin C as an estimate of GFR has now been investigated in multiple clinical studies and has performed comparably or superior to the diagnostic accuracy of serum creatinine for discrimination of normal from impaired kidney function [22, 28]. In addition, cystatin C may be more sensitive to early and mild changes to kidney function compared with creatinine [29–31].

Recently, estimation equations for GFR based on serum cystatin C levels have been formulated [32, 33]. There is suggestion that cystatin C–based estimates of GFR may show superior performance in selected patient populations, in particular those with lower serum creatinine concentrations such as elderly patients, children, renal transplant recipients, cirrhotics, and those who are malnourished [34, 35]. However, the main drawback for use of cystatin C is that there is no widely accepted or available standardized method to measure cystatin C. Thus, whether cystatin C can be incorporated into routine clinical practice and enable improvements in the diagnosis of AKI and have an impact on outcome for critically ill patients requires additional investigations.

3.2.3.6 Equations to Estimate GFR

Several equations to estimate GFR have been developed and validated. The two most commonly used are the Cockcroft-Gault and Modification of Diet in Renal Disease (MDRD) Study Group equations [36, 37]. These equations estimate GFR based on a patient's serum creatinine concentration while at the same time incorporating several recognized demographic and clinical factors that can independently influence serum creatinine concentration such as age, sex, race, and body weight.

The Cockcroft-Gault equation to estimate creatinine clearance [36]:

$$\text{CrCl} = (140 - \text{age}) \times \text{IBW}/\text{SCr}\ (\times\ 0.85 \text{ for women})$$

Where CrCl represents creatinine clearance (ml/min), age is measured in years, IBW represents ideal body weight (kg), and SCr represents serum creatinine (μmol/l).

The abbreviated MDRD equation to estimate GFR [37]:

$$\text{GFR} = 186.3 \times (\text{SCr}/88.4) - 1.15 \times (\text{age}) - 0.203 \times (0.742 \text{ if female}) \times (1.21 \text{ if black})$$

Where GFR represents glomerular filtration rate (ml/min/1.73 cm^2), and SCr represents serum creatinine (μmol/l). The final two terms of the equation are adjustments for patient sex (i.e., female) and race (i.e., black). These formulas can be accessed online at www.kidney.org/professional/kdoqi/gfr_calculator or www.nephron.com where estimates of GFR can be automatically calculated.

In the end, however, use of these GFR estimation equations is limited, in particular for critically ill patients with AKI. First, there are several populations where these equations have not been validated, such as those with liver disease, kidney transplant recipients, morbidly obese, and patients at extremes of age. Second, these equations require stability in kidney function and a stable serum creatinine value. In general, for the critically ill patient with a rapidly changing serum creatinine, data from these equations is not interpretable and would not reflect dynamic changes to GFR. In addition, it is important to highlight that in the critically ill patient, exact knowledge of GFR is generally not necessary and provides little supplementary information. Rather, what is vital is to recognize whether kidney function is stable or acutely changing. This can usually be interpreted by comparisons of changes in serum creatinine from baseline [6]. As an example, an elderly woman who is malnourished may have a baseline creatinine that is well below the lower range of normal (i.e., 35 μmol/l), and whereby a twofold increase would still represent a serum creatinine in the "normal" range. The estimated GFR in this circumstance would yield a normal value, yet, not be valid or interpretable. However, such as change in serum creatinine from baseline would be indicative of a severe reduction in kidney function.

3.2.3.7 Urinary Tests in Acute Kidney Injury

3.2.3.7.1 Urine Output

Urine output is a commonly measured parameter of kidney function in AKI. Following of urine output can be advantageous because it is a dynamic gauge of kidney function and is measured continuously. Urine output can be a more sensitive barometer for changes in renal hemodynamics than biochemical markers of solute clearance. Dynamic changes to urine output have been integrated into the RIFLE classification of AKI [6]. However, the urine output is also of limited sensitivity and specificity, with patients capable of developing severe AKI, as detected by a markedly elevated serum creatinine, while maintaining normal urine output (i.e., so-called nonoliguric AKI). Since nonoliguric AKI has been described as having a better outcome than oliguric AKI, urine output is frequently used to differentiate AKI; however, the value of this distinction is questionable and can be frequently be negated by the use of diuretics [38]. Oliguria has classically been defined (approximately) as urine output < 5 ml/kg/day or 0.5 ml/kg/h.

3.2.3.7.2 Urinary Biochemistry and Derived Indices

Numerous tests of urinary biochemistry and derived indices have been described and traditionally used to aid clinicians for the detection and classification of early AKI into prerenal AKI and so-called ATN or established AKI. These tests and indices are outlined in Table 3.2.2.

Fractional Excretion of Sodium – Traditionally, the fractional excretion of filtered sodium (FE_{Na}) has been advocated for the discrimination between a prerenal and established AKI [39–41]. Filtered sodium is avidly reabsorbed in the renal tubules from glomerular filtrate in the setting of prerenal AKI, resulting in a FE_{Na} <1%, whereas in the setting of renal tubular injury in established AKI, the resulting FE_{Na} is >1%. However, the diagnostic utility of the FE_{Na} has been questioned, and there are several reports indicating that FE_{Na} mandates careful interpretation [42, 43]. For example, FE_{Na} is often >1% in patients having received diuretic therapy regardless of the fluid status of the patient [44, 45]. Furthermore, a FE_{Na} <1% has been shown in conditions associated with parenchymal AKI including sepsis, rhabdomyolysis, and exposure to radiocontrast media, perhaps reflecting nonhomogenous injury to the renal parenchyma and preservation of tubular function in some regions [46–49].

Urinary Sodium Concentration: The urinary sodium (UNa) is a widely cited urinary measure for the classification of AKI with values <10–20 mmol/l generally suggestive of a sodium avid state and prerenal AKI, whereas values >40 mmol/l are more consistent with ATN [40, 50–52]. Several studies have found UNa performs poorly for discriminating prerenal AKI and ATN. In one study, only 33% of patients classified as suffering from prerenal AKI had a UNa <20 mmol/l, whereas, 23% of those classified as ATN had a UNa <20 mmol/l [53]. Fewer still have reported changes to UNa over time. Several small reports have found a UNa <20 mmol/l in critically ill patients with hyperdynamic septic shock [49, 54, 55]. Similar data have been found in a large mammalian model of hyperdynamic septic AKI where there is evidence of an early decline in UNa <20 mmol/l and FE_{Na} <1% despite grossly elevated renal blood flow [46, 56]. These series of experimental studies challenge the prevailing dogma of low UNa and FE_{Na} reflecting a state of prerenal AKI. Moreover, Pru et al. suggested that the UNa and FE_{Na} are poor prognostic predictors for the need for renal replacement therapy (RRT) or recovery of renal function after an episode of AKI [43]. The available data suggests UNa has little diagnostic or prognostic value for critically ill patients with AKI.

Fractional Excretion of Urea: The fractional excretion of urea (FE_U) has been cited as a more precise method for discriminating early AKI, in particular if concomitant diuretic therapy has been given, with a FE_U <35% indicating prerenal AKI and >35% consistent with ATN [52]. In a study by Carvounis et al. where AKI was classified as prerenal AKI by diuretic exposure or ATN, a FE_U <35% was evident in 90%, 89%, and 4% of patients for cases of prerenal, prerenal with diuretics, and ATN, respectively [44]. This study found that FE_U was superior in sensitivity and specificity compared with FE_{Na} for classifying AKI.

Urine to Plasma Creatinine Ratio: The urine to plasma (U/P) creatinine ratio has been cited as a measure to aid in the classification of AKI, with values >40 suggestive of prerenal AKI and <20 indicative of ATN [50, 51]. While studies have described the classic pattern in U/P creatinine ratios [40, 44]; other studies have shown inconsistent results [49, 54, 57]. For example, in one series, 83% of ratios were <20 in the setting of presumed ATN [54]. Likewise, other studies have found ratios >40 in only 33–50% of those classified as prerenal AKI [49, 55, 57]. Moreover, there are numerous examples whereby a ratio <20 appears to contradict the findings of a FE_{Na} <1% in classifying AKI [49, 57, 58]. As a consequence, the value of the U/P creatinine ratio for discriminating AKI remains unproven.

Serum Urea to Creatinine Ratio: A serum urea to creatinine ratio value >20 is considered suggestive of prerenal AKI and <10–15 reflective of ATN [51]. In one study, a serum urea to creatinine ratio <15 was found in 38% of those with presumed prerenal AKI [57]. Likewise, this ratio frequently misclassified AKI in patients in another study [44]. Overall, no studies have evaluated the diagnostic and/or prognostic value of this ratio in AKI.

Additional Biochemistry/Indices: There are numerous additional urinary biochemistry tests and derived indices that have been reported that aim to further improve our capability to discriminate pre-renal AKI from established AKI. These have included U/P urea ratio [40, 57, 59]; urine uric acid to creatinine ratio [60]; fractional excretion of uric acid [57, 60]; fractional excretion of chloride [57]; and the renal failure index (RFI) [40, 57, 61]. However, due to such a few number of small studies, the significance of each of these measures for classifying or making predictions about prognosis in patients with AKI remains unproven.

In summary, considering the evidence available, the clinical utility of these urinary biochemical tests and derived indices in the diagnosis, classification, and for providing prognostic information in hospitalized and/or critically ill patients who often receive massive fluid resuscitation, diuretics, vasopressor infusions, radiocontrast media, and nephrotoxic drugs remains untested and questionable [43, 62]. The significance of these urinary tests and indices in the context of septic AKI was recently reviewed [62]. This study concluded there was no single urinary test that could be reliably used to diagnose, classify, or predict the clinical course of septic AKI. Moreover, it is imperative to recognize that so-called prerenal AKI and established ATN are part of a continuum, and their separation in diagnostic terms is rather arbitrary and has limited clinical implications or prognostic value. In general, targeted therapeutic interventions would be similar, specifically, to address the underlying cause of AKI while ensuring prompt and adequate resuscitation of the patient.

3.2.3.7.3 Urinalysis and Microscopy

Urinalysis and microscopy is an essential and simple noninvasive test that can yield important diagnostic information and patterns suggestive of specific syndromes. Ideally, sterile urine should be collected, centrifuged, and separated. The supernatant should be tested for color, pH, specific gravity, protein, and glucose while the sediment is placed on a slide and examined under a microscope for cells, casts, crystals, and bacteria.

Color: Urine is normally clear with a mild yellow color that varies with concentration. Several factors can influence the color of urine. Urine appears red/brown in many pathologic states. Red color restricted to the urine sediment is suggestive of hematuria. A red supernatant should prompt assessment of heme pigment usually due to myoglobinuria or hemoglobinuria. Red supernatant that is heme negative would suggest other uncommon causes (i.e., porphyria, drugs, beet ingestion). In addition, the urine may appear white due to pyuria, and uncommonly green due to administration of methylene blue, propofol or amitriptyline, or blue/black due to ochronosis.

Protein: Protein is frequently detected in the urine of hospitalized and/or critically ill patients [63]. This can result from several factors and may be transient in response to critically illness, physiologic stress, fever, or persistent and due to new acute or pre-existing kidney disease. An increase in urinary protein excretion is commonly associated with sepsis [54, 61, 64–67]. The urinary protein can generally be classified into glomerular, tubular, or overflow based on its probable site of origin. Glomerular proteinuria results from leakage and filtration of large-molecular-weight protein (i.e., albumin) across the glomerular capillary wall and implies intrinsic injury to this structure (i.e., glomerulonephritis). Tubular proteinuria, on the other hand, is due to filtration of lower-molecular-weight proteins (i.e., immunoglobulin, retinol-binding protein) that are incompletely reabsorbed by proximal renal tubular cells. Overflow proteinuria results from increased excretion of low-molecular proteins that are markedly overproduced (i.e., immunoglobulins in multiple myeloma) and generally exceed the reabsorptive capacity of proximal renal tubular cells. Detecting and quantifying urinary protein in patients may provide not only data on the etiology of AKI but also important prognostic information [68–70]. A urinary dipstick or calculation of a total protein to creatinine or albumin to creatinine ratio can be easily performed at the bedside. However, urinary dipstick primarily detects macroalbuminuria only, and thus would not detect microalbuminuria (i.e., <300–500 mg/day) or the presence of low-molecular-weight proteins. A sulfosalicylic acid (SSA) test can detect all types of protein in the urine and may alternatively be performed. However, radiocontrast media have been shown to cause false positives in both urinary dipstick and SSA tests [71]. In the end, in those patients where there is suspicion of clinically important proteinuria, quantitative assessments of protein excretion should be performed (i.e., timed urine collection). In addition, serum and urine protein electrophoresis can be done to assess for low-molecular-weight proteinuria.

pH: Normal urine pH ranges from 4.5 to 8.0, however, it can vary depending on patient acid–base status and therapeutic interventions (i.e., administration of bicarbonate). Routine monitoring of urinary pH in patients has little practical importance. However, urinary pH can be informative in patients with metabolic acidosis to assess for appropriate urinary acid excretion. In addition, urinary pH monitoring is important during intentional urinary alkalinization (i.e., rhabdomyolysis, salicylate poisoning) to monitor response to sodium bicarbonate loading. Finally, urinary tract infection with urease-splitting pathogens such as *Proteus mirabilis* can be a cause of highly alkaline urine (i.e., pH >7.5).

Urine Specific Gravity and Osmolality: Measurement of the urine specific gravity (USG), defined as the ratio of the weight of a given solution compared with that of an equal volume of distilled water, is generally used as a surrogate for urine osmolality. The USG and osmolality are generally well correlated; however, large molecules in the urine, such as glucose or radiocontrast media, can increase USG with no significant change in osmolality. While serum osmolality is generally regulated within a narrow physiologic range (i.e., 280–290 mOsm/kg), the urine osmolality fluctuates widely in response to changes in serum osmolality and the volume status of the patient. Measurement of USG and osmolality has limited values in hospitalized and/or critically ill patients [72]. However, urine osmolality has traditionally been used as a measure to discriminate prerenal AKI and established AKI and may have value for the diagnosis of diabetes insipidus [40, 67] (Table 3.2.2).

Glucose: Glucose is regularly detected in the urine of hospitalized and/or critically ill patients and in this setting has limited clinical value [67, 73]. The detection of glucose in the urine can signify surplus filtration due to elevated serum glucose concentrations or dysfunctional reabsorption by the proximal renal tubular cells.

Urine Microscopy: While small quantities of cells, casts, crystals, and bacteria can be encountered in healthy patients, for the sick patient with AKI, assessment of urine sediment by microscopy can yield important diagnostic information.

The cells found in urine sediment include red blood cells (RBC), white blood cells (WBC), and epithelial cells. Microscopic hematuria may be commonly encountered in critically ill patients (i.e., severe sepsis), however, evidence of gross hematuria may reflect urogenital trauma or other serious underlying pathology (i.e., bladder cancer) while the presence of dysmorphic RBC or RBC casts are virtually diagnostic of active glomerulonephritis or vasculitis [61, 74, 75]. Pyruia (WBCs in urine) can arise from several conditions, by far the most common being infection. However, sterile (culture-negative) pyruia can occur with tuberculosis infection, severe sepsis, interstitial nephritis, and nephrolithiasis [61, 74]. While many epithelial cells may appear in the urine, only renal tubular epithelial cells have diagnostic significance [54, 65, 74, 75]. The existence of renal tubular epithelial cells in the urine, in particular when present with casts, indicate a kidney source of injury such as with tubular necrosis, tubular apoptosis, or pyelonephritis [76].

There are several types of casts that can occur in the urine. Casts form as a result of conformation to the renal tubule and appear cylindrical in structure. Hyaline casts are common and can be present under normal circumstances or with concentrated urine specimens. On the other hand, the detection of cellular casts (RBC, WBC, or epithelial) is abnormal and typically signifies significant kidney injury. RBC casts are virtually pathognomonic of glomerulonephritis or vasculitis. WBC casts are classically can be seen with acute pyelonephritis or tubulointerstitial diseases.

Epithelial cell casts can be seen in conditions where epithelial cells are necrosed and/or desquamated such as ATN, apoptosis, or loss of renal tubular cell basement membrane integrity [76]. Granular and waxy casts generally represent the progressive degeneration of cellular casts. Such descriptions of the urinary sediment represent additional widely accepted criteria for the discrimination of AKI into prerenal or ATN. The classic urinary sediment description of ATN is evidence of renal tubular epithelial cells with coarse granular, muddy brown, or mixed cellular casts, whereas the sediment in prerenal AKI is rather bland with occasional hyaline or fine granular casts [50–52, 77]. However, the use of urinary microscopy for classifying AKI is imperfect and often fails to correlate with urinary biochemistry or derived indices. For example, in one small study, no significant differences in microscopy could be found based on a FE_{Na} values <1% or >1% [74]. Moreover, while abnormal sediment has been described in ATN, normal microscopy has also been described even days after onset of kidney injury [54, 61, 64–67, 74]. In addition, the urinary sediment may be highly variable and dependent more on the timing of measurement, duration, and the underlying pathophysiology predisposing to AKI (i.e., ischemic vs septic) [62].

The occurrence of crystals in the urine generally has little clinical importance for hospitalized and/or critically ill patients; however, it may be important in select circumstances. For example, the finding of calcium oxylate crystals in a patient with a high anion gap metabolic acidosis and AKI would suggest poisoning with ethylene glycol. Likewise, the presence of uric acid cystalluria and AKI may signify tumor lysis syndrome. Importantly, a normal urinalysis can also yield diagnostic information and suggest that AKI is due to factors extrinsic to the kidney (i.e., prerenal) or has an obstructive etiology.

3.2.3.7.4 Urinary Biomarkers

Several novel biomarkers (i.e., proteins, enzymes, antigens, cytokines) that can be detected in the urine of patients have been suggested as surrogate markers for acute kidney injury. The rationale for characterization of many of these biomarkers has been to further aid in the early diagnosis AKI, to help characterize the potential anatomical site of injury (i.e., proximal tubular, distal tubule, etc.) and provide potentially important prognostic data on the severity and nature of injury (i.e., septic, toxic, ischemic) [78, 79]. A summary and classification of currently available biomarkers is presented Tables 3.2.3–3.2.5. This section will focus on some of the newer biomarkers to be described that show early promise for use in routine clinical practice.

Urinary Na+/H+exchanger isoform 3 (NHE3): NHE3 is the most abundant sodium transporter in the renal tubule and is responsible for the reabsorption of large amounts of filtered sodium from the urine. NHE3 is normally expressed on the apical membrane of proximal renal tubular and thick ascending loop of Henle cells. Normally NHE3 is not detectable in the urine. However, abnormal elevations of NHE3 have been described in the urine of critically ill patients with AKI [80]. In this small

Table 3.2.3 Urinary proteins reported as potential indicators of acute kidney injury

Urinary proteins	Proposed site of nephron injury
Low-molecular-weight proteins:	
α_1-Microglobulin	Proximal renal tubule
B_2-Microglobulin	Proximal renal tubule
Retinol binding protein	Proximal renal tubule
High-molecular-weight proteins:	
Albumin	Glomerulus
Immunoglobulin	Glomerulus
Transferrin	Glomerulus
Other:	
Tamm-Horsfall glycoprotein	Distal renal tubule/ ascending loop of Henle

Source: Adapted from [21]

Table 3.2.4 Urinary enzymes reported as potential surrogate markers of acute kidney injury

Urinary enzymes	Proposed site of nephron injury
Brush border antigens	
Adenosine deaminase binding protein	Proximal renal tubule
Proximal renal tubular epithelial antigen (HRTE-1)	Proximal renal tubule
Carbonic anhydrase	Proximal renal tubule
Urinary enzymes	
Alanine aminopeptidase	Proximal renal tubule
Cathepsin B	Proximal renal tubule
Neutral endopeptidase	Proximal renal tubule
γ-Glutamyl transferase	Proximal renal tubule
Alkaline phosphatase	Proximal/distal renal tubule
β-Glucosidase	Proximal/distal renal tubule
Lactate dehydrogenase	Proximal/distal renal tubule
N-Acetyl-β-glucosaminidase	Proximal/distal renal tubule
Kallikrein	Distal renal tubule

Source: Adapted from [21]

Table 3.2.5 Summary of novel urinary biomarkers and cytokines reported as potential surrogate markers of early acute kidney injury

Urinary biomarker
Actin
Cysteine-rich protein 61 (Cyr61)
Glutathione-S-transferases
Kidney injury molecule-1 (KIM-1)
Na/H Exchanger Isoform 3 (NHE3)
Neutrophil gelatinase-associated lipocalin (NGAL)
Cytokines:
Interleukin-1
Interleukin-6
Interleukin-8
Interleukin-18
Platelet-activating factor (PAF)
Tumor necrosis factor-α

Source: Adapted from [21]

study, AKI was classified as prerenal azotemia, ATN, or intrinsic AKI other than ATN. The urinary NHE3 was significantly higher in those designated as ATN when compared with prerenal azotemia. In addition, urinary NHE3 was not detected in patients with intrinsic AKI other than ATN (i.e., glomerulonephritis or renal transplant rejection). These findings suggest that detection of NHE3 may be a novel early biomarker of AKI and may aid in discrimination of prerenal azotemia, ATN, and AKI due to other intrinsic renal causes. Further prospective studies are necessary to verify the diagnostic and prognostic value of NHE3.

Neutrophil gelatinase-associated lipocalin (NGAL): NGAL belongs to the lipocalin superfamily of >20 structurally related secreted proteins and are thought to participate in ligand transport with a β-barreled calyx [81]. Human NGAL was originally isolated as a 25-kDa protein covalently bound to gelatinase from human neutrophils and was shown to be markedly up-regulated in response to kidney ischemic or nephrotoxic injury [81, 82]. The appearance of NGAL in the urine after injury was rapid and preceded the detection of other known urinary biomarkers. These results suggested that NGAL may be an early and sensitive urinary biomarker of ischemic and nephrotoxic acute kidney injury. Elevations in urinary NGAL early (1–3 h) after cardiac surgery with cardiopulmonary bypass has been shown to be highly sensitive, specific, and predictive for delayed acute kidney injury [83, 84]. Similarly, early elevations in urinary NGAL after kidney transplantation were predictive of delayed graft failure, and need for RRT during the first week posttransplant [85, 86].

Kidney Injury Molecule-1 (KIM-1): KIM-1 is a type 1 transmembrane glycoprotein that is normally minimally expressed in kidney tissue, however, shows marked up-regulation in proximal renal tubular cells in response to ischemic or nephrotoxic acute kidney injury [87–89]. The ectodomain segment of KIM-1 is shed from proximal cells and detected in the urine by immunoassay [90]. Kidney biopsies from patients with ATN show increased and significantly greater KIM-1 tissue expression compared with other acute and chronic kidney diseases [90]. In addition, urinary levels of KIM-1 were significantly higher in ATN compared with other causes of AKI (i.e., prerenal AKI, contrast-induced nephropathy) or CKD. KIM-1 may represent an early, noninvasive biomarker for proximal tubular AKI; however, further prospective studies are needed to characterize its utility in clinical practice.

Urinary Cytokines: Numerous cytokines have now been detected in the urine of patients with AKI including interleukin-1 (IL-1), IL-6, IL-8, IL-18, tumor necrosis factor-α, and platelet-activating factor (PAF) [21, 78, 79, 91]. Inflammatory states characterized by increased production of these cytokines may both be a consequence of and predispose to AKI. In one series of 40 patients undergoing kidney transplant, urinary IL-6, IL-8, and actin were found to be elevated and predictive of early and sustained postoperative AKI [92].

In another small series, increased PAF was detected in the urine of patients with septic AKI [93]. Moreover, urinary PAF was correlated with additional serum and urine inflammatory cytokines (i.e., IL-1, IL-6, IL-8, and TNF-α) leading to speculation as to whether PAF has a role in the pathophysiology of acute kidney injury in sepsis. Experimental studies have shown IL-18 to be a mediator of ischemic AKI. Urinary IL-18 concentrations were found to be significantly increased in the urine of patients with ATN when compared with urine from those with prerenal azotemia, urinary tract infection, CKD, or healthy controls [94]. In addition, raised urinary IL-18 concentrations after kidney transplant have been shown to be predictive of delayed graft failure [86, 94]. Early detection (4–6 h) of urinary IL-18 after cardiac surgery with cardiopulmonary bypass has also been found to be predictive of late increases (48–72 h) in serum creatinine suggestive of acute kidney injury [95]. Recently, in a nested case-control study of critically ill patients with acute respiratory distress syndrome (ARDS), elevated urinary IL-18 values preceded clinical evidence of overt AKI by 24–48 h [96]. Moreover, in this patient population, a high urinary IL-18 concentration at enrollment was an independent predictor of mortality.

The newer urinary biomarkers have generally only recently been developed and have not been assessed in large prospective studies and are not widely available. Therefore, while encouraging, the value of these biomarkers as early noninvasive tests to diagnose kidney injury, guide in classifying AKI, or provide useful prognostic data remains uncertain. Additional investigation will hopefully provide further insights into their role.

3.2.4 Summary

Acute kidney injury is a complex and heterogeneous syndrome. This is all the more evident in the context of critical illness. The hospitalized and/or critically ill patient with AKI frequently has a multitude of factors that can predispose to or worsen kidney function, such as the presenting illness (i.e., sepsis, major surgery, liver disease), preexisting comorbidities (e.g., CKD), ongoing investigations (i.e., radiocontrast media), and/or therapeutic interventions (i.e., mechanical ventilation, antimicrobials and/or diuretics). In these circumstances, accurate measures of kidney function and detection of injury are essential. While many kidney function and urinary tests have been described, it is likely that no one test will ever be considered ideal or have sufficient sensitivity and specificity to be valuable across a broad spectrum of patients with AKI. As a consequence, clinicians generally continue to rely on the measurement of serum creatinine, urea, and urine output as the three pillars to diagnose and classify AKI. Future study will hopefully clarify the role of cystatin C for routine measurement of kidney function. More traditional tests of urinary biochemistry and derived indices used to discriminate prerenal AKI from ATN appear to have limited value and are increasingly supplanted by search for novel noninvasive biomarkers that would allow for early detection of kidney injury across a spectrum of AKI. Many urinary biomarkers require further investigation to clarify their diagnostic and prognostic utility. However, many are promising and hold the potential to guide research in nephrology in exciting new directions.

References

1. Bagshaw SM, Laupland KB, Doig CJ, et al. Prognosis for long-term survival and renal recovery in critically ill patients with severe acute renal failure: a population-based study. *Crit Care*. 2005;9:R700–R709
2. de Mendonca A, Vincent JL, Suter PM, et al. Acute renal failure in the ICU: risk factors and outcome evaluated by the SOFA score. *Intensive Care Med*. 2000;26:915–921
3. Liano F, Junco E, Pascual J, Madero R, Verde E. The spectrum of acute renal failure in the intensive care unit compared with that seen in other settings. The Madrid Acute Renal Failure Study Group. *Kidney Int Suppl*. 1998;66: S16–24
4. Uchino S, Kellum JA, Bellomo R, et al. Acute renal failure in critically ill patients: a multinational, multicenter study. *JAMA*. 2005;294:813–818
5. Metnitz PG, Krenn CG, Steltzer H, et al. Effect of acute renal failure requiring renal replacement therapy on outcome in critically ill patients. *Crit Care Med*. 2002;30:2051–2058
6. Bellomo R, Ronco C, Kellum JA, Mehta RL, Palevsky P. Acute renal failure - definition, outcome measures, animal models, fluid therapy and information technology needs: the Second International Consensus Conference of the Acute Dialysis Quality Initiative (ADQI) Group. *Crit Care*. 2004;8: R204–212
7. Uchino S, Bellomo R, Goldsmith D, Bates S, Kellum J, Ronco C. An Assessment of the RIFLE Criteria for Acute Renal Failure in Hospitalized Patients. *Crit Care Med*. 2006;34:1913–1917
8. Hoste EA, Clermont G, Kersten A, et al. RIFLE criteria for acute kidney injury are associated with hospital mortality in

critically ill patients: a cohort analysis. *Crit Care.* 2006;10:R73
9. Hoste EAJ, Kellum JA. Acute kidney injury: epidemiology and diagnostic criteria. *Curr Opin Crit Care.* 2006;12: 531–537
10. Stevens LA, Levey AS. Measurement of kidney function. *Med Clin North Am.* 2005;89:457–473
11. Shemesh O, Golbetz H, Kriss JP, Myers BD. Limitations of creatinine as a filtration marker in glomerulopathic patients. *Kidney Int.* 1985;28:830–838
12. Grossman RA, Hamilton RW, Morse BM, Penn AS, Goldberg M. Nontraumatic rhabdomyolysis and acute renal failure. *N Engl J Med.* 1974;291:807–811
13. Oh MS. Does serum creatinine rise faster in rhabdomyolysis? *Nephron.* 1993;63:255–2557
14. Molitch ME, Rodman E, Hirsch CA, Dubinsky E. Spurious serum creatinine elevations in ketoacidosis. *Ann Intern Med.* 1980;93:280–281
15. Kaji DM, Lim J, Shilkoff W, Zaidi W. Urea inhibits the Na-K pump in human erythrocytes. *J Membr Biol.* 1998;165: 125–131
16. Lim J, Gasson C, Kaji DM. Urea inhibits NaK2Cl cotransport in human erythrocytes. *J Clin Invest.* 1995;96: 2126–2132
17. Prabhakar SS, Zeballos GA, Montoya-Zavala M, Leonard C. Urea inhibits inducible nitric oxide synthase in macrophage cell line. *Am J Physiol.* 1997;273:C1882–1888
18. Chalasani N, Clark WS, Wilcox CM. Blood urea nitrogen to creatinine concentration in gastrointestinal bleeding: a reappraisal. *Am J Gastroenterol.* 1997;92:1796–1799
19. Sherman DS, Fish DN, Teitelbaum I. Assessing renal function in cirrhotic patients: problems and pitfalls. *Am J Kidney Dis.* 2003;41:269–278
20. Papadakis MA, Arieff AI. Unpredictability of clinical evaluation of renal function in cirrhosis. Prospective study. *Am J Med.* 1987;82:945–952
21. Han WK, Bonventre JV. Biologic markers for the early detection of acute kidney injury. *Curr Opin Crit Care.* 2004; 10:476–482
22. Herget-Rosenthal S, Feldkamp T, Volbracht L, Kribben A. Measurement of urinary cystatin C by particle-enhanced nephelometric immunoassay: precision, interferences, stability and reference range. *Ann Clin Biochem.* 2004;41: 111–118
23. Herget-Rosenthal S, Kribbin A. Urinary cystatin C: preanalytical and analytical characteristics and its clinical application. *Dade Behring J.* 2004:13–15
24. Knight EL, Verhave JC, Spiegelman D, et al. Factors influencing serum cystatin C levels other than renal function and the impact on renal function measurement. *Kidney Int.* 2004; 65:1416–1421
25. Manetti L, Genovesi M, Pardini E, et al. Early effects of methylprednisolone infusion on serum cystatin C in patients with severe Graves' ophthalmopathy. *Clin Chim Acta.* 2005; 356:227–228
26. Manetti L, Pardini E, Genovesi M, et al. Thyroid function differently affects serum cystatin C and creatinine concentrations. *J Endocrinol Invest.* 2005;28:346–349
27. Rule AD, Larson TS. Response to 'Calculation of glomerular filtration rate using serum cystatin C in kidney transplant recipients'. *Kidney Int.* 2006;70:1878–1879
28. Villa P, Jimenez M, Soriano MC, Manzanares J, Casasnovas P. Serum cystatin C concentration as a marker of acute renal dysfunction in critically ill patients. *Crit Care.* 2005;9: R139–143
29. Coll E, Botey A, Alvarez L, et al. Serum cystatin C as a new marker for noninvasive estimation of glomerular filtration rate and as a marker for early renal impairment. *Am J Kidney Dis.* 2000;36:29–34
30. Hoek FJ, Kemperman FA, Krediet RT. A comparison between cystatin C, plasma creatinine and the Cockcroft and Gault formula for the estimation of glomerular filtration rate. *Nephrol Dial Transplant.* 2003;18:2024–2031
31. Dharnidharka VR, Kwon C, Stevens G. Serum cystatin C is superior to serum creatinine as a marker of kidney function: a meta-analysis. *Am J Kidney Dis.* 2002;40:221–226
32. Grubb A, Bjork J, Lindstrom V, Sterner G, Bondesson P, Nyman U. A cystatin C-based formula without anthropometric variables estimates glomerular filtration rate better than creatinine clearance using the Cockcroft-Gault formula. *Scand J Clin Lab Invest.* 2005;65: 153–162
33. Grubb A, Nyman U, Bjork J, et al. Simple cystatin C-based prediction equations for glomerular filtration rate compared with the modification of diet in renal disease prediction equation for adults and the Schwartz and the Counahan-Barratt prediction equations for children. *Clin Chem.* 2005;51:1420–1431
34. Poge U, Gerhardt T, Stoffel-Wagner B, et al. Cystatin C-based calculation of glomerular filtration rate in kidney transplant recipients. *Kidney Int.* 2006;70:204–210
35. Poge U, Gerhardt T, Stoffel-Wagner B, Klehr HU, Sauerbruch T, Woitas RP. Calculation of glomerular filtration rate based on cystatin C in cirrhotic patients. *Nephrol Dial Transplant.* 2006;21:660–664
36. Cockcroft DW, Gault MH. Prediction of creatinine clearance from serum creatinine. *Nephron.* 1976;16:31–41
37. Levey AS, Bosch JP, Lewis JB, Greene T, Rogers N, Roth D. A more accurate method to estimate glomerular filtration rate from serum creatinine: a new prediction equation. Modification of Diet in Renal Disease Study Group. *Ann Intern Med.* 1999;130:461–470
38. Hou SH, Bushinsky DA, Wish JB, Cohen JJ, Harrington JT. Hospital-acquired renal insufficiency: a prospective study. *Am J Med.* 1983;74:243–248
39. Espinel CH. The FENa test. Use in the differential diagnosis of acute renal failure. *JAMA.* 1976;236:579–581
40. Miller TR, Anderson RJ, Linas SL, et al. Urinary diagnostic indices in acute renal failure: a prospective study. *Ann Intern Med.* 1978;89:47–50
41. Espinel CH, Gregory AW. Differential diagnosis of acute renal failure. *Clin Nephrol.* 1980;13:73–77
42. Zarich S, Fang LS, Diamond JR. Fractional excretion of sodium. Exceptions to its diagnostic value. *Arch Intern Med.* 1985;145:108–112
43. Pru C, Kjellstrand CM. The FENa test is of no prognostic value in acute renal failure. *Nephron.* 1984;36:20–23
44. Carvounis CP, Nisar S, Guro-Razuman S. Significance of the fractional excretion of urea in the differential diagnosis of acute renal failure. *Kidney Int.* 2002;62:2223–2229
45. Kaplan AA, Kohn OF. Fractional excretion of urea as a guide to renal dysfunction. *Am J Nephrol.* 1992;12:49–54

46. Langenberg C, Wan L, Bagshaw SM, Egi M, May CN, Bellomo R. Urinary biochemistry in experimental septic acute renal failure. *Nephrol Dial Transplant*. 2006
47. Fang L, Sirota R, Ebert T, Lichtenstein N. Low fractional excretion of sodium with contrast media-induced acute renal failure. *Arch Intern Med*. 1980;140:531–533
48. Corwin HL, Schreiber MJ, Fang LS. Low fractional excretion of sodium. Occurrence with hemoglobinuric- and myoglobinuric-induced acute renal failure. *Arch Intern Med*. 1984;144:981–982
49. Vaz AJ. Low fractional excretion of urine sodium in acute renal failure due to sepsis. *Arch Intern Med*. 1983;143: 738–739
50. Esson ML, Schrier RW. Diagnosis and treatment of acute tubular necrosis. *Ann Intern Med*. 2002;137:744–752
51. Needham E. Management of acute renal failure. *Am Fam Physician*. 2005;72:1739–1746
52. Van Biesen W, Yegenaga I, Vanholder R, et al. Relationship between fluid status and its management on acute renal failure (ARF) in intensive care unit (ICU) patients with sepsis: a prospective analysis. *J Nephrol*. 2005;18:54–60
53. Zager RA, Rubin NT, Ebert T, Maslov N. Rapid radioimmunoassay for diagnosing acute tubular necrosis. *Nephron*. 1980;26:7–12
54. Diamond JR, Yoburn DC. Nonoliguric acute renal failure associated with a low fractional excretion of sodium. *Ann Intern Med*. 1982;96:597–600
55. Cabrera J, Arroyo V, Ballesta AM, et al. Aminoglycoside nephrotoxicity in cirrhosis. Value of urinary beta 2-microglobulin to discriminate functional renal failure from acute tubular damage. *Gastroenterology*. 1982;82:97–105
56. Langenberg C, Wan L, Egi M, May CN, Bellomo R. Renal blood flow in experimental septic acute renal failure. *Kidney Int*. 2006;69:1996–2002
57. Fushimi K, Shichiri M, Marumo F. Decreased fractional excretion of urate as an indicator of prerenal azotemia. *Am J Nephrol*. 1990;10:489–494
58. Smith-Erichsen N. Renal and liver function tests in surgical septicemia. *Acta Anaesthesiol Scand*. 1987;31:208–213
59. Perlmutter M, Grossman SL, Rothenberg S, Dobkin G. Urine serum urea nitrogen ratio; simple test of renal function in acute azotemia and oliguria. *JAMA* 1959;170: 1533–1537
60. Tungsanga K, Boonwichit D, Lekhakula A, Sitprija V. Urine uric acid and urine creatine ratio in acute renal failure. *Arch Intern Med*. 1984;144:934–937
61. Chesney PJ, Davis JP, Purdy WK, Wand PJ, Chesney RW. Clinical manifestations of toxic shock syndrome. *JAMA*. 1981;246:741–748
62. Bagshaw SM, Langenberg C, Bellomo R. 2006 Urinary biochemistry and microscopy in septic acute renal failure – a systematic review. *Am J Kidney Dis*. 48:695–705
63. Thorevska N, Sabahi R, Upadya A, Manthous C, Amoateng-Adjepong Y. Microalbuminuria in critically ill medical patients: prevalence, predictors, and prognostic significance. *Crit Care Med*. 2003;31:1075–1081
64. Gay C, Cochat P, Pellet H, Floret D, Buenerd A. Urinary sediment in acute renal failure. *Pediatrie*. 1987;42:723–727
65. Graber M, Lane B, Lamia R, Pastoriza-Munoz E. Bubble cells: renal tubular cells in the urinary sediment with characteristics of viability. *J Am Soc Nephrol*. 1991;1:999–1004
66. Richmond JM, Sibbald WJ, Linton AM, Linton AL. Patterns of urinary protein excretion in patients with sepsis. *Nephron*. 1982;31:219–223
67. Strauch M, McLaughlin JS, Mansberger A, et al. Effects of septic shock on renal function in humans. *Ann Surg*. 1967;165:536–543
68. Gosling P, Brudney S, McGrath L, Riseboro S, Manji M. Mortality prediction at admission to intensive care: a comparison of microalbuminuria with acute physiology scores after 24 hours. *Crit Care Med*. 2003;31:98–103
69. Gosling P, Czyz J, Nightingale P, Manji M. Microalbuminuria in the intensive care unit: Clinical correlates and association with outcomes in 431 patients. *Crit Care Med*. 2006;34: 2158–2166
70. Gopal S, Carr B, Nelson P. Does microalbuminuria predict illness severity in critically ill patients on the intensive care unit? A systematic review. *Crit Care Med*. 2006;34: 1805–1810
71. Morcos SK, el-Nahas AM, Brown P, Haylor J. Effect of iodinated water soluble contrast media on urinary protein assays. *BMJ*. 1992;305:29
72. Lugo N, Silver P, Nimkoff L, Caronia C, Sagy M. Diagnosis and management algorithm of acute onset of central diabetes insipidus in critically ill children. *J Pediatr Endocrinol Metab*. 1997;10:633–639
73. Zaloga GP, Chernow B, McFadden E, Soldano S, Lyons P, O'Brian JT. Urine glucose testing in the critically ill: a comparison of two enzymatic test strips. *Crit Care Med*. 1984; 12:188–190
74. Brosius FC, Lau K. Low fractional excretion of sodium in acute renal failure: role of timing of the test and ischemia. *Am J Nephrol*. 1986;6:450–457
75. Marotto MS, Marotto PC, Sztajnbok J, Seguro AC. Outcome of acute renal failure in meningococcemia. *Ren Fail*. 1997; 19:807–810
76. Wan L, Bellomo R, Di Giantomasso D, Ronco C. The pathogenesis of septic acute renal failure. *Curr Opin Crit Care*. 2003;9:496–502
77. Klahr S, Miller SB. Acute oliguria. *N Engl J Med*. 1998; 338:671–675
78. Wedeen RP, Udasin I, Fiedler N, et al. Urinary biomarkers as indicators of renal disease. *Ren Fail*. 1999;21:241–249
79. Price RG, Wedeen R, Lichtveld MY, et al. Urinary biomarkers: roles in risk assessment to environmental and occupational nephrotoxins: monitoring of effects and evaluation of mechanisms of toxicity. *Ren Fail*. 1999;21:xiii–xviii
80. du Cheyron D, Daubin C, Poggioli J, et al. Urinary measurement of Na+/H+ exchanger isoform 3 (NHE3) protein as new marker of tubule injury in critically ill patients with ARF. *Am J Kidney Dis*. 2003;42:497–506
81. Mishra J, Ma Q, Prada A, et al. Identification of neutrophil gelatinase-associated lipocalin as a novel early urinary biomarker for ischemic renal injury. *J Am Soc Nephrol*. 2003;14:2534–2543
82. Mishra J, Mori K, Ma Q, Kelly C, Barasch J, Devarajan P. Neutrophil gelatinase-associated lipocalin: a novel early urinary biomarker for cisplatin nephrotoxicity. *Am J Nephrol*. 2004;24:307–315
83. Mishra J, Dent C, Tarabishi R, et al. Neutrophil gelatinase-associated lipocalin (NGAL) as a biomarker for acute renal injury after cardiac surgery. *Lancet*. 2005;365:1231–1238

84. Wagener G, Jan M, Kim M, et al. Association between increases in urinary neutrophil gelatinase-associated lipocalin and acute renal dysfunction after adult cardiac surgery. *Anesthesiology*. 2006;105:485–491
85. Mishra J, Ma Q, Kelly C, et al. Kidney NGAL is a novel early marker of acute injury following transplantation. *Pediatr Nephrol*. 2006;21:856–863
86. Parikh CR, Jani A, Mishra J, et al. Urine NGAL and IL-18 are predictive biomarkers for delayed graft function following kidney transplantation. *Am J Transplant*. 2006;6: 1639–1645
87. Ichimura T, Bonventre JV, Bailly V, et al. Kidney injury molecule-1 (KIM-1), a putative epithelial cell adhesion molecule containing a novel immunoglobulin domain, is up-regulated in renal cells after injury. *J Biol Chem*. 1998;273: 4135–4142
88. Ichimura T, Hung CC, Yang SA, Stevens JL, Bonventre JV. Kidney injury molecule-1: a tissue and urinary biomarker for nephrotoxicant-induced renal injury. *Am J Physiol Renal Physiol*. 2004;286:F552–563
89. Vaidya VS, Ramirez V, Ichimura T, Bobadilla NA, Bonventre JV. Urinary kidney injury molecule-1: a sensitive quantitative biomarker for early detection of kidney tubular injury. *Am J Physiol Renal Physiol*. 2006;290:F517–529
90. Han WK, Bailly V, Abichandani R, Thadhani R, Bonventre JV. Kidney Injury Molecule-1 (KIM-1): a novel biomarker for human renal proximal tubule injury. *Kidney Int*. 2002; 62:237–244
91. D'Amico G, Bazzi C. Urinary protein and enzyme excretion as markers of tubular damage. *Curr Opin Nephrol Hypertens*. 2003;12:639–643
92. Kwon O, Molitoris BA, Pescovitz M, Kelly KJ. Urinary actin, interleukin-6, and interleukin-8 may predict sustained ARF after ischemic injury in renal allografts. *Am J Kidney Dis*. 2003;41:1074–1087
93. Mariano F, Guida G, Donati D, et al. Production of platelet-activating factor in patients with sepsis-associated acute renal failure. *Nephrol Dial Transplant*. 1999;14:1150–1157
94. Parikh CR, Jani A, Melnikov VY, Faubel S, Edelstein CL. Urinary interleukin-18 is a marker of human acute tubular necrosis. *Am J Kidney Dis*. 2004;43:405–414
95. Parikh CR, Mishra J, Thiessen-Philbrook H, et al. Urinary IL-18 is an early predictive biomarker of acute kidney injury after cardiac surgery. *Kidney Int*. 2006;70:199–203
96. Parikh CR, Abraham E, Ancukiewicz M, Edelstein CL. Urine IL-18 is an early diagnostic marker for acute kidney injury and predicts mortality in the intensive care unit. *J Am Soc Nephrol*. 2005;16:3046–3052

Renal Ultrasound

3.3

Vicki E. Noble, Andrew Liteplo, and David F. M. Brown

Core Messages

- Hydronephrosis is the most common application and most easily identified pathologic state for renal ultrasound (US). Because fluid is so readily imaged with ultrasound, dilation of the renal pelvis and central collecting system appears black on the sonogram scan and can be seen readily.
- One of the most common disease processes of the urinary tract is nephrolithiasis causing colic. The overall advantages of computed tomography usually make formal renal US the second choice in diagnostic imaging of suspected renal colic. However, given radiation exposure risk and allergic and nephrotoxic risk of iodinated contrast if used, occasionally US is the test of choice.
- Patients with acute renal vein thrombosis present with flank pain and tenderness, hypertension, and proteinuria. Patients with renal transplants are at particularly high risk for this and this diagnosis should be high on the list of differential diagnoses. Significant improvements in magnetic resonance imaging and magnetic resonance venous phase imaging (MRV) scanning have greatly expanded their role in the evaluation of acute renal vein thrombosis. However US is diagnostic when it includes Doppler studies that show the absence of blood flow in the renal vein.
- Transplanted kidneys are easily imaged because of their relatively superficial location in the iliac fossa. With acute rejection, the kidney loses it ellipsoid shape and can start to appear more lobulated with shortening of the anteroposterior length.

3.3.1 Introduction

There are many diagnostic imaging modalities available to the clinician when evaluating the renal system. Indeed, standards of practice have continued to evolve with developments in imaging techniques. Advances in computed tomography (CT) and magnetic resonance imaging (MRI) have largely supplanted many of the traditional imaging modalities such as intravenous pyelography or plain abdominal X-rays. Newer modalities such as radionuclide renograms give information on renal function that would have been unimaginable in the last decade.

Ultrasound remains a mainstay in the evaluation of the kidney and bladder, however, and is an important complimentary study to both CT and MRI. Partially, this is because both organs are so readily imaged by sonography. In addition, ultrasound of the renal system has the same advantages as ultrasound for other organ systems. Ultrasound does not expose patients to ionizing radiation, does not require intravenous contrast administration, can often be done at the bedside, can provide information about other organ systems if alternative diagnoses are suspect, and can be repeated multiple times without risk to show disease progression or resolution.

This chapter will review how ultrasound works, describe basic renal ultrasound anatomy, discuss how to perform a basic sonography scan, and review scanning

D. F. M. Brown (✉)
Department of Emergency Medicine, Massachusetts General Hospital, 55 Fruit St., Boston, MA 02114-2696, USA
e-mail: dbrown2@partners.org

A. Jörres et al. (eds.), *Management of Acute Kidney Problems*,
DOI: 10.1007/978-3-540-69441-0_3.3, © Springer-Verlag Berlin Heidelberg 2010

protocols for different renal and urologic system complaints. Finally, ultrasound images of both normal and common pathologic conditions will be reviewed.

3.3.2 Ultrasound Basics

Ultrasound works by sending out a pulsed longitudinal wave that is partially reflected, partially absorbed and partially transmitted through tissue. The degree to which the sound is transmitted or reflected depends on the density of the tissue. The strength of the returning echo is sensed by the ultrasound probe and is transcribed onto the screen with a pixel strength corresponding to the echo strength (black for weak echos and white for strong echos). Therefore, tissue that transmits the majority of sound, such as fluid, will appear dark on the ultrasound screen and tissue that transmits little sound, such as bone, will appear bright on the ultrasound screen.

Ultrasound may be performed using a range of frequencies and selection of the proper frequency (and hence of the proper probe) is an important consideration. In general, high frequency probes generate high resolution pictures but are able to penetrate only superficially, whereas lower frequency probes are able to penetrate more deeply into the body but lose some of their resolution as a result.

Finally, Doppler ultrasound assesses flow and velocity by using the Doppler frequency shift principle. This is important in renal imaging as flow velocity can be demonstrated using Doppler, and vascular resistance can be calculated using the resistance index (RI) which quantifies arterial resistance by the following formula:

$$\text{R1} = (\text{peak systolic velocity - lowest diastolic velocity})/\text{peak systolic velocity}.$$

Increased peripheral arterial resistance is defined by an intrarenal RI of greater than 0.7 and is indicative of disease although it is a nonspecific finding and so should always be used in clinical context [1].

3.3.3 Anatomy

The kidneys are located in the retroperitoneum and are surrounded by Gerota's fascia. Because the liver is larger than the spleen, the right kidney is usually more anterior and inferior, while the left kidney is more posterior and superior. The normal adult kidney dimensions range from 10–12 ccm long (superior to inferior axis), 5–6 cm wide (lateral to medial axis), and 3–4 cm deep (anteroposterior axis) [2]. The parenchyma is the renal tissue composed of both the cortex and the medulla and in most patients ultrasound can distinguish between the two through a difference in the echogenicity or brightness. The medulla is typically less echogenic (not as bright) because of the increased presence of plasma filtrate in that part of the kidney [3]. In addition, occasionally the renal pyramids are visible as triangular dark structures within the medulla (Fig. 3.3.1). The overall echogenicity of normal renal parenchyma is less bright or hypoechoic than the spleen or liver tissue nearby, and an alteration in this normal relationship can be indicative of renal failure or chronic infection. The outline of the normal kidney is smooth and if it is noticeably irregular, a pathologic

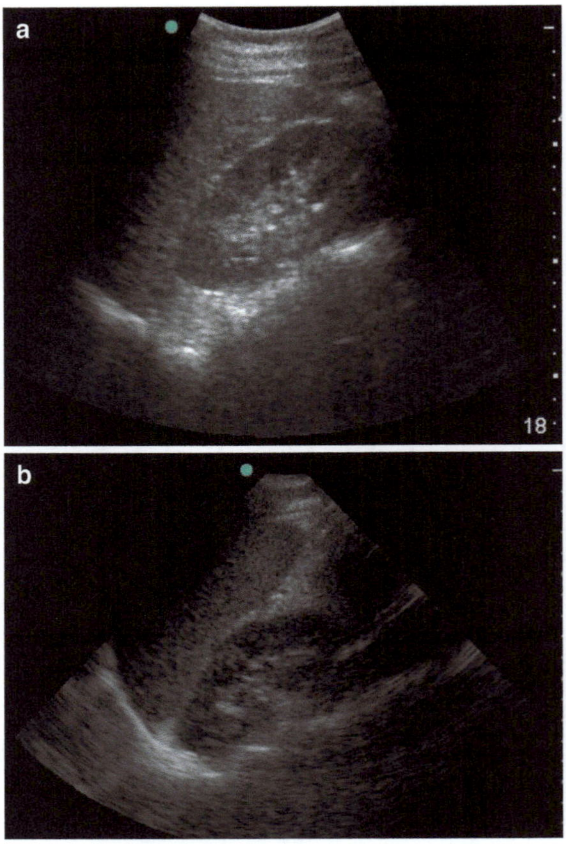

Fig. 3.3.1 Panel **a** shows a normal right kidney with the brighter liver tissue to the left and the bright diaphragm in the lower left corner. Panel **b** shows a normal left kidney

process such as infiltrative disease, scarring, masses, or infection should be suspected. Occasionally patients will have retained fetal lobulations which can cause irregular outlines, but in these cases the thickness of the cortex is preserved. The normal renal sinus or hilum should appear brighter on ultrasound as it is composed of fat and the fibrous tissue of the collapsed collecting system in the normal kidney. In the normal kidney the ureter is not visualized and is only seen as it starts to distend and fill with fluid.

While renal vasculature is seen more readily with angiography, occasionally renal vessels are well seen on ultrasound and can be evaluated with Doppler flow. Although there are limitations to the sensitivity and specificity of ultrasound, it can be useful in diagnosing vascular insufficiency, stenosis, or structural abnormalities such as aneurysmal dilatations.

The bladder is located in the inferoumbilical region of the lower abdomen and upper pelvis. A full bladder can distend so that it becomes intraperitoneal, but usually the bladder is located deep in the pelvis. While other imaging modalities are more sensitive in screening for bladder abnormalities (cystoscopy for polyps or masses, CT or MRI for extrinsic masses or wall thickening), ultrasound can be a safe, efficient, and accurate way to assess bladder volume and to identify larger lesions or abnormal bladder wall thickening.

3.3.4 Scanning Techniques

Renal ultrasound is performed using a B-mode scanner with a lower frequency (2–5 MHz) abdominal probe. The sonographer stands at the bedside on the patient's right with the patient supine. Extending the patient's arms over the head can improve imaging by elevating the ribs and minimizing rib shadow artifact. The right kidney is usually interrogated first as it is generally more easily accessible through the acoustic window the liver provides. The probe should be placed with the probe marker to the patient's head in the mid-axillary line scanning through the liver, just inferior to the ribs in the coronal plane. The image obtained here should be a longitudinal scan of the kidney. Occasionally, when bowel gas is present, the sound waves will scatter obscuring any clear renal image. The probe can be moved anteriorly or posteriorly and angled around the offending loop of bowel. When the optimal longitudinal view is seen, the probe should be rocked back and forth (anterior to posterior) to sweep through the entire parenchyma of the kidney in the longitudinal plane. The probe is then rotated 90° with the probe marker pointing up to the ceiling to visualize the kidney in the transverse plane and is rocked inferiorly and superiorly again to fan through the entire kidney.

The left kidney is more difficult to visualize because the spleen provides a smaller acoustic window. Also, occasionally the gas-filled stomach can obscure the coronal view. For the left kidney the probe is initially placed in the posterior axillary line with the probe marker to the patient's head slightly more superiorly than on the right. Again, if there is bowel gas overlying the kidney, the probe may have to be moved to the patient's flank or the patient put in the right lateral decubitus position so the probe can be slid further toward the back and away from the stomach bubble. Otherwise the technique of fanning forward and back in the longitudinal plane and up and down in the transverse plane is the same.

Scanning the bladder is done by placing the probe in the transverse position (probe marker to the patient's right) just above the symphysis pubis and sliding back and forth to find the fluid-filled bladder. Once the bladder is identified the probe should be rocked superiorly and inferiorly to scan through the whole structure and then rotated 90° to image the bladder sagittally. Once the bladder is identified in the sagittal plan, the probe should be fanned from side to side to see the entirety of the bladder. Color Doppler can be used when scanning the bladder transversely to identify ureteral jets indicating patent ureter excretion capability.

3.3.5 Applications

3.3.5.1 *Hydronephrosis*

This is the most common application and most easily identified pathologic state for renal ultrasound. Because fluid is so readily imaged with ultrasound, dilation of the renal pelvis and central collecting system appears black on the sonogram scan and can be seen readily (Fig. 3.3.2). The degree of hydronephrosis has been

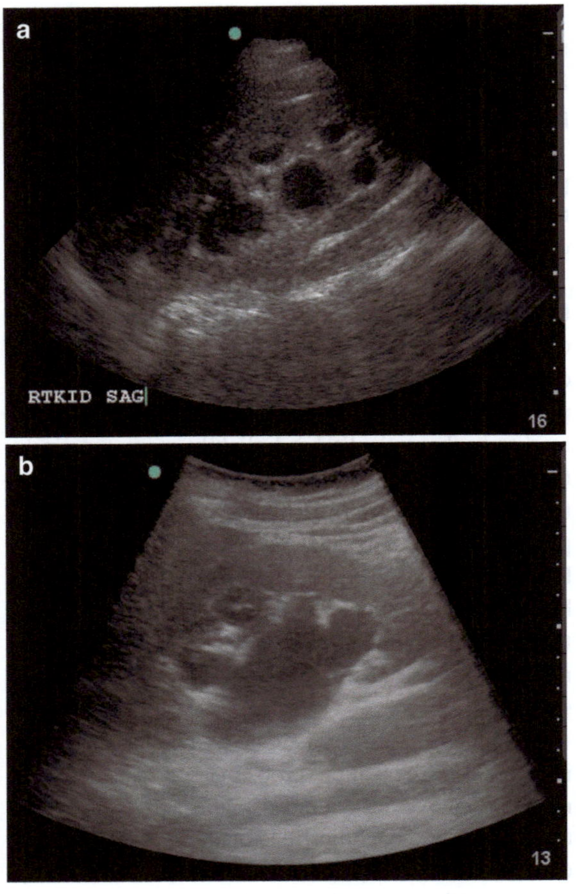

Fig. 3.3.2 Panel **a** shows dilated calyces and dark fluid splaying open the medullary pyramids. Panel **b** shows the connection with a dilated renal pelvis

graded and oftentimes the duration of obstruction can be estimated. In acute obstructions, the thickness of the renal cortex is maintained, while chronic obstructions can lead to cortex destruction and thus appears thinner. The grading of hydronephrosis has had inconsistent clinical prognostic value and so the role for grading clinically is unclear. However, one common grading system is described in Grainger and Allison's *Diagnostic Radiology*, 4th ed as the following:

- Grade I – slight blunting of calyceal fornices
- Grade II – blunting and enlargement of calyceal fornices but easily seen shadows of papillae
- Grade III – rounding of calices with obliteration of papillae
- Grade IV – extreme calyceal ballooning [5]

One benefit of ultrasound is that oftentimes if the hydronephrosis is bilateral, an ultrasound evaluation of the bladder can identify if bladder outlet obstruction is the cause of poor drainage.

3.3.5.2 Renal Colic

One of the most common disease processes of the urinary tract is nephrolithiasis causing colic. Clinically renal stones commonly present as abrupt, sharp, severe flank and low back pain. This is caused by the acute obstruction and distention of the ureter and renal pelvis by the stone. Intravenous pyelography (IVP) was long the radiologic mainstay in the diagnosis of renal colic, but advances in CT scanning have essentially replaced IVP scanning for nephrolithiasis and renal colic. CT has a shorter examination time, provides better visualization of the calculus, and allows for measurement of the stone anywhsere along the urinary tract including the ureter and bladder. The overall advantages of CT usually make formal renal ultrasound the second choice in diagnostic imaging of suspected renal colic. However, given radiation exposure risk and allergic and nephrotoxic risk of iodinated contrast if used, occasionally ultrasound is the test of choice.

Renal ultrasound may identify the actual calculi which are seen as small echogenic structures with posterior shadowing (Fig. 3.3.3), particularly when the calculi are intrarenal. Intraureteral stones are very difficult to demonstrate, and the sensitivity and specificity of ultrasound identification of ureteral stones is very low [6, 7]. More commonly, ultrasound will reveal

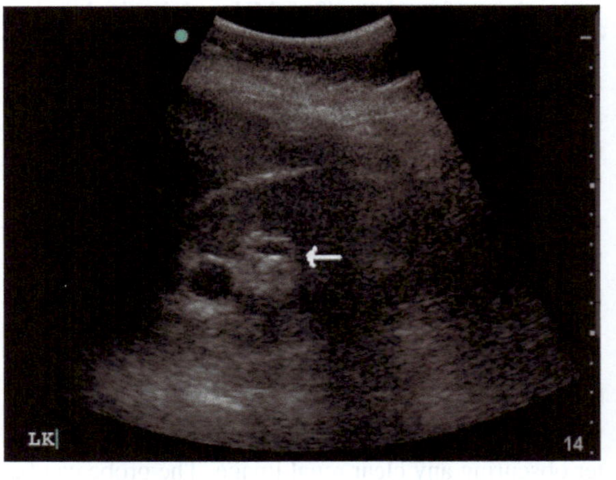

Fig. 3.3.3 The arrow points to a hyperechoic stone in the renal pelvis causing dark shadowing behind it as the ultrasound can not penetrate beyond the calcification

some degree of unilateral hydronephrosis which occurs when the central calyceal system is dilated with urine and appears sonographically as dark black and homogeneously anechoic. The test characteristics for ultrasonographic detection of urinary tract calculi depend on which diagnostic criteria are used (direct visualization of the stone, unilateral hydronephrosis, or both). Using both criteria, Sinclair et al. demonstrated a sensitivity of 85% and a specificity of 100% for ultrasound (compared with 90% and 94%, respectively, for IVP) [8]. Fowler showed that ultrasound identified 24 of 101 calculi seen on CT, for a sensitivity of 24% and a specificity of 90% [9]. Sheafor et al. had similar test characteristics for identifying renal stones by ultrasound (sensitivity 61% and specificity 100%). However, when the presence of stones and the presence of unilateral hydronephrosis were both used to diagnose colic, the sensitivity of ultrasound increased to 92% [10].

Therefore, for renal colic, CT is a better test. However, if ultrasound is used, it has comparable sensitivities if unilateral hydronephrosis and the identification of stones are both used for diagnosis.

3.3.5.3 Pyelonephritis

Pyelonephritis, or an infection of the upper urinary tract, does not always require imaging for diagnosis. As with most inflammatory processes seen by ultrasound, acute pyelonephritis often causes the kidney to appear enlarged and darker, or more hypoechoic than usual. This is best appreciated when compared with the unaffected contralateral kidney. Furthermore, a small subset of patients with pyelonephritis will progress to focal abscess formation. In these patients the involved kidney may have hypoechoic foci at the corticomedullary junction. As the disease progresses, these foci can enlarge and become abscesses which will appear larger and have thicker circumferential borders.

Pyonephrosis is a clinical emergency, and the presence of heterogenous appearing fluid within a dilated collecting system is concerning. The fluid in this case is filled with 'debris' or gray echoes that layer in the most dependent position.

Xanthogranulomatous pyelonephritis is a condition due to chronic infection where lipid-laden histiocytes destroy the normal renal architecture and large abscesses are formed (Fig. 3.3.4).

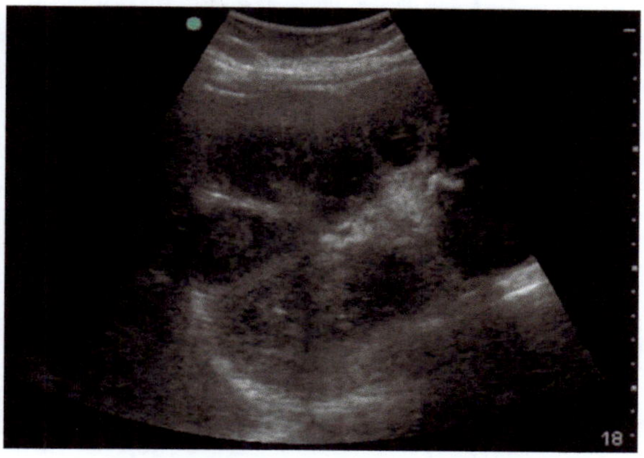

Fig. 3.3.4 Massive cyst formation destroying all normal renal architecture with heterogenous debris visualized within the cyst itself

3.3.5.4 Cysts

The majority of cysts are cortical and tubular in origin – that is they are located in the periphery. However, a minority are located in the parapelvic region and are lymphatic in origin [4]. These parapelvic cysts can often be mistaken for hydronephrosis, and it is important to fully scan through the renal pelvis to identify if the fluid collection is within the pelvis or external to the pelvis. Classically, cysts are smooth-walled with no internal echoes. The anterior and posterior of the walls should be seen clearly, and often there is posterior acoustic enhancement present. Multiple cysts (more than 10) are always abnormal. Multiple cysts that destroy normal renal architecture are findings consistent with polycystic kidney disease.

3.3.5.5 Renal Vein Thrombosis

Patients with acute renal vein thrombosis present with flank pain and tenderness, hypertension, and proteinuria. Patients with renal transplants are at particularly high risk for this and this diagnosis should be high on the list of differential diagnoses. Significant improvements in MRI and MRV scanning have greatly expanded their role in the evaluation of acute renal vein thrombosis. However ultrasound is diagnostic when it includes Doppler studies that show the absence of blood flow in the renal vein [10, 11].

3.3.5.6 Renal Infarction

Acute renal infarctions present very similarly to renal colic with flank pain, tenderness, hypertension, and proteinuria. However, ultrasound imaging in this case will show segmented triangular hypoechoic lesions within the periphery or cortex where decreased arterial supply has caused infarction.

3.3.5.7 Masses

The differential of renal masses is broad and includes carcinoma, lymphoma, adenoma, sarcomas, or metastases. One subset of tumor that sometimes has characteristic ultrasound findings are angiomyolipomas. These are benign tumors that are well-circumscribed and very echogenic as they are composed of blood muscles, smooth muscle, and fat. Otherwise, ultrasound is not generally able to differentiate between benign and malignant masses.

CT is regarded as a superior diagnostic test and any irregularity seen on ultrasound should be referred for further imaging. The great benefit of ultrasound is that given the increasing frequency with which renal ultrasounds are being performed, the opportunity to identify renal masses earlier in their course has increased [13]. This is especially important as early clinical identification of renal tumors is often difficult given their asymptomatic presentation until a large enough tumor burden is present to cause symptoms such as flank pain (Fig. 3.3.5).

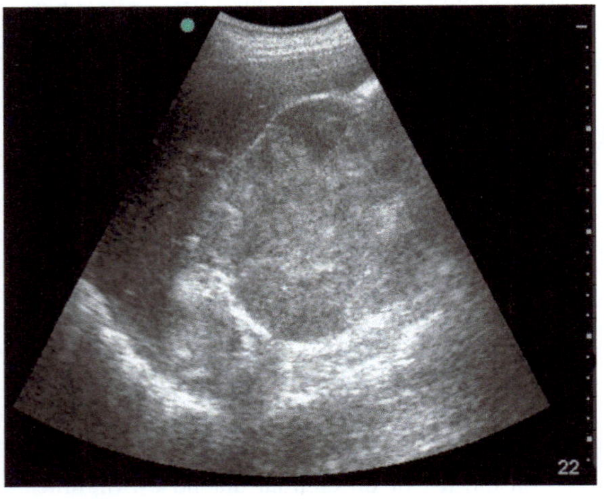

Fig. 3.3.5 The renal parenchyma looks hyperechoic compared with the liver so this is already concerning for an infiltrative process. In addition, there is an irregular contor to the renal capsule and the superior pole (where the adrenal gland should be) destroying the neighboring renal parenchyma. This was a patient with a large adrenal cortical tumor that was invading the surrounding structures

3.3.5.8 Renal Transplant Evaluation

Transplanted kidneys are easily imaged because of their relatively superficial location in the iliac fossa. With acute rejection, the kidney loses it ellipsoid shape and can start to appear more lobulated with shortening of the anteroposterior length [1]. The parenchyma can also increase in thickness with acute rejection although a normal renal sonogram does not rule out acute rejection. Oftentimes Doppler evaluation is performed to assess vascular flow to the transplanted kidney, and, while not specific, an RI from 0.75 to 0.9 is cause for concern for thrombosis and/or rejection [1].

3.3.5.9 Renal Trauma

The traditional role for renal ultrasound in trauma is as a part of the Focused Assessment with Sonography in Trauma (FAST) exam whereby ultrasound is used as a screening tool to look for intraperitoneal fluid. This exam is not designed to pick up specific renal injuries, but to identify abdominal hemorrhage responsible for hemodynamic instability and to predict the need for emergent laparotomy (Fig. 3.3.6). While some research has shown that ultrasound is highly reliable in distinguishing renal contusion from more serious injuries [14, 15], these results have not been reproduced in trauma centers in the United States, and thus contrast-enhanced CT is usually the diagnostic modality of choice to identify specific traumatic kidney injury.

Focal areas of parenchymal hemorrhage and edema may be seen as hypoechoic areas within the kidney. A linear, reproducible absence of echoes suggests renal fracture. If the collecting system has been injured, urine may leak out of the kidney yet be contained between the renal capsule and Gerota's fascia, creating a urinoma. A urinoma should be considered when an anechoic ring is seen around a portion of the kidney. However, the differential for this finding includes lymphocele, hematoma, abscess, cyst, and ascites, and this finding usually requires further imaging.

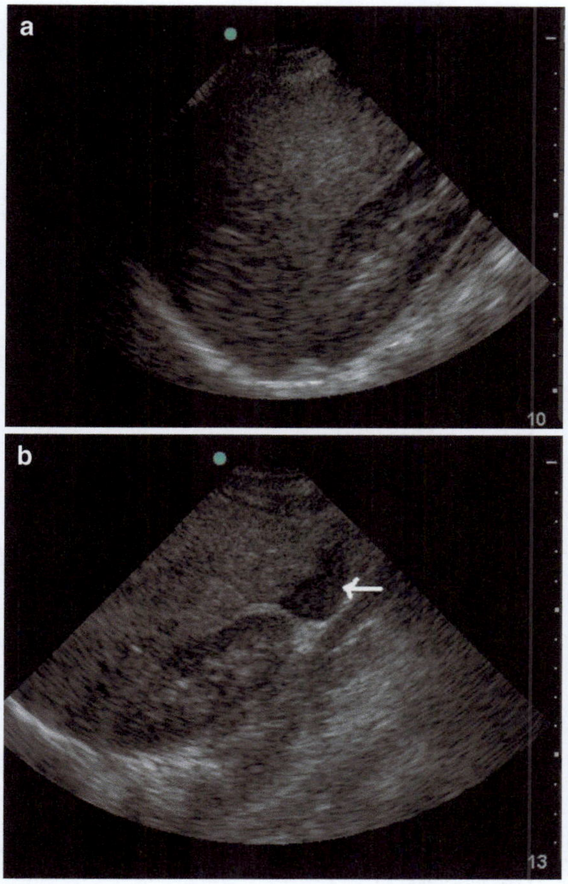

Fig. 3.3.6 In Panel **a** most of Morrison's pouch is seen with no obvious fluid in the potential space between the liver and the kidney. However, by obtaining the view of the inferior pole in Panel **b**, a large fluid collection is seen. The inferior pole of the right kidney is the most posterior aspect in a supine patient, and thus it must be seen to rule out free fluid or hemorrhage

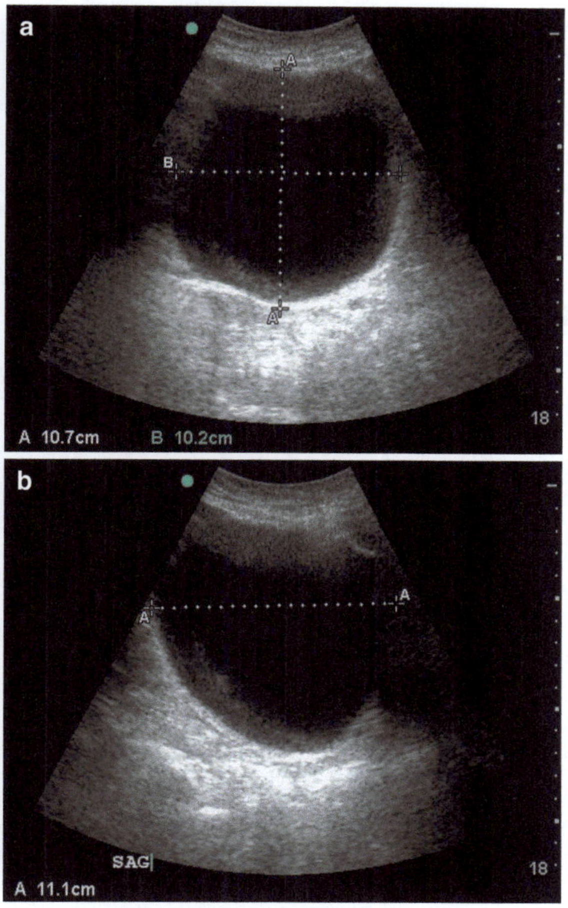

Fig. 3.3.7 Here are the two views of the bladder needed to calculate bladder volume with height and depth (*panel* ***a***) and length (*panel* ***b***)

Finally, new technological advances such as power Doppler may provide alternative diagnostic strategies to CT for renal perfusion injuries. This technique deserves further study in the trauma setting [16].

3.3.5.10 Bladder Evaluation

By using color Doppler techniques on the trigone of the bladder, you may observe a jet of urine entering the bladder. Observing bilateral ureteral jets lends evidence against the diagnosis of obstructive uropathy.

Bladder volume estimation can be calculated by the simple formula: Volume = (Width × Depth × He) × 0.7, where volume is expressed in milliliters (ml), and three orthogonal places are expressed in centimeters (cm) [17] (Fig. 3.3.7). Some ultrasound machines will do this calculation for you if you measure the three variables.

3.3.6 Summary

Renal ultrasound is one of several imaging modalities available to the clinician and in many ways is complimentary to computed tomography or magnetic resonance imaging. It offers excellent anatomic detail without exposure to ionizing radiation or contrast agents and is an important alternative tool for patients with contraindications to other imaging modalities. It is likely that as ultrasound technology advances and power color Doppler and other supplemental ultrasound methodologies add to its capability, renal ultrasound will evolve into the initial screening diagnostic tool for kidney and bladder complaints and may even start to supplant other diagnostic modalities.

References

1. Parisky YR, Yassa NA. Diagnostic use of ultrasound in kidney and bladder. In Shaul G Massry and Richard J Glassock ed. Textbook of Nephrology. Lippincott Williams & Wilkins, Philadelphia, 2001, pp 1821.
2. Brandt T, Neiman H, Dragowski M, et al. Ultrasound assessment of normal renal dimensions. J Ultrasound Med 1982; 1:49.
3. Arthur C Fleischer renal and urological sonography. In Fleischer AC and Kepple DM ed. Diagnostic Sonography. WB Saunders, Philadelphia, 1995, pp 473.
4. Frederick J Doherty. Ultrasound of the kidney. In Jacobsen HR, Striker Gem Klahr S, ed. The Principles and Practice of Nephrology. BC Decker Inc, Philadelphia, 1991, pp 178–179.
5. Cronan JJ. Urinary obstruction. In Grainger RG, Allison DJ, Adam A, Dixon AK ed. Diagnostic Radiology: A Textbook of Medical imaging, 4th ed. Churchill Livingstone, London, 1997, pp 1593–1613.
6. Coleman BG. Ultrasonography of the upper genitourinary tract. Urol Clin N Am 1985;12:633–644.
7. Keller MJ. The genitourinary tract. In Grainger RD, Allison DJ, eds. Diagnostic Radiology: A Textbook of Medical Imaging. Churchill Livingstone, London, 2001, pp 1489–1496.
8. Sinclair D, Wilson S, Toi A, et al. The evaluation of suspected renal colic: ultrasound scan vs excretory urography. Ann Emerg Med 1989;18:556–559.
9. Fowler KA. US for detecting renal calculi with nonenhanced CT as a reference standard. Radiology 2002;222(1): 109–113.
10. Sheafor DH, Hertzberg BS, Freed KS, et al. Nonenhanced helical CT and US in the emergency evaluation of patients with renal colic: a prospective comparison. Radiology 2000; 217:792–797.
11. Williamson M. Renal ultrasound. In: Williamson M. ed. Essentials of Ultrasound. WB Saunders, Philadelphia, 1996, pp 562–579.
12. Zubarev AV. [AU2]Ultrasound of renal vessels. Eur Radiol 2001;11(10):1902–1915.
13. Mandavia DP, Pregerson B, Henderson SO. Ultrasonography of flank pain in the emergency department: renal carcinoma as a diagnostic concern. J Emerg Med 2000;18:83–86.
14. Buchberger W, Penz T, Wicke K et al. Diagnosis and staging of blunt kidney trauma. A comparison of urinalysis, IV urography, sonography and computed tomography. Rofo Fortschr Geb Rontgenstr Neuen Bildgeb Verfahr 1993; 58:507.
15. Furtschegger A, Egender G, Jaske G. The value of sonography in the diagnosis and follow-up of patients with blunt renal trauma. Br J Urol 1988;62:110–116.
16. Swadron S, Mandavia DP. Renal ultrasound. In: Ma OJ, Mateer JR, eds. Emergency Ultrasound.McGraw Hill Professional, New York, 2002, pp 197–220.
17. Walton JM, Irwin KS, Whitehouse GH. Comparison of real-time ultrasonography and magnetic resonance imaging in the assessment of urinary bladder volume. Br J Urol. 1996 Dec;78(6):856–61.

Management of Acute Kidney Problems: Indications for Renal Biopsy in Acute Renal Disease

3.4

Alan D. Salama

Core Messages

- Renal biopsy is the only means of establishing certain diagnoses, many of which may not be suspected from the clinical scenario.
- In most cases, two renal cores should be obtained and should be processed for light microscopy, immunohistochemistry and electron microscopy to optimally interpret the biopsy. In some cases, diagnosis can only be made by electron microscopy or immunohistochemistry.
- Renal biopsy can provide information regarding reversibility of lesions and hence the likely benefit of therapy, but must be of adequate size for accurate interpretation.
- Using real time ultrasound and adhering to strict screening policies, biopsy is safe and results in few complications.
- To properly interpret the pathologic findings, close liaison between nephrologists and pathologists is required.
- Renal biopsies should only be carried out in centres and by individuals experienced in obtaining and processing the material.
- Percutaneous biopsy is the preferred method for renal biopsy, but alternative approaches exist for obtaining renal tissue, which can be used depending on clinical context.

A. D. Salama
Renal Section, Division of Medicine, Imperial College London, Hammersmith Hospital, Du Cane Road, London W12 0NN, UK
email: a.salama@imperial.ac.uk

3.4.1 Introduction

The renal biopsy has become an essential tool in the management of acute and chronic renal disease. Prior to its routine use, pathologists relied on autopsy material for investigation of disease pathophysiology. However, its development and refinement since the late 1950s has been fundamental for the diagnosis and definition of clinical syndromes and the discovery of new pathologic entities [1]. Through their critical analysis, certain key pathophysiologic features of kidney disease have been discovered, which have helped establish new paradigms in nephrology and in turn have led to alterations in patient management. This is true for native renal biopsies and even more so for renal transplant biopsies [2]. In addition, it is fair to say that we are still learning a significant amount about disease pathogenesis through the study of renal biopsy material, which remains a gold standard for disease diagnosis, and this is especially true in the modern era of transplantation, where novel biopsy markers have revolutionised our concepts of rejection mechanisms.

The first percutaneous kidney biopsies were performed over 50 years ago using a liver biopsy needle and intravenous pyelograms for screening, with the patient either sitting or supine. Their success in obtaining renal tissue and in aiding management confirmed the benefit of the procedure [1]. Many innovations such as using real-time ultrasound, spring-loaded needles or needle holders and careful preoperative evaluation of the patient have improved the rate of obtaining renal tissue while minimising the risks of the procedure [3]. Consequently, this has placed percutaneous renal biopsy at the very centre of modern clinical nephrology. A general schema for performing the renal biopsy

A. Jörres et al. (eds.), *Management of Acute Kidney Problems*,
DOI: 10.1007/978-3-540-69441-0_3.4, © Springer-Verlag Berlin Heidelberg 2010

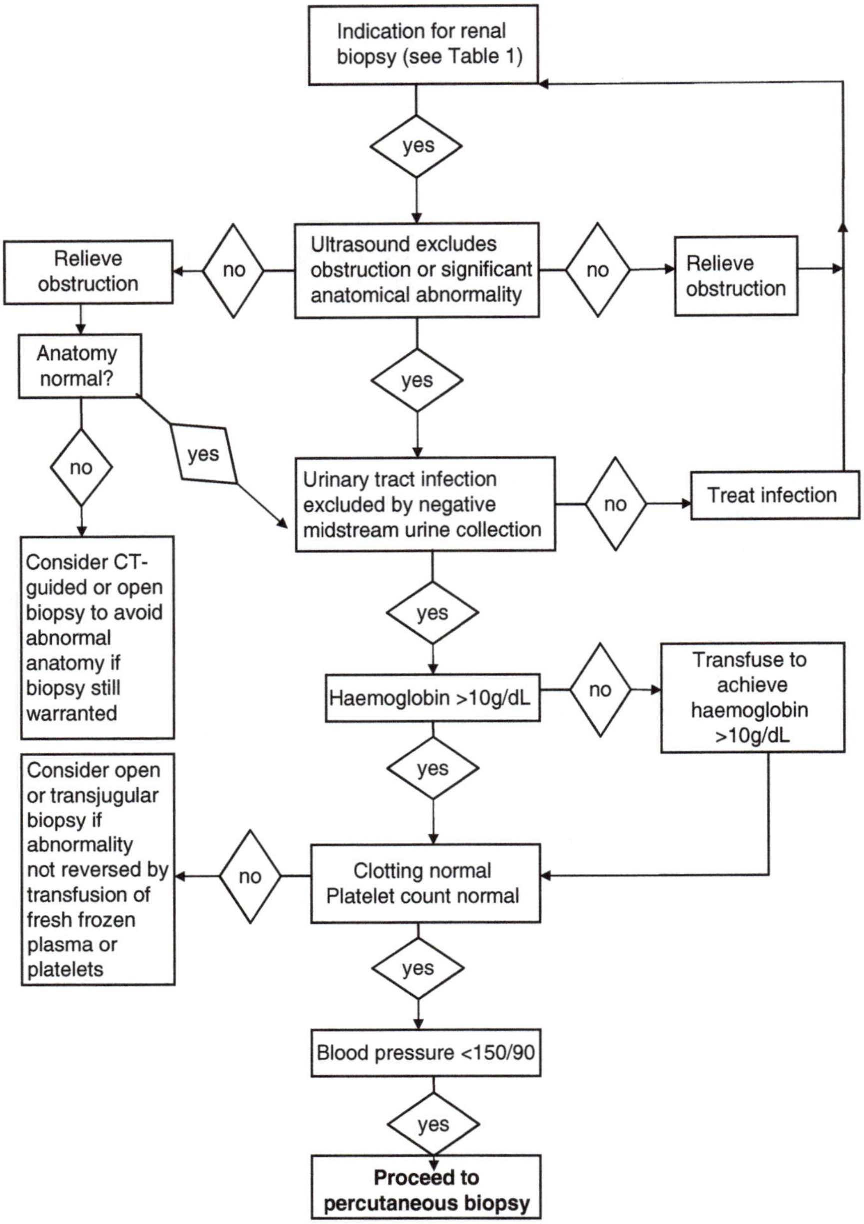

Fig. 3.4.1 Pathway for performing a renal biopsy

is shown in Fig. 3.4.1, while the indications and contraindications are summarised in Tables 3.4.1 and 3.4.2. It should be noted that these will vary from centre to centre, and this will therefore bias the pattern of disease entities found. For example, biopsying all patients with isolated microscopic haematuria will result in a large proportion of patients with IgA disease and thin membrane lesions, while the proportion of biopsies demonstrating diabetic nephropathy will depend on the threshold of biopsying diabetic patients with proteinuria. Finally, local policy regarding re-biopsy of patients following therapy may bias the number of biopsies with certain diagnoses. Figure 3.4.2 demonstrates the proportions of pathologic diagnoses in a series of over 600 biopsies taken at our institution, during a 2-year period.

Table 3.4.1 General indications for renal biopsy

Indications for renal biopsy
Significant proteinuria(> 1 g/day or equivalent spot protein to creatinine ratio)
Microscopic haematuria with any degree of proteinuria
Unexplained renal impairment
Renal manifestations of systemic disease

Table 3.4.2 Contraindications to renal biopsy

Absolute contraindications	*Relative contraindication*
Uncontrolled hypertension	Single kidney
Bleeding diathesis	Anti-platelet agents
Widespread cystic disease or renal	Anatomical abnormalities
Malignancy	Small kidneys
Hydronephrosis	
Uncooperative patient	
Active urinary sepsis	

3.4.2 Renal Biopsy in Acute Renal Failure

Renal biopsy is performed to diagnose the cause of acute renal failure in between 9% and 13% of biopsy series, but makes up a much greater percentage in older patients (>60 years, up to 27% of all biopsies) [4–6], while it appears a relatively uncommon indication in children. In part, the reason for such a relatively low percentage of biopsies being carried out for acute renal failure, is the fact that most acute renal failure is part of an underlying illness such as sepsis, and frequently reversible without specific renal treatment. Thus, treating the underlying condition, such as sepsis or hypovolaemia, and withdrawing nephrotoxic drugs, frequently results in an improvement in renal function. A common presumed diagnosis for acute renal impairment is acute tubular necrosis (ATN). Interestingly, in the Italian registry series of biopsies for acute renal failure (defined as rapidly deteriorating renal function) the incidence of ATN was only 8% of the biopsies, less than necrotising vasculitis, crescentic glomerulonephritis and tubulointerstitial nephritis, demonstrating the potential utility in performing a biopsy in this setting (see Fig. 3.4.3). Other biopsy series have suggested a similar incidence for necrotising vasculitis, and tubulointerstitial nephritis in those patients with more advanced renal impairment (serum creatinine [SCr] > 200 μmol/l). In a series of over 250 biopsies taken from older patients (>60 years) with acute renal failure, the pathologic diagnosis confirmed a pre-biopsy differential diagnosis in 67% of cases, and again demonstrated a frequency of isolated ATN of just under 7% [5]. In this series the most common pathologic finding was pauci-immune glomerulonephritis (with or without arteritis) (31.2%), followed by acute tubulointerstitial nephritis (18.6%), ATN with nephrotic syndrome (7.5%), atheroemboli (7.1%) and lesser frequencies of B cell dyscrasias, postinfectious

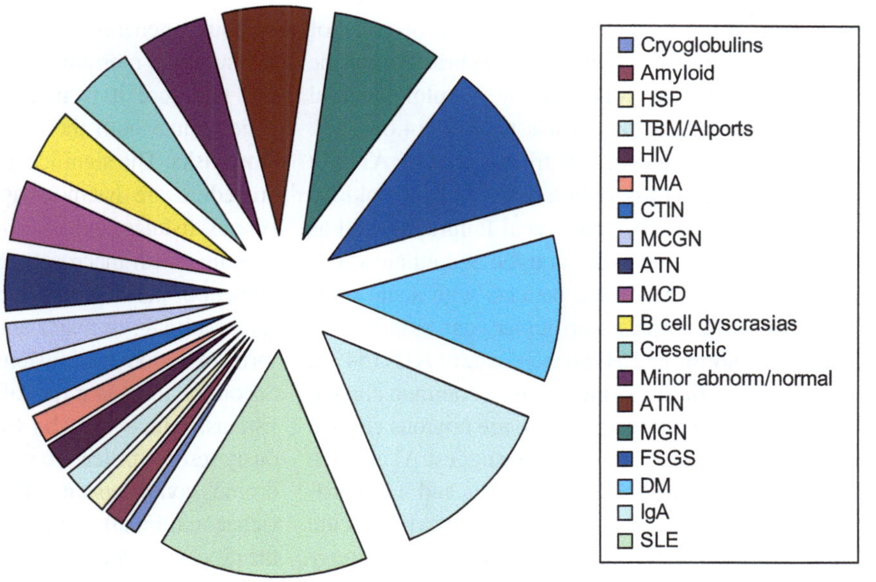

Fig. 3.4.2 Proportion of diagnoses in 634 renal biopsies performed at Hammersmith Hospital over a 2-year period

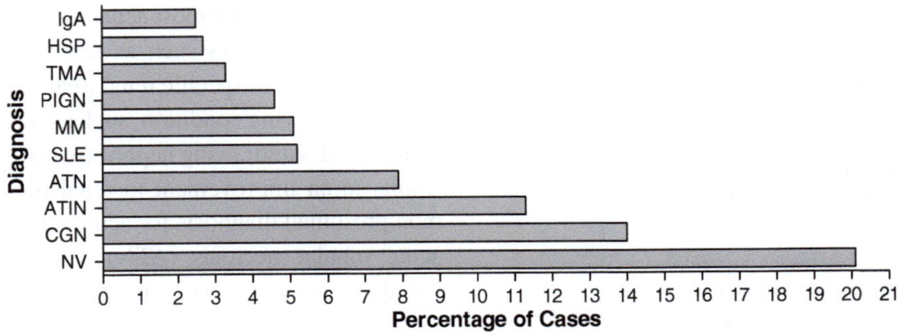

Fig. 3.4.3 Frequency of pathologic diagnoses recorded in renal biopsies obtained for the diagnosis of acute renal failure, adapted from the Italian registry

NV = Necrotizing vasculitis
CGN = Crescentic glomerulonephritis
ATIN = Acute tubulointerstitial nephritis
ATN = Acute tubular necrosis
SLE = Systemic lupus erythematosus
MM = Multiple myeloma
PIGN = Postinfectious glomerulonephritis
TMA = Thrombotic microangiopathy
HSP = Henoch-Schönlein Purpura
IgA = IgA nephropathy

glomerulonephritis, anti-glomerular basement membrane disease and IgA nephropathy. In only 5% of the biopsies was a diagnosis not arrived at, due to inadequate tissue or no obvious pathologic cause of acute renal failure found. By contrast, data from a large cohort of Indian patients with acute renal failure demonstrated that of 1,122 cases, 891 were due to intrinsic renal disease and of these 705 (79.2%) were due to ischaemic or toxic ATN. Thus intrinsic renal diseases other than ATN accounted for only 21% of cases of acute renal failure, with glomerulonephritis being the commonest (9.4%), followed by tubulointerstitial nephritis (7%) and acute cortical necrosis (4.6%) [7]. These marked differences in frequencies of ATN in part reflect local biopsy policies and the threshold for biopsy in the setting of acute renal failure, as well as disease incidence due to geographic and ethnic variations. A series of paediatric patients with acute renal failure from the tropics who underwent biopsy have similarly demonstrated a high incidence of ATN (54%), with diarrhoeal illness being the most common clinical association [8]. Thus, unless there are obvious clinical and laboratory features to strongly suggest ATN (such as a bland urine dipstick, hyaline casts and a low urinary sodium concentration) in the context of acute renal failure with rapidly deteriorating function, biopsy is indicated. This must obviously be tempered by considering the condition of the patient and the presence of any absolute or relative contraindications (see above). A schema detailing the steps required prior to biopsy is shown in Fig. 3.4.1.

3.4.3 Complications of Biopsies

Although generally safe, there is a morbidity and a measureable mortality associated with the procedure, and therefore it is imperative only to subject those patients in whom there will be a potential benefit to those risks. The significant complications related to the procedure are haemorrhage, development of arteriovenous fistulas and to a lesser extent sepsis [9–11]. Bleeding with macroscopic haematuria and the development of perinephric haematomas, may be minor and self-resolving, or major and require intervention in the form of blood transfusions, embolisation or surgery. Secondly, there is a risk of formation of arteriovenous fistulas, which may be asymptomatic and spontaneously resolve or lead to a significant vascular steal syndrome, compromising the rest of the kidney through ischaemia. Finally, there is the risk of sepsis following the procedure, through the introduction of a septic focus or its dissemination. Overall the risks of complication vary from centre to centre, but can be estimated between 3.5% and 13%, with the majority being minor complications (approximately 3–9%) [9–11]. Additionally, there is the chance that an inadequate core is obtained for diagnosis, containing too few glomeruli or insufficient cortical material, and this is reported in up to 5% of cases. The size requirements for accurate diagnosis are discussed below. Mortality from the procedure is generally as a result of undiagnosed bleeding with significant haematoma formation and is reported in up to 0.2% of cases from larger biopsy series [10, 11]. Complications appear to be more common in native than transplanted kidneys, and in patients with more advanced renal impairment (SCr >440 µmol/l) or with lower haemoglobin levels (12 vs 11 g/dl) [10, 11]. In addition, careful selection and management of the patients for the procedure appears to decrease the overall risk. There are certain absolute contraindications, which preclude percutaneous biopsy, while there are a number of relative contraindications (Table 3.4.2) which may be circumvented depending on the importance of the biopsy, the operator's experience and the supportive facilities available. Ideally, all efforts should be made to deal with the relative contraindications; however, in the context of acute renal failure, this is not always possible. The critical preoperative steps are to ensure that blood pressure is controlled, that the patient does not have a bleeding diathesis or a urinary tract infection and that the kidneys are suitably imaged (see Fig. 3.4.4), with no evidence of obstruction, generalised cystic disease or malignancy. As a result, preoperative assessment should allow those patients unsuitable for percutaneous biopsy to be referred for an alternative approach. In these patients, there are other means of obtaining renal tissue which include open biopsies [12], laparoscopic biopsies or transjugular biopsies [13]. Each is associated with certain complications and has particular merits depending on the clinical scenario (see Table 3.4.3). Overall, these are generally only required for a minority of potential biopsy patients.

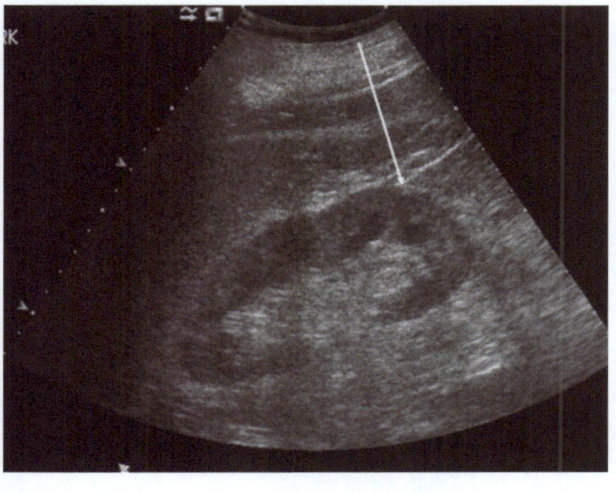

Fig. 3.4.4 Ultrasound of a kidney prior to biopsy. The arrow demonstrates the path taken by the biopsy needle which is visualised in real time

Table 3.4.3 Alternative methods for obtaining real tissue and their risks and benefits compared to a percutaneous approach

Method	Advantage	Disadvantage
Transjugular approach	Can be of use in those with a bleeding diathesis	Risk of capsular perforation
		Inadequate material in up to 24% of procedures
Open approach	High yield of adequate tissue	Requires general/ spinal anaesthesia
	Haemostasis is more secure	
Laparoscopic approach	High yield of adequate tissue	Requires general/ spinal anaesthesia
	Haemostasis is more secure	

3.4.4 Biopsy Processing and Adequacy

Adequate biopsy material allows a complete diagnosis to be made. However, how much tissue is required is variable and dependent on the underlying condition. To confidently diagnose a focal glomerular processes (a common pattern of renal disease), at least 20 glomeruli are required for 90% confidence of finding a focal lesion affecting less than 10% of glomeruli [14]. Fewer glomeruli increases the likelihood of missing the focal lesion and makes the interpretation of the biopsy incomplete. Additionally, certain diagnoses are completely dependent on particular analyses. For example thin basement membrane lesions and IgA nephropathy require electron microscopy and immunohistochemistry, respectively, to make the diagnosis. However, in certain cases, less than adequate material may still allow a definitive diagnosis to be made, if for example, amyloid deposits are found in vessels on Congo red staining, in a sample that may even lack any glomeruli, a diagnosis may be made.

In general, two cores should be taken at biopsy and divided into three parts for light and electron microscopy and immunohistochemistry, either in the form of immunofluorescence or immunoperoxidase, which can be carried out on formalin-fixed tissue. In renal transplant biopsies, it has been shown that taking two cores rather than one increases the chance of diagnosing acute rejection from 91% to 99% [15], demonstrating that the more material the pathologist has available, the greater the confidence of making a correct diagnosis. Processing of the biopsy and obtaining the necessary stains will be dependent on the clinical scenario and the available facilities. Recommendations for best practice have been summarised recently [16].

3.4.5 Conclusions

Percutaneous renal biopsy is generally safe if care is taken to select and prepare the patients. It should be considered in any suitable patient with acute renal failure, in whom ATN is not the most likely diagnosis clinically, or who has abnormal urinary sediment and in whom there are no contraindications.

3.4.6 Take Home Pearls

Renal biopsy is an essential part of modern nephrology and with the correct approach is a safe procedure.

Judicious preoperative assessment is required to minimise complications.

Liaison between pathologists and nephrologists is essential for optimal biopsy interpretation.

References

1. Cameron, JS & Hicks, J: The introduction of renal biopsy into nephrology from 1901 to 1961: a paradigm of the forming of nephrology by technology. *Am J Nephrol*, 17: 347–58, 1997.
2. Pascual, M, Vallhonrat, H, Cosimi, AB, Tolkoff-Rubin, N, Colvin, RB, Delmonico, FL, Ko, DS, Schoenfeld, DA & Williams, WW, Jr.: The clinical usefulness of the renal allograft biopsy in the cyclosporine era: a prospective study. *Transplantation*, 67: 737–41, 1999.
3. Korbet, SM: Percutaneous renal biopsy. *Semin Nephrol*, 22: 254–67, 2002.
4. Covic, A, Schiller, A, Volovat, C, Gluhovschi, G, Gusbeth-Tatomir, P, Petrica, L, Caruntu, ID, Bozdog, G, Velciov, S, Trandafirescu, V, Bob, F & Gluhovschi, C: Epidemiology of renal disease in Romania: a 10 year review of two regional renal biopsy databases. *Nephrol Dial Transplant*, 21: 419–24, 2006.
5. Haas, M, Spargo, BH, Wit, EJ & Meehan, SM: Etiologies and outcome of acute renal insufficiency in older adults: a renal biopsy study of 259 cases. *Am J Kidney Dis*, 35: 433–47, 2000.
6. Liano, F & Pascual, J: Epidemiology of acute renal failure: a prospective, multicenter, community-based study. Madrid Acute Renal Failure Study Group. *Kidney Int*, 50: 811–8, 1996.
7. Prakash, J, Sen, D, Kumar, NS, Kumar, H, Tripathi, LK & Saxena, RK: Acute renal failure due to intrinsic renal diseases: review of 1122 cases. *Ren Fail*, 25: 225–33, 2003.
8. Chugh, KS, Narang, A, Kumar, L, Sakhuja, V, Unni, VN, Pirzada, R, Singh, N, Pereira, BJ & Singhal, PC: Acute renal failure amongst children in a tropical environment. *Int J Artif Organs*, 10: 97–101, 1987.
9. Hergesell, O, Felten, H, Andrassy, K, Kuhn, K & Ritz, E: Safety of ultrasound-guided percutaneous renal biopsy-retrospective analysis of 1090 consecutive cases. *Nephrol Dial Transplant*, 13: 975–7, 1998.
10. Preda, A, Van Dijk, LC, Van Oostaijen, JA & Pattynama, PM: Complication rate and diagnostic yield of 515 consecutive ultrasound-guided biopsies of renal allografts and native kidneys using a 14-gauge Biopty gun. *Eur Radiol*, 13: 527–30, 2003.
11. Whittier, WL & Korbet, SM: Timing of complications in percutaneous renal biopsy. *J Am Soc Nephrol*, 15: 142–7, 2004.
12. Nomoto, Y, Tomino, Y, Endoh, M, Suga, T, Miura, M, Nomoto, H & Sakai, H: Modified open renal biopsy: results in 934 patients. *Nephron*, 45: 224–8, 1987.
13. Mal, F, Meyrier, A, Callard, P, Altman, JJ, Kleinknecht, D, Beaugrand, M & Ferrier, JP: Transjugular renal biopsy. *Lancet*, 335: 1512–3, 1990.
14. Corwin, HL, Schwartz, MM & Lewis, EJ: The importance of sample size in the interpretation of the renal biopsy. *Am J Nephrol*, 8: 85–9, 1988.
15. Colvin, RB, Cohen, AH, Saiontz, C, Bonsib, S, Buick, M, Burke, B, Carter, S, Cavallo, T, Haas, M, Lindblad, A, Manivel, JC, Nast, CC, Salomon, D, Weaver, C & Weiss, M: Evaluation of pathologic criteria for acute renal allograft rejection: reproducibility, sensitivity, and clinical correlation. *J Am Soc Nephrol*, 8: 1930–41, 1997.
16. Furness, PN: Acp. Best practice no 160. Renal biopsy specimens. *J Clin Pathol*, 53: 433–8, 2000.

Part IV

Prevention and Conservative Therapy of Acute Kidney Failure

VI

Volume Resuscitation and Management

4.1

Jean-Louis Vincent and Barbara Ceradini

Core Messages

- Adequate fluid balance and good renal perfusion must be targeted in critically ill patients to reduce the risks of developing acute renal failure.
- Fluid resuscitation and management are complicated in acute renal failure, and these patients must be carefully and closely monitored.
- No intravenous fluid is perfect, and fluid choices should be based on individual patient's requirements.

4.1.1 Introduction

Acute renal failure is common in the intensive care unit (ICU), and ICU patients with acute renal failure have worse mortality and morbidity rates than those without acute renal failure [4, 6, 18]. A large multicenter study in Europe, which included 1,411 patients from 40 ICUs in 16 countries and excluded patients admitted for routine postoperative surveillance, determined that 25% of the ICU patients developed acute renal failure as diagnosed by a serum creatinine of 3.5 mg/dl (300 μmol/l) or more and/or a urine output of less than 500 ml/day; ICU mortality was three times higher in patients with acute renal failure than in other patients (43% vs. 14%, $p < 0.01$), and oliguric renal failure was an independent risk factor for mortality by multivariate analysis [6]. In a multicenter international study, Uchino et al. [25] reported that 6% of ICU patients developed severe renal failure as defined by a urine output of less than 200 ml in 12 h and/or a blood urea nitrogen (BUN) level higher than 84 mg/dl (> 30 mmol/l), or requirement for renal replacement therapy. Despite modern extracorporeal support techniques, mortality rates from acute renal failure remain high [7, 30]. As there are no pharmacological strategies to treat acute renal failure, prevention is an essential factor in trying to limit the impact of this disease process. The maintenance of an adequate renal blood flow in critically ill patients, first by maintaining blood volume and, second, possibly by using vasoactive agents to restore sufficient renal perfusion [2], is a key preventative measure. However, although hypovolemia can compromise renal blood flow, hypervolemia also has its risks, and these patients must be carefully monitored to ensure their volemic balance is optimal at all times.

4.1.2 Risk of Hypervolemia

Hypervolemia can be associated with edema formation, especially in the presence of altered capillary permeability (acute lung injury [ALI]/acute respiratory distress syndrome [ARDS]). Blood volume is unable to expand much, so the hemodiluting effects of fluid infusion are achieved with relatively small amounts of fluid, and any further increase in blood volume is associated with edema formation (Fig. 4.1.1). There is then a direct relationship between the amount of fluid given and the degree of edema.

Edema formation is important because edema can have multiple deleterious effects on organ function (Box 4.1.1). Lung edema is often a primary concern, but

J.-L. Vincent (✉)
Department of Intensive Care, Erasme Hospital, Université libre de Bruxelles, 808, route de Lennik, 1070-Brussels, Belgium
e-mail: jlvincent@ulb.ac.be

A. Jörres et al. (eds.), *Management of Acute Kidney Problems*,
DOI: 10.1007/978-3-540-69441-0_4.1, © Springer-Verlag Berlin Heidelberg 2010

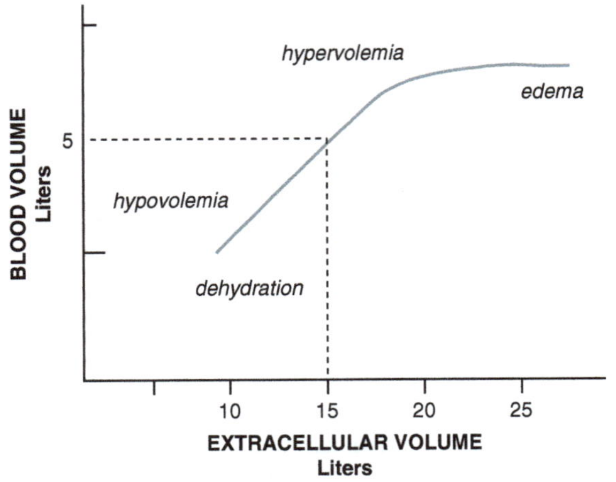

Fig. 4.1.1 The relationship between blood volume and extracellular volume (Adapted from A.C. Guyton)

this is in part because it is easily recognized early on: lung infiltrates are rapidly visible on a chest X-ray and the consequences are immediately apparent in terms of altered gas exchange (hypoxemia). However, edema in other systems can also be harmful. Edema in the brain may contribute to the development of delirium; edema in the heart may contribute to the development of systolic and diastolic dysfunction; edema in the abdominal wall can contribute to abdominal compartment syndrome; edema in the gut may limit tolerance to feeding; edema in the muscle and subcutaneous tissues may contribute to general weakness and can certainly impair mobilization; it is possible that edema in the kidneys could contribute to altered renal function. Taken in isolation, these factors may not sound so important, but it is interesting that in the SOAP study [17], one of the most important prognostic factors for mortality (by multivariate analysis) in patients with acute renal failure was a positive fluid balance (Table 4.1.1).

Table 4.1.1 Cox regression analysis in patients with acute renal failure in the SOAP study [17]

Characteristic	Hazard ratio	95% CI	*p* value
Mean daily fluid balance (l/24 h)	1.21	1.13–1.28	< 0.001
SAPS II score (per point)	1.03	1.02–1.04	< 0.001
Medical admission	1.68	1.35–2.08	< 0.001
Mechanical ventilation	1.55	1.14–2.11	< 0.001
Age	1.02	1.01–1.03	< 0.001
Liver cirrhosis	2.73	1.88–3.95	< 0.001
Heart failure	1.38	1.05–1.81	0.02

95% CI 95% confidence interval, *SAPS II* Simplified Acute Physiology Score II

Box 4.1.1 Potential adverse effects of tissue edema

- Impaired gas exchange
- Altered mental status – delirium
- Gut dysfunction – intolerance to feeding
- Intra-abdominal edema – increased abdominal pressure
- Myocardial dysfunction (systolic and diastolic)
- Risk of decubitus ulcers
- Impaired wound-healing
- Muscle weakness – impaired mobilization

4.1.3 Potential Errors in Fluid Management in the Patient with, or at Risk of, Acute Renal Failure

The relationship between volume status and complications can therefore be considered as a U-shaped curve (Fig. 4.1.2) with both ends of inappropriate volume status - hypervolemia and hypovolemia - being associated with worse outcomes. This makes tackling fluid management in patients with acute renal failure difficult, and there are several potential errors which must be avoided:

- Insufficient fluid administration: In the oliguric patient one may be afraid of inducing lung edema with excessive fluid administration, so that fluid restriction is often adopted, but while limiting edema

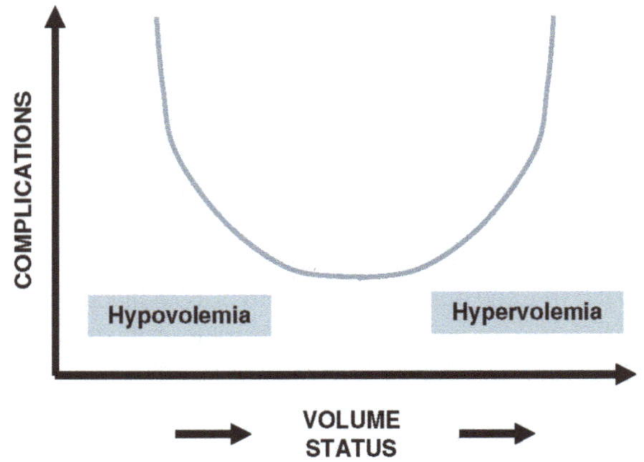

Fig. 4.1.2 The relationship between volume status and the risk of complications

formation, this can maintain kidney hypoperfusion and worsen renal function.

- Excess fluid administration: All too often, fluid is given to oliguric patients without sufficient monitoring or without careful attention to which variables are being monitored, with the focus being only on urine output. As an example, imagine a patient who is given 1 l of crystalloid, which has a small effect on urine output, e.g., urine output increases from 5 to 25 ml in 1 h; this encouraging effect prompts the administration of another liter, and the urine output again seems to increase somewhat, from 25 to 35 ml/h. This fluid administration could therefore be considered a success. But in fact, looking closer at the numbers, we can see that the patient received 2 l of fluid and eliminated only 60 ml in their urine, so where did the rest of the fluid go? Clearly, the excess fluid did not all remain in the circulation, and the patient will slowly be developing edema, with all its negative consequences.
- Excessive use of diuretics: It may be an attractive option to maintain urine output with diuretics. Actually, from a conceptual point of view, diuretics could decrease the oxygen demand of the renal tubules by inhibiting the Na^+-K^+-Cl^- pump. The major risk with use of diuretics is inducing hypovolemia if diuretics are given in the absence of hypervolemia. In the oliguric patient, diuretics often increase urine output regardless of the volume status but may thus aggravate a volume deficit. There are several studies indicating that diuretics may have harmful effects. Mehta et al. [14] studied 552 ICU patients with acute renal failure (defined by a BUN level of at least 40 mg/dl [14.3 mmol/l] or a serum creatinine level of at least 2.0 mg/dl [177 μmol/l] in patients with no existing renal dysfunction, or by a sustained rise in serum creatinine levels of at least 1 mg/dl [88.4 μmol/l] compared with baseline in other patients), categorizing them according to whether or not they received diuretics on the day of nephrology consultation; 326 of the patients (59%) received diuretics, and diuretic use was associated with a 68% increase in in-hospital mortality. Uchino et al. [24] studied 1,743 consecutive ICU patients who were receiving renal replacement therapy and/or had urine output < 200 ml in 12 h, a plasma urea > 30 mmol/l or BUN > 86 mg/dl, or a serum potassium > 6.5 mmol/l. At baseline, about 70% of the patients were receiving diuretics, largely furosemide. Using a confirmatory propensity-adjusted mortality model, these authors proposed that there was no difference in mortality rates among patients who were treated with diuretics and those who were not. However, the odds ratio was 1.21 (95% confidence interval [95% CI], 0.96–1.50) with a p value of 0.10, suggesting that in a larger number of patients, the difference may have been significant with perhaps a 20% worse outcome with diuretics [5]. A recent meta-analysis by Ho and Sheridan [11] evaluating the effects of furosemide to prevent or treat acute renal failure included nine randomized controlled trials and a total of 849 patients with, or at risk of, acute renal failure. Although there were no statistically significant differences in in-hospital mortality rates or need for renal replacement therapy with diuretic use, in patients who received furosemide to prevent an acute deterioration in renal function, the relative risk of mortality was 2.33 (95% CI, 0.75–7.25), again with a p value of 0.15, suggesting a potential harmful effect. This meta-analysis also suggested an increased risk of temporary deafness and tinnitus with use of high doses of furosemide [11], an effect that is often underrecognized [9]. With these studies suggesting a potentially harmful effect of diuretics, is there a need for a further randomized controlled study to evaluate these effects? We do not think so, largely because the patient population is too difficult to define. While in hypervolemic patients, diuretics may indeed help, in normovolemic or hypovolemic patients, they may be harmful; our techniques to determine fluid status are still too imprecise to be able to separate with certainty these groups of patients. We believe the key indication for diuretics in patients with acute renal failure is hypervolemia, and rather than being used routinely in all patients, diuretics should be restricted to those with fluid overload.

4.1.4 How to Assess Fluid Status?

As we have seen, the fluid status of a patient with acute renal failure is important, but assessing fluid status is difficult, particularly in the critically ill patient with sepsis or other conditions associated with capillary leak, because large fluid shifts can occur in the extravascular space, resulting in edema despite ongoing intravascular depletion [13].

Static and dynamic indices have been proposed (Box 4.1.2), but all have their limitations. Static indicators are easy to perform but have many restrictions: Signs such as tachycardia or hypotension are not specific, low cardiac filling pressures do not necessarily mean the patient will respond to fluid administration, and high filling pressures do not necessarily mean that the fluid status is optimized. Measurements of end-diastolic or intrathoracic volumes do not reflect volemia any better and are not superior to pressure measurements. If diuresis is maintained, it can be useful to send a urine sample to the laboratory, as kidney hypoperfusion (prerenal failure) will be associated with concentrated urine (high urine osmolarity) and low sodium content. Persistent metabolic alkalosis may also reflect a reduction in effective blood volume.

Box 4.1.2 Techniques for assessing fluid status and responsiveness

Static techniques

Dehydration: Thirst, dry mouth, dry armpits, diminished skin turgor

Decreased blood volume: Hypotension, tachycardia, skin vasoconstriction

Hemoconcentration: Hypernatremia, high hematocrit, hyperproteinemia

Decreased renal perfusion: Increased urinary osmolality, decreased urinary sodium concentration, elevated blood urea nitrogen/urea, metabolic alkalosis

Dynamic techniques

Orthostatic hypotension

Arterial pressure and stroke volume variation

Response to fluid challenge

The limitations of static indices have led to research into dynamic indices of fluid status or responsiveness - in particular, measurement of pulse pressure from arterial pressure tracings (provided the patient has an arterial catheter) or stroke volume variation (provided the patient has a cardiac output monitor allowing stroke volume calculations from a beat-by-beat analysis of the arterial pressure tracing [PICCO or LiDCO]). However, these measures are only really reliable in patients treated with mechanical ventilation without spontaneous respiratory effort, and in the absence of significant arrhythmias. In spontaneously breathing patients, pulse pressure variation to assess fluid responsiveness is less accurate [10, 21].

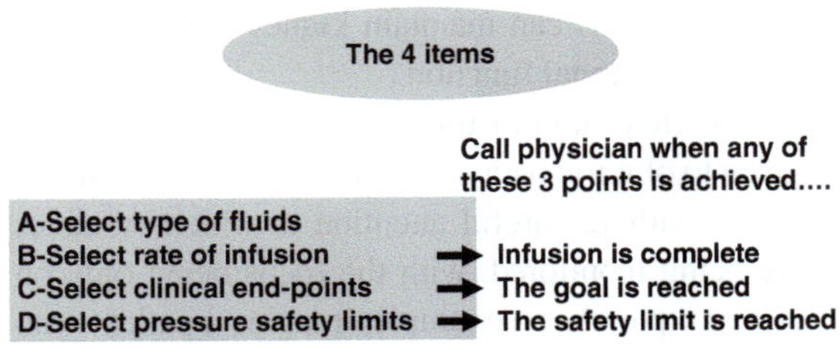

Fig. 4.1.3 The four items of the fluid challenge technique

Ultimately the best method of assessing fluid status and responsiveness is the fluid challenge technique [27] (Fig. 4.1.3); however, the fluid challenge must be done correctly and carefully, so that fluid administration is interrupted immediately if there is no benefit. Hence, patients must be closely monitored at least every 10 min during administration of the fluid and nothing else be done to the patient during the fluid challenge (not even touching the patient!).

4.1.5 Types of Fluids

Many different fluid types are available and it can be difficult to choose among them, particularly as there is little evidence that any one is superior to another in terms of improving outcomes. Indeed, in a patient with hypovolemia, any fluid is probably better than none. Nevertheless, each fluid type has its own advantages and disadvantages, and optimal fluid choices may play a role in maximizing outcomes and limiting renal dysfunction.

It can be argued that as urine is composed of water and small solutes (crystalloids), crystalloids should be administered principally. This is true, initially at least, where crystalloids represent the first choice for intravascular hypovolemia. Crystalloids also have no specific nephrotoxic effects, unlike most of the colloid solutions. However, in patients with reduced urine output and limited capacity to eliminate excess fluids, the higher quantities of crystalloids needed compared with colloids to achieve the same end point may support a greater use of colloid solutions. In addition, if maintenance of blood volume is of paramount importance, colloids may be more effective, although it is important to recognize that hyperoncocity may induce renal failure, so that excessive administration of colloids should be avoided.

Among the crystalloids, excessive saline administration can result in hyperchloremic acidosis [20], and it has been suggested that hyperchloremic acidosis may decrease renal blood flow [28] and thereby increase the risk of renal dysfunction [29]. Ringer's lactate solution has an osmolarity of less than 280 mOsm/l, so it is slightly hypotonic and should be avoided in hypotonic states or in cases of brain edema (including brain trauma) [23]. In addition, even a small amount of potassium may not be desirable in the presence of severe hyperkalemia. However, the hyperlactatemia that may result with administration of large amounts of this solution does not seem to be toxic, and lactate may even serve as a cellular nutrient [19]. Crystalloid solutions containing ethyl pyruvate, an aliphatic ester derived from pyruvate which has antioxidant and antiinflammatory properties, have been shown to have beneficial effects on renal function in animal models of septic shock [15, 22]. However, early clinical trials have not shown similar beneficial effects.

Among the colloids, the use of human albumin has been decreasing following several studies and meta-analyses that failed to demonstrate its superiority over other colloids [1, 8, 26] in addition to its high costs. Several synthetic colloid solutions exist, but none is ideal. Gelatin solutions have a relatively low molecular weight (MW) and as such have a limited effect on volume expansion with limited oncotic effects and relatively short (2–3 h) intravascular persistence. Their superiority over crystalloids in terms of volume expansion is, therefore, restricted. Moreover, gelatin solutions can induce anaphylactic reactions, although they are usually transient and of limited severity, and they may compromise clot formation - although to a lesser degree than some of the other colloids [16]. Gelatin solutions are not available in the United States, but are used in other countries largely because of their relatively low cost.

Dextrans are mixtures of glucose polymers synthesized by the bacteria *Leuconostoc mesenteroides*. Dextran 70 (MW 70,000 Da) has been the most widely used dextran for fluid therapy. Although they are efficient volume expanders, dextran solutions are associated with a substantial risk of anaphylactic reaction, even when hapten prophylaxis is given, and also have antihemostatic effects. Dextran solutions may also precipitate renal failure [12] by accumulation of the molecule in the renal tubules and/or hyperviscosity.

The development of hydroxyethyl starches (HESs) was met with some excitement in the hope that these fluids would prove effective without adverse effects. Synthesized from amylopectin, different HES solutions are available with different molecular weights and different degrees of hydroxyethyl substitutions, which determine their different pharmacokinetic characteristics. However, although associated with fewer anaphylactic reactions, HES solutions can affect hemostasis, may accumulate and persist in host cells, particularly those of the reticuloendothelial system, and may alter renal function. A recent study reported that therapy of septic patients with a particular HES 10% solution (200/0.5) was associated with higher rates of acute renal failure and renal replacement therapy than was Ringer's lactate solution [3]. Newer forms of HES may have fewer adverse effects on renal function, but until more data are available, they should be used with caution in patients with, or at risk of, acute renal failure.

4.1.6 Conclusion

Acute renal failure is common in the ICU and associated with poor outcomes. Adequate intravascular volumes and renal perfusion must be maintained to limit the development of acute renal failure. However, excess volume replacement carries its own risks. We have inadequate tools to assess and monitor fluid balance and responsiveness, especially in patients with capillary leak syndromes, and, currently, carefully conducted, repeated fluid challenges represent the best way of determining ongoing fluid needs. While crystalloids represent a good initial choice of fluid, for large or continuing losses, colloid solutions must also be used. No fluid is ideal, and fluid selection should be individualized depending on specific patient needs and known adverse effects of the different fluid types; in many patients, it may be wiser to infuse smaller amounts of several different types of solution so that the benefits of each type can be maximized while limiting the risks.

4.1.7 Take Home Pearls

- Both *hyper*volemia and *hypo*volemia can be detrimental.
- Diuretic use in patients with acute renal failure should be restricted to patients with *hyper*volemia.
- In many patients, it may be wiser to use smaller amounts of several different types of fluid than a large amount of any single solution.

References

1. Alderson P, Bunn F, Lefebvre C, et al (2004) Human albumin solution for resuscitation and volume expansion in critically ill patients. Cochrane Database Syst Rev CD001208
2. Bellomo R, Wan L, May C (2008) Vasoactive drugs and acute kidney injury. Crit Care Med 36:S179–S186
3. Brunkhorst FM, Engel C, Bloos F, et al (2008) Intensive insulin therapy and pentastarch resuscitation in severe sepsis. N Engl J Med 358:125–139
4. Clermont G, Acker CG, Angus DC, et al (2002) Renal failure in the ICU: comparison of the impact of acute renal failure and end-stage renal disease on ICU outcomes. Kidney Int 62: 986–996
5. De Backer D, Vincent JL (2005) Decreased mortality with the use of the pulmonary artery catheter? Crit Care Med 33: 917
6. de Mendonca A, Vincent JL, Suter PM, et al (2000) Acute renal failure in the ICU: risk factors and outcome evaluated by the SOFA score. Intensive Care Med 26:915–921
7. Eachempati SR, Wang JC, Hydo LJ, et al (2007) Acute renal failure in critically ill surgical patients: persistent lethality despite new modes of renal replacement therapy. J Trauma 63: 987–993
8. Finfer S, Bellomo R, Boyce N, et al (2004) A comparison of albumin and saline for fluid resuscitation in the intensive care unit. N Engl J Med 350:2247–2256
9. Gallagher KL, Jones JK (1979) Furosemide-induced ototoxicity. Ann Intern Med 91:744–745
10. Heenen S, De Backer D, Vincent JL (2006) How can the response to volume expansion in patients with spontaneous respiratory movements be predicted? Crit Care 10:R102
11. Ho KM, Sheridan DJ (2006) Meta-analysis of frusemide to prevent or treat acute renal failure. BMJ 333:420
12. Mailloux L, Swartz CD, Capizzi R, et al (1967) Acute renal failure after administration of low-molecular weight dextran. N Engl J Med 277:1113–1118
13. Mehta RL, Clark WC, Schetz M (2002) Techniques for assessing and achieving fluid balance in acute renal failure. Curr Opin Crit Care 8:535–543
14. Mehta RL, Pascual MT, Soroko S, Chertow GM (2002) Diuretics, mortality, and nonrecovery of renal function in acute renal failure. JAMA 288:2547–2553
15. Miyaji T, Hu X, Yuen PS, et al (2003) Ethyl pyruvate decreases sepsis-induced acute renal failure and multiple organ damage in aged mice. Kidney Int 64:1620–1631
16. Niemi TT, Kuitunen AH (2005) Artificial colloids impair haemostasis. An in vitro study using thromboelastometry coagulation analysis. Acta Anaesthesiol Scand 49:3 73–378
17. Payen D, Sakr Y, Gerlach H, Reinhart K, Sprung C, Vincent JL, Carlet J, Ranieri VM, Le Gall J-R, Moreno R (2003) Early and late renal failure in ICU: Incidence and predictors of mortality and morbidity. Intensive Care Med 29 (Suppl): 614 (abst)
18. Philp A, Macdonald AL, Watt PW (2005) Lactate - a signal coordinating cell and systemic function. J Exp Biol 208: 4561–4575
19. Scheingraber S, Rehm M, Sehmisch C, Finsterer U (1999) Rapid saline infusion produces hyperchloremic acidosis in patients undergoing gynecologic surgery. Anesthesiology 90:1265–1270
20. Soubrier S, Saulnier F, Hubert H, et al (2007) Can dynamic indicators help the prediction of fluid responsiveness in spontaneously breathing critically ill patients? Intensive Care Med 33:1117–1124
21. Su F, Wang Z, Cai Y, et al (2007) Beneficial effects of ethyl pyruvate in septic shock due to peritonitis. Arch Surg 142:166–171
22. Tommasino C, Moore S, Todd MM (1988) Cerebral effects of isovolemic hemodilution with crystalloid or colloid solutions. Crit Care Med 16:862–868
23. Uchino S, Doig GS, Bellomo R, et al (2004) Diuretics and mortality in acute renal failure. Crit Care Med 32:1669–1677
24. Uchino S, Kellum JA, Bellomo R, et al (2005) Acute renal failure in critically ill patients: a multinational, multicenter study. JAMA 294:813–818
25. Veneman TF, Oude NJ, Woittiez AJ (2004) Human albumin and starch administration in critically ill patients: a prospective randomized clinical trial. Wien Klin Wochenschr 116: 305–309
26. Vincent JL, Sakr Y, Sprung CL, et al (2006) Sepsis in European intensive care units: results of the SOAP study. Crit Care Med 34:344–353
27. Vincent JL, Weil MH (2006) Fluid challenge revisited. Crit Care Med 34:1333–1337
28. Wilcox CS (1983) Regulation of renal blood flow by plasma chloride. J Clin Invest 71:726–735
29. Williams EL, Hildebrand KL, McCormick SA, Bedel MJ (1999) The effect of intravenous lactated Ringer's solution versus 0.9% sodium chloride solution on serum osmolality in human volunteers. Anesth Analg 88:999–1003
30. Ympa YP, Sakr Y, Reinhart K, Vincent JL (2005) Has mortality from acute renal failure decreased? A systematic review of the literature. Am J Med 118:827–832

Management of Electrolyte Disorders

4.2

Michael Oppert

Core Messages

- Electrolyte disorders are frequent, especially in the intensive care unit (ICU) and the emergency department. The most important imbalances of electrolyte homeostasis include disorders of sodium, potassium, calcium, and phosphate.
- Hyponatremia and hyperkalemia are certainly the most common disorders and require prompt and safe correction, once the diagnosis is made and the underlying illness is identified. Therefore, the physiology of electrolytes will be covered briefly here, while the main emphasis is on the causes and management of electrolyte abnormalities.
- Patients with hyponatremia are at high risk of cerebral edema, while hyperkalemia may lead to life-threatening cardiac rhythm abnormalities.

4.2.1 Sodium

4.2.1.1 Physiology

Sodium is the principle extracellular cation and the predominant solute regulating the serum osmolality [1]. Sodium salts account for more than 90% of total body osmolality of extracellular fluids, which is kept between 285 and 295 mOsm/kg of water [2]. Therefore, sodium balance regulates the extracellular fluid volume. The serum sodium level under normal conditions is maintained within the narrow range of 135–145 mmol/l, regardless of water and salt intake [3].

Total body sodium balance depends on the dietary intake and the capacity of renal sodium excretion (under normal conditions extrarenal sodium losses are negligible). The kidneys control natriuresis through hormonal mechanisms including atrial natriuretic peptide (ANP) and aldosterone. ANPs can increase glomerular sodium filtration and inhibit sodium reabsorption in the collecting ducts [4].

Osmoreceptors in the hypothalamus detect small changes in serum osmolality and control the secretion of antidiuretic hormone (ADH; vasopressin). An increase in osmolality leads to ADH secretion while a decrease results in the opposite. With maximal ADH secretion the urine volume may be as little as 500 ml/day and the urine osmolality will be 800–1,400 mOsm/kg. In absence of ADH, the urine osmolality will be between 40 and 80 mOsm/kg, and the urine volume may be as much as 20 l/day.

4.2.1.2 Hyponatremia

Hyponatremia, defined as a serum sodium of less than 135 mmol/l, is the most common electrolyte disorder among critically ill patients [3, 5, 6]. In a prospective study hyponatremia (Na <135 mmol/l) was observed in 30% of critically ill patients [7]. A retrospective survey found the incidence of hyponatremia (<130 mmol/l) to be 14% [8]. Hyponatremia carries a substantial morbidity and mortality.

Patients with sodium levels above 120–125 mmol/l are usually asymptomatic. Values below 120 mmol/l

M. Oppert
Nephrology & Medical Intensive Care, Charité Campus Virchow-Klinikum, 13343 Berlin, Germany
e-mail: oppert@charite.de

A. Jörres et al. (eds.), *Management of Acute Kidney Problems*,
DOI: 10.1007/978-3-540-69441-0_4.2, © Springer-Verlag Berlin Heidelberg 2010

Table 4.2.1 Causes of hyponatremia

Hydration status	Disorder
Hypervolemia (TBW↑↑, TBNA⁺↑)	
UNa < 20	• Heart failure • Nephrotic syndrome • Cirrhosis
UNa > 20	• Acute renal failure • Chronic renal failure
Euvolemia (TBW ↔; TBNA⁺↔)	
UNa > 20	• Syndrome of inappropriate ADH secretion • Steroid deficiency • Hypothyroidism • Polydipsia • Drugs etc.
Hypovolemia (TBW↓; TBNA⁺↓↓)	
UNa < 20	*Extrarenal losses* • Sweating • Diarrhea • Vomiting • Third spacing (pancreatitis, peritonitis, etc.)
UNa > 20	*Renal losses* • Diuretics • Mineralocorticoid deficiency • Salt-losing nephropathy • Renal tubular acidosis Type II • Cerebral salt wasting syndrome • Osmotic diuresis etc.

lead to symptoms mainly related to the central nervous system, such as nausea and vomiting, headache, confusion, seizures, and coma. Muscle cramps, rhabdomyolysis, and noncardiogenic pulmonary edema may also occur [9]. Patients are usually more symptomatic when hyponatremia develops rapidly over a few days. Hyponatremic patients can be hypovolemic, hypervolemic, or euvolemic. To better understand the etiology of the hyponatremia, the hydration status of the patient needs to be assessed. Further, it is wise to measure urine osmolality and urine sodium concentration (Table 4.2.1). The most common causes of hyponatremia in adults are thiazide therapy, postoperative state, and other causes of inappropriate ADH secretion and polydipsia in psychiatric patients and after prostate surgery [10, 11].

4.2.1.2.1 Management

The management of hyponatremia depends mainly on the degree of the disorder and the time period over which it has developed. Hyponatremia developing within 48 h has a substantially higher risk of causing cerebral edema [10, 12], especially in patients with serum sodium levels below 120 mmol/l. Although there is little consensus on the general management of hyponatremia, therapeutic options include normal saline infusion, fluid restriction, and occasionally diuretics. Recently, arginine vasopressin (AVP) receptor antagonists offer a new treatment option.

Severe hyponatremia (serum sodium level <120 mmol/l occurring within 48 h) constitutes a medical emergency. Untreated, this extent of hyponatremia can lead to serious neurologic deficits such as coma, downward herniation, raised intracranial pressure, and death. This condition requires prompt intervention under careful monitoring. Here, hypertonic (3%) saline is infused at a rate of 1–2 ml/kg per h. A loop diuretic may be added to enhance free water clearance. Hyponatremia should be corrected quickly by 1–2 mmol/h until the symptoms improve, the sodium concentration is above 120 mmol/l, or an increase in sodium concentration of 20 mmol is reached within 24 h [2]. In a retrospective analysis, rapid correction of hyponatremia to a serum sodium above 120 mmol/l was an independent predictor of improved outcome [13]. Of predominant importance are the correction of possible volume depletion and the targeting of the calculated sodium deficit. A formula may help the clinician to estimate the amount of saline infusion needed to correct the sodium deficit. The following formula is used for the infusion of 3% (513 mmol/l) saline (total body water [TBW] equals the body weight times 0.6 in men and 0.5 in women).

Change in serum Na^+ = (infusate Na^+ − serum Na^+)/(TBW + 1)[10]

Although, this formula is easy to use, it carries certain limitations, as it assumes that the patient's body is a closed system. It can, therefore, not predict shifts of body water. Frequent monitoring of serum sodium is, therefore, mandatory.

The role of AVP receptor antagonists in the management of acute hyponatremia is still under investigation [1, 14–16]. Conivaptan is the only AVP antagonist currently approved in the United States. It blocks the V1a and V2 receptor, induces aquaresis and is used in euvolemic and hypervolemic hyponatremia including syndrome of inappropriate antidiuretic hormone (SIADH), hypothyroidism, and adrenal insufficiency, heart failure, and hepatic cirrhosis [6]. Excessive free water clearance may lead to overcorrection of the hyponatremia with the danger of central pontine myelinolysis.

In *chronic hyponatremia,* patients tend to present with mild symptoms and only subtle neurologic findings. When patients are asymptomatic, treatment with fluid restriction is usually sufficient. Only when patients are symptomatic, saline infusion may be required.

Central pontine myelinolysis is the most feared complication of hyponatremia and the correction itself. Hyponatremia causes entry of water into the brain resulting in cerebral edema. Fortunately, solutes leave the brain tissues within hours inducing a water loss and ameliorating cerebral hypertension. This process develops over a few days and explains why patients with chronic hyponatremia are largely asymptomatic. Pontine demyelination is most often the consequence of over rapid correction of chronic hyponatremia [12]. A correction rate below 12 mmol/day will allow most patients to recover from hyponatremia without neurologic complications [6, 12].

Unfortunately, the duration of the hyponatremia is often difficult to determine. The presence of symptoms rather than laboratory values should therefore guide treatment regimes.

Pitfalls in the management of hyponatremia include fluid restriction in hypovolemic patients. In this situation the sodium deficit should be targeted rather than the presumed water excess. On the other hand, normal saline infusion in SIADH patients may aggravate the symptoms as the infused salt is excreted via the kidneys resulting in a net water retention worsening the hyponatremia. Endocrine disorders such as hypothyroidism and adrenal insufficiency should be looked for, especially in patients with concomitant hyperkalemia. Whereas patients with oligosymptomatic hyponatremia should be corrected slowly, patients with severe hyponatremia require rapid correction. Careful use of hypertonic saline can be life saving, while failure to follow the above recommendations may lead to serious and even lethal complications.

4.2.1.3 Hypernatremia

Hypernatremia (serum sodium >150 mmol/l) only leads to symptoms when it has developed rapidly to levels exceeding 160 mmol/l [2, 12] (Table 4.2.2). In health, thirst will be an important back-up to inhibit rising sodium concentration. In intensive care unit (ICU) patients with altered mental status or under sedation, this defense mechanism may not work. The main cause of hypernatremia in the ICU is iatrogenic. Fluid resuscitation containing saline infusion may eventually lead to hypernatremia. Another important mechanism is the widespread application of steroids (even in low doses) in patients with septic shock. Here the fluid resuscitation containing saline and the steroids may have additive effects. Although, sodium retention is not widely accepted under steroids, all studies investigating low-dose steroids in septic shock found increases in serum sodium [17–20].

Table 4.2.2 Causes of hypernatremia

Hydration status	Disorder
Hypervolemia (TBW↑↑, TBNA⁺↑)	
UNa > 20	*Iatrogenic* • Saline infusion • Bicarbonate infusion • Steroids • Antibiotics-containing sodium etc.
Euvolemia (TBW ↔; TBNA⁺↔)	
UNa variable	*Renal fluid losses* • Diabetes insipidus • Hypodipsia *Extra renal fluid losses* • Fever • Hyperventilation • Mechanical ventilation
Hypovolemia (TBW ↓; TBNA⁺↓↓)	
UNa < 20	*Extrarenal fluid losses* • Sweating • Diarrhea • Vomiting • Burns
UNa > 20	*Renal fluid losses* • Diuretics • Osmotic diuresis • Postobstruction • Acute and chronic renal disease

4.2.1.3.1 Management

Rapid correction of serum sodium in patients when hypernatremia occurred quickly, is warranted and improves prognosis without the risk of cerebral edema [21]. A reduction in serum sodium by 1 mmol/h is without risk [22]. In hypovolemic states alternating infusions of normal saline and glucose should be given, while enteral intake of hypotonic fluids is preferred in euvolemic or hypervolemic patients. Hormonal interventions (such as desmopressin) should be considered in patients with central diabetes insipidus. Here the sodium concentration should be monitored closely.

4.2.2 Potassium

4.2.2.1 Physiology

Potassium is the predominant intracellular cation and has a serum concentration of 3.5–5.5 mmol/l. The intracellular to extracellular ratio is created by an energy-consuming active transport to stabilize membrane potential. Acute changes in serum potassium levels are influenced among others by insulin, beta adrenergic drugs, and changes in acid–base balance. The potassium level is influenced by intake disorders, excretion disorders, or transcellular shifting disorders. The long-term potassium balance is maintained by the interaction of aldosterone and the kidney.

4.2.2.2 Hypokalemia

A decrease of 30–40 mmol (1%) of total body potassium may already interfere with important physiologic functions. On the other hand, serum potassium may be reduced due to intra/extracellular shifts without affecting total body sodium. Mild hypokalemia (3.0–3.5 mmol/l) is usually not associated with major symptoms [23]. In patients with underlying cardiac disease, however, already minor changes in serum potassium may lead to arrhythmias, especially when digoxin is prescribed. Serum levels below 3 mmol/l may lead to serious symptoms, including weakness, arrhythmias (atrial tachycardias, atrioventricular conduction blocks), paralytic ileus, and in severe cases (<2.5 or even 2 mmol/l) may lead to ascending paralysis leading to respiratory failure, and constitutes a medical emergency [24].

4.2.2.2.1 Management

In the management of hypokalemia, one needs to consider the possible pathogenesis of hypokalemia (Table 4.2.3). The history (including drug history) is equally important as to check the acid–base status and urinary potassium. In chronic and/or mild hypokalemia, substitution with oral potassium seems to be a safe approach, as potassium is absorbed slowly and the risk of hyperkalemia is reduced. In patients with symptomatic and/or severe hypokalemia, aggressive emergency treatment is indicated with intravenous substitution. As the amount of potassium depletion may be enormous, an infusion containing high potassium chloride concentrations may be required. This drip should be given via a central line. Due to possible cardiovascular events, close monitoring of cardiac function and laboratory parameters is warranted. Concomitant magnesium repletion should be considered. Special care must be taken in patients with hypokalemia due to transcellular shifts as potassium repletion may lead to rebound hyperkalemia [25].

Table 4.2.3 Causes of hypokalemia

Renal losses	• Diuretics • Drugs
Enteral losses	• Diarrhea • Vomiting • Laxants • Nasogastric drainage • Tumors
Transcellular shifts	• Alkalosis • Drugs (catecholamines, theophylline, etc.) • Insulin • Hypothermia • Thyrotoxicosis
Others	• Renal tubular acidosis (Types I and II) • Diabetic ketoacidosis • Increased sweating

4.2.2.3 Hyperkalemia

It is difficult to differentiate between mild, moderate, and severe hyperkalemia, as not only the absolute serum potassium level is important, but also the timing of the increase and the baseline level. Further the acid–base status and the serum calcium concentration need to be taken into account. Most often hyperkalemia is due to reduced renal potassium excretion or increased endogenous release from cells [26, 27]. In health, hyperkalemia is rare, as the kidney is able to excrete potassium quickly after a relevant potassium load. Therefore, hyperkalemia is the consequence of impaired potassium excretion or transcellular shifts. The differential potential mechanisms of hyperkalemia are given in Table 4.2.4.

Table 4.2.4 Causes of hyperkalemia

Increased potassium load	• Potassium infusions • Red blood cell transfusions • Potassium supplements
Reduced renal excretion	• Renal failure • Drugs (ACE-I, AT 1-blockers, spironolactone, NSAIDs, etc.) • Addison's disease • Uretrojejunostomy
Increased cell release	• Hemolysis • Trauma including rhabdomyolysis • Tumor lysis syndrome • Acidosis • Drugs (beta-blockers, succinylcholine, etc.)

Symptoms of hyperkalemia include general weakness, paralysis, and arrhythmias. Electrocardiographic changes include highly elevated T-waves, changes in the p-wave, and conduction blocks.

4.2.2.3.1 Management

The first step in *managing* a patient with hyperkalemia is to decide whether the disorder is potentially life-threatening so that it requires urgent correction. Potassium levels <6.5–7.0 mmol/l usually lead to few symptoms (unless the potassium level has risen very quickly), although one has to be cautious as considerable interindividual susceptibility to hyperkalemia exists. Further, severe problems may occur without warning and ECG changes do not necessarily correlate with the degree of hyperkalemia. Therefore, any patient with ECG changes consistent with hyperkalemia or with proven potassium levels > 6.0–6.5 mmol/l should be treated immediately.

There are three main options in the management of hyperkalemia, which may be used in the treatment of this disorder. They include antagonizing the toxic effects, shifting potassium from the extracellular to the intracellular space, and enhancing the excretion of potassium.

Calcium gluconate (10 ml of 10% solution intravenous) is the preferred immediate treatment in hyperkalemia, as it directly opposes the membrane toxic effects of potassium. It should be given with caution in patients under co-medication with digoxin, as it may increase digoxin toxicity [28]. An effect may be expected within a few minutes lasting for up to 30–60 min. Calcium is a temporary measure and must always be used with other treatments to lower potassium levels [23].

A shift of potassium from the extracellular to the intracellular space is the next step in the management of hyperkalemia. Within 10–20 min, a shift can be expected with the application of insulin. To prevent hypoglycemia, an insulin/glucose infusion is indicated. Insulin is warranted in all patients with hyperkalemia irrespective of acid–base status and a reliable tool to lower potassium levels. In patients with metabolic acidosis the serum potassium may also be lowered with an infusion of 50–100 mmol of sodium bicarbonate. This approach has some disadvantages over insulin treatment as it is less effective in nonorganic metabolic acidosis (lactic acidosis, ketoacidosis). Also, if repeated doses are needed, patients could receive large amounts of sodium, an undesirable side effect especially in patients with heart failure and renal failure.

One needs to keep in mind, however, that the infusion of calcium, insulin, and bicarbonate are only temporary measures as they do not enhance the excretion of potassium. Most hyperkalemic states, however, are due to excess potassium and this potassium overload must be excreted.

Renal excretion may be promoted using loop diuretics given a preserved diuresis. Oral application of an exchange resin (with a laxans to prevent constipation) or an enema containing exchange resins lead to a significant potassium loss. In severe cases, renal replacement therapy using a diffusive mode is the treatment of choice. Hemodialysis is the preferred option with a dialysate containing 1 mmol potassium/l. Potassium levels can be lowered by as much as 1–2 mmol/l per h. Because hemodialysis affects the extracellular component, only small amounts of total body potassium can be removed. Redistribution of potassium (which may have been shifted to the intracellular space with insulin prior to dialysis therapy) may occur. Therefore, potassium levels need to be checked repeatedly even after a primary successful management of hyperkalemia. Management of hyperkalemia should – if possible – be performed under continuous ECG – and careful potassium monitoring.

4.2.3 Calcium

4.2.3.1 Physiology

Calcium is important for the normal function of many intracellular systems, muscle contraction (including the heart), nerve conduction, and coagulation pathways. It is kept within a narrow range of 2.1 and 2.6 mmol/l. The calcium homeostasis is regulated by complex interaction and feedback loops including parathyroid hormone (PTH) and vitamin D acting on the intestine, kidney, and bone. One percent of total body calcium is in the extracellular fluid, where the physiologic active ionized fraction equals about 50%. The rest is protein bound (mainly albumin).

4.2.3.2 Hypocalcemia

Hypocalcemia is defined as a total serum calcium concentration of less than 2 mmol/l (or ionized less than 1 mmol/l). Its causes are given in Table 4.2.5. Symptomatic hypocalcemia rarely occurs when the ionized calcium is >0.7–0.8 mmol/l. In severe (and acute) hypocalcemia (<0.7 mmol/l), neuropsychiatric and neuromuscular symptoms predominate. The most important sign of increased neuromuscular irritability is tetany. Weakness, cramps, and laryngeal spasm or bronchospasm may also occur. Patients may complain of perioral numbness (often seen in hyperventilation due to respiratory alkalosis) and distal paresthesias. Cardiac symptoms include reduced myocardial contractility, arrhythmias, and a QT interval prolongation. The neuropsychiatric problems may consist of confusion, anxiety, and seizures.

Table 4.2.5 Causes of hypocalcemia and hypercalcemia

Hypocalcemia	• Hypoparathyroidism (postradiation, postsurgery) • Vitamin D deficiency (low sun exposure, malnutrition, liver disease, renal disease) • Drugs (bisphosphonates, calcitonin, citrate, chemotherapeutic drugs) • Others (sepsis, pancreatitis, burns)
Hypercalcemia	• Endocrine: – Hyperparathyroidism – Hypothyroidism – Vitamin D calcidiol intoxication • Paraneoplastic: – Multiple endocrine neoplasia (MEN Types I and II) – Parathyroid hormone-related protein – Non-small-cell lung cancer – Multiple myeloma – Metastatic disease • Excessive intake/increased bone resorption: – Milk-alkali syndrome – Thiazide diuretics – Lithium – Granulomatous disease

4.2.3.2.1 Management

In the management of severe hypocalcemia, intravenous supplements should be given until symptoms cease or the ionized calcium is >0.9 mmol/l [29]. A continuous infusion is preferred as a fast bolus injection carries the risk of sever arrhythmias including asystole, especially in patients with cardiac conditions or under digoxin [29]. In the situation of hyperphosphatemia at the same time, one should be cautious in fast correction of calcium due to the risk of soft tissue calcification. Here, calcium supplementation should be postponed as long as possible, and phosphate binders should be considered. Hemodialysis may be a rational therapeutic option.

4.2.3.3 Hypercalcemia

In hypercalcemia, elevations of serum calcium of <3 mmol/l are usually associated with no or few symptoms [22]. With increasing serum calcium, symptoms may be nonspecific including malaise, nausea, vomiting, weakness, and abdominal pain. Severe hypercalcemia (>4 mmol/l) may lead to acute pancreatitis [30] and relevant cognitive disorders such as hallucinations, stupor, and coma [31].

The most important causes of hypercalcemia are PTH excess and malignant tumors. Other reasons for hypercalcemia are given in Table 4.2.5.

4.2.3.3.1 Management

The management of hypercalcemia is based on adequate (re)hydration, increased calcium excretion via the kidneys, inhibition of bone turnover, and treatment of the underlying disease. The infusion of normal saline in severe hypercalcemia at a rate of 1–2 l/h may be mandatory. A combination with a loop diuretic (but not a thiazide, as it may increase calcium reabsorption in the kidney) is recommended to not only restore hydration but also enhance calcium diuresis. Bisphosphonates are an effective mode of therapy. Repeat dosages should not be given within 7 days. In patients with vitamin D intoxication, lymphoma, or multiple myeloma, steroids are mandatory as they decrease calcitriol production [32]. Treatment effects with both steroids and bisphosphonates may, however, be delayed by 2–4 days. Calcitonin acts very rapidly (usually within 4–6 h) and may be safely given in the meantime. In patients with severe symptomatic hypercalcemia, hemodialysis (containing a low calcium dialysate) may be indicated, especially in patients with renal and/or heart failure.

4.2.4 Phosphate

Less than 1% of total body phosphate is found in the serum. It is essential for the mineralization of the bone and cellular functions including energy metabolism and genetic encoding. The normal phosphate plasma concentration is 0.8–1.45 mmol/l. Ninety percent of the phosphate is secreted via the kidneys.

4.2.4.1 Hyperphosphatemia

Hyperphosphatemia can be found with increased endogenous production, excessive intake, or reduced urinary excretion. Most often chronic hyperphosphatemia is due to acute or chronic renal failure. A summary of causes of hyperphosphatemia is given in Table 4.2.6.

4.2.4.1.1 Management

Hyperphosphatemia is best managed by targeting the underlying disorder. In chronic renal failure, mild hyperphosphatemia can usually be treated with reduced oral intake and/or phosphate-binding salts. In patients with end-stage renal disease and in patients with severe hyperphosphatemia (>2 mmol/l) and acute renal failure, hemodialysis may be indicated. Renal excretion may be enhanced with the infusion of normal saline or insulin.

4.2.4.1.2 Hypophosphatemia

Hypophosphatemia is rare, but some patients are at greater risk. Table 4.2.6 gives a summary of the most relevant causes of hypophosphatemia. After a successful renal transplant, a persistent hyperparathyroidism may lead to profound hypophosphatemia not rarely needing intravenous supplementation. In the ICU, patients under continuous renal replacement therapy (CRRT) may develop a severe decrease in phosphate. In this setting, phosphate should be monitored on a regular basis and supplemented if needed.

Table 4.2.6 Causes of hypophosphatemia and hyperphosphatemia

Hypophosphatemia	• Sepsis • Decreased absorption: – Chronic diarrhea – Vitamin D deficiency • Renal losses: – Osmotic diuresis – Renal transplantation – Hyperparathyroidism – Steroid therapy • Other losses: – Burns – Pancreatitis • Transcellular shifts: – Alkalosis – Hormonal (calcitonin, insulin) – Hungry bone syndrome – Lencemic crisis – Hypothermia
Hyperphosphatemia	• Renal failure • Tumor calcinosis syndrome • Bisphosphonates • Rhabdomyolysis • Tumor lysis syndrome • Malignant hyperthermia • Lactic acidosis

4.2.4.1.3 Management

In general, mild hypophosphatemia can be managed with oral supplements. Severe symptomatic hypophosphatemia (<0.5 mmol/l) requires intravenous application of phosphate. The amount of the possible phosphate deficit is unpredictable, and repletion therapy must be empiric. In the ICU, a single dose of 15–30 mmol over 2 h or a dose of up to 0.08 mmol/kg body weight are considered safe and have been well tolerated [33, 34]. One should be cautious, however, when the serum calcium is grossly elevated, because of the risk of soft tissue calcification. Calcium and phosphate repletion must be strictly separated, as precipitation may trigger anaphylactic reactions. Careful monitoring of phosphate and prevention of hypophosphatemia is therefore much safer than intravenous infusions.

4.2.5 Conclusions

Electrolyte disorders are extremely frequent in the ICU and in the emergency department. The most important imbalances of electrolyte homeostasis include disorders of sodium, potassium, calcium, and phosphate. Hyponatremia and hyperkalemia are the most common disorders and require prompt and safe correction, once the diagnosis is made and the underlying illness is identified. Thus, the main emphasis is on the causes and management of electrolyte abnormalities. Patients with hyponatremia are at high risk of cerebral edema, while hyperkalemia may lead to life-threatening cardiac rhythm abnormalities. Prompt recognition and effective management of these disorders will limit the risk of life-threatening consequences.

References

1. Verbalis JG. Disorders of body water homeostasis. *Best Pract Res Clin Endocrinol Metab* 2003; 17: 471–503
2. Kumar S, Berl T. Sodium. *Lancet* 1998; 352: 220–228
3. Howanitz JH, Howanitz PJ. Evaluation of serum and whole blood sodium critical values. *Am J Clin Pathol* 2007; 127: 56–59
4. Patel GP, Balk RA. Recognition and treatment of hyponatremia in acutely ill hospitalized patients. *Clin Ther* 2007; 29: 211–229
5. Kennedy PG, Mitchell DM, Hoffbrand BI. Severe hyponatraemia in hospital inpatients. *Br Med J* 1978; 2: 1251–1253
6. Verbalis JG, Goldsmith SR, Greenberg A, Schrier RW, Sterns RH. Hyponatremia treatment guidelines 2007: expert panel recommendations. *Am J Med* 2007; 120: S1–21
7. DeVita MV, Gardenswartz MH, Konecky A, Zabetakis PM. Incidence and etiology of hyponatremia in an intensive care unit. *Clin Nephrol* 1990; 34: 163–166
8. Bennani SL, Abouqal R, Zeggwagh AA, et al. Incidence, causes and prognostic factors of hyponatremia in intensive care. *Rev Med Interne* 2003; 24: 224–229
9. Richter S, Betz C, Geiger H. Severe hyponatremia with pulmonary and cerebral edema in an Ironman triathlete. *Dtsch Med Wochenschr* 2007; 132: 1829–1832
10. Adrogue HJ, Madias NE. Hyponatremia. *N Engl J Med* 2000; 342: 1581–1589
11. Chung HM, Kluge R, Schrier RW, Anderson RJ. Postoperative hyponatremia. A prospective study. *Arch Intern Med* 1986; 146: 333–336
12. Reynolds RM, Padfield PL, Seckl JR. Disorders of sodium balance. *BMJ* 2006; 332: 702–705
13. Nzerue CM, Baffoe-Bonnie H, You W, Falana B, Dai S. Predictors of outcome in hospitalized patients with severe hyponatremia. *J Natl Med Assoc* 2003; 95: 335–343
14. Wong F, Blei AT, Blendis LM, Thuluvath PJ. A vasopressin receptor antagonist (VPA-985) improves serum sodium concentration in patients with hyponatremia: a multicenter, randomized, placebo-controlled trial. *Hepatology* 2003; 37: 182–191
15. Gheorghiade M, Niazi I, Ouyang J, et al. Vasopressin V2-receptor blockade with tolvaptan in patients with chronic heart failure: results from a double-blind, randomized trial. *Circulation* 2003; 107: 2690–2696
16. Schrier RW, Gross P, Gheorghiade M, et al. Tolvaptan, a selective oral vasopressin V2-receptor antagonist, for hyponatremia. *N Engl J Med* 2006; 355: 2099–2112
17. Briegel J, Forst H, Haller M, et al. Stress doses of hydrocortisone reverse hyperdynamic septic shock: a prospective, randomized, double-blind, single-center study. *Crit Care Med* 1999; 27: 723–732
18. Annane D, Sebille V, Charpentier C, et al. Effect of treatment with low doses of hydrocortisone and fludrocortisone on mortality in patients with septic shock. *JAMA* 2002; 288: 862–871
19. Oppert M, Schindler R, Husung C, et al. Low-dose hydrocortisone improves shock reversal and reduces cytokine levels in early hyperdynamic septic shock. *Crit Care Med* 2005; 33: 2457–2464
20. Sprung CL, Annane D, Keh D, et al. Hydrocortisone therapy for patients with septic shock. *N Engl J Med* 2008; 358: 111–124
21. Adler SM, Verbalis JG. Disorders of body water homeostasis in critical illness. *Endocrinol Metab Clin North Am* 2006; 35: 873–94, xi
22. Weiss-Guillet EM, Takala J, Jakob SM. Diagnosis and management of electrolyte emergencies. *Best Pract Res Clin Endocrinol Metab* 2003; 17: 623–651
23. Schaefer TJ, Wolford RW. Disorders of potassium. *Emerg Med Clin North Am* 2005; 23: 723–7ix
24. Gennari FJ. Hypokalemia. *N Engl J Med* 1998; 339: 451–458
25. Tassone H, Moulin A, Henderson SO. The pitfalls of potassium replacement in thyrotoxic periodic paralysis: a case report and review of the literature. *J Emerg Med* 2004; 26: 157–161
26. Gennari FJ, Segal AS. Hyperkalemia: an adaptive response in chronic renal insufficiency. *Kidney Int* 2002; 62: 1–9
27. Gennari FJ. Disorders of potassium homeostasis. Hypokalemia and hyperkalemia. *Crit Care Clin* 2002; 18: 273–88, vi
28. Mattu A, Brady WJ, Robinson DA. Electrocardiographic manifestations of hyperkalemia. *Am J Emerg Med* 2000; 18: 721–729
29. Tohme JF, Bilezikian JP. Hypocalcemic emergencies. *Endocrinol Metab Clin North Am* 1993; 22: 363–375
30. Carnaille B, Oudar C, Pattou F, Combemale F, Rocha J, Proye C. Pancreatitis and primary hyperparathyroidism: forty cases. *Aust N Z J Surg* 1998; 68: 117–119
31. Petersen P. Psychiatric disorders in primary hyperparathyroidism. *J Clin Endocrinol Metab* 1968; 28: 1491–1495
32. Gardner DG. Hypercalcemia and sarcoidosis – another piece of the puzzle falls into place. *Am J Med* 2001; 110: 736–737
33. Sedlacek M, Schoolwerth AC, Remillard BD. Electrolyte disturbances in the intensive care unit. *Semin Dial* 2006; 19: 496–501
34. Charron T, Bernard F, Skrobik Y, Simoneau N, Gagnon N, Leblanc M. Intravenous phosphate in the intensive care unit: more aggressive repletion regimens for moderate and severe hypophosphatemia. *Intensive Care Med* 2003; 29: 1273–1278

Acid–Base Balance

4.3

John A. Kellum

Core Messages

- The essence of the physical chemical approach to acid–base balance is the understanding that there are three variables that are essential in determining blood pH: partial pressure of CO_2, strong ion difference (SID), and total weak acid concentration (A_{TOT}). Neither H^+ nor HCO_3^- can change unless one or more of these three variables change.
- Strong ions are completely dissociated in blood plasma; weak acids by contrast alter their ionization with changes in pH.
- While it is possible to describe an acid–base disorder in terms of H^+ or HCO_3^- concentrations or base excess, it is incorrect to analyze the pathology, and potentially dangerous to plan treatment, on the basis of altering these variables.

4.3.1 Introduction

Regulation of blood pH is an essential component of homeostasis. In health, the pH of the arterial blood is maintained between 7.35 and 7.45 by a precise balance of alveolar ventilation and carbon dioxide (CO_2) production matched to nonvolatile acid production and elimination. This nonvolatile or "fixed" component of acid–base balance is traditionally referred to as "metabolic." Recent advances in the understanding of the regulation and interaction of weak acids and strong ions, along with the application of basic physical chemical principles, permit a simpler, yet more comprehensive treatment of acid–base balance. At the same time, this "new" approach is grounded in the same basic principles as more traditional approaches (and is, in fact, entirely consistent with them). What is different with this new approach is a more careful attention to the requirements for thermodynamic equilibrium. The absolute requirement for equilibrium in aqueous solutions such as blood plasma sheds addition light on the understanding of mechanism of acid–base disorders and is also useful for planning treatment.

J. A. Kellum
Department of Critical Care Medicine, University of Pittsburgh, 608 Scaife Hall, 3550 Terrace Street, Pittsburgh, PA 15261, USA
e-mail: kellumja@ccm.upmc.edu

4.3.2 The Henderson–Hasselbalch Equation

Since Hasselbalch adapted the Henderson equation to the pH notation of Sörensen, the following equation has been used to understand the relationship between volatile and nonvolatile acid–base variables:

$$pH = pK \times \log[HCO_3^-/(0.03 \times pCO_2)]$$

where pK is the dissociation constant and pCO_2 is the partial pressure of CO_2.

This is the Henderson–Hasselbalch (HH) equation, and it is important to realize what this equation tells us. An increase in pCO_2 will result in a decrease in pH and an increase in HCO_3^- concentration. Thus, a patient found to have a low blood pH, a condition known as

A. Jörres et al. (eds.), *Management of Acute Kidney Problems*,
DOI: 10.1007/978-3-540-69441-0_4.3, © Springer-Verlag Berlin Heidelberg 2010

acidemia will either have an increased pCO_2 or a pCO_2 that is "not increased." In the former circumstance, the disorder is classified as a "respiratory acidosis." The term "acidosis" is used to describe the process resulting in acidemia and "respiratory" because the apparent cause is an increased pCO_2. This is logical since carbonic acid results when CO_2 is added to water (or blood) and the resultant decrease in pH is entirely expected. In the latter condition, pCO_2 is not increased and thus there cannot be a respiratory acidosis. This condition is referred to as "metabolic" because some nonvolatile acid must be the cause of the acidemia. The above logic can be reversed and used to easily classify simple conditions of alkalemia as either resulting from respiratory or metabolic alkaloses. Thus, the HH equation allows us to classify disorders as to the primary type of acid being increased or decreased. Over time, physiology superimposes its effects on simple chemistry, and the relationship between pCO_2 and HCO_3^- is altered in order to reduce the alterations in pH. However, by carefully examining the changes that occur in pCO_2 and HCO_3^- in relationship to each, one can discern highly conserved patterns. In this way, rules can be established to allow one to discover mixed disorders and to separate chronic from acute respiratory derangements. For example, one such rule is the convenient formula [1] for predicting the expected pCO_2 in the setting of a metabolic acidosis: $pCO_2 = (1.5 \times HCO_3^-) + 8 \pm 5$. This rule tells what the pCO_2 should be secondary to the increase in alveolar ventilation that accompanies a metabolic acidosis. If pCO_2 does not change enough or changes too much, the condition is classified as a "mixed" disorder, with either a respiratory acidosis if the pCO_2 is still too high or a respiratory alkalosis if the change is too great.

It is equally important to understand what the HH equation does not tell us. First, it does not allow us to discern the severity (quantity) of the metabolic derangement in a manner analogous to the respiratory component. For example, when there is a respiratory acidosis, the increase in the pCO_2 quantifies the derangement even when there is a mixed disorder. However, the metabolic component can only be approximated by the change in HCO_3^-.

Second, the HH equation does not tell us about any other acids other than carbonic acid. The relationship between CO_2 and HCO_3^- provides a useful clinical "road map" to guide the clinician in uncovering the etiology of an acid–base disorder. However, the total CO_2 concentration, and hence the HCO_3^- concentration is determined by the pCO_2, which is in turn determined by the balance between alveolar ventilation and CO_2 production. HCO_3^- cannot be regulated independent of pCO_2. The HCO_3^- concentration in the plasma will always increase as the pCO_2 increases, yet this is not an alkalosis. To understand how the pH and HCO_3^- concentration are altered independent of pCO_2, it is necessary to look beyond the HH equation.

4.3.3 Water and Physical Chemistry

Almost all biological solutions share two important characteristics. First, virtually all are aqueous (composed of water) and second, most are alkaline (OH^- concentration > H^+ concentration). Because these characteristics are so universal in human physiology, they are often ignored in reviews of physiology, especially for clinical medicine. Yet, they are extremely important. Aqueous solutions contain a virtually inexhaustible source of H^+. Although pure water dissociates only slightly into H^+ and OH^-, electrolytes, and CO_2 produce powerful electrochemical forces that influence water dissociation. Similarly, aqueous solutions that are alkaline behave very differently compared with acidic solutions in terms of the extent to which changes in their composition influence changes in pH (Fig. 4.3.1).

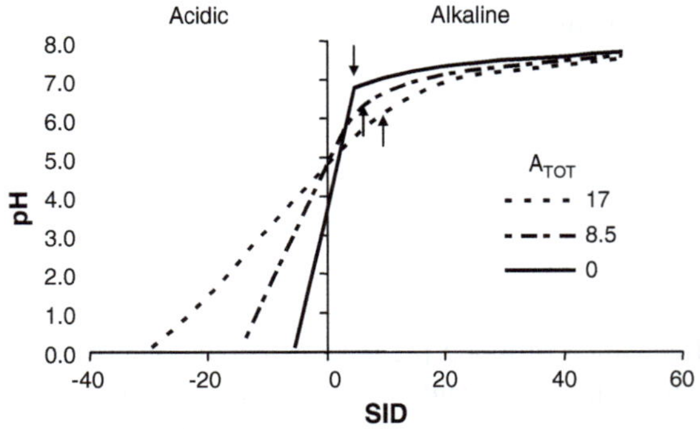

Fig. 4.3.1 Plot of pH versus strong ion difference (SID). For this plot, partial pressure of CO_2 (pCO_2) was held constant at 40 mm Hg. The three curves correspond to three different concentrations of total weak acid concentration (A_{TOT}; normal, 50% of normal, and zero). The plots assume a water dissociation constant for blood of 4.4×10^{-14} (Eq/l). The arrows refer to the point of neutrality ($OH^- = H^+$). To the right of these points $OH^- > H^+$ and the solutions are alkaline. To the left of these points, $H^+ > OH^-$ and the solutions are acidic. Note how different the slopes of these lines are when the solutions are acidic versus alkaline

Importantly, this property of alkaline solutions is often overlooked, and what has often been attributed to the power of buffering systems is merely a physical-chemical property of alkaline solutions.

4.3.4 Strong Ions

Blood plasma contains numerous ions. These ions can be classified both by charge – positive "cations" and negative "anions" – as well as by their tendency to dissociate in aqueous solutions. Some ions are completely dissociated in water, for example, Na^+, K^+, Ca^{++}, Mg^{++}, and Cl^-. These ions are called "strong ions" to distinguish them from "weak ions" (e.g., albumin, phosphate, and HCO_3^-), which can exist both as charged (dissociated) and uncharged forms. Certain ions such as lactate are so nearly completely dissociated that they may be considered strong ions under physiologic conditions. In a neutral salt solution containing only water and NaCl, the sum of strong cations (Na^+) minus the sum of strong anions (Cl^-) is zero (i.e., $Na^+ = Cl^-$). However, in blood plasma, strong cations (mainly Na^+) outnumber strong anions (mainly Cl^-). The difference between the sum of all strong cations and all strong anions is known as the strong ion difference (SID). Since both conservation of mass and conservation of charge must be maintained in macroscopic aqueous solutions, as SID becomes more positive, pH increases (Fig. 4.3.1).

In healthy humans, the plasma SID is between 40 and 42 mEq/l, although it is often quite different in critically ill patients. According to the principle of electrical neutrality, blood plasma cannot be charged so the remaining negative charges balancing the SID come from CO_2 and the weak acids (A^-) and, to very small extent, from OH^-. At physiologic pH, the contribution of OH^- is so small (nEq range) that it can be ignored. The total weak acid concentration (mainly albumin and phosphate) can be considered together and, for convenience, is abbreviated A_{TOT}, where $AH + A^- = A_{TOT}$. The SID of a blood sample can be estimated from the value of the remaining negative charge since $SID - (CO_2 + A^-) = 0$. This estimate of SID has been termed the effective SID (SIDe) [2], but it is really no different from the term "buffer base," first described over a half-century ago [3]. Thus SID and buffer base are mirror images of each other. Furthermore, since the base excess (BE) is the change in buffer base required to return a blood sample to a pH of 7.4 where $pCO_2 = 40$ mm Hg [4], the BE is therefore defines the change in SID from this equilibrium point.

An alternative estimate of SID is $(Na^+ + K^+ + Ca^{++} + Mg^{++}) - (Cl^- + lactate^-)$. This is referred to as the "apparent" SID (SIDa) because some "unmeasured" ions might also be present [2]. Neither SIDe nor SIDa are perfect estimates of the true SID. Blood samples from patients may contain unmeasured strong ions (e.g., sulfate, ketones) making the SIDa an inaccurate estimate of SID. Similarly, these patients may have abnormal weak ions (e.g., proteins) that will make the SIDe inaccurate. However, in healthy humans, SIDa and SIDe are nearly identical and are thus valid estimates of SID [2]. Furthermore, when SIDa and SIDe are not equal, a condition referred to as the strong ion gap (SIG), where SIDa – SIDe = SIG, abnormal strong and/or weak ions must be present [5]. The SIG is positive when unmeasured anions > unmeasured cations, and negative when unmeasured cations > unmeasured anions. Unexplained anions, and in some cases cations, have been found in the circulation of patients with a variety of diseases [5–8] and in animals under experimental conditions [9].

4.3.5 Regulation of Plasma Strong Ion Difference

To alter the SID, the body must affect a change in the relative concentrations of strong cations and strong anions. The kidney is the primary organ that affects this change. However, the kidney can only excrete a very small amount of strong ion into the urine each minute, and several minutes to hours are therefore required to impact significantly on the SID. The handling of strong ions by the kidney is extremely important because every Cl^- filtered but not reabsorbed decreases the SID. Since most of the human diet contains similar ratios of strong cations to strong anions, there is usually sufficient Cl^- available for this to be the primary regulating mechanism. This is particularly apparent, when one considers that renal Na^+ and K^+ handling are influenced by other priorities (e.g., intravascular volume and plasma K^+ homeostasis). Accordingly, "acid handling" by the kidney is generally mediated through Cl^- balance. How the kidney handles Cl^- is obviously very important. Traditional approaches to this problem have focused on

H^+ excretion and emphasized the importance of NH_3 and its conjugate acid NH_4^+. However, NH_4^+ is important not because of its carriage of H^+ or because of its direct action in the plasma (normal plasma NH_4^+ concentration is < 0.01 mEq/l), but because of its "co-excretion" with Cl^-.

Of course NH_4^+ is not only produced in the kidney. Hepatic ammoniagenesis (and also glutaminogenesis) is important for systemic acid–base balance, and, as expected, it is tightly controlled by mechanisms sensitive to plasma pH [10]. Indeed this reinterpretation of the role of NH_4^+ in acid–base balance is supported by the evidence that hepatic glutaminogenesis is stimulated by acidosis [11]. Amino acid degradation by the liver can result in the production of urea, glutamine, or NH_4^+. Normally, the liver does not release more than a very small amount NH_4^+ but rather incorporates this nitrogen into either urea or glutamine. Hepatocytes have enzymes to enable them to produce either of these end-products and both allow for the regulation of plasma NH_4^+ at suitably low levels. However, the production of urea or glutamine has significantly different effects at the level of the kidney. This is because glutamine is used by the kidney to generate NH_4^+ and facilitate the excretion of Cl^-. Thus, the production of glutamine can be seen as having an alkalinizing effect on plasma pH because of the way in which the kidney utilizes it.

Further support for this scenario comes from the recent discovery of an anatomic organization of hepatocytes according to their enzymatic content [12]. Hepatocytes with a propensity to produce urea are positioned closer to the portal venule and thus have the first opportunity to metabolize NH_4^+ delivered from the splanchnic circulation. However, acidosis inhibits ureagenesis and under these conditions more NH_4^+ is available for the downstream hepatocytes which are predisposed to produce glutamine. Thus the leftover NH_4^+ is "packaged" as glutamine for export to the kidney where it is used to facilitate Cl^- excretion and hence increases the SID.

The gastrointestinal (GI) tract also has important effects on the SID. Along its length, the GI tract handles strong ions quite differently. In the stomach, Cl^- is pumped out of the plasma and into the lumen reducing the SID of the gastric juice and thus reducing the pH. On the plasma side, SID is increased by the loss of Cl^- and the pH is increased producing the so-called alkaline tide, which occurs at the beginning of a meal when gastric acid secretion is maximal [13]. In the duodenum, Cl^- is reabsorbed and the plasma pH is restored. Normally, only slight changes in plasma pH are evident because Cl^- is returned to the circulation almost as soon as it is being removed. However, if gastric secretions are removed from the patient, either by suction catheter or vomiting, Cl^- will be progressively lost and the SID will steadily increase. It is important to realize that it is the Cl^- loss not the H^+ that is the determinant of plasma pH. Although H^+ is "lost" as HCl, it is also lost with every molecule of water removed from the body. When Cl^- (a strong anion) is lost without loss of a strong cation, the SID is increased and therefore the plasma H^+ concentration is decreased. When H^+ is "lost" as water rather than HCl, there is no change in the SID and hence no change in the plasma H^+ concentration.

In contrast to the stomach, the pancreas secretes fluid into the small intestine that has a SID much higher than plasma and is very low in Cl^-. Thus, the plasma perfusing the pancreas has its SID decreased, a phenomenon that peaks about an hour after a meal and helps counteract the alkaline tide. If large amounts of pancreatic fluid are lost, for example from surgical drainage, an acidosis will result as a consequence of the decreased plasma SID. In the large intestine, fluid also has a high SID because most of the Cl^- has been removed in the small intestine and the remaining electrolytes are mostly Na^+ and K^+. The body normally reabsorbs much of the water and electrolytes from this fluid, but when severe diarrhea exists, large amounts of cations can be lost. If this loss is persistent, the plasma SID will decrease and acidosis will result. Finally, whether the GI tract is capable of regulating strong ion uptake in a compensatory fashion has not been well studied. There is some evidence that the gut may modulate systemic acidosis in experimental endotoxemia by removing anions from the plasma [4]. However, the full capacity of this organ to affect acid–base balance is unknown.

4.3.6 Pathophysiology of Strong Ion Imbalance

Metabolic acidoses and alkaloses are categorized according to the ions that are responsible. Thus there is lactic acidosis and chloride responsive alkalosis, etc. It is important to recognize that metabolic acidosis is produced by a decrease in the SID which produces an electrochemical force that results in a decrease in blood pH. A decrease in SID may be brought about by the generation of organic anions (e.g., lactate, ketones) the loss of cations (e.g., diarrhea), the mishandling of ions (e.g., renal tubular acidosis), or the addition of exogenous anions (e.g., iatrogenic acidosis, poisonings). By contrast metabolic alkaloses occur as a result of an inappropriately large SID, although the SID need not be greater than the "normal" 40–42 mEq/l. This may be brought about by the loss of anions in excess of cations (e.g., vomiting, diuretics), or rarely by administration of strong cations in excess of strong anions (e.g., transfusion of large volumes of banked blood).

In the acute setting, acidosis is usually more of a problem than alkalosis, and in the critically ill, the most common sources of metabolic acidosis are disorders of (1) chloride homeostasis, (2) lactate, and (3) other anions. Hyperchloremic metabolic acidosis occurs either as a result of chloride administration or secondary to abnormalities in chloride handling or related to movements of chloride from one compartment to another. The effect of chloride administration on the development of metabolic acidosis has been known for many years [14, 15]. Recently, new attention has been paid to this area in light of a better understanding of the mechanisms responsible for this effect [16–20]. It has now been shown in animal models of sepsis [16] and in patients undergoing surgery [17, 18, 20] that saline causes metabolic acidosis not by "diluting" HCO_3^- but rather by its chloride content. From a physical-chemical prospective this is completely expected. HCO_3^- is a dependent variable and cannot be the *cause* of the acidosis. Instead, Cl^- administration decreases the SID (an independent variable) and produces an increase in water dissociation and hence H^+ concentration. The reason this occurs with saline administration is that although saline contains equal amounts of both Na^+ and Cl^-, the plasma does not. When large amounts of salt are added, the Cl^- concentration increases much more than the sodium concentration. For example, 0.9% ("normal") saline contains 154 mEq/l of Na^+ and Cl^-. Administration of large volumes of this fluid will have a proportionally greater effect on total body Cl^- than on total body Na^+. Of note, it is the total body concentrations of these strong ions that must be considered, and although the true volume of distribution of Cl^- is less, like Na^+, the effective volume of distribution (after some time of equilibration) is equal to total body water [16].

There are other important causes of hyperchloremia (renal tubular acidosis, diarrhea, etc.) and in addition, this form of metabolic acidosis is common in critical illness, especially sepsis. Although saline resuscitation undoubtedly plays a role, there appears to be unexplained sources of Cl^-, at least in animal models of sepsis [16]. One possible explanation is that this Cl^- is coming from intracellular and interstitial compartments as a result of the partial loss of Donnan equilibrium due to albumin exiting the intravascular space [16]. However, this hypothesis is as yet unproven.

4.3.7 Weak Acids

The second nonvolatile determinant of blood pH is the total weak acid concentration (A_{TOT}). The weak acids, are mostly proteins (predominantly albumin) and phosphates, and they contribute the remaining charges to satisfy electroneutrality such that $SID - (CO_2 + A^-) = 0$. However, A^- is not an independent variable because it changes with alterations in SID and pCO_2. Rather, A_{TOT} ($AH + A^-$) is the independent variable because its value is not determined by any other. The identification of A_{TOT} as the third independent acid–base variable has led some authors to suggest that a third "kind" of acid–base disorder exists [21]. Thus, along with respiratory and metabolic, there would also be acidosis and alkalosis due to abnormalities in A_{TOT}. However, mathematical and therefore chemical independence does not necessarily imply physiologic independence. Although the loss of weak acid (A_{TOT}) from the plasma space is an alkalinizing process [19], there is no evidence that the body regulates A_{TOT} to maintain acid–base balance. Furthermore, there is no evidence that clinicians should treat hypoalbuminemia as an acid–base disorder. Indeed, a recent trial in 7,000 patients comparing albumin-based fluid resuscitation versus saline found no difference in 28-day survival [22].

Critically ill patients frequently have hypoalbuminemia, and as such their A_{TOT} is reduced. However, these patients are not often alkalemic and their SID is also reduced [23]. When these patients have a normal pH and a normal BE and HCO_3^- concentration, it would seem most appropriate to consider this to be a physiologic compensation for a decreased A_{TOT} [24] rather than classifying this condition as a complex acid–base disorder with a mixed metabolic acidosis/hypoalbuminemic alkalosis. Thus, it seems far more likely that this "disorder" is in fact the normal physiologic response to a decreased A_{TOT}. Furthermore, since changes in A_{TOT} generally occur slowly, the development of alkalemia would require the kidney to continue to excrete Cl^- despite an evolving alkalosis. Most authorities would consider such a scenario to be renal-mediated hypochloremic metabolic alkalosis, the treatment for which would include fluids and/or chloride depending on the clinical conditions. Although the "normal" SID of is approximately 40 mEq/l, this is based on a "normal" CO_2 and A_{TOT}. The "normal" SID for a patient with an albumin of 2 g/dl, for example, would be much lower (e.g., ~32 mEq/l).

4.3.8 Unmeasured Anions

Unmeasured anions can be quantified by the SIG, or less reliably but the anion gap (AG). The AG is calculated from the abundant strong ions and HCO_3^- without regard to weak acids ($AG = [Na^+ + K^+] - [Cl^- + HCO_3^-]$). Normally, the SIG is near zero, while the AG is 8–12 mEq/l. The AG is an estimate of the sum of ($SIG + A^-$). Thus, subtracting A^- from the AG approximates the SIG. A convenient and reasonably accurate way to estimate A^- is to use the following formula [25]:

$$2(\text{albumin g/dl}) + 0.5(\text{phosphate mg/dl})$$

Or for international units:

$$0.2(\text{albumin g/l}) + 1.5(\text{phosphate mmol/l})$$

Note that the "normal" AG for a person with no unmeasured anions or cations in their plasma is equal to A^- such that $AG - A^- = SIG = 0$. This technique allows one to "calibrate" the AG for patients with abnormal albumin and/or phosphate concentrations.

In addition to the "measured anions" (e.g., Cl^-, lactate) several other anions may be present in the blood of critically ill patients. Ketones are perhaps the most important of these, but sulfates and certain poisons (e.g., methanol, salicylate) are important in the appropriate clinical conditions. In addition, unmeasured anions have been shown to be present in the blood of many critically ill patients [5–8]. It is important to emphasize that both strong and weak ions will alter the SIG (and the anion gap for that matter). Thus, the exact chemical makeup of the SIG may vary significantly from patient to patient. Healthy humans and laboratory animals appear to have very little if any unmeasured anions and so their SIG is near zero. One study, citing a previously published laboratory data set, calculated the total unmeasured anions in the blood of exercising humans at 0.3 ± 0.6 mEq/l [5].

However, unlike healthy exercising subjects or normal laboratory animals [9, 16], critically ill patients seem to have much higher SIG values [26–31]. Recently, there has been controversy as to what constitutes a "normal" SIG and as to whether an abnormal SIG is associated with adverse clinical outcomes. Reports from the United States [26, 27, 31] and from Holland [28] have found that the SIG was close to 5 mEq/l in critically ill patients, while studies from England and Australia [29, 30] have found much higher values. The use of resuscitation fluids containing unmeasured anions (e.g., gelatins) could be the explanation for this, but this has not been established. If exogenous anions are administered, the SIG will be a mixture of endogenous and exogenous anions and, quite possibly, of different prognostic significance. Interestingly, these two studies involving patients receiving gelatins [29, 30] have failed to find a correlation between SIG and mortality, while studies in patients not receiving gelatins [26, 27, 32], a positive correlation between SIG and hospital mortality has been found. Indeed one recent study reported that pre-resuscitation SIG predicts mortality in injured patients better than blood lactate, pH, or injury severity scores [27]. Dondorp and colleagues had similar results with pre-resuscitation SIG as a strong mortality predictor in patients with severe malaria [32].

Interestingly, in none of these studies have the anions responsible for the SIG been identified. Given that individual patients may have SIG values of more than 10–15 mEq/l, it seems unlikely that any strong ion could be present in the plasma at these concentrations and be unknown to us. Yet, it seems stranger still for weak acids such as proteins to be the cause, given that they are, in fact, weak. In healthy subjects the total charge concentration of plasma albumin is only about 10–12 mEq/l. For a similarly charged protein to affect a SIG of 15 mEq/l, it would need to be present in very large quantities indeed. The answer, probably, is that the identity of the SIG in these patients is multifactorial. Endogenous strong ions such a ketones and sulfate are added to exogenous ones such as acetate and citrate. Reduced metabolism of these and other ions owing to liver [9] and kidney [33] dysfunction likely exacerbates this situation. The release of myriad of acute phase proteins, principally from the liver, in setting of critical illness and injury likely adds to the SIG. Furthermore, the systemic inflammatory response is associated with the release of a substantial quantity of proteins including cytokines and chemokines some of which, like high-mobility group (HMG) B1 have been linked to mortality [34]. The cumulative effect of all of these factors may well be a reflection of both organ injury and dysfunction. It is perhaps not surprising that there is a correlation between SIG and mortality. Indeed, whatever the source of SIG, it appears that its presence in the circulation, especially early in the course of illness or injury, portends a poor prognosis. While the prognostic significance of SIG is reduced (or abolished) when exogenous unmeasured anions are administered (e.g., gelatins), a SIG acidosis seems to be far worse than a similar amount of hyperchloremic acidosis and more like lactic acidosis in terms of significance [35]. Although it is possible that saline-based resuscitation fluids contaminate the prognostic value of hyperchloremia the same way gelatins appear to confound SIG, there remains strong evidence that not all metabolic acidoses are the same.

4.3.9 Conclusions

Unlike many other areas in clinical medicine, the approach to acid–base physiology has not often distinguished cause from effect. Although it is perfectly reasonable to describe an alteration in acid–base status by the observed changes in H^+ and HCO_3^-, this does not itself imply causation. The essence of the physical-chemical approach to acid–base balance is the understanding that only three variables are important in determining blood pH: pCO_2, SID, and A_{TOT}. Neither H^+ nor HCO_3^- can change unless one or more of these three variables change. Strong ions cannot be created or destroyed to satisfy electroneutrality, but H^+ ions are generated or consumed by changes in water dissociation. Hence, to understand how the body regulates pH one needs only to ask how it regulates these three independent variables. Other approaches to acid–base physiology have ignored the distinction between independent and dependent variables, and while it is possible to describe an acid–base disorder in terms of H^+ or HCO_3^- concentrations or base excess, it is incorrect to analyze the pathology, and potentially dangerous to plan treatment, on the basis of altering these variables.

References

1. Albert M, Dell R, Winters R: Quantitative displacement of acid-base equilibrium in metabolic acidosis. *Ann Intern Med* 1967; 66:312–315
2. Figge J, Mydosh T, Fencl V: Serum proteins and acid-base equilibria: a follow-up. *J Lab Clin Med* 1992; 120:713–719
3. Singer RB, Hastings AB: An improved clinical method for the estimation of disturbances of the acid-base balance of human blood. *Medicine (Baltimore)* 1948; 27:223–242
4. Kellum JA, Bellomo R, Kramer DJ, et al: Fixed acid uptake by visceral organs during early endotoxemia. *Adv Exp Med Biol* 1997; 411:275–279
5. Kellum JA, Kramer DJ, Pinsky MR: Strong ion gap: a methodology for exploring unexplained anions. *J Crit Care* 1995; 10:51–55
6. Gilfix BM, Bique M, Magder S: A physical chemical approach to the analysis of acid-base balance in the clinical setting. *J Crit Care* 1993; 8:187–197
7. Mecher C, Rackow EC, Astiz ME, et al: Unaccounted for anion in metabolic acidosis during severe sepsis in humans. *Crit Care Med* 1991; 19:705–711
8. Kirschbaum B: Increased anion gap after liver transplantation. *Am J Med Sci* 1997; 313:107–110
9. Kellum JA, Bellomo R, Kramer DJ, et al: Hepatic anion flux during acute endotoxemia. *J Appl Physiol* 1995; 78: 2212–2217
10. Bourke E, Haussinger D: pH homeostasis: the conceptual change. *Contrib Nephrol* 1992; 100:58–88
11. Oliver J, Bourke E: Adaptations in urea and ammonium excretion in metabolic acidosis in the rat: a reinterpretation. *Clin Sci Mol Med* 1975; 48:515–520
12. Atkinson DE, Bourke E: pH Homeostasis in terrestrial vertebrates; Ammonium ion as a proton source. In: Comparative and Environmental Physiology. Mechanisms of Systemic Regulation, Acid-Base Regulation, Ion Transfer and Metabolism. Heisler N (Ed). Berlin: Springer, 1995, pp 1–26.
13. Moore EW: The alkaline tide. *Gastroenterology* 1967; 52:1052–1054
14. Cushing H: Concerning the poisonous effect of pure sodium chloride solutions upon the nerve muscle preparation. *Am J Physiol* 1902; 6:77ff
15. Shires GT, Tolman J: Dilutional acidosis. *Ann Intern Med* 1948; 28:557–559
16. Kellum JA, Bellomo R, Kramer DJ, et al: Etiology of metabolic acidosis during saline resuscitation in endotoxemia. *Shock* 1998; 9:364–368
17. Scheingraber S, Rehm M, Sehmisch C, et al: Rapid saline infusion produces hyperchloremic acidosis in patients undergoing gynecologic surgery. *Anesthesiology* 1999; 90: 1265–1270

18. Waters JH, Bernstein CA: Dilutional acidosis following hetastarch or albumin in healthy volunteers. *Anesthesiology* 2000; 93:1184–1187
19. Morgan TJ, Venkatesh B, Hall J: Crystalloid strong ion difference determines metabolic acid-base change during in vitro hemodilution. *Crit Care Med* 2002; 30:157–160
20. Waters JH, Miller LR, Clack S, et al: Cause of metabolic acidosis in prolonged surgery. *Crit Care Med* 1999; 27: 2142–2146
21. Fencl V, Jabor A, Kazda A, et al: Diagnosis of metabolic acid-base disturbances in critically ill patients. *Am J Respir Crit Care Med* 2000; 162:2246–2251
22. Finfer S, Bellomo R, Boyce N, et al: A comparison of albumin and saline for fluid resuscitation in the intensive care unit. *N Engl J Med* 2004; 350:2247–2256
23. Kellum JA: Recent advances in acid-base physiology applied to critical care. In: Yearbook of Intensive Care and Emergency Medicine. Vincent JL (Ed). Heidelberg: Springer-Verlag, 1998, pp 579–587.
24. Wilkes P: Hypoproteinemia, SID, and acid-base status in critically ill patients. *J Appl Physiol* 1998; 84:1740–1748
25. Kellum JA: Determinants of blood pH in health and disease. *Crit Care* 2000; 4:6–14
26. Balasubramanyan N, Havens PL, Hoffman GM: Unmeasured anions identified by the Fencl-Stewart method predict mortality better than base excess, anion gap, and lactate in patients in the pediatric intensive care unit. *Crit Care Med* 1999; 27:1577–1581
27. Kaplan L, Kellum JA: Initial pH, base deficit, lactate, anion gap, strong ion difference, and strong ion gap predict outcome from major vascular injury. *Crit Care Med* 2004; 32: 1120–1124
28. Moviat M, van Haren F, van der Hoeven H: Conventional or physicochemical approach in intensive care unit patients with metabolic acidosis. *Crit Care* 2003; 7: R41–R45
29. Cusack RJ, Rhodes A, Lochhead P, et al: The strong ion gap does not have prognostic value in critically ill patients in a mixed medical/surgical adult ICU. *Intensive Care Med* 2002; 28:864–869
30. Rocktaschel J, Morimatsu H, Uchino S, et al: Unmeasured anions in critically ill patients: can they predict mortality? *Crit Care Med* 2003; 31:2131–2136
31. Gunnerson KJ, Roberts G, Kellum JA: What is normal strong ion gap (SIG) in healthy subjects and critically ill patients without acid-base abnormalities. *Crit Care Med* 2003; 31:A111-Abstract
32. Dondorp AM, Chau TT, Phu NH, et al: Unidentified acids of strong prognostic significance in severe malaria. *Crit Care Med* 2004; 32:1683–1688
33. Rocktaschel J, Morimatsu H, Uchino S, et al: Acid-base status of critically ill patients with acute renal failure: analysis based on Stewart-Figge methodology. *Crit Care* 2003; 7: R60-R66
34. Wang H, Bloom O, Zhang M, et al: HMG-1 as a late mediator of endotoxin lethality in mice. *Science* 1999; 285: 248–251
35. Gunnerson KJ, Saul M, Kellum JA: Lactic versus nonlactic metabolic acidosis: outcomes in critically ill patients. Abstract. *Crit Care* 2003; 7(Suppl 2):S8–S9

Monitoring and Management of Systemic Hemodynamics*

4.4

Non Wajanaponsan and Michael R. Pinsky

> **Core Messages**
>
> › Hemodynamic monitoring is an essential tool for evaluation and management of patients with acute kidney injury (AKI).
>
> › Hemodynamic support includes identification of preload-response, volume resuscitation, vasopressor, and inotropic management.
>
> › An evidence-based management strategy with the goal of increasing tissue oxygen delivery can improve outcome in AKI.

4.4.1 Epidemiology

Acute kidney injury (AKI) occurs in 2–5% of general medical-surgical admissions, but up to 10–30% of intensive care unit (ICU) admissions[12]. ICU patients with AKI have increased mortality of 23%, compared with 11% for patients with chronic renal failure on hemodialysis and 5% for general ICU patients with renal insufficiency. Despite recent medical advances, the mortality for patients with AKI requiring dialysis remains unchanged over the past two decades [8, 23, 39, 40]. Thus, if acute renal injury can be prevented, mortality should be markedly reduced.

*This work was supported in part by NIH grants HL067181 and HL07820

M. R. Pinsky (✉)
Department of Critical Care Medicine, University of Pittsburgh, 606 Scaife Hall, 3550 Terrace Street, Pittsburgh, PA 15261, USA
e-mail: pinskymr@upmc.edu

4.4.2 Renal Hemodynamic Management Perspective

The management of patients with AKI involves rapid identification of its causes, specific treatment, adjustment of medication dosage, and renal replacement therapy. One primary therapy for renal hypoperfusion (so-called prerenal azotemia) is optimization of renal blood flow by optimizing global oxygen delivery (DO_2) to prevent further organ damage and facilitate organ recovery. Hemodynamic profile analysis, including assessment of cardiovascular function, preload responsiveness, DO_2, and tissue organ O_2 demand provide useful information for management of critically ill patients. Although these analyses give additional information, hemodynamic monitoring cannot translate into improvement in patient outcome, unless it is coupled with a treatment that itself improves outcome [11, 28].

We will assess in turn the issues of estimating renal perfusion pressure (RPP), defining resuscitation goals to promote improved outcome, identifying volume responsiveness (preload responsiveness), and the various pharmacotherapies to aid in achieving resuscitation renal perfusion pressure and global DO_2 goals.

4.4.3 Renal Perfusion Pressure

Renal perfusion is very well preserved within a wide range of systemic arterial pressures. This constant of renal perfusion despite varying arterial pressure is

A. Jörres et al. (eds.), *Management of Acute Kidney Problems*,
DOI: 10.1007/978-3-540-69441-0_4.4, © Springer-Verlag Berlin Heidelberg 2010

maintained by an autoregulation from intrinsic properties of the renal vasculature. Renal hypoperfusion starts to develop when mean arterial pressure (MAP) falls <80 mm Hg [3, 4, 7]. However, ischemic renal injury usually only develops at renal perfusion pressures <60 mm Hg. The first goal of organ resuscitation is to provide adequate organ perfusion pressure. In patients with AKI, a goal of keeping renal perfusion pressure >70 mm Hg has been widely accepted. However, patients with prior renal vascular disease may need higher perfusion pressures, and healthy young adults need lower perfusion pressures. Although these target values are often quoted, the only study to systematically examine the impact of varying MAP on renal function found no added benefit on renal function of increasing MAP > 60 mm Hg in critically ill patients [16].

However, renal perfusion pressure (RPP) is the driving pressure across the renal vasculature and, thus, not determined by MAP alone, but also the back-pressure to MAP. Thus, RPP is calculated as the input pressure minus the back-pressure. Under most circumstances the input pressure is the MAP. However, with renal arterial stenosis and in the case of hypertensive renal disease, afferent arteriole pressure can be much lower than MAP. Finally, the vascular back-pressure in the renal veins is usually just slightly higher than central venous pressure (CVP). CVP is also called right atrial pressure (Pra). To simplify matters, RPP is usually calculated at the bedside as MAP minus CVP.

Not only does renal artery stenosis alter RPP, but intra-abdominal hypertension does so as well. Although the kidneys lie in the retroperitoneal space, their venous drainage is into an intra-abdominal inferior vena cava. Thus, changes in intra-abdominal pressure (IAP) will directly alter renal venous pressure. If IAP exceeded CVP, then IAP and not CVP becomes the back-pressure to MAP defining RPP. In a very important subgroup of patients intra-abdominal hypertension develops as a consequence of sepsis, trauma, and prior gut ischemia. Under these conditions, where IAP > CVP, estimating RPP from MAP minus Pra will overestimate RPP. Under these conditions RPP is defined as MAP minus IAP. And unlike renal artery stenosis, which is uncommon, increases in IAP commonly occur in the critically ill, especially after fluid resuscitation for the management of shock. Thus, it is important to accurately measure IAP in assessing RPP in critically ill patients.

IAP can be measured by many techniques, some of which are quite invasive, such as inserting a fluid-filled catheter into the abdominal compartment. One can also use the bladder as a pressure transducer and measure intravesicular pressure using a urinary (Foley) catheter. Although there are many methods of transducing the bladder to estimate IAP, including inserting a t-tube into the drainage system and filling the tubing with sterile water or saline, the simplest one is merely to identify the air–fluid level height of urine from the Foley catheter held upright above the patient, documenting free flow of urine as it reaches its own level above the patient. The height of the column of urine in the tubing in centimeters reflects accurately IAP. The conversion factor for cm H_2O to mm Hg is 1.36 cm H_2O equals 1 mm Hg.

4.4.4 Hemodynamic Management and Resuscitation

Fluid resuscitation is an essential part for management of AKI. History taking, physical examination, and laboratory study such as urinary profile may help the physician evaluate the patient's volume status. However, physical findings are often misleading in unstable patients who may have an expanded total body fluid volume but low intravascular volume. This is a common occurrence in septic patients with capillary leak syndrome or in congestive heart failure patients. Regrettably, except for identifying dehydration by lack of skin turgor or massive volume overload by evidence of pulmonary edema, the finding of peripheral edema does not exclude intravascular volume contraction.

Classically, one can identify subjects who will respond to fluid resuscitation by performing an initial fluid challenge. A fluid challenge is the rapid (e.g., 15 min) intravenous infusion of a bolus (e.g., 250–500 ml crystalloid) and noting the response. Such volume challenges can be safely done in patients with oliguria or who are developing acute renal failure. One measures markers of response to therapy, such as a decrease in heart rate, increase in blood pressure or arterial pulse pressure, or an increase in urine output. If such positive responses are seen, then intravascular volume loading can proceed with a reasonable chance that this further fluid resuscitation will manifest itself as an increase in blood flow. However, only half (52%)

of all critically ill patients receiving a fluid bolus display an increase in cardiac output[21]. Thus, if one performed a fluid challenge in all hemodynamically unstable patients as a primary method of making the diagnosis of functional hypovolemia, it would be beneficial only half the time. Furthermore, in the other half of patients, appropriate treatment would be delayed and potentially unnecessary volume loading performed, which may lead to worsening acute cor pulmonale, pulmonary edema, or heart failure states [29].

Both CVP and pulmonary artery occlusion pressure (PAOP) have been widely used to guide fluid management in critically ill patients. Traditionally, patients with low CVP values are given volume for resuscitation, whereas patients with high CVP values are considered in a "volume overload" state. Similar practices are used for PAOP. Cutoff values for stopping fluid resuscitation based on CVP and PAOP values vary by usually >12 and >18 mm Hg for CVP and PAOP, respectively. Although this practice has been widely accepted, regrettably there is little to no data to support this approach and, if anything, the literature shows that such an approach is wrong [29]. One of the most straightforward studies was reported by Kumar et al. [13] These workers demonstrated that there is no correlation between specific values of CVP or PAOP and right ventricular (RV) or left ventricular (LV) end diastolic volume, respectively, and either stroke volume or its change and any of these estimates of preload (Fig. 4.4.1). In fact, numerous studies have collectively demonstrated that neither CVP, PAOP, nor measures of RV or LV end-diastolic volume predict volume responsiveness. In essence, preload values do not predict preload responsiveness.

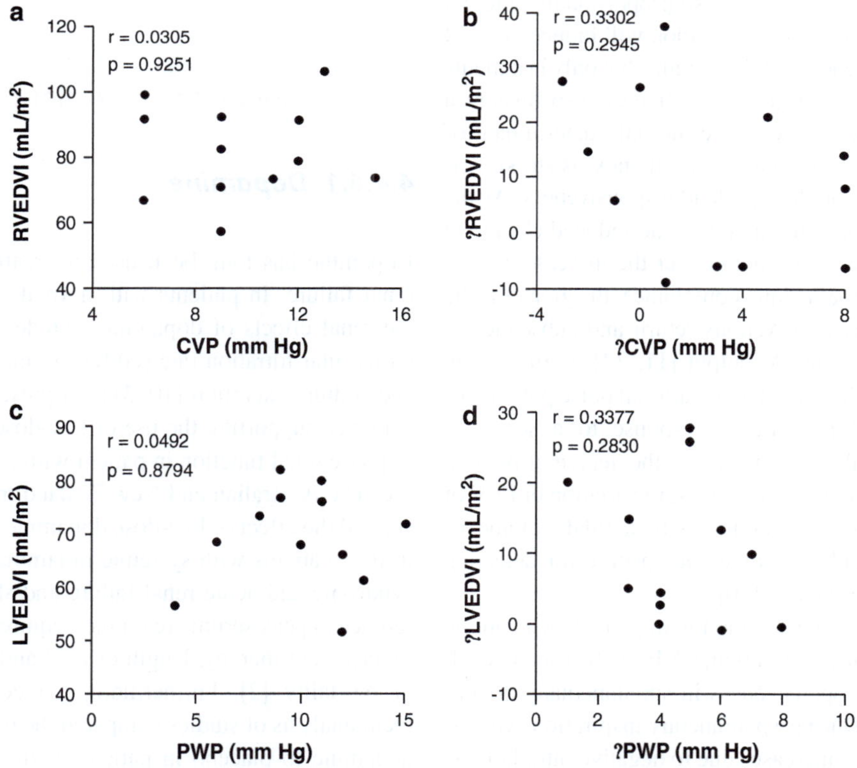

Fig. 4.4.1 Relationship between (**a**) initial central venous pressure (CVP) and right ventricular end-diastolic volume index (RVEDVI); (**b**) changes in central venous pressure and RVEDVI in response to saline; (**c**) initial pulmonary artery occlusion pressure (PWP) and left ventricular end-diastolic volume index (LVEDVI); and (**d**) changes in PWP and LVEDVI in response to saline in group 1 subjects. No significant relationship was found between initial values for CVP and RVEDVI or changes in these variables following 3 l of saline infusion. Similar negative results were found for the relationship between PWP and LVEDVI (From [13])

4.4.5 Evaluation for Preload Responsiveness

Recent studies building on solid physiologic principles of heart–lung interaction have documented that the presence of a minimal threshold level of either arterial pulse pressure variation (PPV) or LV stroke volume variation (SVV) during fixed tidal volume positive-pressure breathing accurately identifies patients whose cardiac output will increase in response to intravascular volume loading, and by how much the cardiac output will subsequently increase. In patients who are passively ventilated with positive-pressure ventilation with fixed tidal volume, arterial waveform and pulse pressure analysis is a good tool for evaluation for preload responsiveness. Why is this the case?

Positive-pressure ventilation cyclically alters the pressure gradient for systemic venous return, proportionally altering RV output on the next beat. Subsequently, LV filling is also proportionally altered. Thus, positive-pressure ventilation will induce cyclical changes in LV end-diastolic volume, but only in patients who are preload responsive will they also display a ventilatory cycle SVV. Since the only determinant of pulse pressure from one beat to the next is stroke volume, PPV also predicts preload responsiveness. As the forcing function is the tidal volume-induced change in intrathoracic pressure, the greater the increase in tidal volume for the same lung compliance, the greater is the transient decrease in venous return and subsequently greater decrease in LV output [11, 33]. Furthermore, the degree of changes in either arterial pulse pressure or systolic blood pressure in response to a series of increasing tidal breath quantifies the degree of preload responsiveness. A systolic pressure variation or PPV of ≥13% in patients breathing with a tidal volume of 8ml/ kg is highly sensitive and specific for detecting preload responsiveness [20].

In contrast to the situation with patients who are on positive-pressure ventilation, CVP can be used to evaluate preload responsiveness in spontaneously breathing patients. During spontaneous inspiration, venous return normally increases due to negative intrathoracic pressure [27]. A normal right ventricle pumps this increased blood flow into the pulmonary circulation. Therefore, CVP will decrease with decreasing intrathoracic pressure with each spontaneous inspiratory effort. An inspiratory decrease in CVP of more than 1 mm Hg when intrathoracic pressure decrease is >2 mmHg has been shown to accurately predict preload responsiveness, whereas those patients whose CVP does not decrease in such a setting do not increase their cardiac output in response to fluid challenge [18].

The alternative approach to prediction for fluid responsiveness is the passive leg-raising test. Venous return is increased by raising lower extremities to 30° above the chest for 1 min [41]. This maneuver causes approximately 300 ml of blood bolus in a 70-kg man that persists for a few minutes before intravascular volume redistribution [5]. The passive leg-raising maneuver is reliable in patients breathing spontaneously and in patients with cardiac arrhythmias [22]. However, in patients who are severely hypovolemic, the blood volume increased by leg-raising which is dependent on total blood volume could be small, which, in turn, can show only minimal to no increase in cardiac output or blood pressure in patients who are fluid responders [11].

4.4.6 Vasopressor Treatment

4.4.6.1 Dopamine

Dopamine has long been used in treatment of acute renal failure. In patients with normal renal function, the renal effects of dopamine include an increase in glomerular filtration rate (GFR) and increase in water and sodium excretion [10, 31]. At present, there is no evidence supporting the use of low-dose dopamine to improve renal function in patient with acute renal failure. The Australian and New Zealand trial (ANZICS) studied the effect of low-dose dopamine (2 µg/kg/min) in ICU patients with systemic inflammatory response syndrome and acute renal failure and showed no difference in peak serum creatinine, requirement for renal replacement therapy, length of ICU and hospital stay, or mortality [2]. Furthermore, a recent large-scale meta-analysis of studies compared the use of low-dose dopamine to placebo in patients with, or at risk for, renal dysfunction and showed no effect of low-dose dopamine on mortality, requirement for renal replacement therapy, or the occurrence of adverse outcomes. There were no changes in serum creatinine level or GFR on days 1, 2, or 3 of therapy [9].

Potential harmful effects of dopamine include tachyarrhythmias, myocardial ischemia, decreased intestinal blood flow, hypothyroidism, and suppressed T cell function [24]. When dopamine was given prophylactically to patients with diabetic nephropathy, it also increased the risk of radiocontrast nephropathy [32, 42].

4.4.6.2 Norepinephrine

Norepinephrine causes potent stimulation at α1 and β1 receptors, but unlike epinephrine, it has minimal effect at -β2 receptors. Blood pressure is reliably increased but the effect on cardiac output is variable. Although β1 receptor simulation has a direct inotropic effect, in the setting of hypovolemia or impaired ventricular function, increased left ventricular afterload due to α1 receptor stimulation can cause cardiac output to fall. Similarly, the effect on heart rate is variable: direct β1 stimulation has a chronotropic effect, but increased blood pressure can cause baroreceptor-mediated bradycardia. Norepinephrine is typically started at dosages of 0.01–0.05 μg/kg/min and titrated to desired blood pressure. Because of potential impaired cardiac output, in general, norepinephrine infusion at dosages above 0.05–0.1 μg/kg/min should be avoided in patients with impaired ventricular function unless cardiac output is being measured. Norepinephrine is commonly combined with an inotropes such as dobutamine or milrinone to support cardiac output [38].

Previously, concern was raised about the use of norepinephrine in the management of patients with shock, because of the fear that it would worsen renal ischemia by inducing renal vasoconstriction. Clearly, norepinephrine causes a reduction in renal blood flow in healthy animals and humans [36]. However, the effect on renal vascular resistance depends on the increase in systemic pressure, with a decreased renal sympathetic tone causing vasodilatation as well as an autoregulatory vasoconstriction secondary to increased perfusion pressure and α1-mediated renal vasoconstriction [31]. In a study of septic patients, Martin et al. demonstrated that norepinephrine infusion resulted in higher blood pressure, systemic vascular resistance, and diuresis than did high-dose dopamine [19].

Both high-dose dopamine and norepinephrine can be used to increase blood pressure via stimulation of adrenergic receptors. However, many studies suggest the use of norepinephrine is preferable to dopamine due to higher rates of ability to achieve hemodynamic goals and may even be associated with decreased mortality. In an observational cohort study of 1,058 patients with shock due to any cause, ICU mortality was greater among patients who received dopamine (odds ratio 1.67; 95% confidence interval [95% CI], 1.19–2.35) [35]. This effect was greater among patients with septic shock (odds ratio 2.05; 95% CI, 1.25–3.37). Just because norepinephrine is stronger does not mean it is better. Dopamine and norepinephrine have been compared in clinical trials. In a double-blind trial 32 patients with septic shock were randomly assigned to receive dopamine (3–25 μg/kg/min) or norepinephrine (35–350 μg/min). An adequate hemodynamic response was achieved in 31% of dopamine and 93% of norepinephrine treated patients; furthermore, over 90% of patients who failed to respond to dopamine responded to norepinephrine [19]. Several large prospective clinical trials comparing dopaime ± norepinephrine to norepionephrine are ongoing, and the interim analyses suggest no clear winner. Still, in all the ongoing studies, if dopamine does not achieve an adequate MAP level, norepinehprine is added. In practice, norepinephrine is added about 70% of the itme to patients in the dopamine arm who also have septic shock. Thus, if norepinephrine is needed as the default vasopressor in both arms of all these studies, then the relative merit of the group differences is mute. Unless there is a clear reason to use dopamine, there appears little logic in its continued use for the treatment of distributive shock.

4.4.6.3 Epinephrine

Epinephrine is a potent catecholamine with actions at both α and β receptors. At lower dosages (0.01–0.03 μg/kg/min) β effects predominate, resulting in an increase in contractility and heart rate. Despite β2 receptor-mediated vasodilatation, a fall in blood pressure is uncommon. As the dose increases, α receptor-mediated vasoconstriction predominates, such that at higher dosages (>0.05–0.1 μg/kg/min) vasoconstriction occurs in most vascular beds. In the acutely failing heart, epinephrine has the advantage of providing increased cardiac output while maintaining coronary perfusion pressure. Epinephrine can cause sinus tachycardia, atrial and ventricular arrhythmias, and marked metabolic disturbance, particularly hypokalemia, hyperglycemia, and lactic acidosis [38]. Recently, Annane et al. performed a study comparing infusion of norepinephrine plus dobutamine versus epinephrine alone in treating patients with septic shock [1]. The study found no difference in outcome including mortality, time to hemodynamic success, time to vasopressor withdrawal, and time course of SOFA score with same rate of serious adverse events. Thus, if the venoconstriction effects of epinephrine are needed, it is a reasonable vasopressor to use.

4.4.6.4 Vasopressin

Vasopressin is secreted by the posterior pituitary gland and increases systemic vascular resistance through the activation of V1 receptors on vascular smooth muscle. In an animal study, Landry et al. demonstrated that after 1 h of hemorragic shock, the stainable hormone by immunohistochemistry was absent in tissuue from animals' neurohypophysis [15, 32]. Studies have supported the role of vasopressin in the management of hypotension in septic shock. Landry et al. reported that an infusin of 0.04 U/min of vasopressin in ten hypotensive patients with severe sepsis increased arterial blood pressure from a mean of 92/52 mm Hg to 146/66 mm Hg [14]. Furthermore, withdrawal of vasopressin resulted in hypotension in six patients in whom it was the only pressor [14]. A study by Patel et al. also showed that vasopressin produced an catecholamine-sparing activity, and its use was accompanied by a larger volume of urine output and improved creatinine clearance [25, 31, 32]. Still, a large multicenter Canadian trial showed minimal benefit when vasopressin was added to routine vasopressor management in patinets in septic shock. Thus, its use is quesitonable, but if used in the low dosages listed above, probably has few side effects.

4.4.7 Inotropic Therapy

Inotropic drug infusions should be considered to augment hemodynamic management in patients who are unable to maintain blood flow despite restoration of MAP with the use of vasopressors. The associated low cardiac output threatens tissue ischemia and carried a high mortality rate. Furthermore, patients who have underlying heart failure may need inotropic support to maintain cardiac output after vasopressor has been started to prevent worsening heart failure from an increased afterload.

4.4.7.1 Dobutamine

Dobutamine is a synthetic catecholamine with relative specificity for β1 receptors. Modest β2 receptor-mediated vasodilatation may occur. Cardiac output is reliably increased, but the effect on blood pressure is unpredictable. The dosage range is 1–10 μg/kg/min. At higher dosages, tachyarrhythmias become common. Metabolic side effects are minimal [38]. Because of its ease of titration, minimal caridovascular side effects and good safety profile, dobutamine is the inotrope of choice in the acute managrment of heart failure. However, if a patient has a reduced intravascular blood volume, the initiation of dobutmaine infusion can be accompanied by profound hypotension. Thus, dobutamine infusions must occur in the presence of an expanded intravascular blood volume.

4.4.7.2 Milrinone

Milrinone inhibits breakdown of cyclic nucleotides, including cAMP and cGMP. Hemodynamic effects include increased cardiac contractility and cause pulmonary and systemic vasodilatation. AS a result, milrinone is useful for treating patients with low cardiac output, particularly in the presence of pulmonary edema or pulmonary hypertension. The inotropic effect is independent of the β1 receptor, which is advantageous in patients with β1 receptor desensitization. Milrinone causes less tachycardia and atrial fibrillation than dobutamine. It is administered as a loading dose of 50 μg/kg over 30 min, followed by an infusion 0.25–0.75 μg/kg/min. In patients at risk for hypotension, the loading dose should be reduced or given very slowly. Milrinone is eliminated via the kidneys, and the rate of infusion should be adjusted in patients with severe renal dysfunction so as to avoid excessive vasodilatation [38].

4.4.8 Improve Patient Outcome with Optimizing Oxygen Delivery

For patients who have an adequate blood pressure or organ perfusion pressure but low tissue DO_2, as manifested by low mixed venous oxygen saturation (SvO_2), inotropic support should be considered to augment cardiac output and DO_2 to prevent organ ischemia despite adequate blood pressure. Although early clinical trials in shock failed to demonstrate an improvement in outcome when resuscitation strategies were driven by measured hemodynamic variables, recent multiple randomized controlled trials demonstrated reduction in mortality and cost when resuscitation was done early in the course of illness [30].

Rivers et al. performed a randomized controlled trial including patients with systemic inflammatory response syndrome who were hypotensive or had an elevated serum lactate concentration, to receive either standard therapy or goal-directed therapy to keep central venous O_2 saturation ($ScvO_2$) at greater than 70% [34]. The control group receive standard treatment with the goal of keeping adequate hemodynamic parameters (CVP ≥8–12 mm Hg, MAP ≥65 mm Hg, and urine output ≥0.5 ml/kg/h), The early goal-directed therapy group were monitored in the emergency department for at least 6 h according to the same end points, but treated in addition with blood transfusion or inotrope, according protocol, to achieve $ScvO_2$ >70%. The goal of $ScvO_2$ >70% was achieved in 60% of the control group and 95% of the treatment group. The total amount of resuscitation fluids given was similar in the treatment and control groups, but the treatment group received more fluid early on during treatment course. This landmark study showed a significant reduction in mortality (in-hospital mortality 46.5% vs. 30.5%), incidence of multiple organ failure, and length of hospital stay [34].

Benefit of resuscitation and optimization of tissue DO_2 were also demonstrated in high-risk surgery patients. Shoemaker et al. demonstrated improved outcome and reduced cost when high-risk surgery patients were resuscitated to achieve oxygen delivery more than 600 ml/min/m^2 prior to surgery [37]. Subsequently, Boyd et al. [6] and Lobo et al. [17] also confirmed benefits of preoperative optimization in high-risk surgery patients. Importantly, Lobo et al. showed that the improved patient outcomes were realized across the entire treatment group of elderly patients, even in those patients who did not achieve the target DO_2 levels. Pearse et al. performed a study design in postoperative high-risk patients. They targeted a postoperative DO_2 of 600 ml/kg/min using arterial pressure–derived estimates of cardiac output. Importantly, the treatment group received more colloid and dopexamine infusions but had similar reductions in hospital length of stay primarily because of a reduced incidence of postoperative complications [26].

These studies demonstrated in high-risk patients, that preoptimization applied prior to surgery and postoptimization therapies applied in the ICU both in a protocolized fashion improve outcomes and reduce cost. However, to improve patient outcomes, resuscitation needs to be done in an early phase of the illness. It is uncertain how long that therapeutic window remains open before such aggressive therapies worsen outcome.

4.4.9 Conclusion

In management of patients with AKI, hemodynamic support plays a fundamental role that includes supplying kidneys with adequate perfusion pressure, identifying patients who are preload responsive, and guiding management of vasopressor and inotropic support. Furthermore, early resuscitation with the goal of improving organ oxygen delivery improves patient outcomes.

References

1. Annane D, Vignon P, Renault A, et al. (2007) Norepinephrine plus dobutamine versus Epinephrine alone for management of septic shock: a randomized trial. Lancet 370:676–84.
2. Bellomo R, Chapman M, Finfer, et al. (2000) Low-dose dopamine in patients with early renal dysfunction: a placebo-controlled randomized trial. Australian and New Zealand Intensive Care Society (ANZICS) Clinical Trials Group. Lancet 356:2139–2143.
3. Bersten AD, Holt AW (1995) Vasoactive drugs and the importance of renal perfusion pressure. New Horizon 3:650–661.
4. Blantz RC (1998) Pathophysiology of prerenal azotemia. Kidney Int 53:512–523.
5. Boulain T, Archard JM, Teboul JL, et al. (2002) Changes in blood pressure induced by passive leg raising predict response to fluid loading in critically ill patients. Chest 121:1245–1252.

6. Boyd O, Grounds M, Bennett ED (1993) A randomized clinical trial of the effect of deliberate perioperative increase of oxygen delivery on mortality in high-risk surgical patients. JAMA 270:2699–2707.
7. Bruns FJ, Fraley DS, Haigh J, et al. (1987) Control of organ blood flow. In: Snyder JV, Pinsky MR (eds) Oxygen Transport in the Critically Ill. Year Book Medical Publishers, Chicago, IL.
8. Clermont G, Acker C, Angus D, et al. (2002) Renal failure in the ICU: comparison of the impact of acute renal failure and end-stage renal disease on ICU outcomes. Kidney Int 62:986–996.
9. Friedrich JO, Adhikari N, Herridge MS, et al. (2005) Meta-analysis: low-dose dopamine increases urine output but does not prevent renal dysfunction or death. Ann Intern Med 142:510–524.
10. Gambaro G, Bertaglia G, Puma G, et al. (2002): Diuretics and dopamine for the prevention and treatment of acute renal failure: a critical reappraisal. J Nephrol 15:213–219.
11. Hadian M, Pinsky MR (2007) Functional hemodynamic monitoring. Curr Opin Crit Care 13:318–323.
12. Hou SH, Bushinsky DA, Wish JB, et al. (1983) Hospital acquired renal insufficiency: a prospective study. Am J Med 74:243–248.
13. Kumar A, Anel R, Bunnell E, et al. (2004) Pulmonary artery occlusion pressure and central venous pressure fail to predict ventricular filling volume, cardiac performance, or the response to volume infusion in normal subjects. Crit Care Med 32:691–699.
14. Landry DW, Levin HR, Gallant EM, et al. (1997) Vasopressin deficiency contributes to the vasodilation of septic shock. Circulation 95:1122–1125.
15. Landry DW, Oliver JA (2001) The pathogenesis of vasodilatory shock. N Engl J Med 345:588–595.
16. LeDoux D, Astiz M, Carpati CM, Rackow EC. (2000) Effects of perfusion pressure on tissue perfusion in septic shock. Crit Care Med 28:2729–32.
17. Lobo S, Salgado P, Castillo VGT, et al. (2000) Effects of maximizing oxygen delivery on morbidity and mortality in high-risk surgical patients. Crit Care Med 28:3396–3404.
18. Madgar SA, Geogiadis G, Tuck C (1992) Respiratory variations in right atrial pressure predict response to fluid challenge. J Crit Care 7:76–85.
19. Martin C, Papzian L, Perrin G, et al. (1993) Norepinephrine or dopamine for treatment of hyperdynamic septic shock. Chest 103:1826–31.
20. Michard F, Boussat S, Chemla D, et al. (2000) Relation between respiratory changes in arterial pulse pressure and fluid responsiveness in septic patients with acute circulatory failure. Am J Respir Crit Care Med 162:134–138.
21. Michard F, Teboul JL (2002) Predicting fluid responsiveness in ICU patients: a critical analysis of the evidence. Chest 121:2000–2008.
22. Monnet X, Rienzo M, Osman D, et al. (2006) Response to leg raising predicts fluid responsiveness during spontaneous breathing or with arrhythmia. Crit Care Med 34:1402–1407.
23. Murray PT, Hall JB (2000) Renal replacement therapy for acute renal failure. Am J Respir Crit Care Med 162: 777–781.
24. Murray PT (2003) Use of dopaminergic agents for renoprotection in the ICU. Yearbook of Intensive Care and Emergency Medicine. Springer-Verlag, New York.
25. Patel BM, Chit tock DR, Russell JA, et al. (2002) Beneficial effects of short-term vasopressin infusion during severe septic shock. Anesthesiology 96:576:582.
26. Pearse R, Dawson D, Fawcett J, et al. (2005) Early goal-directed therapy after major surgery reduces complications and duration of hospital stay: a randomized, controlled trial. Crit Care 9:R687–R693.
27. Pinsky MR (1984) Determinants of pulmonary artery flow variation during respiration. J Appl Physiol 56:1237–1245.
28. Pinsky MR, Payen D (2005) Functional hemodynamic monitoring. Crit Care 9:566–572.
29. Pinsky MR (2005) Assessment of indices of preload and volume responsiveness. Curr Opin Crit Care 11:235–239.
30. Pinsky MR. (2007) Hemodynamic evaluation and monitoring in the ICU. Chest 132:2020–2029.
31. Poole BD, Schrier RW (2005) Acute renal failure. In: Fink MP (ed) Textbook of Critical Care. Elsevier Saunders, Philadelphia.
32. Reddy B, Murray P (2005) Acute renal failure. In: Hall JB (ed) Principles of Critical Care. McGraw Hill, New York.
33. Reuter DA, Bayerlein J, Goepfert MS, et al. (2003) Influence of tidal volume on left ventricular stroke volume variation measured by pulse contour analysis in mechanically ventilated patients. Intensive Care Med 29:476–480.
34. Rivers E, Nguyen B, Havstad S, et al. (2001) Early goal-directed therapy in the treatment of severe sepsis and septic shock. N Engl J Med 345:1368–1377.
35. Sakr Y, Reinhart K, Vincent JL, et al. (2006) Does dopamine administration in shock influence outcome? Result of the sepsis occurrence in acutely ill patients (SOAP) study. Crit Care Med 34:589–597.
36. Schertz M (2002) Vasopressors and the kidney. Blood Purif 20:243–251.
37. Shoemaker WC, Appel PL, Kram HB, et al. (1998) Prospective trial of supranormal values of survivors as therapeutic goals in high-risk surgical patients. Chest 94: 1176–1186.
38. Sniecinsky RM, Wright S, Levy JH (2007) Cardiovascular pharmacology. In Levy JH (ed) Cardiothoracic Critical Care. Elsevier, Philadelphia.
39. Star RA (1998) Treatment of acute renal failure. Kidney Int 54:1817–1831.
40. Tang I, Murray PT (2004) Prevention of perioperative ARF: what works? Best Pract Res Clin Anesthesiol 18:91–111.
41. Thomas M, Shillingford J (1965) The circulatory response to a standard postural change in ischaemic heart disease. Brit Heart J 27:17–27.
42. Weisberg LS, Kurnik PB, Kurnik BR (1994) Risk of radiocontrast nephropathy in patients with and without diabetes mellitus. Kidney Int 45:259–265.

Treatment of Anemia

4.5

Annette Beyea and Howard L. Corwin

Core Messages

- In the absence of acute bleeding or acute ischemic cardiac disease, a transfusion trigger of 7.0 g/dl is appropriate in most critically ill patients including those with acute kidney injury (AKI).
- A transfusion trigger of between 8.0 and 10.0 g/dl is appropriate for patients with acute coronary syndromes until further evidence becomes available.
- Epoetin alpha administration, in the acute setting, will increase the hemoglobin concentration; however, it does not reduce red blood cell (RBC) transfusion in the critically ill.
- In those patients with prolonged dialysis-dependent acute renal failure (ARF) following the acute phase of critical illness (>28 days), epoetin may play a role similar to that in chronic kidney disease.
- In view of the increase in risk of thrombotic events, patients receiving epoetin alpha in the intensive care unit (ICU) should receive prophylactic anticoagulation if possible.

H. L. Corwin (✉)
Departments of Medicine and Anesthesiology, Dartmouth-Hitchcock Medical Center, One Medical Center Drive, Lebanon, NH 03756, USA
e-mail: howard.l.corwin@hitchcock.org

Anemia is common in acute renal failure (ARF) and is associated with frequent red blood cell (RBC) transfusions and worse clinical outcomes [1]. Almost two thirds of ARF patients who require dialysis have a baseline hemoglobin concentration below 9 g/dl, with 78% of these receiving an RBC transfusion. A hemoglobin concentration below 9 g/dl in ARF is independently associated with a significant increase in the risk of death at 28 days (adjusted odds ratio [OR] 2.4; 95% confidence interval [95% CI], 1.1–5.2). Thus, anemia presents an important challenge in the management of the patients with ARF. An understanding of anemia and its management in patient with ARF is inseparable from that of anemia in the critically ill patient in general. It is in this latter population that ARF, particularly ARF requiring renal replacement therapy, most commonly occurs [2]. Therefore much of the following discussion will focus on anemia in the critically ill patient, which includes the patient with ARF.

Anemia is common in critically ill patients and, similar to ARF patients, appears early in their intensive care unit (ICU) course. By day 3 after ICU admission, almost 95% of patients are anemic [3, 4]. The anemia in these critically ill patients persists throughout the duration of their ICU and hospital stay. As a consequence of this anemia, critically ill patients receive a large number of RBC transfusions. Two recent cross-sectional studies conducted in Europe and the United States observed that RBC transfusions were administered in approximately 40% of all patients studied [5, 6]. Similar to the ARF patients, 65–85% of patients in the ICU for more than 1 week are transfused [1, 3, 6]. On average, critically ill patients received almost 5 units of RBCs. This is little changed over the past 2 decades despite the

A. Jörres et al. (eds.), *Management of Acute Kidney Problems*,
DOI: 10.1007/978-3-540-69441-0_4.5, © Springer-Verlag Berlin Heidelberg 2010

scrutiny of transfusion practice. Of note, both recent observational studies [5, 6] found that RBC transfusion was independently associated with worse clinical outcomes.

What is responsible for this anemia? Phlebotomy is an important factor contributing to anemia and the need for blood transfusions in the critically ill patient. In the past, ICU patients could be phlebotomized on average 65 ml/day.[3] Smoller and Kruskall [7] found that almost half of their ICU patients receiving blood transfusions were phlebotomized more than the equivalent of one unit of blood. More recently, phlebotomy losses of 40 ml/day were still noted in ICU patients [5]. It is now becoming clear that the view of anemia in the critically ill as simply the result of excessive phlebotomy by "medical vampires" is not completely accurate [8]. Red blood cell production in critically ill patients is not normal, and decreased RBC production is also important in the development and maintenance of the anemia observed in the critically ill.

Over 90% of ICU patients have low serum iron (Fe), total iron binding capacity (TIBC), and Fe/TIBC ratio, but have a normal or, more usually, an elevated serum ferritin level [4, 9]. Similarly, low iron parameters and elevated ferritin levels are observed in patients with multiple organ dysfunction and ARF [1, 10]. On the other hand, nutritional deficiencies are uncommon [4]. At the same time, serum erythropoietin (EPO) levels are only mildly elevated, with little evidence of reticulocyte response to endogenous EPO [4]. Similarly decreased EPO levels are observed in ARF [11]. Rogiers et al. [12] compared EPO levels in critically ill patients with those in patients with iron-deficiency anemia. Although EPO levels were somewhat elevated compared with those in adults without anemia, they were significantly lower when compared with patients with iron-deficiency anemia despite similar levels of hematocrit.

The blunted EPO response observed in the critically ill appears to result from inhibition of the EPO gene by inflammatory mediators [13, 14]. These same inflammatory cytokines directly inhibit RBC production by the bone marrow and may produce the distinct abnormalities of iron metabolism [15, 16]. Anemia of critical illness therefore is a distinct clinical entity characterized by blunted EPO production and abnormalities in iron metabolism similar to what is commonly referred to as the anemia of chronic disease.

In anemia, O_2 carrying capacity is decreased but tissue oxygenation is preserved at hemoglobin levels well below 10.0 g/dl. Following the development of anemia, adaptive changes include a shift in the oxyhemoglobin dissociation curve, hemodynamic alterations, and microcirculatory alterations. The shift to the right of the oxyhemoglobin dissociation curve in anemia is primarily the result of increased synthesis of 2,3-DPG in red cells. This rightward shift enables more O_2 to be released to the tissues at a given pressure of oxygen (pO_2), offsetting the effect of reduced O_2 carrying capacity of the blood. Several hemodynamic alterations also occur following the development of anemia. The body primarily attempts to preserve O_2 delivery to vital organs through increased cardiac output as well as increased arterial and venous vascular tone mediated through increased sympathetic tone. Central and regional reflexes redistribute organ blood flow.

There is evidence that low levels of hemoglobin can be tolerated in healthy subjects. Hematocrits of 10–20% have been achieved in both dogs and baboons using normovolemic hemodilution without untoward effects to the animals [17, 18]. Similarly, studies in patients with preserved left ventricular function undergoing coronary artery bypass grafting demonstrated that hemodilution to a target hematocrit of 15% was well tolerated [19, 20]. Weiskopf et al. induced normovolemic hemodilutional anemia to hemoglobin levels of 5 g/dl in healthy human patients prior to surgery as well as normal volunteers. They found no evidence for reduced oxygen delivery associated with acute anemia [21]. Similarly, data regarding the ability to tolerate significant levels of anemia comes from studies of Jehovah's Witness patients [22, 23]. It seems clear that hemoglobin levels falling significantly below the "10/30" threshold can be tolerated by individuals who are not critically ill. However, is this applicable to the critically ill patient population?

RBC transfusions are commonly utilized in an attempt to increase oxygen delivery to the tissues and in turn improve tissue oxygenation, especially in shock states. The rationale for this therapeutic approach is that an increase in hemoglobin will increase the oxygen-carrying capacity of blood and thus provide more oxygen delivery to delivery-dependent tissue. However, stored RBCs have a low p50 that increases the affinity of hemoglobin for oxygen and thereby reduces oxygen release to tissues (shifting oxygen dissociation curve to the left). Furthermore, standard CPD-stored blood is rapidly depleted of 2,3-diphosphoglycerate (2,3-DPG) and adenosine triphosphate, with resultant inadequacy of the RBC oxygen transport function.

The best evidence available regarding the efficacy of RBC transfusion among critically ill patients is from a randomized controlled trial commonly referred to as the Transfusion Requirements in Critical Care (TRICC) trial, conducted by the Canadian Critical Care Trials Group [24]. In this study, a liberal transfusion strategy (hemoglobin 10.0–12.0 g/dl, with a transfusion trigger of 10.0 g/dl) was compared with a restrictive transfusion strategy (hemoglobin 7.0–9.0 g/dl, with a transfusion trigger of 7.0 g/dl) in a general medical and surgical critical care population. The TRICC trial documented an overall nonsignificant trend toward decreased 30-day mortality in the restrictive group; however, there was a significant decrease in mortality in the restrictive group among patients who were less acutely ill (APACHE II scores less than 20) and among patients who were less than 55 years of age. The diversity of patients enrolled in the trial and the consistency of the results suggest that the conclusions may be generalized to most critical care patients, with the possible exception of patients with active coronary ischemic syndromes.

Recent observational studies [5, 6] in combination with the TRICC trial [24] have raised questions regarding the validity of the historic assumption that RBC transfusion was beneficial for critically ill patients with anemia. To date, there are no convincing data to support the routine use of RBC transfusion to treat anemia in hemodynamically stable critically ill patients without evidence of acute bleeding. In fact, the data available suggests that RBC transfusions are associated with worse clinical outcomes. In the absence of acute bleeding, hemoglobin levels of 7.0–9.0 g/dl are well tolerated by most critically ill patients, and a transfusion threshold of 7.0 g/dl is appropriate. There is still some controversy as to what the appropriate transfusion threshold should be for critically ill patients with acute ischemic cardiac disease.

Two observational studies have explored the clinical consequences of anemia in patients with acute coronary syndromes or an acute myocardial infarction. Wu et al. [25] used US Medicare records in a retrospective study of 78,974 patients older than age 65 who were hospitalized with a primary diagnosis of acute myocardial infarction. Lower admission hematocrit values were associated with increased 30-day mortality with a mortality rate approaching 50% among patients with a hematocrit of 27% or lower who did not receive an RBC transfusion. However, a number of potential biases severely limited any inferences made from this study. The second study by Rao and colleagues [26] studied patients in three large trials of patients with acute coronary syndromes who received RBC transfusions. They observed that RBC transfusions were not associated with improved survival when nadir hematocrit values were in the range of 20% or 25%, and were clearly associated with worsened outcomes when values were greater than 30%. Importantly, despite their differences, both the Wu and Rao studies consistently demonstrate that patients who receive RBCs at a higher hematocrit appear to be harmed by the transfusions. Further evidence from randomized controlled trials would provide the needed evidence to determine optimal transfusion strategies in this high-risk patient population.

To date, the TRICC trial remains the only large randomized trial that has examined RBC transfusion in the critical care setting [24]. Given the lack of any demonstrated clinical efficacy of RBC transfusion in critically ill patients, in the absence of active bleeding, a transfusion trigger of 7.0 g/dl in most critically ill patients including patients with a history of cardiac disease is appropriate. On the other hand, a transfusion trigger of between 8.0 and 10.0 g/dl would seem reasonable for patients with acute coronary syndromes until further evidence becomes available.

As previously noted, the anemia associated with critical illness is fundamentally similar to the anemia of chronic inflammatory disease. A major feature of the anemia of critical illness is a failure of circulating EPO concentrations to increase appropriately in response to the reduction in hemoglobin levels. These observations have suggested that treatment with pharmacological doses of recombinant human erythropoietin (epoetin alpha) might decrease exposure to allogeneic blood and raise the hemoglobin level in critically ill patients. The rationale for epoetin alpha therapy is that increased erythropoiesis will result in higher hemoglobin levels, a more rapid return to normal hemoglobin levels, and thus a reduced need for RBC transfusions. A corollary to this is the hope that by avoiding the negative effects of transfused RBCs, clinical outcomes would improve.

The above rationale led to a small randomized pilot study (160 patients) which demonstrated a reduction in RBC transfusion with epoetin alpha treatment (300 U/kg daily for 5 days then every other day until ICU discharge) [27]. This was followed by a much larger randomized study (1,302 patients) which confirmed the transfusion findings [28]. Of interest, a post hoc analysis in this latter trial suggested subgroup differences in mortality with epoetin alpha treatment in trauma patients. This led to a third randomized study (1,460 patients) in which the primary outcome was again transfusion reduction. However, because of the prior subgroup differences, the three admitting subgroups were now prospectively identified, and randomization was stratified on these groups. In this prospective analysis, a mortality benefit in the trauma patients receiving epoetin alpha was replicated [29]. Surprisingly, there was no transfusion reduction found with epoetin alpha treatment, although hemoglobin concentration did rise, suggesting that the mortality benefit was independent of transfusion effects. In the last two trials, epoetin alpha was administered at a dosage of 40,000 U/week [28, 29]. The absence of transfusion benefit in the most recent trial likely reflected a change in transfusion practice between the studies. No data was available regarding development of or recovery from ARF in these trials.

An important additional observation was a significant increase in thrombotic events noted with epoetin alpha treatment which was not observed in the earlier studies. Trials in other populations (cancer and chronic renal failure) to achieve target hemoglobin concentrations above 12 g/dl with epoetin alpha have reported an increase in the risk of thrombotic complications and mortality [30–33]. In contrast to studies on EPO in cancer and renal failure, the findings in the critically ill are notable in two respects: first, the increase in thrombotic events occurred with a hemoglobin target below 12 g/dl; and second, the duration of therapy was brief (less than 2 weeks). In a post hoc analysis, the increase in thrombotic events was not observed in epoetin alpha patients receiving heparin (prophylactic or therapeutic). An increase in thrombotic events was not noted in earlier trials [27, 28].

These studies specifically excluded patients with preexisting renal insufficiency, although patients who developed ARF during the study were included. However, there is no reason to suspect that patients with ARF would behave differently from the general critically ill population. No prospective data are available regarding epoetin alpha in ARF. A retrospective cohort study in critically ill patients with ARF did not demonstrate either a transfusion effect or effect on renal recovery [34]. However, the dosing of epoetin alpha was quite variable, with few patients receiving doses comparable to those in the other epoetin alpha trials.

The hypothesis was that improvement in clinical outcome with epoetin alpha would result from avoiding adverse effects from transfused RBCs. However, the mortality benefit observed occurred without transfusion reduction. Similarly, the timing of the mortality benefit and the modest increase in hemoglobin observed makes it unlikely that the hemoglobin rise was responsible for mortality improvement. A more likely explanation for the mortality improvement is related to non-hematopoietic effects of epoetin alpha.

EPO has actions aside from stimulating the bone marrow to produce mature erythrocytes. EPO acts as a cytokine with antiapoptotic activity [35–37]. In this latter role, EPO has been demonstrated in preclinical and small clinical studies to protect cells from hypoxemia/ischemia. Multiple tissues express EPO and the EPO receptor, in response to stress and mediate local stress responses. These "non-hematologic" activities of EPO in protecting cells suggest a role for it in the critically ill [35–37]. Apoptosis is important in the pathogenesis of many critical illnesses such as sepsis and multiorgan failure as well as ARF. Similar mechanisms may also be involved in mediating injury in trauma patients. The recent trials suggest that the antiapoptotic activity of EPO could be responsible for the improved outcomes in the critically ill trauma patient and could possibly improve renal outcome. Further preclinical and clinical studies will be necessary to establish the mechanism responsible for the epoetin alpha effects.

In summary, it is clear that anemia is common in patients with ARF and is similar to the critically population in general. Although there are few data on anemia and its treatment specific to patients with ARF, based on the available data in the critically ill several conclusions can be made:

1. Given the lack of demonstrated clinical efficacy of RBC transfusion in critically ill patients, in the absence of acute bleeding or acute ischemic cardiac disease, a transfusion trigger of 7.0 g/dl is appropriate in most critically ill patients including ARF patients.
2. A transfusion trigger of between 8.0 and 10.0 g/dl is appropriate for patients with acute coronary syndromes until further evidence becomes available.
3. Epoetin alpha administration, in the acute setting, will increase the hemoglobin concentration; however, it does not reduce RBC transfusion in the critically ill. In the acute setting, epoetin alpha is of

little benefit with the possible exception for patients admitted following trauma. No clinical data are available regarding potential for renal protection with epoetin alpha.

4. In those patients with prolonged dialysis-dependent ARF following the acute phase of critical illness (>28 days), epoetin may play a role similar to that in chronic kidney disease. In view of the increase in risk of thrombotic events, patients receiving epoetin alpha in the ICU should receive prophylactic anticoagulation if possible.

References

1. du Cheyron D, Parienti JJ, Fekih-Hassen M, Daubin C, Charbonneau P. Impact of anemia on outcome in critically ill patients with severe acute renal failure. *Intensive Care Med* 2005; 31:1529–1536.
2. Waikar SS, Liu KD, Chertow GM. Diagnosis, epidemiology and outcomes of acute kidney injury. *Clin J Am Soc Nephrol* 2008; 3:844–861.
3. Corwin HL, Parsonnet KC, Gettinger A. RBC transfusion in the ICU. Is there a reason? *Chest* 1995; 108:767–771.
4. Rodriguez RM, Corwin HL, Gettinger A, Corwin MJ, Gubler D, Pearl RG. Nutritional deficiencies and blunted erythropoietin response as causes of the anemia of critical illness. *J Crit Care* 2001; 16:36–41.
5. Vincent JL, Baron J-F, Reinhart K, Gattinoni L, Thijs L, Webb A et al. Anemia and Blood Transfusion in Critically Ill Patients. *JAMA* 2002; 288:1499–1507.
6. Corwin HL, Gettinger A, Pearl RG, Fink MP, Levy MM, Abraham E et al. The CRIT Study: Anemia and blood transfusion in the critically ill--current clinical practice in the United States. *Crit Care Med* 2004; 32:39–52.
7. Smoller BR, Kruskall MS: Phlebotomy for diagnostic laboratory tests in adults: Pattern of use and effect on transfusion requirements. *N Engl J Med* 1986; 314:1233–1235.
8. Burnum JF. Medical vampires. *N Engl J Med* 1986; 314: 1250–1251.
9. van Iperen CE, Gaillard CAM, Kraaijenhagen RJ, Braam BG, Marx JJM, van de Wiel A. Response of erythropoiesis and iron metabolism to recombinant human erythropoietin in intensive care unit patients. *Crit Care Med* 2000; 28: 2773–2778.
10. Gabriel A, Kozek S, Chiari A, Fitzgerald R, Grabner C, Geissler K, Zimpfer M, Stockenhuber F, Bircher NG. High-dose recombinant human erythropoietin stimulates reticulocyte production in patients with multiple organ dysfunction syndrome. *J Trauma* 1998; 44:361–367.
11. Nielsen OJ, Thaysen JH. Erythropoietin deficiency in acute tubular necrosis. *J Intern Med* 1990; 227:373–380.
12. Rogiers P, Zhang H, Leeman M, Nagler J, Neels H, Melot C, Vincent J-L. Erythropoietin response is blunted in critically ill patients. *Intensive Care Med* 1997; 23:159–162.
13. Frede S, Fandrey J, Pagel H, Hellwig T, Jelkmann W. Erythropoietin gene expression is suppressed after lipopolysaccharide or interleukin-1 beta injections in rats. *Am J Physiol* 1997; 273:R1067–R1071.
14. Jelkmann W. Proinflammatory cytokines lowering erythropoietin production. *J Interferon Cytokine Res* 1998; 18: 555–559.
15. Means RT Jr, Krantz SB. Progress in understanding the pathogenesis of the anemia of chronic disease. *Blood* 1992; 80:1639–1647.
16. Krantz SB. Pathogenesis and treatment of the anemia of chronic disease. *Am J Med Sci* 1994; 307:353–359.
17. Levine E, Rosen A, Sehgal L, Gould S, Sehgal H, Moss G. Physiologic effects of acute anemia: Implications for a reduced transfusion trigger. *Transfusion* 1990; 30: 11–14.
18. Geha AS. Coronary and cardiovascular dynamics and oxygen availability during acute normovolemic anemia. *Surgery* 1976; 80:47–53.
19. Kitchens CS. Are transfusions overrated? Surgical outcome of Jehovah's Witnesses. *Am J Med* 1993; 94:117–119.
20. Hebert P, Schweitzer I, Calder L, Blajchman, Giulivi MA. Review of the clinical practice literature on allogeneic red blood cell transfusion. *Can Med Assoc J* 1997; 156: S9–S26.
21. Weiskopf RB, Viele MK, Feiner J, Kelley S, Liebermen J, Noorani M, Leung JM, Fisher DM, Murray WR, Toy P, Moore MA. Human cardiovascular and metabolic response to acute, severe isovolemic anemia. *JAMA* 1998; 279: 217–221.
22. Carson JL, Spence RK, Poses RM. Severity of anaemia and operative mortality and morbidity. *Lancet* 1998; 727–729.
23. Spence RK, Carson JA, Poses R, McCoy S, Pello M, Alexander J, Popovich J, vNorcross E, Camishion RC. Elective surgery without transfusion: Influence of preoperative hemoglobin level and blood loss on mortality. *Am J Surg* 1990; 159:320–324.
24. Hebert PC, Wells G, Blajchman MA, Marshall J, Martin C, Pagliarello G et al. A multicenter, randomized, controlled clinical trial of transfusion requirements in critical care. Transfusion Requirements in Critical Care Investigators, Canadian Critical Care Trials Group. *New Engl J Med* 1999; 340:409–417.
25. Wu WC, Rathore SS, Wang Y, Radford MJ, Krumholz HM. Blood transfusion in elderly patients with acute myocardial infarction. *New Engl J Med* 2001; 345:1230–1236.
26. Rao SV, Jollis JG, Harrington RA, Granger CB, Newby LK, Armstrong PW et al. Relationship of blood transfusion and clinical outcomes in patients with acute coronary syndromes. *JAMA* 2004; 292:1555–1562.
27. Corwin HL, Gettinger A, Rodriguez RM, Pearl RG, Enny C, Colton T, Corwin MJ. Efficacy of recombinant human erythropoietin in the critically ill patient: A randomized double blind placebo controlled trial. *Crit Care Med.* 1999;27: 2346–2350.
28. Corwin HL, Gettinger A, Rodriguez RM, et al. Efficacy of recombinant human erythropoietin in the critically ill patient: A randomized double blind placebo controlled trial. *JAMA* 2002;288:2827–2835.
29. Corwin HL, Gettinger A, Fabian T, May Addison, Pearl RG, Heard S, An R, Bowers P, Burton P, Klausner MA, Corwin MJ.

Efficacy and safety of epoetin alpha in the critically ill. *N Engl J Med* 2007; 357:965–976.
30. Henke M, Laszig R, Rube C, et al. Erythropoietin to treat head and neck cancer patients with anaemia undergoing radiotherapy: randomised, double-blind, placebo controlled trial. *Lancet* 2003; 362:1255–1260.
31. Leyland-Jones B, Semiglazov V, Pawlicki M, et al. Maintaining normal hemoglobin levels with epoetin alfa in mainly nonanemic patients with metastatic breast cancer receiving first-line chemotherapy: A survival study. *J Clin Oncol* 2005; 23:5960–5972.
32. Bohius J, Wilson J, Seidenfeld J, et al. Recombinant human erythropoietins and cancer patients: Updated meta-analysis of 57 studies including 9353 patients. *JNCI* 2006; 98:708–714.
33. Singh AK, Szczech L, Tang KL, et al. Correction of anemia with epoetin alfa in chronic kidney disease. *N Engl J Med* 2006; 355:2085–2098.
34. Park J, Gage BF, Vijayan A. Use of EPO in critically ill patients with acute renal failure requiring renal replacement therapy. *Am J Kidney Dis* 2005; 46:791–798.
35. Colman T, Brines M. Science review: Recombinant human erythropoietin in critical illness: A role beyond anemia. *Critical Care* 2004; 8:337–341.
36. Maiese K, Li F, Chong ZZ. New avenues of exploration for erythropoietin. *JAMA* 2005; 293:90–95.
37. Brines M, Cerani A. Discovering erythropoietin's extra-hematopoietic functions: Biology and clinical promise. *Kidney Int* 2006; 70:246–250.

Metabolic Alterations and Nutrition in AKI 4.6

Wilfred Druml

Core Messages

- Acute kidney injury (AKI) typically results in a catabolic, prooxidative, and proinflammatory state.
- Nutritional support must be viewed as a cornerstone in the treatment of patients with AKI, a specific type of metabolic intervention which must be planned together with renal replacement therapy (RRT) and fluid and electrolyte management.
- Nutritional support for a patient with AKI is not fundamentally different from that in patient without renal dysfunction. However, in a patient who has acquired AKI and needs nutritional support, the nutritional regimen must take into account the multiple metabolic consequences of AKI, of RRT, and of the underlying disease process and/or associated complications.
- Enteral nutrition has become the preferred type of nutritional support also in patients with AKI. Nevertheless, many patients have severe limitations to enteral nutrition and will require supplementary or even total parenteral nutrition.
- Modern nutrition therapy has moved from a quantitatively oriented approach in covering nitrogen and energy requirements, to a more qualitative type of metabolic intervention aimed at modulating the inflammatory state, the oxygen radical scavenger system, supporting immunocompetence and endothelial functions, and taking advantage of specific pharmacologic effects of various nutrients (such as glutamine, fish oil, selenium, antioxidants).

4.6.1 Introduction

The perception of acute kidney injury (AKI) in the critically ill patient has fundamentally changed during recent years. Regarded earlier as a "simple" organ failure which could easily be supported by modern replacement therapies, AKI has recently been recognized as a systemic inflammatory syndrome, a prooxidative, proinflammatory, and hypermetabolic state which exerts a profound impact on the course of disease, the evolution of complications, and which is associated with a high attributable mortality [1, 2]. It is increasingly appreciated that metabolic and nutritional factors play a crucial role in this scenario and are of outmost relevance in the prevention and treatment of AKI.

The metabolic environment in a patient with AKI is complex and is not only affected by the acutely uremic condition per se, but also by the underlying disease process and associated complications, and by the type and intensity of renal replacement therapy (RRT).

W. Druml
Department of Medicine III, Division of Nephrology, Vienna General Hospital, Währinger Gürtel 18–20, 1090 Vienna, Austria
e-mail: wilfred.druml@meduniwien.ac.at

A. Jörres et al. (eds.), *Management of Acute Kidney Problems*,
DOI: 10.1007/978-3-540-69441-0_4.6, © Springer-Verlag Berlin Heidelberg 2010

Depending on the severity of associated illness, nutrient requirements may differ widely between individual patients and also during the course of the disease.

The nutritional and metabolic management must present a cornerstone in the care of these patients [3]. A nutritional program for a patient with AKI is not fundamentally different from that for other critically ill patients but must take into consideration these complex alterations in metabolism and nutrient balances, and nutrition has also to be coordinated with RRT.

Nutrition support has left a merely quantitative approach of provision of energy and nitrogen, to become a more qualitative type of metabolic intervention aimed at modulating the inflammatory state, the oxygen radical scavenger system, and immunocompetence, and at taking advantage of specific pharmacologic effects of various nutrients; this is also relevant for prevention and treatment of AKI.

For many years, parenteral nutrition was the preferred route for nutritional support in AKI patients. Recently, *enteral* nutrition has become the principal type of nutritional support for AKI patients and actually may exert specific beneficial effects on the kidney. Nevertheless, enteral and parenteral nutrition should not be viewed as opposed therapies but rather as complementary methods of nutritional support because it is often impossible to meet requirements by the enteral route alone, so supplementary parenteral nutrition may become necessary.

4.6.2 The Metabolic Environment and Nutritional Requirements in Patients with AKI

AKI presents a complication occurring in a broad spectrum of underlying pathologies. Clinical presentation of a patient with AKI may thus range from uncomplicated mono-organ failure in a noncatabolic patient, to a critically ill patient with multiple organ dysfunction syndrome (MODS). The metabolic changes will be determined not only by AKI per se, but also by the underlying disease process and/or additional complications and organ dysfunction [4].

Nevertheless, AKI in addition to the obvious effects on water, electrolyte, and acid–base balances, affects all metabolic pathways of the body; exerts specific alterations in protein and amino acid, carbohydrate, and lipid metabolism; and induces a proinflammatory, prooxidative, and hypercatabolic state (Table 4.6.1). Moreover, the type and intensity of RRT has a profound effect on nutrient balances.

Table 4.6.1 Important metabolic abnormalities induced by AKI

- Activation of protein catabolism
- Peripheral glucose intolerance/increased gluconeogenesis
- Inhibition of lipolysis and altered fat clearance
- Depletion of the antioxidant system
- Induction of a proinflammatory state
- Impairment of immunocompetence
- Endocrine abnormalities: hyperparathyroidisms, insulin resistance, erythropoietin resistance, resistance to growth factors, etc.

The optimal intake of nutrients in patients is mainly influenced by the nature of the illness causing AKI, the extent of catabolism, and type and frequency of RRT. Again, AKI presents a heterogeneous group of subjects with widely differing nutrient requirements, and it must be noted that these can vary considerably also during the course of disease.

4.6.3 Energy Metabolism and Energy Requirements

In patients with uncomplicated AKI, energy expenditure is within the range of healthy subjects. Energy requirements in patients with AKI are thus rather determined by the underlying disease and associated complications [5].

Energy intake for nutritional support in the critically ill patient should never exceed actual energy requirements. Complications, if any, from slightly underfeeding are less deleterious than those from overfeeding. Increasing energy intake from 30 to 40 kcal/kg body weight [BW] per day in patients with AKI increased the frequency of metabolic complications, such as hyperglycemia and hypertriglyceridemia, but had no beneficial effects [6].

Patients with AKI should receive 20–30 kcal/kg BW per day. Even in hypermetabolic conditions such as sepsis or MODS, energy expenditure rarely is higher than 130% of calculated basic energy expenditure (BEE), and energy intake usually should not exceed 30 kcal/kg BW per day. In several patients actually, “less might be more,” and “permissive underfeeding” might present a preferable approach [7].

4.6.4 Carbohydrate Metabolism

In patients with AKI, hyperglycemia is frequently present. The major cause of elevated blood glucose concentrations is insulin resistance. A second feature of glucose metabolism in AKI is accelerated hepatic gluconeogenesis, mainly from conversion of amino acids released during protein catabolism that cannot be suppressed by exogenous glucose infusions [8].

Hyperglycemia in the critically ill has been recognized as an important determinant in the evolution of complications such as infections or organ failures (also of AKI!) and of prognosis [9]. Thus, maintaining normoglycemia must be strictly observed during nutritional support, and insulin requirements are usually higher in patients with AKI.

4.6.5 Lipid Metabolism

Profound alterations of lipid metabolism occur in patients with AKI which result in hypertriglyceridemia [10]. The triglyceride content of plasma lipoproteins, especially of very low density lipoproteins, is increased, and total cholesterol and in particular high density lipoprotein cholesterol are decreased. The major cause of lipid abnormalities in AKI is an impairment of lipolysis, and this is in sharp contrast to other acute disease states in which lipolysis is usually augmented.

Fat particles of artificial lipid emulsions for parenteral nutrition are degraded similarly to endogenous very low density lipoproteins, and impaired lipolysis in AKI also retards elimination of intravenously infused lipids [11]. Regarding enteral nutrition, it should be noted that intestinal lipid absorption is also retarded in renal failure.

4.6.6 Protein and Amino Acid Metabolism/Protein Requirements

AKI is characterized by an activation of protein catabolism with excessive release of amino acids from skeletal muscle and sustained negative nitrogen balance [12]. Muscular protein degradation and amino acid oxidation is stimulated, and hepatic extraction of amino acids from the circulation, gluconeogenesis, and ureagenesis are increased. In the liver, protein synthesis and secretion of acute phase proteins are also stimulated.

The causes of hypercatabolism in AKI are complex and manifold. They present a combination of nonspecific mechanisms induced by the acute disease process and underlying illness and associated complications, with specific effects induced by the acute loss of renal function and finally, also by the type and intensity of RRT. The dominating mechanism is the stimulation of hepatic gluconeogenesis from amino acids, which – in contrast to healthy subjects but also to patients with chronic kidney disease (CKD) – can be decreased but not halted by exogenous substrate supply. A major stimulus of muscle protein catabolism in AKI is insulin resistance. Moreover, acidosis was identified as an important factor in mediating muscular protein breakdown [4].

Several additional catabolic factors are operative in AKI. The release of inflammatory mediators such as TNF-α, depletion of antioxidative factors, the secretion of catabolic hormones, hyperparathyroidism, suppression and/or decreased sensitivity of growth factors, the release of proteases from activated leukocytes all can stimulate protein breakdown. Moreover, RRT causes a loss of amino acids and protein and may stimulate protein catabolism [4].

Last but not least, inadequate nutrition contributes to the loss of lean body mass in AKI. Starvation can augment the catabolic response of AKI, and malnutrition was identified a major determinant of morbidity and mortality in AKI [13].

4.6.6.1 Amino Acid and Protein Requirements in AKI

The optimal intake of amino acid/protein continues to be the most controversial question relating to nutritional support in critically ill patients with AKI. In noncatabolic patients and during the polyuric recovery phase of AKI, a protein intake of 1–1.3 g/kg BW per day was required to achieve a positive nitrogen balance. In critically ill patients on continuous renal replacement therapy (CRRT), protein catabolic rate accounts on average for 1.4–1.7 g/kg BW per day, and an amino acid/protein intake of 1.4–1.7 g/kg BW per day was recommended [14]. This amount is comparable to that for other critically ill patients. These calculations include amino acid/protein losses induced by RRT.

Recently, some authors have suggested an even higher amino acid intake of up to 2.5 g/kg BW per day [15]. However, there are no proven advantages of such excessive intakes, which can increase uremic toxicity and provoke metabolic complications such as hyperammonemia.

4.6.7 Metabolism and Requirements of Micronutrients

Serum levels of water-soluble vitamins usually are low in AKI patients mainly because of losses induced by RRT, and thus requirements are increased. Intake of ascorbic acid should be kept below 250 mg/day because any excessive supply may precipitate secondary oxalosis.

Despite the fact that there are not relevant losses during RRT, plasma concentrations of lipid soluble vitamins A, D, and E, but not of vitamin K are decreased in patients with AKI [16].

Many alterations of trace element homeostasis are a reflection of an nonspecific acute phase response with redistribution of trace elements within the body. Selenium levels are profoundly decreased, and in addition this is augmented by CRRT-associated selenium losses.

Several micronutrients are important components of the organism's defense mechanisms against free oxygen radical–induced injury. A profound depression in antioxidant status has been documented in patients with AKI, and an adequate supplementation of micronutrients to meet the increased requirements must be strictly observed [17].

4.6.8 Electrolytes

Derangements in electrolyte balance in patients with AKI are affected by a broad spectrum of factors in addition to renal failure, including the type of underlying disease and degree of hypercatabolism, type and intensity of RRT, drug therapy, and also the timing, type, and composition of nutritional support.

Electrolyte requirements do not only vary considerably between patients but can vary during the course of the disease. In nonoliguric patients, in subjects on CRRT, and during the polyuric phase of AKI, electrolyte requirements can be considerably altered. Thus, electrolyte requirements have to be evaluated in patients with AKI on a day-to-day basis and intake has to be adjusted frequently.

4.6.9 Metabolic Impact of Renal Replacement Therapy

The impact of intermittent hemodialysis on metabolism is manifold. Several water soluble substances, such as amino acids, vitamins, and carnitine are lost during hemodialysis. Protein catabolism is caused not only by amino acid losses, but also by activation of protein breakdown. Moreover, it has been shown that generation of reactive oxygen species is augmented during hemodialysis.

In the care of critically ill patients with AKI, CRRT is frequently used, and these are also associated with a broad pattern of metabolic consequences which are especially relevant because of the continuous mode of therapy and the currently recommended high fluid turnover of up to more than 60 l/day [18] (Table 4.6.2).

Table 4.6.2 Metabolic effects renal replacement therapy in acute kidney injury (AKI)

Intermittent hemodialysis
Loss of water-soluble molecules:
Amino acids
Water-soluble vitamins
L-Carnitine etc.
Activation of protein catabolism:
Loss of amino acids
Loss of proteins and blood
Induction of cytokine release (TNF-α, etc.)
Inhibition of protein synthesis
Increase in reactive oxygen species production
Loss of antioxidants
Stimulation of reactive oxygen species formation through bioincompatibility
Continuous renal replacement therapy (CRRT)
Heat loss
Excessive load of substrates (lactate, citrate, glucose)
Loss of nutrients (amino acids, vitamins, selenium, etc.)
Loss of electrolytes (phosphate, magnesium)
Elimination of (short-chain) proteins
(hormones, mediators?, but also albumin)
Metabolic consequences of bioincompatibility (induction/activation of mediator cascades, of an inflammatory reaction, stimulation of protein catabolism)

A major effect of CRRT is the elimination of small- and medium-sized molecules. In the case of amino acids, the loss of amino acids can be estimated from the volume of the filtrate and the average plasma concentrations. Usually, this amounts to approximately 0.2 g/l filtrate and, depending on the filtered volume, results in a total loss of 5–15 g amino acid per day, representing about 10–15% of amino acid intake. Depending on the type of therapy and the membrane material used, additional losses of protein can account for up to 10 g/day.

Water soluble vitamins, such as folic acid, vitamin B6, and vitamin C are also eliminated during CRRT, and an intake above the recommended dietary allowance (RDA) is required to maintain plasma concentrations of these vitamins in these patients. Moreover, selenium losses during CRRT can account for twice the RDA.

4.6.10 Nutrient Administration

The practice of nutritional support in critically ill patients with AKI is not fundamentally different from that in patients without renal dysfunction but has to take into consideration the multiple consequences of AKI and RRT on metabolism and nutrient balances.

Again, the optimal intake of nutrients in patients is mainly influenced by the nature of the illness causing AKI, the extent of catabolism, and type and frequency of RRT. AKI thus presents a heterogeneous group of subjects with widely differing nutrient requirements and these can considerably vary also during the course of disease.

Nutrient requirements of patients with AKI are summarized in Table 4.6.3.

4.6.11 Enteral Nutrition (Tube Feeding)

In the past, parenteral nutrition was the preferred route of nutritional support in patients with AKI. During recent years, enteral nutrition has become the primary type of nutritional support for all critically ill patients and also for patients with AKI [19]. Even small amounts of luminally provided diets can help to support intestinal defense functions, support the intestinal immune system, and reduce infectious complications.

Moreover, enteral nutrition might exert specific advantages in AKI. In experimental AKI, enteral nutrition can augment renal plasma flow and improve renal function. In the clinical situation, enteral nutrition was a factor associated with an improved prognosis in critically ill patients with AKI [2].

Nevertheless, gastrointestinal motility is impaired in many patients with AKI, and frequently it is not possible to meet requirements by the enteral route alone, and parenteral nutrition at least as a supplement and/or temporarily may become necessary.

Unfortunately, few systematic studies on enteral nutrition have been conducted in patients with AKI. In the largest study to date, nutritional effects, feasibility,

Table 4.6.3 Nutrient requirements in acute renal injury (AKI)[a]

Energy intake	20–30 kcal/kg/day (max. 35)
Glucose	<3–5 g/kg/day
Lipids	0.8–1.2 g/kg/day (max. 1.5)
Amino acids/protein	
Conservative Therapy	0.6–1.2 g/kg/day
+ RRT	1.2–1.5 g/kg/day (max. 1.7)
+ Hypercatabolism	
Vitamins (combination products providing RDA)	
Water-soluble	2 × RDA/day (Cave: Vitamin C <250 mg/day)
Lipid-soluble	1–2 × RDA/day (higher for vitamin E?)
Trace Elements (combination products providing RDA)	
1 × RDA/ day (selenium 300 μg/day ?)	
Electrolytes (Requirements must be assessed individually)	
(Cave: hypokalemia and/or hypophosphatemia)	

RDA recommended dietary allowance
[a]Requirements differ between individual patients and may vary considerably during the course of disease

and tolerance of enteral nutrition using either a conventional diet or a preparation adapted to the metabolic needs of hemodialysis patients was investigated in 182 patients with AKI [20]. Side effects of enteral nutrient supply were higher and the amount of nutrient provided was lower in patients with AKI as compared with those with normal renal function, but in general, enteral nutrition was well tolerated, safe, and effective.

4.6.11.1 Enteral Formulas

Essentially, three types of enteral formulas can be used in AKI patients, but none of these diets have been developed specifically for nutrition in AKI:

(a) *Elemental powder diets*: These formulas conform to the concept of a low protein diet supplemented with essential amino acids (EAA) in CKD. These diets are not complete, do not meet the requirements of AKI patients and should be replaced by more complete ready-to-use liquid products.
(b) *Standard enteral formulas designed for nonuremic patients*: In most intensive care patients with AKI, standard enteral formulas as for patients without AKI are used. Potential disadvantages are the amount and type of protein, and the high content of electrolytes. Whether diets enriched in specific substrates such as glutamine, arginine, nucleotides, or omega-3 fatty acids ("Immunonutrition") might exert beneficial effects also in patients with AKI remains to be shown.
(c) *Specific enteral formulas adapted to the metabolic alterations of uremia*: Ready-to-use liquid diets adapted to the nutrient requirements of patients on regular hemodialysis therapy (with a reduced electrolyte and higher protein content plus specific nutrients) present a reasonable approach in enteral nutrition of hypercatabolic intensive care patients with AKI.

4.6.12 Parenteral Nutrition

In the critically ill patient with AKI, it is frequently impossible to cover nutrient requirements exclusively by the enteral route alone, and a supplementary or even total parenteral nutrition may become necessary. Parenteral and enteral nutrition should not be viewed as conflicting but rather as complementary types of nutritional support, a combination which enables an optimal nutrient provision in many critically ill patients [21].

4.6.12.1 Composition of Parenteral Nutrition Solution

Glucose: Glucose should be used as the main energy substrate. In contrast to earlier recommendations, glucose intake must be restricted to <3 to a maximum of 5 g/kg BW per day, because higher intakes are not used for energy but will promote lipogenesis with fatty infiltration of the liver, excessive carbon dioxide production, impair immunocompetence, and increase rates of infections [22].

Glucose tolerance is decreased in AKI, and infusion of insulin is frequently necessary to maintain normoglycemia. Moreover, insulin requirements are approximately 25% higher in parenteral than during enteral nutrition. Strictly maintaining a glucose below 150 mg/dl by insulin therapy must be observed to prevent the evolution of AKI and other complications [9]. By limiting energy intake and providing a portion of the energy by lipid emulsions, the risk of developing hyperglycemia can be reduced.

Lipid emulsions: Changes in lipid metabolism associated with AKI should not prevent the use of lipid emulsions, but the amount infused must be adjusted to the patient's capacity to utilize lipids, and plasma triglyceride concentrations have to be monitored regularly. Usually, 1 g of fat per kg BW per day will not increase plasma triglycerides substantially.

Whether lipid emulsions with a lower content of polyunsaturated fatty acids (replacing soybean oil with olive oil and/or fish oil and/or medium chain triglycerides) to reduce potential proinflammatory side effects of polyunsaturated fatty acids should be preferred in patients with AKI remains to be shown [23].

Amino acid solutions: Three types of amino acid solutions for parenteral nutrition in patients with AKI have been used: exclusively essential amino acids, standard solutions of essential plus nonessential amino acids, and specifically designed "nephro" solutions of adapted proportions of essential and specific

Table 4.6.4 Parenteral nutrition in AKI: "Renal failure fluid" (all-in-one solution)[a]

Component		Quantity	Remarks
Glucose	30–60%	500 ml	In the presence of severe insulin resistance switch to D30W
Fat emulsion	10–20%	500 ml	Start with 10%, switch to 20% if triglycerides are <350 mg/dl
Amino acids	6.5–10%	500 ml	General or special "nephro" amino acid solutions including EAA and NEAA
Water soluble vitamins[b]		2 × RDA	Limit vitamin C intake < 250 mg/day
Fat-soluble vitamins[b]		RDA	Increased requirements of vitamin E?
Trace elements[b]		RDA	Plus selenium 100–300 μg/day?
Electrolytes		As required	Cave: hypophosphatemia or hypokalemia after initiation of TPN
Insulin		As required	Added directly to the solution or given separately

EAA essential amino acid, *NEAA* nonessential amino acid

[a]"All-in-one solution" with all components contained in a single bag, Infusion rate initially 50% of requirements, to be increased over a period of 3 days to satisfy requirements

[b]Combination products containing the recommended dietary allowances (RDA)

nonessential amino acids that might become "conditionally essential" in AKI.

The use of solutions of essential amino acids alone was based on principles established for treating CKD patients with a low protein diet and an amino acid supplement. These solutions should no longer be used, because they are incomplete (several amino acids designated as nonessential amino acids such as histidine, arginine, tyrosine, serine, and cysteine may become indispensable in AKI patients) and have an unbalanced composition.

Thus, solutions including both essential and nonessential amino acids in standard proportions or in special proportions ("nephro" solutions) should be used in patients with AKI. Because of the low water solubility of tyrosine, dipeptides containing tyrosine (such as glycyl-tyrosine) are included in modern "nephro" solutions.

Recently, it was suggested that glutamine exerts important metabolic functions in catabolic patients. Glutamine can improve survival in critically ill patients and may also exert beneficial effects on renal function [24]. Since free glutamine is not stable in aqueous solutions, glutamine containing dipeptides are used as the glutamine source in parenteral nutrition.

"Renal failure fluid": Standard solutions with amino acids, glucose, and lipids contained in a single bag are available ("all in one" solutions) (Table 4.6.4). As required, vitamins, trace elements, and electrolytes can be added to these solutions.

To ensure maximal nutrient utilization and prevent metabolic derangements, the infusion must be started at a low rate (providing about 50% of requirements) and gradually increased over several days.

4.6.13 Complications of Nutritional Support

Technical problems and infectious complications originating from central venous catheters or enteral feeding tubes, metabolic complications of artificial nutrition, and gastrointestinal side effects of enteral nutrition are similar in AKI patients and in non-uremic subjects. However, both metabolic and gastrointestinal complications are far more pronounced and occur more frequently in AKI because the utilization of various nutrients is impaired, the tolerance to electrolytes and volume load is limited, and moreover, gastrointestinal motility is impaired. Because of the high frequency of metabolic complications, nutritional therapy in AKI requires a tighter schedule of monitoring compared with other patient groups.

By gradually increasing the infusion rate and avoiding any infusion above requirements, many adverse effects can be minimized. Moreover, monitoring of nutrition therapy must be more closely observed in patients with AKI than in those with other disease states.

4.6.14 Conclusions

Modified by the clinical context in which it is occurring, AKI presents a catabolic, prooxidative, and proinflammatory syndrome. Nutritional support must be viewed as a cornerstone in the treatment of patients with AKI, with a specific type of metabolic intervention which must be planned together with RRT and fluid and electrolyte management.

RRTs exert a profound impact on electrolyte and nutrient balances. This is especially true for CRRT because of the continuous mode of therapy and with the recommended high fluid turnover.

Basically, a nutritional program for a patient with AKI is not fundamentally different from that in patients without renal dysfunction. However, in a patient who has acquired AKI and needs nutritional support, the nutritional regimen must take into account the multiple metabolic consequences of AKI, RRT, and of the underlying disease process and/or associated complications. In the critically ill patient with AKI, nutritional support must be initiated early and both qualitatively and quantitatively sufficient.

Enteral nutrition has become the preferred type of nutritional support also in patients with AKI. Nevertheless, many patients have severe limitations to enteral nutrition and will require supplementary or even total parenteral nutrition.

Modern nutritional therapy has left a merely quantitatively oriented approach in covering nitrogen and energy requirements, and has moved toward a more qualitative type of metabolic intervention aimed at modulating the inflammatory state, the oxygen radical scavenger system, supporting immunocompetence and endothelial functions, and taking advantage of the specific pharmacologic effects of various nutrients (such as glutamine, fish oil, selenium, and antioxidants). A reduction of the distressingly high mortality rate of patients with AKI will depend also on further improvements in metabolic care.

References

1. Druml W. Acute renal failure is not a "cute" renal failure! Intensive Care Med 2004;30:1886–90.
2. Metnitz PG, Krenn CG, Steltzer H, et al. Effect of acute renal failure requiring renal replacement therapy on outcome in critically ill patients. Crit Care Med 2002;30:2051–8.
3. Druml W. Nutritional management of acute renal failure. J Ren Nutr 2005;15:63–70.
4. Druml W. Nutritional support in patients with acute renal failure. In: Molitoris B, Finn W, eds. Acute renal failure. A Companion to Brenner & Rector's The Kidney. Philadelphia: WB Saunders, 2001.
5. Schneeweiss B, Graninger W, Stockenhuber F, et al. Energy metabolism in acute and chronic renal failure. Am J Clin Nutr 1990;52:596–601.
6. Fiaccadori E, Maggiore U, Rotelli C, et al. Effects of different energy intakes on nitrogen balance in patients with acute renal failure: a pilot study. Nephrol Dial Transplant 2005;20:1976–80.
7. Jeejeebhoy KN. Permissive underfeeding of the critically ill patient. Nutr Clin Pract 2004;19:477–80.
8. Cianciaruso B, Bellizzi V, Napoli R, Sacca L, Kopple JD. Hepatic uptake and release of glucose, lactate, and amino acids in acutely uremic dogs. Metabolism 1991;40:261–9.
9. Schetz M, Vanhorebeek I, Wouters PJ, Wilmer A, Van den Berghe G. Tight blood glucose control is renoprotective in critically ill patients. J Am Soc Nephrol 2008;19:571–8.
10. Druml W, Zechner R, Magometschnigg D, et al. Post-heparin lipolytic activity in acute renal failure. Clin Nephrol 1985; 23:289–93.
11. Druml W, Fischer M, Sertl S, Schneeweiss B, Lenz K, Widhalm K. Fat elimination in acute renal failure: long-chain vs medium-chain triglycerides. Am J Clin Nutr 1992;55: 468–72.
12. Leblanc M, Garred LJ, Cardinal J, et al. Catabolism in critical illness: estimation from urea nitrogen appearance and creatinine production during continuous renal replacement therapy. Am J Kidney Dis 1998;32:444–53.
13. Fiaccadori E, Lombardi M, Leonardi S, Rotelli CF, Tortorella G, Borghetti A. Prevalence and clinical outcome associated with preexisting malnutrition in acute renal failure: a prospective cohort study. J Am Soc Nephrol 1999;10: 581–93.
14. Cano N, Fiaccadori E, Tesinsky P, et al. ESPEN Guidelines on Enteral Nutrition: Adult renal failure. Clin Nutr 2006;25: 295–310.
15. Scheinkestel CD, Kar L, Marshall K, et al. Prospective randomized trial to assess caloric and protein needs of critically Ill, anuric, ventilated patients requiring continuous renal replacement therapy. Nutrition 2003;19:909–16.
16. Druml W, Schwarzenhofer M, Apsner R, Horl WH. Fat-soluble vitamins in patients with acute renal failure. Miner Electrolyte Metab 1998;24:220–6.
17. Metnitz GH, Fischer M, Bartens C, Steltzer H, Lang T, Druml W. Impact of acute renal failure on antioxidant status in multiple organ failure. Acta Anaesthesiol Scand 2000;44: 236–40.
18. Druml W. Metabolic aspects of continuous renal replacement therapies. Kidney Int Suppl 1999;72:S56–61.
19. Druml W, Mitch W. Enteral nutrition in renal disease. In: RH R, ed. Clinical nutrition: enteral and tube feeding. Philadelphia: WB Saunders, 2004.
20. Fiaccadori E, Maggiore U, Giacosa R, et al. Enteral nutrition in patients with acute renal failure. Kidney Int 2004;65: 999–1008.
21. Heidegger CP, Romand JA, Treggiari MM, Pichard C. Is it now time to promote mixed enteral and parenteral nutrition for the critically ill patient? Intensive Care Med 2007;33: 963–9.
22. Dissanaike S, Shelton M, Warner K, O'Keefe GE. The risk for bloodstream infections is associated with increased parenteral caloric intake in patients receiving parenteral nutrition. Crit Care 2007;11:R114.
23. Mayer K, Schaefer MB, Seeger W. Fish oil in the critically ill: from experimental to clinical data. Curr Opin Clin Nutr Metab Care 2006;9:140–8.
24. Griffiths RD, Jones C, Palmer TE. Six-month outcome of critically ill patients given glutamine-supplemented parenteral nutrition. Nutrition 1997;13:295–302.

Glucose, Insulin, and the Kidney

4.7

Miet Schetz, Ilse Vanhorebeek,
Jan Gunst, and Greet Van den Berghe

Core Messages

- Several types of critical illness are associated with hyperglycemia and insulin resistance. This "diabetes of stress" used to be considered an adaptive response, beneficial for survival. This dogma was challenged by two large randomized clinical trials showing that tight glycemic control with intensive insulin therapy improves morbidity and mortality rates in critically ill patients.
- Improved morbidity rates associated with intensive insulin therapy included a beneficial effect on kidney function. Possible mechanisms for this renoprotective effect include prevention or attenuation of oxidative and nitrosative stress, protection of the endothelium, and reduction of inflammation, mitochondrial damage, and apoptosis.

4.7.1 Introduction

Acute kidney injury (AKI) is a frequent complication in intensive care unit (ICU) patients and is associated with a high mortality. Prevention of AKI is therefore an important target in critical care medicine. Besides maintaining adequate hydration and hemodynamics and avoidance of nephrotoxic substances, no intervention has conclusively been demonstrated to protect the kidney of critically ill patients [129]. Recent clinical studies suggest that control of blood glucose levels by intensive insulin therapy (IIT) reduces the incidence of AKI in ICU patients. This chapter will summarize the available evidence on this subject and discuss possible underlying mechanisms.

4.7.2 Hyperglycemia and Insulin Resistance in the Critically Ill

Several types of critical illness are associated with important alterations in carbohydrate metabolism as part of the stress response. This "diabetes of stress" is characterized by hyperglycemia and insulin resistance. Hepatic gluconeogenesis, fueled by proteolytic, glycolytic, and lipolytic metabolites, is increased and not suppressed by insulin or exogenous glucose. Peripheral glucose utilization in insulin-dependent tissues (muscle, fat) is decreased. The increased whole body glucose uptake is accounted for by tissues that do not depend on insulin for their cellular glucose uptake [78, 81, 117]. Stress diabetes results from the integrated action of inflammatory cytokines and counter-regulatory hormones, including catecholamines, glucagon, growth hormone, and cortisol [74, 121, 123]. Since most patients with AKI also have an underlying critical illness, it is not surprising that the same picture is seen in AKI patients [11].

4.7.3 Carbohydrate Metabolism and Transport in the Kidney

The kidney assists in keeping blood glucose levels within normal levels by reabsorbing virtually all of the filtered glucose (± 180 g/day). Ninety percent of this

G. Van den Berghe (✉)
Department of Intensive Care Medicine, University Hospitals, University of Leuven, Herestraat 49, 30000 Leuven, Belgium
e-mail: greet.vandenberghe@med.kuleuven.be

A. Jörres et al. (eds.), *Management of Acute Kidney Problems*,
DOI: 10.1007/978-3-540-69441-0_4.7, © Springer-Verlag Berlin Heidelberg 2010

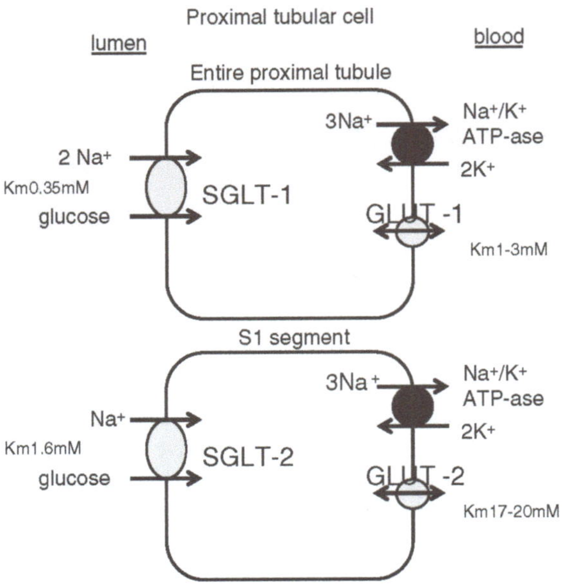

Fig. 4.7.1 Glucose transporters in proximal tubular cells. SGLT = sodium glucose cotransporter

reabsorption occurs in the S1 segment of the proximal tubule, whereas the remaining is completeley reabsorbed in the S3 segment or straight part of the proximal tubule. Two families of transporters are responsible for this reabsorption: the sodium-glucose cotransporters (SGLT or SLC5 gene family) in the apical membrane and the facilitative-diffusion glucose transporters (GLUT or SLC2 gene family) in the basolateral membrane (Fig. 4.7.1). The SGLT-mediated transport is a secondary active transport that uses the sodium gradient, generated by the Na^+,K^+-ATPase located in the basolateral membrane to move glucose into the tubular cell. The rate of apical glucose reabsorption depends on the magnitude of the generated sodium gradient. SGLT-2 is abundantly present in the proximal convoluted tubule, has a lower affinity for glucose (Km = 1.6 mM) and is responsible for the majority of glucose reabsorption in the S1 and S2 segment. SGLT-1 is found along the whole proximal tubule, has a higher affinity (Km = 0.35 mM) and reabsorbs the remaining glucose from the filtrate in the S3 segment. GLUTs speed up the equilibration (bidirectional passive transport) of glucose across the basolateral membrane. GLUT-2 has a low affinity (Km = 17–20 mM) and is the predominant glucose transporter in the basolateral membrane of the S1 segment. GLUT-1 has a higher affinity for glucose (Km = 1–3 mM). Its expression correlates with glycolytic activity which is higher in the S3 segment. GLUT-4 is an insulin-responsive high-affinity glucose transporter that is expressed in the thin ascending limb of the loop of Henle, reflecting the intense oxidative metabolism in this segment (high level of Na^+,K^+-ATPase activity and preferential use of glucose to fuel the activity) [68, 118, 132].

Little is known about factors that modulate the expression of glucose transporters in the kidney. Most experimental settings with high glucose concentrations or streptozotocin-induced diabetes show an increased expression of GLUT-2 [27, 38, 130], which even becomes detectable at the brush border [46, 76], a moderate increase of SGLT [130], and a decreased tubular expression of GLUT-1 [27, 130]. Also human exfoliated proximal tubular epithelial cells in the urine of diabetic patients express more SGLT-2 and GLUT-2 [98]. The effect of critical illness on the expression of glucose transporters in the kidney has not been investigated. Administration of endotoxin or cytokines in mice increases fractional glucose excretion, coinciding with a decreased espression of SGLT-2 and GLUT-2 and increased expression of SGLT-1 and GLUT-1 [105]. It should however be stressed that the animals in this experiment developed hypoglycemia and not hyperglycemia, raising questions regarding its relevance to the critically ill hyperglycemic patient.

Besides glucose reabsorption and using glucose as a metabolic fuel, the kidney also releases glucose via gluconeogenesis, with glutamine and lactate being the major precursors. Renal gluconeogenesis seems even more sensitive to epinephrine than hepatic gluconeogenesis. Defective gluconeogenesis may contribute to the increased risk of hypoglycemia in patients with renal failure [112]. Another factor explaining the susceptibility of renal failure patients to hypoglycemia is the reduced renal insulin clearance. Whereas endogenous insulin is largely metabolized by the liver in its first pass, the kidney is the main organ responsible for metabolizing exogenous insulin, which is metabolized in the proximal tubular cells [55].

4.7.4 Diabetic Nephropathy

Diabetic nephropathy is one of the most serious complications affecting patients with type 1 or type 2 diabetes. It is the most common cause of end-stage renal failure in the Western world. The precise mechanisms that lead to diabetic kidney disease still remain largely unknown. Although early research mainly focused on glomerular abnormalities, recent investigations point to an important or even primary role of tubular damage. Genetic as well as hemodynamic and metabolic factors are thought to be involved and result in trophic, inflammatory, and profibrogenic effects on renal cells. Most hypotheses include poor glycemic control as an important concomitant [106, 109, 133, 137].

Strict glucose control in both type 1 and 2 diabetes has a beneficial effect on the development and progression of diabetic nephropathy [1, 43, 89, 115, 116, 122, 140]. Also the outcome of renal transplants is adversely affected by poor glycemic control [107]. In diabetic animals, pretreatment with insulin, depending on the duration of the treatment, prevents or attenuates the degree of renal ischemia/reperfusion (I/R) injury [80].

4.7.5 Adverse Effects of Acute Hyperglycemia in the Critically Ill

An association between hyperglycemia and mortality has been established in several conditions of acute illness, including acute myocardial infarction (AMI) [19, 32], percutaneous coronary intervention [87], cardiac surgery [37, 44], heart failure [10], chronic obstructive pulmonary disease exacerbation [9], stroke [8, 20, 45, 111], major trauma [12, 66, 114, 144], traumatic head injury [57, 143], burns [49, 54], and critical illness in general [42, 63]. Hyperglycemia has shown deleterious effects on the myocardium [26] and on the brain in stroke patients [7, 8, 18, 111].

Several observational trials have shown an association between pre- or intraoperative hyperglycemia and postoperative AKI after cardiac surgery [44, 72], between hyperglycemia at cardiac catheterization and contrast nephropathy [120] and between hyperglycemia during total parenteral nutrition and the development of AKI [25, 70]. In animal experiments the induction of diabetes or acute hyperglycemia increases the susceptibility to renal I/R injury [53, 86, 94].

4.7.6 Tight Glycemic Control with Intensive Insulin Therapy in Acute Illness

Until recently the hyperglycemia of acute illness used to be considered as an adaptive stress response and as such important for survival by keeping glucose available for vital tissues with insulin-independent glucose uptake such as the brain and for provision of substrate to wounded tissues and reparative cells [81]. The goal of treatment was to prevent excessive hyperglycemia and to avoid ketoacidosis and hyperosmolality-induced fluid shifts, while minimizing the risk of hypoglycemia. Insulin was therefore only administered if the blood glucose level exceeded 200 mg/dl. The association with adverse outcome was interpreted as hyperglycemia being merely a marker of insulin resistance and illness severity. This dogma has recently been challenged by two large clinical trials (hereafter referred to as the Leuven studies) that randomly assigned ICU patients to either intensive or conventional insulin treatment [124, 126]. In the IIT group, the insulin infusion was titrated to achieve blood glucose levels between 80 and 110 mg/dl. In the conventional treatment group, the insulin infusion was only started if blood glucose exceeded 215 mg/dl and it was titrated to keep the level between 180 and 200 mg/dl. In this group, the insulin infusion was decreased and eventually stopped when blood glucose levels fell below 180 mg/dl. This approach resulted in blood glucose levels of approximately 150–160 mg/dl in the conventional and 100 mg/dl in the IIT group. The first study was performed in 1,548 mechanically ventilated surgical ICU patients and found a significant reduction in ICU mortality (from 8.0% to 4.6%) and hospital mortality (from 10.9% to 7.2%) with tight glycemic control (TGC). This benefit was even more pronounced in patients with prolonged ICU stay (>5 days) [126]. The second study was performed in 1,200 medical ICU patients. Although morbidity in these patients was significantly affected, mortality in the intention-to-treat analysis did not show a significant difference. However, the study was statistically powered for patients with prolonged ICU stay, who indeed showed a reduction in ICU (from 38.1 to 31.3%) and hospital (from 52.3 to 43%) mortality [124]. Pooled analysis of the two Leuven studies showed that hospital mortality was significantly reduced from 23.6% to 20.4% in all patients and from 37.9% to 30.1% in the patients with at least 3 days of ICU treatment [125]. This result was not confirmed by a recent, much smaller, multicenter trial in patients with severe sepsis, that was prematurely stopped because of a high incidence of hypoglycemia and was therefore substantially (> sixfold) underpowered [17]. On the other hand, the survival benefit of TGC in critical illness has been confirmed by several observational studies showing a reduced mortality after implementation of a protocol aiming at stricter blood glucose control in ICU or trauma patients [64, 99, 102].

4.7.7 Tight Glycemic Control with Intensive Insulin Therapy and Acute Kidney Injury

4.7.7.1 Clinical Data

The two Leuven studies also found a beneficial effect of TGC with IIT on kidney function [104, 124, 126]. In the pooled data set, the incidence of newly acquired AKI, defined as a least a doubling of admission serum creatinine (corresponding with RIFLE class Injury/Failure or AKIN stage II/III), was reduced from 7.6% to 4.5% (Fig. 4.7.2). In the surgical study the need for renal replacement therapy (RRT) was also reduced from 7.4% to 4.0%. The latter effect was not present in the medical patients nor in the pooled data set, which was at least partially explained a higher initial illness severity of the medical patients, many of whom presented with increased serum creatinine on admission. Since IIT is a protective strategy, which cannot prevent damage that is already present at the start of the treatment, the need for RRT could not be prevented in many of these medical patients. However, when those patients requiring RRT within the first 2 days of their ICU stay were excluded from the pooled analysis, the protective effect of IIT on the need for RRT became significant (decrease from 8.8% to 6.7%) [104]. The renoprotective effect was most pronounced in those patients achieving normoglycemia [104, 125]. The small VISEP study, that did not establish an effect of TGC on mortality, also could not find an effect on AKI or need for RRT [17]. A larger implementation study in 1,600 ICU patients showed a 75% relative reduction in the development of new AKI after implementation of TGC in a mixed medical/surgical ICU [64].

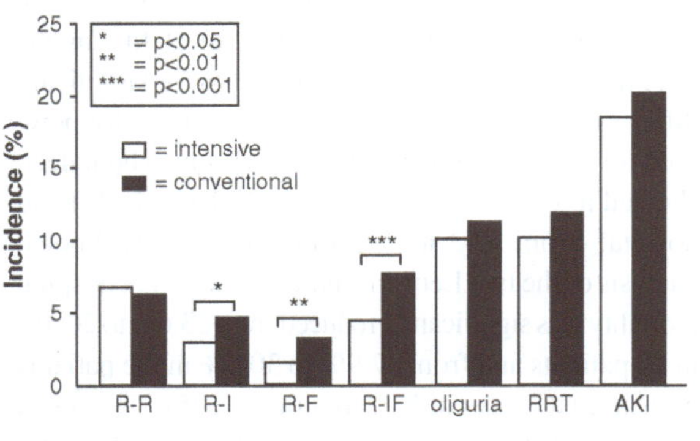

Fig. 4.7.2 Impact of intensive insulin therapy (light bars) versus conventional treatment (dark bars) on the incidence of different renal outcome categories: R-R = RIFLE class Risk, R-I = RIFLE class Injury, R-F = RIFLE class Failure, R-IF = RIFLE class Injury or Failure, RRT = need for renal replacement therapy, AKI = acute kidney injury = any of the adverse renal outcomes *= $p < 0.05$; ** = $p < 0.01$; *** = $p < 0.001$

In an attempt to dissociate the relative impact of maintaining normoglycemia versus glycemia-independent actions of insulin, a multivariate logistic regression analysis of the results of the surgical study was performed. Although the lowered blood glucose level was related to the reduced mortality and most of the morbidity effects, this was not the case for AKI, for which the insulin dose was an independent determinant [127]. This would suggest that the renoprotection is a direct effect of insulin and not related to blood glucose control. Analysis of the pooled data set of the surgical and medical study however could not confirm this finding, since both the insulin dose and the blood glucose level were significantly higher in patients developing AKI [104, 125]. This probably reflects a more severe insulin resistance in the sicker patients and does not allow us to draw conclusions about a direct effect of insulin on the kidney.

4.7.7.2 Experimental Data

Because of the difficulty of dissociating the effect of insulin from that of glucose control in the clinical setting (administering insulin and lowering of blood glucose occur simultaneously with IIT), blood glucose and insulin levels were manipulated independently in a burn-injured parenterally fed rabbit model of critical illness. After suppression of endogenous insulin production, rabbits were randomly allocated to four study groups: normal insulin, normoglycemia (NI/NG); high insulin, normoglycemia (HI/NG); normal insulin, hyperglycemia (NI/HG); or high insulin, hyperglycemia (HI/HG). This model confirmed the survival benefit and the renoprotective effect of TGC and demonstrated the deleterious effect of high blood glucose levels on the kidney, irrespective of the insulin level [41].

4.7.8 Possible Mechanisms of Renoprotection by TGC

Hypoperfusion and sepsis are the most important pathogenic triggers underlying AKI in critically ill patients. Prevention of sepsis might have contributed to the renoprotective effect of TGC. Indeed in the surgical Leuven study, the incidence of bacteremia decreased significantly in the patients treated with TGC [126]. This effect could, however, not be confirmed in the medical study, many of whom were already septic on admission [124].

A direct effect of the prevention of hyperglycemia on the kidney is a more plausible explanation. The cellular mechanisms involved in the development of AKI are complex and not yet fully understood. Experimental data point to an important role of inflammation and oxidative and nitrosative stress that result in mitochondrial damage and necrosis/apoptosis that may affect both endothelial and epithelial renal cells, leading to vascular and tubular dysfunction [13, 14, 23, 82]. Most of these pathways are also affected by hyperglycemia as will be discussed hereafter.

4.7.8.1 Oxidative Stress

Oxidative stress occurs when production of oxidants or reactive oxygen species (ROS) exceeds local antioxidant capacity and results in tissue damage. Oxidative stress has been shown to be involved in the pathophysiology of both AKI [23, 52, 88] and diabetic complications [21, 28]. Prevention of hyperglycemia-induced oxidative stress might therefore be a possible explanation for the observed renoprotective effect of TGC.

Hyperglycemia and, even more so, acute fluctuations of blood glucose levels induce the formation of ROS, such as superoxide and H_2O_2 [28, 83]. The major sources of hyperglycemia-induced ROS are the mitochondrial electron transport chain and activation of nicotinamide adenine dinucleotide phosphate (NADPH) oxidase [69, 138]. According to the "Brownlee hypothesis," these ROS inhibit glycolysis by interference with the activity of the enzyme glyceraldehyde-3-phosphate dehydrogenase (GADPH) through posttranslational modification driving glucose into other pathways responsible for the hyperglycemic damage: increased polyol pathway flux, increased formation of advanced glycation end products (AGE), activation of protein kinase C, and increased hexosamine pathway flux [16, 100] (Fig. 4.7.3). The posttranslational modification of GADPH involves poly (ADP)ribose polymerase (PARP) activation, which has been shown to play an important role in both renal I/R and diabetic complications [34, 92].

In critically ill patients, I/R is the main cause of ROS overproduction, which, together with a compromised antioxidant system, contributes to tissue damage [29, 40]. Whether the combination of hyperglycemia with I/R is additive or even synergistic in this regard remains to be proven. A recent animal study showed more severe kidney damage and more evidence of oxidative stress if renal I/R was preceded by the induction of acute hyperglycemia [53].

4.7.8.2 Nitric Oxide and Nitrosative Stress

Nitric oxide (NO), produced by NO synthase (NOS), plays an important role in both normal and abnormal renal function. The effect of NO on kidney function is complex [23, 62]. Endothelial NO synthase (eNOS)-mediated NO production has a protective effect by preventing vasoconstriction and microvascular thrombosis [50, 134, 142]. Inducible NOS (iNOS) is expressed in proximal tubular cells after exposure to I/R, hypoxia, and inflammatory cytokines [23]. Excessive NO generation by iNOS not only inhibits NO production by eNOS [48, 50], but also contributes to activation of caspases [119] and is a key mediator of I/R-induced damage to the kidney [47, 48, 136]. The concomitant increased ROS production results in the formation of reactive nitrogen species such as peroxynitrite, resulting in further inflammation and damage (nitrosative stress) [23, 48, 131, 141]. Selective iNOS inhibition significantly improves renal function in animal models of I/R [24, 75].

In vitro experiments have shown that high glucose levels decrease eNOS expression [36, 110] or inhibit its activity [39] in endothelial cells and increase cytokine-induced iNOS expression on vascular smooth muscle cells [65]. Insulin on the other hand, induces eNOS upregulation [3, 36, 84]. In a rabbit model of chronic critical illness, endothelial function, as measured by endothelium-dependent vasodilation in isolated perfused aortic

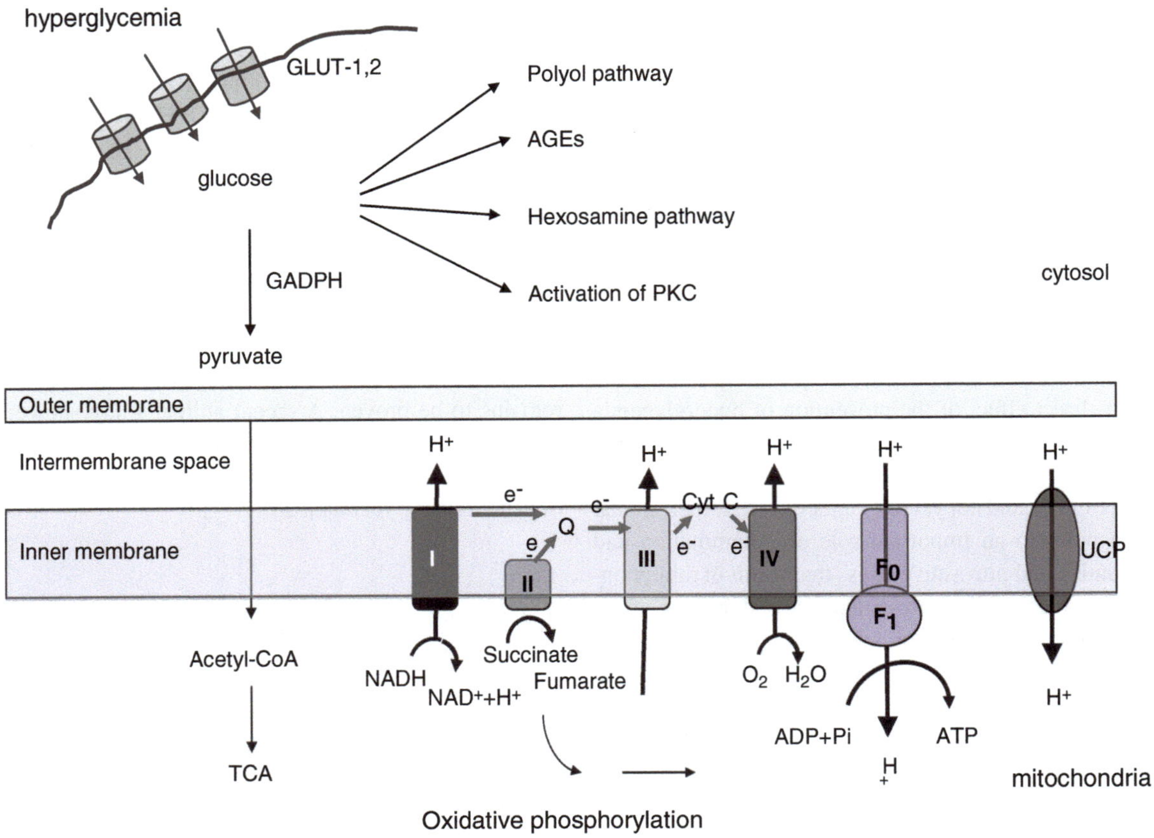

Fig. 4.7.3 Pathways of intracellular glucose metabolism and possible pathways of hyperglycemia-induced damage. AGE = advanced glycation end product, GADPH = glyceraldehyde-3-phosphate dehydrogenase, PKC = protein kinase C, TCA = tricarboxylic acid cycle, UCP = uncoupling proteins, Q = coenzyme Q, Cyt C = cytochrome C, NADH = nicotinamide adenine dinucleotide, ATP = adenosine triphosphate, ADP = adenosine diphosphate, Pi = inorganic phosphate, Acetyl-CoA = acetyl-Coenzyme A, $O^{2}.-$ = superoxide anion

rings, was better maintained in the presence of normoglycemia versus hyperglycemia, irrespective of insulin levels [41].

A subgroup analysis from the surgical Leuven study including patients with prolonged ICU stay showed that TGC with IIT reduced iNOS expression in liver and muscle biopsies from nonsurvivors and attenuated the rise in NO levels [67]. In addition, elevated NO levels appeared to be an independent predictor of AKI [104], suggesting that the effect of TGC on NO may have contributed to its renoprotective effect.

4.7.8.3 Adhesion Molecules

The role of the endothelium in the pathogenesis of I/R-induced AKI is increasingly recognized [82]. Endothelial dysfunction is also the central pathophysiologic denominator for all cardiovascular complications of diabetes [92, 103]. Extensive literature is available on the vascular effects of hyperglycemia and insulin. In general, hyperglycemia causes a provasoconstrictive, prothrombotic, and proinflammatory phenotype, whereas insulin has vasodilatory, antiinflammatory, antioxidant, antithrombotic, and profibrinolytic effects (reviewed by [31, 77]).

Besides the previously mentioned effect on eNOS and endothelium-dependent vasodilation, hyperglycemia also induces endothelin-1 expression and associated vasoconstriction [93]. Another aspect of endothelial dysfunction is the expression of adhesion molecules leading to leukocyte adhesion, activation, and migration. In vitro exposure of endothelial cells to high glucose concentration leads to their activation with increased expression of adhesion molecules [59, 85, 95, 96].

In humans, acute hyperglycemia results in increased Soluble intercellular adhesion molecule (sICAM) levels [4, 22, 73]. Analysis of a subgroup of patients from the surgical Leuven study with prolonged ICU stay showed that TGC with IIT lowered circulating levels of ICAM-1 and tended to reduce E-selectin levels, reflecting reduced endothelial activation [67].

Animal experiments have found a renoprotective effect of antibodies to ICAM-1 and antisense oligonucleotides for ICAM-1 in ischemic injury [51, 61, 97]. A similar effect has been shown for E-selectin inhibition [108, 113]. The reported protective effect of IIT on the endothelium, [67] might therefore be an important pathway of renoprotection, which is suggested by the higher levels of ICAM-1 and E-selectin in patients developing AKI, although the latter might also have resulted from a reduced renal clearance.

4.7.8.4 Inflammation

Renal inflammation is an important contributor to the development of AKI (reviewed in [13, 14, 23]). In diabetes patients, hyperglycemia has been shown to promote inflammation, which is mainly related to oxidative stress and the previously mentioned subsequent damaging pathways [16, 100]. This results in the activation of three key proinflammatory transcription factors: nuclear factor-kappa B (NF-kB), activator protein-1 (AP-1), and early growth response-1 (EGR-1), which, on the other hand, are suppressed by insulin [2, 3, 30]. The stimulatory effect of hyperglycemia and inflammatory cytokines on NF-kB-mediated transcription of inflammatory mediators seems to be additive [56, 65], which could explain the pronounced inflammatory effect of hyperglycemia in critically ill patients. In the experimental setting, hyperglycemia has been shown to counteract the antiinflammatory effect of insulin in a porcine endotoxemic model [15], whereas insulin attenuated the inflammatory response in endotoxemic rats [58].

The surgical Leuven study showed a significant effect of TGC with IIT on markers of inflammation such as C-reactive proteins (CRP) [126]. This finding was confirmed in an animal model of chronic critical illness [135] and in patients with AMI [139]. In the medical Leuven study, the CRP effect was only present in the long-stay patients. Whether the antiinflammatory effect of preventing hyperglycemia contributed to the observed renoprotective effect remains to be investigated. Key players in the inflammatory response, besides oxidative stress, NO, and adhesion molecules, are cytokines. However, in the surgical Leuven study, cytokine levels were only marginally affected [67].

4.7.8.5 Mitochondrial Damage

Analysis of biopsies obtained immediately after death from nonsurvivors in a surgical ICU showed that TGC with IIT protected mitochondria in hepatocytes. Hepatocytic mitochondria in the conventionally treated patients showed severe ultrastructural abnormalities and decreased activities of respiratory chain complexes I and IV [128]. Whether similar protection occurs in the kidney remains to be investigated. Also the pathways underlying mitochondrial damage in hyperglycemic, hyperinsulinemic critically ill patients remain to be explored.

4.7.8.6 Apoptosis

Apoptosis is an active mode of cell death under molecular control. Apoptosis regulation is mediated by death ligands and receptors (e.g., TNF, Fas), by mitochondrial injury and endoplasmatic reticulum stress, and involves proapoptotic and antiapoptotic Bcl-2 family members, caspases, and mitochondrial membrane permeabilization [71]. Evidence suggests that apoptosis is the major mechanism of cell death in AKI (reviewed in [35, 60, 90]) and shows an important relationship to diabetic complications (reviewed in [6]).

In vitro experiments with human proximal tubular epithelial cells have shown that their exposure to high glucose concentrations induces oxidative and nitrosative stress resulting in apoptosis mediated by Bcl-2 family proteins and multiple caspases [5, 91, 101]. High glucose-induced oxidative stress also favors mitochondrial permeability transition pore (PTP) opening and subsequent cell death in several endothelial cell types [33].

On the other hand, insulin inhibits caspase-3 activity in human renal tubular epithelial cells via the phosphatidylinositol 3-kinase/Akt pathway [79].

Depending on the timing of its administration, pretreatment with insulin (resulting in a lowering of blood glucose levels) prevents or attenuates the degree of renal I/R injury and the induction of apoptosis in diabetic animals [80].

4.7.9 Conclusion (Take Home Message)

Hyperglycemia in critically ill patients is associated with adverse outcomes, including AKI. Tight glycemic control with insulin reduces the incidence of AKI. Possible mechanisms include reduced oxidative and nitrosative stress, attenuated inflammation, and endothelial dysfunction, and decreased mitochondrial dysfunction and apoptosis. These mechanisms, however, need to be further explored. New adequately powered randomized trials in heterogeneous ICU populations are necessary to confirm the effect of the Leuven studies and eventually identify subgroups with the greatest benefit.

Acknowledgement Supported by the Fund for Scientific Research (FWO), Flanders, Belgium (G.0533.06 and G.085.09), the Research Council of the Katholieke Universiteit Leuven (GOA2007/14), FWO and KULeuven Research Council Postdoctoral Fellowships to I.V., and FWO Research Assistant Fellowship to J.G. GVdB by the University of Leuven receives structural research financing via the Methusalem program, funded by the Flemish Government.

References

1. ADVANCE Collaborative Group, Patel A, MacMahon S, et al. (2008) Intensive blood glucose control and vascular outcomes in patients with type 2 diabetes. N Engl L Med 358:2560–2572
2. Aljada A, Friedman J, Ghanim H, et al. (2006) Glucose ingestion induces an increase in intranuclear nuclear factor kappaB, a fall in cellular inhibitor kappaB, and an increase in tumor necrosis factor alpha messenger RNA by mononuclear cells in healthy human subjects. Metabolism 55: 1177–1185
3. Aljada A, Ghanim H, Mohanty P, et al. (2002) Insulin inhibits the pro-inflammatory transcription factor early growth response gene-1 (Egr)-1 expression in mononuclear cells (MNC) and reduces plasma tissue factor (TF) and plasminogen activator inhibitor-1 (PAI-1) concentrations. J Clin Endocrinol Metab 87:1419–1422
4. Aljada A, Saadeh R, Assian E, et al. (2000) Insulin inhibits the expression of intercellular adhesion molecule-1 by human aortic endothelial cells through stimulation of nitric oxide. J Clin Endocrinol Metab 85:2572–2575.
5. Allen DA, Harwood S, Varagunam M, et al. (2003) High glucose-induced oxidative stress causes apoptosis in proximal tubular epithelial cells and is mediated by multiple caspases. FASEB J 17:908–910
6. Allen DA, Yaqoob MM, Harwood SM (2005) Mechanisms of high glucose-induced apoptosis and its relationship to diabetic complications. J Nutr Biochem 16:705–713
7. Alvarez-Sabin J, Molina CA, Ribo M, et al. (2004) Impact of admission hyperglycemia on stroke outcome after thrombolysis: risk stratification in relation to time to reperfusion. Stroke 35:2493–2498
8. Baird TA, Parsons MW, Phanh T, et al. (2003) Persistent poststroke hyperglycemia is independently associated with infarct expansion and worse clinical outcome. Stroke 34:2208–2214
9. Baker EH, Janaway CH, Philips BJ, et al. (2006) Hyperglycaemia is associated with poor outcomes in patients admitted to hospital with acute exacerbations of chronic obstructive pulmonary disease. Thorax 61:284–289
10. Barsheshet A, Garty M, Grossman E, et al. Admission blood glucose level and mortality among hospitalized nondiabetic patients with heart failure. Arch Intern Med 166: 1613–1619
11. Basi S, Pupim LB, Simmons EM et al. (2005) Insulin resistance in critically ill patients with acute renal failure. Am J Physiol Renal Physiol 289:F259–264
12. Bochicchio GV, Joshi M, Bochicchio KM, et al. (2007) Early hyperglycemic control is important in critically injured trauma patients. J Trauma 63:1353–1359
13. Bonventre J (2004) Ischemic acute renal failure: an inflammatory disease? Kidney Int 66: 480–485
14. Bonventre JV (2007) Pathophysiology of acute kidney injury: roles of potential inhibitors of inflammation. Contrib Nephrol 156: 39–46
15. Brix-Christensen V, Gjedsted J, Andersen SK, et al. (2005) Inflammatory response during hyperglycemia and hyperinsulinemia in a porcine endotoxemic model: the contribution of essential organs. Acta Anaesthesiol Scand 49: 991–998
16. Brownlee M (2001) Biochemistry and molecular cell biology of diabetic complications. Nature 414:813–820
17. Brunkhorst FM, Engel C, Bloos F, et al. German Competence Network Sepsis (SepNet) (2008) Intensive insulin therapy and pentastarch resuscitation in severe sepsis. N Engl J Med 358:125–139
18. Bruno A, Williams LS, Kent TA (2004) How important is hyperglycemia during acute brain infaction? Neurologist 10:195–200
19. Capes SE, Hunt D, Malmberg K, et al. (2000) Stress hyperglycaemia and increased risk of death after myocardial infarction in patients with and without diabetes: a systematic overview. Lancet 355:773–778
20. Capes SE, Hunt D, Malmberg K, et al. (2001) Stress hyperglycemia and prognosis of stroke in nondiabetic and diabetic patients: a systematic overview. Stroke 32:2426–2432
21. Ceriello A (2006) Oxidative stress and diabetes-associated complications. Endocrine Pract 12(Suppl 1):60–62
22. Ceriello A, Falleti E, Motz E, et al. (1998) Hyperglycemia-induced circulating ICAM-1 increase in diabetes mellitus: the possible role of oxidative stress. Horm Metab Res 30:146–149

23. Chatterjee PK (2007) Novel pharmacological approaches to the treatment of renal ischemia-reperfusion injury: a comprehensive review. Naunyn Schmiedebergs Arch Pharmacol 376: 1–43
24. Chatterjee PK, Patel NSA, Kvale EO, et al. (2002) Inhibition of inducible nitric oxide synthase reduces renal ischemia/reperfusion injury. Kidney Int. 61: 862–871
25. Cheung NW, Napier B, Zaccaria C, et al. (2005) Hyperglycemia is associated with adverse outcomes in patients receiving total parenteral nutrition. Diabetes Care 28: 2367–2371
26. Cheung NW, Wong VW, McLean M (2006) The Hyperglycemia: Intensive Insulin Infusion in Infarction (HI-5) study: a randomized controlled trial of insulin infusion therapy for myocardial infarction. Diabetes Care 29:765–770
27. Chin E, Zamah AM, Landau D, et al. (1997) Changes in facilitative glucose transporter messenger ribonucleic acid levels in the diabetic rat kidney. Endocrinology 138: 1267–1275
28. Choi SW, Benzie IFF, Ma SW, et al. (2008) Acute hyperglycemia and oxidative stress: direct cause and effect? Free Rad Biol Med 44:1217–1231
29. Crimi R, Ignarro J, Napoli C (2007) Microcirculation and oxidative stress. Free Rad Res 41:1364–1375
30. Dandona P, Aljada A, Mohanty P, et al. (2001) Insulin inhibits intranuclear nuclear factor Kappa B and stimulates Ikappa B in mononuclear cells in obses subjects: evidence for an anti-inflammatory effect. J Clin Endocrinol Metab 86: 3257–3265
31. Dandona P, Chaudhuri A, Mohanty P, et al. (2007) Anti-inflammatory effects of insulin. Curr Opin Clin Nutr Metab Care 10:511–517
32. Deedwania P, Kosiborod M, Barrett E, et al. (2008) Hyperglycemia and acute coronary syndrome: A scientific statement from the American heart association diabetes committee of the council on nutrition, physical activity, and metabolism. Circulation 117:1610–1619
33. Detaille D, Guigas B, Chauvin C, et al. (2005) Metformin prevents high-glucose-induced endothelial cell death through a mitochondrial permeability transition-dependent process. Diabetes 54:2179–2187
34. Devalaraja-Narashimha K, Singaravelu K, Padanilam BJ (2005) Poly(ADP-ribose) polymerase-mediated cell injury in acute renal failure. Pharmacol Res 52:44–59
35. Devarajan P (2005) Cellular and molecular derangements in acute tubular necrosis. Curr Opin Pediatr 17:193–199
36. Ding Y, Vaziri ND, Coulson R, et al. (2000) Effects of simulated hyperglycemia, insulin, and glucagon on endothelial nitric oxide synthase expression. Am J Physiol Endocrinol Metab 279:E11–17
37. Doenst T, Wijeysundera D, Karkouti K, et al. (2005) Hyperglycemia during cardiopulmonary bypass is an independent risk factor for mortality in patients undergoing cardiac surgery. J Thorac Cardiovasc Surg 13:1144e1–e7
38. Dominguez JH, Song B, Maianu L, Garvey WT, et al. (1994) Gene expression of epithelial glucose transporters: the role of diabetes mellitus. J Am Soc Nephrol 5 (Suppl 1):S29–36
39. Du XL, Edelstein D, Dimmeler S, et al. (2001) Hyperglycemia inhibits endothelial nitric oxide synthase activity by post-translational modification at the Akt site. J Clin Invest 108: 1341–1348
40. Eaton S (2006) The biochemical basis of antioxidant therapy in critical illness. Proc Nutr Soc 65:242–249
41. Ellger B, Debaveye Y, Vanhorebeek I, et al. (2006) Survival benefits of intensive insulin therapy in critical illness: impact of maintaining normoglycemia versus glycemia-independent actions of insulin. Diabetes 55:1096–1105
42. Finney SJ, Zekveld C, Elia A, et al. (2003) Glucose control and mortality in critically ill patients. JAMA 290:2041–2047
43. Fioretto P, Bruseghin M, Berto I, et al. (2006) Renal protection in diabetes: role of glycemic control. J Am Soc Nephrol 17(Suppl 2):S86–S89
44. Gandhi GY, Nuttall GA, Abel MD, et al. (2005) Intraoperative hyperglycemia and perioperative outcomes in cardiac surgery patients. Mayo Clin Proc 80:862–866
45. Gentile NT, Seftchick MW, Huynh T, et al. (2006) Decreased mortality by normalizing blood glucose after acute ischemic stroke. Acad Emerg Med 13:174–180
46. Goestemeyer AK, Marks J, Srai SK, et al. (2007) GLUT2 protein at the rat proximal tubule brush border membrane correlates with protein kinase C (PKC)-betal and plasma glucose concentration. Diabetologia 50:2209–2217
47. Goligorsky MS, Brodsky SV, Noiri E (2002) Nitric oxide in acute renal failure: NOS versus NOS. Kidney Int 61:855–861
48. Goligorsky MS, Brodsky SV, Noiri E (2004) NO bioavailability, endothelial dysfunction, and acute renal failure: new insights into pathophysiology. Semin Nephrol 24:316–323
49. Gore DC, Chinkes D, Heggers J, et al. (2001) Association of hyperglycemia with increased mortality after severe burn injury. J Trauma 51:540–544
50. Guan Z, Gobe G, Willgoss D, et al. (2006) Renal endothelial dysfunction and impaired autoregulation after ischemia-reperfusion injury result from excess nitric oxide. Am J Physiol Renal Physiol 91:F619–628
51. Haller H, Dragun D, Miethke A, et al. (1996) Antisense oligonucleotides for ICAM-1 attenuate reperfusion injury and renal failure in the rat. Kidney Int 50:473–480
52. Himmelfarb J, McMonagle E, Freedman S et al. (2004) Oxidative stress is increased in critically ill patients with acute renal failure. J Am Soc Nephrol 15:2449–2456
53. Hirose R, Xu F, Dang K, Liu T, Behrends M, et al. (2008) Transient hyperglycemia affects the extent of ischemia-reperfusion-induced renal injury in rats. Anesthesiology 108:402–414
54. Holm C, Horbrand F, Mayr M, et al. (2004) Acute hyperglycaemia following thermal injury: friend or foe? Resuscitation 60:71–77
55. Iglesias P, Diez JJ (2008) Insulin therapy in renal disease. Diabetes, Obesity and Metabolism PMID: 18248491
56. Iwasaki Y, Kambayashi M, Asai M, et al. (2007). High glucose alone, as well as in combination with proinflammatory cytokines, stimulates nuclear factor kappa-B-mediated transcription in hepatocytes in vitro. J Diabetes Complications 21:56–62
57. Jeremitsky E, Omert LA, Dunham CM et al. (2005) The impact of hyperglycemia on patients with severe brain injury. J Trauma 58:47–50
58. Jeschke MG, Klein D, Bolder U, et al. (2004) Insulin attenuates the systemic inflammatory response in endotoxemic rats. Endocrinology 145:4089–4093
59. Kado S, Wakatsuki T, Yamamoto M, et al. (2001) Expression of intercellular adhesion molecule-1 induced by high glu-

cose concentrations in human aortic endothelial cells. Life Sci 68:727–737
60. Kaushal GP, Basnakian AG, Shah SV (2004) Apoptotic pathways in ischemic acute renal failure. Kidney Int 66: 500–506
61. Kelly KJ, Williams WW Jr, Colvin RB, et al. (1994) Antibody to intercellular adhesion molecule 1 protects the kidney against ischemic injury. Proc Natl Acad Sci USA 91:812–816
62. Kone BC (2004) Nitric oxide synthesis in the kidney: isoforms, biosynthesis, and functions in health. Semin Nephrol 24:299–315
63. Krinsley JS (2003) Association between hyperglycemia and increased hospital mortality in a heterogeneous population of critically ill patients. Mayo Clin Proc 78:1471–1478
64. Krinsley JS (2004) Effect of an intensive glucose management protocol on the mortality of critically ill adult patients. Mayo Clin Proc 79:992–1000
65. Lafuente N, Matesanz N, Azcutia V, et al. (2008). The deleterious effect of high concentrations of D-glucose requires pro-inflammatory preconditioning. J Hypertens 26:478–485
66. Laird AM, Miller PR, Kilgo PD, et al. (2004) Relationship of early hyperglycemia to mortality in trauma patients. J Trauma 56:1058–1062
67. Langouche L, Vanhorebeek I, Vlasselaers D, et al. (2005) Intensive insulin therapy protects the endothelium of critically ill patients. J Clin Invest 115:2277–2286
68. Lee YJ, Lee YJ, Han HJ (2007) Regulatory mechanisms of Na(+)/glucose cotransporters in renal proximal tubule cells. Kidney Int Suppl 106:S27–35
69. Leverve X (2003) Hyperglycemia and oxidative stress: complex relationships with attractive prospects. Intensive Care Med 29: 511–514
70. Lin LY, Lin HC, Lee PC, et al. (2007) Hyperglycemia correlates with outcomes in patients receiving total parenteral nutrition. Am J Med 333:261–265
71. Lorz C, Benito-Martin A, Justo P, et al. (2006) Modulation of renal tubular cell survival: where is the evidence? Curr Med Chem 13: 449–454
72. Mangano CM, Diamondstone LS, Ramsay JG, et al. (1998) Renal dysfunction after myocardial revascularization: risk factors, adverse outcomes, and hospital resource utilization. The Multicenter Study of Perioperative Ischemia Research Group. Ann Intern Med 128:194–203
73. Marfella R, Esposito K, Giunta R, et al. (2000) Circulating adhesion molecules in humans: role of hyperglycemia and hyperinsulinemia. Circulation 101:2247–2251
74. Marik PE, Raghaven M (2004) Stress-hyperglycemia, insulin and immunomodulation in sepsis. Intensive Care Med 30:748–756
75. Mark LA, Robinson AV, Schulak JA (2005) Inhibition of nitric oxide synthase reduces renal ischemia/reperfusion injury. J Surg Res 129: 236–241
76. Marks J, Carvou NJ, Debnam ES, et al. (2003) Diabetes increases facilitative glucose uptake and GLUT2 expression at the rat proximal tubule brush border membrane. J Physiol 553:137–145
77. Martini SR, Kent TA (2007) Hyperglycemia in acute ischemic stroke: a vascular perspective. J Cerebr Blood Flow Metab 27:435–451
78. McCowen KC, Malhotra A, Bistrian BR (2001) Stress-induced hyperglycaemia. Crit Care Clin 17:107–124
79. Meier M, Nitschke M, Hocke C, et al. (2008) Insulin Inhibits Caspase-3 Activity in Human Renal Tubular Epithelial Cells via the PI3-Kinase/Akt Pathway. Cell Physiol Biochem.21: 279–286
80. Melin J, Hellberg O, Larsson E, et al. (2002) Protective effect of insulin on ischemic renal injury in diabetes mellitus. Kidney Int 61: 383–392
81. Mizock BA (2001) Alterations in fuel metabolism in critical illness: hyperglycaemia. Best Pract Res Clin Endocrinol Metab 15:533–551
82. Molitoris BA, Sutton TA (2004) Endothelial injury and dysfunction: role in the extension phase of acute renal failure. Kidney Int 66: 496–499
83. Monnier L, Mas E, Ginet C, et al. (2006) Activation of oxidative stress by acute glucose fluctuations compared with sustained chronic hyperglycemia in patients with type 2 diabetes. JAMA 295: 1681–1687
84. Montagnani M, Chen H, Barr VA, et al. (2001) Insulin-stimulated activation of eNOS is independent of Ca^{2+} but requires phosphorylation by Akt at Ser(1179). J Biol Chem 276:30392–30398
85. Morigi M, Angioletti S, Imberti B, et al. (1998) Leukocyte-endothelial interaction is augmented by high glucose concentrations and hyperglycemia in a NF-kB-dependent fashion. J Clin Invest 101:1905–1915
86. Moursi M, Rising CL, Zelenock GB, et al. (1987) Dextrose administration exacerbates acute renal ischemic damage in anesthetized dogs. Arch Surg 122:790–704
87. Muhlestein JB, Anderson JL, Horne BD, et al. Intermountain Heart Collaborative Study Group (2003) Effect of fasting glucose levels on mortality rate in patients with and without diabetes mellitus and coronary artery disease undergoing percutaneous coronary intervention. Am Heart J 146:351–358
88. Nath KA, Norby SM (2000) Reactive Oxygen species and acute renal failure. Am J Med 109: 655–678
89. Ohkubo Y, Kishikawa H, Araki E, et al. (1995) Intensive insulin therapy prevents the progression of diabetic microvascular complications in Japanese patients with non-insulin-dependent diabetes mellitus: a randomized prospective 6-year study. Diabetes Res Clin Pract 28:103–117
90. Ortiz A, Justo P, Catalan MP, et al. (2002) Apoptotic cell death in renal injury: the rationale for intervention. Curr Drug Targets Immune Endocr Metabol Disord 2:181–192
91. Ortiz A, Ziyadeh-FN, Neilson EG (1997) Expression of apoptosis-regulatory genes in renal proximal tubular epithelial cells exposed to high ambient glucose and in diabetic kidneys. J Investig Med 45:50–56
92. Pacher P, Obrosova IG, Mabley JG, et al. (2005). Role of nitrosative stress and peroxynitrite in the pathogenesis of diabetic complications. Emerging new therapeutical strategies. Curr Med Chem 12: 267–275
93. Park JY, Takahara N, Gabriele A, et al. (2000) Induction of endothelin-1 expression by glucose. An effect of protein kinase C activation. Diabetes 49:1239–1248
94. Podrazik RM, Natale JE, Zelenock GB, et al. (1989) Hyperglycemia exacerbates and insulin fails to protect in acute renal ischemia in the rat. J Surg Res 46:572–578
95. Punete Nayazo MD, Chettab K, Duhault J, et al. (2001) Glucose and insulin modulate the capacity of endothelial cells (HUVEC) to express P-selectin and bind a monocytic cell line (U937). Thromb Haemost 86:680–685

96. Quagliaro L, Piconi L, Assaloni R, et al. (2005) Intermittent high glucose enhances ICAM-1, VCAM-1 and E-selectin expression in human umbilical vein endothelial cells in culture: the distinct role of protein kinase C and mitochondrial superoxide production. Atherosclerosis 183:259–267
97. Rabb H, Mendiola CC, Saba SR, et al. (1995) Antibodies to ICAM-1 protect kidneys in severe ischemic reperfusion injury. Biochem Biophys Res Commun 211:67–73
98. Rahmoune H, Thompson PW, Ward JM, et al. (2005) Glucose transporters in human renal proximal tubular cells isolated from the urine of patients with non-insulin-dependent diabetes. Diabetes 54:3427–3434
99. Reed CC, Stewart RM, Sherman M, et al. (2007) Intensive insulin protocol improves glucose control and is associated with a reduction in intensive care unit mortality. J Am Coll Surg 204:1048–1055
100. Rolo AP, Palmeira CM (2006) Diabetes and mitochondrial function: role of hyperglycemia and oxidative stress. Toxicol Appl Pharmacol 212:167–178
101. Samikkannu T, Thomas JJ, Bhat J, et al. (2006) Acute effect of high glucose on long term cell growth: a role for transient glucose increase in proximal tubule cell injury. Am J Physiol Renal Physiol 291:F162–175
102. Scalea TM, Bochicchio GV, Bochicchio KM, et al. (2007) Tight glycemic control in critically injured trauma patients. Ann Surg 246:605–612
103. Schalkwijk CG, Stehouwer CD (2005) Vascular complications in diabetes mellitus: the role of endothelial dysfunction. Clin Sci (Lond) 109:143–159
104. Schetz M, Vanhorebeek I, Wouters P, et al. (2008) Tight glycemic control protects the kidney of critically ill patients. J Am Soc Nephrol 19:571–578
105. Schmidt C, Höcherl K, Bucher M (2007) Regulation of renal glucose transporters during severe inflammation. Am J Physiol Renal Physiol 292:F804–811
106. Schrijvers BF, De Vriese AS, Flyvbjerg A (2004) From hyperglycemia to diabetic kidney disease: the role of metabolic, hemodynamic, intracellular factors and growth factors/cytokines. Endocr Rev 25:971–1010
107. Sezer S, Akgul A, Altinoglu A, et al. (2006) Posttransplant diabetes mellitus: impact of good blood glucose regulation on renal transplant recipient outcome. Translant Proc 38:529–532
108. Singbartl K, Ley K (2000) Protection from ischemia-reperfusion induced severe acute renal failure by blocking E-selectin. Crit Care Med 28:2507–2514
109. Singh DK, Winocour P, Farrington K (2008) Mechanisms of disease: the hypoxic tubular hypothesis of diabetic nephropathy. Nat Clin Pract Nephrol 4:216–226
110. Sorrenti V, Mazza F, Campisi A, et al. (2006) High glucose-mediated imbalance of nitric oxide synthase and dimethylarginine dimethylaminohydrolase expression in endothelial cells. Curr Neurovasc Res 3:49–54
111. Stead LG, Gilmore RM, Bellolio MF, et al. (2008) Hyperglycemia as an independent predictor of worse outcome in non-diabetic patients presenting with acute ischemic stroke. Neurocrit Care PMID: 18357419
112. Stumvoll M, Meyer C, Mitrakou A, et al. (1999) Important role of the kidney in human carbohydrate metabolism. Med Hypotheses 52:363–366
113. Subramanian S, Bowyer MW, Egan JC, et al. (1999) Attenuation of renal ischemia-reperfusion injury with selectin inhibition in a rabbit model. Am J Surg 178:573–576
114. Sung J, Bochicchio GV, Joshi M, et al. (2005) Admission hyperglycemia is predictive of outcome in critically ill trauma patients. J Trauma 59:80–83
115. The Diabetes Control and Complications (DCCT) Research Group (1995) Effect of intensive therapy on the development and progression of diabetic nephropathy in the Diabetes Control and Complications Trial. Kidney Int 47:1703–1720
116. The Diabetes Control and Complications Trial Research Group (1993) The effect of intensive treatment of diabetes on the development and progression of long-term complications in insulin-dependent diabetes mellitus. N Engl J Med 329:977–986
117. Thorell A, Nygren J, Ljungqvist O (1999) Insulin resistance: a marker of surgical stress. Curr Opin Clin Nutr Met Care 21:69–78
118. Thorens B (1996) Glucose transporters in the regulation of intestinal, renal, and liver glucose fluxes. Am J Physiol. 270:G541–553
119. Tiwari MM, Brock RW, Megyesi JK, et al. (2005) Disruption of Renal Peritubular Blood Flow in Lipopolysaccharide-induced Renal Failure: Role of Nitric Oxide and Caspases. Am J Physiol Renal Physiol 289:F1324–1332
120. Turcot DB, Kiernan FJ, McKay RG, et al. (2004) Acute hyperglycemia: implications for contrast-induced nephropathy during cardiac catheterization. Diabetes Care 27:620–621
121. Turina M, Christ-Crain M, Polk HC Jr. (2006) Diabetes and hyperglycemia: strict glycemic control. Crit Care Med 34(Suppl 9):S291–300
122. UK Prospective Diabetes Study (UKPDS) Group (1998) Intensive blood-glucose control with sulphonylureas or insulin compared with conventional treatment and risk of complications in patients with type 2 diabetes (UKPDS 33). Lancet 352:837–853
123. Van den Berghe G (2004) How does blood glucose control with insulin save lives in intensive care? J Clin Invest 9:1187–1195
124. Van den Berghe G, Wilmer A, Hermans G, et al. (2006) Intensive insulin therapy in the medical ICU. N Engl J Med 354:449–461
125. Van den Berghe G, Wilmer A, Milants I, et al. (2006) Intensive insulin therapy in mixed medical/surgical intensive care units: benefit versus harm. Diabetes 55:3151–3159
126. Van den Berghe G, Wouters P, Weekers F, et al. (2001) Intensive insulin therapy in the critically ill patients. N Engl J Med 345:1359–1367
127. Van den Berghe G, Wouters PJ, Bouillon R, et al. (2003) Outcome benefit of intensive insulin therapy in the critically ill: insulin dose versus glycemic control. Crit Care Med 31:359–366
128. Vanhorebeek I, De Vos R, Mesotten D, et al. (2005) Strict blood glucose control with insulin in critically ill patients protects hepatocytic mitochondrial ultrastructure and function. Lancet 365:53–59
129. Venkataraman R, Kellum JA (2007) Prevention of acute renal failure. Chest 131:300–308

130. Vestri S, Okamoto MM, de Freitas HS, et al. (2001) Changes in sodium or glucose filtration rate modulate expression of glucose transporters in renal proximal tubular cells of rat. J Membr Biol 182:105–112
131. Vinas JL, Sola A, Hotter G (2006) Mitochondrial NOS upregulation during renal I/R causes apoptosis in a peroxynitrite-dependent manner. Kidney Int 69:1403–1409
132. Wallner EI, Wada J, Tramonti G et al. (2001) Status of glucose transporters in the mammalian kidney and renal development. Ren Fail 23:301–310
133. Wang S, Mitu GM, Hirschberg R (2008) Osmotic polyuria: an overlooked mechanism in diabetic nephropathy. Nephrol Dial Transplant PMID: 18456680
134. Wang W, Mitra A, Poole B, et al. (2004) Endothelial nitric oxide synthase-deficient mice exhibit increased susceptibility to endotoxin-induced acute renal failure. Am J Physiol Renal Physiol 87: F1044–1048
135. Weekers F, Gifulietti A, Michalaki M, et al. (2003) Metabolic, endocrine and immune effects of stress hyperglycaemia in a rabbit model of prolonged critical illness. Endocrinology 144:5329–5338
136. Weight SC, Nicholson ML (1998) Nitric oxide and renal reperfusion injury: a review. Eur J Vasc Endovasc Surg 16: 98–103
137. Wolf G (2004) New insights into the pathophysiology of diabetic nephropathy: from haemodynamics to molecular pathology. Eur J Clin Invest 34:785–796
138. Wolin MS, Ahmad M, Gupte SA (2005) The sources of oxidative stress in the vessel wall. Kidney Int 67:1659–1661
139. Wong VW, McLean M, Boyages SC, et al. (2004) C-reactive protein levels following acute myocardial infarction: effect of insulin infusion and tight glycemic control. Diabetes Care 27:2971–2973
140. Writing Team for the Diabetes Control and Complications Trial/Epidemiology of Diabetes Interventions and Complications Research Group (2003) Sustained effect of intensive treatment of type 1 diabetes mellitus on development and progression of diabetic nephropathy: the Epidemiology of Diabetes Interventions and Complications (EDIC) study. JAMA 290:2159–2167.
141. Wu L, Gokden N, Mayeux PR (2007) Evidence for the role of reactive nitrogen species in polymicrobial sepsis-induced renal peritubular capillary dysfunction and tubular injury. J Am Soc Nephrol 18:1807–815
142. Yamasowa H, Shimizu S, Inoue T, et al. (2005) Endothelial nitric oxide contributes to the renal protective effects of ischemic preconditioning. J Pharmacol Exp Ther 312: 153–159
143. Yang SY, Zhang S, Wang ML (1995) Clinical significance of admission hyperglycemia and factors related to it in patients with acute severe head injury. Surg Neurol 44: 373–377
144. Yendamuri S, Fulda GJ, Tinkoff GH (2003) Admission hyperglycemia as a prognostic indicator in trauma. J Trauma 55:33–38

Bleeding and Hemostasis

4.8

Herwig Gerlach and Susanne Toussaint

Core Messages

- Coagulation is defined as transition of liquid proteins into the solid state and has to be considered as one of the oldest systems of host response. It depends on a dynamic balance between coagulation and fibrinolysis. During bleedings, the coagulation system is poised to rapidly generate a hemostatic plug at sites of vascular injury. On the other hand, perturbation of the balance can lead to thrombosis or bleeding.
- The endothelial cell emerges as a dynamic regulator maintaining homeostasis in the quiescent state and contributing to the pathogenesis of vascular lesions in the stimulated state. The apparent inertness of the endothelial cell probably results from a complex balance of opposing mechanisms.
- Blood remains liquid in homeostasis via multiple anticoagulant mechanisms, ranging from the protein C/protein S and fibrinolytic pathways to expression of heparin and eicosanoids having anticoagulant activities. Following exposure to appropriate environmental stimuli, such as cytokines or glycosylated proteins, this balance can be shifted and thus promote mechanisms leading to clot formation and escape of fluid from the intravascular space.
- Dysfunctional endothelium could be an important participant in the pathogenesis of vascular lesions. The most common problems of the hemostatic system in the critical care setting are unexpected and/or excessive bleedings, congenital bleeding disorders, venous thromboembolism, and disseminated intravascular coagulation, occurring as a complication of a variety of disorders.
- Thromboprophylaxis and the management of the underlying diseases are indicated to prevent these disorders.

4.8.1 Basics of Hemostasis

Generally, activation of the hemostatic process is proportional to the extent of vascular damage and limited to the site of injury. These features of the coagulant response require that the coagulation mechanism functions in an amplified and localized manner. The response to vascular injury begins when blood is exposed to subendothelial structures, and rapid activation of the hemostatic process is initiated. A sequence of events occurs in the initial formation of platelet thrombi, which includes platelet adhesion to exposed subendothelium, release of platelet granular material, and the aggregation of platelets onto attached platelets. At the same time the coagulation mechanism is activated to support the platelet plug by the formation of thrombin. Thrombin induces more platelets to aggregate and forms fibrin which stabilizes the platelet plug. This cascade arrangement of the blood coagulation reactions is clearly one mechanism by which the initiating stimulus is amplified to obtain a sufficient coagulant response.

H. Gerlach (✉)
Department of Anesthesia, Intensive Care Medicine, and Pain Management, Vivantes–Klinikum Neukölln, Klinik fuer Anaesthesie, Operative Intensivmedizin und Schmerztherapie, Rudower Strasse 48, 12313 Berlin, Germany
e-mail: herwig.gerlach@vivantes.de

A. Jörres et al. (eds.), *Management of Acute Kidney Problems*,
DOI: 10.1007/978-3-540-69441-0_4.8, © Springer-Verlag Berlin Heidelberg 2010

There are two major defense mechanisms against bleeding: fibrin generation (humoral hemostasis) and platelet aggregation (cellular hemostasis). Fibrin and activated platelets constitute the major components of hemostatic plugs. These mechanisms operate in tandem, although fibrin generation may be relatively more important for hemostasis in veins and venules, and platelet aggregation may be relatively more important for hemostasis in arteries, arterioles, and capillaries. In addition, the vascular component was found to play a major role (vascular hemostasis).

4.8.1.1 *Humoral Hemostasis*

Fibrin generation is a series of coordinated and calcium-dependent proenzyme-to-serine protease conversions likely to be localized on the surfaces of activated cells in vivo. It culminates in the conversion of prothrombin to thrombin by the coagulant complex known as prothrombinase. Prothrombinase consists of a serine protease (factor Xa) and its cofactor (factor Va) bound to phospholipid cell membranes in a calcium-dependent manner. Blood coagulation is initiated when the serine protease factor VIIa in blood combines with tissue factor (TF). Tissue factor is a transmembrane receptor for factor VII/VIIa. The apparent end point of blood coagulation is the conversion of the soluble plasma protein, fibrinogen, into insoluble fibrin. This is only one of several necessary reactions that are catalyzed by thrombin.

The traditional concept of the coagulation system consists of a strict cascade which is divided into the extrinsic and intrinsic system (Fig. 4.8.1). In contrast, the current model of blood coagulation differs from the original "cascade" scheme, in which an intrinsic pathway begins with contact activation of factor XII (FXII), leading to factor IX activation, followed by factor X activation, and an extrinsic pathway is initiated by TF and FVII activation, also leading to factor X activation. The primary ambiguity of the old model was the importance of FXII, because clinical bleeding is absent in persons affected by hereditary FXII deficiency. In contrast, patients with FXI deficiency have a severe bleeding disorder when provoked, indicating FXI's importance in normal hemostasis [31]. The current model of coagulation helps reconcile these observations by describing hemostasis as a process involving three overlapping phases (Fig. 4.8.2).

The revised model of hemostasis by Hoffman and Monroe emphasizes the role of different cell surfaces in the localization and control of the coagulation process, rather than a process controlled by the levels and kinetics of the different coagulation proteins [24].

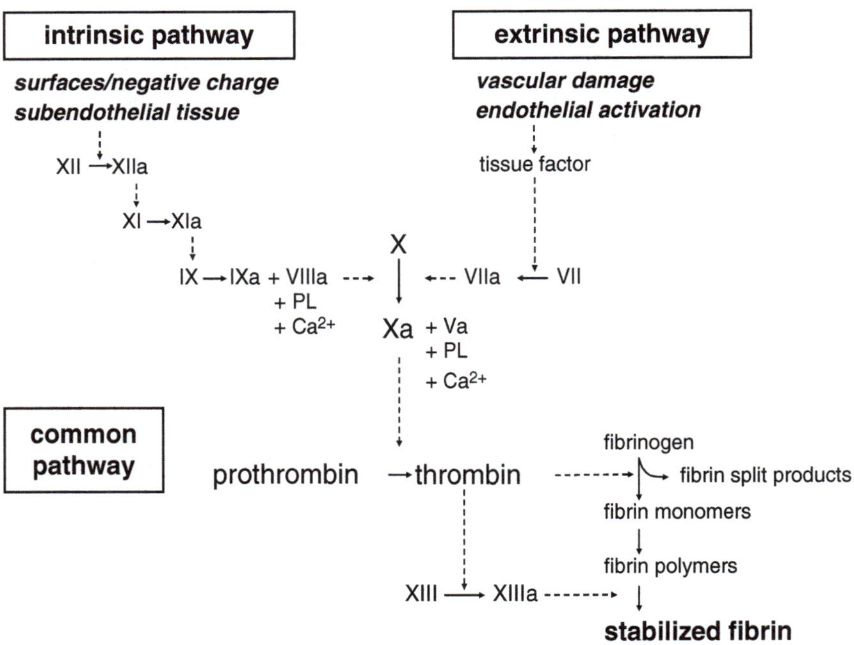

Fig. 4.8.1 The "classical" coagulation cascade is described as a pathway of proteolytic enzymatic reactions, resulting in the formation of fibrin via the cleavage of fibrinogen, a process mediated by the serine protease thrombin. PL, phospholipids

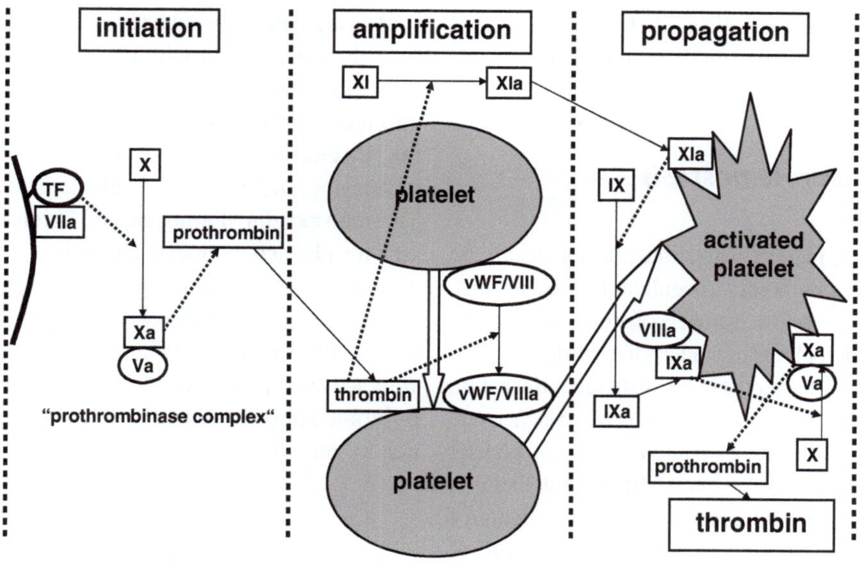

Fig. 4.8.2 The cell-based model of coagulation according to Hoffman and Monroe [24]. Fibrin formation occurs on different cell surfaces in three phases (from *left* to *right*). During the initiation (*left*), only small amounts of thrombin are formed, which coactivates platelets as an amplification step (*middle*). Several factors are cleaved and activated to form the "intrinsic tenase" (IXa/VIIIa) on the surface of activated platelets (*right*). This finally leads to the formation of large amounts of thrombin and subsequent fibrinogen cleavage to form the clot

- *Phase 1 (Initiation):* The clotting cascade is *initiated* when TF is exposed to the blood flow following either the damage or the activation of the endothelium (see also Section 4.8.1.2). This disturbance may be due to perforation of a vessel wall or to activation by chemicals, cytokines, or inflammatory processes. TF is a member of the type II cytokine family of glycoproteins and is expressed on subendothelial cells and smooth muscle cells. Bacterial and viral infections lead to production of cytokines, which stimulate TF synthesis in and expression on endothelial cells and monocytes. The inflammatory responses, e.g., during sepsis, also induce TF synthesis and its expression on endothelial cells. TF, when exposed to blood, complexes with circulating factor VII (FVII). The TF-activated VII complex (TF/VIIa) is the critical *initiating* reaction that ultimately results in fibrin generation. The TF/VIIa complex cleaves the proenzyme FX to FXa. FXa complexes with FVa to form the "prothrombinase" complex. The "prothrombinase" complex converts small amounts of prothrombin to thrombin. Thrombin then cleaves fibrinogen, releasing fibrinopeptides A and B, and generates insoluble fibrin. The initial formation of fibrin at the site of vascular injury is unstable.
- *Phase 2 (Amplification):* As platelets adhere to the initiation site, they become activated and accumulate cofactors on their surfaces *amplifying* the procoagulant stimulus. Thrombin, generated in the initiation phase, binds to platelets enhancing both their binding to matrix and activation. It also activates factors V, VIII, and XI.
- *Phase 3 (Propagation):* Coagulation is *propagated* by TF/FVIIa-catalyzed FIXa generation from FIX and by small amounts of thrombin generated by the initiating coagulation reaction. FIXa complexes with FVIIIa to form the "intrinsic tenase" complex. The "intrinsic tenase" complex promotes FX activation. FXa then activates the "prothrombinase" complex as described. Thrombin causes activation of FXI to FXIa. FXIa cleaves FIX to FIXa. FIXa leads to FXa production from FX, leading to enhanced production of the "prothrombinase" complex. In addition to cleaving fibrinogen and activating FXI, thrombin also activates FVIII, FV, and platelets.

This three-step activation of coagulation is followed by a termination phase, which is mediated by a series of anticoagulant proteins. Tissue factor pathway inhibitor (TFPI) complexes with FVIIa and FXa, which terminates the initiating reaction. Antithrombin III (ATIII) inactivates thrombin and FXa. Activated protein C (APC) and protein S inactivate FVa and FVIIIa.

4.8.1.2 Cellular Hemostasis

As shown above, platelet activation can not strictly be separated from humoral coagulation mechanisms. Platelet activation results from exposure of the platelet to damaged endothelium or underlying components of the vessel wall. Other biologic agonists (e.g., thrombin, ADP, epinephrine, and thromboxane A_2) can activate platelets as well. Platelet activation results in platelet shape change, platelet adhesion to the subendothelium, platelet aggregation, and secretion of the contents of intracellular granules with subsequent formation of fibrin-stabilized platelet aggregates. Platelets contain two major kinds of intracellular granules, the α-granules and the dense bodies. The α-granules contain platelet thrombospondin, fibrinogen, fibronectin, platelet factor 4, von Willebrand factor (vWF), platelet-derived growth factor, β-thromboglobulin, and coagulation factor V. The dense bodies contain adenosine diphosphate (ADP), adenosine triphosphate (ATP), and serotonin.

Platelet activation can be described in the following three steps [37]. Firstly, following vessel injury, there are initial rolling contacts between the platelet receptor glycoprotein Ib (GP Ib) and the Al domain of vWF. vWF is bound to extravascular collagen via its A3 domain. The rolling contacts slow down the flow of platelets to allow their activation to begin. Thus, interaction of vWF with GP Ib initiates hemostatic plug formation. Secondly, the activation of platelets likely consists of two steps. Collagen, located on the subendothelial matrix, binds to its platelet receptor, GP Ia/IIa, and subnanomolar amounts of thrombin (generated on platelets) bind to their main receptor on platelets, known as the protease activated receptor-l (PAR-1). PAR-1 cleavage initiates signaling cascades within platelets that result in platelet shape change, platelet aggregation, and release of platelet α-granule and dense granule contents that help propagate platelet activation.

The platelet receptor, glycoprotein IIb/IIIa (GP IIb/IIIa) also necessarily becomes activated. Glycoprotein IIb/IIIa combines with vWF, fibrinogen, thrombospondin, fibronectin, and vitronectin. Binding of fibrinogen to activated GP IIb/IIIa is necessary for platelet–platelet cohesion and subsequent platelet aggregation during hemostatic plug formation.

Activated platelets secrete several proteins that influence their interaction with other platelets, endothelial cells, and white cells. These proteins include P-selectin, thrombospondin, fibrinogen, fibronectin, and vitronectin. P-selectin facilitates adherence of neutrophils, monocytes, and endothelial cells to activated platelets. Thrombospondin, fibrinogen, and fibronectin are necessary for platelet–monocyte adherence, platelet–platelet cohesion, and subsequent aggregation through GP IIb/IIIa. Vitronectin is required for fibrinogen-dependent and fibronectin-dependent inflammatory cell interactions with activated platelets. Activated platelets also secrete β-thromboglobulin, which inhibits prostacyclin production by endothelial cells.

4.8.1.3 Vascular Hemostasis

The vascular system has a relevant impact on procoagulant and anticoagulant functions [32]. The nature of blood flow within the vascular circuit can help explain fibrin formation in the venous system and platelet thrombus formation in the arterial system. Blood flow is influenced by blood pressure, vessel diameter, vessel compliance, vessel branching, and blood viscosity. Although there may be comparable blood flow (volume/unit time) in the arterial and venous circuits, the flow velocities (distance/unit time) are not comparable. Such differences in blood flow velocities account for venous thrombi being composed of fibrin and red cells ("red thrombus") and arterial thrombi being composed primarily of platelets ("white thrombus").

Arteries have relatively high blood-flow velocities. This results in an elevated shear stress on the vessel wall. Within a roughly tubular vessel, blood flow generates a parabolic flow velocity profile. Blood-flow velocity is maximal and shear stress is minimal at the center of the tube. At the blood–vessel interface, the flow velocity is minimal and the shear stress is maximal. The shear stresses generated by blood flow affect the coagulation reactions taking place at sites of vascular injury. Shear stresses are low in the venous circulation. Thus, activation of the coagulation factors can occur without them being "washed away" by the force of the blood flow on the vessel wall. In the arterial system, the higher shear stresses tend to dilute out certain procoagulant molecules, e.g., fibrinogen, prothrombin, and thrombin. This prevents the formation of insoluble fibrin. However, vWF supports platelet adhesion and aggregation on subendothelial structures exposed on damaged blood vessels, even with such high wall shear stresses. Yet, the arterial thrombus formation is a dynamic process. As arterial diameter decreases, blood flow velocity and shear stress also decrease. This will allow development of fibrin generation, thus being a crucial mechanism to stop bleeding by active vasoconstriction.

4.8.2 The Vascular Endothelium as Central Regulator of Hemostasis

Our current view of the endothelium's role in the coagulation mechanism has evolved radically from the original concept of endothelium as an inert or blood-compatible surface [20]. Until roughly 2 decades ago, the endothelium was considered to be merely a passive barrier that preserved the fluidity of blood by preventing the fluid and cellular elements from coming into contact with interstitial matrix. In the presence of a continuous layer of intact endothelium, blood remains fluid: thus, disruption of endothelial continuity was considered the initial event in clot formation, and indeed clots form most effectively after a vessel injury in which the integrity of the endothelium is clearly compromised. Furthermore, the adherence of platelets to the collagenous subendothelial basement membrane and the ability of interstitial cells, such as fibroblasts and smooth muscle cells, to promote coagulation both lent credence to this view. Based on these considerations, endothelium was termed a "blood-compatible" surface that by virtue of its inertness prevented components in the intravascular space from interacting with deeper layers of the vessel wall and the interstitial tissues.

It was shown, however, that the early stages of vessel wall injury can occur in the presence of a continuous layer of endothelium. This discovery prompted studies of the more subtle changes in endothelial cell function that may precede cell death and/or desquamation. Barrier function of the endothelial monolayer and cell surface coagulant properties are closely linked since activation of coagulation leads to formation of proteases and fibrin, which can, in turn, increase endothelial permeability. Conversely, diminished barrier function and ingress of plasma proteins into the subendothelium promotes clotting. In the "quiescent" state, mechanisms that confine intravascular components to the vessel lumen and promote blood fluidity predominate; in the "perturbed" or "activated" state, transendothelial leakage of plasma factors and passage of cells, along with promotion of clot formation, can occur. A balance of opposing, active endothelial-dependent mechanisms can clearly determine properties of the luminal surface of the vessel wall. Vessel wall dysfunction arising from changes in endothelial cell physiology may play a role in the pathogenesis of venous thrombosis, atherosclerosis, inflammatory vasculitides, shock, and disseminated intravascular coagulation.

4.8.2.1 Modulation of Endothelial Coagulant Properties

Although contact between intact endothelium and blood does not lead to clot formation or adherence of platelets, recent studies have shown that this apparent antithrombogenicity or nonthrombogenicity is not a passive phenomenon. Rather, the effect of endothelium on coagulation is the result of multiple mechanisms, both anticoagulant and procoagulant, operative on the cell surface. Central anticoagulant mechanisms of the endothelial cell include the heparin-antithrombin III, fibrinolytic, and protein C/protein S systems [40]. Another important feature contributing to the anticoagulant properties of normal endothelium is the paucity of procoagulant activities on the cell surface. The current perspective for considering the physiology of perturbed or stimulated endothelium is this: in disturbed or pathologic states, endothelial cell surface receptors and secretory products involved in anticoagulant mechanisms could be down-regulated, and procoagulant activities could be induced [21, 36].

The protein C/protein S pathway consists of two plasma components, the regulatory vitamin K-dependent proteins C and S, and cellular cofactor activities, which allow for effective anticoagulation by this pathway [13]. The pathway is initiated when thrombin, bound to the endothelial cell surface cofactor thrombomodulin, interacts with the zymogen protein C, cleaving the latter and resulting in formation of the enzyme APC. APC is a potent anticoagulant enzyme capable of inactivating clotting factors Va and VIIIa (thereby blocking activation of the coagulation cascade) and inactivating plasminogen activator inhibitor 1, a central inhibitor of the fibrinolytic system [22]. For optimal anticoagulant function, APC requires protein S and an appropriate cellular surface [16].

Thrombomodulin, the endothelial cofactor that facilitates thrombin-mediated protein C activation, is subject to regulation by environmental mediators, and thus alters the function of the protein C/protein S system. Incubation of cultured endothelium with tumor necrosis factor (TNF), for example, leads to a decline in thrombomodulin activity [21]. In addition to these tests in cell culture, interleukin-1, a cytokine many of whose actions are similar to TNF, was infused into animals, and the thrombomodulin activity on vessel segments was then studied at later times. The results of this study [36] also demonstrated suppression of thrombomodulin. Besides decreasing expression of thrombomodulin, TNF suppresses the endothelial fibrinolytic system by promoting synthesis of plasminogen activator inhibitor-l [22]. Thus, two important anticoagulant mechanisms of the vessel surface can be compromised by exposing endothelium to TNF, a central factor in the pathogenesis of the septic shock state.

In the quiescent state there is little expression of procoagulant activity initiating clot formation. To shift effectively the balance of endothelial coagulant properties to a state in which activation of coagulation could be promoted, suppression of anticoagulant mechanisms should be accompanied by induction of procoagulant properties. Studies with cultured endothelial cells and a limited number of in vivo experiments demonstrate that this shift in the phenotype of endothelial coagulant properties can take place. Tissue factor is a cell surface cofactor that promotes the activation of coagulation by binding factor VII/VIIa and allowing the latter enzyme to activate factors IX and X [2]. Endothelium characteristically has little tissue factor, in keeping with its role in promoting the fluidity of blood. Following incubation of endothelium with a cytokine such as TNF, for example, induction of tissue factor is observed [4, 21]. This is the result of de novo transcription and translation, followed by expression of the active procoagulant cofactor on the cell surface. Induction of tissue factor in response to TNF can be modulated by prior exposure of endothelium to other stimuli, such as glycosylated proteins [16]. Recent experiments have shown that advanced glycation end product (AGE) albumin considerably augments the induction of tissue factor in response to TNF. These results indicate that the endothelial response to a single mediator is modified by other factors in the cell's environment.

In addition to tissue factor, other potential procoagulant activities of the endothelial surface can be induced. Certain agents, such as thrombin, can induce the synthesis and cell surface expression of platelet-activating factor by endothelium [50]. Another cofactor that could promote procoagulant events on the vessel surface is the specific cell surface binding site for factor IX/IXa [39, 45]. In contrast to the interaction of factor IX with phospholipids, the factor IX–cell surface interaction is of high affinity and very specific. From the vessel surface the factor X activation complex (factors IXa–VIII–X) can assemble and potentially promote the activation of coagulation.

The formation of activated coagulation enzymes on the endothelial surface can have far ranging consequences. Localized clot formation with thrombosis can occur, as well as severe organ dysfunction such as acute renal failure in severe sepsis. In addition, procoagulants can have "hormonal" effects on endothelium: for example, they can stimulate release of mitogenic activities, induce procoagulants (tissue factor and platelet-activating factor), and elaborate cytokines (interleukin-1). Activation of coagulation on the vessel surface could thus create a positive feedback loop and set into motion events that transform the phenotype of the endothelial surface.

4.8.2.2 Modulation of Endothelial Permeability

Endothelium serves as the cellular barrier retaining blood components within the intravascular space. This function is the result of the tight apposition of cell margins maintained by specialized cell–cell junctions through most of the vascular tree. Barrier function is compromised in many pathophysiologic states, most notably in endotoxic/septic shock, in which profound disturbance in endothelial cell barrier function is specifically induced by host mediators released in response to bacterial lipopolysaccharide.

The cytokine TNF cachectin, one of several host mediators synthesized by macrophages after exposure to lipopolysaccharide, is a central mediator of the shock state in gram-negative sepsis [43]. Infusion of TNF into animals produces many of the abnormalities characteristic of *Escherichia coli* lipopolysaccharide toxemia, including vascular leakage due to loss of barrier function. Vascular endothelium is a direct target for the action of TNF, which modulates many endothelial cell functions such as coagulant activity and immunologic properties [43]. Structurally, decreased barrier function is closely correlated with a retraction of lateral cell margins and the formation of intercellular spaces. A mechanism underlying TNF-induced increase in monolayer permeability was demonstrated by studies with pertussis toxin, an agent that inactivates certain G proteins [5]. These results contribute to an emerging picture in which one pathway by which stimulation of endothelial cell TNF receptor is coupled to effector mechanisms involves signal transduction via regulatory G proteins.

Factors other than cytokines can modulate endothelial permeability. AGE of proteins accumulate in the vasculature with diabetes and aging and are thought to be associated with vascular complications [6]. Exposing the endothelium to AGE-modified albumin increases the permeability of endothelium by inducing a major change in the architecture of the monolayer [16]. Endothelial cells are perturbed by AGE of proteins when these glucose-modified proteins bind to a specific site on the cell surface and thereby create specific changes in cellular physiology.

4.8.3 Physiologic Anticoagulation and Fibrinolysis

A fine and delicate balance that normally exists between anticoagulant mechanisms and the procoagulant response is altered in various diseases. Regulation of coagulation is exerted throughout the pathway either by enzyme inhibition or by modulation of the activity of cofactors. The tissue factor pathway inhibitor (TFPI), antithrombin, and protein C anticoagulant system all participate in this regulation. If fibrin clots are formed, either by proinflammatory processes such as sepsis or by physiologic hemostasis against bleedings, fibrinolysis is activated. This is a proteolytic process to initiate hydrolytic lysis of fibrin to maintain blood flow.

4.8.3.1 Anticoagulant Mechanisms

The TFPI is a protease inhibitor that inhibits the initial reactions of blood coagulation [25]. The surface of endothelial cells houses a major pool of TFPI. Tissue factor pathway inhibitor may also modulate cell proliferation. It contains three domains. The first and second domains inhibit TF/VIIa and Xa, respectively. The third domain has no inhibitory activity toward proteases, but it does contain heparin-binding sites. In addition to endothelial cells, TFPI is also synthesized by mesangial cells, smooth muscle cells, monocytes, fibroblasts, and cardiomyocytes. In the blood stream, TFPI exists in a free form and also in lipoprotein-associated forms. It mediates the permanent down-regulation of cell surface TF in monocytes and fibroblasts via internalization and degradation by low-density lipoprotein (LDL) receptor-related protein. The endothelial cell-associated form of TFPI is released into the blood stream on infusion of heparin. This suggests that TFPI binds to heparan sulfate proteoglycans on endothelial cells. Some studies suggest that TFPI may be a marker of endothelial cell dysfunction. Recombinant TFPI may attenuate thrombosis and prevent restenosis.

Antithrombin is a serine protease inhibitor [10]. It inhibits most of the enzymes generated during activation of coagulation. It preferentially binds free enzymes. Enzymes in the "tenase" and "prothrombinase" complexes are less accessible to antithrombin. Antithrombin limits the coagulation process to sites of vascular injury. It also protects the circulation from liberated enzymes. Antithrombin is in itself an inefficient serine protease inhibitor. Heparin and heparin-like molecules, which are present on the surface of endothelial cells, stimulate its activity.

The protein C anticoagulant pathway serves as a major system for controlling thrombosis, limiting inflammatory responses, and potentially decreasing endothelial cell apoptosis in response to inflammatory cytokines and ischemia. The essential components of the pathway involve thrombin, thrombomodulin, the endothelial cell protein C receptor (EPCR), protein C, and protein S [15]. The protein C anticoagulant pathway converts the coagulation signal generated by thrombin into an anticoagulant response through the activation of protein C by the binding of thrombin to thrombomodulin (TM) [14]. Thrombomodulin is located on the vascular endothelium. APC interacts with protein S on membrane surfaces to catalyze the inactivation of factors Va and VIIIa. It is suggested that the binding of TM to thrombin alters thrombin conformation. This blocks access of normal substrates to thrombin and provides a binding site for protein C. The role of protein S appears to be the alteration of the cleavage site in factor Va that is specific for APC. The thrombin-TM complex also activates thrombin-activated fibrinolysis inhibitor (TAFI) more rapidly than free thrombin. APC resistance has been described and is due to a genetic mutation in factor V (factor V Leiden). This mutation is the most common inherited cause of venous thrombosis.

4.8.3.2 Fibrinolysis

The classic intravascular fibrinolytic system consists of sequential proteolytic events, in which tissue plasminogen activator (t-PA) cleaves and activates plasminogen, resulting in the generation of the serine protease, plasmin. Besides the proenzyme plasminogen and enzymes that activate plasminogen (tissue-type plasminogen activator, urokinase), the fibrinolytic system consists of several inhibitors that control the activity of plasminogen, the activity of plasmin, and degradation of fibrin [11].

Tissue-type plasminogen activator (t-PA) is synthesized and secreted by endothelial cells as a single-chain active enzyme. It consists of five domains, two of which possess distinct fibrin-binding sites. Plasminogen activator inhibitor type-1 (PAI-1) inhibits t-PA. The complex of t-PA and PAI-l retains some affinity to fibrin. Therefore, it can compete with free t-PA for binding to fibrin. Cell membranes and extracellular matrix compounds (e.g., thrombospondin and collagen IV) also increase the rate of activation of plasminogen, but less than the activation rate afforded by fibrin.

Urokinase (u-PA) exists in two forms. The single-chain urokinase-type plasminogen activator (scu-PA) is less active than the 2-chain urokinase-type plasminogen activator (tcu-PA). Plasmin and kallikrein cleave scu-PA to result in a fully active urokinase compound. Scu-PA does not specifically bind fibrin. Urokinase and tissue-type plasminogen activator appear to be complementary activators of plasminogen with functional overlap. It has been suggested that u-PA may mediate cellular activation of plasminogen in tissues, whereas t-PA may be more important for lysis of fibrin clots in the circulation.

Plasminogen activator inhibitors consist of four groups of proteins. Plasminogen activator inhibitor type-l (PAI-1) inhibits t-PA and tcu-PA in normal blood. It is synthesized by endothelium. Plasminogen activator inhibitor type-2 is synthesized by the placenta monocytes and macrophages. It inactivates tcu-PA. It is not detected in normal blood, but appears in various disease states. PAI-3 and PAI-4 inhibit protein C and protease nexin I, respectively. Approximately 90% of the total blood content of PAI-1 is stored in the α-granules of platelets. Activated platelets or membranes of disrupted cells may activate latent PAI-1, which will increase the stability of a thrombus. PAI-l may be considered as a major determinant of fibrinolytic activity in vivo.

Plasminogen is secreted by the liver as a single-chain glycoprotein. It consists of five domains that mediate binding with fibrin, α_2-antiplasmin, and cell receptors. Plasminogen is activated to plasmin by t-PA by cleavage at Arg561. Plasmin cleaves fibrinogen, fibrin, and fibrin-fibrin dimers, thus dissolving the clot and leading to the formation of fibrin split products and D-dimers. These fibrin split products may themselves have an anticoagulant effect by increasing vascular permeability and plasmin activity and by inhibiting thrombin and destroying factors V and VIII.

Fibrinogen has a symmetrical structure formed by three pairs of polypeptide chains. Fibrin is sequentially digested by plasmin, leading to formation of degradation products. α_2-antiplasmin (α_2-AP), α_2-macroglobulin (α_2-MG), and (TAFI) are inhibitors of plasmin. α_2-AP is secreted by the liver as a single-chain glycoprotein. α_2-AP helps regulate the lysis of fibrin matrix within a thrombus. Inactivation of plasmin by α_2-MG is slower than that by α_2-AP and may play an important role in plasmin inactivation after consumption of α_2-AP. Thrombin-activated fibrinolysis inhibitor is secreted by the liver as a single-chain inactive glycoprotein. It is activated by thrombin or plasmin. The mechanism of action of TAFI is the removal of those residues in fibrin that are generated from the inactivation of plasmin by α_2-AP. Inactivation of TAFI occurs spontaneously and is associated with a conformational change.

4.8.4 Bleeding Disorders in Acute Care Patients

The clinical pictures of hemostatic disorders are multiple, and this as well as the following two sections will try to give a short overview. However, including all aspects such as epidemiology, pathogenesis, diagnostics, and therapeutic measures of coagulation disorders is far beyond the scope of this chapter. For details, it is recommended to refer to the specific literature.

4.8.4.1 Congenital Bleeding Disorders

Hemophilia A and B are the most frequent inherited bleeding disorders. Together with von Willebrand disease, a defect of primary hemostasis associated with a secondary defect in coagulation factor VIII, these X-linked disorders include 95–97% of all inherited deficiencies of coagulation factors [30]. The remaining defects, generally transmitted as autosomal recessive traits in both sexes, are rare, with prevalences of the presumably homozygous forms in the general population ranging from approximately 1 in 2 million for factor II (prothrombin) and factor XIII (FXIII) deficiency to 1 in 500,000 for factor VII (FVII) deficiency. The combined performance of the global coagulation tests prothrombin time (PT) and activated partial thromboplastin time (APTT) is usually apt to identify the disorders of clinically significant severity but not FXIII deficiency. A prolonged APTT contrasting with a normal PT is indicative of FXI deficiency, provided hemophilia A and B and the asymptomatic defects of the contact phase are ruled out. The specular pattern (normal APTT and prolonged PT) is typical of FVII deficiency, whereas the prolongation of both tests directs further analysis on the possible deficiencies of FX, FV, prothrombin, or fibrinogen. This paradigm is not valid for disorders due to combined deficiencies, which prolong both the PT and the APTT. Specific assays of factor coagulant activity are necessary when the degree of prolongation of the global tests suggests the presence of severe, clinically significant deficiencies [30].

The most typical symptom, common to all recessively inherited coagulation disorders, is the occurrence of excessive bleeding at the time of invasive procedures such as circumcision and dental extractions. Bleeding in mucosal tracts (particularly epistaxis and menorrhagia) is also a frequent feature, and impaired wound healing is rather typical of FXIII deficiency. Such life-endangering symptoms as umbilical cord and recurrent hemoperitoneum during ovulation, as well as limb-endangering hemarthroses and soft tissue hematomas, occur with higher frequency in patients with prothrombin, FX, and FXIII deficiency. FVII deficiency presents with a wide spectrum of symptom severity that sometimes correlates poorly with FVII levels, a number of patients with undetectable FVII being totally asymptomatic.

The mainstay of treatment, single-donor fresh-frozen plasma (FFP) that contains all coagulation factors, is relatively inexpensive and widely available. However, the risk of volume overload is real when repeated infusions are administered to keep the deficient factor at normal levels. Hence, concentrates should be preferred for major surgical procedures. Only one product produced by recombinant DNA technology is licensed for FVII deficiency (recombinant activated FVII). A few plasma-derived single-factor concentrates (fibrinogen, FVII, FXI, and FXIII) are available or licensed in some European countries but not in the United States. FV deficiency and the combined deficiency of FV and FVIII can only be treated with fresh-frozen plasma; prothrombin and FX deficiencies are often treated with prothrombin complex concentrates containing vitamin K-dependent factors other than those actually deficient.

vWF is a multimeric plasma protein that mediates platelet adhesion at sites of injury, and normal platelet adhesion depends on the largest vWF multimers. Deficiency of vWF causes von Willebrand disease (vWD), a bleeding disorder of variable severity that is divided into several subtypes. vWD type 1 is reported to be common but frequently is difficult to diagnose. Many people have nonspecific mild bleeding symptoms; vWF levels display low heritability, and low VWF levels (15–50% of normal) are weak risk factors for bleeding. Therefore, bleeding and low vWF levels often associate by chance [42]. A low vWF level might yet be useful clinically if it conferred a sufficiently high risk of bleeding, but it does not appear to do so. Patients with undetectable vWF usually do have serious bleeding. Unsurprisingly, screening of asymptomatic persons for low vWF does not have much value. A low vWF level did not predict surgical bleeding in patients, and a prolonged bleeding time (a poor surrogate for low vWF) does not predict surgical bleeding [26]. However, it is reasonable to determine vWF levels in persons with symptomatic bleeding. Desmopressin, or DDAVP, acutely increases the plasma level of vWF and has been used in mild hemophilia [29]. In patients with congenital defects of platelet function, with the hemostatic abnormalities associated with chronic liver disease, and with those induced by the therapeutic use of antiplatelet and anticoagulant agents, desmopressin has been used successfully to prevent or stop bleeding. However, there is still no well-designed clinical trial that truly shows efficacy of the compound in these conditions. Moreover, the use of desmopressin in surgical operations other than cardiac surgery is not warranted at the moment.

4.8.4.2 Acquired Bleeding Disorders

The most common acquired inhibitor of coagulation is the lupus anticoagulant (LA) [47]. LA is a member of the antiphospholipid antibody (APA) family. APAs may be seen in many patient populations, e.g., after infection and in patients with autoimmune disease. Most APAs seen in the setting of infections have no clinical complications. However, a large percentage of APA patients with underlying autoimmune disease present with thrombotic complications involving both the arterial and venous circulation, as well as recurrent fetal loss/spontaneous abortion in women. APA syndrome is diagnosed based on the presence of clinical complications (e.g., thrombosis or recurrent spontaneous abortion) and positive laboratory testing for LA and/or anticardiolipin antibodies [47].

Bleeding during pregnancy is often fulminant and life-threatening for mother and child. Of maternal deaths occurring during pregnancy, 25% are caused by hemorrhaging. All physicians involved in the interdisciplinary treatment of hemorrhaging during pregnancy need to be familiar with the specific pathophysiology of hemostatic changes during pregnancy, e.g., elevated hemostatic capacity, reduced anti-coagulation activity and severe alterations of the fibrinolysis system. Therapists must be able to perform a consequent, goal-directed interdisciplinary approach to prevent adverse maternal and fetal outcomes. The major issues of therapy are causal obstetric treatment of the bleeding, early detection and therapy of hyperfibrinolysis, optimization of fibrinogen and platelet levels, and knowledge of the possibilities of a targeted coagulation therapy [23].

Abnormalities of platelet function are characterized by clinical bleeding of varying severity. In most cases, patients present with mucocutaneous bleeding or excessive hemorrhage following surgery or trauma. A platelet count and careful examination of the peripheral smear is essential in the initial evaluation of patients with mucocutaneous bleeding. When examining the peripheral smear, it is important to evaluate the relative size of platelets. Large platelets may be seen as a result of accelerated marrow production of platelets attributable to a hemorrhagic event or recovery from bone marrow suppression as a result of infections or drugs. Large platelets are also encountered in the setting of patients with accelerated platelet turnover (idiopathic thrombocytopenic purpura) [19, 47]. Platelet aggregation is an important component of laboratory testing in a patient with clinical findings suggestive of a primary hemostatic abnormality.

Increasingly, desmopressin is being used to manage patients with abnormalities of primary hemostasis (e.g., vWD), patients exposed to aspirin, and cirrhotic patients with bleeding complications [48]. Desmopressin triggers the release of VWF from Weibel-Palade bodies of vascular endothelium. Desmopressin has also been used in the management of patients with mild to moderate hemophilia A (deficiencies of factor VIII). In cases of severe thrombocytopenia or iatrogenic inhibition of platelet function, the use of platelet concentrates is indicated. In renal failure patients with hemorrhagic complications, correction of the hematocrit to >30% often will alleviate bleeding problems [27, 47].

4.8.5 Thromboembolic Disorders

4.8.5.1 Venous Thromboembolism and Pulmonary Embolism

Patients in the intensive care unit (ICU) are at a high risk of deep vein thrombosis (DVT), and pulmonary embolism (PE). Patients who develop these thromboembolic complications have a higher risk of both ICU and hospital-acquired morbidity and mortality, including the need for and the duration of mechanical ventilation, the ICU and hospital lengths of stay, and, perhaps, death [8, 46]. It is therefore important that all patients in the ICU receive effective thromboprophylaxis [9]. In the absence of a contraindication, all patients in the ICU should receive some form of pharmacologic thromboprophylaxis. In most cases this will consist of either unfractionated heparin or low-molecular-weight heparin (LMWH). Unfractionated heparin at a dose of 5,000 U subcutaneous twice or three times daily is the preferred anticoagulant in North America, while LMWH at prophylactic doses is used most frequently in Europe [46].

Despite the routine provision of anticoagulant prophylaxis, failures do occur. For example, in a prospective study of 261 patients, 25 patients (9.6%) developed ultrasonographically detected DVT despite routine and protocol-directed provision of thromboprophylaxis [8]. This observation suggests that additional research is required to refine prophylaxis for these very-high-risk patients. Failure of pharmacologic prophylaxis may be due to an overwhelming prothrombotic stimulus or due to inadequate anticoagulant effect. Critically ill patients may harbor ICU-specific characteristics that predispose to failure of thromboprophylaxis. Critically ill patients receiving inotropic support have significantly lower peak LMWH levels than similar patients not exposed to inotropes [12]. It was hypothesized that impaired tissue perfusion as a result of vasoconstriction reduces absorption of LMWH. This reduced anticoagulant effect may in turn predispose to thrombosis. Furthermore, many patients in the ICU have extensive subcutaneous edema. Such edema is due to aggressive fluid resuscitation, reduced colloid oncotic pressure, renal insufficiency, and tissue trauma associated with injury or surgery. It is reasonable to hypothesize that subcutaneous edema may impair absorption of LMWH, thus predisposing to lower peak heparin levels and an increased risk of thrombosis [9].

Acute embolic events can occur without symptoms, and symptomatic PE is often overlooked or misdiagnosed in practice. Autopsy studies frequently show that most cases of fatal PE are unrecognized and/or undiagnosed, and data from studies screening for PE in patients with DVT and in postoperative patients suggest that many patients with PE are asymptomatic and that PE often goes unrecognized [41]. Passarino and colleagues reported that of 546 autopsy-confirmed cases of death associated with PE, correct diagnoses were seen only in 8.4% of cases [38]. Meignan and colleagues performed perfusion lung scans in 622 outpatients with no clinical indication of PE and with proximal DVT confirmed by venography and showed that 40–50% had silent PE [34]. These findings provide compelling evidence that venous thromboembolism (VTE) is extensively overlooked and that PE is frequently undetected by physicians.

Critical care patients recovering from major trauma, spinal cord injury (SCI), or other critical illness share a high risk for VTE, they often have at least a temporary high bleeding risk, and there are relatively few thromboprophylaxis trials specific to these populations. Routine thromboprophylaxis should be provided to major trauma, SCI, and critical care patients based on an individual assessment of their thrombosis and bleeding risks. For patients at high risk for VTE, including those recovering from major trauma and SCI, prophylaxis with LMWH should commence as soon as hemostasis has been demonstrated. For critical care patients at lower thrombosis risk, either LMWH or low-dose heparin is recommended. For those with a very high risk of bleeding, mechanical prophylaxis should be instituted as early as possible and continued until pharmacologic prophylaxis can be initiated. The use of prophylactic inferior vena caval filters is strongly discouraged because their potential benefit has not been shown to outweigh the risks or substantial costs [18].

4.8.5.2 Heparin-Induced Thrombocytopenia

Heparin-induced thrombocytopenia (HIT) is the most significant adverse effect of heparin after bleeding complications. It is defined as a decrease in platelet count during or shortly following exposure to heparin. There are two categories of HIT: a benign form, also called type I, and an immune-mediated form called type II or "white clot syndrome" associated with an increased risk for potentially catastrophic thrombosis. It has been proposed that the term "HIT type I" be changed to "nonimmune heparin-associated thrombocytopenia," and that the term "HIT type II" be changed to "HIT" to avoid confusion between the two syndromes. In accordance with these new recommendations, the term HIT refers strictly to the clinically relevant, immune-mediated (i.e., type II) form [7].

HIT is immunologically mediated. The pathologic mechanism in HIT is antibody-induced platelet activation, leading to platelet loss (thrombocytopenia) and platelet aggregation (thrombosis). The principal antigen is a complex of heparin and platelet factor 4 (PF4). The HIT antibody cannot bind to the platelet in the absence of heparin. Following platelet activation, platelets may aggregate. Activated platelets also release additional PF4, perpetuating the cycle of heparin-induced platelet activation. Because the pathogenesis of HIT predominantly involves platelet activation, the resultant thrombi are platelet-rich with a white appearance, giving rise to the name "white clot syndrome." Recent evidence suggests that up to 8% of heparinized patients will develop the antibody associated with HIT without becoming thrombocytopenic [49]. One percent to 5% of patients on heparin will progress further to HIT with thrombocytopenia, and of those, at least one third will develop venous and/or arterial thrombosis [49].

Thrombocytopenia and thrombosis are the predominant clinical features of HIT. Despite the thrombocytopenia, bleeding complications are uncommon. Although thrombosis occurs in a small fraction of heparin-treated patients, when it occurs it tends to be extensive, with greatly increased morbidity and mortality. In patients receiving heparin for the first time, thrombocytopenia in HIT becomes clinically apparent 4–20 days after initiation of heparin, most commonly between days 5 and 12, with a median of day 10. Heparin-induced thrombocytopenia-associated thrombosis has been reported with normal platelet counts. However, most of thrombosis cases have occurred when the platelet count was decreased by at least 30–50%. Thrombosis in HIT is associated with a mortality of approximately 20–30%, with an equal number becoming permanently disabled by amputation, stroke, or other causes. The thrombosis often involves occlusions of large vessels, particularly the distal aorta and femoral arteries. Thrombosis may also lead to stroke, myocardial infarction, DVT, and PE. In addition, platelet aggregation can cause a disseminated intravascular coagulation-like syndrome in some patients [7].

Either a decrease in platelet count of 30% of the preheparin level or an unexpected thromboembolic event in a patient receiving heparin warrants consideration of the diagnosis of HIT. A heparin/PF4 enzyme-linked immunosorbent assay to detect the HIT antibody is commercially available. Up to 8% of patients on heparin without thrombocytopenia are positive by this assay. If HIT is considered, heparin should be discontinued immediately, and alternative forms of antithrombotic therapy commenced. This may include the use of danaparoid, hirudin, argatroban, vitamin-K antagonists, ancrod, iloprost, aspirin, dipyridamole, or dextran. Most importantly, close monitoring of the platelet count should be maintained in all patients receiving heparin to assure prompt diagnosis of HIT [7].

4.8.6 Sepsis-Associated Hemostatic Disorders

4.8.6.1 Thrombocytopenia

In the ICU, thrombocytopenia occurs in up to 20% of medical and 35% of surgical admissions. While there are many causes of thrombocytopenia in this setting, sepsis is a clear risk factor, with an estimated incidence of 35–59% [1]. In addition, there is an inverse relationship between the severity of sepsis and the platelet count [33]. Thrombocytopenia in sepsis arises from and/or coexists with intense platelet activation, increased platelet–endothelium interactions, and an underlying hypercoagulable state. Furthermore, thrombocytopenia is a predictor of mortality in ICU patients and in patients with severe sepsis. The degree and duration of thrombocytopenia, as well as the net change in the platelet count, are important determinants of survival.

Until recently, the reasons for sepsis-induced thrombocytopenia were unknown. Meanwhile, there are data indicating an immunologic etiology. Nonspecific platelet-associated antibodies can be detected in up to 30% of ICU patients. In these cases, nonpathogenic immunoglobulin G (IgG) presumably binds to bacterial products on the surface of platelets, to an altered platelet surface, or as immune complexes. A subset of patients with platelet-associated antibodies has autoantibodies directed against glycoprotein IIb/IIIa [44]. These antibodies have been implicated in the pathogenesis of immune thrombocytopenic purpura and, although not proven, may play a role in mediating sepsis-induced thrombocytopenia. Patients with sepsis may also develop de novo ethylenediaminetetraacetic acid (EDTA)-dependent antibodies, which cause platelet clumping in the test tube with a resultant pseudothrombocytopenia [35]. Nonimmune destruction of platelets is an important cause of thrombocytopenia in sepsis, a process that is only occasionally associated with underlying disseminated intravascular coagulation (DIC) (see Section 4.8.6.2).

Thrombocytopenia is a common cause of bleeding in the ICU. Patients with thrombocytopenia may have petechiae, purpura, bruising, or frank bleeding. The diagnosis of thrombocytopenia is made from the complete blood count. A peripheral smear may show evidence of platelet clumping. If that is the case, the platelet count should be remeasured in blood drawn into a tube that contains an anticoagulant other than EDTA. If the thrombocytopenia is associated with consumptive coagulopathy, the international normalized ratio (INR), PTT, thrombin time, D-dimers, fibrinogen, and/or thrombin–antithrombin complexes may be abnormal, and the peripheral smear may show schistocytes. Although patients with sepsis may have increased platelet-associated IgG, this test is nonspecific and does not help in guiding therapy.

While guidelines for prophylactic transfusions in patients with chemotherapy-induced thrombocytopenia have been established, the threshold for transfusing the thrombocytopenic patient with sepsis is not clear. Patients with sepsis have an underlying shift in the hemostatic balance toward the procoagulant side. Moreover, platelets are activated in the setting of sepsis and likely contribute in important ways to the pathogenesis of the syndrome. Therefore, when considering the cost-effectiveness of platelet transfusion, it is important to consider the theoretical risk of accelerating the underlying pathophysiology (i.e., "adding fuel to the fire"). This caveat notwithstanding (and in the absence of evidence-based guidelines), most patients are transfused to achieve a platelet count ≥ 10,000/μl. If the patient has concomitant coagulopathy (e.g., DIC or liver disease), active bleeding, or platelet dysfunction (e.g., uremia), it may be prudent to employ a more liberal transfusion strategy with the goal of maintaining an even higher platelet count.

4.8.6.2 Disseminated Intravascular Coagulation

DIC with disseminated fibrin depositions in the microcirculation of various organ systems is a frequent, if not invariable, finding in patients with septic shock [28].

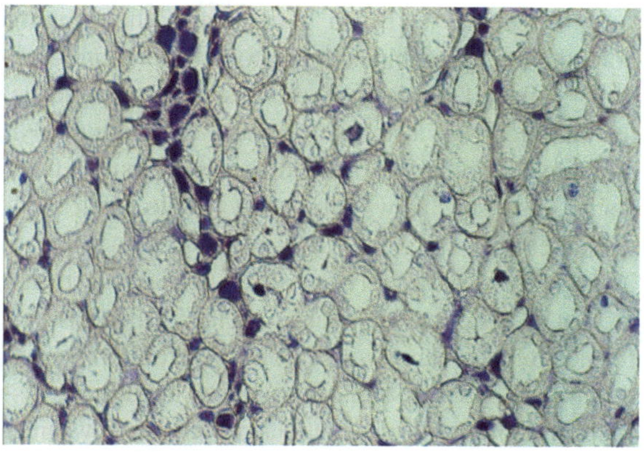

Fig. 4.8.3 Fibrin clot formation in the kidney during severe sepsis (animal model by injection of lipopolysaccharide (LPS) in hamsters. Light microscopy, 300× magnification, fibrin stain). Intravascular clots (blue) induce vascular occlusion and microcirculatory failure, thus leading to the typical acute renal failure (Resource: own laboratory)

This microvascular thrombosis is closely related to the development of multiple organ failure and is therefore linked to the prognosis of patients with septic shock [17]. The microvascular damage is especially pronounced in the lungs and kidneys (see Fig. 4.8.3). DIC is a condition in which the clotting and/or fibrinolytic systems are activated systemically, leading ultimately to the consumption of many coagulation factors and platelets. Such a consumptive state represents the decompensated or acute state of DIC in which the rate of platelet/factor consumption exceeds the body's capacity to synthesize these components. As a consequence, platelet and coagulation factor concentrations decrease steadily, ultimately leading to a breakdown of the physiologic hemostasis system. This results in a diffuse bleeding tendency which is often the first clinical manifestation of DIC. This process is encompassed in the term "consumptive coagulopathy" [28].

This decompensated form of DIC is relatively rare. It is always preceded, however, by a compensated form which is quite common in patients with many disorders and always present in severe sepsis. The compensated form of DIC is characterized by a "slower" generalized activation of the hemostasis system. Although platelets and coagulation factors are consumed more rapidly than normal, compensation can occur by increasing coagulation factor production in the liver, by the release of platelets from reserve storage sites and by the synthesis of inhibitors at an accelerated rate. As the clotting system becomes activated systemically, the inhibitor potential (antithrombin and the protein C/protein S systems) will tend to block this process; as a consequence, the inhibitors will also be consumed. This, in turn, will allow more clotting to proceed so that a positive feedback loop arises that will ultimately lead to the death of the patient.

Most laboratories rely on readily available tests that are not specific for DIC. Table 4.8.1 lists the tests performed by most laboratories. It is, therefore, important to take the patient's clinical situation, underlying disease, and the status of hepatic and bone marrow function into account when interpreting laboratory findings that suggest DIC. Unfortunately, these common laboratory tests only suggest acute (or decompensated) DIC. In patients with compensated (or chronic) DIC these laboratory tests are less reliable. APTT and PT may be normal or reduced, fibrinogen concentrations may be normal or elevated, and FSP and D-dimer concentrations may or may not be elevated. The last two tests are better performed using enzyme-linked immunosorbent assay (ELISA)-based assays; the routinely used latex agglutination tests may not be sufficiently sensitive. Platelet counts may be normal, but are mostly low, especially as time progresses.

The management of patients with DIC, whether compensated or decompensated, has to follow three basic approaches: (i) elimination of the underlying disorder (trigger); (ii) arrest of the intravascular clotting process; and (iii) substitution of coagulation constituents lost to consumption. The first approach is a very important one. In some instances, such as patients with obstetric complications associated with DIC, the underlying cause can be eliminated fairly rapidly. In others, treatment takes time so that the trigger will persist. It must be remembered that DIC will persist as long as the underlying disorder is not controlled.

The second approach should attempt to arrest the intravascular clotting process. The protein C anticoagulant pathway plays an integral part in modulating the coagulation and inflammatory responses to infection. In patients with sepsis, endogenous protein C levels are decreased, shifting the balance toward greater systemic inflammation, coagulation, and cell death. On the basis of a single large randomized phase III trial, drotrecogin alfa (activated), a recombinant form of human APC, was approved for the treatment of adult patients with severe sepsis and a high risk of death [3]. Since its approval, several questions have been raised regarding the appropriate use of this agent. Given the increased risk of serious bleeding and the high cost of treatment, drotrecogin alfa (activated) should be reserved at this time for the most acutely ill patients with severe sepsis who meet the criteria that were used in the phase III trial. In contrast to APC, studies with other anticoagulant drugs (e.g., tissue factor pathway inhibitor, antithrombin, heparin) trying to demonstrate beneficial effect so far failed. In patients with chronic, compensated DIC, such as some cancer patients, low-dose heparin (5,000–7,500 U) may be considered. These patients usually have no serious hemorrhagic disorder and display no symptoms or signs.

The third approach should try to replenish the consumed coagulation constituents. Diffuse hemorrhage in patients with acute, decompensated DIC is due to low concentrations of clotting factors and thrombocytopenia. Attempts must be made to raise the plasma concentrations of these lost constituents so that normal physiologic hemostasis can be achieved. Platelet concentrates and fresh-frozen plasma contain all the procoagulant factors needed for hemostasis and both should be administered in large quantities, depending, of course, on platelet counts and factor concentrations measured by APTT and PT. Clotting factor concentrates may be used to substitute lost components more rapidly but contain only selected factors. In DIC

Table 4.8.1 Laboratory tests used for diagnosis of DIC

Test	Acute, decompensated DIC	Chronic, compensated DIC
Activated partial thromboplastin time (APTT)	Prolonged	Normal or short
Prothrombin time (PT)	Prolonged	Normal or short
Platelet count	Decreased	Normal, elevated, or decreased
Fibrinogen levels	Decreased	Elevated or normal
Fibrin(ogen) split products (FSP)	Elevated	Elevated or normal
Fibrin monomer	Elevated	Elevated or normal
D-Dimer	Elevated	Elevated or normal
Antithrombin levels	Decreased	Decreased or normal
Thrombin–antithrombin complex (TAT)	Markedly elevated	Elevated or normal
Fragments 1 and 2	Markedly elevated	Elevated or normal

DIC disseminated intravascular coagulation

virtually all factors are consumed. Cryoprecipitate can be administered as a source of fibrinogen and other non-vitamin K-dependent factors. Erythrocyte concentrates are indicated to raise the oxygen-carrying potential.

4.8.7 Take Home Pearls

- Hemostasis is initiated by injury to the vascular wall, leading to the deposition of platelets adhering to components of the subendothelium. Platelet adhesion requires the presence of von Willebrand factor and platelet receptors. Additional platelets are recruited to the site of injury by release of platelet granular contents. The "platelet plug" is stabilized by interaction with fibrinogen.
- The protein C pathway is important for the negative control of both coagulation and inflammation. The pathway may be down-regulated in a variety of disease states to such an extent that the down-regulation contributes to the severity of the disease.
- Endothelium regulates both barrier function and coagulant reactions. This regulation occurs in response to environmental stimuli, such as cytokines, which have a central role in inflammation.
- Patients with known coagulation deficiencies, either congenital or acquired, may bleed spontaneously, with trauma or with surgical intervention. Unchallenged patients who bleed in a variety of clinical settings demand rapid diagnosis so that appropriate therapy can be instituted.
- Deep venous thrombosis and pulmonary embolism are major causes of morbidity and mortality in ICU patients. The main treatment objectives are the prevention of recurrent events and removal of thrombus in case of hemodynamic complications. Prevention is accomplished with anticoagulation. Fluid and vasoactive therapy may be indicated for refractory hypotension.
- Coagulation disorders in septic patients are primarily thrombocytopenia and disseminated intravascular coagulation (DIC). DIC contributes to bleeding and microvascular thrombosis, leading to organ dysfunction. Management of DIC must address the underlying disease, interrupt the activated coagulation system, and replace consumed clotting constituents.

References

1. Aird WC (2003) The hematologic system as a marker of organ dysfunction in sepsis. Mayo Clin Proc 78: 869–881
2. Bach R (1988) Initiation of coagulation by tissue factor. CRC Crit Rev Biochem 23: 339–368
3. Bernard GR, Vincent JL, Laterre PF, et al. (2001) Efficacy and safety of recombinant human activated protein C for severe sepsis. N Engl J Med 344: 699–709
4. Bevilacqua M, Pober J, Majeau G, et al. (1986) Recombinant TNF induces procoagulant activity in endothelium. Proc Natl Acad Sci USA 83: 4533–4537
5. Brett J, Gerlach H, Nawroth P, et al. (1989) TNF increases permeability of endothelial cell monolayers by a mechanism involving regulatory G proteins. J Exp Med 169: 1977–1991
6. Brownlee M, Cerami A, Vlassara H (1988) Advanced glycosylation end products in tissue and the biochemical basis of diabetic complications. N Engl J Med 318: 1315–1321
7. Comunale ME, Van Cott EM (2004) Heparin-induced thrombocytopenia. Int Anesthesiol Clin 42: 27–43
8. Cook DJ, Crowther MA, Meade M, et al. (2005) Deep venous thrombosis in medical-surgical critically ill patients: prevalence, incidence, and risk factors. Crit Care Med **33**: 1565–1571
9. Crowther MA, Lim W (2006) Measuring the anticoagulant effect of low molecular weight heparins in the critically ill. Crit Care 10: 150–151
10. Dahlback B (2000) Blood coagulation. Lancet 355: 1627–1632
11. Dobrovolsky AB, Titaeva EV (2002) The fibrinolysis system: regulation of activity and physiologic functions of its main components. Biochem 67: 99–108
12. Dorffler-Melly J, de Jonge E, Pont AC, et al. (2002) Bioavailability of subcutaneous low-molecular-weight heparin to patients on vasopressors. Lancet 359: 849–850
13. Esmon CT (1987) The regulation of natural anticoagulant pathways. Science 235: 1348–1352
14. Esmon CT (2000) Regulation of blood coagulation. Biochem Biophys Acta 1477: 349–360
15. Esmon CT (2003) The protein C pathway. Chest 124 (3 Suppl): 24S–32S
16. Esposito C, Gerlach H, Brett J, et al. (1989) Endothelial receptor-mediated binding of glucose-modified albumin is associated with increased monolayer permeability and modulation of cell surface coagulant properties. J Exp Med 170: 1387–1407
17. Fourrier F, Chopin C, Goudemand J, et al. (1992) Septic shock, multiple organ failure, and disseminated intravascular coagulation. Chest 101: 816–823
18. Geerts WH (2006) Prevention of venous thromboembolism in high-risk patients. Hematol Am Soc Hematol Educ Program 6: 462–466
19. George JN, Raskob GE (1998) Idiopathic thrombocytopenic purpura: diagnosis and management. Am J Med Sci 316: 87–93
20. Gerlach H, Esposito C, Stern DM (1990) Modulation of endothelial hemostatic properties: An active role in the host response. Annu Rev Med 41: 15–24
21. Gerlach H, Lieberman H, Bach R, et al. (1989) Enhanced responsiveness of endothelium in the growing/motile state to tumor necrosis factor/cachectin. J Exp Med 170: 913–931

22. Hekman C, Loskutoff D (1987) Fibrinolytic pathways and the endothelium. Semin Thromb Hemostas 13: 514–527
23. Hofer S, Schreckenberger R, Heindl B, et al. (2007) Hemorrhaging during pregnancy. Anaesthesist 56: 1075–1090
24. Hoffman M, Monroe DM (2001) A cell-based model of hemostasis. Thromb Haemost 85: 958–965
25. Kato H (2002) Regulation of functions of vascular wall cells by tissue factor pathway inhibitor. Basic and clinical aspects. Arterioscler Thromb Vasc Biol 22: 539–548
26. Lind SE (1991) The bleeding time does not predict surgical bleeding. Blood 77: 2547–2552
27. Livio M, Gotti E, Marchesi D, et al. (1982) Uremic bleeding: role of anemia and beneficial effect of red blood cell transfusions. Lancet 2: 1013–1015
28. Mammen EF (1998) The haematological manifestations of sepsis. J Antimicrob Chemother 41(Suppl A): 17–24
29. Mannucci PM (1997) Desmopressin (DDAVP) in the treatment of bleeding disorders: the first 20 years. Blood 90: 2515–2521
30. Mannucci PM, Duga S, Peyvandi F (2004) Recessively inherited coagulation disorders. Blood 104: 1243–1252
31. Mannucci PM, Tuddenbam EG (1999) The hemophiliac: progress and problems. Semin Hematol 36: 104–117
32. Matsuda N, Hattori Y (2007) Vascular biology in sepsis: pathophysiological and therapeutic significance of vascular dysfunction. J Smooth Muscle Res 43: 117–137
33. Mavrommatis AC, Theodoridis T, Orfanidou A, et al. (2000) Coagulation system and platelets are fully activated in uncomplicated sepsis. Crit Care Med 28: 451–457
34. Meignan M, Rosso J, Gauthier H, et al. (2000) Systematic lung scans reveal a high frequency of silent pulmonary embolism in patients with proximal deep venous thrombosis. Arch Intern Med 160: 159–164
35. Mori M, Kudo H, Yoshitake S, et al. (2000) Transient EDTA-dependent pseudothrombocytopenia in a patient with sepsis. Intensive Care Med 26: 218–220
36. Nawroth P, Handley D, Esmon C, et al. (1986) Interleukin 1 induces endothelial cell procoagulant while suppressing cell-surface anticoagulant activity. Proc Natl Acad Sci USA 83: 3460–3464
37. Ofosu FA (2002) The blood platelet as a model for regulating blood coagulation on cell surfaces and its consequences. Biochem 67: 47–54
38. Passarino G, Nobili A, Colombo A, et al. (1982) Pulmonary thromboembolism in medical wards: observations on 546 autopsy cases. G It Cardiol 12: 11–16
39. Rimon S, Melamed R, Savion N, et al. (1987) Identification of a factor IX/IXa binding protein on the endothelial cell surface. J Biol Chem 262: 6023–6031
40. Rosenberg R, Rosenberg J (1984) Natural anticoagulant mechanisms. J Clin Invest 74: 1–4
41. Ryu JH, Olson EJ, Pellikka PA (1998) Clinical recognition of pulmonary embolism: problem of unrecognized and asymptomatic cases. Mayo Clin Proc 73: 873–879
42. Sadler JE (2003) Von Willebrand disease type 1: a diagnosis in search of a disease. Blood 101:2089–2093
43. Sherry B, Cerami A (1988) Cachectin/tumor necrosis factor exerts endocrine, paracrine, and autocrine control of inflammatory responses. J Cell Biol 107: 1269–1277
44. Stephan F, Cheffi MA, Kaplan C, et al. (2000) Autoantibodies against platelet glycoproteins in critically ill patients with thrombocytopenia. Am J Med 108: 554–560
45. Stern D, Nawroth P, Kisiel W, et al. (1985) The binding of factor IXa to cultured bovine aortic endothelial cells. J Biol Chem 260: 6717–6722
46. Tapson VF, Humbert M (2006) Incidence and prevalence of chronic thromboembolic pulmonary hypertension. Proc Am Thorac Soc 3:564–567
47. Triplett DA (2000) Coagulation and bleeding disorders: review and update. Clin Chem 46: 1260–1269
48. Vigano GL, Mannucci PM, Lattuada A, et al. (1985) Subcutaneous desmopressin (DDAVP) shortens the bleeding time in uremia. Am J Hematol 31: 32–35
49. Warkentin TE, Levine MN, Hirsh J, et al. (1995) Heparin-induced thrombocytopenia in patients treated with low-molecular weight heparin or unfractionated heparin. N Engl J Med 332: 1330–1335
50. Whatley R, Zimmerman G, McIntyre T, et al. (1987) Production of platelet activating factor by endothelial cells. Semin Thromb Hemostas 13: 445–453

4.9 Neurological Problems

Raf Brouns and Peter Paul De Deyn

Core Messages

- Neurological complications, whether due to the uremic state or its treatment, contribute largely to the morbidity and mortality in patients with renal failure.
- Despite therapeutic advances, many neurological complications of uremia, such as uremic encephalopathy, atherosclerosis, neuropathy, and myopathy, fail to fully respond to dialysis.
- Moreover, dialysis can directly or indirectly be associated with dialysis dementia, dysequilibrium syndrome, aggravation of atherosclerosis, cerebrovascular accidents due to ultrafiltration-related arterial hypotension, hypertensive encephalopathy, Wernicke's encephalopathy, hemorrhagic stroke, subdural hematoma, osmotic myelinolysis, opportunistic infections, intracranial hypertension, and mononeuropathy.
- Renal transplantation itself can give rise to acute femoral neuropathy, rejection encephalopathy, and neuropathy in graft-versus-host disease. The use of immunosuppressive drugs after renal transplant can cause encephalopathy, movement disorders, opportunistic infections, neoplasms, myopathy, and progression of atherosclerosis.

4.9.1 Introduction

Disease-related and treatment-related neurological complications remain an important source of morbidity in patients with renal failure. With the introduction of dialysis and renal transplantation, the spectrum of neurological complications changed [1]. The incidence and severity of uremic encephalopathy, atherosclerosis, neuropathy, and myopathy have declined, but many patients fail to fully respond to dialytic therapy. Complications that can occur as a direct consequence of dialysis are rare nowadays, thanks to improved dialysis techniques, and can include dialysis dementia, dialysis dysequilibrium syndrome, hypertensive encephalopathy, and cerebrovascular accidents due to ultrafiltration-related arterial hypotension. Furthermore, dialysis is associated with aggravation of atherosclerosis and can contribute to the development of Wernicke's encephalopathy, hemorrhagic stroke, subdural hematoma, osmotic myelinolysis, opportunistic infections, intracranial hypertension, and neuropathy. Patients with renal failure may benefit from kidney transplantation, but the use of immunosuppressive drugs can cause encephalopathy, movement disorders, opportunistic infections, neoplasms, myopathy, and progression of atherosclerosis. A renal transplant itself can give rise to acute femoral neuropathy, rejection encephalopathy, and neuropathy in graft-versus-host disease. In what follows, we will address both central and peripheral nervous system complications in patients with renal failure.

P. P. De Deyn (✉)
Department of Neurology and Memory Clinic, Middelheim General Hospital, Lindenreef 1, 2020 Antwerp, Belgium
e-mail: peter.dedeyn@ua.ac.be

A. Jörres et al. (eds.), *Management of Acute Kidney Problems*,
DOI: 10.1007/978-3-540-69441-0_4.9,

4.9.2 Central Nervous System Complications

4.9.2.1 Encephalopathy

In patients with renal failure, encephalopathy is a common problem that may be caused by uremia, thiamine deficiency, dialysis, transplant rejection, hypertension, fluid, and electrolyte disturbances or drug toxicity (Table 4.9.1). In general, encephalopathy presents with a symptom complex progressing from mild sensorial clouding to delirium and coma. It is often associated with headache, visual abnormalities, tremor, asterixis, multifocal myoclonus, chorea, and seizures. These signs fluctuate from day to day or sometimes from hour to hour. Besides this general symptom complex, focal motor signs and the "uremic twitch-convulsive" syndrome can be seen in uremic encephalopathy [2], and dialysis results in significant improvement. Electroencephalographic findings are nonspecific but in contrast to the level of azotemia [3], they correlate with the degree of neurological dysfunction and therefore may be of diagnostic value especially if serial studies are performed [4]. Typically, an excess of delta and theta waves and sometimes bilateral spike-wave complexes are found (Fig. 4.9.1). With progression of the uremic state, the electroencephalogram displays more slow activity [3]. Cerebral imaging is not necessary for the diagnosis, but is useful to exclude other causes of confusion. The pathophysiology of uremic encephalopathy is complex and poorly understood. Accumulation of numerous organic substances occurs, among which urea and guanidine compounds, hormonal disturbance, disturbance of the intermediary metabolism, and imbalance in excitatory and inhibitory neurotransmitters have been identified as contributing factors, but no single metabolite has been identified as the sole cause of uremia [5–10]. Wernicke's encephalopathy typically presents with the triad of ophthalmoplegia, ataxia, and cognitive symptoms or disturbances of consciousness. Because the complete triad is rarely present and because of similarities with uremic encephalopathy, this disorder often remains unrecognized, with high fatality rates as a consequence. A good outcome, however, can be obtained if thiamine is administrated immediately [11]. Hemodialysis patients especially are at risk because of not only low thiamine intake but probably also accelerated loss of thiamine [3, 11]. Dialysis encephalopathy or dialysis dementia is rare nowadays but sporadically occurs due to errors in dialysis water purification or the use of aluminum hydroxide or aluminum-based phosphate binders [3, 12, 13]. Accumulation of aluminum in many organs results in microcytic anemia, osteomalacia, and subacute progressive neurological symptomatology finally leading to dementia [2, 14]. Chelation with deferoxamine is the treatment of choice [15]. Rejection encephalopathy may be present in patients with systemic features of acute graft rejection [16] and typically occurs within 3 months of transplant, but cases up to 2 years after transplant have been reported. Adequate treatment of the rejection episode results in rapid and complete recovery [17]. In hypertensive

Table 4.9.1 Encephalopathy in renal failure

Encephalopathy	(Presumed) pathophysiology	Therapeutic or preventive measures
Uremic encephalopathy	Accumulation neurotoxins Disturbance intermediary metabolism Hormonal disturbances	Dialysis or kidney transplant
Wernicke's encephalopathy	Thiamine deficiency	Thiamine administration
Dialysis encephalopathy/dementia	Aluminum accumulation	Use of aluminum free dialysate Avoid aluminum-based phosphate binders Administration of deferoxamine
Rejection encephalopathy	Cytokine production due to rejection process	↑ Immunosuppression
Hypertensive encephalopathy	Cerebral vasogenic edema	Antihypertensive treatment
Dysequilibrium syndrome	Reverse urea effect Intracellular acidosis in cerebral cortex	Self-limited
Fluid and electrolyte disturbances	↑ Calcium, magnesium, natrium, osmolality ↓ Natrium, osmolality	Correction of electrolyte imbalance
Drug toxicity	Drugs metabolized or excreted by kidney Immunosuppressive drugs	Dose reduction or cessation

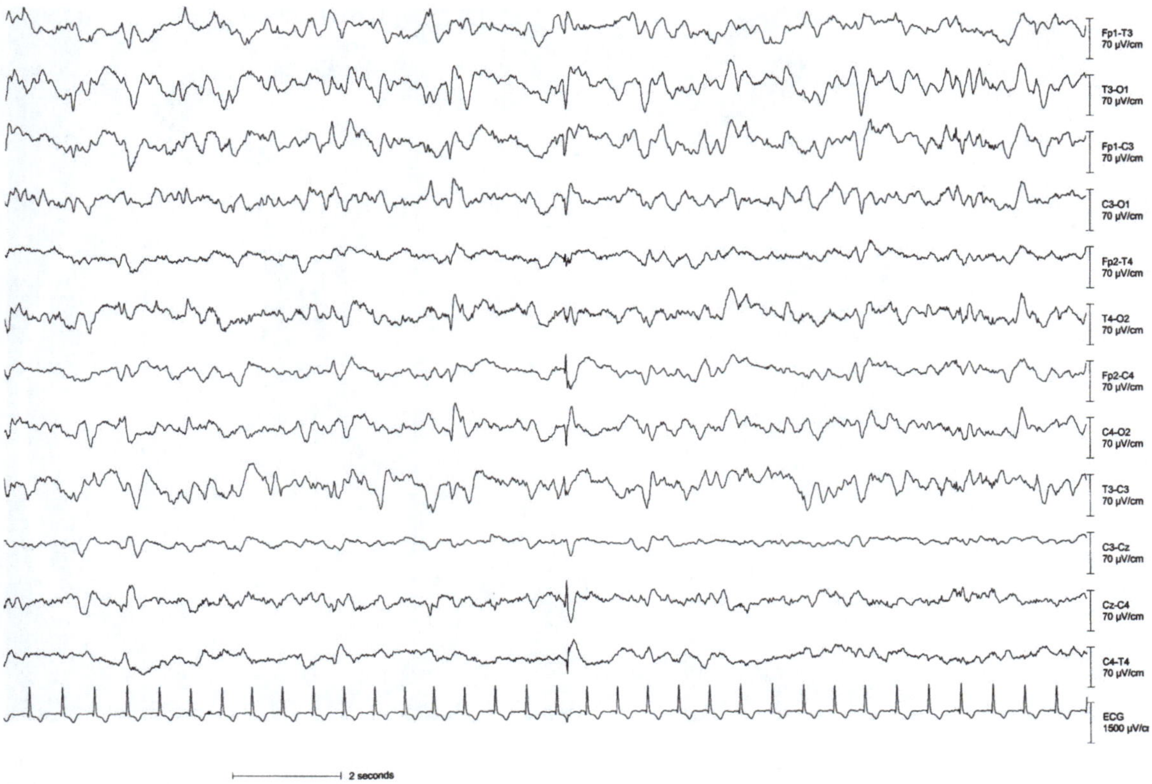

Fig. 4.9.1 Electroencephalographic findings in a patient with uremic encephalopathy, showing generalized slowing with an excess of delta and theta waves and bilateral spikes

encephalopathy, patients display the encephalopathic symptom complex in combination with severe hypertension. Magnetic resonance imaging (MRI) often demonstrates posterior leukoencephalopathy (Fig. 4.9.2). Accurate diagnosis and immediate antihypertensive treatment is regarded as a medical emergency because symptoms and imaging abnormalities may be reversible [18]. Dialytic treatment can be associated with the dialysis dysequilibrium syndrome which typically presents with headache, nausea, muscle cramps and twitching, delirium, and seizures [19]. The dysequilibrium syndrome tends to be self-limiting and subsides over several hours to days. It is thought to be the consequence of transient cerebral edema either due to relative slow clearance of urea from the brain [20], formation of osmoles in the brain [20], or intracellular acidosis in the cerebral cortex. Slow dialysis and addition of osmotically active solute to the dialysate can prevent the condition [3]. Fluid and electrolyte disturbances are common in patients with renal failure and can produce central nervous system depression with encephalopathy as the major clinical manifestation (Table 4.9.2). Especially hypercalcemia, hypermagnesemia, hyponatremia, and hypernatremia, hypoosmolality and hyperosmolality are known to cause this problem [21]. Symptoms subside after correction of the electrolyte imbalance. Encephalopathy due to drug toxicity is often seen in patients with kidney failure, mainly with drugs that are normally metabolized or excreted by the kidney (including acyclovir and radiographic contrast) [22, 23]. Further, protein binding of drugs can be altered in renal failure, which not only might affect the therapeutic effectiveness of the drug, but also could result in neurotoxicity [24]. Immunosuppressant-associated encephalopathy has been described with the calcineurin inhibitors cyclosporine [25] and tacrolimus (FK506) [26] and to a lesser extend with muromonab-CD3 (OKT3) [27]. Neurotoxicity associated with these drugs is more frequent with toxic levels but may be apparent at levels within the therapeutic range. Common manifestations are tremor, headache, cerebellar, or extrapyramidal signs [28].

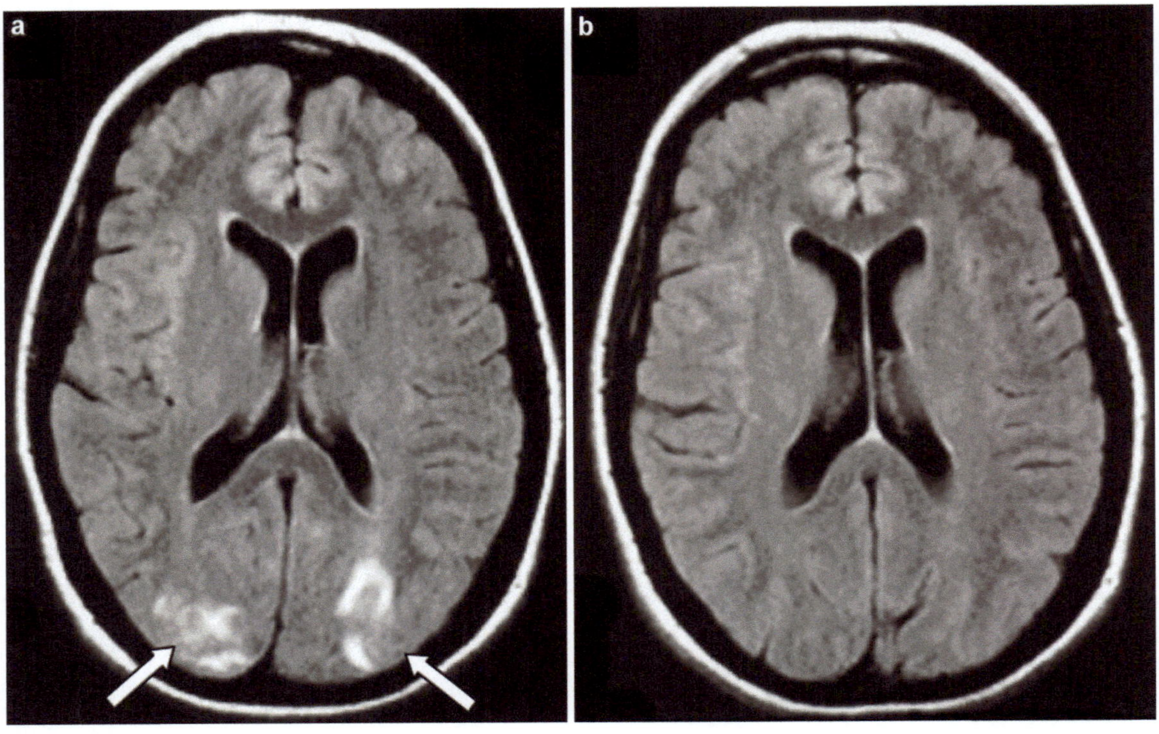

Fig. 4.9.2 Initial magnetic resonance imaging of the brain in a patient with severe hypertension, headache, confusion, and visual disturbances reveals typical subcortical edema in the occipital regions with only minimal cortical involvement (*arrows*) on axial FLAIR sequence (**a**). One week later, after antihypertensive treatment and clinical improvement, follow-up study reveals complete resolution of the lesions (**b**)

The most serious complication is reversible posterior leukoencephalopathy [26] with subcortical and deep white matter changes [18, 29] resembling upon imaging to those found in hypertensive encephalopathy. Dose reduction or discontinuation of immunosuppressive drugs mostly results in resolution of clinical symptoms and neuroimaging abnormalities.

4.9.2.2 Cerebrovascular Disease

Cerebrovascular disease is a predominant cause of morbidity and mortality in patients with renal failure. Ischemic stroke in renal failure mainly results from atherosclerosis, thromboembolic disease, or intradialytic hypotension. Atherosclerosis in patients with chronic renal failure is generally more diffuse and distally located than in the general population, probably because of the combination of traditional atherogenic risk factors with factors more specifically related to renal failure and its treatment [30–32]. In particular, renal failure may be associated with accumulation of guanidino compounds [33, 34], oxidative and carbonyl stress [35], hyperhomocysteinemia [36], and disturbances of the calcium-phosphate metabolism that may hamper endothelial function [37]. Dialysis by itself appears to promote the development of arterial disease [38], and progression of atherosclerosis may be influenced by the use of immunosuppressive agents used in renal transplant recipients [30]. Thromboembolic ischemic stroke may result from either characteristic cardiac disease in renal failure, e.g., dilated cardiomyopathy and arrhythmias [39, 40] or "artery-to-artery embolism" due to severe atherosclerosis. Ultrafiltration-related arterial hypotension is a common complication of hemodialysis, especially in patients with anemia [41] and autonomic neuropathy [42]. Severe arterial hypotension can result in cerebral hypoperfusion and eventually ischemic stroke which is typically located in the boundary zones between the vascular territories of the cerebral arteries [43]. The use of sodium profiling, cool dialysate, midodrine, and possibly sertraline can increase hemodynamic stability during dialysis

Table 4.9.2 Neurological complications related to treatment of renal failure

Neurological complication	Pathophysiology
Wernicke's encephalopathy	Accelerated loss of thiamine in hemodialysis
Dialysis dementia	Aluminum-containing dialysate
	Aluminum-based phosphate binders
Rejection encephalopathy	Cytokine production in renal transplant rejection
Dysequilibrium syndrome	Reverse urea effect in dialysis
	Intracellular acidosis in cerebral cortex
Immunosuppressant-associated encephalopathy	Disruption blood-brain barrier, axonal swelling, extracellular edema, demyelination, drug metabolites, microvascular damage
Ischemic stroke	↑ Atherosclerosis due to unsuitable dialysate calcium concentration, bioincompatibility in dialysis, calcium-containing phosphate binders, immunosuppressive
	Intradialytic hypotension
Hypertensive encephalopathy	Cerebral vasogenic edema due to (intradialytic) hypertension
Intracerebral hemorrhage	Anticoagulation in hemodialysis
Subdural hematoma	Anticoagulation in hemodialysis, rapid ultrafiltration, use of hypertonic dialysate, cerebral atrophy
Osmotic myelinolysis	Rapid correction of chronic hypo- or hyperosmolar state, eventually by dialysis
Movement disorders	Drug-induced in hemodialysis patients
	Immunosuppressive agents (cyclosporine, tacrolimus)
Opportunistic infections	↑ Infection hazard and immunosuppression in dialysis
	Immunosuppressants in renal transplant patients
Neoplasms	Immunosuppression due to dialysis
	Immunosuppressants in transplant patients
Intracranial hypertension	Pseudotumor cerebri secondary to dialysis or steroids
Carpal tunnel syndrome	Compression median nerve by arteriovenous fistula or dialysis-associated amyloidosis
Acute femoral neuropathy	Compression or ischemia during renal transplantation
Non-uremic neuropathy	Graft versus host disease in transplant patients
Steroid-induced myopathy	Use of steroids, especially in transplant patients

[44, 45]. Since renal anemia is an independent risk factor for stroke in chronic renal failure [46], treatment with recombinant human erythropoietin seems an important preventive measure.

The uremic state causes platelet dysfunction and altered platelet–vessel wall interaction resulting in a bleeding tendency and increased risk of hemorrhagic stroke [47]. Hemodialysis can partially correct the bleeding tendency but is associated with a higher incidence of intracerebral hemorrhage and subarachnoidal hemorrhage by itself [48]. Other factors predestinating patients with renal failure for hemorrhagic stroke are hypertension, the use of anticoagulation or platelet antiaggregants, and polycystic kidney disease that associated with a tenfold increased risk for cerebral vascular malformations [48, 49]. Regional or minimal heparinization in patients treated with hemodialysis reduces the bleeding risk. Peritoneal dialysis or heparin-free dialysis may be indicated for patients who are actively bleeding or have recently suffered a cerebral hemorrhage [49, 50]. Systemic anticoagulation in hemodialysis can also be complicated by subdural hematoma, especially if combined with other predisposing factors for this condition such as cerebral atrophy [51], hypertension, rapid ultrafiltration, and the use of hypertonic dialysate [52]. The occurrence of subdural hematoma is well known but frequently overlooked because of clinical similarity with encephalopathy and dementia. However, diagnosis can easily be made by cerebral imaging. Neurosurgical intervention can be done by burr hole aspiration or craniotomy. However, conservative therapy with replacement of hemodialysis by peritoneal dialysis or continuation of hemodialysis without anticoagulation is often sufficient [53].

4.9.2.3 Cognitive Impairment

Patients with renal failure are prone to cognitive impairment and dementia even when uremia is treated adequately [54, 55]. The incidence of dementia in aged patients undergoing dialysis is estimated at 4.2% [56] with predominant occurrence of multi-infarct dementia [57]. Subacute dementia can occur in progressive multifocal leukoencephalopathy [58] and dialysis dementia [3, 13].

4.9.2.4 Osmotic Myelinolysis

Osmotic myelinolysis in patients with renal failure mainly occurs within the basis pontis, but extrapontine regions can be affected as well [59]. Central pontine myelinolysis is clinically characterized by acute progressive quadriplegia, dysarthria, dysphagia, and alterations of consciousness. With expansion of the demyelination through the midbrain, horizontal, and vertical gaze paralysis can be seen. Parkinsonism or ataxia can occur when the basal nuclei or the cerebellum are affected, respectively. T2-weighted MRI demonstrates hyperintense patchy areas of demyelination [60]. The prognosis is often fatal, and in those who survive, maximum recovery may require several months. Treatment is supportive only. Since osmotic myelinolysis after rapid correction of prolonged hyponatremia – or less frequent hypernatremia – by dialysis is well known [61] and since it is thought to be the result of glial edema due to fluctuating osmotic forces, it probably is important to correct chronic hyponatremia slowly and to avoid hypernatremia. On the other hand, rapid serum sodium correction by hemodialysis occurs often, but only a few patients develop demyelination.

4.9.2.5 Movement Disorders and Restless Legs Syndrome

Movement disorders in patients with renal failure can occur as a result of encephalopathy, medication, or structural lesions. A typical movement disorder in uremic encephalopathy is the uremic "twitch-convulsive" syndrome that consists of intense asterixis or "flapping tremor" and myoclonic jerks that are accompanied by fasciculations, muscle twitches, and seizures [1, 2]. Thiamine deficiency is thought to cause a dysfunction of the basal ganglia which may induce chorea [62], and elevated serum manganese levels may be associated with symmetric hyperintensity in the globus pallidus on T1-weighted MRI that may present with parkinsonian symptoms or myoclonus [63]. Involuntary movements secondary to cyclosporine and tacrolimus neurotoxicity mainly present with extrapyramidal signs [28]. Patients with renal failure are prone to structural intracranial lesions secondary to cerebrovascular disease, myelinolysis, neoplasms, and opportunistic infections. Lesions are located in the basal ganglia and may induce extrapyramidal movement disorders. Furthermore, acute movement disorders can be caused by bilateral basal ganglia lesions due to hypoperfusion with global brain ischemia and selective vulnerability of the basal ganglia to hypoxemia and uremic toxins [64]. The restless legs syndrome is a common disorder that is characterized by an imperative need to move the legs because of paresthesias that worsen during periods of inactivity. At least 20% of patients with chronic renal failure suffer from this incapacitating disorder [65, 66]. In general, dialysis does not substantially improve uremic restless legs syndrome but the use of cool dialysate fluid [67], levodopa, dopamine agonists, benzodiazepines (e.g., clonazepam), gabapentin, clonidine, or opioids may bring relief [68]. Substantial improvement after kidney transplant has been described [69].

4.9.2.6 Opportunistic Infections

Neurological infections in patients with renal failure mainly present as acute, subacute, or chronic meningitis, encephalitis, myelitis, or brain abscess [70]. Opportunistic infections often are the consequence of immunosuppression associated with the uremic state itself [71], dialysis, and immunosuppressive agents. Early diagnosis may be difficult in this population because the usual signs of infection are blunted and infection with uncommon opportunistic organisms frequently occurs. Lumbar puncture is often indicated, but should only be performed after exclusion of intracranial space–occupying lesions. Treatment with antimicrobial therapy and reduction of immunosuppressive agents should not be delayed. If a definitive diagnosis cannot be made in a reasonable time, empirical therapy must be started [3].

4.9.2.7 Neoplasms

The immunosuppressive state of patients with renal failure also predisposes to neoplasms [72]. Malignant meningioma [73] and primary central nervous system lymphoma have been described in end-stage renal failure [74–76]. With the increased incidence of urogenital, gastrointestinal, hematological, and endocrine neoplasia in end-stage renal disease [72, 77], one can expect a higher risk of brain metastasis.

4.9.2.8 Intracranial Hypotension

Dehydration and uremia can result in intracranial hypotension, presenting with orthostatic headache that occasionally may be associated with neck stiffness, visual disturbances, and cranial nerve palsy [78]. Accurate diagnosis is important since subdural hematoma may develop [79], and conservative management with bed rest, increased fluid intake, and administration of steroids is quite effective [80]. MRI typically shows diffuse pachymeningeal gadolinium enhancement, often with imaging evidence of descent of the brain [81]. The diagnosis can be confirmed by measuring cerebrospinal fluid pressure [80].

4.9.2.9 Intracranial Hypertension

Intracranial hypertension in patients with renal failure can be idiopathic, or secondary to dialysis, use of steroids, or intracranial lesions [82]. Idiopathic intracranial hypertension can be diagnosed in a patient with symptoms due to elevated intracranial pressure, normal findings on neuroimaging and increased cerebrospinal fluid pressure with a normal composition [83]. Intracranial hypertension results in papilledema and progressive optic atrophy with accompanying visual disturbances and eventually blindness. The treatment goal is to prevent visual impairment by management of the underlying renal disease and if possible use of acetazolamide, furosemide, or corticosteroids [82, 84]. Surgery should be considered in patients with deterioration of visual function despite maximum medical treatment [82].

4.9.3 Peripheral Nervous System Complications

4.9.3.1 Mononeuropathy

Susceptibility of the peripheral nerves to compression and local ischemia is increased in uremia. Damage to the ulnar and median nerve in patients with renal failure typically occurs at Guyon's canal and the carpal tunnel. It may be the consequence of uremic tumoral calcinosis, dialysis-associated amyloidosis, or an arteriovenous shunt for dialysis [85–88]. Renal transplant may bring relief but does not reverse the amyloidosis [89], and dialysis with biocompatible membranes and pure dialysis water slows down disease progression [90]. If conservative treatment with antiinflammatory medication, tricyclic antidepressants, anticonvulsants, and splinting show no response, or if motor deficits develop, surgical neurolysis is indicated. Acute femoral neuropathy is estimated to occur in about 2% of patients undergoing a renal transplant. It is the result of nerve compression by retractors or ischemia [91] and mostly has a good prognosis [92].

4.9.3.2 Polyneuropathy

Well-known causes of polyneuropathy in patients with renal failure are uremic or diabetic polyneuropathy and neuropathy associated with graft-versus-host disease or systemic vasculitides [93]. Uremic polyneuropathy occurs in approximately 60% of patients with chronic renal failure and can affect motor, sensory, autonomic, and cranial nerves [94]. An early finding is elevation of the vibratory threshold and impaired temperature sensibility [95, 96]. Paradoxical heat sensation, paresthesias, or pain are common [97]. Later in the course, ascending hypesthesia, hyporeflexia or areflexia, restless legs, muscle weakness, cramps, and atrophy can be found. The neuropathy usually evolves over several months, but rarely an acute or subacute course is seen. Autonomic neuropathy can play a role in the pathogenesis of intradialytic and orthostatic hypotension [42]. Electrophysiologically, mainly axonal loss and secondary demyelination can be found. In most patients, uremic neuropathy will stabilize or even improve during chronic dialysis [98, 99]. Renal transplant can result in recovery from uremic neuropathy through remyelinization [100], but if extended axonal degeneration has developed and large numbers of axons are lost, results are disappointing [94]. Improvement after supplementation with biotin, pyridoxine, cobalamin, and thiamine has been described [101, 102].

4.9.3.3 Myopathy

Uremic myopathy is common in patients with end-stage renal disease and manifests as proximal limb weakness, with muscle wasting, limited endurance, exercise limitation, and rapid fatigability [103]. In general, physical examination, electromyography, and muscle enzymes are normal [104]. Muscle biopsy occasionally reveals structural alterations, mainly fiber atrophy that predominantly involves type II fibers [105]. No specific treatment exists for uremic myopathy, but aerobic exercise training, prevention, and treatment of secondary hyperparathyroidism, dietary corrections, and treatment of renal anemia may be of use [103, 104, 106]. Conflicting results about L-carnitine supplementation are reported [107]. A successful renal transplant significantly reduces complaints, but does not fully restore physical working capacity [104]. Uremic myopathy should be differentiated from steroid-induced myopathy and ischemic myopathy secondary to atherosclerosis. Moreover, water and electrolyte disturbances with hypermagnesemia, hypocalcemia, or hypercalcemia and hypokalemia or hyperkalemia in particular can mimic myopathy [21].

4.9.4 Conclusion

Neurological complications whether due to the uremic state or its treatment, contribute greatly to the morbidity and mortality in patients with renal failure. Despite continuous therapeutic progress, most neurological complications of uremia fail to fully respond to dialysis and many are elicited or aggravated by dialysis or renal transplant.

References

1. Brouns R, De Deyn PP: Neurological complications in renal failure: a review. Clin Neurol Neurosurg. 2004;107:1–16.
2. De Deyn PP, Saxena VK, Abts H, et al.: Clinical and pathophysiological aspects of neurological complications in renal failure. Acta Neurol Belg. 1992;92:191–206.
3. Burn DJ, Bates D: Neurology and the kidney. J Neurol Neurosurg Psychiatry. 1998;65:810–821.
4. Rohl JE, Harms L, Pommer W: Quantitative EEG findings in patients with chronic renal failure. Eur J Med Res. 2007; 12:173–178.
5. Vanholder R, De SR, Glorieux G, et al.: Review on uremic toxins: classification, concentration, and interindividual variability. Kidney Int. 2003;63:1934–1943.
6. De Deyn PP, D'Hooge R, Van Bogaert PP, Marescau B: Endogenous guanidino compounds as uremic neurotoxins. Kidney Int Suppl. 2001;78:S77–S83.
7. D'Hooge R, Pei YQ, Manil J, De Deyn PP: The uremic guanidino compound guanidinosuccinic acid induces behavioral convulsions and concomitant epileptiform electrocorticographic discharges in mice. Brain Res. 1992;598: 316–320.
8. D'Hooge R, Pei YQ, Marescau B, De Deyn PP: Convulsive action and toxicity of uremic guanidino compounds: behavioral assessment and relation to brain concentration in adult mice. J Neurol Sci. 1992;112:96–105.
9. Meyer TW, Hostetter TH: Uremia. N Engl J Med. 2007; 357:1316–1325.
10. Torremans A, Marescau B, Kranzlin B, et al.: Biochemical validation of a rat model for polycystic kidney disease: comparison of guanidino compound profile with the human condition. Kidney Int. 2006;69:2003–2012.
11. Sechi G, Serra A: Wernicke's encephalopathy: new clinical settings and recent advances in diagnosis and management. Lancet Neurol. 2007;6:442–455.
12. Andrade LG, Garcia FD, Silva VS, et al.: Dialysis encephalopathy secondary to aluminum toxicity, diagnosed by bone biopsy. Nephrol Dial Transplant. 2005;20:2581–2582.
13. Mach JR, Jr., Korchik WP, Mahowald MW: Dialysis dementia. Clin Geriatr Med. 1988;4:853–867.
14. Dunea G: Dialysis dementia: an epidemic that came and went. ASAIO J. 2001;47:192–194.
15. Hernandez P, Johnson CA: Deferoxamine for aluminum toxicity in dialysis patients. ANNA J. 1990;17:224–228.
16. Gross ML, Sweny P, Pearson RM, Kennedy J, Fernando ON, Moorhead JF: Rejection encephalopathy. An acute neurological syndrome complicating renal transplantation. J Neurol Sci. 1982;56:23–34.
17. Gross ML, Pearson R, Sweny P, Fernando ON, Moorhead JF: Rejection encephalopathy. Proc Eur Dial Transplant Assoc. 1981;18:461–464.
18. Port JD, Beauchamp NJ, Jr.: Reversible intracerebral pathologic entities mediated by vascular autoregulatory dysfunction. Radiographics. 1998;18:353–367.
19. Benna P, Lacquaniti F, Triolo G, Ferrero P, Bergamasco B: Acute neurologic complications of hemodialysis. Study of 14,000 hemodialyses in 103 patients with chronic renal failure. Ital J Neurol Sci. 1981;2:53–57.
20. Silver SM, Sterns RH, Halperin ML: Brain swelling after dialysis: old urea or new osmoles? Am J Kidney Dis. 1996; 28:1–13.
21. Riggs JE: Neurologic manifestations of fluid and electrolyte disturbances. Neurol Clin. 1989;7:509–523.
22. Muruve DA, Steinman TI: Contrast-induced encephalopathy and seizures in a patient with chronic renal insufficiency. Clin Nephrol. 1996;45:406–409.
23. Peces R, de la TM, Alcazar R: Acyclovir-associated encephalopathy in haemodialysis. Nephrol Dial Transplant. 1996;11:752.
24. Vanholder R, Van LN, De SR, Schoots A, Ringoir S: Drug protein binding in chronic renal failure: evaluation of nine drugs. Kidney Int. 1988;33:996–1004.
25. Chang SH, Lim CS, Low TS, Chong HT, Tan SY: Cyclosporine-associated encephalopathy: a case report and literature review. Transplant Proc. 2001;33:3700–3701.
26. Parvex P, Pinsk M, Bell LE, O'Gorman AM, Patenaude YG, Gupta IR: Reversible encephalopathy associated with

tacrolimus in pediatric renal transplants. Pediatr Nephrol. 2001;16:537–542.
27. Parizel PM, Snoeck HW, van den HL, et al.: Cerebral complications of murine monoclonal CD3 antibody (OKT3): CT and MR findings. AJNR Am J Neuroradiol. 1997;18: 1935–1938.
28. Bechstein WO: Neurotoxicity of calcineurin inhibitors: impact and clinical management. Transpl Int. 2000;13: 313–326.
29. Inoha S, Inamura T, Nakamizo A, Ikezaki K, Amano T, Fukui M: Magnetic resonance imaging in cases with encephalopathy secondary to immunosuppressive agents. J Clin Neurosci. 2002;9:305–307.
30. Capron L, Grateau G: Accelerated arterial disease in renal transplant recipients. Nephrol Dial Transplant. 1998;13 (Suppl 4):49–50.
31. Cheung AK, Sarnak MJ, Yan G, et al.: Atherosclerotic cardiovascular disease risks in chronic hemodialysis patients. Kidney Int. 2000;58:353–362.
32. Koren-Morag N, Goldbourt U, Tanne D: Renal dysfunction and risk of ischemic stroke or TIA in patients with cardiovascular disease. Neurology. 2006;67:224–228.
33. De Deyn PP, Vanholder R, D'Hooge R: Nitric oxide in uremia: effects of several potentially toxic guanidino compounds. Kidney Int Suppl. 2003;S25–S28.
34. Segarra G, Medina P, Ballester RM, et al.: Effects of some guanidino compounds on human cerebral arteries. Stroke. 1999;30:2206–2210.
35. Peppa M, Uribarri J, Cai W, Lu M, Vlassara H: Glycoxidation and inflammation in renal failure patients. Am J Kidney Dis. 2004;43:690–695.
36. Perna AF, Ingrosso D, Castaldo P, De Santo NG, Galletti P, Zappia V: Homocysteine, a new crucial element in the pathogenesis of uremic cardiovascular complications. Miner Electrolyte Metab. 1999;25:95–99.
37. Locatelli F, Cannata-Andia JB, Drueke TB, et al.: Management of disturbances of calcium and phosphate metabolism in chronic renal insufficiency, with emphasis on the control of hyperphosphataemia. Nephrol Dial Transplant. 2002;17:723–731.
38. Vicca S, Massy ZA, Hennequin C, et al.: New insights into the effects of the protein moiety of oxidized LDL (oxLDL). Kidney Int Suppl. 2003;S125–S127.
39. Parfrey PS: Cardiac and cerebrovascular disease in chronic uremia. Am J Kidney Dis. 1993;21:77–80.
40. Genovesi S, Pogliani D, Faini A, et al.: Prevalence of atrial fibrillation and associated factors in a population of long-term hemodialysis patients. Am J Kidney Dis. 2005;46: 897–902.
41. Agraharkar M, Martinez MA, Kuo YF, Ahuja TS: Hospitalization for initiation of maintenance hemodialysis. Nephron Clin Pract. 2004;97:c54–c60.
42. Chang MH, Chou KJ: The role of autonomic neuropathy in the genesis of intradialytic hypotension. Am J Nephrol. 2001;21:357–361.
43. Weiner DE, Tighiouart H, Levey AS, et al.: Lowest systolic blood pressure is associated with stroke in stages 3 to 4 chronic kidney disease. J Am Soc Nephrol. 2007;18: 960–966.
44. Hoeben H, bu-Alfa AK, Mahnensmith R, Perazella MA: Hemodynamics in patients with intradialytic hypotension treated with cool dialysate or midodrine. Am J Kidney Dis. 2002;39:102–107.
45. Brewster UC, Ciampi MA, bu-Alfa AK, Perazella MA: Addition of sertraline to other therapies to reduce dialysis-associated hypotension. Nephrology (Carlton). 2003;8:296–301.
46. Abramson JL, Jurkovitz CT, Vaccarino V, Weintraub WS, McClellan W: Chronic kidney disease, anemia, and incident stroke in a middle-aged, community-based population: the ARIC Study. Kidney Int. 2003;64:610–615.
47. Di MG, Martinez J, McKean ML, De La RJ, Burke JF, Murphy S: Platelet dysfunction in uremia. Multifaceted defect partially corrected by dialysis. Am J Med. 1985;79:552–559.
48. Iseki K, Kinjo K, Kimura Y, Osawa A, Fukiyama K: Evidence for high risk of cerebral hemorrhage in chronic dialysis patients. Kidney Int. 1993;44:1086–1090.
49. Janssen MJ, van der MJ: The bleeding risk in chronic haemodialysis: preventive strategies in high-risk patients. Neth J Med. 1996;48:198–207.
50. Yorioka N, Oda H, Ogawa T, et al.: Continuous ambulatory peritoneal dialysis is superior to hemodialysis in chronic dialysis patients with cerebral hemorrhage. Nephron. 1994; 67:365–366.
51. Savazzi GM, Cusmano F, Vinci S, Allegri L: Progression of cerebral atrophy in patients on regular hemodialysis treatment: long-term follow-up with cerebral computed tomography. Nephron. 1995;69:29–33.
52. Leonard A, Shapiro FL: Subdural hematoma in regularly hemodialyzed patients. Ann Intern Med. 1975;82:650–658.
53. Inzelberg R, Neufeld MY, Reider I, Gari P: Non surgical treatment of subdural hematoma in a hemodialysis patient. Clin Neurol Neurosurg. 1989;91:85–89.
54. Kurella M, Chertow GM, Luan J, Yaffe K: Cognitive impairment in chronic kidney disease. J Am Geriatr Soc. 2004;52:1863–1869.
55. Murray AM, Tupper DE, Knopman DS, et al.: Cognitive impairment in hemodialysis patients is common. Neurology. 2006;67:216–223.
56. Fukunishi I, Kitaoka T, Shirai T, Kino K, Kanematsu E, Sato Y: Psychiatric disorders among patients undergoing hemodialysis therapy. Nephron. 2002;91:344–347.
57. Lass P, Buscombe JR, Harber M, Davenport A, Hilson AJ: Cognitive impairment in patients with renal failure is associated with multiple-infarct dementia. Clin Nucl Med. 1999;24:561–565.
58. Irie T, Kasai M, Abe N, et al.: Cerebellar form of progressive multifocal leukoencephalopathy in a patient with chronic renal failure. Intern Med. 1992;31:218–223.
59. Kim J, Song T, Park S, Choi IS: Cerebellar peduncular myelinolysis in a patient receiving hemodialysis. J Neurol Sci. 2007;253:66–68.
60. Dervisoglu E, Yegenaga I, Anik Y, Sengul E, Turgut T: Diffusion magnetic resonance imaging may provide prognostic information in osmotic demyelination syndrome: report of a case. Acta Radiol. 2006;47:208–212.
61. Loo CS, Lim TO, Fan KS, Murad Z, Suleiman AB: Pontine myelinolysis following correction of hyponatraemia. Med J Malaysia. 1995;50:180–182.
62. Hung SC, Hung SH, Tarng DC, Yang WC, Huang TP: Chorea induced by thiamine deficiency in hemodialysis patients. Am J Kidney Dis. 2001;37:427–430.

63. da Silva CJ, da Rocha AJ, Jeronymo S, et al.: A preliminary study revealing a new association in patients undergoing maintenance hemodialysis: manganism symptoms and T1 hyperintense changes in the basal ganglia. AJNR Am J Neuroradiol. 2007;28:1474–1479.
64. Wang HC, Brown P, Lees AJ: Acute movement disorders with bilateral basal ganglia lesions in uremia. Mov Disord. 1998;13:952–957.
65. Kawauchi A, Inoue Y, Hashimoto T, et al.: Restless legs syndrome in hemodialysis patients: health-related quality of life and laboratory data analysis. Clin Nephrol. 2006;66: 440–446.
66. Winkelman JW, Chertow GM, Lazarus JM: Restless legs syndrome in end-stage renal disease. Am J Kidney Dis. 1996;28:372–378.
67. Kerr PG, van BC, Dawborn JK: Assessment of the symptomatic benefit of cool dialysate. Nephron. 1989;52: 166–169.
68. Molnar MZ, Novak M, Mucsi I: Management of restless legs syndrome in patients on dialysis. Drugs. 2006;66:607–624.
69. Molnar MZ, Novak M, Ambrus C, et al.: Restless Legs Syndrome in patients after renal transplantation. Am J Kidney Dis. 2005;45:388–396.
70. Gupta SK, Manjunath-Prasad KS, Sharma BS, et al.: Brain abscess in renal transplant recipients: report of three cases. Surg Neurol. 1997;48:284–287.
71. Vanholder R, Ringoir S: Infectious morbidity and defects of phagocytic function in end-stage renal disease: a review. J Am Soc Nephrol. 1993;3:1541–1554.
72. Cengiz K: Increased incidence of neoplasia in chronic renal failure (20-year experience). Int Urol Nephrol. 2002; 33:121–126.
73. Bosmans JL, Ysebaert D, De Cock AM, et al.: Interferon-alpha and the cure of metastasis of a malignant meningioma in a kidney allograft recipient: a case report. Transplant Proc. 1997;29:838.
74. Urasaki E, Yamada H, Tokimura T, Yokota A: T-cell type primary spinal intramedullary lymphoma associated with human T-cell lymphotropic virus type I after a renal transplant: case report. Neurosurgery. 1996;38:1036–1039.
75. Schwechheimer K, Hashemian A: Neuropathologic findings after organ transplantation. An autopsy study. Gen Diagn Pathol. 1995;141:35–39.
76. Gill D, Juffs HG, Herzig KA, et al.: Durable and high rates of remission following chemotherapy in posttransplantation lymphoproliferative disorders after renal transplantation. Transplant Proc. 2003;35:256–257.
77. Maisonneuve P, Agodoa L, Gellert R, et al.: Cancer in patients on dialysis for end-stage renal disease: an international collaborative study. Lancet. 1999;354:93–99.
78. Mokri B: Spontaneous intracranial hypotension. Curr Pain Headache Rep. 2001;5:284–291.
79. Evan RW, Mokri B: Spontaneous intracranial hypotension resulting in coma. Headache. 2002;42:159–160.
80. Thomke F, Bredel-Geissler A, Mika-Gruttner A, et al.: Spontaneous intracranial hypotension syndrome. Clinical, neuroradiological and cerebrospinal fluid findings. Nervenarzt. 1999;70:909–915.
81. Spelle L, Boulin A, Tainturier C, Visot A, Graveleau P, Pierot L: Neuroimaging features of spontaneous intracranial hypotension. Neuroradiology. 2001;43:622–627.
82. Guy J, Johnston PK, Corbett JJ, Day AL, Glaser JS: Treatment of visual loss in pseudotumor cerebri associated with uremia. Neurology. 1990;40:28–32.
83. Chang D, Nagamoto G, Smith WE: Benign intracranial hypertension and chronic renal failure. Cleve Clin J Med. 1992;59:419–422.
84. Korzets A, Gafter U, Floru S, Chagnac A, Zevin D: Deteriorating renal function with acetazolamide in a renal transplant patient with pseudotumor cerebri. Am J Kidney Dis. 1993;21:322–324.
85. Saito A, Gejyo F: Current clinical aspects of dialysis-related amyloidosis in chronic dialysis patients. Ther Apher Dial. 2006;10:316–320.
86. Chary-Valckenaere I, Kessler M, Mainard D, et al.: Amyloid and non-amyloid carpal tunnel syndrome in patients receiving chronic renal dialysis. J Rheumatol. 1998;25:1164–1170.
87. Gousheh J, Iranpour A: Association between carpel tunnel syndrome and arteriovenous fistula in hemodialysis patients. Plast Reconstr Surg. 2005;116:508–513.
88. Garcia S, Cofan F, Combalia A, Campistol JM, Oppenheimer F, Ramon R: Compression of the ulnar nerve in Guyon's canal by uremic tumoral calcinosis. Arch Orthop Trauma Surg. 2000;120:228–230.
89. Mourad G, Argiles A: Renal transplantation relieves the symptoms but does not reverse beta 2-microglobulin amyloidosis. J Am Soc Nephrol. 1996;7:798–804.
90. Floege J, Ketteler M: beta2-microglobulin-derived amyloidosis: an update. Kidney Int Suppl. 2001;78:S164–S171.
91. Vaziri ND, Barton CH, Ravikumar GR, Martin DC, Ness R, Saiki J: Femoral neuropathy: a complication of renal transplantation. Nephron. 1981;28:30–31.
92. Sharma KR, Cross J, Santiago F, Ayyar DR, Burke G, III: Incidence of acute femoral neuropathy following renal transplantation. Arch Neurol. 2002;59:541–545.
93. Amato AA, Barohn RJ, Sahenk Z, Tutschka PJ, Mendell JR: Polyneuropathy complicating bone marrow and solid organ transplantation. Neurology. 1993;43:1513–1518.
94. Galassi G, Ferrari S, Cobelli M, Rizzuto N: Neuromuscular complications of kidney diseases. Nephrol Dial Transplant. 1998;13 (Suppl 7):41–47.
95. Lindblom U, Tegner R: Thermal sensitivity in uremic neuropathy. Acta Neurol Scand. 1985;71:290–294.
96. Tegner R, Lindholm B: Vibratory perception threshold compared with nerve conduction velocity in the evaluation of uremic neuropathy. Acta Neurol Scand. 1985;71:284–289.
97. Yosipovitch G, Yarnitsky D, Mermelstein V, et al.: Paradoxical heat sensation in uremic polyneuropathy. Muscle Nerve. 1995;18:768–771.
98. Hojs-Fabjan T, Hojs R: Polyneuropathy in hemodialysis patients: the most sensitive electrophysiological parameters and dialysis adequacy. Wien Klin Wochenschr. 2006;118 (Suppl 2):29–34.
99. Ogura T, Makinodan A, Kubo T, Hayashida T, Hirasawa Y: Electrophysiological course of uraemic neuropathy in haemodialysis patients. Postgrad Med J. 2001;77:451–454.
100. Hupperts RM, Leunissen KM, van Hooff JP, Lodder J: Recovery of uremic neuropathy after renal transplantation. Clin Neurol Neurosurg. 1990;92:87–89.
101. Okada H, Moriwaki K, Kanno Y, et al.: Vitamin B6 supplementation can improve peripheral polyneuropathy in patients with chronic renal failure on high-flux haemodialysis

and human recombinant erythropoietin. Nephrol Dial Transplant. 2000;15:1410–1413.
102. Kuwabara S, Nakazawa R, Azuma N, et al.: Intravenous methylcobalamin treatment for uremic and diabetic neuropathy in chronic hemodialysis patients. Intern Med. 1999;38:472–475.
103. Moore GE, Parsons DB, Stray-Gundersen J, Painter PL, Brinker KR, Mitchell JH: Uremic myopathy limits aerobic capacity in hemodialysis patients. Am J Kidney Dis. 1993;22:277–287.
104. Campistol JM: Uremic myopathy. Kidney Int. 2002;62: 1901–1913.
105. Diesel W, Emms M, Knight BK, et al.: Morphologic features of the myopathy associated with chronic renal failure. Am J Kidney Dis. 1993;22:677–684.
106. Cheema B, Abas H, Smith B, et al.: Randomized controlled trial of intradialytic resistance training to target muscle wasting in ESRD: the Progressive Exercise for Anabolism in Kidney Disease (PEAK) study. Am J Kidney Dis. 2007;50:574–584.
107. Feinfeld DA, Kurian P, Cheng JT, et al.: Effect of oral L-carnitine on serum myoglobin in hemodialysis patients. Ren Fail. 1996;18:91–96.

Gastrointestinal Complications of Acute Kidney Injury

4.10

Susie Q. Lew, Marie L. Borum, and Todd S. Ing

Core Messages

- Gastrointestinal (GI) complications are commonly encountered in patients with acute kidney injury (AKI) and are the result of uremia.
- Since the degree of uremia varies in AKI, a spectrum of symptoms and GI complications may occur.
- GI complications of AKI include anorexia, hiccups, upper and lower GI hemorrhage, as well as diseases of the small and large intestines.

4.10.1 Introduction

Gastrointestinal (GI) complications in patients with acute kidney injury (AKI) are mostly similar to those with chronic kidney disease. The scarcity of data on the incidence and prevalence of GI complications associated with AKI is related to the wide variability in the definition of AKI, as well as the extent and duration of uremia. GI complications vary with the degree of uremia sustained from the kidney injury, as well as the timing, dose, and modality of renal replacement therapy deployed in the management of uremia. Therefore, GI complications vary in manifestations and in intensity in patients with AKI. AKI of short duration with renal function returning to baseline values and with minimal signs and symptoms of uremia is generally not associated with GI complications.

Patients with AKI requiring short- or long-term renal replacement therapy are more likely to develop GI complications similar to those with chronic kidney disease in most respects or similar to those related to the dialysis treatment itself. Since uremic AKI patients are nowadays frequently treated promptly with renal replacement therapy in most developed countries, the florid GI complications associated with advanced uremia (such as uremic fetor, stomatitis, salivary gland inflammation, and uremic enterocolitis) are less commonly observed these days. However, these previously prevalent complications may still be encountered in less well-developed countries in which facilities for renal replacement therapy are fewer. This chapter will review the common GI complications associated with AKI. It should be noted that some of the older studies mentioned below pertain to levels of urea and/or other waste products that are much higher than those encountered among the present-day AKI patients. Therefore, how much the findings of those older studies apply to our current AKI patients is uncertain.

4.10.2 Uremic Fetor, Dysgeusia, Anorexia, Dyspepsia, Hiccups, Nausea, and Vomiting

Patients with uremia can present with a uriniferous odor to the breath, known as uremic fetor [79]. The latter is often accompanied by dysgeusia (defined as a perversion of the sense of taste) which often presents as an unpleasant metallic or a foul taste in the mouth [79].

T. S. Ing (✉)
Department of Nephrology, Loyola University Medical Center, 2160 First Avenue, Maywood, IL 60153, USA
e-mail: todding@att.net

A. Jörres et al. (eds.), *Management of Acute Kidney Problems*,
DOI: 10.1007/978-3-540-69441-0_4.10, © Springer-Verlag Berlin Heidelberg 2010

Both uremic fetor and dysgeusia are believed to be the result of the breakdown of the large amounts of salivary urea present in the mouth to ammonia [79]. There are no reliable data on the incidence and prevalence of uremic fetor, dysgeusia, anorexia, dyspepsia, hiccups, nausea, or vomiting associated with AKI. Data can hardly be obtained from critically ill patients in the intensive care unit who, deprived of a normal sensorium, are often supported by life-sustaining measures such as mechanical ventilation, vasoactive agents, and parenteral nutrition. In addition, some symptoms such as anorexia, dyspepsia, hiccups, nausea, and vomiting may be the result of underlying comorbidities rather than of AKI. However, there are data from patients with end-stage renal disease (ESRD). Anorexia is present in about one third of ESRD patients [9, 12, 49]. More patients have anorexia on dialysis treatment days (12.7%) compared with nondialysis treatment days (5.4%) [12]. Malnutrition and cachexia are consequences of reduced calorie and protein intakes [8, 9, 49]. In general, food intake is regulated by short-term satiety factors such as gastric distension, certain amino acids and peptide hormones, as well as long-term appetite regulation by agents such as leptin and insulin. In patients with ESRD, anorexia is associated with a higher mortality risk and an increased hospitalization rate [49, 60]. Anorexia is associated with a poor quality of life, a lower physical component scale rating and a lower mental component scale rating of the Medical Outcomes Study Short Form Health Survey (MOS-SF-36) [27]. In AKI, catabolism is a short-term consequence of anorexia. Hospital lengths of stay and mortality risks are consequently raised. With regard to nausea and vomiting, one evitable cause of these symptoms is excessively rapid dialysis. Such an approach can bring about the dialysis disequilibrium syndrome caused by the entry of water into the brain as the result of too abrupt a fall in plasma levels of urea and osmolality [71].

4.10.2.1 Anorexia

The exact pathogenesis of anorexia in uremic patients is unknown. Mediators implicated in dialysis-related anorexia include orexigenic (i.e., appetite-stimulating) substances such as ghrelin, neuropeptide Y, and agouti-related peptide; anorexigenic substances such as leptin, cholecystokinin, insulin, melanocyte stimulating hormone; and other factors such as serotonin, melanocortin, tryptophan, corticotrophin-related hormone, TNF-α, and interleukin-1B [5, 10]. Uremic anorexia is associated with elevated levels of plasma and central nervous system short-term satiety factors (such as cholecystokinin, glucagon, serotonin, and certain middle molecules) [5]. Other satiety factors that can influence the long-range regulation of appetite (such as leptin and insulin) are also elevated in the face of uremic anorexia [5]. Excellent reviews exist on anorexia, eating behaviors, and disorders complicating the uremic syndrome [2, 10].

4.10.2.1.1 Treatment

Uremia-induced uremic fetor, dysgeusia, anorexia, nausea, and vomiting generally improve with frequent dialysis sessions. High-intensity dialysis in ESRD patients leads to improved appetite and food intake, better general feelings of well-being, increased physical activity, fewer dietary restrictions, decreased dose of medications such as phosphate binders and antihypertensive agents [45, 86], and probably better removal of potential anorexic factors. Whether AKI patients respond to high-intensity dialysis to some extent in the same fashion or not is unclear at present. Improvement data are difficult, if not impossible, to obtain in critically ill AKI patients. In the HEMO study on maintenance hemodialysis patients, where high-dose thrice weekly treatments or high-flux membranes were used, there was no difference in dialysis-related anorexia [27].

Megestrol acetate is a synthetic, orally active derivative of the naturally occurring hormone progesterone. Megestrol acetate increases appetite via stimulation of neuropeptide Y in the hypothalamus, modulation of calcium channels in the ventromedial hypothalamus, a well-known satiety center, and inhibition of the activity of proinflammatory cytokines such as IL-1, IL-6, and TNF-α. Megestrol acetate improves appetite as well as protein and energy intakes [7, 74]. However, the adverse effects of megestrol acetate are substantial and limit its use. Noted adverse effects include headaches, dizziness, confusion, diarrhea, hyperglycemia, thromboembolic phenomena, break-through uterine bleeding, peripheral edema, hypertension, adrenal suppression, and adrenal insufficiency [8].

Branched-chain amino acid supplementation in chronic dialysis patients improves appetite as well as protein and caloric intakes [41]. The role of branched-chain amino acid supplementation in AKI to improve appetite as well as protein and caloric intakes is unclear.

A pharmacological approach with antiemetic agents may provide temporary symptomatic relief for uremia-related nausea and vomiting. Antihistamines (diphenhydramine and promethazine) and dopamine receptor antagonists, which include phenothiazines (e.g., prochlorperazine), butyrophenones (e.g., haloperidol), and benzamides (e.g., metoclopramide), may be used safely in patients with renal failure. Some of these drugs can also be given rectally or parenterally if vomiting precludes oral administration.

4.10.2.2 Hiccups

Hiccups are involuntary, intermittent spasmodic contractions of the diaphragm that repeat a number of times per minute. The inspiratory rush of air causes the epiglottis to close, creating the 'hic' noise. Diaphragmatic irritation, hyponatremia, and uremia may result in intractable hiccups. Persistent or intractable hiccups can lead to significant adverse effects including malnutrition, weight loss, fatigue, dehydration, and insomnia. In general, a bout of hiccups resolves by itself without intervention. Pharmacological intervention includes antipsychotics (chlorpromazine, haloperidol), anticonvulsants (phenytoin, valproic acid, carbamazepine, gabapentin), muscle relaxants (baclofen, cyclobenzaprine), central nervous system stimulants (methyphenidate), antiarrhythmic drugs (quinidine sulfate), dopamine antagonists (metoclopramide), tricyclic antidepressants (amitriptyline), and nifedipine. The uremic component in a patient with AKI may be corrected with dialysis.

4.10.3 Stomatitis and Salivary Gland Inflammation

Uremic stomatitis, characterized by a red, thickened buccal mucosa with a gray and gluey exudate can occur in advanced uremia, often in association with a dry burning mouth and poor dental hygiene. Ulceration of the buccal mucosa and glossitis can also be present. Believed to be caused by a high level of salivary ammonia as a result of the breakdown of salivary urea by bacterial urease, the stomatitis may be associated with inflammation of the salivary glands such as parotitis as well [79].

4.10.4 Uremic Lesions in the Alimentary Tract

The mucosal layers of the alimentary tract of uremic patients have been found to show capillary hyperemia, dilatation of submucosal veins, edema, hemorrhage, and subsequent bacterial invasion of the devitalized areas accompanied by fibrinous exudates and necrosis [46]. The involvement of various parts of the alimentary tract by these pathological features can bring about esophagitis, gastritis, duodenitis, enteritis, and colitis of the uremic variety [11, 38, 46, 79, 87]. The descriptions of these uremia-related lesions in AKI patients with advanced renal failure have appeared mostly in the older literature from a time when renal replacement therapies were not available. Whether those lesions are still seen, though possibly in a milder form and at a reduced frequency, among modern-day, less uremic (less uremic on account of early renal replacement therapies) AKI patients in developed countries is uncertain. In addition, should uremia-related lesions still be encountered in current, less uremic AKI patients, whether those lesions have any resemblance at all to those observed in severely uremic AKI patients during the pre–renal replacement therapy era is also unknown. In any case, there exist in uremic patients certain factors that may play a role in fostering uremia-related lesions. These factors are:

(A) *Urea*

Urea can alter gastric defenses against autolysis. Elevated gastric juice urea concentration can lead to dissolution of gastric mucus [29] and increase in gastric permeability [20]. The latter can allow the diffusion of hydrogen ions from the gastric lumen to the mucosa, thus impairing mucosal defense against autolysis [20]. Finally, ammonia produced from the action of urease on urea in the alimentary tract lumen of a uremic individual has been suggested to cause mucosal erosions and ulcerations of the various uremic "-itis" conditions [13, 79].

(B) *Cell renewal*

Impairment of cell renewal and cell division in AKI may reduce the competence of the mucosal barrier and contribute to the initiation and persistence of a uremia-induced lesion by retarding mucosal wound healing [65].

(C) *Gastrin and intragastric pH*

In AKI patients, serum gastrin levels are elevated on account of reduced renal catabolism of the hormone [83]. It is known that gastrin can increase acid secretion from the gastric parietal cells. Possibly because of the high serum gastrin levels, gastric acid secretion studies have found a very significant peak acid output in AKI patients [93]. However, a low basal acid output with a high basal intragastric pH has also been described [93]. The elevated basal intragastric pH may reflect the neutralizing influence of a high gastric juice ammonia level [56]. Moreover, gastrin causes pyloric incompetence by antagonizing the effects of cholecystokinin and secretin on the pyloric sphincter [35]. Bile reflux through an incompetent pyloric sphincter has been found to foster the development of gastric lesions [81]. Because of the multitude of gastrin- and pH-related factors, the resultant effects of their influences on the stomach are still not fully understood.

4.10.5 Gastritis

A classic treatise described the most common gastric lesion in advanced uremia as a progressive, diffuse, erosive gastritis with thinning of the mucosa, diffuse hyperemia, and bleeding [79].

4.10.6 Upper Gastrointestinal Hemorrhage

Prior to the availability of medical renal replacement therapies, acute GI hemorrhage was a frequent and dreaded complication in patients with AKI. GI hemorrhage occurred in as many as a third of these patients and was the second leading cause of death [53]. More recently, the incidence of GI hemorrhage has fallen to 8–13% [34]. The decline in the incidence of GI hemorrhage is likely related to better patient care, especially in the intensive care unit. Patients are receiving renal replacement therapies earlier, more frequently, and at a higher dose. Renal replacement therapies are also often performed without systemic anticoagulation. In addition, proton pump inhibitors and H_2-receptor antagonists can reduce the risk of GI hemorrhage [15]. Proton pump inhibitors are the most potent antisecretory agents, inhibiting the gastric H,K-APTase in the parietal cells, and are capable of raising gastric pH to above 6 [32, 42]. A high intragastric pH can lead to improvement of coagulation and platelet aggregation [6].

Acute GI hemorrhage in patients with AKI is considered to be a risk factor for mortality and increased health resource utilization and hospital stay [34, 83]. In one study of AKI, in-hospital mortality was 64% in patients with acute GI hemorrhage compared with 34% in those without [34].

In a clinical observational study carried out in Italy, acute GI hemorrhage occurred in 13.4% of patients with AKI, with 11.5% in the upper and 1.9% in the lower GI tract [34]. Fifty-eight percent of patients with bleeding had clinically significant bleeding. Upper GI hemorrhage is predominately from erosive lesions such as gastritis or duodenitis, ulcerative lesions such as gastric or duodenal ulcers, or arteriovenous malformations [34]. Erosions and/or ulcers accounted for 71% of cases of upper acute GI hemorrhage as a complication of AKI in this study [34]. Independent risk factors for GI bleeding include thrombocytopenia, chronic liver disease, de novo AKI, increased severity of AKI and APACHI II score [34]. It is noteworthy that whether uremia per se might have played a role in the pathogenesis of the gastric and duodenal erosions and ulcers among the AKI patients in the above study [34] has not been determined.

Some of the gastric and duodenal erosions and ulcers that occur nowadays in AKI patients receiving intensive care, are likely to be manifestations of what is known as stress-related mucosal disease (SRMD), a continuum of conditions ranging from stress-related injury consisting of superficial mucosal damage, to stress ulcers which are focal deep mucosal damage [82]. Believed to be a result of a host of factors including gastric acid, mucosal ischemia, and bile reflux, SRMD is most commonly observed in critically ill, intensive care patients [82]. Patients at very high risk for developing SRMD are those maintained on prolonged mechanical ventilation [82] and suffering from coagulopathy. Additional risk factors comprise renal failure, hepatic failure, hypotension, sepsis, trauma, burns, and myocardial infarction.

Several confounding factors can contribute to GI hemorrhage. More than one factor may be the etiology for an episode of GI hemorrhage.

(A) *Coagulopathy*

Uremic patients have a multiplicity of defects that underlie the uremic bleeding diathesis [16, 25, 28, 30, 40, 47, 59, 61, 62, 71, 73, 75, 78]. Patients have defects in coagulation factors, alteration of the fibrinolytic system, vascular abnormalities, and platelet dysfunction [28, 30, 75, 78]. Uremic platelets show a reduced adhesion to vascular subendothelium and an impaired aggregation response to various stimuli. The altered interaction of adhesive macromolecules such as fibrinogen and von Willebrand factor with platelet membrane glycoproteins such as platelet GP IIb–IIIa has been suggested to contribute to the aggregation and adhesion defects [25, 71, 73, 75]. In a subpopulation of uremic patients, platelet aggregation in response to the platelet-activating factor is selectively abnormal as a consequence of a reduced thromboxane A_2 generation [61].

(B) *Gastrin*

See Section 4.10.4.

(C) *Dialysis Treatment*

The dialysis treatment itself may induce GI hemorrhage. Hypotension during dialysis should be judiciously avoided. Both gastric mucosal permeability and acid secretion increase whenever blood pressure falls and thus might contribute to GI hemorrhage during dialysis [80]. Intradialytic hypotension due to excessive ultrafiltration or other causes can precipitate bowel infarction with resultant hemorrhage [17]. Moreover, systemic anticoagulation use during renal replacement therapy can aggravate any bleeding tendencies.

(D) *Ulcerogenic Drugs*

Gastritis and duodenitis presenting as superficial mucosal lesions can also be associated with the use of ulcerogenic drugs such as salicylates, corticosteroids, nonsteroidal antiinflammatory drugs, and iron [48]. Bleeding can occur from any necrotic or ulcerated areas.

4.10.6.1 Diagnosis and Management of Hemorrhage

The diagnosis of GI hemorrhage is made on clinical findings such as hematemesis, melena, hematochezia, a positive stool occult blood test, or an unaccountable drop in hemoglobin/hematocrit levels. In the face of serious bleeding, consultations with a gastroenterologist, an interventional radiologist and/or an abdominal surgeon should be obtained. Endoscopic evaluation is the best modality for identifying the source of bleeding. Upper endoscopy can enable the identification of lesions in the esophagus, stomach, and proximal duodenum. Double-balloon endoscopy can identify lesions lower in the small intestines. Wireless video capsule endoscopy has recently been employed to facilitate the identification of a small bowel bleeding source that had eluded detection by other endoscopic techniques. Occasionally, an imaging procedure is needed for areas not accessible by conventional endoscopy. Tagged red blood cell scan has a poor sensitivity/specificity. Mesenteric angiography is considered the gold standard for identifying specific vascular bleeding sites not identifiable by endoscopy.

A variety of treatment modalities may be required to manage GI bleeding in the patient with AKI. Hemodynamic stabilization, blood product transfusion, correction of metabolic abnormalities, and elimination of coagulopathy are key components of GI hemorrhage management. Additionally, specific intervention to address renal impairment, including administration of deamino-8-D-arginine vasopressin (DDAVP), cryoprecipitate, estrogen, and dialysis may be necessary. Endoscopic, radiographic, and surgical interventions may also be employed.

Antacids are not as effective and convenient to use as acid-suppressing drugs in the treatment of GI hemorrhage [42]. Aluminum- and magnesium-based antacids are to be avoided due to poor efficacy and the toxic effects of accumulation in the face of renal failure. Acid suppression with proton pump inhibitors and H_2-receptor antagonists assist in healing those mucosal sites damaged by erosive or ulcerative lesions. Nowadays, proton pump inhibitors are typically administered intravenously to the critically ill patients as prophylaxis against, and treatment for, GI hemorrhage [82]. In general, prophylactic acid suppression can reduce the risk of major bleeding by 50% but has little or no effect on mortality [15, 39]. However, in AKI patients, acid suppression alone is commonly not effective in stopping hemorrhage.

Endoscopic intervention is often employed for active GI hemorrhage. Electrocauterization, epinephrine/saline injection, hemoclip, and argon plasma coagulation (APC) have been utilized to achieve hemostasis depending upon the character of the identified lesion [37, 44, 58, 85]. Hemoclips may be preferable for very deep ulcers and large, visible blood vessels. APC is the mainstay of endoscopic treatment for superficial lesions such as angiodysplasia. (APC is a method of electrocoagulation in which there is noncontact application of electrical energy to achieve tissue destruction or hemostasis. APC uses high-frequency electrical currents delivered via ionized argon gas.)

Angiographic therapy is usually reserved for acute bleeding lesions (equivalent to 3 units of blood loss per day) detected during diagnostic angiography. Vasoconstrictive and embolic therapeutic angiographic procedures may be used to halt bleeding [68].

Sandostatin, an octapeptide, mimics natural somatostatin pharmacologically. Natural somatostatin reduces gastric acid secretion and splanchnic blood flow. In severe cases of bleeding, an average success rate of 87% has been achieved [14]. Sandostatin is effective and safe in the control of acute upper GI bleeding and the prevention of rebleeding.

Finally, surgical intervention may be needed to resect the area of hemorrhage. With advances in medical and endoscopic therapies for GI hemorrhage, surgical intervention is seldom required.

Correction of uremia-associated coagulopathy can improve hemostasis. Several specific approaches described below are available to treat uremia-induced hemorrhage [16, 40].

DDAVP can shorten bleeding time in uremic patients. DDAVP at a dose of 0.3 μg/kg is effectively within 0.5 h, and the effect lasts for at least 4 h [62]. The addition of cryoprecipitate corrects any coagulation factor insufficiency [47]. Cryoprecipitate is sometimes favored in acute situations because of its early onset of action.

Administration of estrogen corrects uremia-induced platelet dysfunction, as demonstrated by the reversion of an abnormal bleeding time to normal [59]. A specific case of GI bleeding in a uremic patient was reported to improve with estrogen-progesterone therapy [70a]. Estrogen therapy takes 6 h to be effective [59]. However, its effects are long-lasting. In anemic patients, transfusion of blood to reach a hematocrit level of 26% or higher can shorten bleeding time [33], possibly by enhancing platelet functions, by providing an adequate quantity of red blood cells to form a clot, or by fostering the participation of other factors. Although all of these therapies are effective, each of them carries its own side effects. Thus the choice of therapy depends on the benefit to risk ratio as well as the mode and the duration of action.

Platelet function improves with dialysis by removing certain uremic toxins responsible for the coagulopathy [16, 36, 53, 73]. Partial correction of platelet aggregation and thromboxane B_2 formation can be observed after dialysis [25]. Heparin-induced thrombocytopenia may curtail heparin use during dialysis or continuous renal replacement therapies (CRRTs). It is feasible to perform both hemodialysis and CRRT without systemic anticoagulation [66]. For example, one form of heparin-free dialysis involves the flushing of normal saline at an amount of 250 ml or more into the arterial blood line every 15–30 min (sometimes up to a total of 7 l of saline flushes per dialysis session is used), accompanied by the removal of an appropriate quantity of ultrafiltrate at the same time to maintain euvolemia. The use of a citrate-enriched dialysate fashioned by the addition of a small amount of citric acid to the "acid concentrate" of a dual-concentrate, bicarbonate-based dialysate delivery system, has been advanced. The citrate achieved in the final dialysate, of an amount of 0.8 mmol/l, can reduce the dose of heparin used [3, 89], presumably by minimizing clotting on the blood side of the dialyzing membrane by forming a calcium/citrate chelate with blood calcium. Furthermore, this citrate-enrichment technique can be combined with a normal saline-flushing method in an attempt to minimize or avoid heparin use. Another heparin-free approach relates to the use of a regional citrate anticoagulation regimen by infusing sodium citrate into the arterial blood line and dialyzing with a calcium-containing or a calcium-free dialysate [19, 31]. Should a calcium-free dialysate be used, calcium needs to be replenished by infusing calcium chloride into the venous blood line [19]. Every attempt should be made to avoid hypotension during dialysis to ensure adequate tissue perfusion so that ischemia of the bowels and other vital organs does not occur. To minimize the occurrence of hypotension during dialysis, the use of a bicarbonate-buffered dialysate is preferred [18].

4.10.7 Diseases of the Small Intestines

Both AKI and chronic kidney disease can result in a general inhibition of cell proliferation [65]. Cell population kinetic studies in experimental AKI show a prolongation of the cell generation cycle. Loss of intestinal mucosal integrity allows gut bacteria to gain entrance into the blood. Factors that promote the passage of bacteria from the GI tract include: disruption of the ecologic balance of the normal indigenous microflora resulting in the overgrowth of other bacteria, impaired host immune defenses, physical disruption of the gut mucosal barrier, trauma, endotoxemia, and protein malnutrition [21–24, 70]. Correction of these myriad factors may reduce the risk of developing bacteremia. In this regard, it has been suggested that enteral as compared with parenteral feeding is of benefit with respect to infection episodes in critically ill patients with AKI [69]. The benefit may be a consequence of improvement in some of the factors mentioned above.

Lesions in the small bowels (apart from duodenum) encountered as a result of AKI occur less frequently than lesions in the stomach, duodenum, and colon. It is speculated that hemorrhage from existing arteriovenous malformations in the small bowels can occur in patients with kidney disease. Wireless video capsule endoscopy may be employed to visualize the source of small bowel hemorrhage. Management of hemorrhage from arteriovenous malformations is primarily focused on hemodynamic stabilization, blood product transfusion, correction of metabolic abnormalities, and elimination of coagulopathy. Brisk hemorrhages identified by angiography may be rectified by embolization techniques or by surgical intervention when endoscopic intervention is not possible.

4.10.7.1 *Uremic Enterocolitis*

Uremic enterocolitis has been described in advanced renal failure and in the form of mucosal erosions and necrotizing ulcers in the small and large bowels, particularly in the lymphoid tissue [11]. Manifestations include severe diarrhea with purulent or bloody stools [11]. Uremic enterocolitis may present as an acute abdomen with pain, rigidity, and tenderness as well as nausea, vomiting, and weight loss [87]. It is worthy of note that bleeding originating from the lower intestinal tract is not an infrequent event in patients with advanced uremia [79]. Under such circumstances, apart from the uremic bleeding diathesis, it is conceivable that uremic enterocolitis is a contributory factor to the bleeding. Nevertheless, uremic colitis is a rare event in AKI but is one of the terminal complications of untreated uremia [83]. With regard to the development of experimental uremic colitis, it has been found that germ-free uremic rats do not develop this variety of colitis in the caecum when compared with their non-germ-free counterparts. These findings lend support to the suggestion that the ammonia formed from the action of urease on the urea present in the cecal lumen is the culprit for the colonic injury [13].

4.10.8 Diseases of the Colon

4.10.8.1 *Ileus*

Advanced uremia is a common cause of metabolic ileus of the paralytic type [76]. Paralytic ileus is marked by abdominal distention, absent bowel sounds, and abdominal pain. Intervention is often necessary to avoid the potential complications of perforation, peritonitis, and death. Decompression approaches along with the correction of uremia and metabolic abnormalities should be carried out. Nasogastric tube suction can relieve abdominal distention and vomiting. Endoscopic decompression may be necessary for the management of a markedly dilated colon. Rectal tube placement can also be helpful in sustaining colonic decompression in the face of an acutely dilated colon.

4.10.8.2 *Intestinal Necrosis*

The use of sodium polystyrene sulfonate (Kayexalate), a cation exchange resin used for the treatment of hyperkalemia, in sorbitol enema was reported to cause extensive colitis or enterocolitis with necrosis and sometimes perforation in uremic subjects [1, 4, 57, 77]. Kayexalate crystals were noted in the intestinal lumen and in the intestinal lesions [1, 57, 77]. Since postoperative patients have been found to be affected in this manner, intestinal hypomotility [4] – possibly as a result of anesthesia, surgery, and analgesics (such as opiates) – has been suggested to be a pathogenetic factor. An extremely high mortality rate in clinical cases as well as in animal studies was found [1, 57]. Mucosal injuries in the form of ulcers or erosions were also detected on endoscopic examination of the esophagus, stomach, and duodenum after the ingestion of Kayexalate in sorbitol [1]. The following suggestions have been advanced in an attempt to prevent the above toxic effects of Kayexalate: (a) the avoidance of sorbitol when Kayexalate is used as an enema, (b) the use of lactulose as a laxative instead when Kayexalate is given orally, and (c) the avoidance of Kayexalate in the postoperative setting and in the presence of concomitant GI disturbances [4]. Although sorbitol, on account of its hyperosmolality, has been suggested as a cause for the GI lesions [57, 77], the use of a sorbitol-free Kayexalate enema has also recently been reported to result in intestinal necrosis in an infant [77]. Because of all these difficulties, it would seem prudent to consider using Kayexalate as a means of treating hyperkalemia only when other approaches such as renal replacement therapies are not at hand.

4.10.8.3 Colonic Hemorrhage

Bleeding from existing lesions in the colon, including arteriovenous malformations, can occur in patients with AKI due to the uremic bleeding diathesis. Evaluation by endoscopy can help to identify the lesions. Management of bleeding from arteriovenous malformations is primarily focused up hemodynamic stabilization, blood product transfusion, correction of metabolic abnormalities, and elimination of coagulopathy. Endoscopic intervention with electrocauterization or hemoclip placement can be employed for a single or limited number of actively bleeding lesions. Argon plasma coagulation is frequently employed when multiple lesions are present. Angiography with embolization or surgical intervention may be required for persistently or severely bleeding lesions.

4.10.8.4 Pseudomembranous Colitis

Because of frequent exposures to antibiotics, uremia-related impairment of the immune system and reduction in intestinal motility, patients with AKI are more prone to develop *Clostridium difficile*-associated pseudomembranous colitis [55]. Because some of the patients may be less symptomatic or asymptomatic, it is prudent to hold a high index of suspicion of this serious problem at all times.

4.10.9 Pancreatic Complications

In the "sequential system failure syndrome," acute pancreatitis occurred in approximately 17% of patients with AKI after a ruptured abdominal aortic aneurysm [88]. It is well established that AKI may be a complication of pancreatitis. In addition, hemolysis can bring about both AKI and pancreatitis [26]. Autopsy examination of patients dying after oligemic shock showed a 50% incidence of major pancreatic injury if there was concomitant AKI but only a 9% incidence in those without AKI [92]. Moreover, patients dying after nonoligemic shock had a 35% incidence of pancreatic ischemic injury if AKI was present also but only a 12% incidence in those without AKI. The ischemic injury was mainly in the form of pancreatic necrosis and pancreatitis [92].

Plasma levels of pancreatic secretory trypsin inhibitor, a good indicator of acute pancreatitis in individuals with adequate renal function, were measured in the following patients who were not suffering from pancreatitis: namely, patients with AKI, patients with chronic renal failure, patients undergoing regular hemodialysis treatment or continuous ambulatory peritoneal dialysis, and patients following a successful kidney transplant [43]. The highest levels of plasma pancreatic secretory trypsin inhibitor were found in patients with AKI (2,300 ± 22.3 ng/ml) compared with controls (9.2 ± 0.8 ng/ml), patients with chronic kidney failure not on dialysis (156.9 ± 16.2 ng/ml), patients receiving regular hemodialysis treatment (257.6 ± 22.3 ng/ml) and patients receiving peritoneal dialysis (376.8 ± 57.5 ng/ml).

Both serum levels of amylase and lipase can be several times higher than normal in the face of renal failure without the presence of pancreatitis [94], possibly a result of reduced peripheral clearance, pancreatic overproduction, and/or increased release from the pancreas. However, it has been suggested that a diagnosis of acute pancreatitis in the presence of AKI would ordinarily require an amylase level of more than tenfold the normal value [94]. It is well known that serum amylase may reach extremely high levels in AKI patients [67]. Serum lipase activity rises after hemodialysis because of (a) a heparin-induced release of endothelium-bound lipoprotein lipase (should heparin be used for the dialysis treatment) and (b) presumably, an ultrafiltration-induced hemoconcentration. Therefore, only predialysis serum samples should be used for the measurement of lipase [91]. Since P3 isoamylase is solely of pancreatic origin, the absence of significant elevation of this enzyme often suggests that the diagnosis of pancreatitis is less likely [72].

4.10.10 Hepatic Disease

There are no data suggesting that AKI causes hepatic injury. Hepatic and kidney injuries may coexist due to (a) systemic events such as hypotension ("shock liver"), vasculitis, and infection, or (b) harmful exogenous agents such as medications and toxins.

4.10.11 Cholecystitis

Acute acalculous cholecystitis was reported in 17% of critically ill patients with AKI who had no prior or coincidental biliary tract disease [84]. In another series, a 7.7% prevalence of acute acalculous cholecystitis was reported in patients with surgical AKI [50]. The cause of this complication was considered to be multifactorial. Risk factors for acute acalculous cholecystitis included sepsis, previous surgery, trauma, total parental nutrition, intermittent positive pressure ventilation, opiate sedation, multiple transfusions, and hypotension. Diagnosis was based on clinical suspicion, serial imaging studies, as well as serial laboratory tests of white cell count, liver functions, and C-reactive protein. Treatment included conservative therapy with antibiotics, cholecystotomy, or cholecystectomy. The mortality rate was 46%, which was not significantly different from that for patients with AKI but without acute acalculous cholecystitis [50]. Early diagnosis and judicious management are advocated to reduce morbidity and mortality in a population with an already high mortality rate to begin with [50, 84].

4.10.12 Acid–Base and Electrolyte Abnormalities

Metabolic alkalosis can develop in patients experiencing vomiting or undergoing nasogastric suction in spite of the tendency of AKI to bring about metabolic acidosis. The hydrogen cation that is derived from carbonic acid and secreted by the gastric parietal cells along with the chloride anion in the form of hydrochloric acid is removed from the body. The bicarbonate anion that is left behind in the parietal cells after a hydrogen cation has left its parent compound, carbonic acid, now enters the blood to cause metabolic alkalosis. Prophylactic use of proton pump inhibitors or H_2-blockers in patients undergoing nasogastric suction or experiencing vomiting is effective in preventing metabolic alkalosis, but will not rectify any existing metabolic alkalosis once it has been generated. The administration of antacids in the form of absorbable alkalis such as sodium bicarbonate or calcium carbonate in patients with AKI can also result in metabolic alkalosis. The final acid–base status in patients with AKI depends on (a) the net accumulation of hydrogen ions from excessive production and/or decreased kidney excretion, and (b) the formation of bicarbonate ions (e.g., from vomiting, etc.) that the injured kidney cannot excrete. In patients with AKI, severe metabolic alkalosis can be managed with hemodialysis, peritoneal dialysis, CRRT, hemofiltration, or hemodiafiltration employing bicarbonate (or bicarbonate precursor)-poor and chloride-rich dialysis solutions, and/or replacement fluids [51, 90].

Magnesium-containing laxatives are contraindicated in patients with AKI because of the development of hypermagnesemia. Sodium phosphate-containing laxatives or enemas are also not recommended because of the frequent occurrences of hyperphosphatemia and hypocalcemia [54]. In this respect, it is worth noting that both AKI and chronic renal failure secondary to nephrocalcinosis as a result of calcium phosphate deposition in the kidney have been described in non-renal failure patients (especially those who are elderly), after the consumption of sodium phosphate laxatives in preparation for procedures such as colonoscopy [52, 63]. Suggested contributing factors include inadequate hydration, hypertension, diuretic use, presence of diabetes, angiotensin-converting enzyme inhibitor, and/or angiotensin receptor blocker therapy [52, 63]. Furthermore, in the extreme form of sodium phosphate excess, hypernatremia and an increased serum anion gap have been reported [54]. With regard to phosphorus metabolism, although most AKI patients suffer from hyperphosphatemia as a result of catabolism and reduced renal excretion, hypophosphatemia may result from reduced oral intake, excessive phosphate-binder ingestion, parenteral nutrition infusion, glucose administration, or phosphate removal with intensive renal replacement therapies [54]. Sodium phosphates may be given judiciously: (a) by the oral or the intravenous route, or (b) via the dialysis solution [45] or replacement fluid routes.

4.10.13 Summary

GI disorders are frequent and dreaded complications of AKI. The two main areas of complications are anorexia and GI hemorrhage. Disturbances in the GI tract impact on protein and caloric intakes and can lead to malnutrition and cachexia. The incidence of GI hemorrhage has fortunately fallen recently due to better medical care, use of proton pump inhibitors and H_2-receptor antagonists, and early as well as more effective dialysis treatments to combat uremia and platelet dysfunction. The source of GI hemorrhage is diagnosed earlier and more precisely with improved diagnostic techniques. Management of GI hemorrhage with less invasive procedures and with more powerful pharmacological agents are recent advances. Significant pancreatic and hepatic complications are less common.

GI complications of AKI will continue to fall in frequency and severity as more sophisticated techniques become available in the diagnosis and treatment of uremia. Newer pharmacological agents will make their appearance for the treatment of GI symptoms as the mechanisms for disease are better revealed. Finally, GI diagnostic and therapeutic procedures continue to evolve with earlier and more precise diagnosis resulting in better clinical outcomes.

References

1. Abraham SC, Bhagavan BS, Lee LA, et al. (2001) Upper gastrointestinal tract injury in patients receiving kayexalate (sodium polystyrene sulfonate) in sorbitol: clinical, endoscopic, and histopathologic findings. Am J Surg Pathol 25:637–644
2. Aguilera A, Codoceo R, Bajo MA, et al. (2004) Eating behavior disorders in uremia: a question of balance in appetite regulation. Semin Dial 17:44–52
3. Ahmad S, Callan R, Cole JJ, et al. (2000) Dialysate made from dry chemicals using citric acid increases dialysis dose. Am J Kidney Dis 35:493–499
4. Barri YM, Golper TA (2008) Gastrointestinal disease in dialysis patients. UpToDate. www.uptodate.com. Accessed 15 February 2008
5. Bergstrom J (1999) Mechanisms of uremic suppression of appetite. J Ren Nutr 9:129–132
6. Bjorkman DJ (2004). Gastrointestinal hemorrhage and occult gastrointestinal bleeding. In: Goldman L, Ausiello D (eds) Cecil Textbook of Medicine, 22nd ed. WB Saunders, Philadelphia, PA, pp 795–800
7. Boccanfuso JA, Hutton M, McAllister B (2000) The effects of megestrol acetate on nutritional parameters in a dialysis population. J Ren Nutr 10:36–43
8. Bossola M, Muscaritoli M, Tazza L, et al. (2005) Malnutrition in hemodialysis patients: what therapy? Am J Kidney Dis 46:371–386
9. Bossola M, Muscaritoli M, Tazza L, et al. (2005) Variables associated with reduced dietary intake in hemodialysis patients. J Ren Nutr 15:244–252
10. Bossola M, Tazza L, Giungi S, et al. (2006) Anorexia in hemodialysis patients: an update. Kidney Int 70:417–422
11. Boyd W (1953) A Textbook of Pathology – An Introduction to Medicine, 6th ed. Lea & Fibiger, Philadelphia, PA, p 471
12. Burrowes JD, Larive B, Cockram DB, et al. (2003) Effects of dietary intake, appetite, and eating habits on dialysis and non-dialysis treatment days in hemodialysis patients: cross-sectional results from the HEMO study. J Ren Nutr 13: 191–198
13. Carter D, Einheber A, Bauer H, et al. (1966) The role of the microbial flora in uremia. II. Uremic colitis, cardiovascular lesions, and biochemical observations. J Exp Med 123:251–266
14. Christiansen J, Ottenjann R, Von Arx F (1989) Placebo-controlled trial with the somatostatin analogue SMS 201–995 in peptic ulcer bleeding. Gastroenterology 97:568–574
15. Cook DJ, Reeve BK, Guyatt GH, et al. (1996) Stress ulcer prophylaxis in critically ill patients. Resolving discordant meta-analyses. JAMA 275:308–314
16. Couch P, Stumpf JL (1990) Management of uremic bleeding. Clin Pharm 9:673–681
17. Dahlberg PJ, Kisken WA, Newcomer KL, et al. (1985) Mesenteric ischemia in chronic dialysis patients. Am J Nephrol 5:327–332
18. Davenport A (2001) Dialysate and substitution fluids for patients treated by continuous forms of renal replacement therapy. Contrib Nephrol:313–322
19. Davenport A, Lai KN, Hertel J, et al. (2007) Anticoagulation. In: Daugirdas JT, Blake PG, Ing TS (eds) Handbook of Dialysis, 4th ed. Lippincott Williams & Wilkins, Philadelphia, PA, pp 204–218
20. Davenport HW (1968) Destruction of the gastric mucosal barrier by detergents and urea. Gastroenterology 54:175–181
21. Deitch EA, Berg R, Specian R (1987) Endotoxin promotes the translocation of bacteria from the gut. Arch Surg 122:185–190
22. Deitch EA, Bridges RM (1987) Effect of stress and trauma on bacterial translocation from the gut. J Surg Res 42:536–542

23. Deitch EA, Maejima K, Berg R (1985) Effect of oral antibiotics and bacterial overgrowth on the translocation of the GI tract microflora in burned rats. J Trauma 25:385–392
24. Deitch EA, Winterton J, Li M, et al. (1987) The gut as a portal of entry for bacteremia. Role of protein malnutrition. Ann Surg 205:681–692
25. Di Minno G, Martinez J, McKean ML, et al. (1985) Platelet dysfunction in uremia. Multifaceted defect partially corrected by dialysis. Am J Med 79:552–559
26. Druml W, Laggner AN, Lenz K, et al. (1991) Pancreatitis in acute hemolysis. Ann Hematol 63:39–41
27. Dwyer JT, Larive B, Leung J, et al. (2002) Nutritional status affects quality of life in Hemodialysis (HEMO) Study patients at baseline. J Ren Nutr 12:213–223
28. Eberst ME, Berkowitz LR (1994) Hemostasis in renal disease: Pathophysiology and management. Am J Med 96: 168–179
29. Edward DW, Skoryna SC (1964) Properties of gel mucin of human gastric juice. Proc Soc Exp Biol Med 116:794–799
30. Eknoyan G, Wacksman SJ, Glueck HI, et al. (1969) Platelet function in renal failure. N Engl J Med 280:677–681
31. Evenepoel P, Maes B, Vanwalleghem J, et al. (2002) Regional citrate anticoagulation for hemodialysis using a conventional calcium-containing dialysate. Am J Kidney Dis 39: 315–323
32. Fennerty MB (2002) Pathophysiology of the upper gastrointestinal tract in the critically ill patient: rationale for the therapeutic benefits of acid suppression. Crit Care Med 30:S351–355
33. Fernandez F, Goudable C, Sie P, et al. (1985) Low haematocrit and prolonged bleeding time in uraemic patients: Effect of red cell transfusions. Br J Haematol 59:139–148
34. Fiaccadori E, Maggiore U, Clima B, et al. (2001) Incidence, risk factors, and prognosis of gastrointestinal hemorrhage complicating acute renal failure. Kidney Int 59:1510–1519
35. Fisher RS, Lipshutz W, Cohen S (1973) The hormonal regulation of pyloric sphincter function. J Clin Invest 52:1289–1296
36. Gillum DM, Dixon BS, Yanover MJ, et al. (1986) The role of intensive dialysis in acute renal failure. Clin Nephrol 25:249–255
37. Grund KE, Storek D, Farin G (1994) Endoscopic argon plasma coagulation (APC) first clinical experiences in flexible endoscopy. Endosc Surg Allied Technol 2:42–46
38. Hansen I (1947) Uremigenic gastroenteritis (Lesieur). Electrolyte determinations and pathologic – anatomical findings in a case of gastroenteritis with uremia in an adult. Acta Med Scand 127:17–25
39. Harty RF, Ancha HB (2006) Stress ulcer bleeding. Curr Treat Options Gastroenterol 9:157–166
40. Hedges SJ, Dehoney SB, Hooper JS, et al. (2007) Evidence-based treatment recommendations for uremic bleeding. Nat Clin Pract Nephrol 3:138–153
41. Hiroshige K, Sonta T, Suda T, et al. (2001) Oral supplementation of branched-chain amino acid improves nutritional status in elderly patients on chronic haemodialysis. Nephrol Dial Transplant 16:1856–1862
42. Hoogerwerf WA, Pasricha PJ (2006) Pharmacotherapy of gastric acidity, peptic ulcers, and gastroesophageal reflux disease. In: Brunton LL, Lazo JS, Parker KL (eds) Goodman & Gilman's The Pharmacological Basis of Therapeutics, 11th ed. McGraw-Hill, New York, pp 967–981
43. Horl WH, Wanner C, Schollmeyer P, et al. (1988) Plasma levels of pancreatic secretory trypsin inhibitor in relation to amylase and lipase in patients with acute and chronic renal failure. Nephron 49:33–38
44. Hui AJ, Sung JJ (2005) Endoscopic treatment of upper gastrointestinal bleeding. Curr Treat Options Gastroenterol 8: 153–162
45. Ing TS, Ronco C, Blagg CR (2008) High-intensity hemodialysis: the wave of the future? Int J Artif Organs 31: 201–212
46. Jaffe R, Laing D (1934) Changes of the digestive tract in uremia. Arch Intern Med 53:851–864
47. Janson PA, Jubelirer SJ, Weinstein MJ, et al. (1980) Treatment of the bleeding tendency in uremia with cryoprecipitate. N Engl J Med 303:1318–1322
48. Johnson WJ (1994) The Digestive Tract. In: Daugirdas JT, Ing TS (eds) Handbook of Dialysis, 2nd ed. Little, Brown & Company, Boston, MA, pp 623–634
49. Kalantar-Zadeh K, Block G, McAllister CJ, et al. (2004) Appetite and inflammation, nutrition, anemia, and clinical outcome in hemodialysis patients. Am J Clin Nutr 80:299–307
50. Kes P, Vucicevic Z, Sefer S, et al. (2000) Acute acalculous cholecystitis in patients with surgical acute renal failure. Acta Med Croatica 54:15–20
51. Kheirbek AO, Ing TS, Viol GW, et al. (1979) Treatment of metabolic alkalosis with hemofiltration in patients with renal insufficiency. Nephron 24:91–92
52. Khurana A, McLean L, Atkinson S, et al. (2008) The effect of oral sodium phosphate drug products on renal function in adults undergoing bowel endoscopy. Arch Intern Med 168: 593–597
53. Kleinknecht D, Jungers P, Chanard J, et al. (1972) Uremic and non-uremic complications in acute renal failure: Evaluation of early and frequent dialysis on prognosis. Kidney Int 1:190–196
54. Lau K (1990) Phosphate disorders. In: Kokko JP, Tannen RL (eds) Fluids and Electrolytes, 2nd ed. WB Saunders, Philadelphia, PA, pp 505–595
55. Leung AC, Orange G, McLay A, et al. (1985) Clostridium difficile-associated colitis in uremic patients. Clin Nephrol 24:242–248
56. Lieber CS, Lefevre A (1959) Ammonia as a source of gastric hypoacidity in patients with uremia. J Clin Invest 38: 1271–1277
57. Lillemoe KD, Romolo JL, Hamilton SR, et al. (1987) Intestinal necrosis due to sodium polystyrene (Kayexalate) in sorbitol enemas: Clinical and experimental support for the hypothesis. Surgery 101:267–272
58. Lin HJ, Hsieh YH, Tseng GY, et al. (2002) A prospective, randomized trial of endoscopic hemoclip versus heater probe thermocoagulation for peptic ulcer bleeding. Am J Gastroenterol 97:2250–2254
59. Livio M, Mannucci PM, Vigano G, et al. (1986) Conjugated estrogens for the management of bleeding associated with renal failure. N Engl J Med 315:731–735
60. Lorenzo V, de Bonis E, Rufino M, et al. (1995) Caloric rather than protein deficiency predominates in stable chronic haemodialysis patients. Nephrol Dial Transplant 10:1885–1889
61. Macconi D, Vigano G, Bisogno G, et al. (1992) Defective platelet aggregation in response to platelet-activating factor

in uremia associated with low platelet thromboxane A2 generation. Am J Kidney Dis 19:318–325
62. Mannucci PM, Remuzzi G, Pusineri F, et al. (1983) Deamino-8-D-arginine vasopressin shortens the bleeding time in uremia. N Engl J Med 308:8–12
63. Markowitz GS, Stokes MB, Radhakrishnan J, et al. (2005) Acute phosphate nephropathy following oral sodium phosphate bowel purgative: an underrecognized cause of chronic renal failure. J Am Soc Nephrol 16:3389–3396
64. McCarthy JT (1996) Prognosis of patients with acute renal failure in the intensive-care unit: a tale of two eras. Mayo Clin Proc 71:117–126
65. McDermott FT, Dalton MK, Galbraith AJ (1974) The effect of acute renal failure on mitotic duration of mouse ileal epithelium. Cell Tissue Kinet 7:31–36
66. McGill RL, Blas A, Bialkin S, et al. (2005) Clinical consequences of heparin-free hemodialysis. Hemodial Int 9:393–398
67. Meroney WH, Lawson NL, Rubini ME, et al. (1956) Some observations of the behavior of amylase in relation to acute renal insufficiency. N Engl J Med 255:315–320
68. Miller M, Jr., Smith TP (2005) Angiographic diagnosis and endovascular management of nonvariceal gastrointestinal hemorrhage. Gastroenterol Clin North Am 34:735–752
69. Moore FA, Moore EE, Jones TN, et al. (1989) TEN versus TPN following major abdominal trauma – reduced septic morbidity. J Trauma 29:916–922; discussion 922–913
70. Morehouse JL, Specian RD, Stewart JJ, et al. (1986) Translocation of indigenous bacteria from the gastrointestinal tract of mice after oral ricinoleic acid treatment. Gastroenterology 91:673–682
70a. Mosconi G, Mambelli E, Zanchelli F, et al. (1999) Severe gastrointestinal bleeding in a uremic patient treated with estrogen-progesterone therapy. Int J Artif Organs 22:313–316
71. Mujais SK, Ing T, Kjellstrand C (1996) Acute complications of hemodialysis and their prevention and treatment. In: Jacobs C, Kjellstrand CM, Koch KM, Winchester JF (eds): Replacement of renal function by dialysis, 4th revised ed. Kluwer, Dordrecht, The Netherlands, pp 688–725
72. Panteghini M, Pagani F (1989) Diagnostic value of measuring pancreatic lipase and the P3 isoform of the pancreatic amylase isoenzyme in serum of hospitalized hyperamylasemic patients. Clin Chem 35:417–421
73. Rabiner SF, Drake RF (1975) Platelet function as an indicator of adequate dialysis. Kidney Int Suppl:144–146
74. Rammohan M, Kalantar-Zadeh K, Liang A, et al. (2005) Megestrol acetate in a moderate dose for the treatment of malnutrition-inflammation complex in maintenance dialysis patients. J Ren Nutr 15:345–355
75. Remuzzi G (1988) Bleeding in renal failure. Lancet 1: 1205–1208
76. Rubenstein RB, Lantz J, Stevens K, et al. (1979) Uremic ileus. Uremia presenting colonic obstruction. N Y State J Med 79:248–249
77. Rugolotto S, Gruber M, Solano PD, et al. (2007) Necrotizing enterocolitis in a 850 gram infant receiving sorbitol-free sodium polystyrene sulfonate (Kayexalate): clinical and histopathologic findings. J Perinatol 27:247–249
78. Salzman EW, Neri LL (1966) Adhesiveness of blood platelets in uremia. Thromb Diath Haemorrh 15:84–92
79. Schreiner G, Maher J (1961) Uremia: biochemistry, pathogenesis and treatment. Charles C. Thomas, Springfield, IL, pp 331–347
80. Shapira N, Skillman JJ, Steinman TI, et al. (1978) Gastric mucosal permeability and gastric acid secretion before and after hemodialysis in patients with chronic renal failure. Surgery 83:528–535
81. Sobala GM, O'Connor HJ, Dewar EP, et al. (1993) Bile reflux and intestinal metaplasia in gastric mucosa. J Clin Pathol 46:235–240
82. Spirt MJ (2004) Stress-related mucosal disease: risk factors and prophylactic therapy. Clin Ther 26:197–213
83. Steinman T, Lazarus J (1988) Organ-system involvement in acute renal failure. In: Brenner B, Lazarus J (eds) Acute Renal Failure, 2nd ed. Churchill Livingstone, New York, pp 705–739
84. Stevens PE, Harrison NA, Rainford DJ (1988) Acute acalculous cholecystitis in acute renal failure. Intensive Care Med 14:411–416
85. Sung JJ, Tsoi KK, Lai LH, et al. (2007) Endoscopic clipping versus injection and thermo-coagulation in the treatment of non-variceal upper gastrointestinal bleeding: a meta-analysis. Gut 56:1364–1373
86. Suri RS, Nesrallah GE, Mainra R, et al. (2006) Daily hemodialysis: a systematic review. Clin J Am Soc Nephrol 1: 33–42
87. Thoroughman JC, Peace RJ (1959) Abdominal surgical emergencies caused by uremic enterocolitis: report of twelve cases. Am Surg 25:533–539
88. Tilney NL, Bailey GL, Morgan AP (1973) Sequential system failure after rupture of abdominal aortic aneurysms: an unsolved problem in postoperative care. Ann Surg 178: 117–122
89. Tu A, Ahmad S (2000) Heparin-free hemodialysis with citrate-containing dialysate in intensive care patients. Dial Transplant 29:620–626
90. Vilbar RM, Ing TS, Shin KD, et al. (1978) Treatment of metabolic alkalosis with peritoneal dialysis in a patient with renal failure. Artif Organs 2:421–422
91. Vaziri ND, Kayichian D (2007) Serum enzyme levels. In: Daugirdas JT, Blake PG, Ing TS (eds) Handbook of Dialysis, 4th ed. Lippincott Williams & Wilkins, Philadelphia, PA, pp 482–489
92. Warshaw AL, O'Hara PJ (1978) Susceptibility of the pancreas to ischemic injury in shock. Ann Surg 188:197–201
93. Wesdorp RI, Falcao HA, Banks PB, et al. (1981) Gastrin and gastric acid secretion in renal failure. Am J Surg 141: 334–338
94. Zachee P, Lins RL, De Broe ME (1985) Serum amylase and lipase values in acute renal failure. Clin Chem 31:1237

4.11 Cardiovascular Complications of Acute Kidney Injury

W. Van Biesen and R. Vanholder

Core Messages

- The heart and kidney are closely linked. One should always suspect the presence of the other part of the twin when confronted problems with the first part. Prevention of contrast-induced nephropathy starts with considering renal function. Many cardiac medications (e.g., angiotensin-converting enzyme inhibitors) are nephrotoxic. Cardiorenal cross-talk can explain cardiac failure in patients with acute kidney injury (AKI).
- Correct assessment of volume status is of importance both for cardiac and for renal function. The concept of "volume responsiveness" is the most useful clinic tool to evaluate volume status of patients. The leg-tilt test, using pulse pressure variation might be of help.
- Whereas the use of inotropic and vasoconstrictive medication is the treatment of choice to preserve renal perfusion pressure in volume-replenished patients, care should be given to the potential cardiac negative effects of these agents.

4.11.1 Introduction

The relation between the kidney and the heart is a quite complex one for several reasons. As the kidney behaves as a filter, cleaning the blood pumped out by the heart, there is a clear hemodynamic relation, and this relation is most likely the best understood one. Also, as the kidney fails, uremic waste products will accumulate, with a potential negative influence on cardiac function. Third, there is also more and more evidence for a direct humoral link between the damaged kidney and the heart by the interplay of cytokines and hormonal signaling pathways [1]. Finally, renal replacement therapies can cause additional stress to the heart, as they can disturb the homeostasis both of the milieu intérieur as of the hemodynamic regulation.

At the end, it will appear that in some situations, one of both organs should be artificially supported to spare the other.

4.11.2 Differential Diagnosis of Acute Cardiorenal Dysfunction

4.11.2.1 Cardiac Problems Causing Acute Kidney Injury

4.11.2.1.1 Chronic Cardiac Problems

The heart is the driving force for maintaining kidney perfusion and filtration pressure. Heart failure will thus inevitably result in decreasing renal function, and eventually acute kidney injury (AKI). This condition is explored in more depth in other chapters of this book.

W. Van Biesen (✉)
Renal Division, Department of Internal Medicine, University Hospital Gent, ICU De pintelaan 185, 9000 Gent, Belgium
e-mail: wim.vanbiesen@ugent.be

A. Jörres et al. (eds.), *Management of Acute Kidney Problems*,
DOI: 10.1007/978-3-540-69441-0_4.11, © Springer-Verlag Berlin Heidelberg 2010

As cardiac disease and chronic renal disease are linked, it is clear that those patients at risk for developing cardiac problems, like, e.g., diabetics, are mostly already compromised in their renal function [2]. In addition, most of these patients are treated with medications that inhibit the autoregulation of renal perfusion, such as inhibitors of the renine–angiontensine–aldosterone axis [3, 4] and diuretics. They also tend to undergo tests and interventions that are potentially nephrotoxic, such as angiography [5] and extracorporeal circulation [6, 7]. In patients with even small decreases of glomerular filtration, these interventions involve a quite high risk for development of AKI [8]. On the other hand, patients with chronic renal insufficiency seem to be treated inferiorly for their cardiac disease as compared with patients with normal kidney function, leading to a worse prognosis [9]. This effect is probably related to fear of using potentially nephrotoxic interventions to treat the heart condition.

4.11.2.2 Causes of Concomitant Acute Kidney Injury and Cardiac Problems

In some cases, the combined presentation of cardiac problems and AKI might indicate the presence of one common underlying cause.

4.11.2.2.1 Toxic Causes

A wide variety of toxins and medications can cause both cardiac and renal damage. *Cocaine, heroin, amphetamines*, and some other illegal drugs can cause AKI by different mechanisms, such as glomerulonephritis and acute tubular necrosis, but also rhabdomyolysis, and infectious complications of (intravenous) drug use should be excluded, especially when there is evidence for cardiac valve dysfunction. Most of these drugs also have a negative inotropic effect, leading to congestive heart failure, or they cause arrhythmias. Most of these drugs increase cardiac oxygen consumption, and decrease coronary perfusion by causing tachycardia, which can lead to myocardial infarction.

Ethanol is a legal drug that causes both chronic cardiomyopathy and acute congestive heart failure. Ethanol abuse has been linked to IgA nephropathy, leading to chronic renal failure.

Propofol, a sedative agent widely used in the intensive care unit, has been related to sudden-onset AKI, metabolic acidosis, rhabdomyolysis, and cardiac dysfunction. Although the underlying mechanism is not quite clear, there might be a link with disturbance of mitochondrial energy delivery pathways. Propofol infusion syndrome is a rare but frequently fatal complication in critically patients who are given prolonged high-dose infusions of the drug [10].

Ethylene glycol is a well-known renal toxin, that can, however, also cause severe myocarditis [11].

The nephrotoxic effects of *lithium* have been well recognized [12]. Accumulation of lithium might lead to serious cardiac arrhythmias such as atrioventricular and intraventricular conduction delays and QT-segment elongation.

4.11.2.2.2 Infectious Diseases

Several infectious diseases may cause concomitant cardiac and renal problems.

Patients with infective endocarditis can develop AKI due to embolization of thrombi consisting of microorganism-containing vegetation. Most of these patients will also have other signs of embolization in their extremities, brain, and eyes. Some organisms, such as *Staphylococcus aureus* or beta hemolytic streptococci can induce an immune-mediated type glomerulonephritis, mostly a crescentic rapidly progressive glomerulonephritis. As most of the treatment regimes for infectious endocarditis contain aminoglycosides, the differential diagnosis may not be straightforward.

Viruses and atypical bacteria can be the common cause of pericarditis, myocarditis, and a concomitant renal injury, either a glomerulonephritis or an interstitial nephritis.

4.11.2.2.3 Autoimmune Disease and Vasculitis

In patients presenting with cardiac problems and AKI, an underlying systemic disease should be ruled out. Most frequently, the AKI is the most prominent clinical feature, with secondary cardiac congestion due to anasarca. However, pericarditis, myocarditis, and especially arrhythmias due to disturbed conductance are more frequently seen in vasculitis. These are especially prominent in lupus, but also other causes of vasculitis, such as Wegener's granulomatosis, have been related to, e.g., myocarditis.

4.11.2.2.4 Chronic Diseases

When no data on previous renal function are known, one should ascertain the absence of a chronic underlying illness that decompensates, mimicking an acute failure. Some genetic diseases, such as Fabry disease, or other metabolic diseases, cause both cardiac and renal failure.

Amyloidosis can also present as a congestive heart failure with concomitant diuretic resistant anasarca and renal failure or nephrotic syndrome.

4.11.2.2.5 Cardiorenal Cross Talk

There is accumulating evidence that acute kidney injury as seen during ischemia reperfusion evokes also damage in other organs [13]. Kelly et al. [1] described an increase of mRNA of interleukin-1(IL-1), tumor necrosis factor-a (TNF-a), and intercellular adhesion molecule 1 in the heart. This was accompanied by functional changes such as increased left ventricular diameter and decreased fractional shortening, and by morphologic changes such as apoptosis.

Rabb et al. [14], doing comparable experiments, found up-regulation of pulmonary expression of water channels, again compatible with cross-talk between the injured kidney and other organs. In patients with incipient sepsis, already the first day there is evidence for cardiopulmonary problems in those who will develop AKI later on [15]. Unless there is clear evidence for dehydration, fluid loading should be scrutinized in this type of patient [16].

4.11.3 Cardiovascular Complications of Acute Kidney Injury

Cardiovascular complications of AKI can be divided in volume-mediated, toxicity-mediated, and therapy-mediated causes.

4.11.3.1 Causes and Underlying Pathophysiology

4.11.3.1.1 Volume

Volume overload in patients with AKI might have multiple causes, but is mostly iatrogenic. Intentional fluid overload can be caused by an attempt to preserve renal function by correcting "dehydration" in a patient with oliguria. Volume status in an intensive care unit patient might be difficult to assess, but is in fact not what really matters. The more pertinent question is, would further fluid loading improve organ perfusion and function? [17] Organ perfusion is related to cardiac output and perfusion pressure. According to Starlings law, stroke volume will go up if the preload (end-diastolic volume) goes up (Fig. 4.11.1). This is however only true in a

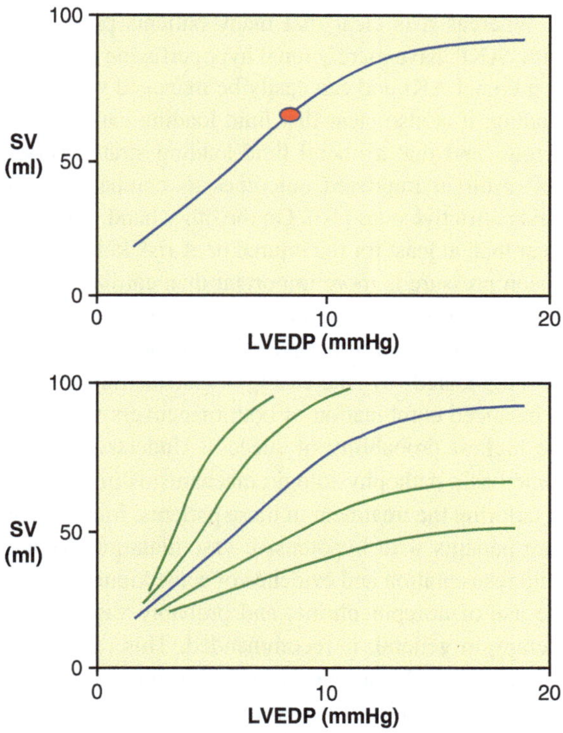

Fig. 4.11.1 *Upper panel*: As left ventricular end-diastolic pressure (LVEDP) increases (*left* to *right* in X-axis), stroke volume (SV) also increases (Y-axis). The relation is not linear, but sigmoidal *Lower panel*: Normal relationship between LVEDP and SV in blue. In patients under inotropic agents, or when afterload decreases (inodilation, or septic shock) the curve shifts to the left upper region of the figure, in patients with heart failure, or when afterload increases (vasoconstriction), the curve shifts to the right under region

limited range of end-diastolic volumes, and if the underlying cardiac muscle is normal. The "preload sensitivity" can accurately be tested by performing the simple bedside leg-tilt test [17]. The premise of this test is that the preload increases by the increased venous return to the right atrium by elevating the legs. If this results in an increase in cardiac output (e.g., measured by aortic flow, or by cardiac ultrasound, or by intra-arterial online blood pressure), the patient is said to be "preload sensitive," and fluid loading will result in improved cardiac output and perfusion pressure. If the left ventricle is overstretched by the excess circulating volume, cardiac output will not further increase at a certain point. The excess blood volume will cause pulmonary congestion, and eventually pulmonary edema. Although the fractional urinary excretion of sodium and/or of urea can be of help to determine the presence of renal hypoperfusion [18], this does not automatically imply that fluid loading will result in better renal function.

Whereas it is clear that many patients presenting with "AKI" have merely renal hypoperfusion resulting in prerenal AKI and can easily be managed with fluid loading, it is also clear that fluid loading can be dangerous, and that a liberal fluid-loading strategy does not result in improved outcomes as compared with fluid restrictive ones [16]. On the other hand, it is also clear that, at least for the injured or at-risk kidney, perfusion pressure is more important than cardiac output per se. As this perfusion pressure is the consequence of cardiac output and of peripheral resistance, it can also be augmented by increasing vasoconstriction [7]. A balanced combination of both maneuvers will have the highest probability of success. Understanding of some basic pathophysiologic mechanisms might help in tailoring the treatment in these patients. In intensive care patients with hypotensive vasodilatation despite fluid resuscitation and evidence of acute kidney injury, the use of norepinephrine, and probably vasopressor therapy in general, is recommended. This concept is based on the physiology of perfusion pressure of the glomerulus, and is further corroborated by experimental and human data [19, 20].

Concept of Diastolic Dysfunction

Volume overload from the point of view of the heart might have multiple causes and underlying mechanisms. As will be clear from the following, it is of utmost importance to understand that "volume overload" has more to do with the manner the heart deals with this volume at hand then with the amount of circulating volume per se. The elasticity of the left ventricle is an important property to allow ventricular filling during diastole. In normal conditions, the largest part of ventricular filling will be induced by the negative pressure generated by the elastic recoil of the ventricle after systolic contraction, and only a minor part will be induced by the contraction of the left atrium, resulting in a typical bimodal pattern of transmitral flow, with a higher first than second peak. Diastolic dysfunction can be the result of ischemia (stunning) or of toxic mediators, e.g., related to sepsis. If the diastolic function is abnormal, the intraventricular pressure will rise more rapidly for the same volume of preload. Again, pulmonary congestion will result. These patients have normal dimensions of the left ventricle, and also present a normal ejection fraction on cardiac ultrasound, which might erroneously lead to the conclusion that cardiac function is normal. Diastolic dysfunction can emerge abruptly, and can be hallmarked by a sudden abrupt increase of left atrial filling pressure and pulmonary congestion, with little or even no preceding fluid load [15]. Often it induces a vicious circle, as diastolic dysfunction caused by ischemia resulting in pulmonary congestion, will rapidly result in a further decrease of oxygenation, and thus stunning. Diastolic dysfunction can be chronic, e.g., in patients with fibrosis, or left ventricular hypertrophy, where it can remain subclinical. In these patients, left ventricular filling is highly dependent upon the atrial kick. When a sudden atrial arrhythmia occurs, this leads to acute preload failure and pulmonary congestion (Fig. 4.11.2).

Diastolic dysfunction can also be the first sign of pericarditis or pericardial effusion, as in both conditions, the normal relaxation of the left ventricle will be impaired. Pericarditis can be caused by uremia itself, but can also be related to the underlying disease itself, e.g., infection, vasculitis, or drugs.

Concept of Diastolic Coronary Perfusion

The coronary circulation, which delivers the oxygen rich blood to the cardial myocytes, is only perfused during the diastole. Conditions that shorten the diastolic perfusion time will thus limit the coronary oxygenation. Also, in conditions of stunning, the myocardial muscle will not completely relax, and a continuous degree of coronary squeezing will be present. The perfusion pressure of the coronaries is generated by the elastic recoil

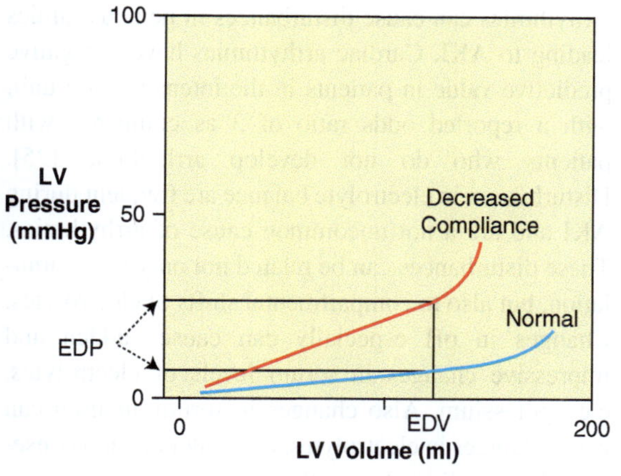

Fig. 4.11.2 *Diastolic dysfunction*: In patients with diastolic dysfunction, the relation between left ventricular volume (end-diastolic volume [EDV], X-axis) and left ventricular pressure (end-diastolic pressure [EDP], Y-axis) is shifted to the upper left part of the figure. This means that the increase in EDP is higher for a smaller EDV. As a consequence, stroke volume will go down

of the large vessels (Windkessel function). In conditions where this elasticity is lost, diastolic coronary perfusion will be jeopardized. Most patients with preexisting cardiovascular disease or with chronic renal failure have a decrease in their vascular wall elasticity. In addition, accumulation of toxins during renal failure might result in an acute stiffening of the vessels by disrupting the regulative role of the endothelium in vascular tone through, e.g., nitric oxide, endothelial hyperpolarizing factor, and prostacyclins.

To cause flow in the coronaries, it is also necessary that the aortic valve seals perfectly. Leakage of the aortic valve during diastole will cause blood flow to go into the ventricle rather than into the coronaries, thus diminishing coronary perfusion. Dilatation of the left ventricle might cause leakage through the aortic valve, as the annular ring also will dilate, so that the valves become insufficient. This is a vicious circle, as the regurgitation of blood from the aorta to the left ventricle during the diastole, and the decreased coronary perfusion with resulting diastolic dysfunction, will result in further dilatation of the left ventricle.

Toxic Causes

During acute kidney injury, toxic mediators with negative impact on cardiovascular function might be released or accumulate in the circulation [1].

4.11.3.1.2 Therapeutic Consequences

Volume Resuscitation

Volume resuscitation should be done rather cautiously, unless overt and clear hypovolemia is present [16]. It should be guided by the preload responsiveness of the patient (leg-tilt test) [17]. The use of pulmonary artery catheters should be avoided, except in patients with complex valvular problems, because they have no proven benefit in avoiding AKI, and because they are a frequent cause of cardiac complications such as arrhythmias and valvular lesions. There is no evidence that colloid are superior to crystalloid osmotic fluids [21], and there is even a suspicion that starches might be detrimental [22]

As vasoconstriction by the use of vasopressive agents is as effective in restoring renal blood flow as volume resuscitation, but in general more easily and rapidly reversible, it should be preferred in not overtly dehydrated patients. The finding of high fractional excretion of urea in the urea nearly excludes hypovolemia, and should bar further volume resuscitation.

Vasopressor Therapy

By increasing vasoconstriction, vasopressors will increase peripheral resistance, and thus perfusion pressure. In addition, preload will be improved by recruitment of fluids in the capacity vessels. All this comes at the expense of an increase of cardiac workload, and potentially increased oxygen consumption. In addition, most of these agents will induce tachycardia, with a negative impact on coronary oxygen delivery, and increased pulse wave reflection, leading to increased ventricular work load. Dopamine should be avoided as it has no proven renal benefit, causes easily arrhythmias, and increases myocardial oxygen consumption [23]. Today, the agent of choice should be norepinephrine [20]. In patients with (septic) shock, vasopressin seems to be a promising agent [24]. It results in a strong vasoconstriction in the splanchnic region, resulting in enhanced preload by redistribution, and causes a vasoconstriction of the efferent glomerular arterioles, increasing filtration pressure. More importantly, it seems to augment blood pressure without jeopardizing cardiac output, causing tachycardia, or increasing cardiac oxygen consumption.

Pericarditis

Uremic pericarditis is a condition which has been reported frequently in chronic renal failure, but that also exists in acute renal failure. There appears to be no clear relation between the degree of retention of uremic waste products, e.g., creatinine, and the occurrence of pericarditis. Despite this, most cases of uremic pericarditis will resolve by starting or augmenting the dose of renal replacement therapy. In patients with AKI where the diagnosis is not 100% clear, and who present pericarditis, an underlying systemic or infectious disease should be excluded.

Pericarditis should actively be searched for in patients with AKI by daily auscultation of the heart, which reveals a typical friction rub in the beginning phase. When the friction sound disappears, either the pericarditis disappears, or a pericardial effusion has emerged. A cardiac ultrasound will easily lead to the correct diagnosis. Pericardial tamponade will lead to pulsus paradoxus, distension of the jugular veins, even during inspiration, and a rapid fall in cardiac output and blood pressure. On cardiac ultrasound, a typical compression of the right atrium and/or ventricle by pericardial fluid will be present.

Cardiac Arrhythmias

In patients with AKI, many reasons can be present to cause cardiac arrhythmias. Vice versa, cardiac arrhythmias can cause disturbances in hemodynamics leading to AKI. Cardiac arrhythmias have a negative predictive value in patients in the intensive care unit, with a reported odds ratio of 3 as compared with patients who do not develop arrhythmia [25]. Disturbances in electrolyte balance are frequent during AKI and are a not uncommon cause of arrhythmias. These disturbances can be related not only to accumulation, but also to compartmental shifts of electrolytes. Changes in pH especially can cause sudden and impressive changes in serum levels of electrolytes, e.g., potassium. Also changes in serum albumin can cause changes in electrolytes, e.g., calcium, and consequently induction of arrhythmias.

In patients with AKI, arrhythmias can also be induced by accumulation of proarrhythmogenic drugs, either by decreased clearance, or by changes in distribution volume. Dose adaptation is warranted for most antiarrhythmic drugs (Table 4.11.1).

Arrhythmias can also be induced by the presence of indwelling lines, such as dialysis catheters or pulmonary artery catheters.

Last, but not least, arrhythmias can be induced by most inotropic agents, such as dopamine [23].

Table 4.11.1 Adaptation of antiarrhythmic agents in renal failure

Drug	Dose adaptation	RRT clearance	Remarks
Disopyramide	Yes	No	
Lidocaine	No	No	Not recommended for long-term administration
Flecainide	Yes	No	
Amiodarone	No	No	
Digoxin	Yes	No	Not to be used when also electrolyte disorders are present
Verapamil	No	Unknown	To be avoided in renal insufficiency
Bretylium	Yes	Yes	
Propafenone	No	No	

4.11.4 Conclusion

The heart and the kidney are closely linked, both by functionally and biochemically. Poor cardiac function will result in renal hypoperfusion, whereas renal dysfunction might lead to volume overload, and finally cardiac failure. Retention of uremic toxins and cytokines can have a negative impact on cardiac function, and electrolyte disturbances caused by renal dysfunction can induce arrhythmias.

A correct volume status is of importance to preserve both cardiac and renal function. This is best evaluated by clinical examination, using pulse pressure variation, during a volume responsiveness test. There is no evidence that liberal fluid loading is better than more restricted volume loading. If patients do not respond to fluid loading, vasopressors should be used to maintain renal perfusion pressure. These agents can, however, cause cardiac ischemia by causing tachycardia, increased afterload, and decreased diastolic coronary perfusion time.

References

1. Kelly KJ. Distant effects of experimental renal ischemia/reperfusion injury. *J Am Soc Nephrol* 2003; 14: 1549–1558
2. Best P, Holmes D. Chronic kidney disease as a cardiovascular risk factor. *Am Heart J* 2003; 145: 383–386
3. Stirling C, Houston J, Robertson S et al. Diarrhoea, vomiting and ACE inhibitors: – an important cause of acute renal failure. *J Hum Hypertens* 2003; 17: 419–423
4. McGuigan J, Robertson S, Isles C. Life threatening hyperkalaemia with diarrhoea during ACE inhibition. *Emerg Med J* 2005; 22: 154–155
5. Dangas G, Iakovou I, Nikolsky E et al. Contrast-induced nephropathy after percutaneous coronary interventions in relation to chronic kidney disease and hemodynamic variables. *Am J Cardiol* 2005; 95: 13–19
6. Kuitunen A, Vento A, Suojaranta-Ylinen R, Pettila V. Acute renal failure after cardiac surgery: evaluation of the RIFLE classification. *Ann Thorac Surg* 2006; 81: 542–546
7. Lameire N, Van Biesen W, Vanholder R. Acute renal failure. *Lancet* 2005; 365: 417–430
8. Lassnigg A, Schmidlin D, Mouhieddine M et al. Minimal changes of serum creatinine predict prognosis in patients after cardiothoracic surgery: a prospective cohort study. *J Am Soc Nephrol* 2004; 15: 1597–1605
9. Beattie JN, Soman SS, Sandberg KR et al. Determinants of mortality after myocardial infarction in patients with advanced renal dysfunction. *Am J Kidney Dis* 2001; 37: 1191–1200
10. Sabsovich I., Rehman Z., Yunen J., Coritsidis G. Propofol infusion syndrome: a case of increasing morbidity with traumatic brain injury. *Am J Crit Care* 2007; 82–85.
11. Guo C MKE. The cytotoxicity of oxalate, metabolite of ethylene glycol, is due to calcium oxalate monohydrate formation. *Toxicology* 2005; 347–355.
12. Hansen HE AA. Lithium intoxication. *Q J Med* 1978; 123–144.
13. Van Biesen W., Lameire N., Vanholder R., MR. Relation between acute kidney injury and multiple-organ failure: the chicken and the egg question. *Crit Care Med* 2007; 316–317.
14. Rabb H, Wang Z, Nemoto T, Hotchkiss J, Yokota N, Soleimani M. Acute renal failure leads to dysregulation of lung salt and water channels. *Kidney Int* 2003; 63: 600–606.
15. Van Biesen W, Yegenaga I, Vanholder R et al. Relationship between fluid status and its management on acute renal failure (ARF) in intensive care unit (ICU) patients with sepsis: a prospective analysis. *J Nephrol* 2005; 18: 54–60.
16. Wiedemann H., Wheeler A., BG, et al Comparison of two fluid-management strategies in acute lung injury. *N Engl J Med* 2006; 2564–2575.
17. Monnet X., Rienzo M., Osman D. et al. Passive leg raising predicts fluid responsiveness in the critically ill. *Crit Care Med* 2006; 1402–1407.
18. Carvounis CP, Nisar S, Guro-Razuman S. Significance of the fractional excretion of urea in the differential diagnosis of acute renal failure. *Kidney Int* 2002; 62: 2223–2229
19. Bellomo R., Wan L., May C. Vasoactive drugs and acute kidney injury. *Crit Care Med* 2008; S179–S186.
20. Leone M., Martin C. Vasopressor use in septic shock: an update. *Curr Opin Anaesthesiol* 2008; 141–147.
21. Alderson P, Bunn F, Lefebvre C, Li WP, Li L, Roberts I, Schierhout G; Albumin Reviewers. *Cochrane Database Syst Rev*. 2004;(4): CD001208. Review
22. Brunkhorst F., Engel C., Bloos F. Intensive insulin therapy and pentastarch resuscitation in severe sepsis. *N Engl J Med* 2008; 125–139.
23. Kellum J., Decker J. Use of dopamine in acute renal failure: a meta-analysis. *Crit Care Med* 2001; 1526–1531.
24. Tsuneyoshi I., Yamada H., Kakihana Y., Nakamura M., Nakano Y., Boyle W. Hemodynamic and metabolic effects of low-dose vasopressin infusions in vasodilatory septic shock. *Crit Care Med* 2001; 487–493.
25. Goodman S., Shirov T., Weissman C. Supraventricular arrhythmias in intensive care unit patients: short and long-term consequences. *Anesth Analg.* 2007;104(4): 880-886.

Acute Kidney Injury: Specific Interventions and Drugs

4.12

John R. Prowle and Rinaldo Bellomo

Core Messages

- Many specific interventions and drugs have been used to protect the kidney in high-risk situations (prophylaxis) or to attenuate loss of function in patients with acute kidney injury (AKI), but very few have been tested in large multicenter double-blind randomized controlled trials (MC-DB-RCTs).
- Nephrotoxins must be removed whenever possible.
- Iso-osmolar nonionic contrast media attenuate the incidence and severity of contrast-induced nephropathy (CIN).
- Fluid loading with intravenous normal saline at 1 ml/kg/h has been shown to attenuate CIN in a large single-center RCT.
- No other prophylactic or therapeutic intervention has been consistently shown to be protective to the kidney.
- Low-dose dopamine has been strongly shown not to deliver any protection from kidney injury in a large MC-DB-RCT.
- A better understanding of the pathogenesis of AKI in different clinical states and the availability of biomarkers which allow the early diagnosis of AKI are both sorely needed if future interventions are to prove more effective.

R. Bellomo (✉)
Department of Intensive Care, Austin Hospital, Studley Rd, Heidelberg, Victoria 3084, Australia
e-mail: rinaldo.bellomo@austin.org.au

4.12.1 Introduction

Multiple specific interventions and drugs have been proposed as protective to the kidney in high-risk situations or in the setting of developing or established acute kidney injury (AKI). In this chapter, we will focus on each specific intervention or drug and discuss our knowledge on their possible efficacy or lack of efficacy in the different clinical contexts where they been used. We will also discuss specific high-risk situations or unique clinical syndromes (contrast-induced nephropathy [CIN], rhabdomyolysis, hepatorenal syndrome, and increased intra-abdominal pressure) as they are the clinical conditions in which some very specific interventions or drugs have been studied. We will conclude by discussing possible explanations for the findings so far in this field and present possible research strategies, which might assist in the future development of effective interventions.

Irrespective of the specific interventions and drugs discussed below, it is the strongly held opinion of the authors that much effort and time is sometimes spent in the pursuit of "magic bullets," or specific drug-based interventions to protect the kidneys, while fundamental aspects or interventions are forgotten or delayed which carry overwhelming physiological and pharmacological weight.

Accordingly, we wish to start this chapter by emphasizing that the following steps must be taken in ALL patients and situations discussed in this chapter before any other intervention is considered:

1. Ensure adequate intravascular filling
2. Ensure adequate mean arterial pressure
3. Ensure adequate cardiac output
4. Ensure adequate hemoglobin
5. Remove all nephrotoxins (if possible)

A. Jörres et al. (eds.), *Management of Acute Kidney Problems*,
DOI: 10.1007/978-3-540-69441-0_4.12, © Springer-Verlag Berlin Heidelberg 2010

In some cases, there will be uncertainty about whether steps 1 to 3 have been achieved. In such cases, if active therapy is contemplated, the necessary information MUST be rapidly obtained (invasively, if necessary). Attempting renal protection without so doing in the appropriate clinical situations is physiologically wrong and will likely lead to clinical failure.

4.12.2 Contrast-Induced Nephropathy

This is the third single most common cause of AKI, and it accounts for approximately 10–30% of cases of AKI, and is discussed in detail elsewhere in this book. In brief, many trials have been conducted testing possible preventive strategies. However, only prehydration with normal saline and the use of iso-osmolar nonionic media have been consistently found to be protective against CIN.

Good evidence exists that isotonic intravenous hydration is effective in reducing the incidence of CIN. A large randomized controlled trial (RCT) [1] showed a reduction in incidence of CIN in patients pretreated with 0.9% saline versus 0.45% saline in dextrose.

Iso-osmolar nonionic media have been shown to be associated with a significantly lower incidence of CIN than ionic high-osmolality media in a multicenter double-blind randomized controlled trials (MC-DB-RCT) [2] of 1,196 patients and are now considered the standard of care. No other interventions for CIN have been shown effective in an MC-DB-RCT and cannot be currently recommended. Smaller trials are discussed in detail in the dedicated chapter.

4.12.3 Nephrotoxins

Circulating exogenous toxins are an important cause of secondary AKI. They may affect glomerular hemodynamics or cause direct tubular injury. Agents such as nonsteroidal antiinflammatory drugs and calcineurin inhibitors increase afferent arteriolar tone reducing renal blood flow and glomerular filtration rate (GFR). This may be one setting where relative renal vasoconstriction is an important factor and, in the setting of systemic hemodynamic instability, may be sufficient to mediate ischemic tubular injury.

Other nephrotoxins, prototypically aminoglycosides, act directly on the tubules. The tubular environment may be uniquely sensitive to filtered or circulating nephrotoxins, particularly via oxidant injury; concentration of filtered toxins in the tubules and the baseline borderline ischemia within these regions may account for this sensitivity.

Interventions in nephrotoxic kidney injury must commence with minimization or elimination of the injurious agent. Specific interventions have then included attempts to dilute toxins or neutralize oxidant species, the effectiveness of such strategies will be dependent on their timing with respect to the nephrotoxic injury.

4.12.4 Specific Interventions for AKI

Interventions for AKI can be classified by their proposed point of action in the pathogenesis of the clinical syndrome, from avoidance of primary injury through to acceleration of renal recovery after sustained acute kidney failure. Table 4.12.1 classifies specific nephroprotective therapies in this fashion. Attempted intervention may be to prevent AKI prior to a predictable renal insult or to limit injury once it has occurred. Discussion of the evidence base for these treatments considers these different scenarios separately.

4.12.4.1 Primary Prevention of AKI

4.12.4.1.1 Fluid Therapy

Intravascular volume depletion is a major risk factor for contrast-induced AKI, and a number of fluid administration-based strategies for the prevention of AKI have been studied with evidence of protective benefit in the setting of CIN; however, there is no formal randomized control trial comparing intravenous volume expansion against no volume expansion.

4.12.4.1.2 Vasodilators

Based on the theory that renal vasoconstriction causes a fall in renal blood flow and ischemic tubular injury,

Table 4.12.1 Specific interventions for acute kidney injury classified by proposed mechanism of action

Strategy	Intervention
Hemodynamic	
Maintenance of cardiac output	Intravenous fluids Inotropic therapy Withdrawal of diuretics and negative inotropes
Maintenance of renal perfusion pressure	Vasopressors Removal of antihypertensives Treatment of raised intra-abdominal pressure Vasopressin analogs in hepatorenal syndrome
Maintenance of glomerular hydrostatic gradient	Avoidance of prostaglandin synthesis inhibitors (nonsteroidal antiinflammatory drugs) and other afferent renal vasoconstrictors Avoidance of renin-angiotensin-aldosterone system inhibitors
Specific renal vasodilators	Dopamine & other selective dopamine agonists Natriuretic peptides Endothelin antagonists Adenosine antagonists
Nephrotoxicity	
Reduction	Iso-osmolar radiological contrast
Prevention of tubular toxicity: dilution	Intravenous fluid Diuretics Natriuretic peptides
Prevention of tubular toxicity: neutralization	Antioxidants including N-acetylcysteine Bicarbonate Iron chelators Caspase inhibitors
Prevention of tubular toxicity: removal	Blood purification techniques including continuous hemofiltration
Cellular Response	
Cytoprotection	Ischemic preconditioning Cooling Thyroxine Insulin and IGFs
Antiinflammatory agents	HMG CoA reductase inhibitors ("statins") Anti-ICAM-1 CD11a Ab Anti-B7-1 Ab IL-10 PAF antagonists A_{2A} Adenosine-R agonists
Agents to promote recovery	Growth factors (including EGF, HGF, BMP-7, etc.)

vasodilatory agents have long been advocated as specific treatments for AKI and many of these agents have been studied in the context of primary prevention.

By action at DA1 receptors low-dose dopamine (0.5–3 μg/kg/min) can cause decreased renal vascular resistance and increased renal blood flow in experimental situations [3]. The clinical significance of this effect in human disease states is questionable. No evidence exists to support a benefit from dopamine as a specific intervention as primary prevention for AKI when studied in the settings of radio-contrast exposure and cardiopulmonary bypass [4, 5] (Fig. 4.12.1).

Fenoldopam, a highly selective DA1 agonist, has also been advocated as a nephroprotective agent and an alternative to dopamine; however, two prospective randomized controlled trials in the prevention of contrast nephropathy [6, 7] and one in cardiac surgery [8] have failed to show any benefit over placebo. Taken together these results form strong evidence against the prophylactic use of DA1 agonists in primary prevention of renal injury.

Natriuretic peptides act as systemic and renal vasodilators and enhance renal salt and water excretion, but their exact physiological role remains uncertain. In a double-bind placebo-controlled trial, infusion of atrial natriuretic peptide did not reduce the risk of contrast nephropathy [9].

Endothelin is a powerful endogenous vasoconstrictor, which has been proposed as another mediator of renal vasoconstriction and ischemic injury; however, in a randomized placebo-controlled trial of a nonselective endothelin antagonist for prevention of contrast nephropathy in high-risk patients there was a significantly

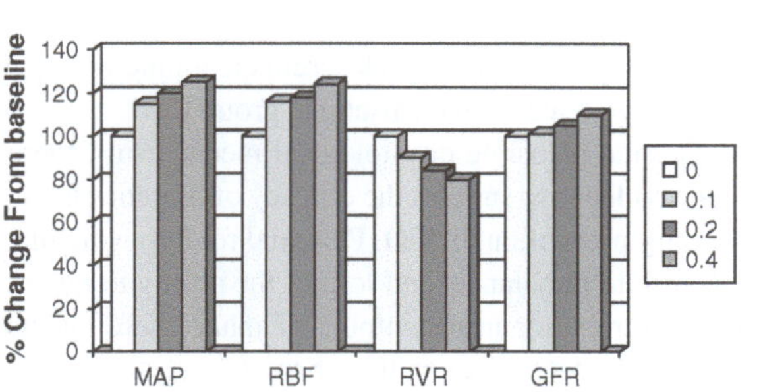

Fig. 4.12.1 Changes in serum creatinine in patients randomized to either placebo or low-dose dopamine begun prior to and continued for 24 h after cardiopulmonary bypass

adverse effect in the treatment group as defined by peak serum creatinine [10].

Adenosine is thought to be a local mediator of tubuloglomerular feedback, a vasoconstrictive autoregulatory response to hyperfiltration. Theophylline an adenosine antagonist has been examined for nephroprotective benefit in contrast nephropathy in a number of small studies. A small benefit in serum creatinine is suggested in a meta-analysis of these studies [11]; however, this is insufficient to recommend use of adenosine antagonists outside of large, well-designed randomized controlled trials.

4.12.4.1.3 Diuretics

Loop diuretics have long been used in attempts to preserve renal function despite having no direct effect on GFR. It has been theorized that an increase in tubular fluid volume might dilute nephrotoxins, that blockage of the NKCC2 cotransporter may reduce tubular oxygen demand, and that reduction of chloride transport to the macula densa may relax tubuloglomerular feedback. Similarly the osmotic diuretic mannitol has been advocated as a method of diluting tubular toxins and maintaining urine output. Clinical experience has not substantiated any meaningful protective effect from either agent, however. In a randomized controlled trial for the prevention of contrast nephropathy in patients with chronic kidney disease, frusemide or mannitol plus 0.45% saline were compared with fluid alone: a detrimental effect was observed with 40% of patients in the frusemide group, 28% with mannitol, and 11% in the control group [12]. In cardiac surgery, intravenous frusemide has been compared as a nephroprotective agent with low-dose dopamine (see 4.12.4.1.2) and placebo, and postoperative peak serum creatinine was significantly greater in the frusemide group [5].

Despite plausible physiological mechanisms, there is no evidence to support the efficacy of diuretics in the primary prevention of AKI. Potential for hypovolemia, electrolyte imbalance, and loss of the ability to meaningfully monitor urine output, all make these agents potentially deleterious in this context.

4.12.4.1.4 Antioxidants

Of the pharmacological agents investigated for the prevention of tubular injury N-acetylcysteine (NAC) has by far the largest literature. A reducing agent, NAC is thought to protect tubular cells from oxidant injury as a result of nephrotoxin exposure and ischemia. An initial randomized controlled trial [13] demonstrated a strong protective effect on the incidence of CIN as defined by rise in serum creatinine. Subsequently there have been a plethora of similar studies, the majority on renal protection in coronary angiography. While a standard dose of 600 mg orally twice daily 24 h either site of the procedure is commonly employed, higher doses [14], and the intravenous route [15] have also been examined. Numerous meta-analyses of these trials have been published [16–25]. There is significant publication bias and heterogeneity between studies [18], and meta-analyses vary in finding no benefit, or small effects in lowering the surrogate end point of peak serum creatinine. Collectively there is no conclusive evidence for true clinical efficacy of NAC. There has been some suggestion that the effects of NAC seen in some trials result from a decrease in serum creatinine by mechanisms unrelated to changes in GFR [26]; a recent randomized controlled trial has refuted this hypothesis, however [27]. Currently the evidence base does not exist to justify routine use of NAC; however, there is clinical equipoise for a large multicenter randomized controlled trial to more definitively determine its true clinical role, if any.

4.12.4.1.5 Statins

HMG CoA reductase inhibitors (statins) have pleiotropic effects beyond lowering serum cholesterol. They may protect against AKI by antioxidant, metabolic, or antiinflammatory effects. Retrospective studies in patients undergoing coronary angiography have found a lower incidence of contrast nephropathy in those patients receiving statin therapy [28]. Statins have also been shown to attenuate inflammatory response to cardiopulmonary bypass in man [29–31] and the severity of experimental AKI in animal models [32–35]. Randomized controlled trials are now required to test these agents in primary and secondary prevention of AKI. A phase II study is currently under way.

4.12.4.1.6 Blood Purification

Prophylactic renal replacement therapy (intermittent hemodialysis or continuous hemofiltration) has been investigated as a method of enhancing toxin removal and thus limiting renal exposure to injury. For prevention of contrast nephropathy in high-risk patients, no benefit has been demonstrated in small trials of prophylactic hemodialysis [36]; however, there is some evidence for a protective effect from hemofiltration [37]. While this approach is not widely applicable, it may be considered in selected patients at high risk, when resources are available.

4.12.4.1.7 Lessons from Primary Prevention

Specific pharmacological interventions for the primary prevention of AKI have been discouraging. This is doubly disappointing given that the intervention is given at the optimal time for prevention of injury. While contrast exposure or cardiopulmonary bypass are not prototypes for all forms of AKI, the failure of an intervention to demonstrate protection against these renal insults at the most favorable time point suggests that beneficial effects when employed later in the course of the clinical syndrome may be unlikely.

4.12.5 Secondary Prevention and Treatment of AKI

In secondary prevention of AKI, intervention is subsequent to the onset of the renal injury and often once biochemical *acute renal failure* has occurred. Given the unpredictable nature of human disease this is the usual clinical scenario. Many of the same agents employed in primary prevention have been utilized in attempts to treat established kidney injury.

4.12.5.1 Hemodynamic Optimization – Cardiac Output

Low cardiac output will reduce renal blood flow and is a risk factor for AKI after cardiac surgery. What constitutes an adequate cardiac output, and by what therapeutic approach this is achieved, will be specific to the individual clinical context. There is no evidence that supramaximal cardiac output is of protective benefit. Adequate volume resuscitation is a cornerstone to achieving acceptable cardiac output and is often the initial response to oliguria. Again what constitutes adequate filling and how to determine this clinically is a subject of debate beyond the scope of this review. As far as choice of resuscitation fluid is concerned, a large multicenter randomized controlled trial comparing crystalloid with albumin in critically ill patients found no significant difference in the incidence of AKI [38]. However, synthetic higher molecular weight colloids, the hydroxyethyl starches, have been associated with an increased incidence of AKI in critically ill patients [39] and may be directly toxic to the kidney. Despite recent development of supposedly less toxic, lower molecular weight starches, at present there is no evidence of safety for these agents and they should be avoided in those at risk of renal injury.

4.12.5.2 Vasopressor Therapy

Maintenance of renal perfusion pressure is required to achieve the glomerular pressure gradient for ultrafiltration and adequate renal blood flow. In context of untreated hypovolemia or low cardiac output, vasopressor therapy can adversely affect renal blood flow. However, in the hypotensive, adequately resuscitated patient, vasopressors will act to restore glomerular perfusion pressure and GFR (Fig. 4.12.2). This has been demonstrated in a clinical study of oliguric patients with septic shock when noradrenaline rapidly restored blood pressure with recovery of urine output [40] and is supported by experimental data (Fig. 4.12.3).

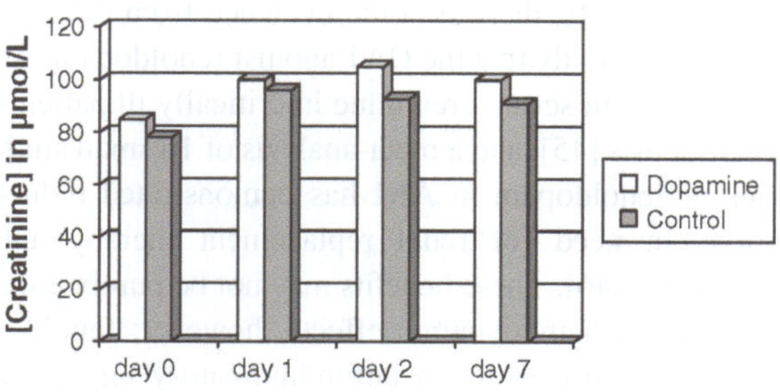

Fig. 4.12.2 Effect of vasopressor therapy on mean arterial pressure (MAP), renal blood flow (RBF), renal vascular resistance (RVR), and glomerular filtration rate (GFR) in the dog. Each value (0, 0.1, 0.2, and 0.4) refers to the dose of noradrenaline (norepinephrine) given at µg/ kg/min

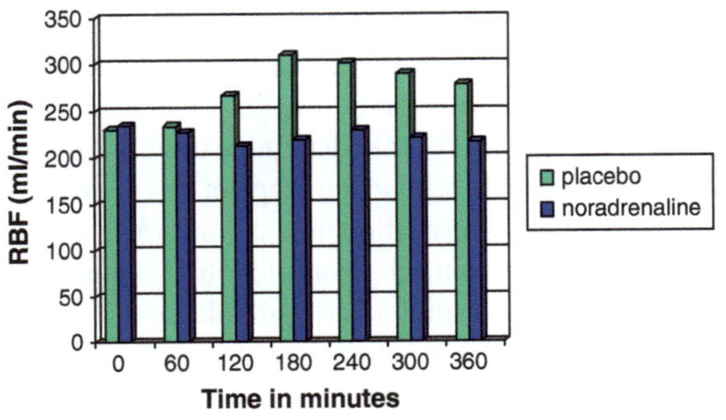

Fig. 4.12.3 Changes in left renal artery blood flow (RBF) during extended noradrenaline (norepinephrine) infusion in sheep

The optimal level of blood pressure to target has not been established and is likely to vary considerably between individuals. There is some evidence that a systolic pressure of <80 mm Hg in hospitalized patients is associated with greatly increased risk of AKI [41]; however, increasing mean arterial blood pressure beyond 65 mm Hg was not beneficial in a small randomized crossover study [42].

4.12.5.3 Renal Vasodilators

Low-dose dopamine has been used extensively to treat oliguric acute renal failure, despite little evidence of efficacy in the literature [43]. Subsequently, a multicenter, placebo controlled, randomized trial of low-dose dopamine (2 μg/kg/min) in patients meeting the criteria for systemic inflammatory response syndrome on admission to the intensive care unit (ICU), has shown that dopamine is no better than placebo in the secondary prevention of AKI [44]. This constitutes strong evidence against the use of low dose dopamine infusion in AKI.

Conversely, there is some evidence from one single-center study that the DA1 agonist fenoldopam can limit rises in serum creatinine in critically ill patients with sepsis [45], and a meta-analysis of 16 small studies of fenoldopam in AKI has demonstrated reductions in need for renal replacement therapy and mortality [46]. These benefits may not be purely attributable to hemodynamic effects, however; fenoldopam may also exert an antiinflammatory effect via blockade of nuclear factor kappa B (NF-κB) signal transduction that may be protective in AKI [47]. Further examination of the agent in larger randomized trials is justified.

Other vasodilatory agents including natriuretic factors, adenosine antagonists, and endothelin antagonists have also been explored for secondary prevention and treatment of acute renal failure. As yet there is no clinical evidence of sufficient quality to justify their use outside of clinical trials.

4.12.5.4 Diuretics

Historically, diuretics have been used for many decades to preserve urine output in acute renal failure. While there are physiological arguments for their use, and a continued flow of urine may be of psychological benefit to the treating physician, there is no evidence for beneficial effects on the course of AKI either for loop or osmotic diuretics.

In an observational study from the United States of patients with AKI, prior use of loop diuretics was associated with delayed referral and increased risk of death or end-stage renal disease [48]. In an international observational study of diuretic use in patients with AKI in intensive care there was no difference in mortality or renal outcome between those receiving diuretics and those who did not [49]. A meta-analysis [50] of five randomized controlled trials of diuretic use in AKI similarly showed no benefit in mortality or renal recovery, although time on renal replacement therapy was shorter; however, these studies were small, heterogeneous, and of poor methodological quality. Of course, diuretics have established clinical indications in the maintenance of fluid, potassium, and acid–base homeostasis, and their use for these indications should not be precluded. The current evidence would suggest that diuretic use for appropriate indications is safe, but that it will not affect the underlying progress of kidney injury. However, indiscriminate use merely to provoke urine output without other indications for diuresis, is not currently justified and is potentially harmful.

4.12.5.5 Cytoprotection

Alteration of renal cellular metabolism may exert protective effects against AKI. In experimental models of AKI, ischemic preconditioning is a powerful mechanism of protection [51]; however, outside of transplantation, this technique is not clinically applicable. Hypothermia, thyroxine, and insulin-like growth factor 1 (IGF-1) have all been suggested as agents that might induce similar protective changes in renal metabolism.

In two randomized controlled trials [52, 53] of hypothermia after cardiac arrest, hypothermia did not affect the course of kidney injury; this does not exclude, however, an effect in situations of primary prevention, such as prior to aortic cross-clamping. Thyroxine has been investigated for protective metabolic effects in AKI in a single-center trial which was stopped after interim analysis, due to increased mortality in the treatment arm [54]. A single-center study of IGF-1 in patients with AKI failed to demonstrate any benefit [55]. However, use of intensive insulin therapy in mechanically ventilated patients following major surgery was associated with a significant decrease in the requirement for renal replacement therapy [56], and in medical ICU patients, with a decreased incidence of new AKI [57]. However, these protocols, from a single center, have proved difficult to institute in general ICU populations, and renal function was not a primary end point of these trials.

Despite promising results from experimental models, thus far strategies to achieve protection by modification renal metabolism have not proven beneficial in treatment of AKI. The putative effects of intensive insulin in prevention of renal injury may be illuminated by the results of forthcoming randomized controlled trials.

4.12.5.6 Antiinflammatory Agents

In multiorgan failure, widespread endothelial activation and inappropriate systemic inflammatory responses are important mediators of organ dysfunction including renal injury. Blockade of these processes might ameliorate AKI. In particular, the complement cascade [58] and cellular adhesion molecules involved in leukocyte recruitment (specifically selectin–glycoside [59, 60] and ICAM–integrin [61] interactions) have been examined with protective benefit in experimental models. As yet these agents have not been examined in humans.

Recombinant activated protein C has been shown to reduce all-cause mortality in patients with severe sepsis and multiorgan failure, including renal failure [62]. A specific role for this anticoagulant and antiinflammatory agent in the prevention or limitation of acute renal failure has not yet been proven.

4.12.6 Specific Situations

4.12.6.1 Hepatorenal Syndrome

Hepatorenal syndrome (HRS) refers to a specific pathophysiological state where renal failure occurs in the context of chronic liver disease and in the absence of other causes of acute impairment. In HRS, the kidney is structurally normal but unable to achieve adequate GFR in an abnormal hemodynamic milieu of systemic hypotension and circulating endogenous vasopressors.

Therapies for HRS are aimed at stabilizing, or partially reversing, the decline in renal function to provide a bridge to a transplant or a period of symptomatic stability. Therapies target effective arterial under-filling and the production of endogenous renal vasoconstrictors by increasing vascular tone in the systemic and splanchnic beds. Vasopressin analogs have been the more successful agents in this context. Ornipressin, a vasopressin-1 agonist, has been shown to increase systemic and splanchnic vascular resistance, redistributing circulating blood volume, and increasing renal perfusion. Clinically it has been shown to suppress renin-angiotensin-aldosterone activity and improve renal function [63]. Long-term infusion is complicated by ischemic complications, however [64]. More recently, terlipressin, another vasopressin analog, has been successful in improving renal function, with a lower complication rate [65]. The effect was particularly marked when combined with volume expansion using intravenous albumin [66].

4.12.6.2 Abdominal Compartment Syndrome

Abdominal compartment syndrome [67] is a complication of critical illness where grossly elevated intra-abdominal pressure occurs in the context of primary abdominal pathology or, more rarely, secondary to massive fluid accumulation. Organ dysfunction occurs through venous congestion, impairment of arterial perfusion, and in the case of the kidney, obstruction to tubular flow. Renal perfusion and urine output may be restored by vasopressors to increase perfusion pressure; however, for definitive treatment, surgical decompression is often required [68].

4.12.6.3 Rhabdomyolysis

Rhabdomyolysis is a complication of major muscle injury from trauma, metabolic, or toxic injury. Myoglobin is vasoconstrictive, and filtered myoglobin may directly block tubules as insoluble pigment casts; however, the majority of toxicity is probably oxidative, principally via iron IV (ferryl)–induced lipid peroxidation [69]. The evidence for treatment is based on retrospective data, case series, and animal studies. No randomized controlled trials have been performed. Precipitants of muscle injury should be identified and corrected. Early and aggressive fluid resuscitation should be commenced aiming to maintain a high urine output (>300 ml/h). Alkalinization of the urine (pH >6.5) may solubilize myoglobin and prevent lipid peroxidation, and intravenous sodium bicarbonate should be infused to achieve this goal. Loop diuretics are not recommended as they acidify the tubular contents, while the role of mannitol is controversial. Myoglobin is not significantly removed by conventional hemofiltration, however a so-called super-high-flux membrane (molecular weight cutoff 100 kDa) can efficiently clear circulating myoglobin [70] and may form a therapeutic approach to critically ill patients with rhabdomyolysis in the future.

4.12.6.4 Limitation of Specific Interventions

This review has sought to place specific therapies for prevention and treatment of acute renal failure within a physiological framework. The importance of adequate resuscitation and arterial blood pressure has been emphasized. However, it is disappointing that many more specific therapies have not proven effective. Delay in diagnosis of AKI and difficulty in identifying those at highest risk in primary prevention may be frustrating attempts to treat or avert kidney injury. Given the complexity of the condition it would be naïve to assume a "magic bullet" for AKI will be identified; however, with the success of many agents in animal models, there is hope that some treatments may be protective if appropriately directed.

Better clinical markers of kidney injury might allow specific measures to be employed much earlier and more accurately during secondary prevention, and may better define high-risk groups, or provide more robust surrogate end points, during primary prevention. It is the development of specific urinary and serum biomarkers of renal cellular injury [61] that is likely to permit development of more effective therapeutic strategies to combat AKI in the future.

4.12.7 Take Home Pearls

- Iso-osmolar contrast media are the standard of care in patients at risk of developing contrast-induced nephropathy (CIN).
- Fluid loading with isotonic crystalloids is recommended in patients at risk of developing CIN.
- The most important specific intervention to protect the kidney from injury is to remove or not to administer nephrotoxins whenever possible.
- Administering more fluid to a patient with adequate central venous pressure (typically 8–12 mm Hg), adequate cardiac output, and adequate blood pressure is unlikely to protect the kidney and may hurt the patient.
- Low-dose dopamine does not protect the kidney from injury.

References

1. Mueller, C., Buerkle, G., Buettner, H. J., Petersen, J., et al. Prevention of contrast media-associated nephropathy: randomized comparison of 2 hydration regimens in 1620 patients undergoing coronary angioplasty. *Arch Intern Med* **162**, 329–336 (2002).
2. Rudnick, M. R., Goldfarb, S., Wexler, L., Ludbrook, P. A., et al. Nephrotoxicity of ionic and nonionic contrast media in 1196 patients: a randomized trial. The Iohexol Cooperative Study. *Kidney Int* **47**, 254–261 (1995).

3. Richer, M., Robert, S. & Lebel, M. Renal hemodynamics during norepinephrine and low-dose dopamine infusions in man. *Crit Care Med* **24**, 1150–1156 (1996).
4. Gare, M., Haviv, Y. S., Ben-Yehuda, A., Rubinger, D., et al. The renal effect of low-dose dopamine in high-risk patients undergoing coronary angiography. *J Am Coll Cardiol* **34**, 1682–1688 (1999).
5. Lassnigg, A., Donner, E., Grubhofer, G., Presterl, E., et al. Lack of renoprotective effects of dopamine and furosemide during cardiac surgery. *J Am Soc Nephrol* **11**, 97–104 (2000).
6. Allaqaband, S., Tumuluri, R., Malik, A. M., Gupta, A., et al. Prospective randomized study of N-acetylcysteine, fenoldopam, and saline for prevention of radiocontrast-induced nephropathy. *Catheter Cardiovasc Interv* **57**, 279–283 (2002).
7. Stone, G. W., McCullough, P. A., Tumlin, J. A., Lepor, N. E., et al. Fenoldopam mesylate for the prevention of contrast-induced nephropathy: a randomized controlled trial. *JAMA* **290**, 2284–2291 (2003).
8. Bove, T., Landoni, G., Calabrò, M. G., Aletti, G., et al. Renoprotective action of fenoldopam in high-risk patients undergoing cardiac surgery: a prospective, double-blind, randomized clinical trial. *Circulation* **111**, 3230–3235 (2005).
9. Kurnik, B. R., Allgren, R. L., Genter, F. C., Solomon, R. J., et al. Prospective study of atrial natriuretic peptide for the prevention of radiocontrast-induced nephropathy. *Am J Kidney Dis* **31**, 674–680 (1998).
10. Wang, A., Holcslaw, T., Bashore, T. M., Freed, M. I., et al. Exacerbation of radiocontrast nephrotoxicity by endothelin receptor antagonism. *Kidney Int* **57**, 1675–1680 (2000).
11. Ix, J. H., McCulloch, C. E. & Chertow, G. M. Theophylline for the prevention of radiocontrast nephropathy: a meta-analysis. *Nephrol Dial Transplant* **19**, 2747–2753 (2004).
12. Solomon, R., Werner, C., Mann, D., D'Elia, J. & Silva, P. Effects of saline, mannitol, and furosemide to prevent acute decreases in renal function induced by radiocontrast agents. *N Engl J Med* **331**, 1416–1420 (1994).
13. Tepel, M., van der Giet, M., Schwarzfeld, C., Laufer, U., et al. Prevention of radiographic-contrast-agent-induced reductions in renal function by acetylcysteine. *N Engl J Med* **343**, 180–184 (2000).
14. Briguori, A., Colombo, A., Violante, P., Balestrieri, F., Manganelli, P., Paolo Elia, B., Golia, S., Lepore, G., Riviezzo, P., Scarpato, A., Focaccio, M., Librera, E., Bonizzoni, B., Ricciardelli, B. Standard vs double dose of N-acetylcysteine to prevent contrast agent associated nephrotoxicity. Eur Heart J. **25**, 206–211 (2004).
15. Webb, J. G., Pate, G. E., Humphries, K. H., Buller, C. E., et al. A randomized controlled trial of intravenous N-acetylcysteine for the prevention of contrast-induced nephropathy after cardiac catheterization: lack of effect. *Am Heart J* **148**, 422–429 (2004).
16. Liu, R., Nair, D., Ix, J., Moore, D. H. & Bent, S. N-acetylcysteine for the prevention of contrast-induced nephropathy. A systematic review and meta-analysis. *J Gen Intern Med* **20**, 193–200 (2005).
17. Bagshaw, S. M. & Ghali, W. A. Acetylcysteine for prevention of contrast-induced nephropathy after intravascular angiography: a systematic review and meta-analysis. *BMC Med* **2**, 38 (2004).
18. Vaitkus, P. T. & Brar, C. N-acetylcysteine in the prevention of contrast-induced nephropathy: publication bias perpetuated by meta-analyses. *Am Heart J* **153**, 275–280 (2007).
19. Gonzales, D. A., Norsworthy, K. J., Kern, S. J., Banks, S., et al. A meta-analysis of N-acetylcysteine in contrast-induced nephrotoxicity: unsupervised clustering to resolve heterogeneity. *BMC Med* **5**, 32 (2007).
20. Zagler, A., Azadpour, M., Mercado, C. & Hennekens, C. H. N-acetylcysteine and contrast-induced nephropathy: a meta-analysis of 13 randomized trials. *Am Heart J* **151**, 140–145 (2006).
21. Bagshaw, S. M., McAlister, F. A., Manns, B. J. & Ghali, W. A. Acetylcysteine in the prevention of contrast-induced nephropathy: a case study of the pitfalls in the evolution of evidence. *Arch Intern Med* **166**, 161–166 (2006).
22. Alonso, A., Lau, J., Jaber, B. L., Weintraub, A. & Sarnak, M. J. Prevention of radiocontrast nephropathy with N-acetylcysteine in patients with chronic kidney disease: a meta-analysis of randomized, controlled trials. *Am J Kidney Dis* **43**, 1–9 (2004).
23. Pannu, N., Manns, B., Lee, H. & Tonelli, M. Systematic review of the impact of N-acetylcysteine on contrast nephropathy. *Kidney Int* **65**, 1366–1374 (2004).
24. Isenbarger, D. W., Kent, S. M. & O'Malley, P. G. Meta-analysis of randomized clinical trials on the usefulness of acetylcysteine for prevention of contrast nephropathy. *Am J Cardiol* **92**, 1454–1458 (2003).
25. Birck, R., Krzossok, S., Markowetz, F., Schnülle, P., et al. Acetylcysteine for prevention of contrast nephropathy: meta-analysis. *Lancet* **362**, 598–603 (2003).
26. Hoffmann, U., Fischereder, M., Krüger, B., Drobnik, W. & Krämer, B. K. The value of N-acetylcysteine in the prevention of radiocontrast agent-induced nephropathy seems questionable. *J Am Soc Nephrol* **15**, 407–410 (2004).
27. Haase, M., Haase-Fielitz, A., Ratnaike, S., Reade, M. C., et al. N-Acetylcysteine does not artifactually lower plasma creatinine concentration. *Nephrol Dial Transplant* (2008).
28. Khanal, S., Attallah, N., Smith, D. E., Kline-Rogers, E., et al. Statin therapy reduces contrast-induced nephropathy: an analysis of contemporary percutaneous interventions. *Am J Med* **118**, 843–849 (2005).
29. Chello, M., Mastroroberto, P., Patti, G., D'Ambrosio, A., et al. Simvastatin attenuates leucocyte-endothelial interactions after coronary revascularisation with cardiopulmonary bypass. *Heart* **89**, 538–543 (2003).
30. Chello, M., Carassiti, M., Agrò, F., Mastroroberto, P., et al. Simvastatin blunts the increase of circulating adhesion molecules after coronary artery bypass surgery with cardiopulmonary bypass. *J Cardiothorac Vasc Anesth* **18**, 605–609 (2004).
31. Chello, M., Goffredo, C., Patti, G., Candura, D., et al. Effects of atorvastatin on arterial endothelial function in coronary bypass surgery. *Eur J Cardiothorac Surg* **28**, 805–810 (2005).
32. Gueler, F., Rong, S., Park, J. K., Fiebeler, A., et al. Postischemic acute renal failure is reduced by short-term statin treatment in a rat model. *J Am Soc Nephrol* **13**, 2288–2298 (2002).
33. Inman, S. R., Davis, N. A., Olson, K. M. & Lukaszek, V. A. Simvastatin attenuates renal ischemia/reperfusion injury in rats administered cyclosporine A. *Am J Med Sci* **326**, 117–121 (2003).

34. Inman, S. R., Davis, N. A., Mazzone, M. E., Olson, K. M., et al. Simvastatin and L-arginine preserve renal function after ischemia/reperfusion injury. *Am J Med Sci* **329**, 13–17 (2005).
35. Yokota, N., O'Donnell, M., Daniels, F., Burne-Taney, M., et al. Protective effect of HMG-CoA reductase inhibitor on experimental renal ischemia-reperfusion injury. *Am J Nephrol* **23**, 13–17 (2003).
36. Vogt, B., Ferrari, P., Schönholzer, C., Marti, H. P., et al. Prophylactic hemodialysis after radiocontrast media in patients with renal insufficiency is potentially harmful. *Am J Med* **111**, 692–698 (2001).
37. Marenzi, G., Marana, I., Lauri, G., Assanelli, E., et al. The prevention of radiocontrast-agent-induced nephropathy by hemofiltration. *N Engl J Med* **349**, 1333–1340 (2003).
38. Finfer, S., Bellomo, R., Boyce, N., French, J., et al. A comparison of albumin and saline for fluid resuscitation in the intensive care unit. *N Engl J Med* **350**, 2247–2256 (2004).
39. Brunkhorst FM, Engel C, Bloos F et al. Intensive insulin therapy and pentastarch resusciation in severe sepsis. *New Engl J Med* **358**, 125–139 (2008).
40. Martin, C., Papazian, L., Perrin, G., Saux, P. & Gouin, F. Norepinephrine or dopamine for the treatment of hyperdynamic septic shock? *Chest* **103**, 1826–1831 (1993).
41. Kohli, H. S., Bhaskaran, M. C., Muthukumar, T., Thennarasu, K., et al. Treatment-related acute renal failure in the elderly: a hospital-based prospective study. *Nephrol Dial Transplant* **15**, 212–217 (2000).
42. Bourgoin, A., Leone, M., Delmas, A., Garnier, F., et al. Increasing mean arterial pressure in patients with septic shock: effects on oxygen variables and renal function. *Crit Care Med* **33**, 780–786 (2005).
43. Kellum, J. A. & M Decker, J. Use of dopamine in acute renal failure: a meta-analysis. *Crit Care Med* **29**, 1526–1531 (2001).
44. Bellomo, R., Chapman, M., Finfer, S., Hickling, K. & Myburgh, J. Low-dose dopamine in patients with early renal dysfunction: a placebo-controlled randomised trial. Australian and New Zealand Intensive Care Society (ANZICS) Clinical Trials Group. *Lancet* **356**, 2139–2143 (2000).
45. Morelli, A., Ricci, Z., Bellomo, R., Ronco, C., et al. Prophylactic fenoldopam for renal protection in sepsis: a randomized, double-blind, placebo-controlled pilot trial. *Crit Care Med* **33**, 2451–2456 (2005).
46. Landoni, G., Biondi-Zoccai, G. G., Tumlin, J. A., Bove, T., et al. Beneficial impact of fenoldopam in critically ill patients with or at risk for acute renal failure: a meta-analysis of randomized clinical trials. *Am J Kidney Dis* **49**, 56–68 (2007).
47. Aravindan, N., Natarajan, M. & Shaw, A. D. Fenoldopam inhibits nuclear translocation of nuclear factor kappa B in a rat model of surgical ischemic acute renal failure. *J Cardiothorac Vasc Anesth* **20**, 179–186 (2006).
48. Mehta, R. L., Pascual, M. T., Soroko, S., Chertow, G. M. & PICARD Study Group Diuretics, mortality, and nonrecovery of renal function in acute renal failure. *JAMA* **288**, 2547–2553 (2002).
49. Uchino, S., Doig, G. S., Bellomo, R., Morimatsu, H., et al. Diuretics and mortality in acute renal failure. *Crit Care Med* **32**, 1669–1677 (2004).
50. Bagshaw, S. M., Delaney, A., Haase, M., Ghali, W. A. & Bellomo, R. Loop diuretics in the management of acute renal failure: a systematic review and meta-analysis. *Crit Care Resusc* **9**, 60–68 (2007).
51. Bonventre, J. V. Kidney ischemic preconditioning. *Curr Opin Nephrol Hypertens* **11**, 43–48 (2002).
52. Bernard, S. A., Gray, T. W., Buist, M. D., Jones, B. M., et al. Treatment of comatose survivors of out-of-hospital cardiac arrest with induced hypothermia. *N Engl J Med* **346**, 557–563 (2002).
53. Hypothermia after Cardiac Arrest Study Group Mild therapeutic hypothermia to improve the neurologic outcome after cardiac arrest. *N Engl J Med* **346**, 549–556 (2002).
54. Acker, C. G., Singh, A. R., Flick, R. P., Bernardini, J., et al. A trial of thyroxine in acute renal failure. *Kidney Int* **57**, 293–298 (2000).
55. Hirschberg, R., Kopple, J., Lipsett, P., Benjamin, E., et al. Multicenter clinical trial of recombinant human insulin-like growth factor I in patients with acute renal failure. *Kidney Int* **55**, 2423–2432 (1999).
56. van den Berghe, G., Wouters, P., Weekers, F., Verwaest, C., et al. Intensive insulin therapy in the critically ill patients. *N Engl J Med* **345**, 1359–1367 (2001).
57. Van den Berghe, G., Wilmer, A., Hermans, G., Meersseman, W., et al. Intensive insulin therapy in the medical ICU. *N Engl J Med* **354**, 449–461 (2006).
58. Yamada, K., Miwa, T., Liu, J., Nangaku, M. & Song, W. C. Critical protection from renal ischemia reperfusion injury by CD55 and CD59. *J Immunol* **172**, 3869–3875 (2004).
59. Singbartl, K. & Ley, K. Protection from ischemia-reperfusion induced severe acute renal failure by blocking E-selectin. *Crit Care Med* **28**, 2507–2514 (2000).
60. Singbartl, K., Green, S. A. & Ley, K. Blocking P-selectin protects from ischemia/reperfusion-induced acute renal failure. *FASEB J* **14**, 48–54 (2000).
61. Kelly, K. J., Williams, W. W., Colvin, R. B. & Bonventre, J. V. Antibody to intercellular adhesion molecule 1 protects the kidney against ischemic injury. *Proc Natl Acad Sci USA* **91**, 812–816 (1994).
62. Bernard, G. R., Vincent, J. L., Laterre, P. F., LaRosa, S. P., et al. Efficacy and safety of recombinant human activated protein C for severe sepsis. *N Engl J Med* **344**, 699–709 (2001).
63. Lenz, K., Hörtnagl, H., Druml, W., Grimm, G., et al. Beneficial effect of 8-ornithin vasopressin on renal dysfunction in decompensated cirrhosis. *Gut* **30**, 90–96 (1989).
64. Guevara, M., Ginès, P., Fernández-Esparrach, G., Sort, P., et al. Reversibility of hepatorenal syndrome by prolonged administration of ornipressin and plasma volume expansion. *Hepatology* **27**, 35–41 (1998).
65. Hadengue, A., Gadano, A., Moreau, R., Giostra, E., et al. Beneficial effects of the 2-day administration of terlipressin in patients with cirrhosis and hepatorenal syndrome. *J Hepatol* **29**, 565–570 (1998).
66. Uriz, J., Ginès, P., Cárdenas, A., Sort, P., et al. Terlipressin plus albumin infusion: an effective and safe therapy of hepatorenal syndrome. *J Hepatol* **33**, 43–48 (2000).
67. de Laet, I. E. & Malbrain, M. Current insights in intra-abdominal hypertension and abdominal compartment syndrome. *Med Intensiva* **31**, 88–99 (2007).

68. De Waele, J. J., Hoste, E. A. & Malbrain, M. L. Decompressive laparotomy for abdominal compartment syndrome – a critical analysis. *Crit Care* **10**, R51 (2006).
69. Holt, S. G. & Moore, K. P. Pathogenesis and treatment of renal dysfunction in rhabdomyolysis. *Intensive Care Med* **27**, 803–811 (2001).
70. Naka, T., Jones, D., Baldwin, I., Fealy, N., et al. Myoglobin clearance by super high-flux hemofiltration in a case of severe rhabdomyolysis: a case report. *Crit Care* **9**, R90–R95 (2005).
71. Bagshaw, S. M. & Bellomo, R. Early diagnosis of acute kidney injury. *Curr Opin Crit Care* **13**, 638–644 (2007).

Drug Dosing in Acute Kidney Injury and During Renal Replacement Therapy

4.13

A. Mary Vilay and Bruce A. Mueller

Core Messages

- Drug dosing in patients with acute kidney injury and those receiving renal replacement therapies is a challenging task since unpredictable and highly variable changes may occur to a drug's pharmacokinetics.
- To complicate matters, glomerular filtration rate is constantly changing, making it difficult to accurately estimate a patient's residual renal function.
- Drug disposition is further affected by the use of renal replacement therapy. The type of renal replacement therapy employed and the operating characteristics all influence drug-dosing regimens.
- Published references may be consulted for an initial dosing recommendation; however, published recommendations are designed for the most part for patients with chronic kidney disease and not acute kidney injury. Thus, it is important to have a working knowledge of pharmacokinetic and pharmacodynamic principles as well as solute removal characteristics of renal replacement therapies.
- As acute kidney injury is a dynamic disease process, vigilant reassessment of drug doses is essential for optimal patient outcomes.

4.13.1 Drug Dosing in Acute Kidney Injury and During Renal Replacement Therapy

The kidneys are a primary site of drug elimination. During acute kidney injury (AKI), clearance of renally eliminated drugs can be substantially decreased. Patients with AKI are often critically ill and experience in-hospital morality rates of 30–60% [1, 66, 87]. Appropriately adjusted drug doses are essential to minimize drug toxicity related to overexposure while providing sufficient doses to derive therapeutic benefit from adequate drug concentrations. However, drug-dosing recommendations specific for AKI rarely exist.

Unfortunately, drug elimination during AKI has not been investigated as extensively as during chronic kidney disease. Studying drug clearance during AKI is challenging. This is in part due to the lack of consensus regarding the definition of AKI and the wide differences in the underlying pathophysiology of AKI. Not only is the presentation of AKI inconsistent, AKI is a dynamic process resulting in a constantly changing glomerular filtration rate (GFR), making it difficult to accurately estimate renal function. Proper drug dose adjustments during AKI are further complicated by the unpredictable and highly variable changes that can occur during AKI to pharmacokinetic parameters such as absorption, distribution, metabolism, and elimination.

B. A. Mueller (✉)
Department of Clinical, Social and Administrative Sciences, College of Pharmacy, University of Michigan, 428 Church Street, Ann Arbor, MI 48109-1065, USA
e-mail: muellerb@umich.edu

A. Jörres et al. (eds.), *Management of Acute Kidney Problems*,
DOI: 10.1007/978-3-540-69441-0_4.13, © Springer-Verlag Berlin Heidelberg 2010

4.13.1.1 Pharmacokinetic Changes During Acute Kidney Injury

4.13.1.1.1 Absorption

Gastrointestinal drug absorption during AKI can be highly unpredictable. Often, patients with renal failure suffer from fluid overload. The resultant edema may impede drug absorption from the gastrointestinal tract. Loop diuretics such as furosemide may be used to treat edema, but alterations in furosemide absorption have been observed with decompensated heart failure, an edematous state [88]. The delayed and decreased rate of furosemide absorption could possibly be related to an edematous bowel and potentially explains the decreased efficacy of oral furosemide during decompensated heart failure. Thus in edematous AKI patients, only parenteral furosemide should be used.

Decreased oral bioavailability in critically ill AKI patients is also caused by changes in blood flow during critical illness due to shunting and vasopressor use. In both cases, gastric blood flow is decreased, resulting in reduced or delayed gastrointestinal absorption. Although low-dose dopamine (<5 μg/kg/min), also called "renal dose" dopamine, may increase renal and mesenteric blood flow and could mitigate shunting, the use of renal dose dopamine to treat AKI has been discredited [7, 34, 48, 52] and is not recommended.

Patients with AKI are commonly admitted into the intensive care unit (ICU). In the ICU, it is customary for patients to be prescribed histamine-2-receptor antagonists or proton pump inhibitors to prevent stress related mucosal damage. Both histamine-2-receptor blockers and proton pump inhibitors increase gastric pH, affecting drugs whose absorption is pH-dependent. The basic environment created by gastric acid–suppressing agents has been shown to decrease the absorption of ketoconazole [14, 53], itraconazole [56], and atazanavir [85].

The association of severe malnutrition with significant increases in morbidity and mortality in AKI [32] underscores the importance of providing adequate nutrition to this subset of patients. Enteral nutrition is the preferred route of administration to maintain gastrointestinal function and integrity. Furthermore, enteral nutrition has been associated with decreased risk of mortality in critically ill patients requiring renal replacement therapy (RRT) [67]. However, decreased absorption of orally administered fluoroquinolones [36, 47, 71] and phenytoin [6, 13] are well-documented interactions that occur with enteral nutrition.

Hyperphosphatemia during AKI may require the administration of phosphate-binding agents. Polyvalent cations, such as calcium, magnesium, and aluminum, found in phosphate binders may bind to orally administered medications and decrease absorption. This interaction typically occurs with fluoroquinolones [58, 74, 77, 82] and tetracyclines [25, 27]. It has been demonstrated that sevelamer, an orally administered nonabsorbable cationic polymer phosphate binder, also decreases the absorption of oral ciprofloxacin by approximately 50% [46].

4.13.1.1.2 Distribution

Fluid overload is a hallmark of AKI. This increased fluid volume may translate into a larger volume in which drugs can disperse and may result in subtherapeutic plasma concentrations. Accordingly, it may be necessary to administer higher medication doses to edematous patients to account for the larger volume of distribution. Similarly, once RRT normalizes a patient's fluid status, dose adjustment to account for volume contraction is essential.

Drugs that are sensitive to changes in fluid status are water-soluble with a fairly small volume of distribution. Aminoglycosides are classic examples of such drugs. The volume of distribution of aminoglycosides is ~0.25 l/kg in patients with normal renal function [38]. However, an increase in volume of distribution to ~0.35 l/kg has been noted in patients with AKI [22, 23, 50]. This observation suggests that larger doses of aminoglycosides may need to be administered to achieve therapeutic serum concentrations in patients with AKI.

In plasma, drugs predominately bind to albumin. Although changes in plasma protein binding with chronic renal failure have been well described, there is limited information about the changes that occur with AKI. However, the available data in AKI suggests that there is decreased drug binding to albumin [2, 4, 13, 35, 51, 73, 84]. Not only is decreased drug binding related to decreased albumin concentration, there is also evidence to suggest a change in albumin-binding capacity during AKI [13]. With recovery of renal function, plasma protein binding appears to return to usual expected values [73]. Additionally, hemodialysis used to treat symptoms associated with AKI may increase plasma protein binding [3].

Alterations in plasma protein binding are particularly important for drugs that are highly protein bound with a narrow therapeutic index. Phenytoin is an example of a highly protein bound drug where a decrease in albumin concentration would result in increased unbound, or free, phenytoin concentration without dramatically affecting total phenytoin concentration. An increase in the free fraction of phenytoin has been noted during AKI [51, 84]. The unbound fraction is responsible for therapeutic and toxic effects of phenytoin. Thus during critical illness, including AKI, it is possible for patients to have total phenytoin concentration within the usual therapeutic range, and yet exhibit clinical signs suggestive of phenytoin toxicity related to an increased phenytoin free fraction [28, 57]. In these situations, it is important to monitor the free concentration of drugs, if readily available, and for clinical signs of drug toxicity.

4.13.1.1.3 Metabolism

AKI may alter both the renal and hepatic metabolism of drugs. In general, drug clearance associated with the kidneys is mostly due to filtration and secretion rather than drug metabolism. To date, studies demonstrating clinically significant changes in renal drug metabolism in patients with AKI have not been published.

Nonrenal clearance refers to the aggregate of drug clearance by all organ pathways excluding the kidneys. Numerous studies have confirmed changes in nonrenal drug clearance in patients with acute and chronic kidney disease. However, the degree that nonrenal clearance is affected by acute kidney disease may be different from chronic kidney disease. Evidence with imipenem [70] and vancomycin [60] established that nonrenal clearance in the early phase of AKI is not depressed to the same extent as in patients with chronic kidney disease (Table 4.13.1). Furthermore, decline in nonrenal drug clearance was dependent on duration of AKI; as duration of AKI increased, nonrenal clearance of vancomycin decreased and approached values found in chronic kidney disease [60].

Even though it is known that nonrenal drug clearance is affected by kidney dysfunction, the exact pathways affected are unknown. Considering that hepatic metabolism is a major route of drug clearance and that alterations in clearance of highly hepatically metabolized drugs occur with chronic kidney disease, the change in drug clearance with renal dysfunction is possibly related to decreased activity of various isoforms of the cytochrome P-450 metabolic enzyme [75]. Animal studies suggest changes in CYP-450 activity with AKI [75]. Transient improvement of hepatic CYP3A4 metabolic activity related to decreased plasma blood urea nitrogen concentration during hemodialysis [76] provides further evidence of the impact renal failure and RRT have on drug metabolism.

AKI will not only result in decreased renal clearance of renally eliminated compounds, but will also affect drug metabolites normally removed by the kidneys. Accumulation of metabolites needs to be considered, as metabolites may exert a pharmacologic effect. This effect may be therapeutic or toxic, and the retention of active metabolites must be taken into account when designing a drug regimen for patients with AKI. Examples of drugs that should be used with caution in AKI because of metabolite accumulation appear in Table 4.13.2.

4.13.1.1.4 Elimination

Many drugs are eliminated by the kidneys through filtration and secretion. The influence of AKI on tubular secretion is poorly defined. GFR is constantly changing

Table 4.13.1 Nonrenal clearance of selected drugs [35, 60, 64, 70]

	Normal kidney function	Acute kidney Injury	Chronic kidney failure
Acyclovir	65 ml/min/70 kg	–	29 ml/min/70 kg
Aztreonam	40 ml/min/70 kg	–	27 ml/min/70 kg
Cefotaxime	217 ml/min/70 kg	–	130 ml/min/70 kg
Imipenem	128 ml/min/70 kg	81 ml/min/70 kg	54 ml/min/70 kg
Procainamide	257 ml/min/70 kg	–	102 ml/min/70 kg
Vancomycin	40 ml/min/70 kg	16.2 ml/min/patient[a]	6 ml/min/70 kg

[a]Weight not reported in this study

Table 4.13.2 Renally eliminated active or toxic drug metabolites [16, 42, 43, 59, 65, 68]

Drug	Drug class	Concern with renal dysfunction	Clinical consequence
Codeine	Opioid analgesic	Accumulation of renally eliminated active metabolite	Apnea, narcosis, seizure, hypotension
Meperidine	Opioid analgesic	Accumulation of renally eliminated toxic metabolite, normeperidine	Anxiety, agitation, tremors, twitches, myoclonus, seizure
Midazolam	Benzodiazepine	Accumulation of renally eliminated active metabolites	Apnea, sedation, drowsiness
Morphine	Opioid analgesic	Renally eliminated active metabolite	CNS depression, respiratory depression
Mycophenolate mofetil/ mycophenolic acid	Immunosuppressant	Accumulation of inactive glucuronide metabolite displacing mycophenolic acid from albumin and resulting in increased free mycophenolic acid concentration	Leukopenia
Procainamide	Antiarrhythmic	Accumulation of renally eliminated active metabolite, *N*-acetyl procainamide (NAPA)	Sinus bradycardia, sinus node arrest, Q-T interval prolongation
Propoxyphene	Opioid analgesic	Renally eliminated active metabolite	Cardiotoxicity resulting in dysrhythmias

in AKI. Consequently, the notion of achieving "steady state" is impossible. Being able to determine the degree of renal impairment would assist in making drug-dosing adjustments. However during AKI, it is difficult to accurately determine renal function. This is related principally to constantly changing serum creatinine concentrations and a lack of correlation between serum creatinine levels and creatinine clearance during periods of rapidly changing renal function [15].

The Cockcroft-Gault [20] and Modified Diet in Renal Disease (MDRD) study [54, 55] equations are the most commonly used methods of estimating creatinine clearance and GFR respectively. However, it may not be ideal to use the Cockcroft-Gault or the MDRD equation to estimate renal function during AKI, as both of these formulas were developed and validated in populations with stable renal function, not in critically ill AKI patients. Several equations have been developed to estimate renal function during AKI and other situations when serum creatinine concentrations are not at steady state [15, 37]. However these equations are not widely used, and nearly all dose adjustment recommendations are developed using the Cockcroft-Gault equation. Thus a simple clinically useful means to estimate renal function quickly and efficiently in AKI is not currently available.

4.13.1.2 Drug Dosing in Acute Kidney Injury

Drug dosing during AKI is challenging as outlined above. When deciding whether a dose adjustment is required, several fundamental questions must be considered. The first thing that needs to be considered is whether a dose adjustment of the drug is required at all (Fig. 4.13.1). Once it has been determined that a dose adjustment is indicated, references on this topic should be consulted. Several dosing guides have been published that provide drug-dosing recommendations for renal failure and RRT [5, 65, 68].

Even published dose adjustments for renal disease differ between sources [90]. Most published recommendations are customarily designed for patients with chronic kidney disease and not AKI, thus the pharmacokinetics issues previously described in this chapter

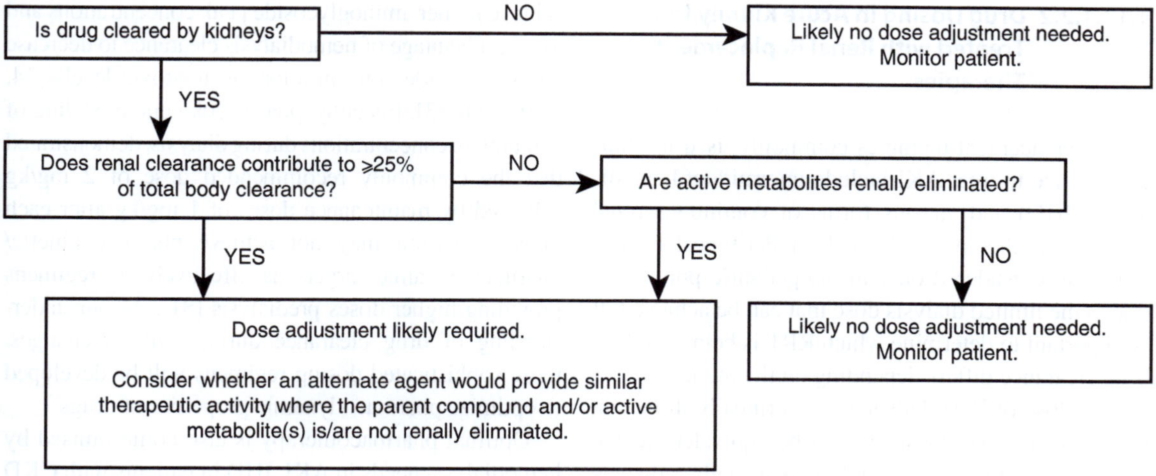

Fig. 4.13.1 Flow diagram to determine whether drug dosage adjustment should be considered

still must be considered by the clinician before determining a final dose.

4.13.1.2.1 Drug Dosing in Acute Kidney Injury with No Renal Replacement Therapy

The most difficult part of drug dosing in AKI patients is determining the patient's actual GFR. Conventional equations used to estimate renal function such as Cockcroft-Gault or MDRD should not be applied to patients with changing serum creatinine or changing GFR, as these equations were not developed for this purpose. Alternative methods to estimate creatinine clearance include a timed measured urine collection or the use of non-steady state creatinine clearance equations [15, 37]. These equations appear in Table 4.13.3. Even with these estimates the clinician must recognize that GFR in critically ill AKI patients may be changing continually, so even use of measured creatinine clearance or use of non-steady state equations to predict dosing is like looking into the rearview mirror of a car. You know what the creatinine clearance was, but it does not predict where it is going in the future. Consequently, monitoring parameters such as urine output and frequent reassessment of creatinine clearance are critical.

Table 4.13.3 Equations for estimating creatinine clearance with rapidly changing serum creatinine concentrations

Reference	Males	Females
Chiou et al. (ml/min) [15]	$\text{CrCl} = \frac{2\text{IBW} \times [28 - 0.2 \times (\text{age})]}{14.4 \times (\text{SCr}_1 + \text{SCr}_2)} + \frac{2V \times (\text{SCr}_1 - \text{SCr}_2)}{(\text{SCr}_1 + \text{SCr}_2) \times \Delta t \text{ min}} - (\text{CLnr})$ IBW = 50 kg + (2.3 kg × each inch of height over 5 ft) $V = 0.6$ l/kg × IBW CLnr = 0.048 ml/kg/min × IBW	$\text{CrCl} = \frac{2\text{IBW} \times [22.4 - 0.16 \times (\text{age})]}{14.4 \times (\text{SCr}_1 + \text{SCr}_2)} + \frac{2V \times (\text{SCr}_1 - \text{SCr}_2)}{(\text{SCr}_1 + \text{SCr}_2) \times \Delta t \text{ min}} - (\text{CLnr})$ IBW = 45.5 kg + (2.3 kg × each inch of height over 5 ft) $V = 0.6$ l/kg × IBW CLnr = 0.048 ml/kg/min × IBW
Jelliffe and Jelliffe (ml/min/1.73 m²) [37]	Ess = IBW × [29.3 – 0.203 × (age)] IBW = 50 kg + (2.3 kg × each inch of height over 5 ft) $\text{Ess(corr)} = \text{Ess} \times \{1.035 - 0.0337 \times [(\text{SCr}_2 + \text{SCr}_1)/2]\}$ $E = \text{Ess(corr)} - \frac{[4\text{IBW} \times (\text{SCr}_2 - \text{SCr}_1)}{\Delta t \text{ day}}$ $\text{CrCl} = \frac{E}{14.4 \times [(\text{SCr}_2 + \text{SCr}_1)/2]}$	Ess = IBW × [25.1 – 0.175 × (age)] IBW = 45.5 kg + (2.3 kg × each inch of height over 5 ft) $\text{Ess(corr)} = \text{Ess} \times \{1.035 - 0.0337 \times [(\text{SCr}_2 + \text{SCr}_1)/2]\}$ $E = \text{Ess(corr)} - \frac{[4\text{IBW} \times (\text{SCr}_2 - \text{SCr}_1)]}{\Delta t \text{ day}}$ $\text{CrCl} = \frac{E}{14.4 \times [(\text{SCr}_2 + \text{SCr}_1)/2]}$

SCr = mg/dl (to convert mmol/l to mg/dl divide by 88.4); CrCl = creatinine clearance; IBW = ideal body weight; SCr_1 = previous SCr value; SCr_2 = most current SCr value; V = volume of distribution; Δt = time between SCr_1 and SCr_2; CLnr = nonrenal clearance; Ess = creatinine excretion at steady state; E = creatinine excretion

4.13.1.2.2 Drug Dosing in Acute Kidney Injury Treated with Renal Replacement Therapies

Renal replacement therapies commonly used in clinical practice to treat AKI include intermittent hemodialysis (IHD) and various forms of continuous renal replacement therapies (CRRT) [69]. Peritoneal dialysis is largely considered only in the pediatric population due to the limited dialysis dose that can be achieved. It is important to determine which RRT is being used, as drug clearance differs depending on the modality.

The dose of IHD delivered in a critically ill patient usually cannot be considered to be equivalent to the IHD dose provided to a stable patient with end-stage renal disease. Dialysis that occurs during AKI typically occurs with a temporary catheter while chronic dialysis patients typically have fistulas and grafts. Therefore, the rate of blood flow achieved at the access site during critical illness may be limited. Additionally, decreased peripheral vascular resistance, a common situation during critical illness, may potentially further contribute to poor blood flow through the dialysis access.

Comparative studies of hemodialysis drug removal during acute and chronic kidney failure are rarely carried out. However a recent comparison of aminoglycoside pharmacokinetics during IHD in patients with AKI and chronic kidney disease found a significant difference in clearance between the two populations [23]. Aminoglycoside clearance between hemodialysis sessions was significantly higher in AKI patients than chronic kidney disease patients. This is likely due to some degree of preserved renal function among patients with AKI. Conversely, aminoglycoside clearance during hemodialysis was significantly lower in AKI patients. Although the authors did not explore explanations for this observation, several other investigators have noted that the delivered dose of dialysis by IHD during AKI is significantly lower than the prescribed dose [29, 30, 80]. Achieving lower than prescribed blood flow may be a major contributing factor in failing to deliver the prescribed dialysis dose [29, 30].

Dager suggested that gentamicin and tobramycin peak and prehemodialysis serum concentrations of 7–10 mg/l and 3.5–5 mg/l, respectively, appear effective for eradicating infections [23]. However, aminoglycosides exhibit concentration-dependent pharmacodynamic activity. Thus, several authors have suggested dosing aminoglycosides immediately before hemodialysis to achieve higher aminoglycoside peak concentrations and to take advantage of hemodialysis clearance to decrease aminoglycoside concentrations to nontoxic levels [24, 41, 63, 81, 83]. Recently, pharmacokinetic modeling of gentamicin concentrations during dialysis, demonstrated that the commonly recommended dose of 2 mg/kg followed by maintenance doses of 1 mg/kg after each dialysis session may not achieve pharmacokinetic/pharmacodynamic targets as effectively as regimens providing higher doses predialysis [81]. As our understanding of drug clearance during dialysis changes, more sophisticated dosing regimens will be developed to optimize pharmacodynamic properties of drugs.

Optimal pharmacotherapy is also compromised by hemodialysis needs in AKI. IHD in patients with CKD typically occur on a regular schedule three times weekly. In the ICU, more frequent hemodialysis may be warranted to maintain azotemic control [18, 19]. Schiffl et al. demonstrated that daily dialysis resulted in better metabolic control as well as reduced mortality and time to renal function recovery among patients with AKI requiring RRT [80]. Published drug-dosing guidelines for IHD are based on a thrice weekly hemodialysis schedule. More frequent hemodialysis likely will necessitate different dosing regimens than those designed for stable chronic kidney disease patients.

New hybrid modes of hemodialysis have been developed to take advantage of the rapid solute removal characteristics of IHD while preserving the improved patient hemodynamic tolerance and fluid removal characteristics of CRRT. These hybrid therapies go by many names, including sustained low-efficiency dialysis (SLED), slow low-efficiency daily dialysis (SLEDD), extended daily dialysis (EDD), and go-slow dialysis. Since the dialysate flow rates of these hybrid therapies are much different than those employed in IHD or CRRT, the solute clearance rates differ as well. When hybrid RRT flow rates and durations differ from IHD, drug removal properties are also different [26, 72]. Little is known about how to dose drugs with these hybrid RRTs. To date, the only pharmacokinetic studies with these hybrid techniques have been conducted with gentamicin [61], meropenem [49], moxifloxacin [21], levofloxacin [21], linezolid [33], and vancomycin [49]. The paucity of pharmacokinetic studies conducted with hybrid RRTs may be the most important impediment to the growth of hybrid RRT in clinical practice.

In CRRT, where the blood flow rate is usually substantially greater than the dialysate flow rate or ultrafiltrate formation rate, the most important rate-limiting step for drug clearance is effluent rate (ultrafiltrate formation rate + dialysate flow rate, if any). Ronco et al. demonstrated that effluent rates greater than 35 ml/kg/h are associated with better patient outcomes [79]. Contemporary CRRT is usually performed with effluent rates greater than 35 ml/kg/h and this reflects a change from previous practices where much slower effluent rates were used [89]. Prior to 2000, pharmacokinetic studies in CRRT generally used effluent rates far below 35 ml/kg/h. As a result, drug-dosing recommendations based on those studies may result in drug underdosing when applied to patients receiving therapy with higher effluent rates [72]. New dosing guidelines accounting for higher effluent rates have recently been published [5].

Worldwide clinical practice shows great variability in CRRT practices. CRRT commonly employed include continuous venovenous hemofiltration (CVVH), continuous venovenous hemodialysis (CVVHD), and continuous venovenous hemodiafiltration (CVVHDF). The merits of each of these modalities are discussed elsewhere in this book, but there are drug removal differences between them. As a general rule, drug removal at any given effluent rate will be greatest with CVVH, followed by CVVHDF, and then CVVHD, especially for drugs with a higher molecular weight. CVVHD is purely a diffusive therapy, and CVVHDF less so. Diffusive clearance is particularly dependent on solute molecular weight, where higher molecular weight substances are cleared more slowly than lower ones. Alternatively, convective solute clearance is independent of molecular weight as long as the solute can traverse the membrane. Numerous examples of decreased drug clearance with CVVHD as compared with CVVH have been published [11, 17 39]. The higher the molecular weight of the drug, the more pronounced the difference between CVVH and CVVHD/CVVHDF clearance. Typically, highly permeable membranes are used in CRRT. Therefore, drugs with molecular weight less than 2,000 Da may be readily cleared at any ultrafiltrate formation rate in CVVH, and at slow dialysate flow rates (less than 1 l/h) in CVVHD. However, with higher effluent rates, such as the rate studied by Ronco and colleagues, it is likely that a larger clearance difference between CVVH and CVVHD/CVVHDF will occur [11, 17 39].

As dialysate flow rate increases in CVVHD or CVVHDF, the time available for the dialysate to become saturated is reduced. Drug clearance increases as dialysate rate is increased to a point where increasing dialysate rate no longer has much of an effect on solute clearance. The dialysate flow rate where this occurs is surprisingly low. Brunet et al. reported that beta2-microglobulin (molecular weight 11,800 Da) clearance did not increase appreciably once dialysate flow rate increased past 1 l/h in CVVHD and CVVHDF with M-60 and M-100 AN69 diafilters [11]. This reduction in clearance is membrane dependent. Joy et al. reported a similar CVVHD ceiling clearance effect with vancomycin and AN69 membranes (surface area 0.6 m^2) once dialysate flow rates reached 1.5 l/h, but no ceiling effect was observed with high permeability polysulfone (surface area 0.65 m^2) or polymethylmethacrylate (surface area 2.1 m^2) membranes [39]. Churchwell et al. reported a ceiling affect with daptomycin at 3 l/h of dialysate flow with M-100 AN69 dialyzers [17].

Drug clearance differs depending on where the replacement fluid is infused during CVVH and CVVHDF. Prefilter infusion, common in the United States, dilutes the blood before the hemodiafilter and may result in lower small solute clearance rates than when replacement solutions are administered postfilter. In the case of CVVHDF, the diffusional component of the overall drug clearance may also be impaired with prefilter fluid replacement because it dilutes the solute concentration and reduces the concentration gradient at the filter membrane. In general, the use of predilutional fluid replacement results in a solute clearance difference of approximately 15–25% [11, 86].

4.13.1.3 Approach to Patient Care

Much has been written describing different approaches to adjusting drug doses for RRT [5, 10, 12, 39]. Once the CRRT operating characteristics are known, initial drug doses can be determined using tables and calculations from any of these references. However further dose individualization may be necessary depending on the clinical status of the patient and the pharmacodynamic properties of the drug. For example, a massively fluid overloaded patient with hepatic failure in addition to AKI likely will require a drug dosage adjustment to the dose that one of the references [5, 65, 68] initially recommends. The loading dose of the drug might have to be larger if it is a water-soluble drug with a small volume of distribution is used, to account for the edema related increase in volume of distribution. Moreover, the dosing interval used may need to be extended if hepatic insufficiency substantially reduces nonrenal drug clearance.

Similarly, pharmacodynamic factors should be considered when determining a dose for an AKI patient. Empiric dose adjustments may be unnecessary when the drug dose is already being titrated to maintain a particular therapeutic effect, for example, adjusting doses of inotropes or vasopressors to achieve a target blood pressure or heart rate. Antibiotic dose titration should be largely dependent on the pharmacodynamic profile of the drug. Aminoglycosides, fluoroquinolones, and daptomycin are examples of drugs that exhibit concentration-dependent antibacterial activity. Better antibacterial efficacy is seen with these antibiotics with higher peak to minimum inhibitory concentration (MIC) ratios. Dosing adjustments with these medications should involve doses that achieve relatively high peaks if possible. Less frequent, higher doses will yield better outcomes than more frequent, smaller doses. In contrast, beta-lactam antibiotics (penicillins and cephalosporins), carbapenems, and vancomycin exhibit time-dependent killing. As long as the antibiotic concentration at the site of infection exceeds the MIC, bacterial growth is inhibited. Concentrations much greater than the MIC do not enhance antibacterial activity with these latter drugs; more frequent smaller doses would be the appropriate renal adjustment. Indeed, some have suggested that continuous infusion of these agents would be optimal [9, 44, 45, 62].

Pharmacotherapeutic management requires vigilant monitoring for efficacy and toxicity. When possible, drugs plasma concentrations should be obtained regularly. Less frequent monitoring may be instituted once the patient is stabilized and has reached euvolemia. However, as the patient recovers renal function and changes are made to RRT, continual dosage adjustments will be necessary.

Clinicians face their greatest challenge when managing pharmacotherapy for critically ill patients with AKI. The traditional concept of dosing at steady state simply does not exist in this patient population. Changes in pharmacokinetic parameters and differing RRT operating characteristics preclude the use of "cookbook" doses for these patients. Pharmacotherapy in these patients requires a working knowledge of pharmacokinetic and pharmacodynamic principles as well as solute removal characteristics of RRTs. Published dosing guidelines give sufficient initial dosing estimates but dosing individualization is often necessary in these dynamic patients. Vigilant and aggressive monitoring is essential to achieve optimal patient outcomes.

4.13.2 Take Home Pearls

- Drug dosing in acute kidney injury patients needs to take into account that acute kidney injury is a dynamic disease process during which glomerular filtration rate may undergo rapid changes in both directions.
- In acute kidney injury, highly variable changes may occur to a drug's pharmacokinetics.
- Drug disposition is further affected by the type, dosing, and operating characteristics of renal replacement therapy.
- As published dosing recommendations are mostly designed for patients with chronic kidney disease, it is important to have a working knowledge of pharmacokinetic and pharmacodynamic principles, as well as solute removal characteristics of renal replacement therapies.

References

1. Ali T, Khan I, Simpson W, et al. (2007) Incidence and outcomes in acute kidney injury: a comprehensive population-based study. J Am Soc Nephrol 18: 1292–1298
2. Andreasen F (1973) Protein binding of drugs in plasma from patients with acute renal failure. Acta Pharmacol Toxicol (Copenh) 32: 417–429
3. Andreasen F (1974) The effect of dialysis on the protein binding of drugs in the plasma of patients with acute renal failure. Acta Pharmacol Toxicol (Copenh) 34: 284–294
4. Andreasen F, Jakobsen P (1974) Determination of furosemide in blood plasma and its binding to proteins in normal plasma and in plasma from patients with acute renal failure. Acta Pharmacol Toxicol (Copenh) 35: 49–57
5. Aronoff GR, Bennett WM, Berns JS, et al. (2007) Drug prescribing in renal failure: dosing guidelines for adults and children, 5th edn. American College of Physicians, Philadelphia, PA
6. Bauer LA (1982) Interference of oral phenytoin absorption by continuous nasogastric feedings. Neurology 32: 571–572
7. Bellomo R, Chapman M, Finfer S, et al. (2000). Low-dose dopamine in patients with early renal dysfunction: a placebo-controlled randomized trial. Lancet 356: 2139–2143
8. Belpaire FM, Bogaert MG, Mussche MM (1977) Influence of acute renal failure on the protein binding of drugs in animals and in man. Eur J Clin Pharmacol 11: 27–32

9. Bodey GP, Ketchel SJ, Rodriguez V (1979) A randomized study of carbenicillin plus cefamandole or tobramycin in the treatment of febrile episodes in cancer patients. Am J Med 67: 608–616
10. Böhler J, Donauer J, Keller F (1999) Pharmacokinetic principles during continuous renal replacement therapy: drug and dosage. Kidney Int 56: S24-S28
11. Brunet S, Leblanc M, Geadah D, et al. (1999) Diffusive and convective solute clearances during continuous renal replacement therapy at various dialysate and ultrafiltration flow rates. Am J Kidney Dis 34: 486–492
12. Bugge JF (2004) Influence of renal replacement therapy on pharmacokinetics in critically ill patients. Best Pract Res Clin Anaesthesiol 18: 175–187
13. Campion DS (1973) Decreased drug binding by serum albumin during renal failure. Toxicol Appl Pharmacol 25: 391–397
14. Chin TW, Loeb M, Fong IW (1995) Effects of an acidic beverage (Coca-Cola) on absorption of ketoconazole. Antimicrob Agents Chemother 39: 1671–1675
15. Chiou WL, Hsu FH (1975) A new simple and rapid method to monitor the renal function based on pharmacokinetic consideration of endogenous creatinine. Res Commun Chem Pathol Pharmacol 10: 315–330
16. Churchwell MD, Mueller BA (2007) Selected pharmacokinetic issues in patients with chronic kidney disease. Blood Purif 25: 133–138
17. Churchwell MD, Pasko DA, Mueller BA (2006) Daptomycin clearance during modeled continuous renal replacement therapy. Blood Purif 24: 548–554
18. Clark WR, Mueller BA, Alaka KJ, et al. (1994) A comparison of metabolic control by continuous and intermittent therapies in acute renal failure. J Am Soc Nephrol 4: 1413–1420
19. Clark WR, Mueller BA, Kraus MA, et al. (1997) Extracorporeal therapy requirements for patients with acute renal failure. J Am Soc Nephrol 8: 804–812
20. Cockcroft DW, Gault MH (1976) Prediction of creatinine clearance from serum creatinine. Nephron 16: 31–41
21. Czock D, Hüsig-Linde C, Langhoff A, et al. (2006) Pharmacokinetics of moxifloxacin and levofloxacin in intensive care unit patients who have acute renal failure and undergo extended daily dialysis. Clin J Am Soc Nephrol 1: 1263–1268
22. Dager WE (1994) Aminoglycoside pharmacokinetics: volume of distribution in specific adult patient subgroups. Ann Pharmacother 28: 944–951
23. Dager WE, King JH (2006) Aminoglycosides in intermittent hemodialysis: pharmacokinetics with individual dosing. Ann Pharmacother 40: 9–14
24. Dang L, Duffull S (2006) Development of a semimechanistic model to describe the pharmacokinetics of gentamicin in patients receiving hemodialysis. J Clin Pharmacol 46: 662–673
25. D'Arcy PF, McElnay JC (1987) Drug-antacid interactions: assessment of clinical importance. Drug Intell Clin Pharm 21: 607–617
26. Decker BS, Mueller BA, Sowinski KM (2007) Drug dosing considerations in alternative hemodialysis. Adv Chronic Kidney Dis 14: e17-e26
27. Deppermann KM, Lode H, Höffken G, et al. (1989) Influence of ranitidine, pirenzepine, and aluminum magnesium hydroxide on the bioavailability of various antibiotics, including amoxicillin, cephalexin, doxycycline, and amoxicillin-clavulanic acid. Antimicrob Agents Chem 33: 1901–1907
28. Driscoll DF, McMahon M, Blackburn GL, et al. (1988) Phenytoin toxicity in a critically ill, hypoalbuminemic patient with normal serum drug concentrations. Crit Care Med 16: 1248–1249
29. Evanson JA, Himmelfarb J, Wingard R, et al. (1998) Prescribed versus delivered dialysis in acute renal failure patients. Am J Kidney Dis 32: 731–738
30. Evanson JA, Ikizler TA, Wingard R, et al. (1999) Measurement of the delivery of dialysis in acute renal failure. Kidney Int 55: 1501–1508
31. Faraji B, Yu PP (1998) Serum phenytoin levels of patients on gastrostomy tube. J Neurosci Nurs 30: 55–59
32. Fiaccadori E, Lombardi M, Leonardi S, et al. (1999) Prevalence and clinical outcome associated with preexisting malnutrition in acute renal failure: a prospective cohort study. J Am Soc Nephrol 10: 581–593
33. Fiaccadori E, Maggiore U, Rotelli C, et al. (2004). Removal of linezolid by conventional intermittent hemodialysis, sustained low-efficiency dialysis, or continuous venovenous hemofiltration in patients with acute renal failure. Critical Care Med 32: 2437–2442
34. Friedrich JO, Adhikari N, Herridge MS, et al. (2005) Meta-analysis: low-dose dopamine increases urine output but does not prevent renal dysfunction or death. Ann Intern Med 142: 510–524
35. Gibson TP (1986) Renal disease and drug metabolism: an overview. Am J Kidney Dis 8, 7–17
36. Healy DP, Brodbeck MC, Clendening CE (1996) Ciprofloxacin absorption is impaired in patients given enteral feedings orally and via gastrostomy and jejunostomy tubes. Antimicrob Agents Chemother 40: 6–10
37. Jelliffe RW, Jelliffe SM (1972) A computer program for estimation of creatinine clearance from unstable serum creatinine levels, age, sex, and weight. Math Biosci 14: 17–24
38. Jhee SS, Burm JP, Gill MA (1994) Comparison of aminoglycoside pharmacokinetics in Asian, Hispanic, and Caucasian patients by using population pharmacokinetic methods. Antimicrob Agents Chemother 38: 2073–2077
39. Joy MS, Matzke GR, Armstrong DK, et al. (1998) A primer on continuous renal replacement therapy for critically ill patients. Ann Pharmacother 32: 362–375
40. Joy MS, Matzke GR, Frye RF, et al. (1998) Determinants of vancomycin clearance by continuous venovenous hemofiltration and continuous venovenous hemodialysis. Am J Kidney Dis 31: 1019–1027
41. Kamel Mohamed OH, Wahba IM, Watnick S, et al. (2007) Administration of tobramycin in the beginning of the hemodialysis session: a novel intradialytic dosing regimen. Clin J Am Soc Nephrol 2: 694–699
42. Kaplan B, Gruber SA, Nallamathou R, et al. (1998) Decreased protein binding of mycophenolic acid associated with leukopenia in a pancreas transplant recipient with renal failure. Transplantation 65: 1127–1129
43. Kaplan B, Meier-Kriesche HU, Friedman G, et al. (1999) The effect of renal insufficiency on mycophenolic acid protein binding. J Clin Pharmacol 39: 715–720
44. Kasiakou SK, Lawrence KR, Choulis N, et al. (2005) Continuous versus intermittent intravenous administration of

antibacterials with time-dependent action: a systematic review of pharmacokinetic and pharmacodynamic parameters. Drugs 65: 2499–2511
45. Kasiakou SK, Sermaides GJ, Michalopoulos A, et al. (2005) Continuous versus intermittent intravenous administration of antibiotics: a meta-analysis of randomised controlled trials. Lancet Infect Dis 5: 581–589
46. Kays MB, Overholser BR, Mueller BA, et al. (2003) Effects of sevelamer hydrochloride and calcium acetate on the oral bioavailability of ciprofloxacin. Am J Kidney Dis 42: 1253–1259
47. Kays MB, Overholser BR, Lagvankar S, et al. (2005) Effect of Ensure on the oral bioavailability of gatifloxacin in healthy volunteers. Pharmacotherapy 25: 1530–1535
48. Kellum JA, Decker JM (2001) Use of dopamine in acute renal failure: a meta-analysis. Crit Care Med 29: 1526–1531
49. Kielstein JT, Czock D, Schöpke T, et al. (2006) Pharmacokinetics and total elimination of meropenem and vancomycin in intensive care unit patients undergoing extended daily dialysis. Crit Care Med 34: 51–56
50. Kihara M, Ikeda Y, Takagi N, et al. (1995) Pharmacokinetics of single-dose intravenous amikacin in critically ill patients undergoing slow hemodialysis. Intensive Care Med 21: 348–351
51. Lau AH, Kronfol NO (1994) Effect of continuous hemofiltration on phenytoin elimination. Ther Drug Monit 16: 53–57
52. Lauschke A, Teichgräber UK, Frei U, et al. (2006) "Low-dose" dopamine worsens renal perfusion in patients with acute renal failure. Kidney Int 69: 1669–1674
53. Lelawongs P, Barone JA, Colaizzi JL, et al. (1988) Effect of food and gastric acidity on absorption of orally administered ketoconazole. Clin Pharm 7: 228–235
54. Levey AS, Bosch JP, Lewis JB, et al. (1999) A more accurate method to estimate glomerular filtration rate from serum creatinine: a new prediction equation. Ann Intern Med 130: 461–470
55. Levey AS, Greene T, Kusek JW, et al. (2000) A simplified equation to predict glomerular filtration rate from serum creatinine. J Am Soc Nephrol 11: 155A.
56. Lim SG, Sawyerr AM, Hudson M, et al. (1993) Short report: the absorption of fluconazole and itraconazole under conditions of low intragastric acidity. Aliment Pharmacol Ther 7: 317–321
57. Lindow J, Wijdicks EF (1994). Phenytoin toxicity associated with hypoalbuminemia in critically ill patients. Chest 105: 602–604
58. Lober S, Ziege S, Rau M, et al. (1999) Pharmacokinetics of gatifloxacin and interaction with an antacid containing aluminum and magnesium. Antimicrob Agents Chemother 43: 1067–1071
59. Lund-Jacobsen H (1978) Cardio-respiratory toxicity of propoxyphene and norpropoxyphene in conscious rabbits. Acta Pharmacol Toxicol (Copenh) 42: 171–178
60. Macias WL, Mueller BA, Scarim SK (1991) Vancomycin pharmacokinetics in acute renal failure: preservation of nonrenal clearance. Clin Pharmacol Ther 50: 688–694
61. Manley HJ, Bailie GR, McClaran ML, et al. (2003) Gentamicin pharmacokinetic during slow daily home hemodialysis. Kidney Int 63: 1072–1078
62. Mariat C, Venet C, Jehl F, et al. (2006) Continuous infusion of ceftazidime in critically ill patients undergoing continuous venovenous haemodiafiltration: pharmacokinetic evaluation and dose recommendation. Crit Care 10: R26
63. Matsuo H, Hayashi J, Ono K, et al. (1997) Administration of aminoglycosides to hemodialysis patients immediately before dialysis: a new dosing modality. Antimicrob Agents Chemother 41: 2597–2601
64. Matzke GR, McGory RW, Halstenson CE, et al. (1984) Pharmacokinetics of vancomycin in patients with various degrees of renal function. Antimicrob Agents Chemother 25: 433–437
65. McEvoy GK, Snow EK, Kester L, et al. (eds)(2007)AHFS drug information. American Society of Health-System Pharmacists Inc., Bethesda, MD
66. Mehta RL, Pascual MT, Soroko S, et al. (2004) Spectrum of acute renal failure in the intensive care unit: the PICARD experience. Kidney Int 66: 1613–1621
67. Metnitz PG, Krenn CG, Steltzer H, et al. (2002) Effect of acute renal failure requiring renal replacement therapy on outcome in critically ill patients. Crit Care Med 30: 2051–2058
68. Micromedex® Healthcare Series (electronic version). Thomson Micromedex, Greenwood Village, Colorado, USA. Available at: http://www.thomsonhc.com (cited: 03/04/08)
69. Monti G, Herrera M, Kindgen-Milles D, et al. (2007) The DOse REsponse Multicentre International collaborative initiative (DO-RE-MI). Contrib Nephrol 156: 434–443
70. Mueller BA, Scarim SK, Macias WL (1993) Comparison of imipenem pharmacokinetics in patients with acute or chronic renal failure treated with continuous hemofiltration. Am J Kidney Dis 21: 172–179
71. Mueller BA, Brierton DG, Abel SR, et al. (1994) Effect of enteral feeding with Ensure on oral bioavailabilities of ofloxacin and ciprofloxacin. Antimicrob Agents Chemother 38: 2101–2105
72. Mueller BA, Pasko DA, Sowinski KM (2003) Higher renal replacement therapy dose delivery influences on drug therapy. Artif Organs 27: 808–814
73. Mussche MM, Belpaire FM, Bogaert MG (1975) Plasma protein binding of phenylbutazone during recovery from acute renal failure. Eur J Clin Pharmacol 9: 69–71
74. Nix DE, Watson WA, Lener ME, et al. (1989) Effects of aluminum and magnesium antacids and ranitidine on the absorption of ciprofloxacin. Clin Pharmacol Ther 46: 700–705
75. Nolin TD, Frye RF, Matzke GR (2003) Hepatic drug metabolism and transport in patients with kidney disease. Am J Kidney Dis 42: 906–925
76. Nolin TD, Appiah K, Kendrick SA, et al. (2006) Hemodialysis acutely improves hepatic CYP3A4 metabolic activity. J Am Soc Nephrol 17: 2363–2367
77. Pletz MW, Petzold P, Allen A, et al. (2003) Effect of calcium carbonate on bioavailability of orally administered gemifloxacin. Antimicrob Agents Chemother 47: 2158–2160
78. Roberts JA, Paratz J, Paratz E, et al. (2007) Continuous infusion of beta-lactam antibiotics in severe infections: a review of its role. Int J Antimicrob Agents 30: 11–18
79. Ronco C, Bellomo R, Homel P, et al. (2000) Effects of different doses in continuous veno-venous haemofiltration on outcomes of acute renal failure: a prospective randomised trial. Lancet 356: 26–30
80. Schiffl H, Lang SM, Fischer R (2002) Daily hemodialysis and the outcome of acute renal failure. N Eng J Med 346: 305–310

81. Sowinski KM, Magner SJ, Lucksiri A, et al. (2008) Influence of hemodialysis on gentamicin pharmacokinetics, removal during hemodialysis, and recommended dosing. Clin J Am Soc Nephrol 3: 355–361
82. Stass H, Bottcher MF, Ochmann K (2001) Evaluation of the influence of antacids and H2 antagonists on the absorption of moxifloxacin after oral administration of a 400 mg dose to healthy volunteers. Clin Pharmacokinet 40: S39–S48
83. Teigen MM, Duffull S, Dang L, et al. (2006) Dosing of gentamicin in patients with end-stage renal disease receiving hemodialysis. J Clin Pharmacol 46: 1259–1267
84. Tiula E, Haapanen EJ, Neuvonen PJ (1987) Factors affecting serum protein binding of phenytoin, diazepam and propranolol in acute renal diseases. Int J Clin Pharmacol Ther Toxicol 25: 469–475
85. Tomilo DL, Smith PF, Ogundele AB, et al. (2006) Inhibition of atazanavir oral absorption by lansoprazole gastric acid suppression in healthy volunteers. Pharmacotherapy 26: 41–346
86. Uchino S, Cole L, Morimatsu H, et al. (2002) Clearance of vancomycin during high-volume haemofiltration: impact of pre-dilution. Intensive Care Med 28: 1664–1667
87. Uchino S, Kellum JA, Bellomo R, et al. (2005) Acute renal failure in critically ill patients: a multinational, multicenter study. JAMA 294: 813–818
88. Vasko MR, Cartwright DB, Knochel JP, et al. (1985) Furosemide absorption altered in decompensated congestive heart failure. Ann Intern Med 102: 314–318
89. Venkataraman R, Kellum JA, Palevsky P (2002) Dosing patterns for continuous renal replacement therapy at a large medical center in the United States. J Crit Care 17: 246–250
90. Vidal L, Shavit M, Fraser A, et al. (2005) Systematic comparison of four sources of drug information regarding adjustment of dose for renal function. BMJ 331: 263–266

4.14 Anesthesia in Patients with Kidney Failure

Dinah Jörres and Achim Jörres

Core Messages

- › The preoperative evaluation of patients with acute kidney failure should encompass
  - Volume status
  - Cardiovascular status
  - Systemic hemodynamics
  - Neurological status
  - Laboratory investigations
- › The development of perioperative or postoperative acute kidney failure is associated with poor outcome of the patients, especially if dialysis is required. Thus, the correct appraisal of the individual patient's risk to develop acute kidney failure is important to develop and apply potential strategies for prevention.
- › The intraoperative monitoring and management of patients with kidney failure is not fundamentally different from that of general patients; however, it needs to be kept in mind that many anesthetic drugs have altered pharmacokinetics and thus prolonged duration of effects in patients with kidney failure.

4.14.1 Introduction

In general, the risk of anesthesia in patients with (acute or chronic) kidney failure is higher than in an average population without renal diseases. For this reason, the careful preoperative evaluation of these patients is of utmost importance. There is no principal difference in the anesthesiology management on the basis of the different etiologies of kidney failure; however, the anesthesiologist needs to establish the degree and severity of kidney failure (e.g. as determined by the glomerular filtration rate) and also take into consideration the typical comorbid conditions often suffered by patients with kidney problems. This will be crucial in deciding on the optimal intraoperative management, the ideal choice of anesthetic drugs, and potential measures for prevention of postoperative complications such as further deterioration of kidney function, electrolyte disorders, or volume overload.

D. Jörres (✉)
Department of Anaesthesiology and Intensive Care Medicine, Charité University Campus Virchow-Klinikum, Augustenburger Platz 1, 13353 Berlin, Germany
e-mail: dinah.joerres@charite.de

4.14.2 Preoperative Evaluation

In the phase of preoperative evaluation there are general and specific aspects the anesthesiologist has to include in the planning of the anesthesia.

Signs of either hypovolemia or fluid overload must be investigated. In patients already on renal replacement therapy, the timing of the surgery in relation to the last dialysis procedure must be carefully weighed, and the following aspects must be considered:

- How is the current body weight of the patient as compared with his or her typical postdialysis "dry weight"? How much residual urine output is present? This will give an indication of how much additional volume the patient may tolerate.
- Particularly in acute patients without established "dry weight," great care must be taken to correctly assess volume status. In addition to careful clinical examination this may include chest X-ray, ultrasound of inferior vena cava diameter, and central venous pressure.

A. Jörres et al. (eds.), *Management of Acute Kidney Problems*,
DOI: 10.1007/978-3-540-69441-0_4.14, © Springer-Verlag Berlin Heidelberg 2010

- When was the last renal replacement therapy (RRT) procedure performed, and with what type/amount of anticoagulation? Even in the absence of overt coagulation abnormalities, platelet function may be impaired in uremic patients and/or patients shortly after RRT as a consequence of blood–membrane interactions [3].
- How is the kinetics of acid–base/electrolyte status in between RRTs? This will give an indication if the patient is likely to develop, e.g., acute hyperkalemia during surgery or shortly afterwards and may prompt readiness for extracorporeal treatment after (or even during) surgery.

Another key point is the evaluation of cardiac function and systemic hemodynamics. Chronic kidney patients suffer from an excess morbidity in terms of coronary heart disease, hypertension, congestive heart failure, and central/peripheral vascular disease. Thus, further preoperative examination may be required, including an electrocardiogram (ECG) and/or stress ECG, echocardiography, or Doppler ultrasound of peripheral and/or cranial vessels. Conversely, acute patients may have developed kidney failure as a consequence of shock and hypotension, requiring inotropes and/or vasopressors. Accordingly, there is not only an increased risk for hypotension (particularly during anesthesia induction, but also in the intraoperative course) but also for cardiac arrhythmias and electrolyte/acid–base disorders (hypokalemia/hyperkalemia and metabolic acidosis). The last must be identified and, if present, corrected prior to anesthesia induction.

The assessment of peripheral venous and arterial status of the patient is important for cannulation planning. In chronic kidney patients, arterial cannulation of the upper extremity arteries should be generally avoided as these vessels may serve as a crucial lifeline in terms of future dialysis access. Future arteriovenous (AV) fistula construction may also be impeded by damage to peripheral veins, thus peripheral venous access should only be made through dorsal hand veins, not through forearm or elbow veins. Stay away from existing AV fistulas and avoid using central venous access on the equilateral side of an established fistula, as there is a relevant risk of central venous thrombosis which may render the fistula nonfunctional. These general rules also apply to patients with acute or acute-on-chronic kidney failure, as these have a relevant risk to remain dialysis dependent or else to retain a substantial chronic kidney injury subsequent to the acute disease episode, eventually requiring dialysis access in the future.

Both patients with chronic and acute uremia may suffer from neurological comorbidities (see Chapter 5.7). Information about peripheral neurological problems is particularly important if regional anesthesia is planned. On the other hand, autonomic neurological disturbances such as gastropathy with delayed gastric emptying are relevant for the type of anesthesia induction (rapid sequence induction).

Concerning the preoperative laboratory evaluation, a current hematology and blood cell count are indispensable to detect anemia or thrombocytopenia. A fresh coagulation profile is of particular importance in patients where regional anesthesia is planned. Current electrolytes (especially potassium and calcium), glucose, and acid–base status need to be determined (and repeated during surgery). Likewise, creatinine and blood urea concentrations should be available for estimation of current kidney function and drug dosing. Total protein/albumin levels may help to better appraise blood viscosity and may guide the strategy for fluid management and the selection of replacement fluids (colloids/crystalloids).

Finally, if oral premedication is possible, a short-acting benzodiazepine (e.g. midazolam) should be preferred.

4.14.2.1 Intraoperative Management in Renal Failure Patients

4.14.2.1.1 Monitoring

Subject to the planned surgical procedure the intraoperative monitoring of patients with kidney failure is not fundamentally different from general patients. During general anesthesia, the minimum standard for monitoring includes:

- Heart rate
- Blood pressure
- Peripheral oxygen saturation
- Expiratory CO_2 concentration
- Narcotic gas concentration

In patients with severe cardiovascular comorbidities and/or in case of planned major surgery, blood pressure should be monitored continuously via an arterial cannula. In patients with kidney failure, a femoral arterial access should be preferred over an upper extremity arterial access to spare vessels for potential future AV fistula construction. If non-invasive blood pressure measurement is sufficient, care should be taken not to place the blood pressure cuff on the side of an existing AV fistula in chronic kidney patients.

If the planned surgical procedure involves major fluid shifts and/or patients will require temporary parenteral nutrition after surgery, the placement of a central venous catheter will be necessary, thus enabling continuous monitoring of central venous pressure during the procedure.

Before starting the anesthesia, the function of an existing AV fistula must be checked (palpation and auscultation) and documented. During surgery, the fistula must be handled with special care (e.g., protecting the extremity with a layer of pads), and function controls should be repeated regularly.

4.14.2.2 Selection of Anesthetic Drugs

As reviewed extensively in Chapter 4.13, many drugs have altered pharmacokinetics and thus prolonged duration of effects in patients with kidney failure. Moreover, a detailed overview of anesthetic drug disposition in advanced kidney failure was recently presented by Craig and Hunter [5]. Beyond that, some additional points of particular relevance for the selection of anesthetic drugs should be considered:

- Anesthetic drugs in general are known to effect the systemic hemodynamics, sympathic nervous system activity, and other humoral regulation mechanisms. This can be particularly relevant in anemic patients who already need a higher cardiac output to compensate the anemia. If possible, subject to the surgical procedure, regional anesthesia or combined regional/general anesthesia should be preferred.
- For induction of general anesthesia, it is possible to use any of the established drugs like thiopental, disoprivan, or etomidate. However, in critically ill patients, dose reduction is often necessary.
- Patients with nausea, vomiting, or other gastrointestinal problems should generally receive rapid sequence induction. In such cases a current potassium blood value is mandatory. If serum potassium is <5 mEq/l, succinylcholine may be used. If serum potassium is >5 mEq/l, however, a nondepolarizing muscle relaxant should be used instead. Atracurium and Cisatracurium should be preferred as they are not subject to relevant metabolism by the kidney. Alternatively, drugs undergoing partial renal metabolism such as Rocuronium, Mivacurium, or Vecuronium may be used. In any case, the continuous assessment of the relaxant status of the patient using relaxometry should be performed.
- Maintenance of anesthesia is possible in the form of total venous anesthesia or balanced anesthesia, using volatile anesthetics. Isoflurane and desflurane have the least effect on cardiac output and may therefore be preferred. Sevoflurane is metabolized in the liver via the cytochrome P450 system to fluoride as the resulting degradation product. Fluoride, in turn, may react to compound A together with the breathing lime in the ventilatory system. As compound A has shown nephrotoxicity in animal models, the use of Sevoflurane should be avoided, especially if low gas flow is used or an extended duration of surgery is expected [8].
- The sensitivity for opioids is substantially higher in patients with kidney failure. Especially the repetition of Fentanyl boli must be handled with care. There is no renal metabolization of Remifentanil or Alfentanil. In contrast, Sufentanil has an active metabolite that is undergoing renal elimination and may thus accumulate in kidney failure. For total intravenous anesthesia, the combination of continuous Propofol and Remifentanil infusion may be considered [6].

4.14.2.3 Fluid Management

The strategy for intraoperative fluid management must be based both on patient-related factors (e.g., preoperative volume status and residual urine excretion) and on surgery-related factors (extent, duration, and type of procedures). There may be preoperative fluid depletion because of the routine nil-by-mouth regimens. In abdominal surgery the patient's gastrointestinal tract has to be cleaned before surgery, potentially resulting in additional (unnoticed) fluid losses on the day before surgery is scheduled. Finally, intraoperative fluid losses may occur which have to be taken into account, caused by, e.g., bleeding, nonhumidified mechanical ventilation, or bowel exterioration. Urinary excretion should be closely monitored via bladder catheter.

4.14.3 Postoperative Management

The postoperative monitoring of patients with renal failure is not fundamentally different from that of general patients. In the postoperative care unit they should be monitored for heart rate, blood pressure, and peripheral oxygen saturation. Blood gas analyses should be performed together with serum potassium and glucose levels.

Patients with kidney failure undergoing extended surgical procedures should be monitored in an intensive care unit for at least 24 h after the operation.

4.14.4 Prevention of Perioperative Acute Kidney Failure

The development of perioperative or postoperative acute kidney failure is associated with poor outcome for patients especially if dialysis is required. Thus, the correct appraisal of the individual patient's risk to develop acute kidney failure is important to develop and apply potential strategies for prevention. The risk stratification should be based both on patient-related factors and risks associated to specific surgical procedures:

4.14.4.1 *Patient-Related Factors*

- Preexisting renal dysfunction
- Diabetes mellitus
- Cardiovascular disease, especially congestive cardiac failure
- Liver cirrhosis
- Sepsis
- Crush injury
- Perioperative cardiac dysfunction
- Hepatic failure
- Electrolyte disorders
- Metabolic acidosis
- Hypovolemia
- Hypotension

4.14.4.2 *Surgical Procedures*

- Cardiopulmonary bypass surgery (discussed extensively in the respective chapter)
- Surgery involving aortic cross-clamp
- Increased intra-abdominal pressure
- Generalized embolization
- Liver or kidney transplant
- Use of radiocontrast agents

4.14.5 Management of High-Risk Patients

Given the substantial heterogeneity of surgical cohorts regarding underlying disease, comorbid conditions, current clinical status, and the large variety of surgical interventions, the perioperative management will have to be aligned with the individual patient's present situation. However, some general rules for the prevention of perioperative kidney failure apply.

4.14.5.1 *Fluid and Electrolyte Homeostasis*

- Crystalloid solutions may best be provided as balanced salt solutions or Ringer's lactate, as large volumes of normal (0.9%) saline may result in hyperchloremic metabolic acidosis. In anuric and/or hyperkalemic patients, however, potassium-free fluids should be preferred.
- Colloid solutions may be provided as low-molecular-weight hydroxyl-ethyl-starch fluids with a low grade of substitution. However, recommended daily maximum doses should not be exceeded, as further impairment of kidney function may result [4]. Alternatively, human serum albumin solution may be used for partial fluid replacement, particularly in patients with preexisting low total protein/albumin levels and subsequent low oncotic pressure.
- Packed red blood cells (RBCs) should be transfused with the aim to maintain the preoperative hemoglobin level to which the patient is adapted. During surgical procedures involving substantial blood

loss, this may be difficult to steer; in such cases, the development of central venous pressure levels may be used as one parameter to direct volume replacement.
- Fresh frozen plasma (FFP) units should be transfused if a greater number (e.g., 5 or more units) of packed red blood cells are required. From there on, RBC and FFP units should be transfused at a 1:1 ratio.

4.14.5.2 Pharmacological Therapy

In patients at risk, potentially nephrotoxic drugs and radiocontrast media must be applied with great caution. In this context, not only typical nephrotoxins such as aminoglycoside antibiotics but also other drugs warrant thoughtful indications: diuretics may induce or aggravate severe electrolyte or acid–base imbalances; nonsteroidal antiinflammatory drugs may interfere with renal autoregulation by blocking intrarenal prostaglandins; angiotensin-converting enzyme inhibitors and angiotensin receptor blockers may alter the vascular tone of intrarenal vessels and impair glomerular filtration pressure.

The problems associated with radiocontrast media are discussed in greater detail in the respective chapter. If contrast media cannot be avoided in high-risk patients, adequate preventive measures must be undertaken. As a first step, (re-)hydration without the use of diuretics is of paramount importance. An infusion rate of 1 ml/kg body weight for 24 h around the intervention is recommended [16, 19]. In addition, *N*-acetylcysteine (600 mg twice daily before and after the contrast media application) has been shown to have preventive effects [1, 17, 20]. In emergency procedures leaving no sufficient room or time for hydration and *N*-acetylcysteine administration, theophylline, given at a dose of 200 mg intravenously 30 min prior to the intervention, may have prophylactic effects [9, 10]. In contrast, 'prophylactic' hemodialysis is not generally recommended (unless for the treatment of complications such as hyperhydration) and may even turn out to be harmful [21].

Likewise, there are no sound recommendations for active pharmacological interventions for the prevention of kidney failure, as none of the proposed strategies were consistently shown to be successful. Examples are calcium channel entry blockers, angiotensin-converting enzyme inhibitors, Fenoldopam, or atrial natriuretic peptides [11]. Importantly, there is also no general indication for the administration of loop diuretics. While these may transform oliguric to normuric kidney failure, this usually fails to improve renal or overall outcome [18]. On the other hand, the unreflected use of diuretics may aggravate undetected dehydration, lead to further impairment of kidney function, and even increase mortality [13, 15]. Similarly, 'renal-dose' dopamine (at a dose of 2–4 μg/kg/min) has never been proven to be clinically beneficial but may lead to increased cardiac oxygen consumption and provoke cardiac arrhythmias [2, 7, 14] Instead, noradrenaline should be considered as the preferred vasopressor, e.g., in septic patients with sustained hypotension despite sufficient fluid resuscitation [12].

4.14.6 Take Home Pearls

- The preoperative evaluation of patients with kidney failure needs to carefully establish fluid, electrolyte and acid–base status; moreover, potential comorbidities as well as treatment-related factors (cardiovascular problems, clotting abnormalities, anemia, and neurological disorders) must be evaluated.
- The intraoperative monitoring is not fundamentally different from that of other patients; however, the selection of anesthetic drugs must be adapted to kidney function.
- The basis for successful prevention of perioperative acute kidney failure is a proper risk stratification followed by adequate prophylactic strategies; key points are to maintain fluid and electrolyte homeostasis and to avoid nephrotoxins whenever possible. In contrast, pharmacological interventions for the prevention of kidney failure were not consistently shown to be successful.

References

1. Alonso A, Lau J, Jaber BL, Weintraub A, Sarnak MJ. Prevention of radiocontrast nephropathy with N-acetylcysteine in patients with chronic kidney disease: a meta-analysis of randomized, controlled trials. Am J Kidney Dis 2004; 43(1): 1–9.

2. Bellomo R, Chapman M, Finfer S, Hickling K, Myburgh J. Low-dose dopamine in patients with early renal dysfunction: a placebo-controlled randomised trial. Australian and New Zealand Intensive Care Society (ANZICS) Clinical Trials Group. Lancet 2000; 356(9248): 2139–2143.
3. Boldt J, Menges T, Wollbruck M, Sonneborn S, Hempelmann G. Continuous hemofiltration and platelet function in critically ill patients. Crit Care Med 1994; 22:1155–1160.
4. Brunkhorst FM, Engel C, Bloos F, Meier-Hellmann A, Ragaller M, Weiler N, et al. Intensive insulin therapy and pentastarch resuscitation in severe sepsis. N Engl J Med 2008; 358(2):125–139.
5. Craig RG, Hunter JM. Recent developments in the perioperative management of adult patients with chronic kidney disease. Br J Anaesth 2008.
6. Dahaba AA, von Klobucar F, Rehak PH, List WF. Total intravenous anesthesia with remifentanil, propofol and cisatracurium in end-stage renal failure. Can J Anaesth 1999; 46(7):696–700.
7. Denton MD, Chertow GM, Brady HR. 'Renal-dose' dopamine for the treatment of acute renal failure: scientific rationale, experimental studies and clinical trials. Kidney Int 1996; 50(1):4–14.
8. Gentz BA, Malan TP Jr. Renal toxicity with sevoflurane: a storm in a teacup? Drugs 2001; 61(15):2155–2162.
9. Huber W, Schipek C, Ilgmann K, Page M, Hennig M, Wacker A, et al. Effectiveness of theophylline prophylaxis of renal impairment after coronary angiography in patients with chronic renal insufficiency. Am J Cardiol 2003; 91(10): 1157–1162.
10. Ix JH, McCulloch CE, Chertow GM. Theophylline for the prevention of radiocontrast nephropathy: a meta-analysis. Nephrol Dial Transplant 2004; 19(11):2747–2753.
11. Kellum JA, Leblanc M, Gibney RT, Tumlin J, Lieberthal W, Ronco C. Primary prevention of acute renal failure in the critically ill. Curr Opin Crit Care 2005; 11(6):537–541.
12. Lameire N, Van BW, Vanholder R. Acute renal failure. Lancet 2005; 365(9457):417–430.
13. Lassnigg A, Donner E, Grubhofer G, Presterl E, Druml W, Hiesmayr M. Lack of renoprotective effects of dopamine and furosemide during cardiac surgery. J Am Soc Nephrol 2000; 11(1):97–104.
14. Lauschke A, Teichgraber UK, Frei U, Eckardt KU. 'Low-dose' dopamine worsens renal perfusion in patients with acute renal failure. Kidney Int 2006; 69(9):1669–1674.
15. Mehta RL, Pascual MT, Soroko S, Chertow GM. Diuretics, mortality, and nonrecovery of renal function in acute renal failure. JAMA 2002; 288(20):2547–2553.
16. Mueller C, Buerkle G, Buettner HJ, Petersen J, Perruchoud AP, Eriksson U, et al. Prevention of contrast media-associated nephropathy: randomized comparison of 2 hydration regimens in 1620 patients undergoing coronary angioplasty. Arch Intern Med 2002; 162(3):329–336.
17. Pannu N, Manns B, Lee H, Tonelli M. Systematic review of the impact of N-acetylcysteine on contrast nephropathy. Kidney Int 2004; 65(4):1366–1374.
18. Shilliday IR, Quinn KJ, Allison ME. Loop diuretics in the management of acute renal failure: a prospective, double-blind, placebo-controlled, randomized study. Nephrol Dial Transplant 1997; 12(12):2592–2596.
19. Solomon R, Werner C, Mann D, D'Elia J, Silva P. Effects of saline, mannitol, and furosemide to prevent acute decreases in renal function induced by radiocontrast agents (see comments). N Engl J Med 1994; 331(21):1416–1420.
20. Tepel M, van der GM, Schwarzfeld C, Laufer U, Liermann D, Zidek W. Prevention of radiographic-contrast-agent-induced reductions in renal function by acetylcysteine. N Engl J Med 2000; 343(3):180–184.
21. Vogt B, Ferrari P, Schonholzer C, Marti HP, Mohaupt M, Wiederkehr M, et al. Prophylactic hemodialysis after radiocontrast media in patients with renal insufficiency is potentially harmful. Am J Med 2001; 111(9):692–698.

Part V

Long-Term Outcome of Acute Kidney Injury

V

Long-Term Outcome of Acute Kidney Injury

5.1

Michael Joannidis and Philipp G.H. Metnitz

Core Messages

- Hospital survival of acute kidney injury (AKI): requiring RRT 38–58%
- 1-year survival of AKI: 21–53%
- 5-year survival of AKI: 15–52%
- 80–90% of surviving patients do not require further renal replacement therapy
- Most patients surviving AKI report satisfying quality of life
- History of chronic renal disease is the major risk factor for dialysis dependency after AKI

5.1.1 Introduction

Acute kidney injury (AKI) is associated with significant morbidity and mortality. Consequently, the diagnosis of this entity has significant impact on the patient's prognosis especially in the intensive care unit (ICU). However, patients who survive AKI are mainly concerned with questions such as whether they will be dependent on dialysis and whether they must consider an increased risk of dying during the following years. The present chapter will focus on these issues.

M. Joannidis (✉)
Medical Intensive Care Unit, Department of General Internal Medicine, Medical University Innsbruck, Anichstrasse 35, 6020 Innsbruck, Austria
e-mail: michael.joannidis@i-med.ac.at

5.1.2 ICU and Hospital Mortality

On the basis of currently available data, the occurrence of AKI is associated with an increase in mortality in excess of predicted mortality by using conventional ICU scores such as SAPS II, APACHE II, or APACHE III [16, 21, 22, 25, 27, 32, 38, 40]. ICU mortality is reported to be between 20% and 70%. Hospital mortality is slightly higher, between 25% and 80%.

There is an ongoing debate on whether excess mortality is already occurring in mild cases of AKI not requiring renal replacement therapy [30]. Nash and coworkers could establish a positive correlation between an increase in serum creatinine and mortality in their prospective study including 4,622 consecutive patients admitted to the medical and surgical services of an urban tertiary care hospital [36]. These findings are supported by two recent studies including patients undergoing cardiovascular surgery in two major academic centers where already a moderate rise in serum creatinine (≥0.5 mg/dl) was associated with a more than 10- to 18-fold increase in 30-day mortality (i.e., 18% and 36%, respectively) [19, 20]. Further support of this hypothesis results from a large US study on 19,982 patients, where a relative modest increase in serum creatinine between 0.3 and 0.4 mg/dl was associated with a 70% increased risk for death [9].

Nevertheless, the need for renal replacement therapy (RRT) appears to be a crucial factor with regard to prognosis. A study from the PICARD program in ICU patients demonstrated significantly lower mortality in AKI not requiring dialysis, in comparison with patients who underwent RRT (24% vs 45%, respectively) [33]. Furthermore, patients with AKI classified by an increase in creatinine [14] but not requiring RRT had a hospital mortality of 31%, compared with 57% for

A. Jörres et al. (eds.), *Management of Acute Kidney Problems*,
DOI: 10.1007/978-3-540-69441-0_5.1, © Springer-Verlag Berlin Heidelberg 2010

those requiring dialysis. One of the largest trials including 17,126 patients admitted to 30 ICUs in Austria showed a roughly fourfold increase in mortality in AKI even compared with subjects with the same level of severity of illness assessed by SAPS II score (62.8% vs 15.8%, $p < 0.01$) [34]. Even after adjusting for age, severity of illness, and treatment center, AKI still conferred about a 1.7-fold higher mortality compared with matched controls without renal failure. Similar results were found in a study performed in the United States where ICU patients suffering from AKI had about a 50% higher mortality when compared with patients with preexistent end-stage renal disease despite comparable APACHE III scores. Interestingly, ICU patients with end-stage renal disease showed mortality rates similar to patients without renal failure [10]. This finding demonstrates that mortality in acute renal failure is not just a matter of organ loss. This assumption is further undermined by the findings that AKI in the ICU is highly associated with the development of multiple organ failure. A multicenter trial performed in forty ICUs in 16 countries, including 1,411 patients, using SOFA scores revealed that about 70% of patients with AKI developed multiple organ failure; whereas, this was only the case in 10% of the patients not suffering from AKI [12].

In some instances the occurrence of AKI requiring RRT is associated with an extremely bad prognosis as described for ICU patients with underlying liver cirrhosis [2], hematological malignancy [7], and after cardiac arrest requiring cardiopulmonary resuscitation [28], with reported mortalities of 89%, 88%, and 94%, respectively.

5.1.3 Factors Predicting Hospital Survival

Very few studies have investigated the factors influencing outcome of AKI in a systematic and prospective manner. In a Canadian study [48] 38% of the 87 patients with AKI requiring RRT survived to discharge. Absence of oliguria, a better premorbid renal function, as well as a shorter period of dependence on RRT were factors associated with better prognosis. In those patients who survived to discharge from hospital dependency on RRT persisted in less then 10%. An Australian study including 299 patients with AKI in an ICU setting showed a mortality rate of roughly 47%. Survival was associated with lower age, absence of mechanical ventilation, as well as less need for vasoactive drugs. Only about 16% of patients discharged from hospital needed further dialysis treatment [42]. Similar mortality rates (49%) were obtained from another Australian multicenter trial including 116 ICU patients requiring RRT. Only 19% of the surviving patients needed dialysis after discharge from hospital [11].

The choice of initial treatment modality of RRT and its possible impact on survival remain a constant matter of debate. A recent prospective multinational study analyzed data of 1,218 patients [44] and compared outcome of AKI in patients treated with continuous renal replacement therapy (CRRT) and those treated with intermittent renal replacement therapy (IRRT). In 80% of the cases, CRRT was the initial treatment form chosen, and these patients presented with higher SAPS II scores, lower mean blood pressure, required higher doses of vasoactive drugs, and showed higher rates of mechanical ventilation compared to those patients treated with IRRT. Not surprisingly, mortality in patients receiving CRRT was higher, but after adjusting for severity of illness, no difference in survival was found. This corresponds to findings from several larger prospective randomized trials, which were unable to prove a significant survival benefit provided by continuous over intermittent RRT [31, 39, 46, 47].

5.1.4 Long-Term Prognosis

Although in-hospital survival of critically ill patients with AKI is poor, long-term prognosis for those patients who survive is not that bad (Table 5.1.1). After discharge from hospital, mortality increases only slightly and renal function recovers in the majority of the cases. The number of studies investigating long-term outcome after AKI, however, is relatively low. A German study including 979 ICU patients treated with CRRT [35] found that although only 31% of the patients survived to hospital discharge, the probability of surviving the first 6 months after discharge was 77%. In patients who survived this period, the probability of surviving also the next 6 months increased to 89%. Five-year survival probability, however, did not surpass 50%. Etiology of AKI had no impact on long-term survival probability, whereas age and comorbidity before hospitalization were associated

Table 5.1.1 Publications on long-term outcome of AKI treated with renal replacement therapy (RRT)

Publication	Patients (n)	Hospital survival (%)	28-day survival (%)	90-day survival (%)	Independence from RRT at hospital discharge (% of survivors)	6-month survival (%)	1-year survival (%)	5-year survival (%)
Jones 1998 [17]	408	38			97	36		
Korkeila 2000 [18]	62	55			82	45		35
Morgera 2002 [35]	979	31			90	24	21	15
Bagshaw 2005 [4]	240	40	49	40	68		36	
Ahlstrom 2005 [1]	703		59		95		43	30
Luckraz 2005 [26]	92	58			98		53	52
Lins 2006 [23]	293		49		90		38	
Wald 2006 [48]	87	38			90			
Schiffl 2006 [41]	443	53			90		35	
Bell 2007 [6]	2,642			42				

with worse outcome. Septic patients had the highest hospital mortality (up to 75%) and required RRT significantly longer than patients who did not suffer from sepsis. Similar numbers resulted from an investigation in 33,375 patients with sepsis-associated AKI using the large database of the Australian and New Zealand Intensive Care Society with increased ICU and hospital length of stay as an additional finding [3]. Interestingly, patients with sepsis and AKI showed a tendency toward better long-term outcome. Fifty-nine percent of the surviving patients regained normal renal function, of the remaining 41% with residual renal impairment, only 10% required chronic dialysis. Seventy-seven percent of the surviving patients reported good-to-excellent health status. Bagshaw et al. [4] investigated the epidemiology and long-term outcomes of 240 patients with AKI requiring RRT. ICU and hospital mortality in these patients were 50% and 60%, respectively. Of the surviving patients, 38% were independent from RRT at discharge from ICU, 68% at the time of hospital discharge. There was only a minor increase in mortality after 1 year from 60% to 64%, whereas 28% of the patients were alive and independent from RRT. Factors independently associated with 1-year mortality were preexisting comorbidities, liver disease, need for CRRT, septic shock, age, and a higher APACHE II score upon ICU admission. Schiffl and coworkers [41] reported similar 1-year survival rates of roughly 35% in patients with AKI treated with RRT. A Finnish study [1] investigating 703 patients with AKI receiving RRT reported a mortality rate of 41% at 28 days, 57% at 1 year and 70% at 5 years. There was a significant difference in the 1-year mortality between patients treated in the ICU (57%) and patients treated on hospital wards (47%). Independent predictors for 1-year mortality were SOFA score, age, and need for CRRT. Korkeila et al. [18] found the mortality of 62 studied patients with AKI to be 45% at hospital discharge, 55% at 6 months and 65% at 5 years. Renal function was restored in 82% of the survivors. Three days after start of RRT, oliguria was present in 82% of the nonsurvivors but in only 43% of the surviving patients, implying oliguria is a risk factor for unfavorable outcome. Eighty percent of the patients who died within 6 months had multiple organ dysfunctions at the time RRT was initiated. Outcome appeared to be slightly better in patients who experienced AKI after cardiac surgery, with complexity of procedure, increased cross-clamp time, and advanced age being the major risk factors for fatal outcome [26].

Four studies also investigated the effect of moderate renal functional impairment on long-term prognosis. In the setting of cardiac surgery, perioperative/postoperative deterioration in renal function, characterized by an increase in serum creatinine of at least 25%, carried a significant risk of increased mortality over an observation period of 8 years, i.e., a hazard ratio of 1.83 compared with the patient group who did not show perioperative deterioration in renal function [24]. Similar results were obtained from a retrospective cohort study on 87,094 patients admitted to 4,473 non-federal US hospitals for acute myocardial infarction. An increase in serum creatinine between 0.1 and 3.0 mg/dl during the hospitalization was associated with increases in hazard ratio for mortality ranging from 1.14 (0.1 mg/dl increase) to 1.39 (0.6–3.0 mg/dl increase) [37]. Hazard ratios for end-stage renal failure in these patients were found to be even higher, ranging from 1.45 to 3.26, respectively, as compared to those patients without creatinine increase.

A study by Bagshaw et al. [5] analyzed 1-year mortality in critically ill patients according to severity of kidney dysfunction at ICU admission in a large cohort consisting of 5,693 patients. Kidney function was stratified as no renal failure (serum creatinine <1.7 mg/dl), mild renal dysfunction (serum creatinine 1.7–3.4 mg/dl), moderate renal dysfunction (serum creatinine ≥ 3.4 mg/dl), severe renal failure (requirement for RRT), and end-stage kidney disease requiring long-term RRT before ICU admission. Hospital mortalities were 13%, 40%, 41%, 60%, and 34%, respectively. Although AKI requiring RRT was associated with a significantly higher hospital mortality, 1-year survival rates of patients discharged from hospital were comparable for all groups, i.e., 89% in patients with mild renal dysfunction, 87% in moderate renal dysfunction, and 90% in severe AKI with requirement for RRT as well as in end-stage kidney disease. Similar findings were reported by Lins and coworkers [23] who showed that there was no difference in 1-year survival after discharge from hospital in patients with AKI treated with RRT compared with those who were not.

5.1.5 Recovery of Renal Function

All of the above-mentioned studies show that the majority of the patients who survive AKI can be discharged from hospital and remain independent from further RRT (Table 5.1.1). In the two Australian studies less than 20% of the patients required further renal support upon discharge from hospital, most of them (80%) having a history of chronic renal impairment [11, 42]. Bagshaw et al. [4, 5] reported an independence from RRT 1 year after diagnosis of AKI, in 78% of the surviving patients. Renal recovery appeared to peak by 90 days with the number of patients requiring RRT being more or less the same at 1 year. The majority of patients remaining dependent on RRT were found to have suffered from preexisting chronic renal dysfunction. Analyzing the data regarding renal function at 90 days showed that a diagnosis of sepsis and septic shock, lower serum creatinine and urea levels prior to RRT, male sex, and fewer comorbidities were independently associated with renal recovery. Patients with cardiac disease, diabetes mellitus, peripheral vascular disease, and chronic kidney disease were less likely to regain renal function. No impact on renal recovery was found for type of admission, severity of illness, need for mechanical ventilation and vasopressor therapy, oliguria, and exposure to nephrotoxins. One study investigated patients who did not regain renal function after AKI [8], which was the case for 16% of the surviving patients. According to the cause of AKI, they found a frequency of dialysis dependency of 3–41% with the highest rate occurring in AKI due to parenchymal disease.

Two studies investigated recurring dependency on RRT after initial recovery of renal function. In the first study this was reported for one patient (<1%) with incomplete recovery of renal function at hospital discharge [41]. In a much larger Swedish study by Bell et al. [6] late development of end-stage renal disease was found in 2.3% (after intermittent hemodialysis [IHD]) and 3.6% (CRRT) of 998 patients with AKF who had initially recovered renal function at 90 days.

Since the choice of technique of RRT remains controversial, several studies investigated the impact of RRT modality on renal recovery. Although mortality in patients treated with CRRT tends to be higher due to the feasibility of this modality also in unstable and more severely ill patients, initial CRRT was found to be associated with significantly higher rates of renal recovery in surviving patients compared with patients treated with IHD (92% in CRRT vs 59% in IHD) [31]. This finding is supported by results obtained from the study by Uchino et al. [45] who demonstrated that CRRT as initial treatment predicted renal recovery in surviving patients, suggesting that hypotension, which was more frequently observed during IHD, might contribute to persistence of renal dysfunction and subsequent higher dependence on RRT in patients treated intermittently. Similar findings were reported by the already mentioned Swedish study in which roughly 50% less patients regained renal function when AKI was treated with IHD as compared with CRRT [6]. The very unbalanced distribution of patient numbers treated with the two modalities (994 CRRT vs 158 IHD), however, prevents reliable conclusions based on this finding.

5.1.6 Quality of Life

In addition to survival and dialysis dependency, quality of life is of major importance to patients with AKI. Korkeila et al. [18] tried to evaluate quality of life by sending a questionnaire to patients having survived AKI 6 months after ICU admission. The majority reported an acceptable quality of life (QOL) as assessed by Nottingham Heath Profile (NHP). The most frequent complaints mentioned were loss of energy and a limited physical mobility. Nearly all of the patients were able to manage everyday life on their own, with only 36% being dependent on external help. Another Finnish study [1] evaluated QOF by the Euro QOL (EQ-5d) instrument including a visual analog scale (VAS) score to assess the patient's perceived health. Although survivors had a lower health-related QOL compared with age- and sex-matched controls, patients themselves were as satisfied with their health as the general population.

Gopal et al. [13] reported that survivors of combined multiple organ failure and AKI treated with RRT have a relatively good state of health and an acceptable QOL. The majority of the patients mentioned that they would undergo the same treatment again, if necessary. Maynard et al. [29] evaluated the health-related QOL among 12 survivors treated with RRT, 6 months following hospital discharge by using the Medical Outcomes Study Short Form 36-item Health Survey (SF-36). Although health status was not perceived to be very good, health-related QOL, however, was fairly satisfying. No correlation was found between SF-36 and APACHE III Score at ICU admission, indicating that severity of illness does not predict QOL in survivors, corresponding to findings from other studies [15, 43].

5.1.7 Conclusion

Although patients with AKI show a very high ICU and hospital mortality, those who survive to hospital discharge have a reasonable, long-term prognosis. Most of the patients regain renal function, along with an acceptable health status. Those patients who remain on dialysis frequently have a history of chronic renal disease before ICU admission. The majority of patients having survived AKI are capable of managing everyday life independently from external help and perception of QOL is comparable to the age- and sex-matched general population.

References

1. Ahlstrom A, Tallgren M, Peltonen S, Rasanen P, Pettila V (2005) Survival and quality of life of patients requiring acute renal replacement therapy. Intensive Care Med 31: 1222–1228
2. Arabi Y, Ahmed QA, Haddad S, Aljumah A, Al Shimemeri A (2004) Outcome predictors of cirrhosis patients admitted to the intensive care unit. Eur J Gastroenterol Hepatol 16: 333–339
3. Bagshaw SM, George C, Bellomo R (2008) Early acute kidney injury and sepsis: a multicentre evaluation. Crit Care 12: R47
4. Bagshaw SM, Laupland KB, Doig CJ, Mortis G, Fick GH, Mucenski M, Godinez-Luna T, Svenson LW, Rosenal T (2005) Prognosis for long-term survival and renal recovery in critically ill patients with severe acute renal failure: a population-based study. Crit Care 9: R700–R709
5. Bagshaw SM, Mortis G, Doig CJ, Godinez-Luna T, Fick GH, Laupland KB (2006) One-year mortality in critically ill patients by severity of kidney dysfunction: a population-based assessment. Am J Kidney Dis 48: 402–409
6. Bell M, Granath F, Schon S, Ekbom A, Martling CR (2007) Continuous renal replacement therapy is associated with less chronic renal failure than intermittent haemodialysis after acute renal failure. Intensive Care Med 33: 773–780
7. Benoit DD, Vandewoude KH, Decruyenaere JM, Hoste EA, Colardyn FA (2003) Outcome and early prognostic indicators in patients with a hematologic malignancy admitted to the intensive care unit for a life-threatening complication. Crit Care Med 31: 104–112
8. Bhandari S, Turney JH (1996) Survivors of acute renal failure who do not recover renal function. QJM 89: 415–421
9. Chertow GM, Burdick E, Honour M, Bonventre JV, Bates DW (2005) Acute kidney injury, mortality, length of stay, and costs in hospitalized patients. J Am Soc Nephrol 16: 3365–3370
10. Clermont G, Acker CG, Angus DC, Sirio CA, Pinsky MR, Johnson JP (2002) Renal failure in the ICU: comparison of the impact of acute renal failure and end-stage renal disease on ICU outcomes. Kidney Int 62: 986–996
11. Cole L, Bellomo R, Silvester W, Reeves JH (2000) A prospective, multicenter study of the epidemiology, management, and outcome of severe acute renal failure in a "closed" ICU system. Am J Respir Crit Care Med 162: 191–196
12. de Mendonca A, Vincent JL, Suter PM, Moreno R, Dearden NM, Antonelli M, Takala J, Sprung C, Cantraine F (2000) Acute renal failure in the ICU: risk factors and outcome evaluated by the SOFA score. Intensive Care Med 26: 915–921
13. Gopal I, Bhonagiri S, Ronco C, Bellomo R (1997) Out of hospital outcome and quality of life in survivors of combined acute multiple organ and renal failure treated with continuous venovenous hemofiltration/hemodiafiltration. Intensive Care Med 23: 766–772
14. Hou SH, Bushinsky DA, Wish JB, Cohen JJ, Harrington JT (1983) Hospital-acquired renal insufficiency: a prospective study. Am J Med 74: 243–248

15. Hurel D, Loirat P, Saulnier F, Nicolas F, Brivet F (1997) Quality of life 6 months after intensive care: results of a prospective multicenter study using a generic health status scale and a satisfaction scale. Intensive Care Med 23: 331–337
16. Joannidis M, Metnitz PG (2005) Epidemiology and natural history of acute renal failure in the ICU. Crit Care Clin 21: 239–249
17. Jones CH, Richardson D, Goutcher E, Newstead CG, Will EJ, Cohen AT, Davison AM (1998) Continuous venovenous high-flux dialysis in multiorgan failure: a 5-year single-center experience. Am J Kidney Dis 31: 227–233
18. Korkeila M, Ruokonen E, Takala J (2000) Costs of care, long-term prognosis and quality of life in patients requiring renal replacement therapy during intensive care. Intensive Care Med 26: 1824–1831
19. Lassnigg A, Schmid ER, Hiesmayr M, Falk C, Druml W, Bauer P, Schmidlin D (2008) Impact of minimal increases in serum creatinine on outcome in patients after cardiothoracic surgery: do we have to revise current definitions of acute renal failure? Crit Care Med 36: 1129–1137
20. Lassnigg A, Schmidlin D, Mouhieddine M, Bachmann LM, Druml W, Bauer P, Hiesmayr M (2004) Minimal changes of serum creatinine predict prognosis in patients after cardiothoracic surgery: a prospective cohort study. J Am Soc Nephrol 15: 1597–1605
21. Levy EM, Viscoli CM, Horwitz RI (1996) The effect of acute renal failure on mortality. A cohort analysis. JAMA 275: 1489–1494
22. Lins RL, Elseviers M, Daelemans R, Zachee P, Zachee P, Gheuens E, Lens S, De Broe ME (2000) Prognostic value of a new scoring system for hospital mortality in acute renal failure. Clin Nephrol 53: 10–17
23. Lins RL, Elseviers MM, Daelemans R (2006) Severity scoring and mortality 1 year after acute renal failure. Nephrol Dial Transplant 21: 1066–1068
24. Loef BG, Epema AH, Smilde TD, Henning RH, Ebels T, Navis G, Stegeman CA (2005) Immediate postoperative renal function deterioration in cardiac surgical patients predicts in-hospital mortality and long-term survival. J Am Soc Nephrol 16: 195–200
25. Lohr JW, McFarlane MJ, Grantham JJ (1988) A clinical index to predict survival in acute renal failure patients requiring dialysis. Am J Kidney Dis 11: 254–259
26. Luckraz H, Gravenor MB, George R, Taylor S, Williams A, Ashraf S, Argano V, Youhana A (2005) Long and short-term outcomes in patients requiring continuous renal replacement therapy post cardiopulmonary bypass. Eur J Cardiothorac Surg 27: 906–909
27. Martin C, Saran R, Leavey S, Swartz R (2002) Predicting the outcome of renal replacement therapy in severe acute renal failure. ASAIO J 48: 640–644
28. Mattana J, Singhal PC (1993) Prevalence and determinants of acute renal failure following cardiopulmonary resuscitation. Arch Intern Med 153: 235–239
29. Maynard SE, Whittle J, Chelluri L, Arnold R (2003) Quality of life and dialysis decisions in critically ill patients with acute renal failure. Intensive Care Med 29: 1589–1593
30. Mehta RL, Kellum JA, Shah SV, Molitoris BA, Ronco C, Warnock DG, Levin A (2007) Acute Kidney Injury Network: report of an initiative to improve outcomes in acute kidney injury. Crit Care 11: R31
31. Mehta RL, McDonald B, Gabbai FB, Pahl M, Pascual MT, Farkas A, Kaplan RM (2001) A randomized clinical trial of continuous versus intermittent dialysis for acute renal failure. Kidney Int 60: 1154–1163
32. Mehta RL, Pascual MT, Gruta CG, Zhuang S, Chertow GM (2002) Refining predictive models in critically ill patients with acute renal failure. J Am Soc Nephrol 13: 1350–1357
33. Mehta RL, Pascual MT, Soroko S, Savage BR, Himmelfarb J, Ikizler TA, Paganini EP, Chertow GM (2004) Spectrum of acute renal failure in the intensive care unit: the PICARD experience. Kidney Int 66: 1613–1621
34. Metnitz PG, Krenn CG, Steltzer H, Lang T, Ploder J, Lenz K, Le Gall JR, Druml W (2002) Effect of acute renal failure requiring renal replacement therapy on outcome in critically ill patients. Crit Care Med 30: 2051–2058
35. Morgera S, Kraft AK, Siebert G, Luft FC, Neumayer HH (2002) Long-term outcomes in acute renal failure patients treated with continuous renal replacement therapies. Am J Kidney Dis 40: 275–279
36. Nash K, Hafeez A, Hou S (2002) Hospital-acquired renal insufficiency. Am J Kidney Dis 39: 930–936
37. Newsome BB, Warnock DG, McClellan WM, Herzog CA, Kiefe CI, Eggers PW, Allison JJ (2008) Long-term risk of mortality and end-stage renal disease among the elderly after small increases in serum creatinine level during hospitalization for acute myocardial infarction. Arch Intern Med 168: 609–616
38. Paganini EP, Halstenberg WK, Goormastic M (1996) Risk modeling in acute renal failure requiring dialysis: the introduction of a new model. Clin Nephrol 46: 206–211
39. Palevsky PM, Zhang JH, O'Connor TZ, Chertow GM, Crowley ST, Choudhury D, Finkel K, Kellum JA, Paganini E, Schein RM, Smith MW, Swanson KM, Thompson BT, Vijayan A, Watnick S, Star RA, Peduzzi P (2008) Intensity of renal support in critically ill patients with acute kidney injury. N Engl J Med 359: 7–20
40. Schafer JH, Maurer A, Jochimsen F, Emde C, Wegscheider K, Arntz HR, Heitz J, Krell-Schroeder B, Distler A (1990) Outcome prediction models on admission in a medical intensive care unit: do they predict individual outcome? Crit Care Med 18: 1111–1118
41. Schiffl H (2006) Renal recovery from acute tubular necrosis requiring renal replacement therapy: a prospective study in critically ill patients. Nephrol Dial Transplant 21: 1248–1252
42. Silvester W, Bellomo R, Cole L (2001) Epidemiology, management, and outcome of severe acute renal failure of critical illness in Australia. Crit Care Med 29: 1910–1915
43. Tian ZM, Miranda DR (1995) Quality of life after intensive care with the sickness impact profile. Intensive Care Med 21: 422–428
44. Uchino S, Bellomo R, Kellum JA, Morimatsu H, Morgera S, Schetz MR, Tan I, Bouman C, Macedo E, Gibney N, Tolwani A, Oudemans-van Straaten HM, Ronco C (2007) Patient and kidney survival by dialysis modality in critically ill patients with acute kidney injury. Int J Artif Organs 30: 281–292
45. Uchino S, Bellomo R, Morgera S, Schetz M, Tan I, Bouman C, Macedo E, Gibney N, Tolwani A, Oudemans-van Straaten H, Ronco C, Kellum JA (2007) Continuous renal replacement therapy: A worldwide practice survey. Intensive Care Med 33: 1563–1570

46. Uehlinger DE, Jakob SM, Ferrari P, Eichelberger M, Huynh-Do U, Marti HP, Mohaupt MG, Vogt B, Rothen HU, Regli B, Takala J, Frey FJ (2005) Comparison of continuous and intermittent renal replacement therapy for acute renal failure. Nephrol Dial Transplant 20: 1630–1637
47. Vinsonneau C, Camus C, Combes A, Costa de Beauregard MA, Klouche K, Boulain T, Pallot JL, Chiche JD, Taupin P, Landais P, Dhainaut JF (2006) Continuous venovenous haemodiafiltration versus intermittent haemodialysis for acute renal failure in patients with multiple-organ dysfunction syndrome: a multicentre randomised trial. Lancet 368: 379–385
48. Wald R, Deshpande R, Bell CM, Bargman JM (2006) Survival to discharge among patients treated with continuous renal replacement therapy. Hemodial Int 10: 82–87

Part VI

Diagnosis and Management of Specific Disorders

Acute Kidney Injury in Sepsis

6.1

Robert W. Schrier, Shweta Bansal, and Wei Wang

Core Messages

- Sepsis is the most common cause of acute kidney injury (AKI) in the intensive care unit. Mortality of AKI is much higher in septic patients compared with nonseptic patients.
- Septic patients frequently present with a hyperdynamic circulation including primary arterial vasodilation and a secondary increase in cardiac output; renal hemodynamics are often characterized by early vasoconstriction.
- The elucidation of key components of pathogenesis of sepsis and septic shock has suggested several potential therapies for sepsis, and significant progress has been made in understanding the biology and mechanisms of endotoxin-related AKI; however, translation of this knowledge into improved management and outcome for patients with AKI has not been optimal.
- This chapter summarizes the hemodynamic and biochemical alterations in sepsis which lead to AKI and addresses the currently available and potential future therapies for the management of sepsis to prevent and treat AKI.

R. W. Schrier (✉)
University of Colorado School of Medicine, 4200 East Ninth Avenue B173, Biomedical Research Building, Room 723, Denver, CO 80262, USA
e-mail: robert.schrier@uchsc.edu

6.1.1 Hemodynamics and Hormones During Sepsis and Acute Kidney Injury

The septic patient frequently presents with a hyperdynamic circulation including primary arterial vasodilation and a secondary increase in cardiac output [22]. A consistent finding in sepsis secondary to gram-negative bacteremia and endotoxemia is an induction of nitric oxide synthase (iNOS) [22]. The resultant increase in circulating nitric oxide (NO) contributes to the arterial vasodilation. In experimental endotoxemia, the increase in renal iNOS and serum NO that occurs in wild-type mice is not observed in iNOS knockout mice [19]. As shown in Fig. 6.1.1, the resultant NO-mediated arterial vasodilatation decreases stretch on the arterial baroreceptors with increased sympathetic nervous system (SNS), renin-angiotensin-aldosterone system (RAAS), and arginine vasopressin (AVP) activity [37]. In experimental endotoxemia and septic patients, an increase in circulating catecholamines has been reported [5, 10]. While activation of this neurohumoral axis counteracts the arterial vasodilation, thereby maintaining blood pressure, this occurs at the expense of renal vasoconstriction with sodium and water retention. The increase in cardiac index also contributes to maintenance of blood pressure during sepsis. It has been noted, however, that this secondary increase in cardiac index during sepsis may be attenuated by depressed myocardial contractility secondary to increased cytokines, e.g., tumor necrosis factor alpha (TNF-α), interstitial myocarditis, and diastolic dysfunction [9]. In fact, the progression from severe sepsis to septic shock may occur not only secondary to more profound arterial vasodilation, but also may be due to an inadequate cardiac output response.

A. Jörres et al. (eds.), *Management of Acute Kidney Problems*,
DOI: 10.1007/978-3-540-69441-0_6.1, © Springer-Verlag Berlin Heidelberg 2010

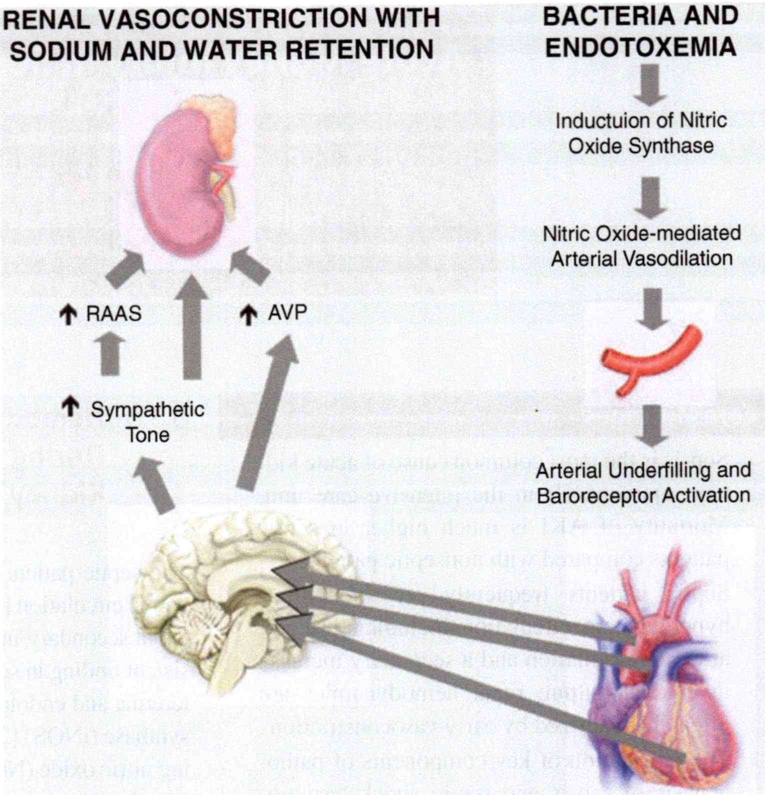

Fig. 6.1.1 Hemodynamic and renal effects of bacteremia and endotoxin (Modified from [7])

In patients with septic shock, a relative resistance to vasopressor agents, particularly norepinephrine, has been reported [41]. The increase in hydrogen ion concentration and circulating lactate and decrease in cellular adenosine triphosphate (ATP) appears to be involved in this decreased vascular response, including the arterial vasodilation during sepsis. These perturbations are associated with an increased opening of ATP-activated potassium channels (K_{ATP}) which hyperpolarizes the vascular membrane secondary to increased K efflux. The membrane hyperpolarization leads to a decrease in voltage-activated channels and diminished cellular calcium influx with relative resistance to norepinephrine and angiotensin. Exogenous AVP has been shown to partially reverse this vascular resistance and thus may have a role in treating septic shock [22].

6.1.2 Sodium and Water Balance During Sepsis

Isotonic saline is most frequently used for resuscitating patients with severe sepsis or septic shock. In the presence of acute kidney failure (AKI) associated with sepsis, the administered resuscitation fluid is largely retained by the patient. A recent study of resuscitation in critically ill patients demonstrated that an average 8–10 l of isotonic saline is generally administered [52]. Arterial vasodilation has been shown in experimental studies to be associated with a tendency for the administered fluid to preferentially move into the interstitium [35]. This is in part due to an increase in albumin distribution space and alterations in Starling forces favoring translocation of intravascular fluid into the interstitium. Thus, noncardiogenic pulmonary edema and hypoxia frequently occur in septic patients with AKI during resuscitation. The patients then are diagnosed as having adult respiratory distress syndrome (ARDS), and mechanical ventilation is instituted. Many of these septic patients, however, do not demonstrate a decrease in pulmonary compliance, i.e., stiff lungs. Moreover, they tolerate judicious fluid removable by ultrafiltration with hemodynamic stability and improved oxygenation. We have used the term pseudo-ARDS as the diagnosis in these patients [36], since it seems unlikely that the classical lung pathology of ARDS is present. As much as 10–20 l of fluid can be removed over several days in

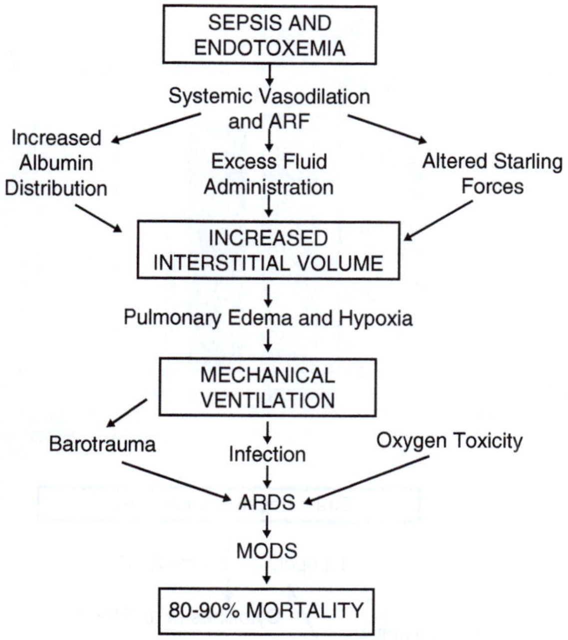

Fig. 6.1.2 Pathway whereby sepsis and endotoxemia can lead to mechanical ventilation and subsequent acute respiratory distress syndrome (ARDS) and multiorgan dysfunction syndrome (MODS)

these patients and mechanical ventilation prevented or discontinued. Thus, knowledge of the accumulated fluid balance in these resuscitated septic patients is critical. Whereas large volumes of fluid may have been necessary during the initial resuscitation, the persistence of an excessive fluid balance necessitating prolonged mechanical ventilation predisposes the patient to pulmonary oxygen toxicity, barotrauma, and infection, and ultimately bona fide ARDS may occur (Fig. 6.1.2) [37]. The combination of AKI, ARDS, and prolonged mechanical ventilation has a mortality greater than 80%. The most common cause of death in patients with AKI is infection, with the lungs as the primary source of sepsis. In this regard, the more prolonged the mechanical ventilation, the higher the mortality [25].

There has been debate about the optimal fluid, saline versus colloid, to be administered for resuscitating critically ill patients. The recent results of the SAFE study indicated that there was no significant difference in mortality between patients resuscitated with saline versus albumin [14]. In a subanalysis, however, there was a better survival with albumin administration in septic shock patients (relative risk [RR] = 0.87, $p < 0.09$). Results of a smaller study indicated a better survival with albumin than saline resuscitation in critically ill patients who were hypoalbuminuric (serum albumin less than 2.5 mg/dl) [13]. These results are in need of verification in prospective randomized studies which are adequately powered. It should be mentioned, however, that the hyperdynamic circulation in cirrhotic patients mimics that of septic patients, and a randomized prospective study clearly demonstrated the beneficial effect of albumin with antibiotics as compared to antibiotics alone in cirrhotic patients with spontaneous bacterial peritonitis [39]. Moreover, in patients with hepatorenal syndrome, the beneficial effect of V1 vasopressin agonists, e.g., terlipressin, necessitates the concomitant administration of albumin [26].

6.1.3 Early Renal Vasoconstriction in Septic AKI

As noted earlier, the SNS and RAAS are activated early in severe sepsis and endotoxemia. In experimental endotoxemia in mice, plasma renin, epinephrine, and norepinephrine are elevated in the absence of any fall in blood pressure (BP) [42]. The role of the SNS in maintaining the BP in this setting has, however, been shown. Alpha adrenergic blockade with phentolamine lowered BP significantly in the endotoxemia, but not wild-type mice. Moreover, the role of increased renal nerve stimulation in endotoxemic-related AKI was demonstrated by the protective effect of renal denervation [42]. Plasma endothelin has also been shown to be increased during endotoxemia (ET) and intrarenal administration of an endothelin antiserum afforded renal protection, as assessed by glomerular filtration rate (GFR) [20].

Studies in endotoxemic-related AKI in mice have indicated a potential renal protective effect of endothelial NOS (eNOS) [44]. There is no specific eNOS inhibition, but eNOS knockout mice are available. These knockout mice have higher BP, but increased renal vascular resistance as compared with wild-type mice. With administration of a small dose (1 mg/kg) of endotoxin, which does not alter GFR in wild-type mice, a profound fall in GFR occurs in the eNOS knockout mice. These results support the importance of intact eNOS in the kidney in preventing or attenuating endotoxin-related AKI. Further evidence of the importance of the integrity of the renal endothelium in protecting against AKI in sepsis was obtained in mice treated with indomethacin, a cyclooxygenase inhibitor [44]. The rise in urine 6-keto PGF 1 alpha, the metabolic product of

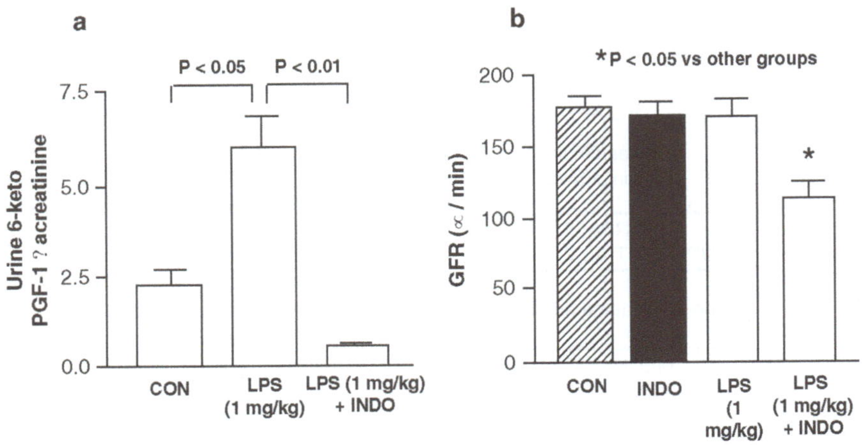

Fig. 6.1.3 Effect of indomethacin (INDO) on urinary 6-keto PGF-1a (**a**) and GFR (**b**) during endotoxemia (lipopolysaccharide [LPS]) in wild-type mice (CON – control) (Used with permission of [23])

prostacyclin, which occurred during endotoxemia, was totally blocked by indomethacin (Fig. 6.1.3a). Moreover, a 1 mg/kg dose of endotoxin which did not alter GFR in untreated mice was associated with a significant fall in indomethacin-treated animals (Fig. 6.1.3b). These results would indicate that septic patients receiving nonsteroidal antiinflammatory agents (NSAIDs) are more prone to develop AKI. Nonspecific inhibitors of NOS, such as LMMA, have been studied in septic patients. Unfortunately, this treatment was associated with increased mortality [17]. The explanation for these disappointing results most likely relates to the nonspecificity of LMMA which inhibits both iNOS and eNOS. In experimental studies using a specific iNOS inhibitor, L-NIL, the integrity of eNOS was preserved and renal protection occurred during endotoxemia [38]. Studies in septic patients using specific iNOS inhibitors need to be undertaken.

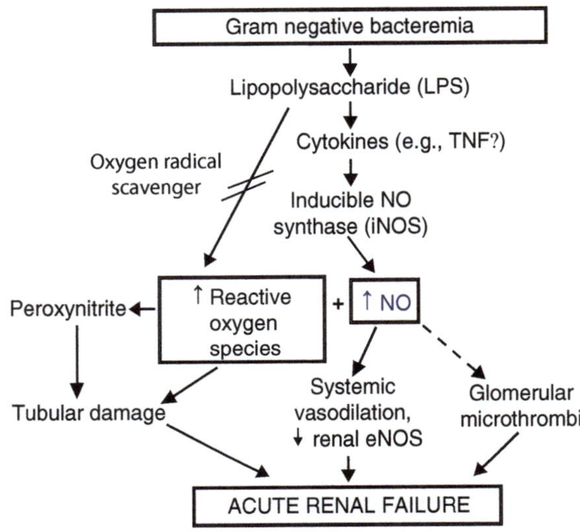

Fig. 6.1.4 Pathogenetic schema whereby endotoxemia leads to tubular and vascular damage. Protective effect of nitric oxide (NO) as indicated by dashed line

6.1.4 Role of Oxygen Radicals and Cytokines in Renal Tubular and Vascular Injury During Sepsis

Sepsis and endotoxemia are known to be associated with generation of reactive oxygen species (ROS) and oxidant injury [43]. Recent experimental mice studies have shown that endotoxemia is associated with decreased extracellular, but not mitochondrial or cystoplasmic, superoxide dismutase (SOD). Moreover, administration of chemically dissimilar SOD mimetics were shown to afford renal protection during endotoxemia as assessed by GFR and renal blood flow (RBF) [43]. In addition to the effect of endotoxemia to increase ROS, cytokine stimulation is a hallmark of sepsis. TNF-α has been examined as a stimulator of iNOS (Fig. 6.1.4). Pentoxifylline is known to block TNF-α production [53], and renal dendritic cells appear to be an important source of TNF-α during ischemia/reperfusion injury [12]. With pentoxifylline treatment during endotoxemia, a major decrease in serum NO and interleukin 1 beta occurred in association with a decrease in renal iNOS and intercellular adhesion molecule (ICAM) [45]. In these endotoxemia studies serum TNF-a did not increase (Fig. 6.1.5a), and GFR was significantly improved compared with untreated animals (Fig. 6.1.5b). There have also been experimental studies in which erythropoietin, independent of an effect on hemoglobin synthesis, has been

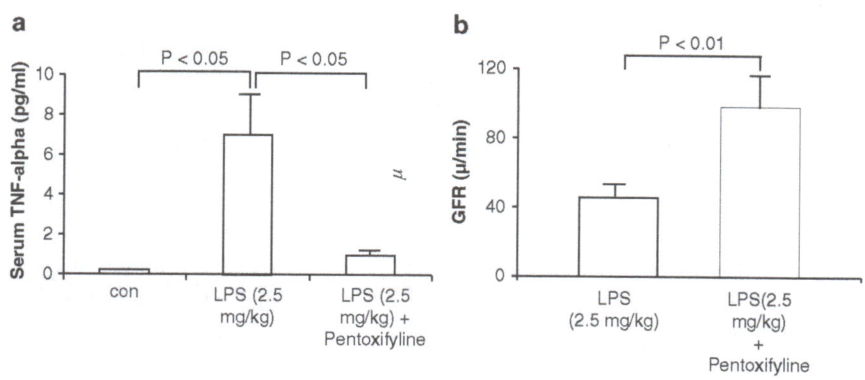

Fig. 6.1.5 Effect of pentoxifylline on serum TNF-a level (**a**) and renal protective effect of pentoxifylline on glomerular filtration rate (GFR) (**b**) during endotoxemia (Used with permission of [29])

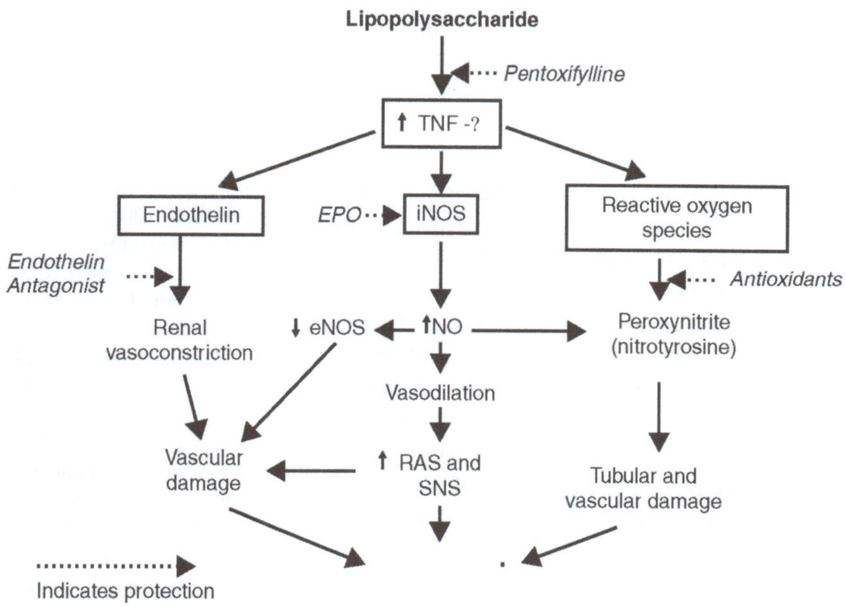

Fig. 6.1.6 Proposed pathogenetic sites where interventions could potentially alter the course of endotoxin-related acute kidney injury

shown to attenuate the kidney injury during ischemia/reperfusion [1, 28]. In experimental endotoxemia in mice, erythropoietin also has been shown to protect against AKI [24]. While the mechanism is unclear, antioxidant and antiapoptotic effects may be involved. In Fig. 6.1.6 are summarized various potential interventions in endotoxin-related AKI.

6.1.5 Prospective Randomized Clinical Studies in Sepsis

An early goal-directed therapy prospective, randomized study examined early resuscitation (0–6 h) in the emergency department at Henry Ford Hospital in patients with severe sepsis and septic shock [32]. The patients had a systolic BP <90 mm Hg or plasma lactate ≥ 4 mmol/l; central venous oxygen saturation ($SCVO_2$) <50%; and mean serum creatinine of 2.6 mg/dl. The standard versus early goal-directed therapy protocol are shown in Table 6.1.1 and the results at 0–6 h are shown

Table 6.1.1 Early goal-directed therapy of severe sepsis and septic shock (0–6 h)

Standard therapy (n = 133)	Early goal-directed therapy for ≥ 6 h (n = 130)
	$SCOV_2$ monitoring
CVP ≥ 8–12 mm Hg	500 ml bolus NS for CVP 8–12 mm Hg
MAP ≥ 65 mm Hg	Vasopressors to maintain MAP ≥ 65 mm Hg
Urine output ≥ 0.5 ml/kg/h	$SCOV_2$ < 70% transfuse to HCT > 30%
	Dobutamine

Source: Modified from [33]

Table 6.1.2 Sepsis and septic shock (0–6 h)

	Standard	Early goal	*P* value
MAP (mm Hg)	81 ± 16	88 ± 16	<0.001
$SCVO_2 \geq 70\%$	60.2%	94.9%	<0.001
CVP, MAP, and UO goals	86.1%	99.2%	<0.001

Source: Modified from [33]

Table 6.1.3 Beneficial effects of early goal-directed therapy of severe sepsis and septic shock (7–72 h)

	Standard	Early goal	*P* value
In-hospital mortality (%)	46.5	30.5	<0.009
$SCOV_2$ (%)	65.3	70.4	<0.02
Lactate (mmol/l)	3.9	3.0	<0.02
pH	7.36	7.4	<0.02
Mechanical ventilation (%)	16.8	2.6	<0.001
Fibrin split product (µg/dl)	62	39	<0.001

Source: Modified from [33]

in Table 6.1.2 and demonstrate better BP, oxygenation, and urine flow than the standard therapy. The results from 7–72 h are shown in Table 6.1.3. The in-hospital mortality was the primary end point and was significantly lower in the early goal-directed than the standard group (30.5 vs 46.5%, $p < 0.009$). A longer term follow-up study confirmed the efficacy of this approach [27]. Earlier studies initiated interventions only after the septic patients had reached the intensive care unit (ICU) and monitoring of $SCOV_2$ also was not undertaken [16, 18]. A more recent study of the same protocol-driven therapy in patients who had septic shock and were transferred to an ICU from either the emergency department and the in-patient ward, demonstrated reduced mortality, decreased ICU length of stay, and decreased ventilator days. Of relevance to the kidney, the incidence of AKI fell from 55.2% in the standard group to 38.9% in goal-directed therapy group ($p = 0.015$) [23].

A prospective randomized study from Belgium examined the effects of intensive insulin therapy in critically ill patients [48]. The initial study was undertaken in 1,548 patients receiving mechanical ventilation in a surgical ICU. The intensive insulin treatment patients had their blood glucose concentrations maintained between 80–100 mg/dl, while the control patients only received insulin when their blood glucose level exceeded 215 mg/dl, then it was maintained between 180–220 mg/dl. The results are shown in Table 6.1.4 with the significant decrease in ICU mortality in the intensive insulin therapy group as the primary end point. A similar randomized protocol of 1,200 patients was followed for a study in the medical ICU [47]. The primary end point of in-hospital mortality was not significantly different between the experimental groups. However, similar to the surgical ICU study, in-hospital mortality was lower in patients in whom the medical ICU stay was 3 days or longer (43.0 vs 52.5%, $p < 0.009$). Acute kidney injury was also significantly less in this same group of patients (8.3 vs 12.5%, $p < 0.05$). Subsequent results would suggest that the control of blood glucose rather than insulin is the most important factor in these results [15, 49]. It is important to note, however, that a recent study assessing aggressive insulin therapy was discontinued on the basis of safety and efficacy [21]. Similarly in another recent prospective randomized study, there was no significant difference in 28- and 90-day mortality and

Table 6.1.4 Beneficial effect of intensive insulin therapy in critically ill patients

- **ICU mortality**
  - 4.6% vs 8.0%, $p < 0.04$
- **Mortality in patients in ICU for more than 5 days**
  - 10.6% vs 20.2%, $p = 0.005$
- **34% decrease in overall hospital mortality**
  - Cause of death from MOF with proven septic focus
  - 8 vs 33, $p = 0.02$
- **41% decrease in acute kidney injury requiring dialysis or hemofiltration**
- **Patients requiring > 14 days of ventilatory support**
  - 7.5% vs 11.9%, $p = 0.003$

Source: Modified from [38]

sequential organ failure assessment score between intensive and conventional insulin therapy in patients with severe sepsis. The trial was discontinued early because of safety reasons relating to the frequency of severe hypoglycemia [8].

The Vasopressin in Septic Shock Trial (VASST) analyzed 779 patients in septic shock requiring vasopressors for at least 6 h and having at least one additional organ dysfunction present for less then 24 h [33, 34]. The patients were randomized to either norepinephrine or AVP. There was no overall difference in 28-day survival between these groups. However, in patients with stratification according to severity of hypotension on enrollment, as assessed by a dosage of greater or less than 15 µg/min of norepinephrine, the patients with the lower norepinephrine dosage had improved survival with AVP (26.5 vs 35.7%, $p = 0.05$). These results persisted at 90 days (35.8 vs 46.1%, $p = 0.04$). There were no differences in BP, but the addition of AVP to the baseline norepinephrine led to a lower dosage of norepinephrine. Digital ischemia was more frequent with AVP, and cardiac arrest was more frequent with norepinephrine, but these differences were not significant.

In 2002 a prospective double-blind randomized study from France examined the effect of daily 50 mg intravenous hydrocortisone and oral 50 µg fludrocortisone for 7 days in septic patients [4]. The patients were analyzed based on their response to adrenocorticotropic hormone (ACTH) stimulation. Nonresponders (n = 229) exhibited less than a 9 mg/ml increment in plasma cortisol, and responders had larger rises in plasma cortisol (N = 70). In nonresponders, the 28-day mortality rate was lower in the corticosteroid than in the placebo group (53 vs 63%, $p < 0.02$) and the vasopressor withdrawal at 28 days was higher in the corticosteroid group (57 vs 40%, $p < 0.001$). There were no differences in the responders.

The recent CORTICUS randomized controlled study of 500 patients enrolled over 3 years from 52 European centers also compared the effects of hydrocortisone versus placebo using a similar protocol [40]. There was no difference in 28-day mortality (33 vs 31%, NS), but the duration of shock was shorter in the hydrocortisone-treated patients. Analysis of nonresponders, as defined in the earlier study by Annane et al. [4], also showed no difference in 28-day mortality between the hydrocortisone and placebo-treated patients. However, patients in the CORTICUS study were enrolled up to 72 h after fulfilling entry criteria as compared with the 8-h window in the Annane study. Moreover, in a subanalysis of the CORTICUS study, patients who had a systolic BP that persisted below 90 mm Hg at 1 day after fluid resuscitation and vasopressor support, showed an absolute reduction in mortality of 11.2% in the hydrocortisone group compared with placebo group. The role of corticosteroid therapy in septic patients thus remains controversial.

What has become clear in monitoring severely ill septic patients is that pulmonary artery catheters do not improve outcomes as compared with a standard central venous catheter [30, 51]. Septic patients with acute lung injury on mechanical ventilation should utilize a tidal volume of 6 ml/kg of predicted body weight to keep plateau airway pressures < 30 cm H_2O [50]. A randomized study has also shown that aggressive fluid administration in patients with acute lung injury, i.e., 8–10-l positive fluid balance, does not diminish the incidence of acute kidney injury as compared with moderate fluid administration, i.e., 2–3-l positive fluid balance [52]. Moreover, the patients receiving the larger fluid volumes exhibited worse pulmonary and central nervous system function.

The randomized LIPOS Trial failed to show a benefit for an antiendotoxin emulsion in the treatment of patients with severe sepsis [11]. While the PROWESS trial demonstrated a beneficial effect of activated human protein C (Drotrecogin alpha) in adult patients with severe sepsis [6], a benefit has not been documented in children or adults with a lower severity of illness and surgical patients with only one organ dysfunction [2]. Because of this latter data and the agent's high cost, the Surviving Sepsis Campaign (SSC) now recommends the use of Drotrecogin alfa only in treating severely ill septic patients with APACHE score ≥ 25 and/or two or more organ dysfunctions.

In summary, AKI in sepsis is a common illness which is associated with high morbidity and mortality. Much has been learned about the pathogenesis of this disorder which has led to several important translational clinical trials. Excess fluid administration with prolonged mechanical ventilation bodes a poor prognosis. While there is some support for a role of albumin and vasopressin in septic patients, more clinical studies are needed. As in spontaneous bacterial peritonitis, in cirrhotic patients, early antibiotics and resuscitation with colloid may prevent the occurrence of AKI and decrease mortality in septic patients. This, however, remains to be proven. Monitoring central venous oxygen saturation and avoidance of pulmonary arterial catheters are recommended. Potential experimental therapies for sepsis, such as oxygen radical scavengers, erythropoietin, and pentoxifylline, alone or in combination, are in need of study in human clinical trials.

6.1.6 Take Home Pearls

- AKI in sepsis is a common illness with a complex pathophysiology and is associated with high morbidity and mortality.
- Better understanding of the pathogenesis of sepsis has led to several important translational clinical trials, including the administration of vasopressin, activated protein C, low-dose corticosteroids, and tight glycemic control. Some of these interventions remain, however, controversial.
- Potential experimental therapies for sepsis, such as oxygen radical scavengers, erythropoietin, and pentoxifylline, are still in need of study in human clinical trials.

Acknowledgments The authors' research papers cited in the article were supported by NIH Grant 2 RO1 DK052599-09A2. The authors appreciate the editorial assistance of Jan Darling.

Acute kidney injury (AKI) is frequently associated with sepsis. In severe sepsis and septic shock, the incidence of AKI has been reported to be 23% and 51%, respectively [31]. Sepsis is the most common cause of AKI in intensive care units, accounting for approximately 50% of cases [29]. The mortality of AKI is reported to be much higher in septic, as compared with nonseptic, patients (73 vs 45%) [7]. The incidence of sepsis is increasing, in part due to the aging of the population worldwide. In the United States the annual mortality secondary to sepsis is an estimated 210,000, a number which equals or exceeds that due to heart attacks [3].

The management of the patient with sepsis and AKI necessitates an understanding of the multifactorial pathogenesis as discussed in this chapter.

References

1. Abdelrahman M, Sharples E, McDonald M, et al. (2004) Erythropoietin attenuates the tissue injury associated with hemorrhagic shock and myocardial ischemia. Shock 22(1): pp. 63–9.
2. Abraham E, Lattere F, Garg E, et al. (2005) Drotrecogin alfa (activated) for adults with severe sepsis and a low risk of death. N Engl J Med 353(13): pp. 1332–41.
3. Angus DC, Linde-Zwirble WT, Lidicker J, et al. (2001) Epidemiology of severe sepsis in the United States: analysis of incidence, outcome, and associated costs of care. Crit Care Med 29(7): pp. 1303–10.
4. Annane D, Sebille V, Charpentier C, et al. (2002) Effect of treatment with low doses of hydrocortisone and fludrocortisone on mortality in patients with septic shock. JAMA 288(7): pp. 862–71.
5. Benedict CR, Rose JA (1992) Arterial norepinephrine changes in patients with septic shock. Circ Shock 38(3): pp. 165–72.
6. Bernard GR, Vincent JL, Laterre PF, et al. (2001) Efficacy and safety of recombinant human activated protein C for severe sepsis. N Engl J Med 344(10): pp. 699–709.
7. Brivet FG, Kleinknecht DJ, Loirat P, et al. (1996) Acute kidney failure in intensive care units – causes, outcome, and prognostic factors of hospital mortality; a prospective, multicenter study. French Study Group on Acute Renal Failure. Crit Care Med 24(2): pp. 192–8.
8. Brunkhorst F, Engel C, Bloss F, et al. (2008) Intensive insulin therapy and pentastarch resuscitation in severe sepsis. N Engl J Med 358(2): pp. 125–139.
9. Court O, Kumar A, Parrillo JE (2002) Clinical review: Myocardial depression in sepsis and septic shock. Crit Care 6(6): pp. 500–8.
10. Cumming A, Driedger A, McDonald J, et al. (1988) Vasoactive hormones in the renal response to systemic sepsis. Am J Kidney Dis 11(1): pp. 23–32.
11. Dellinger R (2007) Update on clinical trials in severe sepsis. LIPOS antiendotoxin trial. in Society of Critical Care Medicine 36th Critical Care Congress, Orlando, FL.
12. Dong X, Swaminathan S, Bachman LA, et al. (2007) Resident dendritic cells are the predominant TNF-secreting cell in early renal ischemia-reperfusion injury. Kidney Int 71(7): pp. 619–28.
13. Dubois M-J, Orellan-Jimeniz C, Melot C, et al. (2006) Albumin administration improves organ function in critically ill hypoalbuminemic patients: A prospective, randomized, controlled, pilot study. Crit Care Med 34(10); pp. 2536–2540.
14. Finfer S, Bellomo F, Boyce N, et al. (2004) A comparison of albumin and saline for fluid resuscitation in the intensive care unit. N Engl J Med 350(22): pp. 2247–56.
15. Finney SJ, Zekveld C, Elia A, et al. (2003) Glucose control and mortality in critically ill patients. JAMA 290(15): pp. 2041–7.
16. Gattinoni L, Brazzi L, Pelosi P, et al. (1995) A trial of goal-oriented hemodynamic therapy in critically ill patients. SvO2 Collaborative Group. N Engl J Med 333(16): pp. 1025–32.
17. Grover R, Zaccarddelli D, Colice G, et al. (1999) An open-label dose escalation study of the nitric oxide synthase inhibitor, N(G)-methyl-L-arginine hydrochloride (546C88), in patients with septic shock. Glaxo Wellcome International Septic Shock Study Group. Crit Care Med 27(5): pp. 913–22.
18. Hayes MA, Timmins AC, Yau EHS, et al. (1994) Elevation of systemic oxygen delivery in the treatment of critically ill patients. N Engl J Med 330(24): pp. 1717–22.

19. Knotek M, Esson M, Gengaro P, et al. (2000) Desensitization of soluble guanylate cyclase in renal cortex during endotoxemia in mice. J Am Soc Nephrol 11(11): pp. 2133–7.
20. Kon V, Badr KF. (1991) Biological actions and pathophysiologic significance of endothelin in the kidney. Kidney Int 40(1): pp. 1–12.
21. Lacherade J, Jabre P, Bastuji-Garin S, et al. (2007) Failure to achieve glycemic control despite intensive insulin therapy in a medical ICU: incidence and influence on ICU mortality. Intensive Care Med 33(5): pp. 814–21.
22. Landry DW, Oliver JA (2001) The pathogenesis of vasodilatory shock. N Engl J Med 345(8): pp. 588–95.
23. Lin SM, Huang CD, Lin HC, et al. (2006) A modified goal-directed protocol improves clinical outcomes in intensive care unit patients with septic shock: A randomized controlled trial. Shock 26: pp. 551–557.
24. Mitra A, Bansal S, Wang W, et al. (2007) Erythropoietin ameliorates renal dysfunction during endotoxaemia. Nephrol Dial Transplant 22(8): pp. 2349–53.
25. Neveu H, Kleinknecht D, Brivet F, et al. (1996) Prognostic factors in acute kidney failure due to sepsis. Results of a prospective multicentre study. The French Study Group on Acute Renal Failure. Nephrol Dial Transplant 11(2): pp. 293–9.
26. Ortega R, Gines P, Uriz J, et al. (2002) Terlipressin therapy with and without albumin for patients with hepatorenal syndrome: results of a prospective, nonrandomized study. Hepatology 36(4 Pt 1): pp. 941–8.
27. Otero R, Nguyen B, Huang D, et al. (2006) Early goal-directed therapy in severe sepsis and septic shock revisited: concepts, controversies, and contemporary findings. Chest 130(5): pp. 1579–95.
28. Patel N, Sharples E, Cuzzocrea S, et al. (2004) Pretreatment with EPO reduces the injury and dysfunction caused by ischemia/reperfusion in the mouse kidney in vivo. Kidney Int 66(3): pp. 983–9.
29. Rangel-Frausto MS, Pittet D, Costigan M, et al. (1995) The natural history of the systemic inflammatory response syndrome (SIRS). A prospective study. JAMA 273(2): pp. 117–23.
30. Richard C, Warszawski J, Anguel N, et al. (2003) Early use of the pulmonary artery catheter and outcomes in patients with shock and acute respiratory distress syndrome: a randomized controlled trial. JAMA 290(20): pp. 2713–20.
31. Riedemann NC, Guo RF, Ward PA (2003) The enigma of sepsis. J Clin Invst 112(4): pp. 460–7.
32. Rivers E, Nguyen B, Havstad S, et al. (2001) Early goal-directed therapy in the treatment of severe sepsis and septic shock. N Engl J Med 345(19): pp. 1368–77.
33. Russell JA (2007) Hemodynamic support of sepsis. Vasopressin versus norepinephrine for septic shock. in Society of Critical Care Medicine 36th Critical Care Congress Orlando, Florida.
34. Russell JA (2007) Vasopressin in septic shock. Crit Care Med 35(9 Suppl): pp. S609–15.
35. Sanz E, Lopez N, Linares M, et al. (1990) Intravascular and interstitial fluid dynamics in rats treated with minoxidil. J Cardiovasc Pharmacol 15(3): pp. 485–92.
36. Schrier RW, Abraham E (1995) Aggressive volume expansion and pseudo-ARDS. Hosp Pract (Minneap) 30(6): pp.19, 23.
37. Schrier RW, Wang W (2004) Acute kidney failure and sepsis. N Engl J Med 351(2): pp. 159–69.
38. Schwartz D, Mendonca M, Schwartz I, et al. (1997) Inhibition of constitutive nitric oxide synthase (NOS) by nitric oxide generated by inducible NOS after lipopolysaccharide administration provokes renal dysfunction in rats. J Clin Invest 100(2): pp. 439–48.
39. Sort P, Navasa M, Arroya V, et al. (1999) Effect of intravenous albumin on renal impairment and mortality in patients with cirrhosis and spontaneous bacterial peritonitis. N Engl J Med 341(6): pp. 403–9.
40. Sprung C, Annane D, Keh D, et al. (2008) Hydrocortisone therapy for patients with septic shock. N Engl J Med 358(2): pp. 111–24.
41. Thiemermann C, Szalbo C, Mitchell J, et al. (1993) Vascular hyporeactivity to vasoconstrictor agents and hemodynamic decompensation in hemorrhagic shock is mediated by nitric oxide. Proc Natl Acad Sci USA 90(1): pp. 267–71.
42. Wang W, Falk S, Jittikanont S, et al. (2002) Protective effect of renal denervation on normotensive endotoxemia-induced acute kidney failure in mice. Am J Physiol Renal Physiol 283(3): pp. F583–7.
43. Wang W, Jittikanont S, Falk S, et al. (2003) Interaction among nitric oxide, reactive oxygen species, and antioxidants during endotoxemia-related acute renal failure. Am J Physiol Renal Physiol, 284(3): pp. F532–7.
44. Wang W, Poole B, Mitra A, et al. (2004) Endothelial nitric oxide synthase-deficient mice exhibit increased susceptibility to endotoxin-induced acute renal failure. Am J Physiol Renal Physiol. 287(5): pp. F1044–8.
45. Wang W, Zolty E, Falk S, et al. (2006) Pentoxifylline protects against endotoxin-induced acute kidney failure in mice. Am J Physiol Renal Physiol 291(5): pp. F1090–5.
46. Wang W, Zolty E, Falk S, et al. (2007) Prostacyclin in endotoxemia-induced acute kidney injury: cyclooxygenase inhibition and renal prostacyclin synthase transgenic mice. Am J Physiol Renal Physiol 293(4): pp. F1131–6.
47. Van den Berghe G, Wilmer A, Hermans G, et al. (2006) Intensive insulin therapy in the medical ICU. N Engl J Med 354(5): pp. 449–61.
48. Van den Berghe G, Wouters P, Weekers F, et al. (2001) Intensive insulin therapy in the critically ill patients. N Engl J Med 345(19): pp. 1359–67.
49. Vanhorebeek I, De Vos R, Mesotten D, et al. (2005) Protection of hepatocyte mitochondrial ultrastructure and function by strict blood glucose control with insulin in critically ill patients. Lancet 365(9453): pp. 53–9.
50. Ventilation with lower tidal volumes as compared with traditional tidal volumes for acute lung injury and the acute respiratory distress syndrome. The Acute Respiratory Distress Syndrome Network (2000) N Engl J Med 342(18): pp. 1301–8.
51. Wheeler A, Bernard G, Thompson B, et al. (2006) Pulmonary-artery versus central venous catheter to guide treatment of acute lung injury. N Engl J Med 354(21): pp. 2213–24.
52. Wiedemann H, Wheeler A, Bernard G, et al. (2006) Comparison of two fluid-management strategies in acute lung injury. N Engl J Med 354(24): pp. 2564–75.
53. Zabel P, Schade FU, Schlaak M (1993) Inhibition of endogenous TNF formation by pentoxifylline. Immunobiology 187(3–5): pp. 447–63.

Kidney in Acute Heart Failure and Cardiogenic Shock

6.2

Vijay Karajala and John A. Kellum

Core Messages

- There is increasing awareness of the complex interplay between the kidney and the heart. Acute kidney injury (AKI) is common in acute heart failure and cardiogenic shock states, and worsening renal failure is associated with increased morbidity and mortality.
- The most important goal in the management of cardiogenic shock is a rapid restoration of cardiopulmonary stability and assessment of the underlying disease process.
- When pharmacologic therapy fails to produce adequate organ perfusion, mechanical circulatory support such as intra-aortic balloon counter-pulsation or ventricular assistance devices need to be considered to serve as a bridge to revascularization or other cardiac surgical interventions.
- Continuous renal replacement therapy is thought to be the best way to support patients with advanced AKI and cardiogenic shock.

6.2.1 Introduction

Acute kidney injury (AKI) is an independent predictor of mortality in the intensive care unit [1, 2]. Unfortunately, AKI often develops as a component of multiple organ system dysfunction in critically ill patients and may lead to mortality rates in excess of 60%, depending on the setting [2, 3]. The exact pathophysiologic mechanisms responsible for AKI in cardiogenic shock and in acute heart failure syndrome (AHFS) are still not well understood, and there is extensive ongoing research on these complex interorgan interactions [3, 4]. AKI arising in these settings may occur either secondary to hypoperfusion itself, as a part of systemic inflammatory response or due to other neurohormonal responses. Renal deterioration in these states can further aggravate and perpetuate not only the cardiac damage (increased fatal arrhythmias, etc.) but other organs as well. Thus, it is imperative that renal function is promptly restored.

6.2.2 Brief Review of Renal Neurohormonal Regulation

Apart from excreting metabolic end products, kidneys closely regulate fluid and electrolyte homeostasis via complex neurohormonal mechanisms. This function of the kidney is closely associated with the vascular supply of the kidney. Two mutually dependent, but opposing neurohormonal systems maintain blood pressure, intravascular volume, and salt and water homeostasis. The sympathoadrenal axis, the renin-angiotensin-aldosterone axis system (RAAS) and arginine-vasopressin (AVP) defend against hypotension and hypovolemia by promoting vasoconstriction, and salt and water retention. The prostaglandins, bradykinins, and atrial natriuretic peptide defend against hypertension and hypervolemia by promoting vasodilation, salt, and water excretion.

Although the kidneys receive about 20% of the cardiac output, blood flow distribution within the kidney is very heterogeneous. The cortex receives more than 85%

J. A. Kellum (✉)
Department of Critical Care Medicine, University of Pittsburgh, 608 Scaife Hall, 3550 Terrace Street, Pittsburgh, PA 15261, USA
e-mail: kellumja@ccm.upmc.edu

A. Jörres et al. (eds.), *Management of Acute Kidney Problems*,
DOI: 10.1007/978-3-540-69441-0_6.2, © Springer-Verlag Berlin Heidelberg 2010

of the blood flow, even though the medulla is highly active metabolically. Tissue partial pressure of oxygen (pO_2) is approximately 50–100 mm Hg in the cortex, whereas it can be as low as 10–15 mm Hg in the medullary thick ascending limb. This progressive fall in tissue pO_2 from the cortex to the medulla is secondary to countercurrent oxygen exchange. Energy is required for the various active transport mechanisms, especially in the metabolically active thick ascending limb of the loop of Henle. Therefore, the medulla is thought to be more prone to ischemic injury. During periods of ischemia, sympathoadrenal activation redistributes blood preferentially to the medulla to attenuate medullary ischemia.

Under normal circumstances, renal blood flow and glomerular filtration rate (GFR) are maintained by autoregulation (i.e., at a constant rate over a wide range of renal perfusion pressures) [5]. The afferent arterioles dilate and the efferent arterioles constrict in response to a decrease in perfusion pressure to maintain the transglomerular pressure. Only when the mean arterial pressure drops below about 70 mm Hg does the transglomerular pressure and GFR decrease as well. It is thought that afferent arterioles contain myogenic stretch receptors that cause vasoconstriction in response to stretch secondary to an increase in perfusion pressure. However, the exact mechanism of renal autoregulation is not completely understood.

Tubuloglomerular feedback (TGF) is a negative feedback loop that induces preglomerular arteriolar constriction in response to increased solute delivery to the distal nephron, thereby reducing GFR and solute resorptive demands. Adenosine, which is a systemic vasodilator, acts as a vasoconstrictor in the kidney, and is thought to mediate TGF. These mechanisms that redistribute blood flow from cortex to medulla are also important in maintaining oxygen balance by decreasing oxygen utilization. However, there is a limit to the extent autoregulation can preserve renal medullary oxygen balance.

6.2.3 Clinical Aspects in the Management of AHFS and Cardiogenic Shock

AHFS is a complex clinical syndrome and is characterized by abnormal hemodynamics, including increase in pulmonary capillary wedge pressure and peripheral vasoconstriction, and is associated with severe morbidity and mortality. Analysis of the ADHERE database has shown that renal dysfunction is an independent risk factor for in-hospital mortality regardless of the extent of left ventricular function [6]. There is growing evidence that early restoration of renal dysfunction is associated with significant improvement in outcomes [7–9].

Standard medical therapy for heart failure such as diuretics, beta blockers, angiotensin-converting enzyme inhibitors (ACE-Is), or angiotensin receptor blockers should be started or maximized in patients in the setting of AHFS when they present with pulmonary congestion but with adequate systemic perfusion pressures [10]. Although beneficial effect of ACE-Is and digoxin in chronic heart failure is well established, evidence is lacking regarding the use of these drugs in acute situations, and caution is advised. Renal functions should be carefully monitored and dosage should be adjusted when these drugs are used.

The Heart Failure Society of America has approved the use of intravenous nitroglycerin, nitroprusside, and nesiritide along with diuretics to attain hemodynamic and symptomatic improvement. The exact effect of nitroglycerin on kidney is not completely known, and the role of B-type natriuretic peptide (nesiritide) in AHFS management remains controversial. Nesiritide may have a role in moderate to severe heart failure in the absence of hypotension. However, large prospective randomized clinical trials are needed to further clarify safety of this agent and what place in AHFS management it will occupy. Two studies have questioned the safety of the drug. The first meta-analysis showed increased risk of worsening renal failure at any time after exposure to the drug. A second analysis showed increased mortality at day 30 after treatment with nesiritide [11, 12]. Subsequent analysis of pooled data showed that the risk of in-hospital mortality was similar for nesiritide and nitroglycerin. Studies show that infusions for longer than 24 h were associated with worsening renal failure [13]. In a study that analyzed the ADHERE database [14], mortality rates with nitroglycerin, nesiritide, and diuretics were all similar. The use of nesiritide with diuretics was associated with greater worsening of AKI compared with diuretics plus nitroglycerin. This study also noted higher mortality rates with inotrope use. The ASCEND-HF study is currently underway to further clarify the utility of nesiritide in AHFS.

Similar to that for AHFS, the etiology of cardiogenic shock is multifactorial (Table 6.2.1). Cardiogenic shock is predominantly seen in the setting of large

Table 6.2.1 Causes of cardiogenic shock

Systolic dysfunction
Diastolic dysfunction
Valvular dysfunction
Cardiac arrhythmias
Coronary artery disease / myocardial infarction
Mechanical complications:
– Ventricular septal defect
– Acute valve dysfunction
– Free wall rupture
– Pericardial tamponade
Others:
– Sepsis (rare in adults)
– Prolonged cardiopulmonary bypass

myocardial infarction. Studies have shown that patients requiring emergency coronary arterial bypass graft surgery (CABG) as a life-saving strategy in the setting of ischemic cardiogenic shock have an in-hospital mortality as high as 20%, and also a high incidence of stroke (8%), renal failure requiring dialysis (8.3%), and bleeding (63.3%) [15]. Cardiogenic shock in patients with chronic renal disease is associated with an increased risk of recurrent hospitalization, subsequent CABG, and mortality. This increased risk of death is independent [2] and additive to the risk associated with diabetes [16].

Management of patients with cardiogenic shock can be challenging because of the limited effectiveness of pharmacologic therapy and the severity of illness in the setting of systemic organ hypoperfusion. The most important goal in the management of cardiogenic shock is a rapid restoration of cardiopulmonary stability and assessment of the underlying disease process. Intravascular volume guided by invasive monitoring is an important tool and remains critical to achieve therapeutic goals in tissue oxygenation and organ function. It is very important to rapidly determine the etiology of cardiogenic shock, and echocardiography is perhaps the most useful tool, particularly if a mechanical cause is suspected.

Inotropic support remains the main therapy for depressed myocardial function, and correction of the underlying cause such as ischemia will improve outcomes and result in less kidney injury. It is important to remember that when pharmacologic therapy fails to produce adequate organ perfusion to maintain renal function, then multiple organ failure will rapidly ensue [17]. In this clinical situation, mechanical circulatory support such as intra-aortic balloon counter-pulsation (IABP) or even ventricular assistance devices need to be considered to serve as a bridge to percutaneous or surgical revascularization or other cardiac surgical interventions.

6.2.4 Mechanical Circulatory Support in Cardiogenic Shock and its Effects on Renal Function

IABP is indicated for medically refractory cardiogenic shock during acute myocardial infarction or after cardiac surgery and for refractory angina, or malignant arrhythmias [18–20]. The physiologic effects of IABP include increasing coronary perfusion pressure by increasing diastolic pressure and increasing cardiac output primarily by a reduction in left ventricular afterload that occurs after balloon deflation just before systole. The net effect is to greatly improve the balance between myocardial oxygen supply and demand while creating a modest improvement in systemic perfusion and blood pressure [21, 22]

Main indications for a ventricular assist device (VAD) include stabilization of patients in postcardiotomy shock, bridging patients with refractory heart failure to heart transplant, and, to a limited extent in myocardial infarction with cardiogenic shock [23, 24]. The development and progression of renal dysfunction helps to identify patients with an acutely deteriorating condition that would benefit most from stabilization with early institution of mechanical circulatory support. Use of VADs has been shown to lead to resolution of severe renal dysfunction in most cardiogenic shock patients with long-term outcomes comparable to those for patients without renal dysfunction [25]. The improvements in renal function are likely explained by not only improved cardiac function but also subsequent correction of abnormal neurohormonal imbalance found in cardiogenic shock [26].

Extracorporeal membrane oxygenation (ECMO) constitutes the last option for circulatory and/or pulmonary support for refractory postoperative cardiopulmonary failure. A venoarterial ECMO-based approach can be used for temporary, complete circulatory support while awaiting myocardial recovery, or determining suitability for heart transplantation. Mortality rates are comparable to those for other cardiac assist devices, with approximately 30% of patients able to be discharged form the hospital [27].

6.2.5 Role of Continuous Renal Replacement Therapy in Cardiogenic Shock

Currently, continuous renal replacement therapy (CRRT) is the best way to support patients with advanced AKI and cardiogenic shock. CRRT allows for control of circulating plasma volume, electrolyte, and acid–base balance and has far less hemodynamic impact compared with hemodialysis. In recent years, other forms of extracorporeal fluid removal have been developed (e.g., aquapheresis), but existing data provide no evidence of advantage relative to CRRT and the absence of solute clearance is a significant disadvantage.

6.2.6 Take Home Pearls

- Renal impairment confers a clinically significant risk for excess mortality in patients with AHFS or cardiogenic shock, and the magnitude of increased mortality is comparable to that associated with traditional prognostic indicators in AHFS, such as ejection fraction.
- Worsening renal function leads to fluid retention and further cardiac decompensation.
- The role of pharmacologic therapy is controversial. Inotropes are useful acutely, whereas diuretics and natriuretics can be effective for treating volume overload but can worsen shock.
- Fluid can also be removed with extracorporeal therapy, and CRRT may be the best way to support patients with advanced AKI and cardiogenic shock.

References

1. Hoste, E.A. and J.A. Kellum, *Acute kidney injury: epidemiology and diagnostic criteria*. Curr Opin Crit Care, 2006;12(6): 531–7.
2. Uchino, S., et al., *Acute renal failure in critically ill patients: a multinational, multicenter study*. JAMA, 2005;294(7): 813–8.
3. Elapavaluru, S. and J.A. Kellum, *Why do patients die of acute kidney injury?* Acta Clin Belg Suppl, 2007;(2):326–31.
4. Kelly, K.J., *Distant effects of experimental renal ischemia/reperfusion injury*. J Am Soc Nephrol, 2003;14(6):1549–58.
5. Loutzenhiser, R., et al., *Renal autoregulation: new perspectives regarding the protective and regulatory roles of the underlying mechanisms*. Am J Physiol Regul Integr Comp Physiol, 2006;290(5): R1153–67.
6. Yancy, C.W., et al., *Clinical presentation, management, and in-hospital outcomes of patients admitted with acute decompensated heart failure with preserved systolic function: a report from the Acute Decompensated Heart Failure National Registry (ADHERE) Database*. J Am Coll Cardiol, 2006;47(1):76–84.
7. Smith, G.L., et al., *Renal impairment and outcomes in heart failure: systematic review and meta-analysis*. J Am Coll Cardiol, 2006;47(10):1987–96.
8. Metra, M., et al., *Worsening renal function in patients hospitalised for acute heart failure: Clinical implications and prognostic significance*. Eur J Heart Fail, 2008;10(2):188–95.
9. Dries, D.L., et al., *The prognostic implications of renal insufficiency in asymptomatic and symptomatic patients with left ventricular systolic dysfunction*. J Am Coll Cardiol, 2000; 35(3):681–9.
10. Feldman, D., et al., *Management Strategies for Stage-D Patients with Acute Heart Failure*. Clin Cardiol, 2008 July; 31(7): 297–301.
11. Sackner-Bernstein, J.D., et al., *Short-term risk of death after treatment with nesiritide for decompensated heart failure: a pooled analysis of randomized controlled trials*. JAMA, 2005;293(15):1900–5.
12. Sackner-Bernstein, J.D., H.A. Skopicki, and K.D. Aaronson, *Risk of worsening renal function with nesiritide in patients with acutely decompensated heart failure*. Circulation, 2005; 111(12):1487–91.
13. Chow, S.L., et al., *Effect of nesiritide infusion duration on renal function in acutely decompensated heart failure patients*. Ann Pharmacother, 2007;41(4):556–61.
14. Costanzo, M.R., et al., *The safety of intravenous diuretics alone versus diuretics plus parenteral vasoactive therapies in hospitalized patients with acutely decompensated heart failure: a propensity score and instrumental variable analysis using the Acutely Decompensated Heart Failure National Registry (ADHERE) database*. Am Heart J, 2007;154(2): 267–77.
15. Moscucci, M., et al., *Reducing costs and improving outcomes of percutaneous coronary interventions*. Am J Manag Care, 2003;9(5):365–72.
16. Szczech, L.A., et al., *Outcomes of patients with chronic renal insufficiency in the bypass angioplasty revascularization investigation*. Circulation, 2002;105(19):2253–8.
17. Goldberg, R.J., et al., *Recent magnitude of and temporal trends (1994–1997) in the incidence and hospital death rates of cardiogenic shock complicating acute myocardial infarction: the second national registry of myocardial infarction*. Am Heart J, 2001;141(1):65–72.
18. Papaioannou, T.G. and C. Stefanadis, *Basic principles of the intraaortic balloon pump and mechanisms affecting its performance*. Asaio J, 2005;51(3):296–300.
19. Torchiana, D.F., et al., *Intraaortic balloon pumping for cardiac support: trends in practice and outcome, 1968 to 1995*. J Thorac Cardiovasc Surg, 1997;113(4):758–64; discussion 764–9.

20. Cowell, R.P., V.E. Paul, and C.D. Ilsley, *The use of intra-aortic balloon counterpulsation in malignant ventricular arrhythmias*. Int J Cardiol, 1993;39(3):219–21.
21. Taguchi, I., et al., *Comparison of hemodynamic effects of enhanced external counterpulsation and intra-aortic balloon pumping in patients with acute myocardial infarction*. Am J Cardiol, 2000;86(10):1139–41, A9.
22. Dekker, A., et al., *Efficacy of a new intraaortic propeller pump vs the intraaortic balloon pump: an animal study*. Chest, 2003;123(6):2089–95.
23. Castells, E., et al., *Acute myocardial infarction with cardiogenic shock: treatment with mechanical circulatory assistance and heart transplantation*. Transplant Proc, 2003; 35(5):1940–1.
24. Chen, J.M., et al., *Improved survival rates support left ventricular assist device implantation early after myocardial infarction*. J Am Coll Cardiol, 1999;33(7):1903–8.
25. Khot, U.N., et al., *Severe renal dysfunction complicating cardiogenic shock is not a contraindication to mechanical support as a bridge to cardiac transplantation*. J Am Coll Cardiol, 2003;41(3):381–5.
26. James, K.B., et al., *Plasma volume and its regulatory factors in congestive heart failure after implantation of long-term left ventricular assist devices*. Circulation, 1996;93(8): 1515–9.
27. Doll, N., et al., *Temporary extracorporeal membrane oxygenation in patients with refractory postoperative cardiogenic shock--a single center experience*. J Card Surg, 2003;18(6):512–8.

6.3 Acute Kidney Problems in Congestive Heart Failure

Andrew Davenport

Core Messages

- In cardiac failure, arterial underfilling leads to neurohumeral activation and renal sodium and water retention, thus increasing both the preload and afterload, potentially setting up a vicious cycle leading to a cardiorenal syndrome.
- During acute decompensated heart failure, a deterioration in renal function is associated with a markedly increased risk of patient mortality.

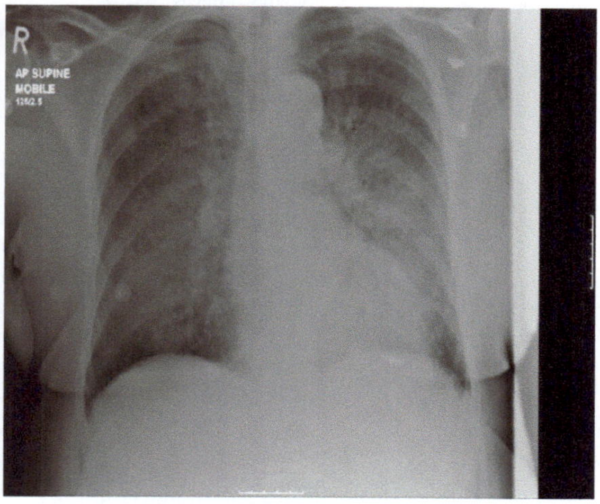

Fig. 6.3.1 Chest X-ray showing left ventricular failure, with upper lobe blood diversion, Kerley B lines, and alveolar air space shadowing

6.3.1 Introduction

Heart failure is the only cardiovascular disease in the United States with an increasing prevalence, currently around 5 million, with an annual incidence of 400,000 new cases/year, and carries a high mortality of around 250,000/year. Typically patients with congestive cardiac failure present with a history of fatigue, increasing dyspnea on exertion, orthopnea, and paroxysmal dyspnea, and on clinical examination are found to have peripheral edema, tachypnea with inspiratory crackles on chest auscultation (Fig. 6.3.1), an elevated jugular venous pulse, tachycardia, arrhythmias, S3 or S4 gallop, cool extremities, and/or diffuse apical impulse. In terms of making a clinical diagnosis of heart failure, then, dyspnea on exercise is the most sensitive symptom, whereas orthopnea and paroxysmal nocturnal dyspnea the most specific, and an elevated jugular venous pressure is the most specific physical finding.

The commonest cause of heart failure is due to ischemic heart disease, often associated with primary risk factors, including family history of ischemic heart disease, smoking, hypertension, hypercholesterolemia, hyperhomocysteinemia, and diabetes mellitus.

However, other conditions can potentially mimic some of the symptoms and signs of heart failure, including major pulmonary emboli, severe anemia, nutritional deficiencies such as beriberi, endocrine disorders including thyrotoxicosis, pheochromocytoma and carcinoid tumors, chronic liver disease with

A. Davenport
Royal Free Hospital, Pond Street, London NW3 2QG, UK
e-mail: andrew.davenport@royalfree.nhs.uk

A. Jörres et al. (eds.), *Management of Acute Kidney Problems*,
DOI: 10.1007/978-3-540-69441-0_6.3, © Springer-Verlag Berlin Heidelberg 2010

Table 6.3.1 Causes of renal dysfunction in patients with cardiac disease

Cause	Disease condition	Cardiac dysfunction	Renal dysfunction
Genetic			
	Fabry's disease	Valvular heart disease	CKD
		IHD	
	Sickle cell disease	Cardiomyopathy	Papillary necrosis
		Iron overload	FSGS/CKD
	PCKD	Valvular heart disease	CKD
Acquired			
Metabolic	Diabetes	IHD	CKD
	Hypothyroid	Pericardial effusion	↑Serum creatinine
	Thyrotoxicosis	Cardiomyopathy	
	Amyloid	Cardiomyopathy	Nephrotic syndrome
Infection	Trypanosomiasis	Cardiomyopathy	Glomerulonephritis
	Malaria		Nephrotic syndrome
			AKI
	Tuberculosis	Pericarditis	TIN
			Obstruction
	Staph/Strep	Endocarditis	Glomerulonephritis
	mycoplasma		
	Syphilis	Endocarditis	Glomerulonephritis
	Coxsackie	Cardiomyopathy	TIN
	HIV	Cardiomyopathy	FSGS
Autoimmune	SLE	Endocarditis	Lupus nephritis
		CAD	
	Wegener's	Endocarditis	Renal vasculitis
	Polyarteritis	CAD	Renal vasculitis
	Anticardiolipin	CAD	Renal infarction
	Scleroderma	Hypertension	HUS
	Sarcoid	Cardiomyopathy	TIN
Macrovascular	Atheroma	CAD	RAS
			Cholesterol emboli
	Thrombus	Atrial thrombus	Renal emboli
Microvascular	Post partum	Cardiomyopathy	HUS
Drugs	Cocaine	Coronary artery spasm	Rhabdomyolysis
	Alcohol	Cardiomyopathy	IgA nephropathy
Malignancy	Atrial myxoma	Cardiac obstruction	Renal emboli

CAD coronary artery disease, *CKD* chronic kidney disease, *FSGS* focal segmental glomerulonephritis, *HUS* hemolytic uremic syndrome, *IHD* ischemic heart disease, *PCKD* polycystic kidney disease, *RAS* renal artery stenosis, *TIN* tubulointerstitial nephritis

ascites, nephrotic syndrome, flash pulmonary edema secondary to renovascular disease, neurogenic pulmonary edema, and marked gastrointestinal associated malabsorption and/or hypoalbuminemia (Table 6.3.1). Unfortunately, in the younger patient, both cocaine and ecstasy self-administration can cause severe sympathetic nervous system overactivation, leading to a combination of acute cardiac ischemia, pulmonary edema, and acute kidney injury (AKI), which may be exacerbated by skeletal muscle ischemic damage.

6.3.2 Congestive Heart Failure

The fall in cardiac output in patients with heart failure leads to arterial underfilling, which is sensed by high pressure baroreceptors in the left ventricle, carotid sinus, and aortic arch, and then leads to compensatory neurohumeral activation of the cardioregulatory centers in the brain [2]. This increased sympathetic nervous system activity stimulates renin release, so activating the renin-angiotensin-aldosterone system. Simultaneously vasopressin is released due to sympathetic nervous system stimulation of the supraoptic and paraventricular nuclei in the hypothalamus. In addition, sympathetic activation also causes peripheral vasoconstriction, and in particular renal vasoconstriction. It is now realized that congestive cardiac failure causes an inflammatory state, with increased cytokine and production, and other inflammatory mediators [18]. The combination of these effects is to reduce renal glomerular filtration, with reduced renal tubular filtrate flow, leading to increased filtrate sodium reabsorption, and reduced urinary sodium losses, further lowered by increased aldosterone secretion. In addition vasopressin impairs renal water excretion and promotes hypotonic hyponatremia. In rats with uncompensated heart failure, aquaporin-2 water channels increase in the distal collecting duct principal cells as a consequence of increased plasma vasopressin. Hyponatremia is common in patients with severe congestive cardiac failure (New York Heart Association classes 3 and 4). In such patients, serum sodium lower than 130 mmol/l (130 mEq/l) is associated with a shortened life expectancy, unless cardiac function improves.

6.3.3 Cardiorenal Syndrome

Acute decompensated heart failure [9] is defined as new or worsening symptoms or signs of dyspnea, fatigue, or edema that lead to hospital admission or unscheduled medical care and are consistent with an underlying worsening of left ventricular function. During hospital admission with acute decompensated heart failure, then, a deterioration in renal function, as assessed by a rise in the serum creatinine, is associated with a marked increase risk in patient mortality [10].

As many of the treatments used to treat heart failure, such as diuretics, can lead to an increase in serum creatinine, then almost a third of patients admitted with acute decompensated heart failure have a rise in serum creatinine > 0.3 mg/dl (27 µmol/l) during their hospital admission [10]. As AKI commonly occurs in this group of patients and is associated with increased mortality, the term cardiorenal syndrome has been proposed [23]. Unlike hepatorenal syndrome, where there is a consensus definition, there is as yet no agreed definition for the cardiorenal syndrome. However, many cardiologists accept the presence of renal dysfunction, defined as a glomerular filtration rate (GFR) of < 60 ml/min/1.73 m^2 in patients with heart failure or an increase in serum creatinine of 0.3 mg/dl (27 µmol/l) during treatment of acute decompensated heart failure [23], (Table 6.3.2).

Table 6.3.2 Risk factors for cardiorenal syndrome

Hemodynamic factors	Renal factors	Drugs
Low cardiac output	Diabetes	NSAIDs
Vasodilatation	Hypertension	ACEIs/ARBs
High vascular resistance	Renovascular disease	Diuretics
Hypovolemia		Cyclosporin A
Ascites		Calcium channel blockers
Increased renal verses pressure		

ACEIs angiotensin-converting enzyme inhibitors (), *ARBs* angiotensin receptor blockers (), *NSAIDs* nonsteroidal antiinflammatories ()

6.3.4 Deterioration in Renal Function During Management of Acute Decompensated Heart Failure

The prevalence of chronic kidney disease in heart failure trials is around 50%, with some 20% of patients having a high serum creatinine, and 80% an estimated GFR < 60 ml/min (chronic kidney disease stage 3 or greater) [10, 22]. The average North American heart failure patient with chronic kidney disease is a 66-year-old diabetic male, with underlying ischemic heart disease, a reduced left ventricular ejection fraction of 26%, and a raised brain natriuretic peptide (BNP), plasma renin activity, aldosterone, and C-reactive protein (CRP) [1].

Standard treatment with loop diuretics may lead to a further deterioration in renal function, as any additional reduction in effective circulating volume will exacerbate arterial underfilling, thus further increasing the compensatory neurohumeral response (Fig. 6.3.2). So although diuretics increase urine output, they may significantly decrease the GFR [8].

This may then lead to so-called diuretic resistance, as additional loop diuretics then fail to establish a diuresis. Loop diuretic resistance may be overcome by the addition of amiloride, a distal renal tubular epithelial sodium channel blocker, but the use of this agent may be contraindicated due to concomitant hyperkalemia, due to previous diuretic therapy with spironolactone or eplerenone [14]. In cases of hyperkalemia, then thiazide

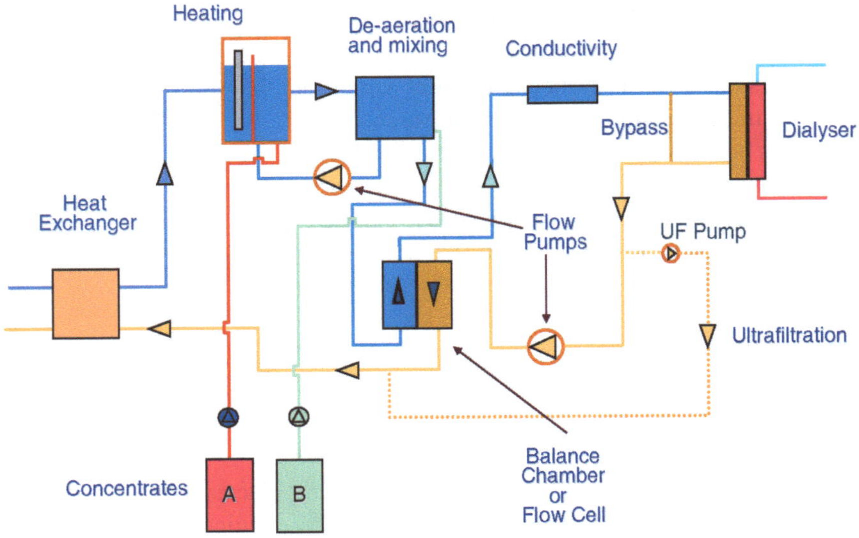

Fig. 6.3.2 The "iatrogenic" cardiorenal syndrome of heart failure

diuretics such as metolazone may have an additional effect in combination with loop diuretics. Thus diuretics should be used cautiously to prevent sudden reductions in the effective arterial volume, which will result in abrupt deterioration in renal function.

Any rise in serum creatinine has to be distinguished from the rise in creatinine that accompanies the introduction of angiotensin-converting enzyme inhibitors/angiotensin receptor blockers and other antihypertensives, as a fall in systemic pressure may lead to a corresponding fall in glomerular filtration pressure, and so a reduction in glomerular filtration [21] (Table 6.3.3). Patients with preexisting hypertension are more likely to have impaired renal autoregulation (Fig. 6.3.3), and are therefore more susceptible to changes in renal perfusion pressure. This response to a lowering of blood pressure can be further exacerbated by underlying renovascular disease, which has been reported to increase with age in patients with coronary artery disease, from < 5% in those aged < 64 years to 42% in those aged > 72 years [15]. Thus angiotensin-converting enzyme inhibitors/angiotensin receptor blockers and β-blockers have to be introduced cautiously to minimize any reduction in systemic blood pressure, so as to prevent an acute deterioration in renal function (Table 6.3.4).

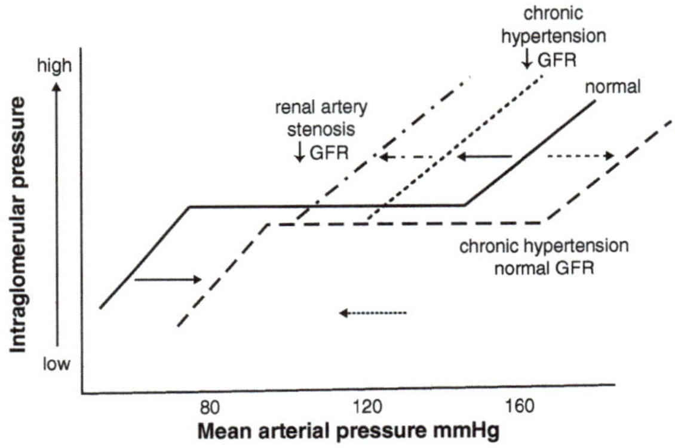

Fig. 6.3.3 Schematic diagram of the changes which occur in intraglomerular pressure over a range of mean arterial blood pressures, depicting the normal autoregulation curve, which is moved to the right by essential hypertension, and then the upper portion moved to the left in patients with intrinsic renal disease, and those with macrovascular renal artery stenosis

Table 6.3.3 Risk factors for acute kidney injury by angiotensin-converting enzyme inhibitors and angiotensin receptor blockers

Renal artery stenosis
Polycystic kidney disease
Decreased absolute and/or effective arterial blood volume
Sepsis
Intra-abdominal compartment syndrome
Nonsteroidal antiinflammatory drugs
Calcineurin inhibitors (cyclosporin A, tacrolimus)

When the intravascular volume increases, this leads to atrial dilatation and release of natriuretic peptides, which cause the kidney to increase sodium losses. Natriuretic peptides therefore increase in cases of congestive cardiac failure, and BNP levels have been advocated as a diagnostic test for heart failure. Although a BNP of > 100 pg/ml was reported as having greater diagnostic accuracy for cardiac failure compared with clinical examination, BNP values are affected by age, female sex, obesity, and renal function [20, 21]. Similarly, cutoff values for terminal pre-BNP

Table 6.3.4 Evidence for improving clinical outcomes with heart failure medications

Drug	GFR < 30 ml/min	GFR > 30 < 60 ml/min	GFR > 60 ml/min
ACEI or ARB*	Possible	Definite	Definite
β-Blocker	Unknown	Definite	Definite
Spironolactone	Unknown	Possible	Definite
Digoxin	Unknown	Possible	Definite
Hydralazine/nitrates	Unknown	Possible	Definite

ACEIs angiotensin-converting enzyme inhibitors, *ARBs* angiotensin receptor blockers, *GFR* glomerular filtration rate
*Only when ACEIs not tolerated

of 450 pg/ml and 900 pg/ml have been suggested for patients aged < 50 and > 50 years, respectively [12]. As natriuretic peptides are part of the compensatory response to congestive cardiac failure, recombinant natriuretic peptides such as nesiritide have been used in the management of acute decompensated heart failure. Unfortunately, several of the trials currently reported have shown that nesiritide when combined with diuretics can also result in an acute deterioration in renal function, which is dose dependent [11].

Adenosine levels increase in congestive cardiac failure and are associated with a reduced renal blood flow in heart failure. Adenosine-1 receptor blockers could potentially improve renal function by regulating renal tubuloglomerular feedback, and by blocking proximal tubular receptors, increase sodium excretion, and by blocking distal tubular receptors, cause a potassium neutral natriuresis. Early trials suggested that adenosine antagonists [8] preserved renal function but allowed a diuresis.

Vasopressin is increased in heart failure, and activation of vasopressin 1a receptors (V1aR) leads to vasoconstriction with increased afterload, and thus exacerbates arterial underfilling, whereas activation of vasopressin 2 receptors (V2R) causes increased renal distal tubular and collecting duct water retention, with hyponatremia and increased preload. Vasopressin receptor blockers are now available. Preliminary trials with tolvaptan and lixivaptan, predominantly V2R blockers, showed an improvement in hyponatremia, with a modest weight loss, but without any deterioration in renal function [6]. Potentially, the increase in serum sodium could increase endogenous vasopressin secretion by increasing plasma osmolality, and this could cause activation of the V1aRs. Therefore there may be advantages to using a combined V1aR and V2R blocker, such as conivaptan. Early results were encouraging, and longer term studies are currently underway [7].

Whereas diuretic therapy may potentially exacerbate the neurohumeral response, removing excess sodium and water by ultrafiltration may be beneficial, by returning patients to the top of their Starling curve, maximizing cardiac output, with a reduction in both sympathetic nervous system activity and the renin-angiotensin system [3].

6.3.5 Risk of Rhabdomyolysis with Statins

Many patients with coronary artery disease are prescribed 3-hydroxy 3-methyl glutaryl coenzyme A inhibitors (statins). The metabolism of the statins varies, with some predominantly metabolized via cytochrome P (CYP) 450 3A4, such as lovastatin and atorvastatin, whereas simvastatin, is also metabolized via CYP 2C8, and fluvastatin by CYP 2CP9. Pravastatin and rosuvastatin are excreted mainly unchanged. The risk of rhabdomyolysis is increased in the older diabetic patient, and also by polymorphisms of CYP 2D6. However, drugs which compete with the hepatic CYP enzyme system, particularly inhibitors of CYP 3A4, or those which delay statin excretion can markedly increase the risk of rhabdomyolysis and AKI (Table 6.3.5).

Table 6.3.5 Risk factors for acute kidney injury due to rhabdomyolysis in patients prescribed 3-hydroxy 3-methyl glutaryl coenzyme A inhibitors

Fibrates – gemfibrozil
Ezetimibe
Diltiazem, verapamil
Amiodarone
Colchicine
Itraconazole, ketoconazole, fluconazole
Protease inhibitors: atazanavir, lopinavir, nelfinavir, ritonavir
Quinine
Fucidic acid
Danazol
Nefazodone
Hypothyroidism
Glycogen storage diseases – McArdle's, acid maltase deficiency
Grape fruit & pomegranate juice

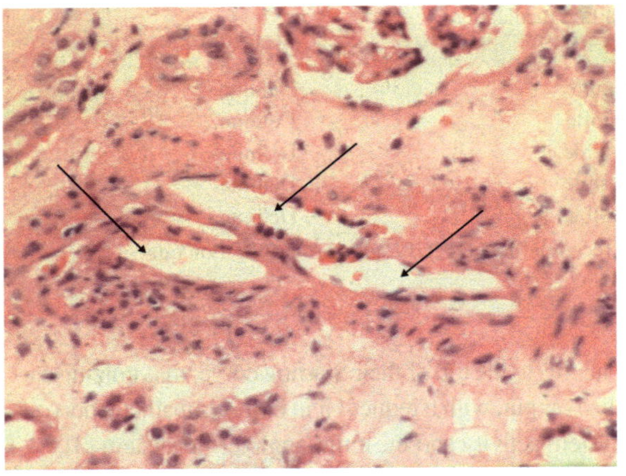

Fig. 6.3.4 Hematoxylin and eosin–stained renal biopsy sample showing an occluded renal arteriole due to cholesterol emboli (black arrows). The fat content of the cholesterol embolus has dissolved during the histological processing (Courtesy of Dr P Dupont)

6.3.6 Cholesterol Embolization

Cholesterol emboli can be dislodged from the aorta following femoral artery cannulation for coronary angiography or positioning of an aortic balloon pump [5], leading to a shower of cholesterol emboli causing AKI (Fig. 6.3.4). If this occurs, then treatment should be supportive, although some reports have suggested a benefit in giving both low-dose and also high-dose pulsed steroids [24], whereas others have suggested a benefit from prostacyclin, and there is a conflicting debate as to whether heparinization exacerbates or ameliorates renal injury. Cholesterol embolization has also been reported post urokinase, streptokinase, and recombinant tissue plasminogen activator therapy.

6.3.7 Radiocontrast Nephropathy

The risk of iodine-based radiocontrast nephropathy is greater following coronary angiography compared with standard computed tomography scanning, due to the greater dose used for coronary angioplasty and/or stenting. The risk of contrast nephropathy can be reduced by using the minimum dose of a hypo-osmolar contrast medium, ensuring adequate preprocedural and periprocedural hydration with saline, and/or isotonic sodium bicarbonate, avoiding repeated investigations within 48 h, and ensuring that potential nephrotoxic concomitant medications are withdrawn (Table 6.3.6).

Table 6.3.6 Risk of developing contrast-induced nephropathy depends on both patient factors and comorbidities, and procedure factors

Patient factors	Cardiac/vascular factors	Procedural factors	Concomitant medications
Age	IABP	Volume > 100 mL	Ciclosporin
Hypovolemia	↓ LVej fraction	Hyperosmolar media	Tacrolimus
Diabetes	CCF	Charged media	NSAIDs
CKD	Previous CABG	Repeated imaging	Aminoglycosides
Myeloma	Previous CA stent	Arterial injection	Cisplatinum
Cirrhosis	Previous stroke	Renal angiography	Amphotericin B
Hypovolemia	Previous MI	Interventional	Vancomycin
RAS	PVD	Blood loss	Diuretics
Nephrotic syndrome		Cholesterol emboli	Nesiritide
Hypoalbuminemia			Bosanten
Hyponatremia			ACEIs/ARBs
			Dipyridamole

ACEIs/ARBs angiotensin-converting enzyme inhibitors/angiotensin receptor blockers, *CABG* coronary artery bypass surgery, *CA stent*coronary artery stenting, *CCF* congestive cardiac failure, *CKD* chronic kidney disease, *IABP* intra-aortic balloon pump, *LVej* left ventricular ejection fraction, *MI* myocardial infraction, *NSAIDs* nonsteroidal anti-inflammatories, *PVD* peripheral vascular disease, *RAS* renal artery stenosis

6.3.8 Special Circumstances

6.3.8.1 Renovascular-Induced Heart Failure

The majority of patients who develop "flash pulmonary edema," due to renal artery stenosis do so on a clinical background of hypertension and expanded extracellular fluid volume. However, during episodes of imminent renal artery occlusion, the extreme sympathetic overdrive with activation of the renin-angiotensin system can lead to severe vasoconstriction with reduced cardiac output and sudden pulmonary edema. The typical patient with renal artery stenosis is an elderly hypertensive, with concomitant vascular atheroma affecting coronary arteries and/or aorta and peripheral arteries, and with chronic kidney disease, although beading due to fibromuscular dysplasia may occur in the younger patient (Fig. 6.3.5).

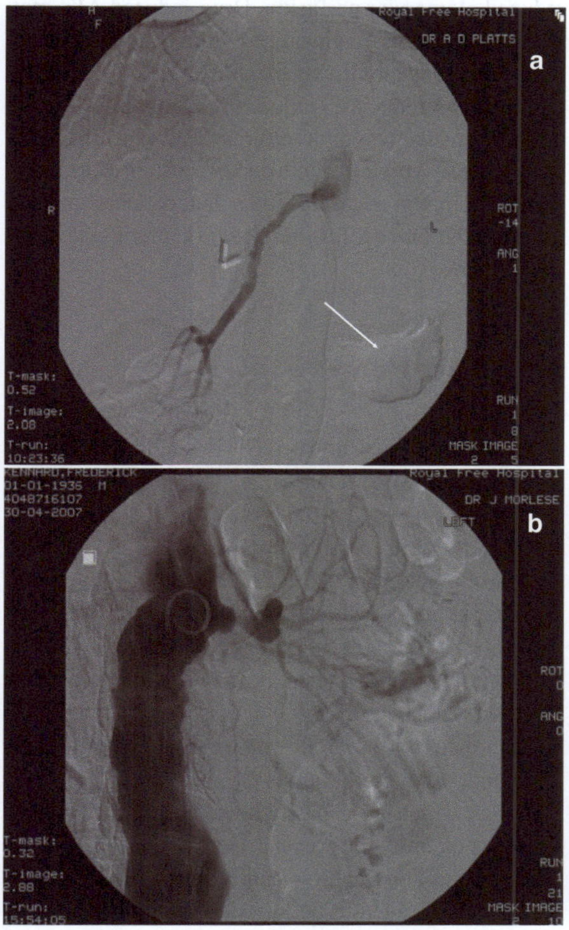

Fig. 6.3.5 Renovascular disease may be due to fibromuscular dysplasia (**a** – left renal artery – white arrow) or atheromatous renal artery stenosis (**b** – severe stenosis due to plaque at origin of right renal artery – white arrow) (Courtesy of Dr D Yu)

6.3.8.2 Scleroderma-Induced Heart Failure

Scleroderma renal crisis usually presents with malignant phase hypertension, complicated by pulmonary edema and AKI. Typically, patients have a past history of Raynaud's, and may have the classical skin changes of scleroderma and antitopisomerase-1 antibodies (Scl70). However, a minority of patients can present sine scleroderma, with antinuclear and anticentromere autoantibody staining. As a consequence of severe hypertension, there may be signs of a microangiopathic hemolytic anemia, characterized by red cell fragmentation, raised lactate dehydrogenase, and reduced haptoglobins, with intra-renal fibrin deposition (Fig. 6.3.6). Classically these patients have intense vasoconstriction with a markedly reduced cardiac output. Treatment is supportive and designed to slowly reduce systemic blood pressure, using vasodilatory prostanoids and angiotensin-converting enzyme inhibitors, which relieve arterial vasospasm, treating pulmonary edema and arterial underfilling.

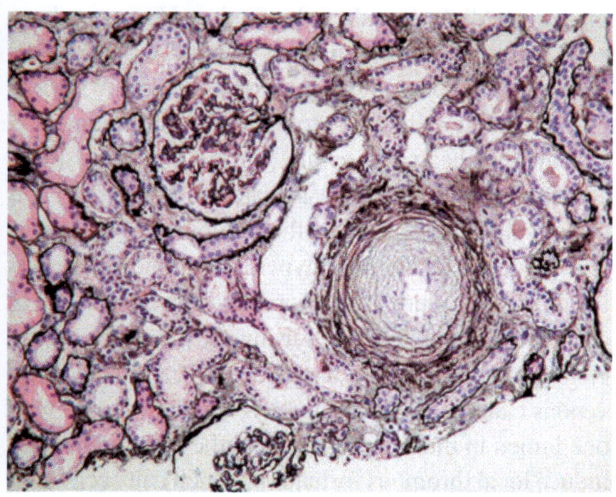

Fig. 6.3.6 Renal biopsy from a patient with scleroderma renal crisis, hematoxylin and eosin–stained section showing "onion ring" appearance of medium sized arteries and ischemic collapse of glomerulus (Courtesy of Dr A Burns)

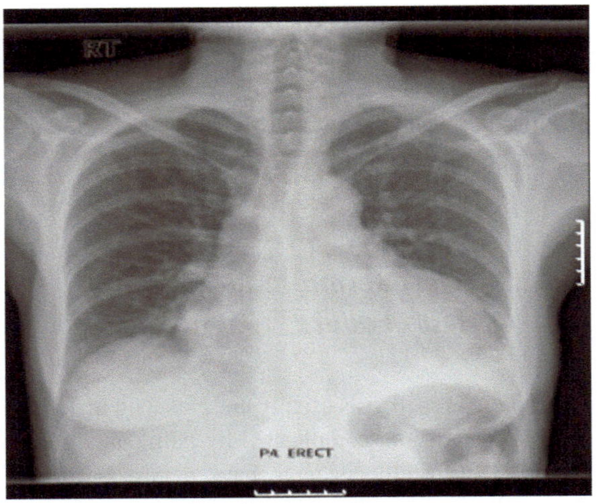

Fig. 6.3.7 Pericardial effusion in a dialysis patient, who presented with dyspnea and peripheral edema

6.3.8.3 Heart Failure in Dialysis and Renal Transplant Patients

Congestive heart failure in the dialysis patient is usually due to excess extracellular fluid retention and failure to achieve target "dry" or postdialysis weight. However, ischemic heart disease is more prevalent in both the dialysis and renal transplant recipient, and heart failure may be induced by acute myocardial ischemia and/or arrhythmia.

Dialysis patients are prone to developing pericardial effusions (Fig. 6.3.7), typically in the setting of inadequate dialysis and viral infection. However, those with active systemic lupus erythematosus and infections such as tuberculosis may also present with low output cardiac failure due to pericardial effusions.

Calcified heart valves are more common in longstanding dialysis patients associated with increased soft tissue calcification, due to the combination of hyperphosphatemia and tertiary hyperparathyroidism, resulting in heart failure due to critical aortic stenosis. In addition, patients dialyzing using central venous catheters are more prone to bacterial endocarditis. Central venous catheters used for dialysis are often placed with one lumen in the right atrium, and the catheter tip may induce local thrombus formation, which can occasional progress to form a right atrial thrombus, and potentially become infected or embolize [16].

As with native kidneys, renal artery stenosis may develop at the site of arterial anastomosis with the transplanted kidney, resulting in hypertension and reduced renal transplant urinary sodium excretion, and congestive cardiac failure. "Flash pulmonary edema" is occurs much less frequency compared with that observed with native renal artery stenosis.

6.3.8.4 Renal Dysfunction in the Heart Transplant Recipient

Renal impairment is a common finding in heart transplant recipients due to calcineurin inhibitor (cyclosporin A and tacrolimus)–induced interstitial fibrosis, and may progress to chronic kidney disease requiring dialysis. These patients are predisposed to developing AKI due to prerenal factors, due to the combination of a denervated heart and relative renal ischemia, and due to reduced glomerular perfusion. Drug-induced AKI may also occur during treatment of cytomegalovirus infections with ganciclovir/valganciclovir, and occasionally HMG CoA 3 reductase–induced rhabdomyolysis.

Posttransplant lymphoproliferative disease, typically a B cell lymphoma induced by Epstein-Barr virus, is more common in cardiac transplant patients, and can infiltrate the kidney, resulting in proteinuria and renal impairment.

6.3.9 Take Home Pearls

- Preexisting renal impairment is a common finding in patients with ischemic and hypertensive cardiac failure.
- Cardiac failure with arterial underfilling leads to neurohumeral activation, causing renal sodium and water retention, which exacerbates cardiac function by increasing both the preload and afterload, thus potentially setting up a vicious cycle leading to a cardiorenal syndrome.
- Treatment with diuretics may cause a deterioration in underlying renal function.
- Drugs which have been shown to improve longer term outcome, such as angiotensin-converting enzyme inhibitors, angiotensin receptor blockers, and β-blockers, need to be introduced cautiously, so as not to reduce intrarenal perfusion, because the normal renal autoregulation compensatory mechanisms may be defective.
- Known potential nephrotoxic insults should be avoided or at least minimized.

References

1. Anand IS, Kuskowski MA, Rector TS et al. (2005) Anemia and change in hemoglobin over time related to mortality and morbidity in patients with chronic heart failure: results from Val-HeFT. Circulation 112:1121–1127.
2. Chen HH, Schrier RW (2006) Pathophysiology of volume overload in acute heart failure syndromes. Am J Med 119:S11–S16.
3. Costanzo MR, Guglin ME, Saltzberg et al. (2007) Ultrafiltration versus intravenous diuretics for patients hospitalized for acute decompensated heart failure. J Am Coll Cardiol 49:675–683.
4. Forman DE, Butler J, Wang Y et al. (2004) Incidence, predictors at admission and impact of worsening renal function among patients hospitalized with heart failure. J Am Coll Cardiol 43:61–67.
5. Funabiki K, Masuoka H, Shimizu H et al. (2003) Cholesterol crystal embolization (CCE) after cardiac catheterization: a case report and a review of 36 cases in the Japanese literature. Jpn Heart J 44:767–774.
6. Gheorghiade M, Niazi I, Ouyang J et al. (2003) Vasopressin V2-receptor blockade with tolvaptan in patients with chronic heart failure: results from a double-blind, randomized trial. Circulation 107:2690–2696.
7. Goldsmith SR (2006) Is there a cardiovascular rationale for the use of combined vasopressin V1a/V2 receptor antagonists? Am J Med 119(Suppl 1):S93–S96.
8. Gottlieb SS, Brater DC, Thomas I et al. (2002) BG9719 (CVT-124), an A1 adenosine receptor antagonist, protects against the decline in renal function observed with diuretic therapy. Circulation 105:1348–1353.
9. Felker GM, Adams KF Jr, Konstam MA et al. (2003) The problem of decompensated heart failure: nomenclature, classification, and risk stratification. Am Heart J 145(Suppl 2):S18–25.
10. Heywood JT, Fonarow GC, Costanzo MR et al. (2007) High prevalence of renal dysfunction and its impact on outcome in 118,465 patients hospitalized with acute decompensated heart failure: a report from the ADHERE database. J Card Fail 13:422–430.
11. Iglesias J, Hom D, Antoniotti M et al. (2006) Predictors of worsening renal function in adult patients with congestive heart failure receiving recombinant human B-type brain natriuretic peptide (nesiritide). Nephrol Dial Transplant 21:3458–3465.
12. Januzzi JL Jr, Camargo A, Anwarruddin S et al. (2005) The N terminal pro-BNP investigation of dyspnoea in the emergency department (PRIDE) study. Am J Cardiol 95: 1625–1633.
13. Jessup M, Brozena S (2003) Heart failure. N Engl J Med 348:2007–2018.
14. Juurlink DN, Mamdani MM, Lee DS et al. (2004) Rates of hyperkalemia after publication of the Randomized Aldactone Evaluation Study. N Engl J Med. 351:543–551.
15. Kalra P, Guo H, Kausz AT et al. (2005) Atherosclerotic renovascular disease in United States patients aged 67 years or older: risk factors, revascularization, and prognosis. Kid Int 62:293–301.
16. Kingdon EJ, Holt SG, Davar J et al. (2001) Atrial thrombus and central venous dialysis catheters. Am J Kidney Dis 38: 631–639.
17. Krumholz HM, Chen Y-T, Vaccarino V et al. (2000) Correlates and impacts on outcomes of worsening renal function in patients ³ 65 years of age with heart failure. Am J Cardiol 139:72–77.
18. Libetta C, Sepe V, Zucchi M et al. (2007) Intermittent haemodiafiltration in refractory congestive heart failure: BNP and balance of inflammatory cytokines. Nephrol Dial Transplant 22:2013–2019.
19. Maisel AS, Krishnaswamy P, Nowak RM et al. (2002) Breathing Not Properly Multinational Study Investigators. Rapid measurement of B-type natriuretic peptide in the emergency diagnosis of heart failure. N Engl J Med 347:161–167.
20. Maisel AS, Krishnaswamy P, Nowak RM et al. (2004) BNP Multinational Study Investigators. Impact of age, race, and sex on the ability of B-type natriuretic peptide to aid in the emergency diagnosis of heart failure: results from the Breathing Not Properly (BNP) multinational study. Am Heart J 147:1078–1084.
21. Palmer BF (2002) Renal dysfunction complicating the treatment of hypertension. N Engl J Med 347:1256–1261.
22. Saltzman HE, Sharma K, Mather PJ et al. (2007) Renal dysfunction in heart failure patients: what is the evidence ? Heart Fail Rev 12:37–47.
23. Schrier RW (2007) Cardiorenal versus renocardiac syndrome: is there a difference? Nat Clin Pract Nephrol. 3:637.
24. Takahashi T, Konta T, Nishida W et al. (2003) Renal cholesterol embolic disease effectively treated with steroid pulse therapy. Intern Med 42:1206–1209.

Hepatorenal Syndrome

6.4

Dietrich Hasper and Thomas Berg

Core Messages

- The hepatorenal syndrome (HRS) is a functional renal failure characterized by renal vasoconstriction in a patient who has advanced acute or chronic liver disease.
- The diagnosis of HRS is one of exclusion. New diagnostic criteria were published in 2007 by the International Ascites Club.
- Once established, the prognosis for hepatorenal syndrome is extremely poor. Therefore, the prevention of HRS should be an important goal in patients with advanced cirrhosis and ascites. Treatment strategies in established HRS may be only successful in the early course of the disease.
- For most patients liver transplant is the only causative therapy. Therefore, all patients developing HRS should be checked for suitability for a liver transplant.
- The application of vasoconstrictors is the treatment of choice in HRS. Although terlipressin is the standard of care, norepinephrine and midodrine are possible alternatives.
- Transjugular intrahepatic portosystemic shunt may be a therapeutic option in selected patients. However, contraindications of the procedure must be considered, which excludes a significant proportion of patients.
- Renal replacement therapy should be initiated in patients with HRS according to the common guidelines for renal failure. Although the results of pilot studies are promising, there is not enough evidence to recommend extracorporeal liver therapy as a standard procedure in patients with HRS.

6.4.1 Definition

The hepatorenal syndrome (HRS) refers to the development of functional acute renal failure in a patient who has advanced acute or chronic liver disease characterized by renal vasoconstriction. Based on the speed of onset of renal failure, two forms of HRS can be distinguished:

- Type I HRS is defined as at least 50% decrease of the creatinine clearance or at least a twofold increase in serum creatinine to a level higher than 2.5 mg/dl in less than a 2-week period. This type of HRS presents as acute renal failure.
- Type II HRS is defined as a more gradual development of renal failure, mostly developing over weeks to months. The typical clinical pattern of HRS type II is refractory ascites.

Both types of HRS often present in the same patient. Elevated serum creatinine (HRS type II) is a frequent

D. Hasper (✉)
Nephrology & Medical Intensive Care,
Charité-Universitätsmedizin Berlin, Campus
Virchow-Klinikum, 13353 Berlin, Germany
e-mail: dietrich.hasper@charite.de

A. Jörres et al. (eds.), *Management of Acute Kidney Problems*,
DOI: 10.1007/978-3-540-69441-0_6.4,

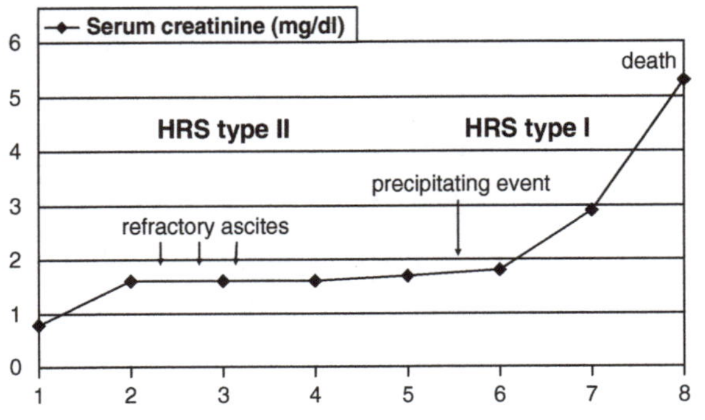

Fig. 6.4.1 Typical clinical course of a patient with cirrhosis and progressive renal failure

finding in patients with advanced liver disease. These patients are susceptible to a rapidly progressive reduction of renal function (HRS type I) when a precipitating event occurs. A typical course of a patient with HRS is shown in Fig. 6.4.1.

HRS is not a rare disease. About 39% of cirrhotic patients develop HRS at 5 years. Independent predictors of HRS are low serum sodium, high renin activity, and low cardiac output, but not the Child-Pugh Score. Once established the prognosis for untreated HRS is extremely poor. In patients without liver transplant, the median survival time for HRS type I has been calculated to be 2 weeks and for type II 6 months [15].

6.4.2 Pathophysiology

Although the complex pathophysiology of HRS is not fully understood, recent studies suggest two key aspects: The first one is intense arterial vasodilation. This may be a consequence of the local release of vasodilatory substances (nitric oxide and/or prostaglandins) due to advanced liver disease [14]. This vasodilation occurs mainly in the splanchnic circulation. The result is a hyperdynamic circulation with high cardiac output and low vascular resistance. The second step is a reduction of cardiac output in end-stage liver disease. This impaired cardiac function may be due to specific cardiac abnormalities termed cirrhotic cardiomyopathy [22]. Additionally, the reduction of cardiac output may be aggravated by events such as infection or fluid losses. The result is the retention of sodium and marked vasoconstriction in extra-splanchnic blood vessels including the kidney due to activation of the renin-angiotensin system, the sympathetic nerve system, and the excretion

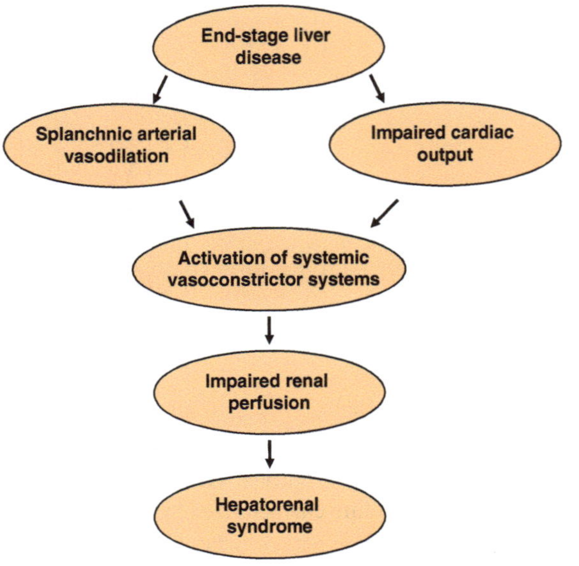

Fig. 6.4.2 Simplified pathophysiology of hepatorenal syndrome (HRS)

of antidiuretic hormone. Initially, renal function can be preserved by the local production of vasodilators (mainly prostaglandins and natriuretic peptides). However, every insult leading to an imbalance of systemic vasoconstriction and local renal vasodilation will result in renal failure – the patient develops HRS due to impaired renal perfusion (Fig. 6.4.2). With restoration of renal perfusion, the functional renal failure disappears. Transplanted kidneys from donors with HRS show a normal renal function in recipients.

It should be outlined that advanced liver failure is a systemic disease affecting almost any organ. Intense vasoconstriction has been also demonstrated for the muscular, cerebral, and intrahepatic circulation. Therefore, HRS can be regarded as a part of a specific multiple organ failure in end-stage liver disease rather than a simple kidney problem [5]. A detailed description of the pathophysiologic changes in liver disease was published by Arroyo and Colmenero [4].

6.4.3 Diagnosis

6.4.3.1 Diagnostic Criteria

HRS should be suspected in patients with acute or chronic liver disease and progressive renal failure. It should be kept in mind that significant renal

Table 6.4.1 New International Ascites Club's diagnostic criteria for hepatorenal syndrome (2007)

- Cirrhosis with ascites
- Serum creatinine > 1.5 mg/dl
- No improvement in serum creatinine after at least 2 days with diuretic withdrawal and volume expansion with albumin. The recommended dose of albumin is 1 g/kg of body weight per day up to a maximum of 100 g/day
- Absence of shock
- No current or recent treatment with nephrotoxic drugs
- Absence of parenchymal kidney disease as indicated by proteinuria > 500 mg/day, microhematuria and/or abnormal renal ultrasonography

insufficiency may be present despite normal serum creatinine and serum urea, because these patients are frequently malnourished with a reduced muscle mass and low urea production rate due to liver failure.

There is no specific diagnostic test for HRS – the diagnosis of HRS is one of exclusion. Diagnostic criteria are first published in 1996 by the International Ascites Club [6] and are now available in a modified version [32] (Table 6.4.1). These criteria should be regarded as the diagnostic standard.

6.4.3.2 Renal Biopsy

Due to the functional nature of HRS, there is no specific glomerular and tubular abnormality. Therefore, renal biopsy is generally not necessary in the diagnosis of HRS. However, in cirrhotic patients with marked proteinuria or nephritic sediment, renal biopsy may be desirable to exclude intrarenal diseases. In these patients, percutaneous biopsy is often a high-risk procedure due to the accompanying coagulation disorder. Transjugular renal biopsy should be considered in these patients if available.

6.4.3.3 Differential Diagnosis

Both systemic vasculitis and glomerulonephritis can occur in patients with cirrhosis and should be suspected in patients with marked proteinuria or active urine sediment. Fluid depletion induced by gastrointestinal losses, bleeding, or diuretic therapy can lead to "simple" prerenal failure with rapid improvement after fluid resuscitation. Therefore, a trial of volume expansion with albumin should be performed to exclude this condition.

6.4.4 Treatment

By definition, HRS is a reversible condition. Recent advances have offered effective treatment strategies in a significant portion of patients. However, it has to be emphasized that successful treatment of HRS has to start in the early stages – even minor changes in serum creatinine or a decrease in urine volume should be treated promptly.

6.4.4.1 Prevention

Once established, the prognosis for patients with HRS is extremely poor. Therefore, the prevention of HRS should be an important goal in patients with advanced cirrhosis and ascites. There are typical insults in these patients precipitating the development of HRS: gastrointestinal bleeding, bacterial infections especially spontaneous bacterial peritonitis (SBP), and fluid losses by forced paracentesis or inadequate diuretic therapy. The following points might contribute to the prevention of HRS in these situations: Gastrointestinal bleeding and SBP should be treated early and aggressively (and every patient with HRS should undergo diagnostic paracentesis to exclude SBP). The diuretic-induced weight loss in patients with tense ascites/peripheral edema should not exceed 500 g/day. If ascites is treated by paracentesis, patients should receive volume expansion using 8 g albumin/l ascites removed, to prevent renal impairment [16]. Importantly, beneficial effects are only seen in patients treated with albumin but not with other colloidal solutions [25]. This may be related to the ability of albumin to bind nitric oxide and proinflammatory cytokines [12].

Tense ascites is a major clinical problem in patients with advanced cirrhosis. As mentioned above, refractory ascites is a typical symptom of HRS type II. In a randomized study, transjugular portosystemic intrahepatic shunting (TIPS) could reduce the progression of renal failure or development of HRS type I compared with repeated paracentesis [17]. Therefore, if suitable, such patients should be treated with TIPS.

In the future the use of nonpeptide vasopressin receptor antagonists (vaptans) may be a therapeutic option in patients with refractory ascites [10]. The efficacy of their use in patients with HRS is still not determined.

Patients with advanced cirrhosis are predisposed to acute renal failure when treated with nephrotoxic drugs. This includes aminoglycosides, nonsteroidal antiinflammatory drugs, radiographic contrast media, and vasodilators (e.g., angiotensin-converting enzyme inhibitors). These drugs should be avoided in this setting.

Infections are a typical complication in patients with advanced liver disease. In a recent study, infection was diagnosed in 45% of 309 patients admitted with liver cirrhosis. Interestingly, the development of progressive renal failure was associated with SBP, biliary tract/gastrointestinal, or urinary tract infections but not with pneumonia and other infections [13]. As a consequence such infections should be searched for and treated aggressively in patients with cirrhosis.

Oral antibiotic prophylaxis with norfloxacin was effective in the prevention of both SBP and HRS in patients with severe liver failure in a randomized study [27]. However, the widespread use of antibiotic prophylaxis over a long period is debatable with regard to the development of antibiotic resistance. Nevertheless, this approach may be acceptable in selected patients awaiting liver transplant.

Regarding treatment of SBP, a randomized trial has proven that albumin not only prevents the development of HRS (10% incidence vs 33% in the control group), but also reduces mortality (22% after 3 months vs 41% in the control group) [35]. Therefore, the addition of albumin (1.5 g/kg of body weight at the time of diagnosis, followed by 1 g/kg on day 3) to antibiotic treatment should be the standard of care.

Preventive strategies in patients with advanced liver disease are summarized in Table 6.4.2.

Table 6.4.2 Preventive strategies in patients with advanced liver disease

- Serum creatinine should be monitored closely
- Avoid or treat fluid losses aggressively
- Use albumin as the preferred plasma expander in these patients
- Consider TIPS in patients with refractory ascites
- Search for infections closely
- Avoid nephrotoxic drugs including contrast media
- Treat spontaneous bacterial peritonitis with a combination of antibiotics plus albumin
- Consider antibiotic prophylaxis in patients at high risk for spontaneous bacterial peritonitis awaiting liver transplantation

TIPS transjugular intrahepatic portosystemic shunt

6.4.4.2 Pharmacologic Interventions

HRS is characterized by intense splanchnic vasodilation with consecutive renal vasoconstriction. Paradoxically, the application of vasoconstrictors is the mainstay of therapy in this situation. The induction of splanchnic and systemic vasoconstriction increases the effective arterial blood volume with consecutive reduction of renal vasoconstrictor systems.

Vasopressin is a potent vasoconstrictor but rarely used due to ischemic side effects (gastrointestinal/myocardial). Terlipressin is a synthetic vasopressin analog with a more favorable safety profile. It is a prodrug which is converted into the active form after cleavage of three glycyl groups. The plasma half-life is 25 min. Terlipressin is degradated by different endopeptidases and exopeptidases. Therefore, dose reduction in case of severe renal or hepatic impairment is not necessary [33].

In historical (mostly uncontrolled) studies, terlipressin has been proven as an effective therapy of HRS [9]. It is now widely used, and most studies do not report relevant ischemic adverse effects. Due to the large experience with terlipressin, some experts state that terlipressin is the drug of choice in the treatment of HRS [7]. A beneficial effect on renal recovery was also documented in the two first randomized controlled studies published recently. Surprisingly, in these trials, terlipressin treatment had no significant effect on survival at 2 or 3 months [23, 34]. The reason for this finding is unclear. However, it should be noted that in both studies, mortality was much lower than expected.

Terlipressin treatment should be started with a dosage of 1 mg every 6 h. If serum creatinine does not respond in the first 3 days the dosage can be increased up to 12 mg/24 h. A beneficial response to terlipressin treatment combined with albumin can be achieved in about 60% of patients [26]. In these cases, treatment should be continued until normalization of serum creatinine. In patients not responding to the bolus application or developing adverse effects (mostly diarrhea), a continuous infusion starting with 3 mg/day may be an option.

Oral vasoconstrictor therapy is possible with the α-adrenergic agonist midodrine. In a randomized trial, oral therapy with midodrine (3 × 10 mg) for 7 days increased both sodium excretion and glomerular filtration rate in patients with ascites, whereas no effect was seen in the placebo group [20]. In several uncontrolled studies, midodrine was given in combination with subcutaneous octreotide to inhibit endogenous vasodilator release. According to the published regimen, midodrine should be titrated to increase the mean arterial pressure by at least 15 mm Hg (dose range 5–15 mg three times a day) [3]. Octreotide was given in a dose of 100–200 µg three times a day; however, the efficacy of octreotide in this regimen is still under debate [29].

Norepinephrine may be also useful for the treatment of HRS. Norepinephrine combined with albumin appeared effective and safe for the treatment of HRS type I [11]. In a small pilot study in patients with both HRS type I and type II, norepinephrine and terlipressin had comparable efficacy in improving renal function [1]. Although these results should be confirmed by large randomized trials, norepinephrine may be an interesting alternative to the expensive vasopressin analogs in the intensive care setting.

Albumin is the second component of therapy. In a prospective study, terlipressin was effective to improve renal function only when combined with albumin [28]. Therefore every pharmacologic intervention in patients with HRS should be accompanied by albumin (1 g/kg starting dose, than 20–40 g/day).

Pharmacologic therapy of HRS is summarized in Table 6.4.3.

Table 6.4.3 Pharmacologic therapy of hepatorenal syndrome: terlipressin combined with albumin should be regarded as the standard of care

Drug	Dose	Expected reversal of HRS[a]
Albumin	Start dose 1 mg/kg, then 20–40 g/day	–
Terlipressin	1 mg every 6 h i.v. (up to 12 mg/day)	60%
Midodrine	10 mg every 8 h	49%
Norepinephrine	0.5–3 mg/h i.v.	(70% – limited data)

[a]Adapted from Angeli P et al. Pathogenesis and management of hepatorenal syndrome in patients with cirrhosis. J Hepatol 2008;48:S93–S103.

6.4.4.3 Transjugular Intrahepatic Portosystemic Shunt

Portal hypertension is a typical problem in cirrhotic patients. An interventional technique to lower portal hypertension is the creation of a channel between the hepatic vein and the portal vein. Although TIPS has primarily been used to treat the major complications of portal hypertension (i.e., variceal bleeding), there is a lot of interest in the role of TIPS in the treatment of HRS. As discussed in Section 6.4.4.1 Prevention, TIPS is a beneficial intervention in patients with refractory ascites/HRS type II. Unfortunately, only three small pilot studies with 52 patients included have evaluated TIPS with focus on type I HRS [8, 19, 38]. An increasing renal function over weeks to months was observed in the majority of patients after TIPS insertion. Best results may be achieved in patients who responded to vasoconstrictor treatment prior to TIPS insertion. However, a number of restrictions were proposed: bilirubin > 5 mg/dl, Child-Pugh Score > 12, or hepatic encephalopathy. Therefore, TIPS could not be used in a significant proportion of patients. Furthermore, a high rate of de novo encephalopathy or deterioration of previous encephalopathy was reported in one of these studies. Deterioration of hepatic encephalopathy may be reduced when using new covered stents [37]. In summary, patients for TIPS insertion should be selected carefully. However, in suitable patients, TIPS may be an effective procedure for the reversal of HRS.

6.4.4.4 Renal Replacement Therapy

Patients with HRS who progress to renal failure can be successfully treated with dialysis until liver transplant or improvement of hepatic function. However, hemodialysis is often difficult to perform in patients with HRS. Dialysis catheters may cause harm due to bleeding complications and increased risk of blood stream infections. Arterial hypotension is a typical problem in patients with HRS, limiting the required ultrafiltration rate. With regard to this continuous renal replacement therapy (either continuous venovenous hemodiafiltration [CVVHDF] or sustained low-efficiency dialysis [SLED]) may be superior to conventional intermittent dialysis. Due to rapid changes in serum osmolality with intermittent hemodialysis, patients with hepatic encephalopathy may be susceptible to critical rises of intracranial pressure.

Anticoagulation during extracorporeal therapy should be minimized or avoided totally due to the preexisting coagulopathy. Regional citrate anticoagulation is useful to reduce bleeding complications but may lead to metabolic acidosis caused by unmetabolized citrate in patients with liver failure.

6.4.4.5 Extracorporeal Liver Support

The majority of toxins accumulating in liver failure are albumin-bound and poorly cleared by conventional renal replacement therapy. Therefore new techniques have been developed removing both water-soluble and protein-bound toxins. Today two systems are commercially available: the Molecular Adsorbents Recirculation System (MARS) [36] and the Fractionated Plasma Separation and Adsorption (FPSA or Prometheus) [31]. In a small randomized trial, MARS treatment both improved renal function and prolonged survival in patients with acute liver failure and HRS type I [24]. Although the results are promising, there is still a lack of robust data from randomized studies to evaluate the impact of these expensive strategies on renal function and patient outcome [21].

6.4.4.6 Liver Transplantation

By definition HRS is a functional renal failure. Therefore renal recovery can be achieved by improving hepatic function. Unfortunately, in most of the patients with advanced liver failure there is no therapeutic option other than liver transplantation. Therefore, all patients developing HRS should be checked for suitability for a liver transplant. The introduction of the MELD score, which now includes serum creatinine, may shorten the time of allocation for patients with HRS. However, many patients with HRS still die on the waiting list due to limited organ availability.

Patients who are transplanted with concomitant HRS have a lower 5-year survival than patients without HRS. Although renal function improved after liver transplant, most of the patients showed some persistent degree of renal impairment. This may be due to greater nephrotoxicity of calcineurin inhibitors in patients with impaired renal function prior to transplant. The incidence of need of dialysis was 7% in patients with HRS compared with 2% in patients without HRS [18].

However, in patients with HRS who were successfully treated before liver transplant, there was no difference in renal outcome compared with patients who never had HRS, in a case–control study [30]. This underlines the importance of adequate therapy of HRS even in patients awaiting liver transplant.

A treatment algorithm for HRS is shown in Fig. 6.4.3.

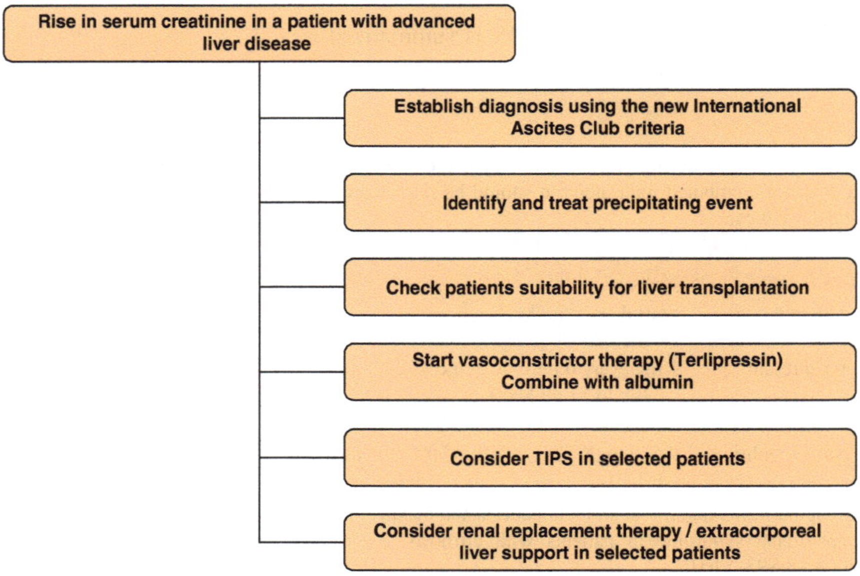

Fig. 6.4.3 Treatment algorithm for hepatorenal syndrome (HRS) type I

6.4.5 Take Home Pearls

- Typical insults in patients with advanced liver disease precipitating the development of HRS are gastrointestinal bleeding, spontaneous bacterial peritonitis, fluid losses by forced paracentesis, or inadequate diuretic therapy or lactulose-induced diarrhea. Be watchful and alert.
- The diagnosis of HRS is one of exclusion. Use the New International Ascites Club's diagnostic criteria.
- Due to the extremely poor prognosis, patients with HRS should be checked for suitability for liver transplantation.
- Pharmacologic standard treatment is terlipressin 1 mg every 6 h. Midodrine or norepinephrine are alternative drugs.
- Every pharmacologic intervention should be accompanied by albumin (1 g/kg starting dose, than 20–40 g/day).
- Transjugular intrahepatic portosystemic shunt may be beneficial in selected patients.

References

1. Alessandria C, Ottobrelli A, bernardi-Venon W, Todros L, Cerenzia MT, Martini S, Balzola F, Morgando A, Rizzetto M, Marzano A. Noradrenalin vs terlipressin in patients with hepatorenal syndrome: a prospective, randomized, unblinded, pilot study. J Hepatol 2007;47:499–505.
2. Angeli P, Merkel C. Pathogenesis and management of hepatorenal syndrome in patients with cirrhosis. J Hepatol 2008; 48 (Suppl 1:) S93-103.
3. Angeli P, Volpin R, Gerunda G, Craighero R, Roner P, Merenda R, Amodio P, Sticca A, Caregaro L, Maffei-Faccioli A, Gatta A. Reversal of type 1 hepatorenal syndrome with the administration of midodrine and octreotide. Hepatology 1999;29:1690–1697.
4. Arroyo V, Colmenero J. Ascites and hepatorenal syndrome in cirrhosis: pathophysiological basis of therapy and current management. J Hepatol 2003;38 (Suppl 1):S69–S89.
5. Arroyo V, Fernandez J, Gines P. Pathogenesis and treatment of hepatorenal syndrome. Semin Liver Dis 2008;28:81–95.
6. Arroyo V, Gines P, Gerbes AL, Dudley FJ, Gentilini P, Laffi G, Reynolds TB, Ring-Larsen H, Scholmerich J. Definition and diagnostic criteria of refractory ascites and hepatorenal syndrome in cirrhosis. International Ascites Club. Hepatology 1996;23:164–176.
7. Arroyo V, Terra C, Gines P. Advances in the pathogenesis and treatment of type-1 and type-2 hepatorenal syndrome. J Hepatol 2007;46:935–946.
8. Brensing KA, Textor J, Perz J, Schiedermaier P, Raab P, Strunk H, Klehr HU, Kramer HJ, Spengler U, Schild H, Sauerbruch T. Long term outcome after transjugular intrahepatic portosystemic stent-shunt in non-transplant cirrhotics with hepatorenal syndrome: a phase II study. Gut 2000;47: 288–295.
9. Cardenas A, Gines P. Therapy insight: management of hepatorenal syndrome. Nat Clin Pract Gastroenterol Hepatol 2006;3:338–348.
10. Decaux G, Soupart A, Vassart G. Non-peptide arginine-vasopressin antagonists: the vaptans. Lancet 2008;371:1624–1632.
11. Duvoux C, Zanditenas D, Hezode C, Chauvat A, Monin JL, Roudot-Thoraval F, Mallat A, Dhumeaux D. Effects of noradrenalin and albumin in patients with type I hepatorenal syndrome: a pilot study. Hepatology 2002;36:374–380.
12. Evans TW. Review article: albumin as a drug – biological effects of albumin unrelated to oncotic pressure. Aliment Pharmacol Ther 2002;16 (Suppl 5):6–11.
13. Fasolato S, P, Dallagnese L, Maresio G, Zola E, Mazza E, Salinas F, Dona S, Fagiuoli S, Sticca A, Zanus G, Cillo U, Frasson I, Destro C, Gatta A. Renal failure and bacterial infections in patients with cirrhosis: epidemiology and clinical features. Hepatology 2007;45:223–229.
14. Gatta A, Bolognesi M, Merkel C. Vasoactive factors and hemodynamic mechanisms in the pathophysiology of portal hypertension in cirrhosis. Mol Aspects Med 2008;29:119–129.
15. Gines A, Escorsell A, Gines P, Salo J, Jimenez W, Inglada L, Navasa M, Claria J, Rimola A, Arroyo V,. Incidence, predictive factors, and prognosis of the hepatorenal syndrome in cirrhosis with ascites. Gastroenterology 1993;105:229–236.
16. Gines A, Fernandez-Esparrach G, Monescillo A, Vila C, Domenech E, Abecasis R, Angeli P, Ruiz-del-Arbol L, Planas R, Sola R, Gines P, Terg R, Inglada L, Vaque P, Salerno F, Vargas V, Clemente G, Quer JC, Jimenez W, Arroyo V, Rodes J. Randomized trial comparing albumin, dextran 70, and polygeline in cirrhotic patients with ascites treated by paracentesis. Gastroenterology 1996;111:1002–1010.
17. Gines P, Uriz J, Calahorra B, Garcia-Tsao G, Kamath PS, Del Arbol LR, Planas R, Bosch J, Arroyo V, Rodes J. Transjugular intrahepatic portosystemic shunting versus paracentesis plus albumin for refractory ascites in cirrhosis. Gastroenterology 2002;123:1839–1847.
18. Gonwa TA, Klintmalm GB, Levy M, Jennings LS, Goldstein RM, Husberg BS. Impact of pretransplant renal function on survival after liver transplantation. Transplantation 1995;59:361–365.
19. Guevara M, Gines P, Bandi JC, Gilabert R, Sort P, Jimenez W, Garcia-Pagan JC, Bosch J, Arroyo V, Rodes J. Transjugular intrahepatic portosystemic shunt in hepatorenal syndrome: effects on renal function and vasoactive systems. Hepatology 1998;28:416–422.
20. Kalambokis G, Fotopoulos A, Economou M, Pappas K, Tsianos EV. Effects of a 7-day treatment with midodrine in non-azotemic cirrhotic patients with and without ascites. J Hepatol 2007;46:213–221.
21. Karvellas CJ, Gibney N, Kutsogiannis D, Wendon J, Bain VG. Bench-to-bedside review: Current evidence for extracorporeal albumin dialysis systems in liver failure. Crit Care 2007;11:215.
22. Ma Z, Lee SS. Cirrhotic cardiomyopathy: getting to the heart of the matter. Hepatology 1996;24:451–459.
23. Martin-Llahi M, Pepin MN, Guevara M, Diaz F, Torre A, Monescillo A, Soriano G, Terra C, Fabrega E, Arroyo V, Rodes J, Gines P. Terlipressin and albumin vs albumin in patients with cirrhosis and hepatorenal syndrome: a randomized study. Gastroenterology 2008;134:1352–1359.

24. Mitzner SR, Stange J, Klammt S, Risler T, Erley CM, Bader BD, Berger ED, Lauchart W, Peszynski P, Freytag J, Hickstein H, Loock J, Lohr JM, Liebe S, Emmrich J, Korten G, Schmidt R. Improvement of hepatorenal syndrome with extracorporeal albumin dialysis MARS: results of a prospective, randomized, controlled clinical trial. Liver Transpl 2000;6:277–286.
25. Moreau R, Durand F, Poynard T, Duhamel C, Cervoni JP, Ichai P, Abergel A, Halimi C, Pauwels M, Bronowicki JP, Giostra E, Fleurot C, Gurnot D, Nouel O, Renard P, Rivoal M, Blanc P, Coumaros D, Ducloux S, Levy S, Pariente A, Perarnau JM, Roche J, Scribe-Outtas M, Valla D, Bernard B, Samuel D, Butel J, Hadengue A, Platek A, Lebrec D, Cadranel JF. Terlipressin in patients with cirrhosis and type 1 hepatorenal syndrome: a retrospective multicenter study. Gastroenterology 2002;122:923–930.
26. Moreau R, Durand F, Poynard T, Duhamel C, Cervoni JP, Ichai P, Abergel A, Halimi C, Pauwels M, Bronowicki JP, Giostra E, Fleurot C, Gurnot D, Nouel O, Renard P, Rivoal M, Blanc P, Coumaros D, Ducloux S, Levy S, Pariente A, Perarnau JM, Roche J, Scribe-Outtas M, Valla D, Bernard B, Samuel D, Butel J, Hadengue A, Platek A, Lebrec D, Cadranel JF. Terlipressin in patients with cirrhosis and type 1 hepatorenal syndrome: a retrospective multicenter study. Gastroenterology 2002;122:923–930.
27. Navasa M, Rodes J. Management of ascites in the patient with portal hypertension with emphasis on spontaneous bacterial peritonitis. Semin Gastrointest Dis 1997;8:200–209.
28. Ortega R, Gines P, Uriz J, Cardenas A, Calahorra B, De Las HD, Guevara M, Bataller R, Jimenez W, Arroyo V, Rodes J. Terlipressin therapy with and without albumin for patients with hepatorenal syndrome: results of a prospective, nonrandomized study. Hepatology 2002;36:941–948.
29. Pomier-Layrargues G, Paquin SC, Hassoun Z, Lafortune M, Tran A. Octreotide in hepatorenal syndrome: a randomized, double-blind, placebo-controlled, crossover study. Hepatology 2003;38:238–243.
30. Restuccia T, Ortega R, Guevara M, Gines P, Alessandria C, Ozdogan O, Navasa M, Rimola A, Garcia-Valdecasas JC, Arroyo V, Rodes J. Effects of treatment of hepatorenal syndrome before transplantation on posttransplantation outcome. A case-control study. J Hepatol 2004;40:140–146.
31. Rifai K, Ernst T, Kretschmer U, Bahr MJ, Schneider A, Hafer C, Haller H, Manns MP, Fliser D. Prometheus – a new extracorporeal system for the treatment of liver failure. J Hepatol 2003;39:984–990.
32. Salerno F, Gerbes A, Gines P, Wong F, Arroyo V. Diagnosis, prevention and treatment of hepatorenal syndrome in cirrhosis. Gut 2007;56:1310–1318.
33. Saner FH, Canbay A, Gerken G, Broelsch CE. Pharmacology, clinical efficacy and safety of terlipressin in esophageal varices bleeding, septic shock and hepatorenal syndrome. Expert Rev Gastroenterol Hepatol 2007;1:207–217.
34. Sanyal AJ, Boyer T, Garcia-Tsao G, Regenstein F, Rossaro L, Appenrodt B, Blei A, Gulberg V, Sigal S, Teuber P. A randomized, prospective, double-blind, placebo-controlled trial of terlipressin for type 1 hepatorenal syndrome. Gastroenterology 2008;134:1360–1368.
35. Sort P, Navasa M, Arroyo V, Aldeguer X, Planas R, Ruiz-del-Arbol L, Castells L, Vargas V, Soriano G, Guevara M, Gines P, Rodes J. Effect of intravenous albumin on renal impairment and mortality in patients with cirrhosis and spontaneous bacterial peritonitis. N Engl J Med 1999;341:403–409.
36. Stange J, Mitzner SR, Risler T, Erley CM, Lauchart W, Goehl H, Klammt S, Peszynski P, Freytag J, Hickstein H, Lohr M, Liebe S, Schareck W, Hopt UT, Schmidt R. Molecular adsorbent recycling system (MARS): clinical results of a new membrane-based blood purification system for bioartificial liver support. Artif Organs 1999;23:319–330.
37. Tripathi D, Ferguson J, Barkell H, Macbeth K, Ireland H, Redhead DN, Hayes PC. Improved clinical outcome with transjugular intrahepatic portosystemic stent-shunt utilizing polytetrafluoroethylene-covered stents. Eur J Gastroenterol Hepatol 2006;18:225–232.
38. Wong F, Pantea L, Sniderman K. Midodrine, octreotide, albumin, and TIPS in selected patients with cirrhosis and type 1 hepatorenal syndrome. Hepatology 2004;40:55–64.

Malignant Hypertension

6.5

Bert-Jan H. van den Born and Gert A. van Montfrans

Core Messages

- Malignant hypertension (MHT) is a hypertensive emergency characterized by severe hypertension and acute ischemic damage to end organs (retina, kidney, brain).
- The most important risk factor for MHT is a history of poorly controlled hypertension; however, secondary causes (primary renal disease or renovascular hypertension) are more frequent.
- Secondary activation of the renin-angiotensin system is common in MHT because of renovascular ischemia and volume depletion.
- Treatment of MHT involves an immediate but controlled blood pressure reduction of mean arterial pressure (MAP) by 25–30% to prevent cerebral hypoperfusion.
- Administration of either sodium nitroprusside, labetalol, or nicardipine in a medium or intensive care setting is the treatment of choice.

6.5.1 Introduction

Malignant hypertension (MHT) is a hypertensive emergency characterized by severe hypertension (diastolic blood pressure [BP] often exceeding 120 mm Hg) and ischemic lesions of the retina, kidney, and brain as a result of microvascular damage. Bilateral retinal abnormalities consistent with grade III or IV hypertensive retinopathy are required for the diagnosis of MHT, where grade III denotes the presence of flame-shaped hemorrhages or exudates, and grade IV the presence of papilledema with or without grade III retinopathy. In the 1940s and 1950s, the 1-year survival of MHT was less than 20%, with most patients dying of renal failure, stroke, myocardial infarction, or heart failure. Nowadays, the survival of MHT has considerably improved because of the availability of antihypertensive drugs and kidney replacement therapy. Despite these advances, renal dysfunction is an important cause of morbidity: one in five patients are on kidney replacement therapy after 4 years [74]. Acute renal failure, thrombotic microangiopathy (TMA), and hypertensive encephalopathy frequently complicate MHT and mandate an immediate but controlled BP reduction. In that sense, the ischemic retinal abnormalities that corroborate MHT, point to ischemic complications elsewhere. Still, the clinical spectrum of MHT varies widely: patients may present with a hypertensive encephalopathy, TMA, and acute renal failure, but may also present without symptoms. Since asymptomatic presentation is rare and MHT may be associated with impaired cerebral autoregulation, it is prudent to admit all MHT patients for controlled intravenous BP reduction. Finally, a hypertensive emergency must also be considered in patients with severe hypertension who lack retinal abnormalities as hypertensive encephalopathy can be present in the absence of retinal abnormalities. Admitting patients for a timely and controlled reduction of BP should therefore not rely on the presence of retinal abnormalities alone, but should include a careful clinical assessment and laboratory evaluation. A decision model incorporating selected clinical and biochemical parameters may be

Bert-Jan H. van den Born (✉)
Department of Internal and Vascular Medicine, Academic Medical Centre, Meibergdreef 9, 1105 AZ Amsterdam, The Netherlands
e-mail: b.j.vandenborn@amc.uva.nl

A. Jörres et al. (eds.), *Management of Acute Kidney Problems*,
DOI: 10.1007/978-3-540-69441-0_6.5, © Springer-Verlag Berlin Heidelberg 2010

Table 6.5.1 Working definition of malignant hypertension

Severe hypertension (diastolic blood pressure usually above 120 mm Hg) and 1 or more of the following:
1. Clinical symptoms consistent with cerebral complications: unexplained lowering of consciousness or delirium, lethargy, confusion, generalized or focal seizures, or (cortical) blindness.
2. Bilateral retinal abnormalities consistent with grade III or IV retinopathy according to the Keith, Wagener, and Barker classification.
3. Coombs negative hemolysis as evidenced by two of the following: low platelet count, elevated LDH, and/or presence of schistocytes

preferred to better identify patients with this hypertensive emergency (Table 6.5.1). For research purposes, however, the original WHO definition, severe hypertension together with grade III or IV hypertensive retinopathy, may be preferred to ensure adequate comparison of patients. In this chapter, the histopathology, pathophysiology, and epidemiology of MHT will be discussed first, followed by the clinical presentation and management of MHT and its associated complications.

6.5.2 Histopathologic Findings

The pathologic characteristics of MHT consist of fibrinoid necrosis and myointimal proliferation of small arteries and arterioles. Fibrinoid necrosis is caused by seepage of fibrin and serum proteins through a necrotic vessel wall into surrounding viable tissue. Myointimal proliferation is characterized by smooth muscle cell hyperplasia of the subintimal layer and results in narrowing of the arterial lumen. Fibrinoid necrosis and myointimal proliferation are often observed together. Their presence is sometimes accompanied by obliteration of the arterial lumen because of thrombosis (Fig. 6.5.1) [36, 61]. Fibrinoid necrosis is not always present and can also be observed in other conditions characterized by microvascular occlusions, such as scleroderma, TTP-HUS, and antiphospholipid antibody syndrome. Myointimal proliferation can also be found in severely hypertensive patients without retinal abnormalities [36, 61]. In one autopsy series, the pathologic findings in the kidney paralleled the histopathologic findings in the retina and brain with regard to the presence of fibrinoid necrosis and myointimal hyperplasia

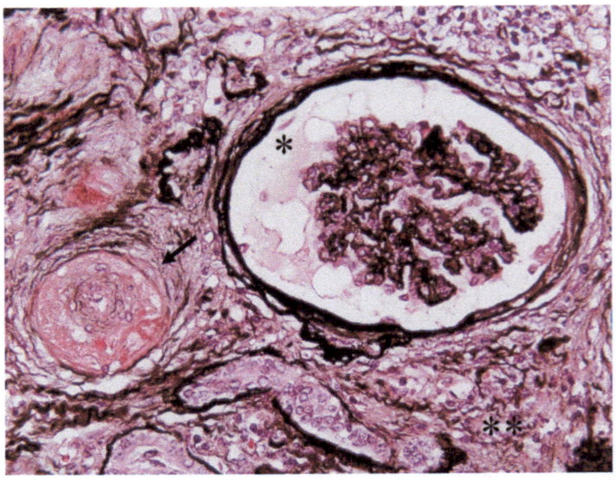

Fig. 6.5.1 Renal microscopic changes in MHT. These include myointimal hyperplasia and fibrinoid necrosis with near occlusion of the lumen of an arteriole (*arrow*), ischemic wrinkling of the glomerulus with widening of Bowman's space (*asterixis*), and tubular atrophy with interstitial fibrosis and chronic inflammation (*double asterisk*) (Courtesy of Dr. J.H. von der Thüsen, pathologist)

[8]. Fibrinoid necrosis and myointimal proliferation have also been described in the vasculature of the heart, pancreas, adrenal glands, intestine, and liver [38]. In the kidney, fibrinoid necrosis and myointimal proliferation are predominantly localized in afferent arterioles and distal interlobular arteries [61]. As a result, the glomerulus becomes ischemic as evidenced by collapsed glomerular tufts due to wrinkling of the capillary basement membrane and thickening of Bowman's capsule with collagen depositions in Bowman's space (Fig. 6.5.1). Tubules may be atrophic with interstitial fibrosis and with blood and fibrin depositions in the lumina. Tubular cells may show patchy necrosis [33, 36]. Finally, hyperplasia and hypergranularity of juxtaglomerular cells may be observed, which is consistent with activation of the renin-angiotensin system in these patients [36, 50].

6.5.3 Pathophysiology

Because of the often marked activation of the renin-angiotensin system, MHT is considered a renin-mediated type of hypertension. However, activation of the renin-angiotensin system is not an exclusive feature of MHT, nor is it a primary event. In experimental models it has been demonstrated that, apart from angiotensin II (ATII), other BP-stimulating factors may lead to MHT [19, 44, 69]. In humans, this is best demonstrated in patients with an aldosterone-producing adenoma (Conn's syndrome). Although rare, these patients may develop MHT with high levels of renin and ATII despite initially suppressed renin secretion [29]. The mechanisms responsible for the (paradoxical) activation of the renin-angiotensin system include sodium depletion due to pressure-induced natriuresis and renovascular ischemia resulting from vascular damage.

6.5.3.1 Sodium Depletion and Pressure-Induced Natriuresis

Animal experiments have shown that MHT is preceded by sodium depletion and activation of the renin-angiotensin system. In uninephrectomized dogs, a modest BP increase elicited by chronic intrarenal infusion of either norepinephrine or ATII will lead to sodium retention [11, 43]. However, intrarenal infusion of increasing doses of norepinephrine results in natriuresis and weight loss, followed by MHT with intravascular hemolysis and activation of the renin-angiotensin system [44]. The same has been demonstrated in rats with a unilateral clip on the renal artery and an untouched contralateral kidney. In these animals, sodium excretion and weight loss precede the development of MHT and activation of the renin-angiotensin system [52]. Administration of isotonic saline ameliorates the malignant course compared with rats receiving only water, likely by suppression of renin release due to restoration of intravascular volume. Uninephrectomized rats with a clip on the renal artery also exhibit activation of the renin-angiotensin system [54]. However, activation of the renin-angiotensin system in these animals is not as great as in unilaterally clipped rats with an intact contralateral kidney. In this case, sodium retention will restore renal perfusion in the uninephrectomized clipped rats,aborting further renin stimulation. Although balance studies are lacking, patients with MHT are often sodium depleted at the time of admission with a history of weight loss in the weeks prior to their presentation. The factors that influence pressure natriuresis have been well established; however, the exact mechanisms responsible for the pressure-induced natriuresis are not fully understood. Renal autoregulation is well preserved in cortical nephrons despite large differences in BP or ATII [37, 59]. In contrast to renal cortical blood flow, however, renal medullary blood flow is less well autoregulated. Therefore, the pressure-induced natriuresis preceding the development of MHT may principally result from enhanced sodium excretion via augmentation of blood flow in medullary nephrons [49, 59]. Contraregulatory tubuloglomerular feedback mechanisms may be overruled in this process.

6.5.3.2 Renovascular Ischemia and Vascular Damage

There is both histologic and angiographic evidence that the severity of vascular damage in patients with MHT is associated with the degree of renin release [27, 50]. The acute vascular damage, together with preexisting arteriolar narrowing, may lead to renovascular ischemia and stimulation of renin release from juxtaglomerular cells. Activation of the renin-angiotensin system in turn may further enhance vasoconstriction and endothelial damage, thereby inducing a vicious circle as previously proposed by Wilson and Byrom [80]. Although the exact mechanisms leading to the vascular damage of MHT are incompletely understood, it is likely that normal vasodilating mechanisms are overruled by exposure of the endothelium to high levels of shear stress and humoral factors such as ATII, norepinephrine, aldosterone, and vasopressin (antidiuretic hormone; ADH) [78]. Initially the endothelium may adapt to the BP changes by shear induced stimulation of nitric oxide (NO) and prostacyclin (PGI_2). However, with increasing levels of shear force and ATII procoagulant and proinflammatory pathways are activated. Shear stress has been shown to (1) stimulate nuclear factor kappa beta (NF-κβ)– a transcription factor which regulates the expression of adhesion molecules and proinflammatory cytokines – via mechanoreceptors [72], (2) stimulate the production of tissue factor – a key factor of coagulation – via transcription factor Egr-1 [28], and (3) help unfold von Willebrand factor (VWF), thereby facilitating platelet adhesion and aggregation. The increasing levels of ATII will further increase BP

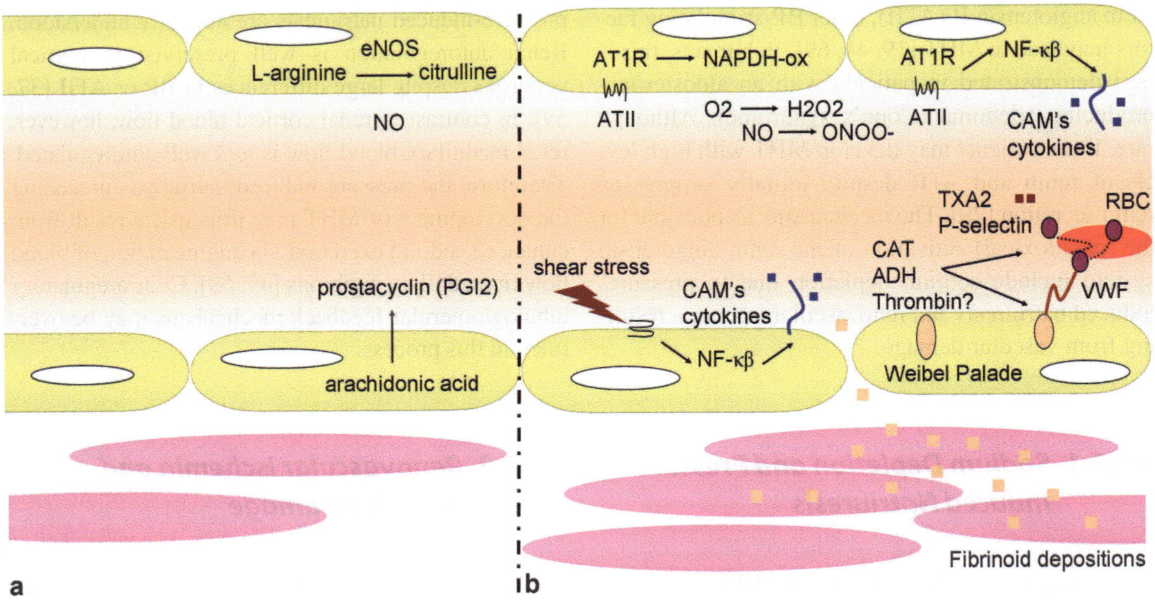

Fig. 6.5.2 (**a**) Vascular homeostasis in healthy normotensive subjects: endothelial cells release vasoactive substances such as nitric oxide (NO) and prostacyclin (PGI2). (**b**) In malignant hypertension normal vasodilatory responses are overwhelmed and proinflammatory pathways are stimulated by vasoactive substances such as angiotensin II (ATII), vasopressin (ADH), catecholamines (CAT), and high levels of shear stress. ATII-mediated stimulation of NADPH oxidase on endothelial and vascular smooth muscle cells results in scavenging of NO (*left upper panel*). Both ATII and shear stress can stimulate nuclear factor kapp beta (NF-κβ), a key regulator of endothelial proinflammatory and procoagulant pathways (*right upper panel* and *left lower panel*). Vasoactive substances (ADH and catecholamines) stimulate the release of von Willebrand factor (VWF) from Weibel-Palade bodies and activate platelets. The VWF can adhere to collagen on the subendothelial surface. Platelets may form fibrin cross-links leading to clot formation with entrapment and destruction of red blood cells (*right lower panel*). Ultimately, these processes of endothelial activation and damage will lead to TMA and fibrinoid necrosis (Modified from Vaughan et al., Lancet, 2000)

and shear stress by various mechanisms including (1) smooth muscle contraction, (2) scavenging of NO by stimulation of nicotinamide adenine dinucleotide phosphate (NADPH) oxidase, and (3) stimulation of ADH, norepinephrine, and aldosterone release. Apart from these BP-mediated effects, ATII also stimulates NF-κβ. Ultimately these processes may lead to the endothelial activation and damage observed in experimental and human MHT (Fig. 6.5.2). Rats, double transgenic for the human renin and angiotensinogen genes, develop severe hypertension and TMA similar to that observed in humans with MHT. In these double transgenic rats, increased expression of adhesion molecules (ICAM, VCAM), plasminogen activator inhibitor-1 (PAI-1), and fibronectin are present in the interstitium, intima, and adventitia of small renal arteries. The increased expression of adhesion molecules is followed by monocyte and macrophage infiltration [51]. Either BP-lowering treatment directed at the renin-angiotensin system or inhibition of NF-κβ leads to attenuation of these vascular changes [53]. In humans with MHT, circulating levels of adhesion molecules, and VWF are markedly increased pointing toward endothelial activation and damage [76, 79]. VWF can adhere to collagen on the subendothelial surface. These platelets may form fibrin cross-links leading to clot formation with entrapment and destruction of red blood cells. Ultimately these processes of endothelial activation and damage will lead to (1) consumption of platelets and intravascular hemolysis characteristic of TMA and (2) increased endothelial permeability with insudation of plasma proteins typical for fibrinoid necrosis.

6.5.4 Epidemiology

The incidence of MHT has declined with increased awareness, treatment possibilities, and control of hypertension in the population at large. However, in

Table 6.5.2 Conditions associated with malignant hypertension

Essential hypertension
Renal parenchymal disease
Primary renal disease (glomerulonephritis, glomerulopathy, tubulointerstitial nephritis)
Systemic disorders with renal involvement (scleroderma, SLE, TTP-HUS syndrome, vasculitis)
Inherited kidney diseases (FPKD, Alport's syndrome)
Renovascular disease
Atherosclerotic
Fibromuscular dysplasia
Vasculitis (Takayasu, PAN)
Endocrine disorders
Pheochromocytoma
Cushing's syndrome
Renin-secreting tumors
Juxtaglomerular cell tumor
Mineralocorticoid hypertension
Drugs and intoxications
Cocaine, amphetamines, licorice, cyclosporine, erythropoietin, MAO interactions, clonidine withdrawal
Autonomic hyperreactivity
Guillain-Barre syndrome
Spinal cord injury
Baroreflex failure
Eclampsia

SLE = Systemic lupus erythematosus
HUS = Hemolytic uremic syndrome
TTP = Thrombotic thrombocytopenic purpura
FPKD = Familial polycystic kidney disease
PAN = Polyarteritis nodosa
MAO = Monoamine-oxidase

large multiethnic Western communities and in urban sub-Saharan African populations, it remains relatively common. The estimated annual incidence rate of MHT is 1–2 cases per 100,000 inhabitants in multiethnic populations in the United Kingdom and The Netherlands [42, 74]. Patients with MHT often have a history of poorly controlled or untreated hypertension [42, 74]. This may also explain why MHT is more frequent among those with lower socioeconomic status and in ethnic minorities [42, 74]. In general an underlying cause can be identified in 20–30% of unselected patients presenting with MHT at the emergency room (Table 6.5.2). However, the prevalence of these secondary causes varies strongly between studies depending on the efforts which were undertaken to demonstrate an underlying cause, selection of patients, and – genuine – differences associated with demographic characteristics and the control of hypertension in the population at large. This may also explain the seemingly low prevalence of secondary causes in black patients with MHT [35, 74]. Most secondary causes are due to primary renal disease and renal artery stenosis [74]. MHT is associated with Conn's syndrome and pheochromocytoma, but in most series they account for less than 5% of the total number of cases. Although rare, oral contraceptives have been associated with MHT including those with low estrogen content (the so-called sub-30 pill) [40]. In some of these patients, normal BP values have been recorded just prior to the prescription of oral contraceptives, and cessation of the pill has led to a remarkable BP improvement in some of these women [40, 56].

6.5.5 Clinical Perspectives

Patients with chronic hypertension can tolerate much higher BP elevations than patients without preexisting hypertension. In other words, the rate of change over time rather than the absolute BP level determines whether MHT will develop [17]. This is likely a result of adaptive vascular changes (e.g., smooth muscle cell hyperplasia) protecting end organs against the high arterial pressures. In adult men and nonpregnant women, MHT is rarely seen below a diastolic BP of 120 mm Hg. The most common presenting complaints are headache and visual disturbances. Other frequent complaints include gastrointestinal symptoms (nausea, vomiting, and abdominal pain), dyspnea, peripheral edema, and dizziness which is believed to result from an impaired cerebral autoregulation.

Hypertensive encephalopathy is present in 10–15% of unselected MHT patients [32, 74]. Because these patients may lack retinal abnormalities, a careful neurologic assessment should be performed in every patient with an extreme BP elevation [5]. Patients with hypertensive encephalopathy may present with altered consciousness, delirium, agitation, stupor, seizures, and cortical blindness. Focal neurologic signs are uncommon and should raise the suspicion of an ischemic or hemorrhagic stroke. Untreated, hypertensive encephalopathy leads to irreversible neurologic damage and death [8]. The cause of hypertensive encephalopathy is a breakthrough of cerebral autoregulation as a result of the high arterial pressures [68], leading to hyperperfusion, increased intracranial pressure, and cerebral edema [20, 64]. The edema in hypertensive encephalopathy is typically (but not exclusively) localized in the posterior regions of the brain and best visible as areas with increased signal intensity on T2-weighted magnetic resonance imaging (MRI) or FLAIR images, or as hypodense areas on computed tomography or T1-weighted MRI [23, 64]. The reason for the posterior involvement is likely the scarce innervation of the sympathetic nervous system in the supply area of the vertebral arteries resulting in a lower damping of BP oscillations compared with flow in the middle cerebral artery [15, 22]. Hypertensive encephalopathy and the cerebral white matter lesions can be fully reversible with timely and appropriate BP treatment. Therefore, this syndrome has also been described as reversible posterior leukoencephalopathy syndrome (RPLS) in the literature [23]. Besides hypertension, RPLS has also been associated with thrombotic thrombocytopenic purpura (TTP), carotid endarteriectomy hyperperfusion syndrome, cytotoxic therapy (e.g., cyclosporine and tacrolimus), and with antiangiogenic and proapoptotic drugs such as bevacizumab and bortezomib. In many of these cases, hypertension was also present. Therefore, the causes of this syndrome appear to be multifactorial including, apart from hypertension, sudden increases in cerebral perfusion and endothelial damage.

MHT is frequently complicated by TMA which can be demonstrated in 30% of unselected patients [32, 73]. TMA is characterized by a Coombs-negative hemolysis with thrombocytopenia and the presence of fragmented red blood cells in a peripheral blood smear. Lactic dehydrogenase (LDH) levels are usually elevated in patients with TMA and may serve as an indicator to assess TMA severity. The presence of TMA can be considered a reflection of vascular damage in patients with MHT and it is associated with the presence of fibrinoid necrosis in kidney biopsies and activation of the renin-angiotensin system [41, 75]. Apart from MHT there are a few other conditions associated with TMA, notably TTP-HUS syndrome, antiphospholipid antibody syndrome, HELLP syndrome, and severe sepsis. Especially, TTP syndrome may closely resemble MHT. A markedly elevated BP, the presence of grade III or IV hypertensive retinopathy, and a less severe TMA with typically only a few schistocytes, and mild thrombocytopenia may point toward MHT. More definite proof can be acquired by measuring ADAMTS13 activity – in general absent in patients with TTP and low to normal in MHT – and by evaluating the response to therapy. If the TMA is associated with MHT, it should quickly resolve after institution of antihypertensive therapy as demonstrated by a decline in LDH levels and an increase in platelet count.

Renal insufficiency may be both a cause and consequence of MHT. Recognition of underlying renal pathology may be difficult in the acute phase of MHT because urinalysis may reveal proteinuria, hematuria, and hyaline, granular, or red blood cell casts in this phase. Increased density of the renal parenchyma on ultrasound examination is suggestive of renal parenchymal disease, but also observed in renal dysfunction related to MHT. Nevertheless, an ultrasound examination is useful to assess kidney size, left to right differences and postrenal obstruction. The urine abnormalities and the amount of proteinuria should quickly improve after BP-lowering therapy. Persistent urine abnormalities and proteinuria > 1 g/24 h despite adequate BP control should raise suspicion of primary renal disease and warrants further examination. Although in general the degree of renal insufficiency at presentation is an important determinant of future renal failure, a subset of patients presenting with MHT and renal dysfunction have a marked recovery of renal function [33, 47, 73]. These patients more often present with oliguric renal failure, normal sized kidneys, and evidence of TMA at presentation [33, 47, 73]. Loss of tubular cells suggestive of acute tubular necrosis and evidence of tubular regeneration in renal biopsies seem to be indicative of potential recovery of renal function [33]. Renal improvement, even in patients who needed kidney replacement therapy after they presented with MHT, usually occurs within the first 3–6 months, but can be seen after up to 2 years [47, 73].

6.5.6 Management

6.5.6.1 General Recommendations

MHT is considered a hypertensive emergency mandating an immediate and controlled BP reduction to a safe level [7]. The recommended initial target is a 25–30% reduction in mean arterial pressure (MAP] within minutes to hours depending on the severity of the presentation. This is based on the assumption that such a BP reduction would place these patients on the plateau phase of the cerebral autoregulation curve, which is shifted toward higher BP levels in these patients. However, the plateau phase of the cerebral autoregulation curve may be lacking in MHT patients, suggesting that the recommended strategy may be based on an incorrect assumption [31]. Nonetheless, a 25–30% reduction in MAP is generally well tolerated and has not been associated with an adverse outcome. In contrast, a reduction in MAP by more than 50% in patients with MHT has been associated with ischemic stroke and death [21, 39, 46]. Most studies examining the efficacy and safety of oral and parenteral BP-lowering agents have included both patients with severe and MHT. Therefore it is difficult to establish the optimal therapy for MHT per se. Oral therapy (e.g., with nifedipine or captopril) is not preferred because the BP-lowering effect is unpredictable in patients with a hypertensive crises [12, 26]. Various parenteral drugs can be used to lower BP in a safe and controlled way (Tables 6.5.3 and 6.5.4). All agents need close monitoring, preferably with an intra-arterial line, in a medium or intensive care setting, as the magnitude of the BP-lowering effect cannot be predicted. Although there is agreement about the initial management of MHT, there is no evidence on how BP should be treated after the initial episode. It is recommended to keep BP at the initial target level for one to several days and then gradually reduce to normotensive values within several weeks [7].

6.5.6.2 Specific Therapy

Sodium nitroprusside (SNP) is an arterial and venous dilator with a short half-life and therefore most suitable

Table 6.5.3 Drugs commonly used for the treatment of a hypertensive emergency

Drug	Dose	Onset	Duration	Adverse effects	Contraindications
Nitroprusside	0.5 μg/kg/min, increase with 0.5 μg/kg/ min every 2–3 min (max. 10 μg/kg/min)	Immediate	1–2 min	Cyanide intoxication	Liver and renal insufficiency (relative CI)
Labetalol	0.5 mg/kg bolus every 10 min until target BP (max 200 mg), maintenance dosage 5–20 mg/h	5–10 min	3–6 h	Bradycardia	COPD, 2nd degree AV block, sick sinus, heart failure
Nicardipine	2.5 mg/h, increase with 2.5 mg/h every 5 min (max. 15 mg/h)	5–10 min	2–4 h	Reflex tachycardia, flushing	
Enalaprilat	0.625–5 mg bolus, repeat every 6 h in responders, switch to other drug in nonresponders	15 min	4–6 h	Precipitous BP falls in volume depleted states	Angioedema with ACE inhibitors
Urapidil	12.5–25 mg bolus every 10 min until goal BP, maintenance dosage 0.06 mg/kg/h	5–10 min	3–5 h	Reflex tachycardia, drowsiness	
Fenoldopam	0.1 μg/kg/min, increase with 0.1 μg/kg/min every 15 min (max. 1.6 μg/kg/min)	5–15 min	30–60 min	Headache	Constriction of cerebral arterioles?
Nitroglycerin	10 μg/min, increase with 10 μg/min every 5 min until target BP	1–5 min	3–5 min	Tachyphylaxis	
Phentolamine	2–5 mg bolus every 5–10 min until target BP, 0.5–1.0 mg/h maintenance dosage	1–2 min	3–5 min	Tachycardia	Heart failure, myocardial ischemia
Ketanserin	5–10 mg bolus, every 10–20 min until target BP, maintenance 4–12 mg/h	1–2 min		Tachycardia	2nd degree AV block, prolonged QT interval, bradycardia < 50 min

Table 6.5.4 Indications for the treatment of specific conditions associated with malignant hypertension (MHT)

Associated condition	Urgency of BP reduction	Drug	Alternative
MHT with or without TMA	Within hours	Nitroprusside	Labetalol
Hypertensive encephalopathy	Immediately	Labetalol	Nitroprusside
MHT with heart failure	Immediately	Nitroprusside	Urapidil, nitroglycerin
MHT with coronary ischemia	Immediately	Nitroglycerin (+ beta blockade)	Labetalol
Scleroderma renal crisis	Immediately	Nitroprusside or labetalol with short-acting oral ACE inhibitor	Enalaprilat
Adrenergic crisis	Immediately	Phentolamine	Urapidil
MHT in pregnancy or eclampsia	Immediately	Ketanserin, labetalol	Nicardipine

TMA = thrombotic microangiopathy

for an immediate and controlled reduction of BP [2]. In spite of its superior pharmacokinetics, SNP has some disadvantages. First, SNP increases intracranial pressure in patients with an intracranial mass [10]. However, in patients with MHT, SNP actually decreases cerebral blood flow, likely because blood flow is redirected to the systemic circulation ("cerebral steal") [30]. Second, SNP has been shown to reduce regional coronary blood flow in patients with ischemic heart disease and to increase ischemic injury compared with nitroglycerin in patients with myocardial infarction [9, 48]. This is explained by the redistribution of blood away from ischemic areas as a result of more potent dilatation of resistance vessels ("coronary steal"). However, the greater BP reduction induced by SNP may compensate for the redistribution of coronary blood flow by decreasing myocardial oxygen demand. Third, after infusion, SNP rapidly dissociates into NO and cyanide [66]. Cyanide immediately reacts with methemoglobin to form the nontoxic cyanomethemoglobin or is converted to thiocyanate in the liver. Thiocyanate is much less toxic than cyanide, but may accumulate to toxic levels in patients with renal failure. The conversion to thiocyanate requires sufficient amounts of thiosulphate. A fasting state, surgery, hepatic failure, and diuretic therapy adversely affect whole body thiosulphate concentrations and may increase the risk of cyanide toxicity [34]. Cyanide toxicity related to SNP for the treatment of hypertensive crises were in most cases observed after prolonged administration (>24 h) or in amounts exceeding the recommended dose [58]. Based on red blood cell cyanide concentrations, treatment with SNP is safe if the average dose does not exceed 2.5 mg/kg/min in 24 h. Dosages between 5 and 10 mg/kg/min should not be given for more than 4–5 h and dosages exceeding 10 mg/kg/min should be avoided [63]. Timely institution of oral antihypertensive agents limits the risk of cyanide or thiocyanate toxicity. *Labetalol*, a combined alpha- and beta-blocking agent, is effective in the treatment of hypertensive emergencies [60], but therapeutic goals may not be achieved in all patients [81]. Its long half-life limits the ability to promptly correct hypotension with cessation of the drug [60, 67]. In these cases intravenous saline may be warranted to restore BP to the desired target level. *Nicardipine*, a calcium-blocker for intravenous use, is equally effective in lowering BP compared to SNP and with a similar increase in heart rate [55]. Nicardipine, and other calcium antagonists, have a vasodilatory effect on cerebral blood vessels. As with SNP, it is possible that systemic vasodilatation counterbalances the vasodilatory action of nicardipine on the cerebral vasculature. Nicardipine may preserve renal blood flow despite its BP-lowering action by decreasing renal vascular resistance [4]. However, there are no comparative data on renal outcome in patients presenting with a hypertensive crisis and renal insufficiency. The BP-lowering action of *enalaprilat*, an intravenous angiotensin-converting enzyme (ACE) inhibitor, is variable and unpredictable because it depends on volume status and ATII before treatment [25]. The use of ACE inhibitors in patients with a hypertensive crisis should therefore be limited to scleroderma renal crisis, which is always associated with a high renin state. *Urapidil* is a combined alpha-1-adrenoreceptor antagonist with central sympatholytic properties. It is effective and safe in the treatment of severe hypertension and in hypertensive patients with pulmonary edema [24, 82]. However, the time to reach the targeted BP with urapidil is longer compared with SNP [24]. Urapidil increases renal blood flow in hypertensive patients [13]. As with nicardipine, comparative trials on renal outcome are lacking. There is evidence that urapidil may increase intracranial pressure directly after intravenous bolus injections [65]. Hypotensive episodes are not immediately corrected after cessation of urapidil because of its long half-life [77]. *Fenoldopam*, a short-acting selective dopamine-1 agonist, has equivalent efficacy compared to SNP in patients with hypertensive crises and enhances urinary sodium excretion [16]. A possible beneficial effect of fenoldopam on renal outcome has not been established. In healthy volunteers, fenoldopam decreases cerebral blood flow despite normalization of BP with phenylephrine, likely by constriction of cerebral arterioles [57]. Therefore, this drug may not be suitable for the management of patients with hypertensive encephalopathy.

6.5.6.3 Specific Conditions

In patients with hypertensive encephalopathy, antihypertensive treatment should be started immediately to lower BP in a controlled way to prevent further neurologic deterioration. Labetalol may be preferred in these patients because cerebral blood flow appears to be better preserved in patients receiving labetalol than in those receiving SNP [30]. Next to BP-lowering treatment, provoking factors (e.g., cytotoxic therapy) should be removed. In case of seizures (temporary) anticonvulsant therapy is reasonable, albeit not evidence-based, and will help lower BP [14]. If neurologic deterioration occurs during the initial BP-lowering phase the presence of an intracranial hemorrhage or ischemic stroke should be considered. In these cases, BP-lowering therapy may adversely affect neurologic outcome, and treatment should be withheld unless BP > 220/120 mm Hg or thrombolytic therapy is indicated [1]. Other causes for neurologic deterioration include cerebral hypoperfusion caused by (excessive) BP reduction, SNP toxicity, and obstructive hydrocephalus due to compression of the cerebral aqueduct as a result of edema (rare).

In patients with MHT and pulmonary edema, SNP is the drug of choice by its ability to immediately decrease ventricular preload and afterload. Nitroglycerin may be a good alternative, although dosages in excess of 200 μg/min may be required to achieve the desired BP-lowering effect. Compared to nitroglycerin, urapidil gives a better BP reduction and improvement of arterial oxygen content without reflex tachycardia. Concomitant administration of loop diuretics decreases volume overload and may further help lower BP.

In MHT, myocardial ischemia may develop as a result of an increase in myocardial oxygen demand associated with an increased afterload. The presence of left ventricular hypertrophy may further diminish coronary flow reserve [62]. In these patients, therapy should be aimed at lowering BP without causing reflex tachycardia because this will reduce diastolic filling time and increase myocardial oxygen demand. Both nitroglycerin or labetalol may safely reduce BP in patients with hypertension and myocardial ischemia [18, 48]. Additional beta blockade may be indicated for patients receiving nitroglycerin, especially if tachycardia is present.

In patients with MHT and acute renal failure, the goal is to lower BP without compromising renal perfusion. This is especially true for patients who also have evidence of TMA. Large BP reductions may further compromise renal blood flow to an already ischemic kidney; however, an insufficient BP reduction may lead to new thrombotic occlusions in the renal microcirculation. Close BP monitoring and a timely response to excessive BP reductions may prevent further renal deterioration. Although not evidence-based, patients presenting with MHT and renal failure may benefit from volume expansion as it will help maintain renal perfusion and will inhibit renin release. Both SNP and labetalol can be used safely for the initial BP-lowering phase without the need for dose adjustments. SNP has the advantage of inhibiting platelet aggregation, which may be beneficial in patients having TMA with renal failure. Patients with TMA and renal dysfunction may benefit from a slightly more vigorous BP reduction to stop ongoing intravascular hemolysis [6]. Patients with a scleroderma renal crisis may be treated with enalaprilat or given a combination of SNP or labetalol with a short-acting oral ACE inhibitor (e.g. captopril) [71]. The combination may be preferred to prevent sudden BP drops elicited by ACE-inhibitor therapy. Although patients with MHT may present with acute renal failure, immediate dialysis is rarely necessary. Fluid overload is rarely present because of previous sodium wasting, and potassium levels are often remarkably low given the degree of renal failure as a result of secondary hyperaldosteronism. If dialysis is needed, only excess fluid should be removed in the first few weeks. In this way, hypoperfusion of the kidney and stimulation of the renin-angiotensin system are avoided. In theory, patients with MHT and TMA might benefit from anticoagulant or antiinflammatory therapy next to BP-lowering treatment to help ameliorate ischemic renal damage. Currently, there is no evidence for a possible beneficial effect of such therapy on renal function.

In MHT associated with an adrenergic crises (e.g., cocaine intoxication and pheochromocytoma), phentolamine or phenoxybenzamine are the drugs of choice. Urapidil has been shown effective and safe in the perioperative management of pheochromocytoma and may alternatively be used [70]. Labetalol has been associated with hypertensive surges in some patients with pheochromocytoma. As the beta-blocking effect of labetalol is larger than its alpha-blocking effect, especially when administered intravenously, it is not the preferred drug for the management of an adrenergic crisis.

MHT may also develop in pregnancy with or without a secondary cause or previous hypertension. As with (pre)eclampsia, therapy should be aimed at lowering BP without harm to the fetus. Labetalol, ketanserin, and nicardipine can be safely used for the initial management. In patients with (pre)eclampsia, magnesium sulphate is the treatment of choice to prevent the evolution of seizures and encephalopathy [3]. Treatment with hydralazine is associated with poorer maternal and perinatal outcome compared with labetalol or nicardipine and may therefore not be the drug of choice for the treatment of preeclampsia [45]. SNP is relatively contraindicated because of the risk of maternal and fetal cyanide toxicity.

6.5.7 Take Home Pearls

- Malignant hypertension (MHT) is a hypertensive emergency characterized by acute ischemic complications and requires an immediate but controlled reduction of blood pressure to limit or prevent damage to the retina, kidney, and brain.

Abbreviations

HUS	Hemolytic uremic syndrome
ICAM	Intracellular adhesion molecule
VCAM	Vascular cell adhesion molecule
WHO	World Health Organization
ADH	Antidiuretic hormone
PGI2	Prostaglandin I2
ATII	Angiotensin II
FLAIR	Fluid attenuated inversion recovery
HELLP	Hemolysis-elevated liver enzymes low platelets
ACE	Angiotensin-converting enzyme
RBC	Red blood cell

References

1. Adams HP, Jr., del ZG, Alberts MJ, et al. (2007) Guidelines for the early management of adults with ischemic stroke. Stroke 38:1655–1711.
2. Ahearn DJ, Grim CE (1974) Treatment of malignant hypertension with sodium nitroprusside. Arch Intern Med 133:187–191.
3. Altman D, Carroli G, Duley L, et al. (2002) Do women with pre-eclampsia, and their babies, benefit from magnesium sulphate? The Magpie Trial: a randomised placebo-controlled trial. Lancet 359:1877–1890.
4. Baba T, Boku A, Ishizaki T, et al. (1986) Renal effects of nicardipine in patients with mild-to-moderate essential hypertension. Am Heart J 111:552–557.
5. Bakker RC, Verburgh CA, van Buchem MA, et al. (2003) Hypertension, cerebral oedema and fundoscopy. Nephrol Dial Transplant 18:2424–2427.
6. Beutler JJ, Koomans HA (1997) Malignant hypertension: still a challenge. Nephrol Dial Transplant 12:2019–2023.
7. Calhoun DA, Oparil S (1990) Treatment of hypertensive crises. N Engl J Med 323:1177–1183.
8. Chester EM, Agamanolis DP, Banker BQ, et al. (1978) Hypertensive encephalopathy: a clinicopathologic study of 20 cases. Neurology 28:928–939.
9. Chiariello M, Gold HK, Leinbach RC, et al. (1976) Comparison between the effects of nitroprusside and nitroglycerin on ischemic injury during acute myocardial infarction. Circulation 54:766–773.
10. Cottrell JE, Patel K, Turndorf H, et al. (1978) Intracranial pressure changes induced by sodium nitroprusside in patients with intracranial mass lesions. J Neurosurg 48:329–331.
11. Cowley AW, Jr., Lohmeier TE (1979) Changes in renal vascular sensitivity and arterial pressure associated with sodium intake during long-term intrarenal norepinephrine infusion in dogs. Hypertension 1:549–558.
12. Damasceno A, Ferreira B, Patel S, et al. (1997) Efficacy of captopril and nifedipine in black and white patients with hypertensive crisis. J Hum Hypertens 11:471–476.
13. de Leeuw PW, van Es PN, de Bruyn HA, et al. (1988) Renal haemodynamic and neurohumoral responses to urapidil in hypertensive man. Drugs 35(Suppl 6):74–77.

14. Delanty N, Vaughan CJ, French JA (1998) Medical causes of seizures. Lancet 352:383–390.
15. Edvinsson L, Owman C, Sjoberg NO (1976) Autonomic nerves, mast cells, and amine receptors in human brain vessels. A histochemical and pharmacological study. Brain Res 115:377–393.
16. Elliott WJ, Weber RR, Nelson KS, et al. (1990) Renal and hemodynamic effects of intravenous fenoldopam versus nitroprusside in severe hypertension. Circulation 81:970–977.
17. Finnerty FA, Jr. (1972) Hypertensive encephalopathy. Am J Med 52:672–678.
18. Frishman WH, Strom JA, Kirschner M, et al. (1981) Labetalol therapy in patients with systemic hypertension and angina pectoris: effects of combined alpha and beta adrenoceptor blockade. Am J Cardiol 48:917–928.
19. Gavras H, Brunner HR, Laragh JH, et al. (1975) Malignant hypertension resulting from deoxycorticosterone acetate and salt excess: role of renin and sodium in vascular changes. Circ Res 36:300–309.
20. Griswold WR, Viney J, Mendoza SA, et al. (1981) Intracranial pressure monitoring in severe hypertensive encephalopathy. Crit Care Med 9:573–576.
21. Haas DC, Streeten DH, Kim RC, et al. (1983) Death from cerebral hypoperfusion during nitroprusside treatment of acute angiotensin-dependent hypertension. Am J Med 75:1071–1076.
22. Haubrich C, Wendt A, Diehl RR, et al. (2004) Dynamic autoregulation testing in the posterior cerebral artery. Stroke 35:848–852.
23. Hinchey J, Chaves C, Appignani B, et al. (1996) A reversible posterior leukoencephalopathy syndrome. N Engl J Med 334:494–500.
24. Hirschl MM, Binder M, Bur A, et al. (1997) Safety and efficacy of urapidil and sodium nitroprusside in the treatment of hypertensive emergencies. Intensive Care Med 23:885–888.
25. Hirschl MM, Binder M, Bur A, et al. (1997) Impact of the renin-angiotensin-aldosterone system on blood pressure response to intravenous enalaprilat in patients with hypertensive crises. J Hum Hypertens 11:177–183.
26. Hirschl MM, Seidler D, Zeiner A, et al. (1993) Intravenous urapidil versus sublingual nifedipine in the treatment of hypertensive urgencies. Am J Emerg Med 11:653–656.
27. Hollenberg NK, Epstein M, Basch RI, et al. (1969) Renin secretion in essential and accelerated hypertension. Am J Med 47:855–859.
28. Houston P, Dickson MC, Ludbrook V, et al. (1999) Fluid shear stress induction of the tissue factor promoter in vitro and in vivo is mediated by Egr-1. Arterioscler Thromb Vasc Biol 19:281–289.
29. Ideishi M, Kishikawa K, Kinoshita A, et al. (1990) High-renin malignant hypertension secondary to an aldosterone-producing adenoma. Nephron 54:259–263.
30. Immink RV, van den Born BJ, van Montfrans GA, et al. (2008) Cerebral and systemic hemodynamics during treatment with sodium nitroprusside and labetalol in malignant hypertension. Hypertension 52:236–240.
31. Immink RV, van den Born BJ, van Montfrans GA, et al. (2004) Impaired cerebral autoregulation in patients with malignant hypertension. Circulation 110:2241–2245.
32. Isles CG (1994) Malignant hypertension and hypertensive encephalopathy. In: Swales JD (ed) *Textbook of Hypertension*. Oxford: Blackwell.
33. Isles CG, McLay A, Jones JM (1984) Recovery in malignant hypertension presenting as acute renal failure. Quart J Med 53:439–452.
34. Ivankovich AD, Braverman B, Stephens TS, et al. (1983) Sodium thiosulfate disposition in humans: relation to sodium nitroprusside toxicity. Anesthesiology 58:11–17.
35. Jhetam D, Dansey R, Morar C, et al. (1982) The malignant phase of essential hypertension in Johannesburg Blacks. A prospective study. S Afr Med J 61:899–902.
36. Jones DB (1974) Arterial and glomerular lesions associated with severe hypertension. Light and electron microscopic studies. Lab Invest 31:303–313.
37. Kaloyanides GJ, DiBona GF (1976) Effect of an angiotensin II antagonist on autoregulation in the isolated dog kidney. Am J Physiol 230:1078–1083.
38. Kincaid-Smith P, McMichael J, Murphy EA (1958) The clinical course and pathology of hypertension with papilloedema (malignant hypertension). Quart J Med 27: 117–153.
39. Ledingham JG, Rajagopalan B (1979) Cerebral complications in the treatment of accelerated hypertension. Quart J Med 48:25–41.
40. Lim KG, Isles CG, Hodsman GP, et al. (1987) Malignant hypertension in women of childbearing age and its relation to the contraceptive pill. Br Med J (Clin Res Ed) 294: 1057–1059.
41. Linton AL, Gavras H, Gleadle RI, et al. (1969) Microangiopathic haemolytic anaemia and the pathogenesis of malignant hypertension. Lancet 1:1277–1282.
42. Lip GY, Beevers M, Beevers G (1994) The failure of malignant hypertension to decline: a survey of 24 years' experience in a multiracial population in England. J Hypertens 12:1297–1305.
43. Lohmeier TE, Cowley AW, Jr. (1979) Hypertensive and renal effects of chronic low level intrarenal angiotensin infusion in the dog. Circ Res 44:154–160.
44. Lohmeier TE, Tillman LJ, Carroll RG, et al. (1984) Malignant hypertensive crisis induced by chronic intrarenal norepinephrine infusion. Hypertension 6:I177–I182.
45. Magee LA, Cham C, Waterman EJ, et al. (2003) Hydralazine for treatment of severe hypertension in pregnancy: meta-analysis. BMJ 327:955–960.
46. Mak W, Chan KH, Cheung RT, et al. (2004) Hypertensive encephalopathy: BP lowering complicated by posterior circulation ischemic stroke. Neurology 63:1131–1132.
47. Mamdani BH, Lim VS, Mahurkar SD, et al. (1974) Recovery from prolonged renal failure in patients with accelerated hypertension. N Engl J Med 291:1343–1344.
48. Mann T, Cohn PF, Holman LB, et al. (1978) Effect of nitroprusside on regional myocardial blood flow in coronary artery disease. Results in 25 patients and comparison with nitroglycerin. Circulation 57:732–738.
49. Mattson DL, Lu S, Roman RJ, et al. (1993) Relationship between renal perfusion pressure and blood flow in different regions of the kidney. Am J Physiol 264:R578–R583.
50. McLaren KM, MacDonald MK (1983) Histological and ultrastructural studies of the human juxtaglomerular apparatus in benign and malignant hypertension. J Pathol 139:41–55.
51. Mervaala EM, Muller DN, Park JK, et al. (1999) Monocyte infiltration and adhesion molecules in a rat model of high human renin hypertension. Hypertension 33:389–395.

52. Mohring J, Petri M, Szokol M, et al. (1976) Effects of saline drinking on malignant course of renal hypertension in rats. Am J Physiol 230:849–857.
53. Muller DN, Dechend R, Mervaala EM, et al. (2000) NF-kappaB inhibition ameliorates angiotensin II-induced inflammatory damage in rats. Hypertension 35:193–201.
54. Munoz-Ramirez H, Chatelain RE, Bumpus FM, et al. (1980) Development of two-kidney Goldblatt hypertension in rats under dietary sodium restriction. Am J Physiol 238:H889–H894.
55. Neutel JM, Smith DH, Wallin D, et al. (1994) A comparison of intravenous nicardipine and sodium nitroprusside in the immediate treatment of severe hypertension. Am J Hypertens 7:623–628.
56. Petitti DB, Klatsky AL (1983) Malignant hypertension in women aged 15 to 44 years and its relation to cigarette smoking and oral contraceptives. Am J Cardiol 52:297–298.
57. Prielipp RC, Wall MH, Groban L, et al. (2001) Reduced regional and global cerebral blood flow during fenoldopam-induced hypotension in volunteers. Anesth Analg 93:45–52.
58. Rindone JP, Sloane EP (1992) Cyanide toxicity from sodium nitroprusside: risks and management. Ann Pharmacother 26:515–519.
59. Roman RJ, Cowley AW, Jr., Garcia-Estan J, et al. (1988) Pressure-diuresis in volume-expanded rats. Cortical and medullary hemodynamics. Hypertension 12:168–176.
60. Rosei EA, Trust PM, Brown JJ, et al. (1975) Letter: Intravenous labetalol in severe hypertension. Lancet 2:1093–1094.
61. Sanerkin NG (1971) Vascular lesions of malignant essential hypertension. J Pathol 103:177–184.
62. Scheler S, Motz W, Strauer BE (1994) Mechanism of angina pectoris in patients with systemic hypertension and normal epicardial coronary arteries by arteriogram. Am J Cardiol 73:478–482.
63. Schulz V, Gross R, Pasch T, et al. (1982) Cyanide toxicity of sodium nitroprusside in therapeutic use with and without sodium thiosulphate. Klin Wochenschr 60:1393–1400.
64. Schwartz RB, Jones KM, Kalina P, et al. (1992) Hypertensive encephalopathy: findings on CT, MR imaging, and SPECT imaging in 14 cases. AJR Am J Roentgenol 159:379–383.
65. Singbartl G, Metzger G (1990) Urapidil-induced increase of the intracranial pressure in head-trauma patients. Intensive Care Med 16:272–274.
66. Smith RP, Kruszyna H (1974) Nitroprusside produces cyanide poisoning via reaction with hemoglobin. J Pharmacol Exp Ther 191:557–563.
67. Solomons R (1979) Hemiparesis after single minibolus of labetalol for hypertensive encephalopathy. Br Med J 2:672.
68. Strandgaard S, Olesen J, Skinhoj E, et al. (1973) Autoregulation of brain circulation in severe arterial hypertension. Br Med J 1:507–510.
69. Sventek P, Li JS, Grove K, et al. (1996) Vascular structure and expression of endothelin-1 gene in L-NAME-treated spontaneously hypertensive rats. Hypertension 27:49–55.
70. Tauzin-Fin P, Sesay M, Gosse P, et al. (2004) Effects of perioperative alpha1 block on haemodynamic control during laparoscopic surgery for phaeochromocytoma. Br J Anaesth 92:512–517.
71. Thurm RH, Alexander JC (1984) Captopril in the treatment of scleroderma renal crisis. Arch Intern Med 144:733–735.
72. Tzima E, Irani-Tehrani M, Kiosses WB, et al. (2005) A mechanosensory complex that mediates the endothelial cell response to fluid shear stress. Nature 437:426–431.
73. van den Born BJ, Honnebier UP, Koopmans RP, et al. (2005) Microangiopathic hemolysis and renal failure in malignant hypertension. Hypertension 45:246–251.
74. van den Born BJ, Koopmans RP, Groeneveld JO, et al. (2006) Ethnic disparities in the incidence, presentation and complications of malignant hypertension. J Hypertens 24:2299–2304.
75. van den Born BJ, Koopmans RP, van Montfrans GA (2007) The renin-angiotensin system in malignant hypertension revisited: plasma renin activity, microangiopathic hemolysis, and renal failure in malignant hypertension. Am J Hypertens 20:900–906.
76. van den Born BJ, van der Hoeven NV, Groot E, et al. (2008) Association between thrombotic microangiopathy and reduced ADAMTS13 activity in malignant hypertension. Hypertension 51:862–866.
77. van der Stroom JG, van Wezel HB, Langemeijer JJ, et al. (1997) A randomized multicenter double-blind comparison of urapidil and ketanserin in hypertensive patients after coronary artery surgery. J Cardiothorac Vasc Anesth 11:729–736.
78. Vaughan CJ, Delanty N (2000) Hypertensive emergencies. Lancet 356:411–417.
79. Verhaar MC, Beutler JJ, Gaillard CA, et al. (1998) Progressive vascular damage in hypertension is associated with increased levels of circulating P-selectin. J Hypertens 16:45–50.
80. Wilson C, Byrom FB (1939) Renal changes in malignant hypertension. Lancet I:136–139.
81. Wilson DJ, Wallin JD, Vlachakis ND, et al. (1983) Intravenous labetalol in the treatment of severe hypertension and hypertensive emergencies. Am J Med 75:95–102.
82. Woisetschlager C, Bur A, Vlcek M, et al. (2006) Comparison of intravenous urapidil and oral captopril in patients with hypertensive urgencies. J Hum Hypertens 20:707–709.

Toxic Nephropathy Due to Drugs and Poisons

6.6

Pieter Evenepoel

Core Messages

- Drug-induced acute renal failure (ARF) is increasingly encountered, especially in hospitalized patients as a result of a more aggressive diagnostic and therapeutic measures in an ageing and multimedicated patient population that is increasingly vulnerable.
- Potentially nephrotoxic drugs include nonsteroidal antiinflammatory drugs, radiocontrast agents, antimicrobial, and anesthetic agents.
- Endogenous compounds such as myoglobin and hemoglobin may also cause toxic nephropathy.
- Tubular injury initiated by toxins often results from a combination of acute renal vasoconstriction and direct cellular toxicity due to intracellular accumulation of the toxin, or, alternatively, may be mediated immunologically in case of interstitial nephritis.
- Patients with reduced renal functional reserve, cardiovascular comorbidity, diabetes mellitus, and advanced age are at increased risk.
- Awareness of the range of toxins on the one hand, and simple measures such as adequate prehydration of the patient and drug monitoring, on the other hand, may be sufficient to avoid drug-induced ARF or minimize its clinical severity in susceptible patients.

6.6.1 Introduction

Acute renal failure (ARF) is a syndrome characterized by a sudden decrease in the glomerular filtration rate (GFR) accompanied by azotemia. More than 30 definitions of ARF exist in literature. This lack of standardized definition has made comparative assessment difficult. Efforts, such as the Acute Dialysis Quality Initiative, are being undertaken to establish a consensus definition of ARF, and to distinguish between varying degrees of acute kidney injury. The reported frequency of ARF among all patients at the time of admission to hospital has been estimated at 1%, however, an estimated 2–5% of total admissions subsequently develop hospital-acquired ARF. Recent epidemiologic data show an increasing incidence rate of ARF over the years [1]. Surgical patients are particularly predisposed to ARF due to the physiologic insult induced by major surgical procedures, preexistent comorbidity, and sepsis [2–4]. Other risk factors include a reduced renal functional reserve, arterial hypertension, cardiac or peripheral vascular disease, diabetes mellitus, jaundice, and advanced age [5–8].

Mortality from ARF varies from 20% to 90% depending on the definition of ARF, the patient population, and the type of surgery [9]. In a recent study, the overall in-hospital death rate for the period 1992 to 2001 was 15.2% in discharges with ARF coded as the principal diagnosis, 32.6% in discharges with ARF as a secondary diagnosis, and 4.6% in discharges without ARF. In-hospital death rate was 32.9% in discharges with ARF that required dialysis and 27.5% in those with ARF that did not require dialysis. In-hospital death rate declined from 1992 to 2001 [1]. In addition to effects on patient mortality, ARF prolongs hospitalization by an average of 10 days [10]. In those who survive,

P. Evenepoel
Department of Nephrology, University Hospital Gasthuisberg, Herestraat 49, 3000 Leuven, Belgium
e-mail: Pieter.evenepoel@uz.kuleuven.ac.be

A. Jörres et al. (eds.), *Management of Acute Kidney Problems*,
DOI: 10.1007/978-3-540-69441-0_6.6, © Springer-Verlag Berlin Heidelberg 2010

the prognosis remains poor with need for maintenance dialysis treatment in as much as 16.6% [11]. Last but not least, treating ARF is expensive.

Community-based statistics estimate the incidence of ARF attributed to drug nephrotoxicity as between 0 and 7% [12, 13] and the incidence of in-hospital drug-induced ARF at about 20% of all ARF [6, 14, 15]. Drug-induced acute renal failure is encountered in a growing number of (hospitalized) patients as a result of a more aggressive diagnostic and therapeutic approach in an ageing and multimedicated patient population that is increasingly vulnerable (increased comorbidity, etc.). Drug–drug interactions may result in increased toxicity. The mechanisms involved are an increase in blood and/or tissue half-life of the nephrotoxic drug (through interference with its metabolism and/or elimination) and/or an additive nephrotoxicity. The kidney is extremely susceptible to drug-induced toxicity because of its high blood flow (approximately 25% of the resting cardiac output), its capacity to concentrate drugs to levels considerably exceeding those in blood, and its ability to degrade drugs, often resulting in the formation of reactive metabolites. Common risk factors are summarized in Table 6.6.1.

The purpose of this article is to summarize current knowledge on toxic ARF. Before discussing nephrotoxins that are relevant in the intensive care and emergency unit, the most important pathophysiologic mechanisms of drug-induced nephrotoxicity will be rehearsed. These include altered renal hemodynamics, immunologic damage, tubular toxicity, vascular toxicity, tubular obstruction, and osmotic nephrosis (Table 6.6.2) [16]. Knowledge of the pathophysiologic mechanism underlying the drug toxicity is a prerequisite to understanding risk factors and clinical presentation, and provides a rationale for the preventive and therapeutic measures that have to be taken.

Table 6.6.1 Common risk factors for acute toxic renal failure

Risk factors for acute toxic renal failure
Pretreatment renal function impairment
Older age
Cardiovascular disease
Diabetes mellitus
Reduced effective arterial volume
Jaundice
Concomitant use of several potentially nephrotoxic agents

Table 6.6.2 Common nephrotoxic agent leading to acute renal failure, categorized according to underlying pathophysiologic mechanism (alphabetical order)

Altered renal hemodynamics
ACEI or ARB
Calcineurin inhibitors
Cocaine
NSAIDs
Norepinephrine
Radiocontrast agents
Acute tubular necrosis
Amphotericin
Aminoglycoside
Cisoplatinum
Foscarnet
Heavy metals
Herbal remedies
Herbicides (paraquat)
Ifosfamide
Intravenous immunoglobulin
Organic solvents
Pentamidine
Radiocontrast agents
Tenofovir, cidofovir, adenofovir
Acute interstitial nephritis
Allopurinol
Antibiotics (penicillins, cephalopsporins, rifampicin, sulfamethoxazole, ciprofloxacin)
Cimetidine
Diuretics
Mesalazine
NSAIDs
Phenytoin
Proton pump inhibitors
Vasculopathy
Calcineurin inhibitor
Clodiprogel
Mitomycin C
Oral contraceptives
Quinine
Obstructive tubulopathy (crystal formation)
Acyclovir
Ethylene glycol
Indinavir
Methotrexate
Sulfonamide antibiotic
Triamterene
Glomerular disease (rapidly progressive glomerulonephritis)
D-Penicillamine
Hydralazine
Organic solvents
Propylthiouracil

ACEI: angiotensin-converting enzyme inhibitor; ARB: angiotensin II receptor blocker; NSAID: nonsteroidal antiinflammatory drug

6.6.2 Pathophysiologic Mechanisms

6.6.2.1 Altered Renal Hemodynamics

In normal circumstances, several mechanisms operate to maintain GFR and renal blood flow at an optimal, stable level, the most important being renal autoregulation by intrinsic mechanisms. However, in situations of decreased renal perfusion pressure (e.g., depleted 'true' or 'effective' circulatory volume) hormonal mechanisms come into action, of which the renin-angiotensin and renal prostaglandin systems are the most important. Angiotensin II causes predominantly vasoconstriction of the efferent arteriole, thus preserving GFR in case of lowered renal blood flow, whereas prostaglandins act as vasodilators of the afferent arteriole. In view of the above-mentioned regulatory functions, it is not surprising that drugs that interfere with either hormonal system can have an in important influence on renal function. These include the nonsteroidal antiinflammatory drugs, angiotensin-converting enzyme inhibitors and angiotensin II receptor antagonists, and calcineurin inhibitors. Hemodynamic-mediated (or functional) renal dysfunction is characterized by a rather abrupt decline of the GFR in the absence of proteinuria and abnormalities of the urinary sediment. After discontinuation of the offending drug and restoration of the effective circulatory volume, the renal failure usually can be reversed quickly. If the reduction of renal blood flow and GFR is more profound and sustained, however, ischemic ATN may ensue.

6.6.2.2 Acute Tubular Necrosis

A substantial body of evidence attests to the involvement of reactive oxygen species (ROS) in the pathogenesis of nephrotoxic acute tubular necrosis (ATN), including heme protein–induced ATN as occurs in severe rhabdomyolysis and hemolysis, and drug-induced ATN [17–20]. ROS commonly incriminated in the pathogenesis of renal and other forms of tissue injury include the superoxide anion (O_2-), hydrogen peroxide (H_2O_2), hypochlorous acid (HOCl), and the hydroxyl radical (OH). Possible sources of ROS include increased xanthine and NADH/NADPH oxidase activity, and disabled mitochondrial respiration. Irons salts play a catalytic role in the generation of the highly reactive hydroxyl radical through the metal-catalyzed Haber-Weiss-Fenton reaction. Oxidative stress is the result of enhanced generation of ROS and/or deficient neutralization by antioxidant defenses such as superoxide dismutase, catalase, and glutathione peroxidase.

The basic constituents of cells and their organelles – lipids, carbohydrates, proteins, and nucleic acids – can all be altered by ROS. Such oxidant-induced alterations can profoundly affect cellular function and viability. ROS, in addition, exert a variety of vasoactive effects, depending on the specific ROS, its rate of generation, and the vascular bed to which it is exposed. Oxidative stress, furthermore, can provoke inflammatory responses, which are increasingly believed to be critical participants in the pathogenesis of ATN. Finally, ROS may not only contribute to the pathogenesis of ATN, but, surprisingly, may also be involved in the reparative and regenerative events that nurse the kidney with ATN back to normality. Such considerations, as yet largely unexplored, raise the cautionary note that antioxidant strategies may not necessarily be beneficial when introduced after ATN is already established [17].

6.6.2.3 Allergic Interstitial Nephritis

Acute interstitial nephritis (AIN) was formerly related to a variety of infections, but is now increasingly associated with drug therapy [21]. Although many drugs have been implicated in clinical cases of AIN, the frequency with which individual drugs are implicated varies widely. The prototype agent for drug-induced AIN is methicillin. As a result of its propensity to cause AIN (up to 17% of patients who have been treated for more than 10 days), it is rarely used anymore in clinical practice. The number of drugs associated with AIN exceeds 50, and is still increasing. Medication groups most commonly implicated in drug-induced AIN include penicillins, cephalosporins, sulfonamides and NSAIDs [21–23]. Acute interstitial nephritis usually occurs on an allergic basis in a idiosyncratic and non-dose-dependent manner. The pathogenesis of the majority of cases involves a cell-mediated hypersensitivity reaction. This is supported by the observation that T cells are the predominant cell type comprising the interstitial infiltrate. A humoral response underlies rare cases of AIN in which a portion of a drug (i.e., methicillin) may act as a hapten, bind to the tubular basement membrane (TBM), and elicit anti-TBM antibodies [24]. Patients with AIN typically present with the following findings: an acute rise in the plasma creatinine temporally related to an offending drug; a urine sediment that reveals white cells, red cells, and white cell casts; normal or only mildly increased protein excretion; and signs of tubulointerstitial damage. The full picture of an allergic reaction (fever, rash, eosinophilia, and eosinophiluria) is not always present [21]. The mainstay of treatment of AIN is supportive therapy. AIN is usually self-limiting, and spontaneous recovery occurs after withdrawal of the offending drug. In patients in whom drug discontinuation does not produce improvement in renal function, the diagnosis of AIN should be confirmed by renal biopsy, and steroids should be considered [23, 25]. In general, if drug-induced AIN is detected early, and the offending drug is promptly discontinued, the long-term outcome is favorable with a return to baseline serum creatinine values [21, 22].

6.6.2.4 Vasculopathy

An variety of drugs including antineoplastics, immunotherapeutics, and antiplatelet agents have been associated with thrombotic microangiopathy (TMA). In many instances, it is difficult to separate the effect of the drug from the role of the underlying disorder (e.g., cancer). Although a direct causal effect has usually not been proven, the cumulative evidence linking several drugs with TMA is strong. Basic scientific discoveries in the late 1990s suggest that the probable mechanisms by which these agents lead to a TMA include either an immune-mediated phenomenon involving the ADAMTS13 metalloprotease (quinine/quinidine, ticlopidine, and clopidogrel) or direct endothelial toxicity (mitomycin C and calcineurin inhibitor) [26–28].

6.6.2.5 Obstructive Tubulopathy

Several mediations, notably acyclovir, sulfonamides, methotrexate, indinavir, foscarnet, ciprofloxacine, and triamterene, are associated with the production of crystals that are insoluble in human urine [19, 29]. Intratubular precipitation of these crystals can lead to ARF through obstructive tubulopathy. Many patients who require treatment with these medications have additional risk factors, such as true or effective intravascular volume depletion, underlying renal insufficiency, and metabolic perturbation (acidosis and electrolyte depletion), that increase the likelihood of drug-induced intrarenal crystal deposition [19, 30]. The occurrence of crystal toxicity is moreover related to the dosage and infusion rate of the drug. Major preventive measures include adequate (pre)hydration and induction of high urinary flow rates (100–150 ml/h), dose adjustment for renal function, and slowing down the infusion rate. Oliguric ARF typically occurs within a few days of treatment and may be associated with abdominal or loin pain. Management of established renal insufficiency includes volume repletion, alkalinization of the urine, dialytic support if necessary, adjustment of drug doses, and avoidance of further exposure to nephrotoxins [30]. There is no evidence that gancyclovir provokes crystalluria.

6.6.2.6 Osmotic Nephrosis

Osmotic nephrosis describes a morphologic pattern with vacuolization and swelling of the renal proximal tubular cells. The term refers to a nonspecific histopathologic finding rather than defining a specific entity [31, 32]. Reports of osmotic nephrosis in the literature are rare compared with the frequency of use of causative agents (sucrose, mannitol, intravenous immunoglobulin, radiocontrast agents, dextran, and hydroxethyl starch). There might, however, be a significant bias. Indeed, in a series of 251 autopsies, Janssen observed significant osmotic nephrosis in 69 cases (27%) [33]. Thus, osmotic nephrosis, regardless of whether it is clinically relevant, might be a more common event than generally realized. Patients with preexisting kidney disease are at greatest risk because of their decreased ability to degrade and excrete the causative agent. Cellular injury begins with the uptake of nonmetabolizable molecules by pinocytosis into proximal tubule cells. Osmotic nephrosis can be accompanied by renal impairment, and intermittent renal replacement therapy may be necessary in up to 40% of patients. Urinalysis may show tubular proteinuria or characteristic vacuolated tubular cells. Osmotic nephrosis usually is reversible, and functional and structural recovery takes place after discontinuation of the agent. However, persistent chronic or even end-stage renal disease has occurred in rare cases of preexisting severe kidney disease. To prevent osmotic nephrosis, preparations with a low concentration of the therapeutic agents and slow infusion rates are advocated. A stable hemodynamic situation and sufficient hydration before the start of therapy are recommended as well.

6.6.3 Common Nephrotoxins

6.6.3.1 Aminoglycoside Antibiotics

Aminoglycoside antibiotics, despite their nephrotoxicity, continue to be a mainstay in the clinical management of gram-negative infections. Gram-negative organisms account for the majority of hospital-acquired infections, and the occurrence of aminoglycoside-induced ARF remains commonplace. The incidence of ARF with aminoglycoside therapy varies with the definition used, but ranges from 5% to 25% [34, 35]. ATN is the most frequent mechanism of toxicity, but different patterns of tubular dysfunction have been described as well. The ATN is largely confined to the proximal convoluted tubule and pars recta. After being filtered and taken up by the proximal renal tubular cell, aminoglycosides reside in a poorly exchangeable pool and can reach concentrations up to 1,000 times their serum concentration; they therefore have prolonged tissue half-lives. This prolonged storage accounts for the observation that renal failure may become clinically apparent as late as several days after the drug has been discontinued [34]. The precise mechanism(s) of aminoglycoside-induced ATN remains largely unknown. Aminoglycosides cause phospholipid accumulation in the proximal tubular cells and induce alterations at the basolateral membrane and mitochondria. Reactive oxygen metabolites are increasingly acknowledged to mediate the tubular toxicity of aminoglycosides [18]. Recent evidence indicates that aminoglycosides besides causing tubular toxicity may also affect glomerular function directly [35].

Aminoglycoside nephrotoxicity typically is associated with nonoliguric renal failure. Decline in GFR and elevations of serum creatinine usually are not apparent until after 5–10 days of aminoglycoside treatment. The urine sediment is benign or shows granular and epithelial cell casts [36]. A variety of risk factors have been identified that increase the risk of aminoglycoside nephrotoxicity including the dose and duration of drug treatment, preexisting renal insufficiency or liver disease, elderly age, volume depletion and sepsis, potassium and magnesium depletion [34]. The nephrotoxic effects of aminoglycosides may be potentiated when they are associated with diuretics, calcineurin inhibitors (CNIs), vancomycin, amphotericin B, nonsteroidal antiinflammatory drugs (NSAIDs), angiotensin-converting enzyme inhibitors (ACEIs), or angiotensin II receptor blockers (ARBs) [37–39]. There is some evidence that divided dose regimens are more likely to produce toxicity than once-daily regimens [40]. Amikacin, containing fewer amino groups per molecule, may be less nephrotoxic as compared with gentamycin, tobramycin, and netilmicin. During treatment with aminoglycosides, every effort should be made to avoid those factors that provoke toxicity. Dose recommendations must be followed and serum drug levels should be carefully monitored. In patients with established aminoglycoside-induced ATN, the plasma creatinine concentration usually returns to the prior baseline level within 21 days after cessation of the aminoglycoside therapy [34]. Irreversible damage, however, may occur, especially with prolonged therapy, even with low doses [41].

6.6.3.2 Amphotericin B

Invasive aspergillosis and disseminated candidiasis are the two major manifestations of opportunistic invasive mycoses. Their incidence has risen considerably during the past decades, due to more intensive anticancer chemotherapy, organ transplants, intensive care, and aggressive surgical interventions [42].

The therapeutic options for these infections are limited. Flucytosine is associated with adverse effects and drug resistance. Fluconazole and itraconazole are safer, though emergence of resistance and innate resistance in some fungal pathogens is a concern for their use. Amphotericin B therefore continues to be the treatment of choice in many cases of severe disseminated mycosis. A common complication of amphotericin B therapy is renal dysfunction, occurring in 5–80% of cases [43, 44]. The clinical manifestations include renal insufficiency and various electrolyte disorders (hypokalemia, hypomagnesemia, renal tubular acidosis, and nephrogenic diabetes insipidus), related to tubular dysfunction. The mechanism by which renal insufficiency occurs is incompletely understood. Amphotericin B may induce changes in renal hemodynamics. By changing vascular smooth muscle cell permeability, amphotericin B may lead to cell depolarization with the resultant opening of voltage-dependent calcium channels and muscle contraction. Increased intracellular calcium concentration may activate arachidonic acid metabolism and lead to the accumulation of vasoactive substances with net vasoconstrictive effect. Renal vasoconstriction and recurrent ischemia may lead to structural and tubular damage and permanent nephrotoxic effects [43]. Increased membrane permeability moreover leads to increased Na^+,K^+-ATPase activity and depletion of cellular energy stores. Additionally, the standard amphotericin B formulation is suspended in the bile salt deoxycholate, which has a detergent effect on cell membranes [44]. Risk factors for amphotericin B–associated nephrotoxicity include total accumulated dose (nephrotoxicity usually occurs after administration of 2–3 g), duration of therapy, dehydration and diuretic use, abnormal baseline renal function, and association with other nephrotoxins [45, 46]. Slow recovery of renal function follows drug withdrawal, but recovery is often incomplete; magnesium wasting, in particular, may be chronic. Studies in humans and animals have shown that salt loading can protect against or ameliorate amphotericin B–induced renal dysfunction [5, 43]. In addition, the severity and incidence of nephrotoxicity can be minimized by administering lipid formulations of amphotericin B [44, 47]. Three lipid formulations of amphotericin B have been developed: amphotericin B colloidal dispersion, amphotericin B lipid complex, and liposomal amphotericin B. These three compounds differ by their lipid composition and therefore by their physical characteristics, their pharmacokinetics, and their safety and efficacy profile [48]. Several mechanisms may contribute to the reduced nephrotoxicity of lipid formulations of amphotericin B, including absence of deoxycholate and preferential distribution to the reticuloendothelial system, where amphotericin B can be transferred directly to trapped fungi, thereby diminishing the delivery to other cholesterol-containing cells such as those in the kidney [49].

Finally, recent literature indicates that the ecchinocandins, a novel class of antifungal agents, may represent a valuable alternative in patients with amphotericin B–induced renal function impairment or in patients at increased risk [50]. It should however be stressed that ecchinocandins are not active against *Cryptococcus neoformans*.

6.6.3.3 Angiotensin-Converting Enzyme Inhibitors and Angiotensin II Receptor Blockers

It has been demonstrated that patients chronically treated with ACEI have an increased risk of postoperative renal dysfunction [54], most probably as a consequence of intraoperative hypotensive episodes [55, 56]. These hypotensive episodes often do not respond to sympathicomimetic agents and as such may require vasopressin receptor agonists. The risks of postoperative renal dysfunctions should at all time be weighed against the benefits of continuing ACEI and ARB in maintaining control of hypertension and/or preventing exacerbation of congestive heart failure [57].

6.6.3.4 Calcineurin Inhibitors

CNIs may cause an acute, functional, and dose-dependent decrease in renal blood flow and GFR. The current hypothesis is that CNIs cause predominantly afferent arteriolar vasoconstriction and thereby alter renal hemodynamics. The vasoconstriction is in part related to an imbalance of prostaglandin E2 (vasodilation) and thromboxane A2 (vasoconstriction). In addition, cyclosporine may interfere with the production of nitric oxide and increase systemic vascular resistance with activation of the sympathetic nervous system. Following discontinuation of CNI, renal function returns to baseline without any major histologic or cytologic abnormalities. However, prolonged vasoconstriction may cause ATN and lead to tubulointerstitial lesions consistent with chronic and irreversible nephrotoxicity [58]. One should be aware that drugs that inhibit cytochrome P450 isoenzyme CYP3A4 may cause kidney injury by enhancing the serum levels of CNI (drug–drug interactions).

6.6.3.5 Colloids

Absolute and relative blood volume deficits often occur in patients undergoing surgery and in the intensive care unit. The preoperative medical status of the patient, medication, anesthesia, surgical trauma, and inflammatory reactions may all alter intravascular volume status. Appropriate intravascular volume replacement is a fundamental component of critical care management because failure to treat hypovolemia may lead to multiple organ dysfunction syndrome or death. There is controversy as to whether crystalloids or colloids are preferred for intravascular volume replacement. Because colloids with different physiochemical characteristics are now available in several countries, a debate around the optimal type of colloid has now been added to the already existing crystalloid versus colloid fluid replacement controversy [59]

Information on the influence of the different colloids (human albumin, dextran, gelatin, or different hydroxyethyl starch [HES] solutions) on renal function is fairly incomplete. All colloids, including hyperoncotic human albumin, may cause osmotic nephrosis and thus induce ARF. Of all colloids, albumin and gelatin seem to have the lowest risk profile as far as renal dysfunction is concerned. Multiple HES solutions are available and differ in their molecular weight and degree of substitution (hydroxyethylations at carbon position C2, C3, C6) [32, 60]. These characteristics determine the toxicity profile as they affect the time to elimination from the intravascular space and the degree of macromolecule accumulation [60]. Studies comparing the renal toxicity of gelatine and HES have provided conflicting results. In patients with severe sepsis, the use of HES 200/0.6 was associated with a significantly increased risk of ARF as compared with gelatin [61]. Conversely, similar (limited) alterations in renal function and structural cell injury were observed in elderly patients undergoing cardiac surgery treated with either HES 130/0.4 or gelatin [62]. The use of different HES preparations with different toxicity profiles may explain at least partly this controversy. It is probably wise to employ low-molecular-weight HES with low degree of substitution (e.g., HES 130/0.4) and to administer doses below their recommended upper limit (50 ml/kg/day) in at risk patients.

6.6.3.6 Ethylene Glycol

Ethylene glycol found in antifreeze, remains a cause of both accidental and deliberate injury. It is rapidly metabolized by alcohol dehydrogenase to glycoaldehyde and glyoxylate, which are toxic to tubular cells. Further metabolism generates oxalic acid, which can precipitate in renal tubules, leading to intratubular obstruction. Symptoms and signs associated with ethylene glycol poisoning include a severe anion gap metabolic acidosis, a serum osmolal gap, and crystalluria. Rapid decision-making is critical in the management of the patient poisoned with methanol or ethylene glycol. The clinician must often make treatment decisions without definitive serum drug levels, based only upon clinical suspicion and readily available laboratory data. Management includes inhibition of alcohol dehydrogenase with intravenous ethanol or the specific alcohol dehydrogenase inhibitor fomepizole [63]. Hemodialysis should be performed to remove the ethylene glycol and metabolites when the level >20 mg/dl and continued until it is <5 mg/dl. In patients with ethylene glycol poisoning presenting with normal renal function and no metabolic acidosis, fomepizole therapy may obviate the need for hemodialysis [64].

Methanol intoxication may present with similar metabolic derangements, but rarely causes ARF[16, 65].

6.6.3.7 Myoglobin (Pigment)

Rhabdomyolysis is the breakdown of striated muscle with release of constitutive components into the extracellular fluid and circulation. One of the key compounds released is myoglobin, an 18.8-kDa oxygen carrier. Normally, myoglobin is loosely bound to plasma globulins and only small amounts reach the urine. When massive amounts of myoglobin are released, the binding capacity of plasma protein is exceeded. Myoglobin is then filtered by the glomeruli and subsequently reaches the tubules [66, 67].

The mechanisms by which rhabdomyolysis provokes ATN are multiple. First, iron in the heme protein may be a mediator of proximal tubular toxicity. (See Section 6.6.2.2). Second, myoglobin may form obstructing tubular casts, especially in acid urine. Finally, myoglobin may provoke intrarenal acute vasoconstriction both as a nitric oxide scavenger and through extensive third spacing of fluid in the damaged muscle, which causes hypovolemia. Muscular trauma is the most common cause of rhabdomyolysis. Less common causes include muscle enzyme deficiencies, electrolyte abnormalities, infectious causes, drugs, toxins, and endocrinopathies. Rhabdomyolysis as a cause of ARF should always be suspected in the perioperative setting, especially after surgical interventions necessitating specific positions (e.g., exaggerated lithotomy position and prone position) for prolonged periods [68–70], or as a complications of malignant hyperthermia [71–73]. Malignant hyperthermia is an inheritable condition that is characterized by a rapid rise of body temperature (1°C/5 min), typically after anesthesia with halogenated hydrocarbons and succinylcholine. Rhabdomyolysis, finally, should also be considered in illicit drug users (cocaine, opiates, phencyclidine, and amphetamines) presenting with ARF [16].

Weakness, myalgia, and tea-coloured urine are the main clinical manifestations. The most sensitive laboratory finding of muscle injury is an elevated plasma creatine kinase level. Myoglobin is rapidly and unpredictably eliminated by hepatic metabolism. Therefore, tests for myoglobin in plasma and urine are not sensitive diagnostic procedures. Release of constituents of necrotic muscle results in increased serum concentrations of several other inorganic and organic compounds, including potassium, phosphate, uric acid, and protons. The accumulation of these compounds is aggravated by the simultaneous development of renal failure. Furthermore, hypocalcemia may occur as result of calcium phosphate deposition in injured muscle. In the presence of hyperkalemia, severe hypocalcemia may lead to cardiac arrhythmia, muscular contraction, or seizures [66].

The primary therapeutic goal is to prevent the factors that predispose to rhabdomyolysis-induced ARF, i.e., hypovolemia, hypotension, hypokalemia, tubular obstruction, aciduria, and free radical release [66]. Mannitol and bicarbonate, although commonly recommended, are of unproven benefit. The amount of fluid required may be as high as 10 l or more per day. Allopurinol may be useful because it reduces the production of uric acid and also acts as a free radical scavenger. Once overt renal failure has developed, the only reliable therapeutic modality is extracorporeal blood purification. The metabolic consequences of rhabdomyolysis, being often profound and life-threatening, require intensive dialysis [66, 67, 74].

6.6.3.8 Nonsteroidal Antiinflammatory Drugs

NSAIDs possess antipyretic and antiinflammatory effects and are effective in the management of mild-to-moderate pain. The analgesic effect of NSAIDs relies on the inhibition of peripheral hyperalgesia mediated by their antiinflammatory properties, possibly supplemented by centrally mediated actions that attenuate central sensitization [39]. Their opioid-sparing effect and availability for parenteral use render them ideal for day-only and short-stay administration in the setting of elective surgery. Acute renal failure can occur with any NSAID, including the parenteral analgesic ketorolac [75]. An overall incidence of ARF of only 1.1% was observed in a recent retrospective study including over 10,000 courses of ketolorac in 35 hospitals. Only patients treated for more than 5 days had an increased risk of ARF as compared with controls [76]. NSAIDs mainly cause functional ARF by inhibiting cyclooxygenase (COX), the enzyme that converts arachidonic acid into prostaglandins (see above). NSAIDs have also been associated with salt and water retention and may cause papillary necrosis and interstitial nephritis [77, 78]. More than 80% of patients with acute interstitial nephritis related to NSAIDs develop a nephrotic syndrome due to a concomitant minimal change type injury.

Spontaneous recovery generally occurs within weeks to a few months after therapy is discontinued. A course of prednisone may be considered in patients whose renal failure persists more than 1–2 weeks after the NSAID has been discontinued [79].

The selective COX-2 inhibitors have a lower incidence of gastrointestinal side effects but appear to offer no advantage with respect to renal regulation of sodium excretion, blood pressure, and occurrence of (functional and inflammatory) ARF [78, 80–83]. Recently, agents with combined lipooxygenase/COX inhibition and agents that combine NSAIDs with a nitric oxide (NO) donor have been reported to reduce adverse renal effects [84, 85].

6.6.3.9 Paraquat

Paraquat is a widely used broad-spectrum and fast-acting herbicide. However, it is extremely toxic, causing fatalities due to accidental or intentional poisoning. Paraquat poisoning causes severe multiple organ failure, with the degree of poisoning dependent on the route of administration, the amount administered, and the duration of exposure. It is rapidly distributed within the body with highest concentrations accumulating within the kidneys, where it produces early and severe nephrotoxicity. Additionally, as it is primarily excreted unchanged via the kidneys, the consequent reduction in renal function increases plasma concentrations by up to fivefold, which contributes to paraquat toxicity in other organs, especially the lungs. Ultimately, respiratory failure, in the presence of nephrotoxic acute renal failure, is responsible for most deaths caused by paraquat. Therefore, maintaining renal function in patients suffering from paraquat poisoning remains a therapeutically important treatment strategy [20]. Symptoms of paraquat poisoning may be delayed for up to 48 h after ingestion in humans. Generation of ROS, such as superoxide anions, plays a major part in the development of paraquat-induced toxicity and especially nephrotoxicity [20, 86]. The diagnosis can rapidly be confirmed using a qualitative urine test. Management is directed at removing paraquat from the gastrointestinal tract, increasing its excretion from blood, and preventing pulmonary damage with antiinflammatory agents. Gut decontamination may be considered in patients who present within 1 h of a life-threatening ingestion. Hemoperfusion provides better clearance of paraquat than hemodialysis, and the use of hemoperfusion within 12 h of poisoning may reduce mortality. Although there is controversy relating to the efficacy of extracorporeal therapy, most clinicians, initiate a 4- to 6-h hemodialysis or hemoperfusion treatment soon after the patient is admitted to the hospital. Daily treatment is continued, with intermittent assessment of pulmonary function and plasma and urinary concentrations of paraquat [87, 88].

6.6.3.10 Radiocontrast Agents

Within the last 2 decades, radiologic procedures utilizing contrast media are being increasingly applied for both diagnostic and treatment purposes. This has resulted in a rising incidence of renal function impairment caused by the exposure to contrast material – an iatrogenic disorder known as radiocontrast nephropathy (RCN). Acute RCN is the third leading cause of new-onset renal failure in hospitalized patients. RCN is associated with prolonged in-hospital stay and increased morbidity, mortality, and costs [89]. Alterations in renal hemodynamics and direct tubular epithelial cell toxicity (probably mediated by oxygen free radicals) are the primary factors believed to be responsible for the development of RCN [90, 91]. Given its clinical relevance, RCN is discussed in extenso elsewhere in this book.

6.6.3.11 Vancomycin

Staphylococci and enterococci are the most common pathogens in surgical-site and bloodstream infections. The emergence of drug resistance among these gram-positive bacteria poses a substantial threat to patients with surgical infections. Resistance to methicillin/oxacillin is frequently observed in *Staphylococcus aureus* isolates and is often accompanied by multidrug resistance. Vancomycin is usually the treatment of choice for infections caused by methicillin-resistant *S. aureus* (MRSA). Vancomycin, however, may induce renal dysfunction. Renal toxicity is reported to be a relatively infrequent complication of vancomycin administration, occurring in approximately 5% of patients [92]. Aggressive vancomycin dosing and prolonged vancomycin administration may be associated with greater risk for renal toxicity [93].

The mechanism of vancomycin-induced renal dysfunction is not known. Recent animal data suggest that oxidative stress underlies the pathogenesis of vancomycin-induced nephrotoxicity and that targeting superoxide dismutase and/or related antioxidants to renal proximal tubule cells might permit the administration of higher doses of vancomycin sufficient for eradication of MRSA without causing renal injury [94]. Pharmacokinetic monitoring and dosage adjustment are effective methods for reducing the toxicity of vancomycin in intensive care patients, especially for those receiving concomitant nephrotoxins [38, 95, 96]. The antimicrobial armantarium has recently been expanded with antibiotics that are also effective against multiresistant organisms including MRSA (linezolid and quinupristin/dalfopristin). These antibiotics provide a reasonable therapeutic alternative for patients infected with MRSA who cannot tolerate vancomycin [97].

6.6.4 Conclusion

Toxic nephropathy should always be considered as a cause of ARF, especially in in-hospital patients. Both exotoxins and endotoxins may be involved. Awareness of the range of toxins and the high-risk clinical settings in which they become important is vital in avoiding toxic ARF and in minimizing its clinical severity. Before prescribing a potentially nephrotoxic drug, the risk-to-benefit ratio and the availability of alternative drugs should be considered. Simple prophylactic measures include therapeutic drug monitoring, avoidance of concomitant use of several potentially nephrotoxic drugs, and restoration/maintenance of adequate hydration. Studies are needed to further elucidate the mechanisms of nephrotoxicity to design more rational prevention and treatment strategies. Computer-based prescriber order entry and an appropriately trained intensive care unit pharmacist are particularly helpful to minimize medication errors and adverse drug events. Frequent monitoring of the glomerular filtration rate during the administration of a potentially nephrotoxic drug may help to recognize the complication of drug-induced ARF at an early stage.

Once established, drug-induced ARF must be handled like any other type of ARF, with stringent fluid and electrolyte management and, if necessary, dialysis. Obviously, all nephrotoxic drugs should be withdrawn where possible. In general, a spontaneous restoration of the renal function ensues. Irreversible damage, however, may occur in some patients.

6.6.5 Take Home Pearls

- Toxic nephropathy is a frequent cause of acute kidney failure.
- Both exogenous and endogenous toxins may be involved.
- Key measures in preventing toxic nephropathy are therapeutic drug monitoring, avoidance of concomitant use of several potentially nephrotoxic drugs, and restoration/maintenance of adequate hydration.
- Once established, the clinical management of drug-induced acute kidney failure is not fundamentally different from any other type of ARF.

Acknowledgments The author thanks B. Sprangers, MD, for his helpful comments and suggestions.

References

1. Xue JL, Daniels F, Star RA, Kimmel PL, Eggers PW, Molitoris BA, et al. Incidence and mortality of acute renal failure in medicare beneficiaries, 1992 to 2001. J Am Soc Nephrol 2006 Apr 1;17(4):1135–42.
2. Novis BK, Roizen MF, Aronson S, Thisted RA. Association of preoperative risk factors with postoperative acute renal failure. Anesth Analg 1994 Jan 1;78(1):143–9.
3. Chertow GM, Lazarus JM, Christiansen CL, Cook EF, Hammermeister KE, Grover F, et al. Preoperative renal risk stratification. Circulation 1997 Feb 18;95(4):878–84.
4. Lote CJ, Harper L, Savage COS. Mechanisms of acute renal failure. Br J Anaesth 1996 July 1;77(1):82–9.
5. Block CA, Manning HL. Prevention of acute renal failure in the critically ill. Am J Respir Crit Care Med 2002 Feb 1;165(3):320–4.
6. Carmichael P, Carmichael AR. Acute renal failure in the surgical setting. ANZ J Surg 2003;73(3):144–53.
7. Conlon P, Stafford-Smith M, White W, Newman M, King S, Winn M, et al. Acute renal failure following cardiac surgery. Nephrol Dial Transplant 1999 May 1;14(5):1158–62.
8. Kellerman PS. Perioperative care of the renal patient. Arch Int Med 1994;154(15):1674–88.
9. Levy EM, Viscoli CM, Horwitz RI. The effect of acute renal failure on mortality. A cohort analysis. JAMA 1996;275(19):1489–94.
10. Corwin HL, Sprague SM, DeLaria GA, Norusis MJ. Acute renal failure associated with cardiac operations. A case-control study. J Thorac Cardiovasc Surg 1989;98(6):1107–12.
11. Bhandari S, Turney JH. Survivors of acute renal failure who do not recover renal function. QJM 1996 June 1;89(6):415–21.
12. Khan IH, Catto GR, Edward N, Macleod AM. Acute renal failure: factors influencing nephrology referral and outcome. QJM 1997 Dec 1;90(12):781–5.
13. Feest TG, Round A, Hamad S. Incidence of severe acute renal failure in adults: results of a community based study. BMJ 1993;306:481–3.
14. Hou SH, Bushinsky DA, Wish JB, Cohen JJ, Harrington JT. Hospital-acquired renal insufficiency: a prospective study. Am J Med 1983;74(2):243–8.
15. Rasmussen HH, Ibels LS. Acute renal failure. Multivariate analysis of causes and risk factors. Am J Med 1982; 73(3):211–8.
16. Jefferson JA, Schrier RW. Pathophysiology and etiology of acute renal failure. InFeehally J, Floege J, Johnson RJ Comprehensive Clinical Nephrology, 3rd ed. Mosby, Philadelphia, PA; 2007, pp. 755–70.
17. Nath KA, Norby SM. Reactive oxygen species and acute renal failure. Am J Med 2000 Dec 1;109(8):665–78.
18. Baliga R, Ueda N, Walker PD, Shah SV. Oxidant mechanisms in toxic acute renal failure. Am J Kidney Dis 1997; 29(3):465–77.

19. Izzedine H, Launay-Vacher V, Deray G. Antiviral drug-induced nephrotoxicity. Am J Kidney Dis 2005;45(5): 804–17.
20. Samai M, Hague T, Naughton DP, Gard PR, Chatterjee PK. Reduction of paraquat-induced renal cytotoxicity by manganese and copper complexes of EGTA and EHPG. Free Rad Biol Med 2008 Feb 15;44(4):711–21.
21. Michel DM, Kelly CJ. Acute interstitial nephritis. J Am Soc Nephrol 1998 Mar 1;9(3):506–15.
22. Rossert J. Drug-induced acute interstitial nephritis. Kidney Int 2001;60:804–17.
23. Gonzalez E, Gutierrez E, Galeano C, Chevia C, de Sequera P, Bernis C, et al. Early steroid treatment improves the recovery of renal function in patients with drug-induced acute interstitial nephritis. Kidney Int 2008 Jan 9;73(8): 940–6.
24. Markowitz GS, Perazella MA. Drug-induced renal failure: a focus on tubulointerstitial disease. Clin Chim Acta 2005 Jan;351(1–2):31–47.
25. Appel GB. The treatment of acute interstitial nephritis: more data at last. Kidney Int 2008;73(8):905–7.
26. Zakarija A, Charles MD. Drug-induced thrombotic microangiopathy. Semin Thromb Hemost 2005;(06):681–90.
27. Medina PJ, Sipols JM, George JN. Drug-associated thrombotic thrombocytopenic purpura-hemolytic uremic syndrome. Curr Opin Hematol 2001;8(5):286–93.
28. Dlott JS, Danielson CF, Blue-Hnidy DE, McCarthy LJ. Drug-induced thrombotic thrombocytopenic purpura/hemolytic uremic syndrome: a concise review. Ther Apher Dial 2004;8(2):102–11.
29. Stratta P, Lazzarich E, Canavese C, Bozzola C, Monga G. Ciprofloxacin Crystal Nephropathy. Am J Kidney Dis 2007 Aug;50(2):330–5.
30. Perazella MA. Crystal-induced acute renal failure. Am J Med 1999 Apr;106(4):459–65.
31. Ebcioglu Z, Cohen DJ, Crew RJ, Hardy MA, Ratner LE, D'Agati VD, et al. Osmotic nephrosis in a renal transplant recipient. Kidney Int 2006;70(10):1873–6.
32. Dickenmann M, Oettl T, Mihatsch MJ. Osmotic nephrosis: acute kidney injury with accumulation of proximal tubular lysosomes due to administration of exogenous solutes. Am J Kidney Dis 2008 Mar;51(3):491–503.
33. Janssen CW. Osmotic nephrosis. A clinical and experimental investigation. Acta Chir Scand 1968;134(6):481–7.
34. Humes HD. Aminoglycoside nephrotoxicity. Kidney Int 1988;33(4):900–11.
35. Martinez-Salgado C, Lopez-Hernandez FJ, Lopez-Novoa JM. Glomerular nephrotoxicity of aminoglycosides. Toxicol Appl Pharmacol 2007 Aug 15;223(1):86–98.
36. Humes HD, Hunt DA, White MD. Direct toxic effect of the radiocontrast agent diatrizoate on renal proximal tubule cells. Am J Physiol Renal Physiol 1987 Feb 1;252(2): F246–F255.
37. Jaquenod M, Ronnhedh C, Cousins MJ, Eckstein RP, Jordan V, Mather LE, et al. Factors influencing ketorolac-associated perioperative renal dysfunction. Anesth Analg 1998 May 1;86(5):1090–7.
38. Goetz MB, Sayers J. Nephrotoxicity of vancomycin and aminoglycoside therapy separately and in combination. J Antimicrob Chemother 1993 Aug 1;32(2):325–34.
39. Kim H, Xu M, Lin Y, Cousins MJ, Eckstein RP, Jordan V, et al. Renal dysfunction associated with the perioperative use of diclofenac. Anesth Analg 1999 Oct 1;89(4):999.
40. Prins JM, Buller HR, Speelman P, Kuijper EJ, Tange RA. Once versus thrice daily gentamicin in patients with serious infections. Lancet 1993 Feb 6;341(8841):335–9.
41. Rose B, Zaleznik D. Manifestations and risk factors for aminoglycoside nephrotoxicity. In: Rose B (ed.) UptoDate 2003.
42. Kullberg BJ, Oude Lashof AM. Epidemiology of opportunistic invasive mycoses. Eur J Med Res 2002;31(7(5)):183–91.
43. Sawaya BP, Briggs JP, Schnermann J. Amphotericin B nephrotoxicity: the adverse consequences of altered membrane properties. J Am Soc Nephrol 1995 Aug 1;6(2): 154–64.
44. Deray G. Amphotericin B nephrotoxicity. J Antimicrob Chemother 2002 Jan 1;49(Suppl 1):37–41.
45. Fisher MA, Talbot GH, Maislin G, McKeon BP, Tynan KP, Strom BL. Risk factors for Amphotericin B-associated nephrotoxicity. Am J Med 1989;87(5):547–52.
46. Furrer K, Schaffner A, Vavricka SR, Halter J, Imhof A, Schanz U. Nephrotoxicity of cyclosporine A and amphotericin B-deoxycholate as continuous infusion in allogenic stem cell transplantation. Swiss Med Wkly 2002;132(23–24):316–20.
47. Saliba F, Dupont B. Renal impairment and Amphotericin B formulations in patients with invasive fungal infections. Med Mycol 2008;46(2):97–112.
48. Ullmann AJ, Sanz MA, Tramarin A, Barnes RA, Wu W, Gerlach BA, et al. Prospective study of amphotericin B formulations in immunocompromised patients in 4 European countries. Clin Infect Dis 2006;43(4):e29–e38.
49. Walsh TJ, Finberg RW, Arndt C, Hiemenz J, Schwartz C, Bodensteiner D, et al. Liposomal Amphotericin B for empirical therapy in patients with persistent fever and neutropenia. N Engl J Med 1999 Mar 11;340(10):764–71.
50. Rogers TR. Optimal use of existing and new antifungal drugs. Curr Opin Crit Care 2001;7(4):238–41.
51. Schoolwerth AC, Sica DA, Ballermann BJ, Wilcox CS. Renal considerations in angiotensin converting enzyme inhibitor therapy: a statement for healthcare professionals from the Council on the Kidney in Cardiovascular Disease and the Council for High Blood Pressure Research of the American Heart Association. Circulation 2001 Oct 16;104(16):1985–91.
52. Palmer BF. Renal dysfunction complicating the treatment of hypertension. N Engl J Med 2002 Oct 17;347(16):1256–61.
53. Cruz CS, Cruz LS, Silva GR, Marcillio de Souza CA. Incidence and predictors of development of acute renal failure related to treatment of congestive heart failure with ACE inhibitors. Nephron Clin Pract 2007;105(2):c77–c83.
54. Cittanova ML, Zubicki A, Savu C, Montalvan C, Nefaa N, Zaier K, et al. The Chronic Inhibition of angiotensin-converting enzyme impairs postoperative renal function. Anesth Analg 2001 Nov 1;93(5):1111–5.
55. Brabant SM, Bertrand M, Eyraud D, Darmon PL, Coriat P. The hemodynamic effects of anesthetic induction in vascular surgical patients chronically treated with angiotensin II receptor antagonists. Anesth Analg 1999 Dec 1;89(6):1388.
56. Ryckwaert F, Colson P. Hemodynamic effects of anesthesia in patients with ischemic heart failure chronically treated with angiotensin-converting enzyme inhibitors. Anesth Analg 1997 May 1;84(5):945–9.
57. Shammash JB, Ghali WA. Preoperative assessment and perioperative management of the patient with nonischemic heart disease. Med Clin North Am 2003;87(1):137–52.

58. Olyaei AJ, de Mattos AM, Bennett W. Nephrotoxicity of immunosuppressive drugs: new insight and preventive strategies. Curr Opin Crit Care 2001;7(6):384–9.
59. Moran M, Kapsner C. Acute renal failure associated with elevated plasma oncotic pressure. N Engl J Med 1987;317(3):150–3.
60. Jungheinrich C, Neff TA. Pharmacokinetics of hydroxyethyl starch. Clin Pharmacokinet 2005;44(7):681–99.
61. Schortgen F, Lacherade JC, Bruneel F, Cattaneo I, Hemery F, Lemaire F, et al. Effects of hydroxyethylstarch and gelatin on renal function in severe sepsis: a multicentre randomised study. Lancet 2001 Mar 24;357(9260):911–6.
62. Boldt J, Priebe HJ. Intravascular volume replacement therapy with synthetic colloids: is there an influence on renal function? Anesth Analg 2003 Feb 1;96(2):376–82.
63. Brent J, McMartin K, Phillips S, Burkhart KK, Donovan JW, Wells M, et al. Fomepizole for the treatment of ethylene glycol poisoning. N Engl J Med 1999 Mar 18;340(11):832–8.
64. Sivilotti MLA, Burns MJ, McMartin KE, Brent J, For the Methylpyrazole for Toxic Alcohols Study Group. Toxicokinetics of ethylene glycol during fomepizole therapy: implications for management. Ann Emerg Med 2000 Aug;36(2):114–25.
65. Sivilotti MLA, Winchester JF. Methanol and ethylene glycol intoxication. In: Rose B (ed.) UpToDate 2008.
66. Vanholder R, Sever MS, Erek E, Lameire N. Rhabdomyolysis. J Am Soc Nephrol 2000 Aug 1;11(8):1553–61.
67. Huerta-Alardin AL, Varon J, Marik PE. Bench-to-bedside review: rhabdomyolysis – an overview for clinicians. Crit Care 2005;9(2):158–69.
68. Bocca G, van Moorselaar JA, Feitz WFJ, van der Staak FH, Monnens LA. Compartment syndrome, rhabdomyolysis and risk of acute renal failure as complications of the lithotomy position. J Nephrol 2002;15(2):183–5.
69. Kikuno N, Urakami S, Shigeno K, Kishi H, Tgawa M. Traumatic rhabdomyolysis resulting from continuous compression in the exaggerated lithotomy position for radical perineal prostatectomy. Int J Urol 2002;9(9):521–4.
70. Gabrielli A, Caruso L. Postoperative acute renal failure secondary to rhabdomyolysis from exaggerated lithotomy position. J Clin Anesth 1999;11(3):257–63.
71. Riess FC, Fiege M, Moshar S, Bergmann H, Bleese N, Kormann J, et al. Rhabdomyolysis following cardiopulmonary bypass and treatment with enoximone in a patient susceptible to malignant hyperthermia. Anesthesiology 2001;94(2):355–7.
72. McKenney KZ, Holman SJ. Delayed postoperative rhabdomyolysis in a patient subsequently diagnosed as malignant hyperthermia susceptible. Anesthesiology 2002;96(3):764–5.
73. Green G. A fatal case of malignant hyperthermia complicated by generalized compartment syndrome and rhabdomyolysis. Acta Anaesthesiol Scand 2003;47(5):619–21.
74. Schenk MR, Beck DH, Nolte M, Kox WJ. Continuous venovenous hemofiltration for the immediate management of massive rhabdomyolysis after fulminant malignant hyperthermia in a bodybuilder. Anesthesiology 2001;94(6):1139–41.
75. Sivarajan M, Wasse L. Perioperative acute renal failure associated with preoperative intake of ibuprofen. Anesthesiology 1997;86:1390–2.
76. Feldman HI, Kinman JL, Berlin JA, Hennessy S, Kimmel SE, Farrar J, et al. Parenteral ketorolac: the risk for acute renal failure. Ann Intern Med 1997 Feb 1;126(3):193–9.
77. Clive DM, Stoff JS. Renal syndromes associated with nonsteroidal antiinflammatory drugs. N Engl J Med 1984;310(9):563–72.
78. Wali RK, Henrich WL. Recent developments in toxic nephropathy. Curr Opin Nephrol Hypertens 2002;11(2):155–63.
79. Rose B. NSAIDs: acute renal failure and nephrotic syndrome. In: Rose B (ed.) UptoDate 2003.
80. Dunn MJ. Are COX-2 selective inhibitors nephrotoxic? Am J Kidney Dis 2000;35(5):976–7.
81. Perazella MA, Eras J. Are selective COX-2 inhibitors nephrotoxic? Am J Kidney Dis 2000;35(5):937–40.
82. Woywodt A, Schwarz A, Mengel M, Haller H, Zeidler H, Köhler L. Nephrotoxicity of selective COX-2 inhibitors. J Rheumatol 2001;28(9):2133–5.
83. Szeto CC, Chow KM. Nephrotoxicity related to new therapeutic compounds. Ren Fail 2005;27(3):329–33.
84. Cheng HF, Harris RC. Renal effects of non-steroidal antiinflammatory drugs and selective cyclooxygenase-2 inhibitors. Curr Pharm Des 2005;11(14):1795–804.
85. Gambaro G. Strategies to safely interfere with prostanoid activity while avoiding adverse renal effects: could COX-2 and COX-LOX dual inhibition be the answer? Nephrol Dial Transplant 2002 July 1;17(7):1159–62.
86. Van Vleet TR, Schnellmann RG. Toxic nephropathy: environmental chemicals. Semin Nephrol 2003;23(5):500–8.
87. Winchester J. Dialysis and hemoperfusion in poisoning. Adv Ren Replace Ther 2002 Jan;9(1):26–30.
88. Winchester JF. Paraquat intoxication. In: Rose B (ed.) UpToDate 2008.
89. Nikolsky E, Aymong ED, Dangas G, Mehran R. Radiocontrast nephropathy: identifying the high-risk patient and the implications of exacerbating renal function. Rev Cardiovasc Med 2003;4(Suppl 1):7–14.
90. Rudnick MR, Berns JS, Cohen RM, Goldfarb S. Contrast media-associated nephrotoxicity. Semin Nephrol 1997; 17(1):15–26.
91. Katholi RE, Woods WT, Taylor GJ, Deitrick CL, Womack KA, Katholi CR, et al. Oxygen free radicals and contrast nephropathy. Am J Kidney Dis 1998;32(1):64–71.
92. Farber BF, Moellering RC, Jr. Retrospective study of the toxicity of preparations of vancomycin from 1974 to 1981. Antimicrob Agents Chemother 1983 Jan 1;23(1):138–41.
93. Jeffres MN, Isakow W, Doherty JA, Micek ST, Kollef MH. A retrospective analysis of possible renal toxicity associated with vancomycin in patients with health care-associated methicillin-resistant *Staphylococcus aureus* pneumonia. Clin Therapeut 2007 June;29(6):1107–15.
94. Nishino Y, Takemura S, Minamiyama Y, Hirohashi K, Ogino T, Inoue M, et al. Targeting superoxide dismutase to renal proximal tubule cells attenuates vancomycin-induced nephrotoxicity in rats. Free Radic Res 2003;37(4):373–9.
95. Darko W, Medicis JJ, Smith A, Guharoy R, Lehmann DE. Mississippi mud no more: cost-effectiveness of pharmacokinetic dosage adjustment of vancomycin to prevent nephrotoxicity. Pharmacotherapy 2003;23(5):643–50.
96. Rybak MJ, Albrecht LM, Boike SC, Chandrasekar PH. Nephrotoxicity of vancomycin, alone and with an aminoglycoside. J Antimicrob Chemother 1990 Apr 1;25(4):679–87.
97. Khare M, Keady D. Antimicrobial therapy of methicillin resistant Staphylococcus aureus infection. Expert Opin Pharmacother 2003;4(2):165–77.

6.7 Toxic Nephropathy Due to Radiocontrast Media*

Peter A. McCullough

Core Messages

- Contrast-induced acute kidney injury (AKI) is a common and potentially serious complication following the administration of contrast media in patients at risk for AKI.
- The risk of contrast-induced AKI is elevated and of clinical importance in patients with chronic kidney disease (glomerular filtration rate <60 ml/min/1.73 m^2); this is particularly important in patients with diabetes mellitus.
- Current evidence suggests that the use of non-ionic, iso-osmolar contrast media is associated with the lowest risk of contrast-induced AKI.
- In patients at risk, adequate intravenous volume expansion with isotonic crystalloid has been shown to reduce the probability of contrast-induced AKI.
- In contrast, no adjunctive medical or dialytic treatment has been conclusively proven to be efficacious for the prophylaxis of AKI after exposure to iodinated contrast medium.

6.7.1 Definition of Toxic Nephropathy After Iodinated Contrast Medium

Contrast-induced acute kidney injury (AKI), previously known as contrast-induced nephropathy (CIN), is an important complication after the intravascular administration of iodinated contrast [1–3]. The most commonly used definition in clinical trials was a rise in serum creatinine (Cr) of 0.5 mg/dl or a 25% increase from the baseline value, assessed at 48 h after the procedure. In 2007, the Acute Kidney Injury Network proposed the definition of a rise in serum Cr ≥0.3 mg/dl with oliguria, which is compatible with the older definitions. It is expected that in addition to this signal of reduced filtration function, markers of acute nephron injury in the blood and urine will be used to establish a diagnosis of AKI.

6.7.2 Consensus Statements on Contrast-Induced Acute Kidney Injury

Table 6.7.1 gives the basic consensus statements on contrast-induced AKI agreed upon by multidisciplinary panels [4]. These statements deal with the issues of screening, risk stratification, high-risk scenarios, and reasonable preventive measures. Fortunately, the frequency of contrast-induced AKI has decreased over the past decade from a general incidence of ~15% to ~7% of patients [5]. As of this writing, there are no approved diagnostic tests or preventive therapies for contrast-induced AKI.

*Prepared For Text "Management of Acute Kidney Problems" to be published by Springer

P. A. McCullough
Division of Nutrition and Preventive Medicine, William Beaumont Hospital, 4949 Coolidge Highway,Royal Oak, MI 48073, USA
e-mail: pmc975@yahoo.com

A. Jörres et al. (eds.), *Management of Acute Kidney Problems*,
DOI: 10.1007/978-3-540-69441-0_6.7, © Springer-Verlag Berlin Heidelberg 2010

Table 6.7.1 Consensus statements concerning contrast-induced AKI (Adapted from [4])

Consensus Statement 1 Contrast-induced AKI is a common (5–15%) and potentially serious complication following the administration of contrast media in patients at risk for acute renal injury.
Consensus Statement 2 The risk of contrast-induced AKI is elevated and of clinical importance in patients with chronic kidney disease (particularly when diabetes is also present), recognized by an estimated glomerular filtration rate (eGFR) <60 ml/min/1.73 m^2.
Consensus Statement 3 When serum creatinine or estimated glomerular filtration rate is unavailable, then a history of kidney disease risk factors can identify patients at higher risk for contrast-induced AKI than the general population.
Consensus Statement 4 In the setting of emergency procedures, where the benefit of very early imaging outweighs the risk of waiting, the procedure can be performed without knowledge of serum creatinine or eGFR.
Consensus Statement 5 The presence of multiple contrast-induced AKI risk factors in the same patient or high risk clinical scenarios can create a very high risk (~50%) for contrast-induced AKI and (~15%) acute renal failure requiring dialysis after contrast exposure.
Consensus Statement 6 In patients at increased risk for contrast-induced AKI undergoing intra-arterial administration of contrast, ionic high-osmolality agents pose a greater risk for contrast-induced AKI than low-osmolality agents. Current evidence suggests that for intra-arterial administration in high-risk patients with chronic kidney disease, particularly those with diabetes mellitus, nonionic, iso-osmolar contrast is associated with the lowest risk of contrast-induced AKI.
Consensus Statement 7 Higher contrast volumes (>100 ml) are associated with higher rates of contrast-induced AKI in patients at risk. However, even small (~30 ml) volumes of iodinated contrast in very high risk patients can cause contrast-induced AKI and acute renal failure requiring dialysis, suggesting the absence of a threshold effect.
Consensus Statement 8 Intra-arterial administration of iodinated contrast appears to pose a greater risk of contrast-induced AKI above that with intravenous administration.
Consensus Statement 9 Adequate intravenous volume expansion with isotonic crystalloid (1.0–1.5 ml/kg/h) for 3–12 h before the procedure and continued for 6–24 h afterwards can lessen the probability of contrast-induced AKI in patients at risk. The data on oral as opposed to intravenous volume expansion as a contrast-induced AKI prevention measure are insufficient.
Consensus Statement 10 No adjunctive medical or mechanical treatment has been proven to be efficacious in reducing the risk of AKI after exposure to iodinated contrast. Prophylactic hemodialysis or hemofiltration has not been validated as an effective strategy

6.7.3 Pathophysiology

Chronic kidney disease (CKD) is both necessary and sufficient for the development of contrast-induced AKI. In patients with CKD, identified by an estimated glomerular filtration rate (eGFR) <60 ml/min/1.73 m^2 (which roughly corresponds in the elderly to a serum Cr >1.0 mg/dl in a woman and >1.3 mg/dl in a man), there is a considerable loss of nephron units, and the residual renal function is vulnerable to declines with renal insults (sepsis, intravascular iodinated contrast, cardiopulmonary bypass, renal-toxic medications, atheroembolism, etc.). Thus, the pathophysiology of contrast-induced AKI assumes baseline reduced nephron number, with superimposed acute vasoconstriction caused by the release of adenosine, endothelin, and other renal vasoconstrictors triggered by iodinated contrast (Fig. 6.7.1). After a very brief increase in renal blood flow, via the above mechanisms, there is an overall ~50% sustained reduction in renal blood flow lasting for several hours. There is concentration of iodinated contrast in the renal tubules and collecting ducts, resulting in a persistent nephrogram on fluoroscopy or repeated X-rays. This nephrogram, representing iodinated contrast in the peritubular and interstitial space, can last for up to 8 days after the original contrast administration in patients with severely reduced renal filtration at baseline (Fig. 6.7.2). This stasis of contrast in the kidney allows for direct cellular injury

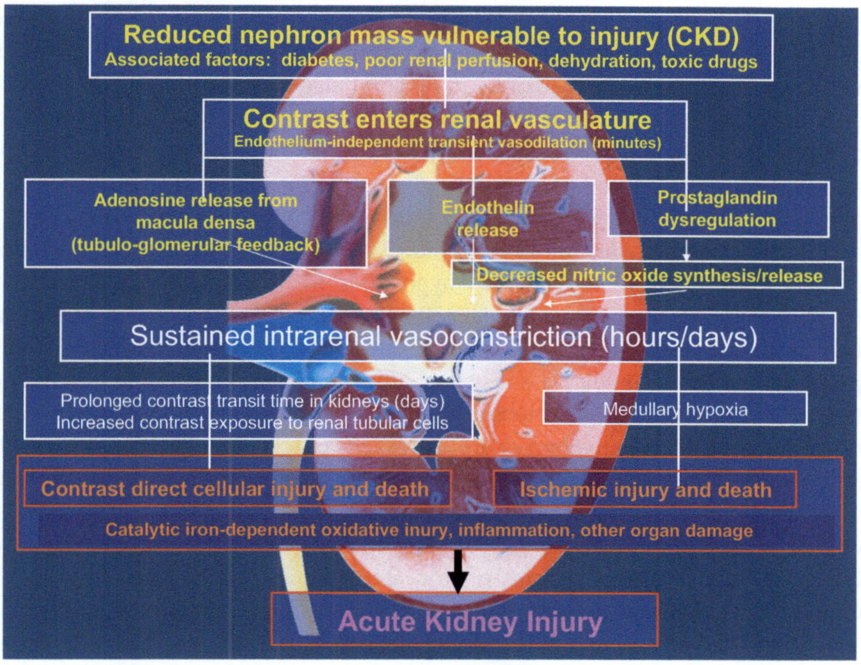

Fig. 6.7.1 Pathophysiology of contrast-induced AKI demonstrating in the presence of a reduced nephron mass, that the remaining nephrons are vulnerable to injury. Iodinated contrast, after causing a brief (minutes) period of vasodilation, causes sustained (hours to days) intrarenal vasoconstriction and ischemic injury. The ischemic injury sets off a cascade of events largely driven by catalytic iron-dependent oxidative injury causing death of renal tubular cells. If a sufficient mass of nephron units are affected, then a recognizable rise in serum creatinine will occur

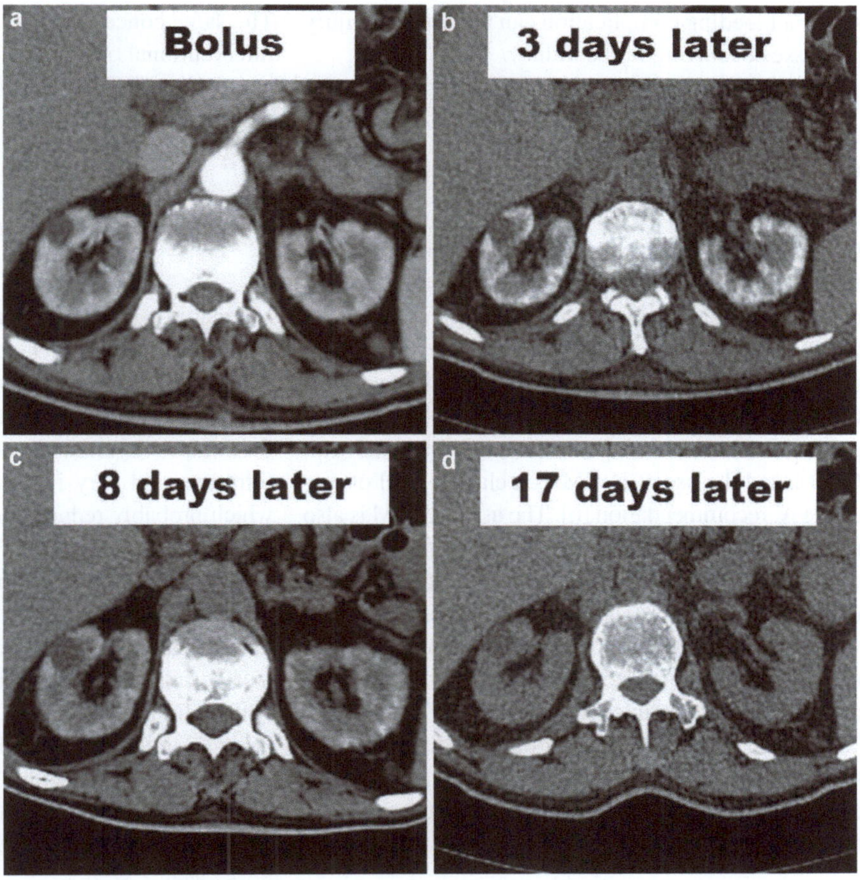

Fig. 6.7.2 Persistent nephrogram demonstrated up to 8 days after administration of intravenous contrast for computed tomography in a 73-year-old patient with a creatinine clearance of 23 ml/min: (**a**) immediately after contrast bolus, (**b**) 3 days later, (**c**) 8 days later, (**d**) 17 days later with final clearing of iodinated contrast (Adapted from [37])

and death to renal tubular cells and explains the variability in the rise in serum creatinine over the following days. The degree of cytotoxicity to renal tubular cells is directly related to the length of exposure those cells have to iodinated contrast, hence, the importance of high urinary flow rates before, during, and after contrast procedures to reduce contrast dwell time. The sustained reduction in renal blood flow to the outer medulla leads to medullary hypoxia, ischemic injury, and death of renal tubular cells. By these two mechanisms, it is believed that other organ injury processes including oxidative stress and inflammation may play a further role. Importantly, many reactions involved in oxidative stress are dependent on sources of intracellular labile iron, including the cytochrome p450 chain and mitochondria. The generation of oxygen free radicals is dependent on catalytic iron, and thus, labile forms of iron are being considered as future therapeutic targets in AKI. Any superimposed insult such as sustained hypotension in the catheterization laboratory, microshowers of atheroembolic material from catheter exchanges, the use of intra-aortic balloon counterpulsation (IABP), sepsis, or a bleeding complication can amplify the injury processes occurring in the kidney.

6.7.4 Classes of Iodinated Contrast

Contrast media can be categorized according to osmolality (high-osmolal [HOCM] ~2,000 mOsm/kg, low-osmolal [LOCM] 600–800 mOsm/kg, and isosmolal [IOCM] 290 mOsm/kg) with decreasing levels of renal toxicity according to these classifications. The American College of Cardiology–American Heart Association guidelines for the management of ACS patients with CKD listed the use of IOCM as a class I, level of evidence A, recommendation [6]. The use of IOCM is also recommended in renal dialysis patients to minimize the chances of volume overload and complications prior to the next dialysis session. Most other societies concur with these recommendations for intra-arterial administration and allow the use of LOCM in lower risk patients and intravenous administration.

Contrast volume is an important predictor of contrast-induced AKI. Even small volumes (~30 ml) of contrast medium can have adverse effects on renal function in patients at particularly high risk [7]. As a general rule, the volume of contrast received should not exceed twice the baseline level of eGFR in milliliters [8]. This means for patients with significant CKD, reasonable goals would be: <30 ml for diagnostic cardiac catheterization and <100 ml for percutaneous coronary intervention (PCI), computed tomography (CT), and other intravascular studies.

The risk of contrast-induced AKI is generally higher following intra-arterial than after intravenous injection [9–10]. However, in CT studies, where a comparatively large volume of contrast medium is given as a compact intravenous (80–120 ml) bolus rather than an infusion, the risk of AKI may be increased.

Finally, it is believed that serial exposures to contrast medium and subsequent administration in the setting of AKI further worsen renal function and may be more likely to cause persistent renal dysfunction. This is particularly true when a persistent nephrogram is present, and iodinated contrast is still present within the kidneys. Therefore, when faced with the option, a limited diagnostic catheterization and PCI in the same setting is favored over a diagnostic catheterization and then a scheduled PCI within 10 days. The same concept applies for diagnostic followed by interventional radiologic procedures. It should be noted, there are no published sources of comparative data on this topic.

6.7.5 Importance of Volume Expansion

Volume expansion and treatment of dehydration has a well-established role in the prevention of contrast-induced AKI, although few studies address this theme directly. Expansion of blood volume with intravenous fluid improves renal blood flow, increases glomerular filtration, and very importantly, increases urine flow which probably reduces the duration of toxic contrast exposure to the kidneys. There are limited data on the most appropriate choice of intravenous fluid, but the evidence indicates that isotonic crystalloid (saline or bicarbonate solution) is probably more effective than half-normal saline [11]. Additional confirmatory trials with sodium bicarbonate [12] are needed because the largest trial to date showed no benefit of sodium bicarbonate over normal saline [13]. There is also no clear evidence to guide the choice of the optimal rate and duration of infusion. However, good urine output

(>150 ml/h) in the 6 h after the procedure has been associated with reduced rates of AKI in one study [14]. Conversely, oliguria in the face of intravenous hydration can be a sign of AKI. Since not all of the intravenously administered isotonic crystalloid remains in the vascular space, to achieve a urine flow rate of at least 150 ml/h, ≥1.0–1.5 ml/kg/h of intravenous fluid has to be administered for 3–12 h pre-contrast exposure and 6–12 h afterwards.

6.7.6 Dialysis and Hemofiltration

Iodinated contrast is water soluble and removed by dialysis, but there is no clinical evidence that prophylactic dialysis reduces the risk of AKI, even when carried out within 1 h or simultaneously with contrast administration. Hemofiltration, however, performed 6 h before and 12–18 h after contrast deserves consideration given reports of reduced mortality and need for hemodialysis in the postprocedure period in very high-risk patients (serum Cr 3.0–4.0 mg/dl, eGFR 15–20 ml/min/1.73 m^2) [15–16]. Specialists should be aware that hemofiltration calls for a 5,000 IU heparin bolus before initiation followed by a continuous heparin infusion of 500–1,000 IU/h through the inflow side of the catheter. At the time of the cardiac procedure, the hemofiltration treatment should be stopped, and the circuit temporarily filled with a saline solution and short-circuited to exclude the patient without interruption of the flow.

6.7.7 Pharmacologic Prophylaxis

There are no currently approved pharmacologic agents for the prevention of AKI. With iodinated contrast, the pharmacologic agents tested in small trials that deserve further evaluation include the antioxidants ascorbic acid and N-acetylcysteine (NAC), statins, aminophylline/theophylline, and prostaglandin E_1. Although popular, NAC has not been consistently shown to be effective. To date, 11 meta-analyses have been published on this subject [17–27], seven of these reports found a net benefit for NAC in the prevention of AKI. However, a recent review by Bagshaw and colleagues found marked heterogeneity in study results in 10 of the 11 meta-analyses [28]. Importantly, only in those trials where NAC reduced serum Cr below baseline values because of decreased skeletal muscle production, did renal injury rates appear to be reduced. Thus, NAC appears to falsely lower Cr and not fundamentally protect against AKI. However, NAC as an antioxidant has been shown to lower rates of AKI and mortality after primary PCI in one trial [29]. Dosing of NAC has varied in the trials; however, the most successful approach has been with 1,200 mg orally twice daily on the day before and after the procedure [30].

The vast majority of cardiovascular patients should be on statin therapy with a common low-density lipoprotein cholesterol (LDL-C) target of <70 mg/dl. It has been demonstrated that patients continued on statins during cardiovascular procedures including PCI and coronary artery bypass graft have lower rates of AKI [31]. Small randomized trials published to date support this concept as well [32–33]. Preservation of endothelial function at the level of the glomerulus and reductions in systemic inflammatory factors are postulated mechanisms by which statins may have renoprotective effects [33].

Nephrotoxic drugs including nonsteroidal antiinflammatory agents, gentamicin, amphotericin, and cyclosporine should be discontinued 72 h prior to contrast exposure if possible. In addition, metformin should be withheld to minimize the risk of lactic acidosis should AKI develop.

6.7.8 Follow-Up

All patients at risk for contrast-induced AKI should have follow-up Cr and electrolyte monitoring daily while in hospital, and then at 48–96 h after discharge (Fig. 6.7.3). Rehospitalization is reasonable for uremic symptoms, hyperkalemia, and volume overload in the setting of AKI.

6.7.9 Biomarkers for Contrast-Induced AKI

Neutrophil gelatinase-associated lipocalin (NGAL), a member of the lipocalin family, is readily excreted and detected in urine, due to its small molecular size

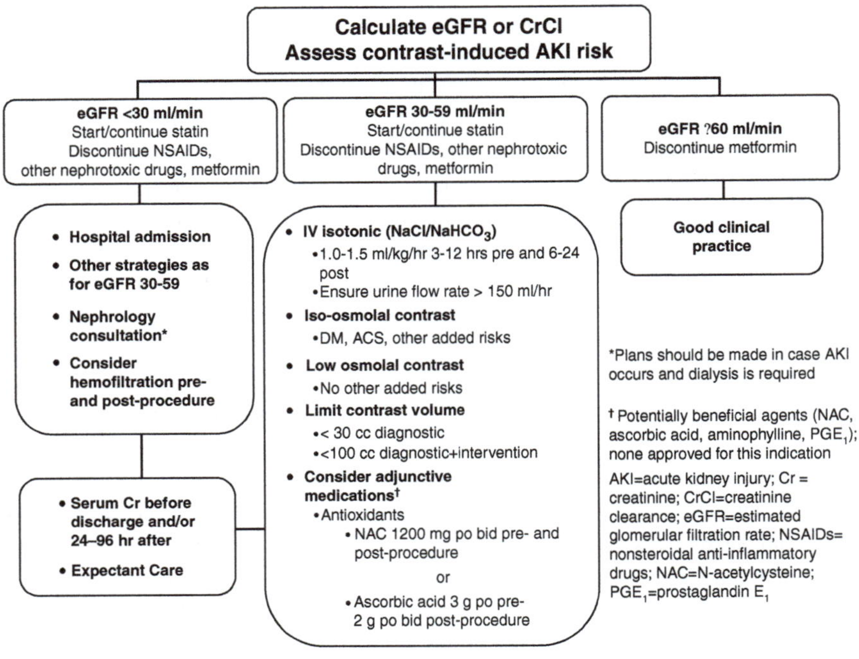

Fig. 6.7.3 Algorithm for management of patients receiving iodinated contrast media suggesting a multidimensional approach with assessment of risk based on eGFR and then volume expansion and use of cytoprotective drugs in patients at risk. Discontinuation of metformin is advised to reduce the risk of lactic acidosis if AKI develops (AKI = acute kidney injury; Cr = creatinine; CrCl = creatinine clearance; eGFR = estimated glomerular filtration rate; NSAIDs = nonsteroidal antiinflammatory drugs; NAC = N-acetylcysteine; PGE_1 = prostaglandin E_1) (Adapted from [36])

(25 kDa) and resistance to degradation. Produced by leukocytes and many somatic cells, NGAL is highly accumulated in the human kidney cortical tubules, blood and urine, after nephrotoxic and ischemic injuries such as exposure to iodinated contrast. Thus, whole blood and/or urinary NGAL might represent an early, sensitive, biomarker for AKI being developed for point-of-care use in the catheterization laboratory and radiology suite, analogous to the use of troponin for myocardial injury [34–35].

6.7.10 Future Approaches

Future approaches include large planned studies of oral and intravenous antioxidants (including a potent labile iron chelator, deferiprone), intrarenal infusions of renal vasodilators using flow-directed catheters in the procedural suite or intensive care unit, forced hydration using a balancing pump with marked elevations of urine output to reduce the transit time of iodinated contrast in the renal tubules and avoid persistent nephrograms, and novel, hopefully less toxic forms of radiopaque contrast agents.

6.7.11 Take Home Pearls

- Contrast-induced AKI is predictable and is partially preventable
- In patients at risk, adequate intravenous volume expansion with isotonic crystalloid (1.0–1.5 ml/kg/h) for 3–12 h before the procedure and continued for 6–24 h afterwards can lessen the probability of contrast-induced AKI
- Novel diagnostic and therapeutic approaches are needed to manage the ever-increasing numbers of patients undergoing interventions using iodinated contrast media [36]

References

1. McCullough PA, Soman SS: Contrast-induced nephropathy. *Crit Care Clin* 2005; 21(2):261–280.
2. Gleeson TG, Bulugahapitiya S: Contrast-induced nephropathy. *AJR Am J Roentgenol* 2004; 183(6):1673–1689.
3. Nash K, Hafeez A, Hou S: Hospital-acquired renal insufficiency. *Am J Kidney Dis* 2002; 39(5):930–936.
4. McCullough PA, Stacul F, Davidson C, et al.: Overview. *Am J Cardiol* 2006; 98:2K–4K.

5. Bartholomew BA, Harjai KJ, Dukkipati S, et al: Impact of nephropathy after percutaneous coronary intervention and a method for risk stratification. *Am J Cardiol* 2004; 93(12): 1515–1519.
6. Anderson JL, Adams CD, Antman EM, Bridges CR, Califf RM, Casey DE Jr, Chavey WE 2nd, Fesmire FM, Hochman JS, Levin TN, Lincoff AM, Peterson ED, Theroux P, Wenger NK, Wright RS, Smith SC Jr, Jacobs AK, Adams CD, Anderson JL, Antman EM, Halperin JL, Hunt SA, Krumholz HM, Kushner FG, Lytle BW, Nishimura R, Ornato JP, Page RL, Riegel B. ACC/AHA 2007 Guidelines for the Management of Patients With Unstable Angina/Non-ST-Elevation Myocardial Infarction-Executive Summary A Report of the American College of Cardiology/American Heart Association Task Force on Practice Guidelines (Writing Committee to Revise the 2002 Guidelines for the Management of Patients With Unstable Angina/Non-ST-Elevation Myocardial Infarction) Developed in Collaboration with the American College of Emergency Physicians, the Society for Cardiovascular Angiography and Interventions, and the Society of Thoracic Surgeons Endorsed by the American Association of Cardiovascular and Pulmonary Rehabilitation and the Society for Academic Emergency Medicine. J Am Coll Cardiol. 2007 Aug 14; 50(7):652–726.
7. Manske CL, Sprafka JM, Strony JT, et al.: Contrast nephropathy in azotemic diabetic patients undergoing coronary angiography. *Am J Med* 1990; 89(5):615–620.
8. Laskey WK, Jenkins C, Selzer F, Marroquin OC, Wilensky RL, Glaser R, Cohen HA, Holmes DR Jr; NHLBI Dynamic Registry Investigators. Volume-to-creatinine clearance ratio: a pharmacokinetically based risk factor for prediction of early creatinine increase after percutaneous coronary intervention. *J Am Coll Cardiol.* 2007 Aug 14;50(7):584–90. Epub 2007 Jul 30.
9. Campbell DR, Flemming BK, Mason WF, et al.: A comparative study of the nephrotoxicity of iohexol, iopamidol and ioxaglate in peripheral angiography. *Can Assoc Radiol J* 1990; 41(3):133–137.
10. Moore RD, Steinberg EP, Powe NR, et al.: Nephrotoxicity of high-osmolality versus low-osmolality contrast media: randomized clinical trial. *Radiology* 1992; 182(3):649–655.
11. Mueller C, Buerkle G, Buettner HJ, et al.: Prevention of contrast media-associated nephropathy: randomized comparison of 2 hydration regimens in 1620 patients undergoing coronary angioplasty. *Arch Intern Med* 2002; 162(3):329–336.
12. Merten GJ, Burgess WP, Gray LV, et al.: Prevention of contrast-induced nephropathy with sodium bicarbonate: a randomized controlled trial. *JAMA* 2004; 291(19):2328–2334.
13. Brar S: A randomized controlled trial for the prevention of contrast induced nephropathy with sodium bicarbonate vs. sodium chloride in persons undergoing coronary angiography (the MEENA trial). Abstract 209–9. *Presentation at the 56th Annual Scientific Session of the American College of Cardiology, New Orleans, LA, USA, 24–27 March 2007.*
14. Stevens MA, McCullough PA, Tobin KJ, et al.: A prospective randomized trial of prevention measures in patients at high risk for contrast nephropathy: Results of the P.R.I.N.C.E. study. *J Am Coll Cardiol* 1999; 33(2):403–411.
15. Marenzi G, Marana I, Lauri G, et al.: The prevention of radiocontrast-agent-induced nephropathy by hemofiltration. *N Engl J Med* 2003; 349(14):1333–1340.
16. Marenzi G, Lauri G, Campodonico J, Marana I, Assanelli E, De Metrio M, Grazi M, Veglia F, Fabbiocchi F, Montorsi P, Bartorelli AL. Comparison of two hemofiltration protocols for prevention of contrast-induced nephropathy in high-risk patients. *Am J Med.* 2006 Feb; 119(2):155–62.
17. Birck R, Krzossok S, Makowetz F, Schnulle P, van der Woude F, Braun C. Acetylcysteine for prevention of contrast nephropathy: Meta-analysis. *Lancet.* 200(3); 362:598–603.
18. Isenbarger D, Kent S, O'Malley P. Meta-analysis of randomized clinical trials on the usefulness of acetylcysteine for prevention of contrast nephropathy. *Am J Cardiol.* 2003; 92: 1454–1458.
19. Alonso A, Lau J, Jaber B, Weintraub A, Sarnak M. Prevention of radiocontrast nephropathy with N-acetylcysteine in patients with chronic kidney disease: A meta-analysis of randomized, controlled trials. *Am J Kidney Dis.* 2004; 43: 1–9.
20. Kshirsagar A, Poole C, Mottl A, Shoham D, Franceschini N, Tudor G, Agrawal M, Denu-Ciocca C, Magnus Ohman E, Finn WF. N-acetylcysteine for the prevention of radiocontrast induced nephropathy: A meta-analysis of prospective controlled trials. J *Am Soc Nephrol.* 2004;15:761–769.
21. Pannu N, Manns B, Lee H, Tonelli M. Systematic review of the impact of N-acetylcysteine on contrast nephropathy. *Kidney Int.* 2004; 65:1366–1374.
22. Guru V, Fremes S. The role of N-acetylcysteine in preventing radiographic contrast-induced nephropathy. *Clin Nephrol.* 2004; 62:77–83.
23. Bagshaw S, Ghali WA. Acetylcysteine for prevention of contrast-induced nephropathy: A systematic review and meta-analysis. *BMC Med.* 2004; 2:38.
24. Misra D, Leibowitz K, Gowda R, Shapiro M, Khan I. Role of N-acetylcysteine in prevention of contrast-induced nephropathy after cardiovascular procedures: a meta-analysis. *Clin Cardiol.* 2004; 27:607–610.
25. Nallamothu BK, Shojania KG, Saint S, Hofer TP, Humes HD, Moscucci M, Bates ER. Is acetylcysteine effective in preventing contrast-related nephropathy? A meta-analysis. *Am J Med.* 2004; 117:938–947.
26. Liu R, Nair D, Ix J, Moore D, Bent S. N-acetylcysteine for prevention of contrast-induced nephropathy: A systematic review and meta-analysis. *J Gen Intern Med.* 2005; 20: 193–200.
27. Duong M, MacKenzie T, Malenka D: N-Acetylcysteine prophylaxis significantly reduces the risk of radiocontrastinduced nephropathy. *Catheter Cardiovasc Interv.* 2005; 64: 471–479.
28. Bagshaw SM, McAlister FA, Manns BJ, Ghali WA. Acetylcysteine in the prevention of contrast-induced nephropathy: A case study of the pitfalls in the evolution of evidence. *Arch Intern Med.* 2006; 166:161–166.
29. Marenzi G, Assanelli E, Marana I, Lauri G, Campodonico J, Grazi M, De Metrio M, Galli S, Fabbiocchi F, Montorsi P, Veglia F, Bartorelli AL. N-acetylcysteine and contrast-induced nephropathy in primary angioplasty. *N Engl J Med.* 2006 Jun 29; 354(26):2773–2782.
30. Briguori C, Airoldi F, D'Andrea D, et al.: Renal insufficiency following contrast media administration Trial (REMEDIAL): a randomized comparison of 3 preventive strategies. *Circulation* 2007; 115(10):1211–1217.
31. Khanal S, Attallah N, Smith DE, Kline-Rogers E, Share D, O'Donnell MJ, Moscucci M. Statin therapy reduces contrast-induced nephropathy: an analysis of contemporary

percutaneous interventions. *Am J Med*. 2005 Aug; 118(8): 843–849.

32. Welten GM, Chonchol M, Schouten O, Hoeks S, Bax JJ, van Domburg RT, van Sambeek M, Poldermans D. Statin use is associated with early recovery of kidney injury after vascular surgery and improved long-term outcome. *Nephrol Dial Transplant*. 2008 Dec; 23(12):3867–73.
33. McCullough PA, Rocher LR. Statin therapy in renal disease: Harmful or protective. *Curr Atheroscler Rep*. 2007 Jan; 9(1): 18–24.
34. Bachorzewska-Gajewska H, Malyszko J, Sitniewska E, Malyszko JS, Dobrzycki S. Neutrophil-gelatinase-associated lipocalin and renal function after percutaneous coronary interventions. *Am J Nephrol*. 2006; 26(3):287–92. Epub 2006 Jun 13.
35. Mishra J, Dent C, Tarabishi R, Mitsnefes MM, Ma Q, Kelly C, Ruff SM, Zahedi K, Shao M, Bean J, Mori K, Barasch J, Devarajan P. Neutrophil gelatinase-associated lipocalin (NGAL) as a biomarker for acute renal injury after cardiac surgery. *Lancet*. 2005 Apr 2–8; 365(9466): 1231–1238.
36. McCullough PA. Contrast-induced acute kidney injury. *J Am Coll Cardiol*. 2008 Apr 15; 51(15):1419–1428.
37. Koneth I, Weishaupt D, Bachli EB. Persistent nephrogram after administration of an isoosmolar contrast medium. *Nephrol Dial Transplant*. 2004 Jun; 19(6):1654–1655.

Acute Glomerulonephritis, Vasculitis, and Pulmonary Renal Syndrome

6.8

Jai Prakash

Core Messages

- Inflammatory diseases of glomeruli (glomerulonephritis [GN]) and renal vessels (vasculitis) are important causes of intrinsic acute kidney failure (ARF), accounting for approximately 10% of cases.
- Both acute glomerulonephritis and vasculitis (particularly ANCA-associated vasculitis) are more common in the elderly while poststreptococcal GN causing ARF is relatively more common in children than in adults.
- The clinical presentation is often that of a rapidly progressive glomerulonephritis (RPGN) with or without signs and symptoms of extrarenal manifestations.
- The diagnostic workup must include an immunologic screening for autoantibodies (ANA, anti-ds DNA antibodies, ANCA, anti-GBM antibodies, and cryoglobulins).
- Patients with hematuria/proteinuria, active urinary sediment, and/or acute renal dysfunction with or without systemic symptoms must be subjected to renal biopsy for the precise diagnosis.
- Early recognition is essential because treatment may result in preservation or recovery of renal function.

6.8.1 Introduction

Acute renal failure (ARF) is a syndrome characterized by rapid (hours to weeks) decline in glomerular filtration rate (GFR) and retention of nitrogenous waste products such as urea and creatinine [1]. Inflammatory diseases of the renal microvasculature and glomeruli (glomerulonephritis and vasculitis) are important causes of intrinsic ARF [2, 3]. About 10% of cases of ARF are caused by glomerulonephritis (GN) [4, 5], and its incidence is similar in Europe, North America, and developing countries like India [6–8]. However, GN-associated ARF is relatively more common in children and the elderly [9–12]. Similarly, vasculitis is also the most common cause of ARF in the biopsies of elderly patients, with a prevalence from 31% to 50% of the cases [10, 13, 14]. Early recognition is essential, because treatment may result in preservation or recovery of renal function.

This review article will focus on ARF due to GN/vasculitis, ARF occurring in patients with underlying glomerular diseases and, finally, acute kidney injury (AKI) complicating nephrotic syndrome.

6.8.2 Causes of ARF Due to Glomerulonephritis/Vasculitis

Acute renal failure associated with GN is common in small vessel vasculitis and systemic lupus erythematosus (SLE), and is uncommon in other multisystem diseases. It is rare in association with primary glomerular diseases. From a clinical point of view, I shall classify the ARF in patients with GN/vasculitis in four categories:

1. ARF due to GN
2. ARF due to vasculitis
3. ARF in patients with preexisting glomerular disease
4. ARF complicating nephrotic syndrome

J. Prakash
Department of Nephrology, Institute of Medical Sciences, Banaras Hindu University, Varanasi-221005, India
e-mail: jpojha555@hotmail.com; jprakash53@gmail.com

A. Jörres et al. (eds.), *Management of Acute Kidney Problems*,
DOI: 10.1007/978-3-540-69441-0_6.8, © Springer-Verlag Berlin Heidelberg 2010

In Europe and North America small vessel vasculitis (polyangiitis), SLE and anti-glomerular basement membrane (anti-GBM) disease are the usual cause of ARF due to GN/vasculitis. However, infection-associated GN is probably the most common cause worldwide. The major categories of GN and systemic vasculitis causing ARF are shown in Tables 6.8.1 and 6.8.2, and their classification is based on the pathogenetic mechanisms. Several vasculitic diseases can affect the kidney and lead to a syndrome of ARF. Vasculitis accounts for approximately 5% of total ARF cases, and it can be associated with severe morbidity and sometimes death. Rapidly progressive GN (RPGN) is a clinical syndrome that is often associated with histologic findings of glomerular crescent and usually presents as anuric ARF.

Table 6.8.1 Acute renal failure (ARF) due to glomerulonephritis GN (e.g. carcinoma, lymphoma, leukemia)

1.	**Immune complex (IC)–mediated diseases**
	Postinfectious glomerulonephritis[a]
	Systemic lupus erythematosus
	Cryoglobulinemia
	Henoch-Schönlein purpura
2.	**Anti-GBM antibody associated**
	• Goodpasture's syndrome
	• Anti-GBM disease
3.	**Pauci-immune glomerulonephritis**
	• Microscopic polyangiitis (MP)
	• Wegener's granulomatosis
	• Churg-Strauss syndrome
	• Renal limited vasculitis
4.	**Miscellaneous**
	• Primary systemic vasculitis
	• Mesangial IgA nephropathy
	• Mesangiocapillary glomerulonephritis
	• Focal segmental sclerosis
	• Membranous nephropathy
	• Neoplasia-associated GN (Carcinoma, lymphoma, leukemia)

[a]Postinfectious glomerulonephritis includes a spectrum of proliferative glomerulonephritis associated with poststreptococcal disease, infective endocarditis, shunt nephritis, and visceral abscess

Table 6.8.2 Causes of acute renal failure (ARF) due to vasculitis

1.	**Immune complex-mediated vasculitis**
	Systemic lupus erythematosus
	Cryoglobulinemic vasculitis
	Henoch-Schönlein purpura
2.	**Anti-GBM antibody–mediated vasculitis**
	• Goodpasture syndrome
	• Anti-GBM disease
3.	**Pauci-immune small vessel vasculitis**
	• Microscopic polyangiitis (MPA)
	• Wegener's granulomatosis
	• Churg-Strauss Syndrome
	• Renal limited vasculitis

6.8.3 Causes of ARF Due to Glomerulonephritis

The causes of ARF associated with GN and crescents are listed in Table 6.8.1. The histologic findings in ARF associated with GN include endocapillary proliferative lesions, crescentic GN, and focal necrotizing GN. The term rapidly progressive glomerulonephritis (RPGN) is often used to describe the clinical syndrome of ARF developing over a period of weeks to a few months (but occasionally days) in patients found to have a proliferative and often crescentic and necrotizing GN [15, 16]. Acute poststreptococcal GN is the most common form of postinfectious GN, accounting for 10–20% of the ARF due to glomerular diseases. It is more frequent in children than in adults, in whom idiopathic forms of RPGN occur more often [17, 18]. Several nonstreptococcal agents can cause similar GN, usually milder and which resolves with infection eradication [19, 20]. However, severe cases of acute proliferative GN have been described in septic patients, primarily related to chronic localized infection such as visceral abscesses, infective endocarditis, and infected ventriculoatrial shunts [21–23]. Eradication of abscesses or localized infection with appropriate antibiotic therapy, has resulted in clinical resolution of nephritis in most reported cases. However, steroid and cyclophosphamide have been given with apparent success because of the intense glomerular inflammation seen in some patients [24].

Crescentic GN (extracapillary cell proliferation within Bowman's space) clinically present as RPGN and can be classified into three groups on the basis of the underlying immunopathology: (i) type I, approximately 20% of cases are mediated by anti-GBM antibodies; (ii) type II, 40% of cases are immune complex related; and (iii) type III, which accounts for approximately 40% of cases, is characterized by absence of immune deposits (pauci-immune). All patients who present clinically with RPGN or evidence of vasculitis should be submitted to renal biopsy and appropriate serologic investigations as a matter of urgency [25–27]. Assays for anti-GBM antibodies, antineutrophil cytoplasmic antibody (ANCA), lupus serology, and complements are particularly important. Making an accurate diagnosis of the cause of RPGN is critically important, as both the nature of the therapy and the response to treatment will be very different, depending on the precise diagnosis.

6.8.4 Acute Renal Failure in Vasculitis

Vasculitis is a heterogeneous group of disorders characterized by inflammation, necrosis, and cellular infiltration of blood vessels. This process can affect large, medium, or small vessels leading to destruction of the integrity of the vessel wall. The kidney is chiefly involved when smaller vessels (arterioles, capillaries, and venules) are affected. Renal vasculitis may be limited to kidney (renal limited vasculitis) or be a part of systemic diseases. ANCA, either directed to myeloperoxidase (P-ANCA), or proteinase 3 (C-ANCA) can be detected in 80–90% of cases of renal vasculitis. About 5–10% of otherwise typical cases of renal vasculitis do not have detectable ANCA (ANCA-negative), and about 5% of specimens may have anti-GBM antibodies along with positive ANCA (double positive type IV renal vasculitis). Systemic vasculitis accounts for only a small minority of cases of ARF (about 5%), but they can be associated with severe morbidity. Most often, the clinical presentation is that of RPGN with or without signs and symptoms of extrarenal manifestation. The working classification of the glomerular and vasculitis syndrome associated with ARF is based on their pathogenetic mechanisms (Table 6.8.2). Active disease is usually associated with ANCA, elevated C-reactive protein, elevated erythrocyte sedimentation rate, and active urinary sediments (dysmorphic erythrocytes and red blood cell casts). Proteinuria per se is a less reliable indicator of active disease. ANCA-associated vasculitis (AAV) includes: microscopic polyangiitis (MP), Wegener's granulomatosis (WG), Churg-Strauss syndrome (CSS), and renal limited vasculitis (RLV). The vasculitis can occur in young or middle-aged patients, while now-a-days, more cases are seen in the elderly. According to the Spanish Register of Glomerulonephritis data (1994–1999), AAV is observed in 7% of all renal biopsies and in 18% of the biopsies in patients over 65 years of age [14]. Twenty-five percent of the patients with AAV have precipitating events (infection, vaccines, and pervious history of drug intake), and another 25% have associated diseases, mainly diabetes mellitus, neoplasm, and stroke [28, 29]. The associated diseases are more common in elderly patients than younger ones. The presentation of MP is usually extrarenal (arthritis, skin lesions, and/or respiratory tract involvement) or a combination of renal and extrarenal involvement. Isolated renal involvement is an uncommon presentation in MP except in the elderly [29, 30]. The presentation of WG is usually extrarenal, always being extrarenal in CSS, and always renal in RLV. ARF is the most common form of renal presentation of ANCA-associated vasculitis. Oliguric ARF is more frequent in elderly patients than in young and middle-aged patients [28, 31]. Renal biopsy is very helpful in the diagnosis of AAV and is also useful in the selection of treatment and in predicting the renal prognosis of the disease. All patients with ARF, should principally undergo biopsy when ARF is accompanied by microhematuria and/or proteinuria and/or positive ANCA. The characteristic feature of the glomerular lesion in pauci-immune small vessel vasculitis is focal necrotizing glomerulonephritis associated with cellular or fibrocellular crescents that usually involve more than 50% of glomeruli. The GNs associated with AAV and anti-GBM disease are characterized predominantly by necrosis rather than hypercellularity. The reverse is true for immune-complex GN which tends to have prominent proliferative changes.

The outcome of renal vasculitis depends on the initial severity of disease, duration of disease before treatment is commenced, the age of the patient, the number of organs involved, the nature of underlying disease (WG, MP, RVL, or CSS), and the result of treatment (initial response and relapse). The current standard treatment of AAV consists of oral prednisone and cyclophosphamide [32]. Immunosuppressive drugs should be adjusted according to age and renal function. Other possible therapies include the use of mycophenolate mofetil and intravenous immunoglobulin [31, 33]. The duration of treatment is not standardized with most groups recommending at least 18 months. In RLV patient who require dialysis, immunosuppressive drugs can be discontinued after 3 months. A balance must be maintained between the complications of treatment and disease remission. The main complications of treatment are infection (24–47%), neoplasm (2.5–12%), diabetes mellitus (5.8%), and bone fracture. Elderly patients have the same percentage of infection as younger patients, but have more severe infections (sepsis). Using conventional treatment with cyclophosphamide and steroids, the prognosis is worse for WG and with high-titer of anti-PR3 activity. Older age at onset and the elevated serum creatinine concentration at diagnosis also confer a worse prognosis [34]. While most ANCA-positive renal vasculitis is associated with pauci-immune necrotizing and crescentic GN, the concomitant presence of immune complex deposit seems to aggravate the severity of the renal lesion by augmenting proliferation and crescent formations [35, 36].

6.8.5 Pathogenesis of ARF in Glomerulonephritis/Vasculitis

The precise mechanism of ARF in these patients is not known but seems to be multifactorial. Glomerular capillary obliteration by influx and proliferation of cells leads to reduction of filtration surface area and subsequently reduced GFR. This is particularly true in case of crescentic and diffuse proliferative GN. Reduced GFR may result from vasculitis of larger vessels causing distal ischemia. Vascular endothelial cell damage results in the generation of endothelins and a reduction of nitric oxide production, both of which will reduce glomerular blood flow [37, 38]. Hemoglobin binds nitric oxide strongly, which may cause vasoconstriction, potentiating medullary hypoxia, and leading to acute tubular necrosis [39]. In addition, direct tubular toxicity may be caused by red blood cells or their contents (haem pigment or free iron). It is suggested that acute tubular damage and/or tubular obstruction by red blood cell casts should be suspected in any patient with proliferative GN, who develops ARF soon after a hematuric episode [40, 41].

6.8.6 Clinical Features

The history and physical examination often provide clues to the diagnosis of ARF due to GN, particularly when associated with systemic disorders. It is important to question patients about fever, possible preceding infection, travel, and their medication history. The systemic review should include enquiries about myalgia, arthralgia/arthritis, skin rashes, mouth ulcers, upper respiratory tract problems, chest pain, hemoptysis, and symptoms of neuropathy. Certain signs/symptoms strongly indicate a single diagnosis or a small number of differential diagnosis. For instance, the presence of a vasculitic rash with arthritis/arthralgia suggests the possibility of vasculitis either of the primary small-vessel type or secondary to lupus, Henoch-Schönlein purpura, cryoglobulinemia, or infective endocarditis. Hypertension is common in renal failure with fluid overload whatever be the cause, and severe hypertension is well recognized in SLE and systemic sclerosis. Hemoptysis commonly occurs in Goodpasture's diseases, primary small vessel vasculitis, and lupus. However, it has been reported occasionally in patient with cryoglobulinemia, systemic sclerosis, and rheumatoid diseases. Oliguria is usual in GN associated with ARF. Complete anuria is reported in patients with crescentic GN in association with anti-GBM diseases and pauci-immune GN. Urine microscopy of freshly voided urine may reveal dysmorphic erythrocytes, particularly acanthocytes, which are indicative of glomerular bleeding [40]. Red cell casts are highly suggestive of proliferative GN. However, they are occasionally seen in acute interstitial nephritis and rarely in acute tubular necrosis. Leukocytes and abundant granular and cellular casts are found in the urine of patients with active GN.

The differential diagnosis of GN-associated ARF requires a combined approach consisting of clinical features, laboratory investigations, imaging, and renal biopsy. Results of immunologic assay of ANCA, anti-GBM, and Anti-dsDNA antibodies and complement abnormalities in all patients with acute GN are essential. Table 6.8.3 lists important investigations relevant to GN/vasculitis-associated ARF. Ultrasound examination of kidney is carried out before kidney biopsy. Renal biopsy has diagnostic, prognostic, and therapeutic value in patients with GN [42]. Diffuse alveolar air-space shadowing on chest X-ray may suggest pulmonary edema, pulmonary hemorrhage, or infection. Hemorrhage and edema may be difficult to differentiate from each other particularly in the absence of hemoptysis. Computed tomography (CT) may help resolve the difference. Round homogeneous lesions with or without cavities on the chest radiograph suggest a diagnosis of WG, but are also manifestations of infection (staphylococcal abscess). Sinus disease is

Table 6.8.3 Laboratory investigation in patients with acute renal failure (ARF) caused by glomerulonephritis/vasculitis

Baseline measurements	Significance
Serum urea, creatinine, glomerular filtration rate (GFR), urinalysis and 24-h protein excretion	Determine current status of renal function and help to monitor progress and response to treatment
Diagnostically important test	
Specific Assay	**Significance**
Anti-GBM antibodies	Anti-GBM diseases
ANCA	Systemic vasculitis
C3 Nephritic factor	Type II MPGN
Anti-ds DNA antibodies	Positive in SLE
Anti-sm antibodies	Positive in SLE
ASO titer	Poststreptococcal GN
Nonspecific assay	**Significance**
Low C4, normal C3	SLE, MEC
Low C4 and C3	Type I MPGN, MEC, SLE
Low C3, normal C4	Type II MPGN, post infectious GN, sometimes SLE
Raised C3 and C4	Systemic vasculitis
Cryoglobulin	Mixed essential cryoglobulinemia
Raised IgG, IgM	SLE, systemic vasculitis, post infectious GN,
Raised IgE	Churg-Strauss Syndrome
Raised IgA	IgA nephropathy/Henoch-Schönlein purpura
Para-protein (usually IgM)	MEC, myeloma
Raised alkaline phosphatase	Systemic vasculitis
Eosinophilia	Churg-Strauss syndrome
Thrombocytopenia	SLE
Positive bacteriological culture	Infection-related GN, particularly endocarditis

ASO antistreptolysin titer, *GBM* glomerular basement membrane, *GN* glomerulonephritis, *MEC* mixed essential cryoglobulinemia, *MPGN* membranoproliferative glomerulonephritis, *SLE* systemic lupus erythematosus

found in WG, but is also common in the general population, although actual bone destruction strongly support the diagnosis of WG. Transesophageal echocardiography is an essential investigation in patients in whom infective endocarditis is suspected.

Acute GN with or without systemic vasculitis must always be considered in the differential diagnosis of ARF. The history and examination often provide clues to the underlying cause of renal failure, and a number of laboratory and radiologic tests will add further diagnostic information. In the absence of a clear-cut cause of ARF, a renal biopsy provides the most rapid route to the diagnosis. However, the wider availability of ANCA assay (ELISA) to detect anti-MPO and anti-PR3 antibodies has resulted in earlier recognition of small vessel vasculitis.

6.8.7 Acute Renal Failure in Patients with Underlying Glomerulonephritis

The development of acute or acute-on-chronic renal failure in a patient already known to have an underlying GN needs careful assessment as the differential diagnosis is wide. ARF associated with crescents in the renal biopsy has been described in mesangial IgA nephropathy, mesangiocapillary GN, and membranous nephropathy [43–45]. Rapid deterioration of renal function, especially during prolonged episodes of macroscopic hematuria has been reported in patients with IgA nephropathy [46, 47]. Rapid development of renal failure is sometimes associated with crescent formation in the renal biopsy in patients with mesangiocapillary GN [48, 49]. Superimposed crescentic change in primary membranous nephropathy causing ARF has also been described [49–51]. Acute interstitial nephritis related to various drugs (nonsteroidal antiinflammatory drugs, antibiotics, diuretics, cimetidine, and allopurinol) may cause ARF in patients with GN [52]. The diagnosis is suggested by the presence of fever, rash, arthralgia, and eosinophilia. A renal biopsy is necessary to confirm the diagnosis. Acute oliguric ARF occurs in less than 5% of patients with mixed essential cryoglobulinemia. The diagnosis is suggested by the association of vasculitic skin rash, arthralgia, peripheral neuropathy, and Raynaud's phenomenon with GN [53]. Acute oliguric renal failure is infrequent, but may occur in patients with Henoch-Schönlein purpura. Renal biopsy usually reveals a high proportion of crescents [54].

6.8.8 Acute Renal Failure Complicating Nephrotic Syndrome

ARF complicates nephrotic syndrome more often than is generally appreciated. Renal failure may develop in the absence of glomerular inflammation, and may occur either around the time of presentation or much later. The possible causes of ARF in nephrotic syndrome include hypovolemia, drug-induced interstitial nephritis, renal vein thrombosis, acute tubular necrosis secondary to sepsis, and crescentic transformation of underlying glomerular diseases. However, most cases of ARF are believed to be secondary to the abnormal renal hemodynamics associated with the nephrotic syndrome itself. Most reported cases are in adults, although children may also be affected [55–57]. Seventy-nine episodes of ARF were reviewed in 75 patients in the English literature since 1966 [58]. The incidence of a significant fall in GFR is more common than dialysis-dependent renal failure and may occur in up to 30% of children and adults [59, 60]. ARF occurred mostly in older patients (mean age 58 ± 2 years), two thirds were male, and proteinuria was usually heavy (11.6 ± 0.6 g/day) with low serum albumin concentration (19 ± 1 g/l). Renal failure developed a mean of 29 days after the onset of nephrotic syndrome and persisted for 7 weeks. The renal failure was irreversible in some patients. The underlying glomerular disease was membranoproliferative GN or focal segmental glomerulosclerosis in the majority. There are reports of only minimal or minor glomerular lesion as well [61]. Features consistent with acute tubular necrosis are the most common histopathologic finding, being observed in 60% of patients [58]. However, variable severity of tubular damage, from mild to very severe damage, is reported in the literature [62–65].

Hypovolemia resulting from a reduced plasma oncotic pressure is the obvious mechanism proposed to explain prerenal and established ARF in severe nephrosis. However, the majority of patients with nephrotic syndrome do not have reduced plasma volume [66]. Hypovolemia becomes a contributory factor in situations like diuretic therapy, diarrhea and vomiting, hemorrhage, or surgery. Diuretic treatment of severely nephrotic patients should be carefully monitored with weight loss aiming for not more than 3 kg per day. Nephrotics are particularly susceptible to ARF induced by nonsteroidal antiinflammatory drugs, and recovery of renal function is usual after withdrawal of drugs [67–69]. The filtration fraction is reduced in nephrotic syndrome, which is attributed to increased intratubular or interstitial pressure secondary to interstitial edema [70, 71]. Sometimes renal failure reverses with aggressive treatment of edema with diuretics and recurs with reaccumulation of edema [72].

Intratubular obstruction caused by intratubular protein casts is another hypothesis for ARF in nephrotic syndrome [53, 73, 74]. Drugs used in managing the nephrotic syndrome, including antibiotics, diuretics, and cimetidine, can cause ARF by inducing interstitial nephritis. These are well-documented causes of interstitial nephritis in minimal change nephropathy [75, 76]. The hypercoagulable state, which accompanies the nephrotic syndrome, predisposes to renal vein thrombosis (RVT). It rarely presents acutely with ARF [77, 78]. Epigastric or loin pain with hematuria are suggestive of RVT. Color Doppler ultrasound may be diagnostic, while confirmation or exclusion of diagnosis usually requires angiography or magnetic resonance venography.

6.8.9 Treatment and Prognosis of Glomerulonephritis/Vasculitis – Associated Acute Renal Failure

General measures: Dialysis and ultrafiltration may be carried out for an acute uremic state or fluid overload if indicated. Antibiotics are indicated if there is evidence of infection. The prophylactic oral nystatin, amphotericin, or fluconazole for fungal infection, and cotrimoxazole for infection with *Pneumocystis* are logical treatments for those who are immunosuppressed. Although routine, this practice is not evidence-based in this setting. The use of H_2 antagonists or proton-pump inhibitors has become standard practice as prophylaxis against stress ulcer in patients with ARF and for those given high-dose steroids. Antihypertensive drugs and diuretics are used for control of hypertension and edema.

Specific treatment: Three major vasculitic syndromes have a common therapeutic protocol. Corticosteroid and intermittent intravenous cyclophosphamide remain the mainstay of therapy of proliferative (severe class III & IV) lupus nephritis, anti-GBM disease, and ANCA-associated vasculitis. It is reasonable to minimize inflammation with prompt aggressive therapy. Typically, patients are given methylprednisolone (07 mg/kg daily for 3 days) followed by daily oral prednisone. Prednisone is started at a dose of 1 mg/kg/day for the first month, tapered to an alternate-day regimen during the second month, and discontinued by the end of 3–4 months. Cyclophosphamide is administered either orally (2 mg/kg/day) or monthly as an intravenous pulse at a starting dose of 0.5 g/m^2 body surface area for 6 months. The dosage is titrated upward during the first 6 month, increasing by 0.25 g/m^2 on successive treatment (not exceeding 1.0 g/m^2), provided that the 2-week leukocyte count remains above 3,000 $cell/mm^3$. After the first 6 months, pulse cyclophosphamide is given every 3 months for a total of 18–24 months. Several recent controlled trials have examined the role of mycophenolate mofetil (MMF) in the induction of remission of severe lupus nephritis. Patients treated with MMF had greater reduction in proteinuria, fever, and infections, and the complete remission rate was higher in the MMF arm [79, 80]. In addition, MMF was also found to be superior during the maintenance phase of severe lupus nephritis, once remission was achieved [81]. The dose of MMF is 2–3 g/day in two divided doses in the induction phase and 0.5–1 g twice daily during the maintenance phase of treatment.

Pulmonary hemorrhage in patients with anti-GBM disease and pauci-immune vasculitis is treated with plasmapheresis. It is typically performed daily until the pulmonary hemorrhage ceases and then every other day for a total of 7–10 treatments. Once remission is attained, an alternative maintenance regimen consists of switching cyclophosphamide to oral azathioprine at the end of 3 months [82]. Azathioprine is then continued for a total of 12–24 months. In pauci-immune vasculitis, the rate of remission is between 70% to 85% with use of an alkylating agent. Patients who *do* recover sufficient renal function, do so within the first 3 months of treatment. For that reason, and in the absence of active extrarenal vasculitis, immunosuppression may be stopped after 3 months if no sign of renal recovery has occurred. Relapse of ANCA-associated small vessel vasculitis occurs in about 30% of patients [83]. Relapsing ANCA-associated small vessel vasculitis responds to immunosuppression with corticosteroids and cytotoxic agents with a similar response rate to that for the initial disease. The survival rates of AAV patient have improved in recent years (from 54% to 84% survival in the first year, and from 38% to 80% survival in the *fifth year*) [84]. Elderly patients have worse survival curves than younger ones. Most death occurs in the acute phase of the disease, usually within the first 2 years, mainly due to lack of response to treatment, sepsis (2–20% of death), or severe associated disease (hemorrhage, thrombosis, and heart disease).

The use of aggressive plasmapheresis with corticosteroids and cyclophosphamide has improved patient and renal survival to approximately 85% and 60%, respectively, in patients with anti-GBM disease [85, 86]. The major prognostic marker of the progression to end-stage renal disease is the serum creatinine level at the time treatment is initiated. Patients with a serum creatinine level above 7 mg/dl are unlikely to recover sufficient renal function to discontinue renal replacement therapy [87]. For those patients with an elevated serum creatinine level, and who yet have active crescentic GN on biopsy, aggressive treatment should be continued for at least 4 weeks and discontinued in the absence of recovery of renal function by 8 weeks. In patients who have both circulating anti-GBM-Ab and ANCA, the chance of recovery of renal function is better when compared with that of patients with anti-GBM-Ab alone. In these patients, immunosuppressive therapy should not be withheld, even with serum creatinine level above 7 mg/dl, because the concomitant presence of ANCA may be associated with a more favorable renal outcome [88]. Recurrence of anti-GBM disease is rare, once remission is achieved [89, 90]. Similarly, the recurrence of anti-GBM disease after a renal transplant is also rare, provided the transplant is delayed until after disappearance or substantial diminution of anti-GBM antibody titer [91].

In summary, acute GN and vasculitis syndrome account for only a small minority of ARF cases. They represent a heterogeneous group of diseases with protean clinical presentation and disparate etiologies and pathogenetic mechanisms. However, they share a common clinical feature and lead to rapid deterioration of renal function and, if left untreated, may be fatal. Combined immunosuppressive therapy with prednisone and cyclophosphamide has improved outcomes for these patients in recent years. The most prominent adverse effects of this form of therapy are infection, bone disease, cataract, ovarian failure, and carcinoma of the urinary bladder. Infectious complications of immunosuppression account for nearly 20% of deaths among patients with SLE.

6.8.10 The Pulmonary Renal Syndrome

The pulmonary renal syndrome is characterized by the coexistence of life-threatening pulmonary hemorrhage and renal disease in individuals without any concomitant destructive pulmonary disease or coagulopathy

[92]. The association of fatal pulmonary hemorrhage and GN was originally observed at autopsy by Goodpasture in 1919 [93]. The treatment of patients with anti-GBM antibody disease is often debated. Bilateral nephrectomy resulted in cessation of the pulmonary hemorrhage in seven of 19 patients, as reported by Wilson and Dixon [94]. In recent years repeated plasmapheresis along with immunosuppressive therapy with steroids and cyclophosphamide has improved the prognosis of Goodpasture's disease [95, 96].

Pulmonary renal syndrome is a potentially life-threatening disorder characterized by a combination of diffuse pulmonary hemorrhage and rapidly progressive GN. Pulmonary renal syndromes are not a single entity, but caused by a wide variety of systemic immune diseases. AAVs account for approximately 60% and Goodpasture's syndrome for approximately 20% of the cases [97, 98]. The other disorders responsible for pulmonary renal syndromes include SLE, Henoch-Schönlein purpura, and various forms of primary systemic vasculitis. However, pulmonary hemorrhage is rarely reported in SLE [99]. The diagnosis rests on the identification of particular patterns of clinical, radiologic, pathologic, and laboratory features. Serologic testing is important in the diagnostic work-up of patients presenting with pulmonary renal syndrome. The majority of cases of pulmonary renal syndrome are associated with ANCAs, either C-ANCA or P-ANCA. The antigen target in Goodpasture's syndrome is type IV collagen, the major component of basement membrane. Diffuse alveolar hemorrhage is characterized by the presence of a hemorrhagic bronchoalveolar lavage (BAL) in serial BAL samples. In the clinical setting of an acute nephritic syndrome or rapidly progressive GN, percutaneous renal biopsy is commonly performed for histopathology and immunofluorescence studies of renal tissue.

The therapy of pulmonary renal syndrome is determined by the underlying disease. Plasmapheresis is always performed when alveolar hemorrhage is present and in most cases where the patient presents with need for immediate dialysis. Intense immunosuppression with cyclophosphamide and glucocorticoids, along with plasmapheresis in the event of Goodpasture's syndrome, is the mainstay of therapy. Supportive measures such as temporary ventilation and hemodialysis have further reduced mortality. Recent evidence suggests that patients with severe AAV and/or severe renal failure (serum creatinine >5.7 mg/dl) might benefit from plasma exchange in combination with cyclophosphamide and corticosteroids [100, 101]. Diffuse pulmonary hemorrhage and rapidly developing renal failure mimicking Goodpasture's syndrome as the initial manifestation of WG have been reported [102].

6.8.11 Take Home Pearls

- Acute glomerulonephritis and vasculitis are responsible for 10% and 5% of cases of total ARF, respectively.
- Acute poststreptococcal glomerulonephritis is the most common form of postinfectious GN, accounting for 10–20% of ARF cases due to glomerular diseases. It is still a common entity in tropical and developing countries, while its incidence is low in Europe and North America.
- In Europe and North America, small vessel vasculitis, systemic lupus erythematosus and anti-GBM disease are the usual causes of ARF due to glomerulonephritis/vasculitis.
- ANCA-associated vasculitis (AAV) is more common in the elderly than young persons.
- Immunologic study for ANCA, ANA, anti-ds DNA antibodies, anti-GBM antibodies, and complements are essential in the diagnostic work-up of ARF associated with glomerulonephritis/vasculitis.
- Renal biopsy is mandatory in all patients with acute glomerulonephritis/vasculitis for precise diagnosis. Kidney biopsy has diagnostic, therapeutic, and prognostic significance in these patients.
- Early diagnosis and immediate institution of immunosuppressive treatment or plasmapheresis is associated with favorable outcome.
- Corticosteroids and intravenous cyclophosphamide therapy remains the mainstay of treatment for severe proliferative lupus nephritis, anti-GBM disease and ANCA small vessel vasculitis.
- The most prominent adverse effects of immunosuppression therapy are infection, bone disease, cataract, ovarian failure, and carcinoma of the urinary bladder.
- Mycophenolate mofetil (MMF) has emerged as a promising therapeutic approach for both the induction and maintenance phase in patients with lupus nephritis.

- Pulmonary renal syndromes are not a single entity, but are caused by a wide variety of diseases. AAV accounts for 60% and Goodpasture's syndrome for approximately 20% of cases.
- The treatment of pulmonary renal syndrome is determined by the underlying disease. Plasmapheresis is always performed when pulmonary hemorrhage is present.

References

1. Anderson RJ, Schrier RW (1980): Clinical spectrum of oliguric and non-oliguric acute renal failure. In Brenner BM, Stein JH (eds) *Contemporary Issues in Nephrology*, Vol. 6. New York, Churchill Livingston.
2. Hou SH, Bushinsky DA, Wish JB, et al. (1983): Hospital acquired renal insufficiency: A prospective study. *Am. J. Med.* 74(2): 243–248.
3. Rasmussen HH, Ibels LS (1982): Acute renal failure: multivariate analysis of causes and risk factors. *Am. J. Med.* 73: 211–218.
4. Espinel CH, Gregory AW (1980): Differential diagnosis of acute renal failure. *Nephrology*. 13(2): 73–77.
5. Turney JH, Marshall DH, Brownjohn AM, et al. (1990): The evolution of acute renal failure (1956–1988). *Q, J. Med.* 74: 83–104.
6. Bamgboye EL, Mabayoje MO, Odutola TA, et al. (1993): Acute renal failure at the Lagos University Teaching Hospital: A 10 years review. *Renal Failure*. 15: 77–80.
7. Chugh KS, Sakhuja V, Malhotra HS, et al. (1989): Changing trends in acute renal failure in third-world countries – Chandigarh Study *Q. J. Med.* 73: 1117–1123.
8. Prakash J, Sen D, Saratkumar N, et al. (2003): Acute renal failure due to intrinsic renal diseases: Review of 1122 cases. *Renal Failure*. 25: 225–233.
9. Kandoth PW, Agrawal GJ, Dharnidharka VR (1994): Acute renal failure in children requiring dialysis therapy. *Indian Pediatrics*. 31: 305–309.
10. Haas M, Spargo BN, Wit EJ, Meehan SM (2000): Etiologies and outcome of acute renal insufficiencies in older adults: A renal biopsy study of 259 cases. *Am. J. Kid. dis.* 25: 433–437.
11. Prakash J, Gupta A, Malhotra V, et al. (1997): Acute renal failure in the elderly: A demographic and clinical study of patients in Eastern India. *Geriatric Nephrol. Urol.* 7: 67–72.
12. Prakash J, Singh AK, Saxena RK, et al. (2003): Glomerular disease in the elderly in India. *Int, Urol. Nephrol.* 35: 283–288.
13. Falk RJ, Hogan S, Carey TS, Jennette JC (1990): Clinical course of antineutrophil cytoplasmic antibody – associated glomerulo nephritis and systemic vasculitis. The Glomerular Disease collaborative Network. *Ann. Int. Med.* 113: 656–663.
14. Pascual J, Liano F, Ortuno J (1995): The elderly patient with renal failure. *J. Am. Soc. Nephrol.* 6: 144–153.
15. Couser WG (1982): Idiopathic rapidly progressive glomerulonephritis. *Am. J, Nephrology*. 2: 57–69.
16. Neild GH, Cameron JS, Ogg CS, et al. (1983): Rapidly progressive glomerulonephritis with extensive glomerular crescents formation. *Q, J, Med.* 52: 395–416.
17. Lieberman E (1973): Management of acute renal failure in infants and children. *Nephron*. 11: 193–208.
18. Stilmant MN, Balton WK, Sturgill BC, et al. (1979): Crescentic glomerulonephritis without immune deposit: clinico-pathologic features. *Kidney Int.* 15: 184–195.
19. Levine JS, Leiberthal W, Bernard DB, Salant DJ, et al. (1993): Acute renal failure associated with renal vascular disease, vasculitis, glomerulonephritis, and nephrotic syndrome. In Lazarus JM, Brenner BM (eds) *Acute Renal Failure*. New York, Churchill Livingston, pp. 247–356.
20. Conlon PJ, Jefferies F, Krigman HR, et al. (1998): Predictors of prognosis and risk of acute renal failure in bacterial endocarditis. *Clin. Nephrol.* 49: 96–101.
21. Beaufils M, Morel-Maroger L, Sraer JD, et al. (1976): Acute renal failure of glomerular origin during visceral abscesses. *N. Engl. J. Med.* 295: 185–189.
22. Saiz Garcia F, Zubimendi Herranz A, Silva Gonzaliz C (1982): Nephritis caused by shunt: care of nephropathy without the need of a surgical replacement of the ventriculo-atrial valve. *Rev. Clin. Esp.* 164–123.
23. Neugarten J, Baldwin DS (1984): Glomerulonephritis in bacterial endocarditis. *Am. J. Med.* 77(2): 297–304
24. Montseny JJ, Meyrier A, Kleinknecht D, Callard P (1995): The current spectrum of infectious glomerulonephritis. Experience with 76 patients and review of the literature. *Medicine*. 74: 63–73.
25. Adler SG, Cohen AN, Glassock RJ (1996): Secondary glomerular diseases. In Brenner BM (ed). *The Kidney*, 5th ed. Philadelphia, WB Saunders. pp.1498–1596.
26. Pusey CD, Rees AJ (1996): Rapidly progressive glomerulonephritis and antiglomerular basement membrane disease. In Weatherall DJ, Ledingham JGG, Warrell DA(eds) *Oxford Textbook of Medicine*, 3rd ed. Oxford, Oxford University Press. pp.3162–3166.
27. Ferrario F, Rastaldi MP, D'Amico G (1996): The crucial role of renal biopsy in the management of ANCA-associated renal vasculitis. *Nephrol. Dial. Transplant.* 11(4): 726–728.
28. Serra A, Martinez-Ocana JC (1997): Vasculitis con afectacion renal predominate en pacientes mayors de 65 anos. *Nefrologia*. 17(Suppl 3): 51–59.
29. Serra A, Cameron JS, Turner DR, et al. (1984): Vasculitis affecting the kidney: Presentation, histopathology and long-term outcome. *Q.J. Med.* 53: 181–207.
30. Higgins RM, Goldsmith DJA, Connolly J, et al. (1996): Vasculitis and rapidly progressive glomerulonephritis in the elderly. *Postgrad Med. J.* 72: 41–44.
31. Jayne DRW, Rasmussen N (1997): For the European Community Systemic Vasculitis Clinical Trials Study Group (ECSYSVASTRIAL). *Mayo Clin. Proc.* 72: 737–747.
32. Haubitz M, Schellong S, Göbel U, et al. (1998): Intravenous pulse administration of cyclophosphamide versus daily oral treatment in patients with antineutrophil cytoplasmic antibody-associated vasculitis and renal involvement: a prospective, randomized study. *Arthritis and Rheumatism*. 41: 1835–1844.
33. Nowack R, Göble U, Klooker P, et al. (1999): Mycophenolate Mofetil for maintenance therapy of Wegener's granulomatosis and microscopic polyangiitis: A pilot study in 11 patients with renal involvement. *J. Am. Soc. Nephrol.* 10: 1965–1971.

34. Weidner S, Geuss S, Hafezi-Rachti S, et al. (2004): ANCA-associated vasculitis with renal involvement: An outcome analysis. *Nephrol. Dial. Transplant.* 19: 1403–11.
35. Hass M, Eustace JA (2004): Immune complex deposits in ANCA-associated crescentic glomerulonephritis: A study of 126 cases. *Kidney Int.* 65: 2145–2152.
36. Wu Q, Jinde K, Endoh M, et al. (2003): Co-stimulatory molecules CD80 and CD86 in human crescentic glomerulonephritis. *Am. J. Kidney Dis.* 41: 950–961.
37. Evans DJ, Savage COS, Winearls CG, et al. (1987): Renal biopsy in prognosis of treated "glomerulonephritis with crescents". *Abstract of the 10th International Congress of Nephrology.* pp.60.
38. Heyman SN, Brezis M (1995): Acute renal failure in glomerular bleeding: a puzzling phenomenon. *Nephrol. Dial. Transplant.* 10: 591–593.
39. Brezis M, Heyman SN, Dinur D (1991): Role of nitric oxide in renal medullary oxygen balance, Studies in isolated and intact rat kidneys. *J. Clinic. Invest*, 88: 390–395.
40. Delclaux C, Jacquot C, Callard P, Kleinknecht D (1993): Acute reversible renal failure with macroscopic hematuria in IgA nephropathy. *Nephrol. Dial. Transplant.* 8: 195–199.
41. Fairley KF, Birch DF (1982): Hematuria: A simple method for identifying glomerular bleeding. *Kid. Int.* 21: 105–108.
42. Prakash J, Tripathi K, Usha, Kumar P (1992, Nov.): Clinical significance of kidney biopsy in Acute Renal Failure. *Indian J. Med. Sci.* 46(11): 328–331.
43. Nicholls KM, Fairley KS, Dowling JP, et al. (1984): The clinical course of Mesangial IgA nephropathy in adults. *Q. J. Med.* 53: 227–256.
44. Welch TR, McAdams AJ, Berry A (1988): Rapidly progressive IgA nephropathy. *Am. J. Diseases Childhood.* 41: 789–793.
45. Packham DK, Hewitson TD, Yan HD, et al. (1994): Acute renal failure in IgA Nephropathy. *Clin. Nephrol.* 42: 349–353.
46. Praga M, Millet VG, Navas JJ, et al. (1985): Acute worsening of renal function during episodes of macroscopic hematuria in IgA nephropathy. *Kidney Int.* 28: 69–74.
47. Kim Y, Michael AF, Fish AJ (1982): Idiopathic membranoproliferative glomerulonephritis. In Brenner BM, Stein J (eds) *Nephrotic Syndrome*. New York, Churchill Livingston. pp. 237–257.
48. Korzets A, Bernheim J, Bernheim J (1987): Rapidly progressive glomerulonephritis (crescentic GN) in the course of Type I idiopathic membranoproliferative glomerulonephritis. *Am. J. Kid. dis.* 10: 56–61.
49. Abreo K, Abero F, Mitchell B, et al. (1986): Idiopathic crescentic membranous glomerulonephritis. *Am. J. Kidney dis.* 8: 257–261.
50. Moorthy AV, Zimmerman SW, Burkholder PM, et al. (1976): Association of crescentic glomerulonephritis with membranous nephropathy: a report of three cases. *Clin. Nephrol.* 6: 319–325.
51. James SH, Lien Y, Ruffenach SJ, et al. (1995): ARF in membranous glomerulopathy: a result of superimposed crescentic glomerulo-nephritis. *J. Am. Soc. Nephrol.* 6: 1541–1546.
52. Cameron JS (1988): Allergic interstitial nephritis: clinical feature and pathogenesis. *Q. J. Med.* 66: 97–115.
53. D'Amico G, Colasanti G, Ferrario F, et al. (1989): Renal involvement in essential mixed cryoglobulinemia. *Kidney Int.* 35: 1004–1014.
54. Habib R, Niaudet P, Levy M (1993): Schonlein-Henoch-Purpura nephritis and IgA nephropathy. In Tisher C, Brenner BM (eds) *Renal Pathology with Clinical and Functional Correlation.* Philadelphia, PA, Lippincott. pp. 472–523.
55. Steele BT, Bacheyic GS, Baumal R, et al. (1982): Acute renal failure of short duration in minimal change nephrotic syndrome. *Int. J. Pediatr. Nephrol.* 3: 59–62.
56. Spingate JE, Coyne JF, Karp MP (1987): Acute renal failure in minimal change nephrotic syndrome. *Pediatrics.* 80: 946–948.
57. Sakarcan A, Timmnons C, Seikaly MG (1994): Reversible idiopathic acute renal failure in children with primary nephrotic syndrome. *J. Pediatrics.* 125:723–727.
58. Smith JD, Hayslett JP (1992): Reversible renal failure in nephrotic syndrome. *Am. J. Kid. Dis.* 19: 201–213.
59. ISKD (1978): Nephrotic syndrome in children: Prediction of histopathology from clinical and laboratory characteristic at time of diagnosis. A report of the international study of Kidney Disease in children. *Kid. Int.* 13: 159–165.
60. Nolasco F, Cameron JS, Heywood EF, et al. (1986): Adult onset minimal change nephrotic syndrome: a long-term follow-up. *Kid. Int.* 29: 1212–1223.
61. Raij L, Keane WF, Leonard A, et al. (1976): Irreversible acute renal failure in idiopathic nephrotic syndrome. *Am. J. Med.* 61:207–214.
62. Cameron JS, Turner DR, Ogg CS, et al. (1974): The nephrotic syndrome in adults with "minimal change" glomerular lesions. *Q. J. Med.* 43: 461–488.
63. Lowenstein J, Schacht RG, Baldwin DS (1981): Renal failure in minimal change nephrotic syndrome. *Am. J. Med.* 70: 227–233.
64. Esparza AR, Khan SI, Garella S, et al. (1981): Spectrum of acute renal failure in nephrotic syndrome with minimal (or minor) glomerular lesion; role of hemodynamic factors. *Lab. Invest.* 45: 510–521.
65. Jennette JC, Falk RJ (1990): Adult minimal change glomerulopathy with acute renal failure. *Am. J. Kid. Dis.* 16: 432–437.
66. Dorhout Mees EJ, Geers AB, Koomans HA (1984): Blood volume and sodium retention in the nephrotic syndrome: A controversial pathophysiological concept. *Nephron.* 36: 201–211.
67. Clive DM, Stoff JS (1984): Renal syndrome associated with non-steroidal anti-inflammatory drugs. *N. Engl. J. Med.* 310: 563–572.
68. Arisz L, Donker AJM, Brentjens JRH, et al. (1976): The effect of indomethacin on proteinuria and kidney function in the nephrotic syndrome. *Acta. Medico. Scandinavica.* 199: 121–125.
69. Vriesendorp R, Donker AJ, De Zeeuw D, et al. (1986): Effect of non-steroidal anti-inflammatory drugs on proteinuria. *Am. J. Med.* 81: 84–94.
70. Furuya R, Kumagai H, Ikegaya N, et al. (1993): Reversible acute renal failure in idiopathic nephrotic syndrome. *Intern. Med.* 32: 31–35.
71. Geers AB, Koomans HA, Roos JC (1984): Functional relationship in nephrotic syndrome. *Kid. Int.* 26: 324–331.
72. Stephens VJ, Yates AP, Lechler RI, et al. (1979): Reversible uremia in normotensive nephrotic syndrome. *BMJ.* 11: 705–706.
73. Kuroda S, Aynedjian NS, Bank N (1979): A micropuncture study of renal sodium retention in nephrotic syndrome in

rats: evidence for increased resistance to tubular fluid flow. *Kid. Int.* 16: 561–571.
74. Imbasciati E, Ponticelli C, Case N, et al. (1981): Acute renal failure in idiopathic nephrotic syndrome. *Nephron.* 28: 186–191.
75. Finkelstein A, Fraley DS, Stachural L, et al. (1982): Fenoprofen nephropathy: lipoid nephrosis and interstitial nephritis. A possible T-Lymphocyte disorder. *Am. J. Med.* 72: 81–87.
76. Van Ypersele de Strihou C (1979): Acute oliguric interstitial nephritis (Nephrology Forum). *Kid. Int.* 16: 751–765.
77. Duffy JL, Letteri J, Cinque T, et al. (1973): Renal vein thrombosis and the nephrotic syndrome: Report of two cases with successful treatment of one. *Am. J. Med.* 54: 663–672.
78. Llach F, Pappes S, Massary SG (1980): The clinical spectrum of renal vein thrombosis: Acute write chronic. *Am. J. Med.* 69: 819–827.
79. Ginzler EM, Dooley MA, Aranow C, et al. (2005): Mycophenolate mofetil or intravenous cyclophosphamide for lupus nephritis. *N. Engl. J. Med.* 353: 2219–2228.
80. Chan TM, Tse KC, Tang CS, et al. (2005): Long term study of mycophenolate mofetil as continuous induction and maintenance treatment for diffuse proliferative lupus nephritis. *J. Am. Soc. Nephrol.* 16; 1076–1084.
81. Sinclair A, Appel GB, Dooler MA, et al. (2005): The Aspreva Lupus Management-ALMS trial. *J. Am. Soc. Nephrol.* 16: 528A.
82. Pusey CD, Rees AJ, Evan DJ, et al. (1991): Plasma exchange in focal necrotizing glomerulonephritis without anti-GBM Antibodies. *Kid. Int.* 40: 757–763.
83. Nachman PH, Hogan SL, Jennette JC, et al. (1996): Treatment response and relapse in ANCA-associated microscopic polyangiitis and glomerulonephritis. *J. Am. Soc. Nephrol.* 7: 33–39.
84. Fuiano G, Cameron JS, Raftery M, et al. (1988): Improved prognosis of renal microscopic polyarteritis in recent years. *Nephrol. Dial. Transplant.* 3: 383–391.
85. Peters DK, Rees AJ, Lockwood CM, et al. (1982): Treatment and prognosis in antibasement membrane antibody-mediated nephritis. *Trans. Proc.* 14: 513–521.
86. Madore F, Lazarus JM, Brady HR, (1996): Therapeutic plasma exchange in renal disease. *J. Am. Soc. Nephrol.* 7: 367–386.
87. Merkel F, Pulling O, Marx M, et al. (1994): Course and prognosis of antibasement membrane antibody mediated disease: report of 35 cases. *Nephrol. Dial. Transplant.* 9: 372–376.
88. Jayne DR, Marshall PD, Jones SJ, et al. (1990): Autoantibodies to GBM and neutrophil cytoplasm in rapidly progressive glomerulonephritis. *Kid. Int.* 37: 965–970.
89. Dahlberg PJ, Kurtz SB, Donadio JV, et al. (1978): Recurrent Goodpasture's syndrome. *Mayo. Clin. Proc.* 53: 533–537.
90. Wu MJ, Moorthy AV, Beirne GJ (1980): Relapse in Anti glomerular basement membrane antibody-mediated crescentic glomerulo nephritis. *Clin. Nephrol.* 13: 97.
91. Almkuist RD, Buckalew VM Jr, Hirszel P, et al. (1981): Recurrence of Anti-GBM-mediated glomerulonephritis in an isograft. *Clin. Immunol. Immunopathol.* 18: 54–60.
92. Herman PG, Balikian JP, Seltzer SE, Ehrie M (1978): The pulmonary-renal syndrome. *Am. J. Roentgenol.* 130: 1141–1148.
93. Goodpasture EW (1919): The significance of certain pulmonary lesions in relation to the etiology of influenza. *Am. J. Med. Sci.* 158: 863–870.
94. Wilson CB, Dixon FJ (1973): Anti-glomerular basement membrane antibody-induced glomerulonephritis. *Kidney Int.* 3: 74–89.
95. Lockwood CM, Rees AJ, Pearson TA, et al. (1976): Immuno suppression and plasma exchange in the treatment of Goodpasture's syndrome. *Lancet.* 1: 711–715.
96. Kopelman R, Hoffsten P, Kahr S (1975): Steroid therapy in Good pasture's syndrome. *Ann. Intern. Med.* 83: 734–735.
97. Dixon FJ (1971): Glomerulonephritis and immunopathology. In Good R.A., Fisher D.W (eds) *Immunobiology.* Stamford Conn. Sinauer. pp. 167–173.
98. Wolff SM, Fauci AS, Horn RG, Dale DC (1974): Wegener's Granulomatosis. *Ann, Intern. Med.* 81: 513–525.
99. Matthay RA, Schwartz MI, Petty TL, et al. (1974): Pulmonary manifestation of systemic lupus erythromatosus: review of twelve cases of acute lupus pneumonitis. *Medicine.* 54: 397–409.
100. Brusselle GG (2007): Pulmonary renal syndrome. *Acta. Clin. Belg.* 62: 88–96.
101. Sugimoto T, Deji N, Kume S, et al. (2007): Pulmonary renal syndrome, diffuse pulmonary hemorrhage and glomerulonephritis associated with Wegener's Granulomatosis effectively treated with early plasma exchange therapy. *Intern. Med.* 46: 49–53.
102. Hensley MJ, Feldman NT, Lazarus JM, Galvanek EG (1979): Diffuse pulmonary hemorrhage and rapidly progressive renal failure. An uncommon presentation of Wegener's Granulomatosis. *Am. J. Med.* 66: 894–898.

6.9 Hemolytic Uremic Syndrome/Thrombotic Thrombocytopenic Purpura

Marina Noris, Miriam Galbusera, and Giuseppe Remuzzi

Core Messages

- Hemolytic uremic syndrome (HUS) and thrombotic thrombocytopenic purpura (TTP) are thrombotic microangiopathies (TMAs) manifesting with thrombocytopenia and microangiopathic hemolytic anemia.
- TMA have either an acquired or a genetic origin.
- The most common form of TMA is Shigatoxin-associated HUS, which is caused by certain strains of bacteria that produce exotoxins, the Shiga-like toxins causing endothelial damage. This form has generally a good outcome with supportive therapy.
- Immune-mediated HUS and TTP are caused by the formation of autoantibodies against complement factor H or ADAMTS-13, respectively. These forms benefit from plasma exchange combined with immunosuppressive treatments.
- Treatment of forms secondary to systemic diseases rests on specific treatments of the underlying condition.
- Genetic predisposition to HUS is determined by mutations in genes encoding complement regulatory proteins. The outcome is poor. Some forms respond to plasma treatment.
- Genetic deficiency of ADAMTS13 is associated with congenital TTP. This form benefits from plasma therapy.

G. Remuzzi (✉)
Clinical Research Center for Rare Diseases "Aldo e Cele Daccò", Mario Negri Institute for Pharmacological Research, Bergamo, Via Gavazzeni, 11, 24125 Bergamo, Italy
e-mail: gremuzzi@marionegri.it

6.9.1 Introduction

The term thrombotic microangiopathy (TMA) defines a lesion of vessel wall thickening (mainly arterioles or capillaries), intraluminal platelet thrombosis, and partial or complete obstruction of the vessel lumina. Laboratory features of thrombocytopenia and microangiopathic hemolytic anemia are almost invariably present in patients with TMA lesions and reflect consumption and disruption of platelets and erythrocytes in the microvasculature. Depending on whether renal or brain lesions prevail, two pathologically indistinguishable, but somehow clinically different entities have been described: the hemolytic uremic syndrome (HUS) and thrombotic thrombocytopenic purpura (TTP).

Injury to the endothelial cell is the central and likely inciting factor in the sequence of events leading to TMA. Loss of physiologic thromboresistance, leukocyte adhesion to damaged endothelium, complement consumption, abnormal von Willebrand factor processing, and increased vascular shear stress may then sustain and amplify the microangiopathic process. Intrinsic abnormalities of the complement system and of the von Willebrand factor pathway may account for a genetic predisposition to the disease that may play a paramount role in particular in familial and recurrent forms.

6.9.2 Acquired Forms

6.9.2.1 Shigatoxin (Stx)–Associated-HUS

Shigatoxin (Stx)–associated HUS – the most frequent form of TMA – may follow infection by certain strains of *Escherichia coli or Shigella dysenteriae* which produce a powerful exotoxin (Shigatoxin [Stx]) [59].

A. Jörres et al. (eds.), *Management of Acute Kidney Problems*,
DOI: 10.1007/978-3-540-69441-0_6.9, © Springer-Verlag Berlin Heidelberg 2010

The term Shigatoxin (Stx) was initially used to describe the exotoxin produced by *S. dysenteriae* type 1. Then, some strains of *E. coli* (mostly the serotype 0157:H7) isolated from human cases with diarrhea were found to produce a toxin similar to the one of *S. dysenteriae.* After food contaminated by Stx-producing *E. coli* or *S. dysenteriae* is ingested, the toxin is released in the gut and may cause watery or, most often, bloody diarrhea because of a direct effect on the intestinal mucosa. When Stx through the intestinal mucosa reaches the systemic circulation, full-blown HUS may develop. Stx-associated HUS is usually considered a disease with a good outcome, with complete recovery in about 90% of cases. However, a recent meta-analysis of 49 studies including 3,476 patients showed that 12% of patients die during the acute phase of the disease or remain dialysis dependent, 16% have residual kidney insufficiency with glomerular filtration rate (GFR) values ranging from 5 to 80 ml/min/1.73 m^2, 15% are proteinuric, and 10% hypertensive [25].

Diagnosis rests on detection of *E. coli* 0157:H7 in stool cultures. Serologic tests for antibodies to Stx and O157 lipopolysaccharide can be done in research laboratories, and tests are being developed for rapid detection of *E. coli* O157:H7 and Shigatoxin in stools.

Undercooked ground beef is the commonest source of infection, but ham, turkey, cheese, unpasteurized milk, juice, and water have also been implicated. Secondary person-to-person contact is an important way of spread in institutional centers, particularly day-care centers and nursing homes. Infected patients should be excluded from day-care centers until two consecutive stool cultures are negative for *E. coli* O157:H7 to prevent further transmission. However, the most important preventive measure in child-care centers is supervised hand-washing.

6.9.2.1.1 Supportive Therapy

In typical Stx-associated HUS of children, the mortality rate has significantly decreased over the last 40 years probably as the result of better supportive management of anemia, renal failure, hypertension, and electrolyte and water imbalance. Intravenous isotonic volume expansion as soon as an *E. coli* O157:H7 infection is suspected – that is within the first 4 days of illness, even before culture results are available – may limit the severity of kidney dysfunction and the need for renal replacement therapy [1]. Bowel rest is important for the enterohemorrhagic colitis associated with Stx-HUS. Anti-motility agents should be avoided since these may prolong the persistency of *E. coli* in the intestinal lumen and therefore increase patient exposure to its toxin. The use of antibiotics should be restricted to the very limited number of patients presenting with bacteremia [10], because in children with gastroenteritis they may increase the risk of HUS by 17-fold [75]. A possible explanation is that antibiotic-induced injury to the bacterial membrane might favor the acute release of large amounts of preformed toxin. Alternatively, antibiotic therapy might give *E. coli* O157:H7 a selective advantage if these organisms are not as readily eliminated from the bowel as are the normal intestinal flora. Moreover, several antimicrobial drugs, particularly the quinolones, trimethoprim, and furazolidone, are potent inducers of the expression of the Stx 2 gene and may increase the level of toxin in the intestine. Although the possibility of a cause-and-effect relationship between antibiotic therapy and increased risk of HUS has been challenged by a recent meta-analysis of 26 reports [61], there is no reason to prescribe antibiotics, since they do not improve the outcome of colitis, and bacteremia is only exceptionally found in Stx-associated HUS. However, when hemorrhagic colitis is caused by *Shigella dysenteria* type 1, early and empirical antibiotic treatment shortens the duration of diarrhea, decreases the incidence of complications, and reduces the risk of transmission by shortening the duration of bacterial shedding. Thus, in developing countries where Shigella is the most frequent cause of hemorrhagic colitis, antibiotic therapy should be started early and even before the involved pathogen is identified.

Careful blood pressure control and renin-angiotensin system blockade may be particularly beneficial on the long-term for those patients who suffer chronic renal disease after an episode of Stx-HUS. A study in 45 children with renal sequelae of HUS followed for 9–11 years documented that early restriction of proteins and use of angiotensin-converting enzyme (ACE) inhibitors may have a beneficial effect on long-term renal outcome, as documented by a positive slope of 1/creatinine values over time in treated patients [6]. In another study, 8–15 year treatment with ACE inhibitors after severe Stx-HUS, normalized blood pressure, reduced proteinuria, and improved GFR [70].

6.9.2.1.2 Shigatoxin-Binding Agents

An oral Shigatoxin-binding agent composed of repeated synthetic carbohydrate determinants linked to colloidal silica that may compete with endothelial and epithelial receptors for Shigatoxin in the gut (SYNSORB Pk) has been developed with the rational of limiting target organ exposure to the toxin. However, after preliminary studies showing that the drug is well tolerated and effectively binds the toxin, a prospective, randomized, double blind, placebo-controlled, clinical trial of 145 children with diarrhea-associated HUS failed to demonstrate any beneficial effect of treatment on disease outcome [67].

6.9.2.1.3 Plasma Manipulation and Other Specific Treatments

No specific therapy aimed at preventing or limiting the microangiopathic process has been proven to affect the course of Stx-HUS in children. Two prospective controlled trials found that plasma therapy may limit short-term renal lesions, but does not affect long-term renal outcome and patients' survival [40, 54]. Heparin and antithrombotic agents may increase the risk of bleeding and should be avoided. Whether tissue type plasminogen activator (t-PA), discriminating between fibrin and fibrin-bound plasminogen, gives a better risk-to-benefit profile in the treatment of HUS is worth investigating.

Efficacy of specific treatments in adult patients is difficult to evaluate, since most information is derived from uncontrolled series that may include also non-Stx-HUS cases. In particular no prospective randomized trials are available to definitely establish whether plasma infusion or exchange may offer some specific benefit as compared with supportive treatment alone. However, comparative analyses of two large series of patients treated [15] or not [9] with plasma suggest that plasma therapy may dramatically decrease overall mortality of Stx-*E. coli* 0157:H7–associated HUS. These findings lead us and others to consider plasma infusion or exchange suitable for adult patients, in particular in those with severe renal insufficiency and central nervous system involvement.

6.9.2.1.4 Kidney Transplantation

Kidney transplant should be considered as an effective and safe treatment for those children who progress to end-stage renal disease (ESRD). Indeed the outcome of renal transplantation is good in children with Stx-HUS: recurrence rates range from 0% to 10% [2, 39] and graft survival at 10 years is even better than in control children with other diseases [17].

6.9.2.2 Neuraminidase Associated–HUS

This is a rare but potentially fatal disease that may complicate pneumonia, or less frequently, meningitis caused by *Streptococcus pneumoniae*. Neuraminidase produced by *S. pneumoniae*, by removing sialic acid from the cell membranes, exposes Thomsen-Friedenreich antigen to preformed circulating IgM antibodies [43]. Then, binding of circulating preformed IgM antibodies to this cryptic antigen exposed on platelet and endothelial cell surfaces causes platelet aggregation and endothelial damage. Binding of IgM antibodies to the antigen expressed on circulating erythrocytes may also explain why Coombs positive hemolytic anemia is so frequently reported in patients with neuraminidase-induced HUS. The clinical picture is usually severe, with respiratory distress, neurologic involvement, and coma.

6.9.2.2.1 Therapy

The outcome is strongly dependent on the effectiveness of antibiotic therapy. In theory, plasma either infused or exchanged, is contraindicated, because adult plasma contains antibodies against the Thomsen-Friedenreich antigen that may accelerate poly agglutination and hemolysis [43]. Thus, patients should be treated only with antibiotics and washed red cells. In some cases, however, plasma therapy, occasionally in combination with steroids, has been associated with recovery.

6.9.2.3 HUS Associated with Immune-Mediated Defective Activity of Complement Regulatory Proteins

Recurrent, atypical HUS has been recently reported [14] in three children with circulating IgG autoantibodies against complement factor H (CFH), a circulating glycoprotein that modulates the activity of the alternative complement pathway (see paragraph on HUS associated with genetic abnormalities in complement regulatory proteins). Subsequent studies in five unrelated patients found that the binding epitopes for CFH autoantibodies localize in the C terminus of CFH [35].

Of interest, the children showed an increased titer of circulating antinuclear antibodies, a finding that supports the possibility of an autoimmune pathogenesis of the disease. One child had two recurrences with pancreas and liver involvement, progressed to ESRD, and eventually required a bilateral nephrectomy to control refractory hypertension. The other two children recovered from the first episode with plasma exchange, then had four and three relapses, respectively, with heart involvement in one case that again recovered with plasma exchange. These two children were maintained on chronic therapy with steroid or azathioprine, respectively.

6.9.2.3.1 Treatment

Available information is insufficient to provide clear-cut guidelines to treatment of this so rare form of HUS. Conceivably, however, when anti-CFH autoantibodies are detected, plasma exchange and steroid, or other immunosuppressive agents, should be considered with the rationale of removing as soon as possible the pathogenic antibody from the circulation, and inhibiting its synthesis.

6.9.2.4 TTP Associated with Immune-Mediated Deficiency of VWF-Cleaving Protease (ADAMTS13) Activity

This is a recently categorized immune-mediated, nonfamilial form of TMA that most likely accounts for the majority of cases so far reported as acute idiopathic or sporadic TTP. The disease is characterized by a severe deficiency of a plasma metalloprotease, ADAMTS13, that in normal individuals cleaves ultralarge von Willebrand factor (ULVWF) multimers as soon as they are secreted [21] and in TTP patients is inhibited by a specific autoantibody that develops transiently and tends to disappear during remission [20, 24, 68, 72]. These inhibitory anti-ADAMTS13 antibodies, characterized either as IgG or IgM and IgA, have been detected in 50–90% of patients with acquired TTP [16, 24]. Evidence of the pathogenetic role of these autoantibodies is derived from the finding that they usually disappear from the circulation when remission is achieved by effective treatment, and that this occurs in parallel with the normalization of ADAMTS13 activity. In patients with acquired ADAMTS13 deficiency, a risk as high as 50% to develop relapses has been reported [29], and undetectable ADAMTS13 activity and persistence of anti-ADAMTS13 inhibitors during remission are predictors of recurrences [16]. Of note, autoantibodies against ADAMTS13 have also been observed in patients developing TTP during treatment with antiplatelet drugs such as ticlopidine (see Section 6.9.2.7 Drug-Associated TMA).

In comparison with patients without autoantibodies, patients with anti-ADAMTS13 inhibitors experience a more severe manifestation of the disease and have a higher mortality rate [41]. Neurologic symptoms usually dominate the clinical picture and may be fleeting and fluctuating, probably because of continuous thrombi formation and dispersion in the brain microcirculation. Coma and seizures complicate more severe forms.

6.9.2.4.1 Supportive Therapy, Plasma Manipulation, and Other Specific Treatments

In the early 1960s, TTP was almost invariably fatal, but nowadays, thanks to earlier diagnosis, improved intensive care facilities, and new techniques such as plasma therapy, survival may reach 90% [4, 55].

Plasma manipulation is a cornerstone in the therapy of the acute episode. Plasma may serve to induce remission of the disease by replacing defective protease activity. In theory, as compared with infusion, exchange may offer the advantage of also rapidly removing anti-ADAMTS13 antibodies. This, however, needs to be proven in controlled trials. In patients with acquired ADAMTS13 deficiency, adjunctive immunosuppressive treatment with corticosteroids might be beneficial in inhibiting the synthesis of antiprotease autoantibodies [29]. The rationale of combined treatment is that plasma exchange will have only a temporary effect on the presumed autoimmune basis of the disease, and additional immunosuppressive treatment may cause a more durable response.

6.9.2.4.2 Rescue Treatments

Rituximab – Recently, the infusion of rituximab, an antibody directed against B cells, administered as adjunctive treatment, has been proven to be effective in inducing remission in TTP patients with anti-ADAMTS13 antibodies refractory to any other treatment [24] and in maintaining patients in remission when used as prophylactic therapy. Longitudinal evaluation of ADAMTS13 activity and autoantibodies levels may help in monitoring patient response to treatment.

Splenectomy – After contrasting results obtained in studies on small series of TTP patients [4, 12, 32], splenectomy was no longer considered for treating TTP refractory to plasma therapy. The above studies, however, were far from conclusive because of their retrospective design and because they included unselected series of patients. Most likely, splenectomy might have a specific indication just in the subset of patients with autoantibodies against ADAMTS13 that persist in the circulation despite immunosuppressive therapy [20]. In this setting, splenectomy might achieve persistent remission by removing a major site of antibody synthesis. Three patients with TTP and high levels of anti-ADAMTS13 autoantibodies entered remission after splenectomy. Splenectomy was followed by disappearance of the inhibitor and normalization of the protease activity [20, 23]. The above reports, however, are far from conclusive and further studies with a larger number of patients are needed to prove the therapeutic value of this irreversible procedure.

Platelet transfusions – The severe thrombocytopenia in TTP has led many physicians to administer platelet transfusions with the aim of preventing severe bleeding complications. However, reports of sudden death, decreased survival, and delayed recovery after platelet transfusion dramatically document the danger of giving platelets to patients with active TTP. Thus, platelet transfusions are contraindicated in acute TTP, with the sole exception of cases of life-threatening bleeding.

6.9.2.5 Pregnancy Associated-TMA

TMA associated with pregnancy includes TTP (usually in the early phases of pregnancy), hemolysis, elevated liver enzymes and low platelet (HELLP) syndrome (usually near term), and HUS (usually postpartum) [73]. The disease is considered a specific complication of pregnancy, but reports of women with familial recurrence or defective ADAMTS13 activity without a demonstrable inhibitor provide convincing evidence that, at least in a proportion of cases, an underlying genetic predisposition plays a central role in the pathogenesis of TMA and pregnancy may just represent a precipitating event [28]. Changes observed during normal pregnancy, such as progressively decreasing fibrinolytic activity, loss of endothelial thrombomodulin, increasing levels of procoagulant factors, and, also, decreasing ADAMTS13 activity, may contribute to precipitate the disease in those at risk.

6.9.2.5.1 TTP

TTP develops during the antepartum period in 89% of cases, usually within 24 weeks. Later in the course of pregnancy, clinical features of TTP and preeclampsia may overlap. Despite limited experience, available series show that the maternal mortality rate has fallen from 68% to almost zero with the institution of plasma therapy [73]. Delivery is recommended only for those patients who do not respond to plasma therapy. However, delivery is the treatment of choice for preeclampsia/HELLP syndrome.

Measurement of plasma antithrombin III (ATIII) activity has been suggested as a useful tool to differentiate TTP and preeclampsia. Before gestational week 28 and when ATIII plasma activity is normal, TTP is most likely. Plasma therapy could be tried, and, if effective, it should be continued until term and/or complete remission of the disease. Delivery can be considered as "rescue" after failure of plasma therapy. The role of other treatments often employed in idiopathic TTP remains elusive.

After week 34 of gestation, preeclampsia is most likely and is usually associated with decreased plasma ATIII activity. Delivery is the treatment of choice and is usually followed by complete recovery within 24–48 h. Persistent disease may be an indication to attempt a course of plasma therapy. Between 28 and 34 weeks, the optimal treatment is controversial. It is sometimes held that delivery should always be considered as first-line therapy, whereas others believe that if there is no evidence of fetal distress and plasma ATIII activity is normal, a course of plasma therapy can be reasonably attempted before inducing delivery [60].

6.9.2.5.2 The HELLP Syndrome

The HELLP syndrome (an acronym for hemolysis, elevated liver enzymes and low platelet count) is simply a form of severe preeclampsia in which besides hypertension and renal dysfunction, there is evidence of microangiopathic hemolysis and liver involvement. The syndrome is most common in white multiparous women with a history of poor pregnancy outcome. It arises in the antepartum period in 70% of cases. Symptoms usually arise within 24–48 h postpartum, occasionally after an uncomplicated pregnancy [73].

Diagnosis is based on: (1) hemolysis (defined as fragmented erythrocytes in the circulation and lactic dehydrogenase $\geq$ 600 U/l), (2) elevated liver enzymes (serum glutamic oxaloacetic transaminase > 70 U/l), and (3) low platelets (platelet count < $100 \times 10^3/\text{mm}^3$) [23]. Overt disseminated intravascular coagulation (DIC) is reported in 25% of cases. Intrahepatic hemorrhage, subcapsular liver hematoma, and liver rupture are rare, life-threatening complications. The maternal and perinatal mortality rates range from 0 to 24% and from 7.7% to 60%, respectively. Most of the perinatal deaths are related to abruptio placentae, intrauterine asphyxia, and extreme prematurity. As many as 44% the infants are growth-retarded.

Termination of pregnancy is the only definitive therapy. Hydralazine or dihydralazine are the first-choice drugs to control pregnancy-induced hypertension, magnesium sulfate to prevent and treat convulsions. Both peritoneal dialysis and hemodialysis have been used to treat acute renal failure. Platelet transfusions are needed for clinical bleeding or severe thrombocytopenia (platelet count < 20,000/μl).

In approximately 5% of patients with HELLP syndrome, symptoms, and laboratory abnormalities do not improve after delivery. These are cases with central nervous system abnormalities, associated with renal and cardiopulmonary dysfunction and activation of coagulation. Uncontrolled studies suggest that plasma exchange may help recovery in patients with persistent evidence of disease 72 h or more after delivery. However, plasma therapy is ineffective during pregnancy and may increase fetal and maternal risk when used to delay delivery. Preliminary evidence suggests that, postpartum, corticosteroids may speed up disease recovery and, antepartum, may postpone delivery of pre viable fetuses and reduce the mother's need for blood products.

6.9.2.5.3 Postpartum HUS

By definition, postpartum HUS follows a normal delivery by no more than 6 months [59]. The clinical course is usually fulminant. Supportive care including dialysis, transfusions, and careful fluid management remains the most important form of treatment. Whether plasma therapy improves survival or limits renal sequelae has not been established so far. Antiplatelet agents, heparin, and antithrombotic therapy may enhance the risk of bleeding and have no proven efficacy.

6.9.2.6 Systemic Disease–Associated TMA

Prevention and treatment of TMA associated with systemic diseases (antiphospholipid syndrome, systemic lupus erythematosus, scleroderma, malignant hypertension, HIV, cancer) largely rests on specific treatment of the underlying conditions.

Plasma therapy should always be attempted in TMA associated with systemic diseases even if its efficacy in this setting is poorly defined.

6.9.2.7 Drug-Associated TMA

6.9.2.7.1 Mitomycin and Anticancer Drugs

A form of TMA resembling HUS has been described in cancer patients treated with mitomycin C. Disease manifestation is dose related, with renal dysfunction reported in less than 2% of patients given a cumulative dose lower than 50 mg/m^2 and in more than 28% of those given more than 50 mg/m^2 or receiving more than one course of therapy. Platinum- and bleomycin-containing combinations have also been reported to induce HUS. The fatality rate is close to 79%, and median time to death is about 4 weeks. Patients surviving the acute phase often remain on chronic dialysis, or die later of recurrence of the tumor or metastases. The possibility of preventing the syndrome by giving steroids during mitomycin treatment has been suggested and needs to be confirmed in prospective controlled trials. Plasma exchange is usually attempted, but its effectiveness is unproved.

6.9.2.7.2 Antiplatelet Drugs

TMA has been reported in 1 every 1,600–5,000 patients treated with ticlopidine. Neurologic abnormalities occur within 1 month of treatment in 80% of cases. The overall survival rate is 67% and is improved by early treatment withdrawal and plasma therapy. Generation of an autoantibody against ADAMTS13 may be involved in the pathogenesis of ticlopidine-associated TTP [69]. The deficiency resolved after ticlopidine therapy was discontinued and plasmapheresis was instituted. Eleven cases have been reported during treatment with clopidogrel, a new antiaggregating agent that has achieved widespread clinical use for its safety profile. All patients had neurologic involvement and were treated with plasma exchange: eight fully recovered, two had relapses that rapidly recovered after re-treatment with plasma exchange, and one died. Half the patients were concomitantly treated with cholesterol-lowering drugs. Conceivably, these drugs should be avoided in clopidogrel-treated patients.

6.9.2.7.3 Quinine

Quinine is one of the drugs more frequently associated with TMA. The disease typically occurs in patients presensitized by prior exposure to quinine and rapidly follows reingestion of the drug. Quinine is generally used to treat muscle cramps, but it is also contained in beverages (tonic water and bitter lemon drinks). Quinine dependent antiplatelet, antierythrocyte, and antigranulocyte antibodies have been involved in the pathogenesis of the disease. Presenting symptoms are often severe, and death or irreversible kidney failure are common outcomes unless quinine is immediately withdrawn and plasma exchange is promptly provided. Avoidance of successive quinine use is necessary to prevent recurrences.

6.9.2.8 Bone Marrow and Solid Organ Transplant Associated HUS

Among acquired forms of HUS, posttransplant HUS is being reported with continuously increasing frequency and appears to affect a progressively increasing number of patients worldwide. Albeit poorly defined, the incidence of the disease is remarkably higher in the transplant than in the general population, most likely because of the clustering of several risk factors in this particular setting of patients. In renal transplants, HUS may ensue for the first time in patients who never suffered the disease *(de novo post transplant HUS)* or may affect patients whose primary cause of ESKD was HUS (*recurrent post transplant HUS* see Section 6.9.3 on TMA associated with congenital defects). Treatment of posttransplant HUS rests on removal of the inciting factor(s), relief of symptoms, and plasma infusion or exchange. No other approach has proven effective.

6.9.2.8.1 De Novo Posttransplant HUS

This form occurs in renal and extrarenal transplant recipients and is usually triggered by immunosuppressive drugs such as calcineurin inhibitors [55], or less frequently, by virus infections and, specifically in renal transplant recipients, by acute vascular rejection. A peculiar form of *de novo* posttransplant HUS may affect the recipients of a bone marrow transplant (BMT), usually in the setting of graft-versus-host disease (GVHD) or of intensive GVHD prophylaxis, including total body irradiation (TBI).

Therapy – Drug withdrawal or dose reduction is the first-line therapy for *de novo* cyclosporin A (CsA)– or tacrolimus-associated forms, but is effective *per se* in less than 50% of cases [66]. A remarkably higher success rate (84%) has been reported with adjunctive plasma infusion or exchange. A similar response rate, but in much smaller series, has been reported with intravenous IgG infusion given with the rationale of neutralizing hypothetical circulating cytotoxic or platelet agglutinating factors. Once remission is achieved, patient rechallenge with decreased doses of CsA or tacrolimus, a switch from one drug to the other one, or, finally, replacement of both drugs with mycophenolate mofetil have been anecdotally reported to maintain adequate immunosuppression without further disease recurrences. Very recently, compassionate treatment with rapamycin has been associated with a remarkably good outcome in 15 patients with CsA- or tacrolimus-associated posttransplant HUS, with no patient requiring rapamycin withdrawal because of disease recurrence [58]. Monoclonal anti-IL-2 receptor antagonists may also be a valid option to maintain adequate immunosuppression, avoiding the toxic effects of calcineurin inhibitors. The outcome of *de novo* forms occurring in the setting of viral infection parallels the response to treatment of the underlying disease. Despite intensive plasma therapy or rescue treatment with plasma cryosupernatant or protein A immune adsorption, the outcome of *de novo* forms complicating BMT is still dramatically poor, with a mortality rate closed to 90%. In addition to the severity of the microangiopathic process – quantified on the basis of serum lactate dehydrogenase levels and percentage of circulating fragmented erythrocytes – infection, progressive GVHD, or relapse of the underlying disease may account for these so discouraging figures.

6.9.3 Genetic (TMA Associated with Congenital Defects)

These forms are rare, often occur in families, mainly but not exclusively in children, and frequently relapse even after complete recovery of the presenting episode. Genetic counseling is therefore of paramount importance. In cases with recognized genetic mutations, antenatal diagnosis by amniocentesis or chorionic villous biopsy is possible, and the carrier state can be identified.

6.9.3.1 HUS Associated with Genetic Abnormalities in Complement Regulatory Proteins

More then 80 different mutations in the gene encoding complement factor H (*CFH*) have been reported so far in patients with HUS [63]. In sporadic forms, the mutation was either inherited from a healthy parent or, more rarely – only four cases reported – ensued de novo in the proband [49]. The mutation frequency is around 30% [8, 45].

CFH is a plasma glycoprotein that plays an important role in the regulation of the alternative pathway of complement. It serves as a cofactor for the C3b-cleaving enzyme, factor I (CFI), in the degradation of newly formed C3b molecules, and controls decay, formation, and stability of the C3b convertase C3bBb. CFH consists of 20 homologous short consensus repeats (SCRs). The complement regulatory domains needed to prevent fluid-phase alternative pathway amplification have been localized within the N-terminal SCR-4 [56]. The inactivation of surface-bound C3b is dependent on the binding of the C-terminal domain of CFH to polyanionic molecules that increases CFH affinity for C3b and exposes its complement regulatory N-terminal domain [34].

The vast majority of *CFH* mutations in HUS patients are heterozygous and cause either single amino acid changes or premature translation interruptions, mainly clustering in the C-terminal domains and are commonly associated with normal CFH plasma levels. Expression and functional studies demonstrated that CFH proteins carrying HUS-associated mutations have a severely reduced capability to interact with polyanions and with surface-bound C3b [34], which results in a lower density of mutant CFH molecules bound to endothelial cells surface and a diminished complement regulatory activity on the cell membrane [34]. In contrast, these mutants have a normal capacity to control activation of the complement in plasma, as indicated by data that they retain a normal cofactor activity in the proteolysis of fluid-phase C3b.

Abnormalities in two additional genes encoding for complement regulatory proteins (membrane cofactor protein, *MCP* and factor I, *CFI*) have been recently involved in predisposition to HUS. MCP is a widely expressed transmembrane glycoprotein that serves as a cofactor for CFI to cleave C3b and C4b deposited on host cell surface [31]. Until now around 40 *MCP* mutations in HUS have been reported, with a mutation frequency of 10–15% [8, 46, 53]. Evaluation of mutant protein expression and function showed either severely reduced protein expression on the cell surface, or reduced C3b-binding capability and/or capacity to prevent complement activation [8].

Twenty-four mutations in *CFI*, encoding a plasma serine protease that cleaves and inactivates C3b and C4b, have been reported in patients with HUS, with a frequency of 5–12% in different studies [8, 18, 36]. All of them are heterozygous mutations, 80% cluster in the serine-protease domain and either cause severely reduced protein secretion or result in mutant proteins with decreased cofactor activity.

The list of published and unpublished mutations within *CFH*, *MCP*, and *CFI* is continuously updated in the fh-HUS database (http://www.fh-hus.org). More recently, two gain-of-function mutations in the gene encoding complement factor B (CFB), a zymogen that carries the catalytic site of the complement alternative pathway convertase, have been found in two families [30].

HUS associated with *CFH* mutations often present early in childhood, although adult onset is reported in around 30% of cases [7, 8, 45, 47]. The clinical course is characterized by a high rate of relapse, and 60–80% of patients die or develop ESKD following the presenting episode or progress to ESKD as a consequences of relapse. HUS associated with *MCP* mutations presents mostly in childhood, the acute episode is in general milder than in *CFH* mutation carriers and 80% of patients undergo complete remission. Recurrences are very frequent but their effect on long-term outcome is rather mild, with around 60–70% of patients remaining dialysis free even after several recurrences. However, there are some exceptions, with a subgroup of patients who lost renal function either during the first episode or later in life. The clinical course of *CFI* mutated patients is more variable. The onset is in childhood in half of the patients. Fifty eight percent of patients develop ESRD in the long term.

6.9.3.1.1 Therapy

Genetic characterization of patients could potentially help tailoring treatment. Plasma infusion or exchange has been used in patients with HUS and *CFH* mutations, with the rationale to provide the patients with normal CFH to correct the genetic deficiency. Some patients with *CFH* mutations did not respond at all to plasma and died or developed ESRD. Others required infusion of plasma at weekly intervals to rise CFH plasma levels enough to maintain remission [11, 37]. Stratton et al. [64] were able to induce sustained remission in a patient with a *CFH* mutation, by 3-month weekly plasma exchange in conjunction with intravenous immunoglobulins. At 1 year after stopping plasma therapy, the patient remained disease-free and dialysis-independent. In our series, around 50% of patients with *CFH* mutations treated with plasma [8] underwent either complete or partial remission (hematologic normalization with renal sequelae). However half of the patients did not respond at all to plasma, and 20% died during the acute episode.

Since CFI and CFB are plasma proteins, plasma infusion and plasma exchange could be theoretically of value in patients with defects in the corresponding genes. Published data in small number of patients document that about half of patients with either *CFI* [8] or *CFB* mutations [30] underwent remission following plasma infusion, exactly as observed in *CFH* mutated patients.

The rationale for using plasma in patients with *MCP* mutations is not so clear, since MCP is a transmembrane protein and theoretically plasma infusion or exchange would not correct the MCP defect. Published data [8, 53] indicate that the majority (70–80%) of patients undergo remission following plasma infusion or exchange; however, complete recovery from the acute episode was also observed in 70–80% of patients not treated with plasma.

6.9.3.1.2 Transplantation

Whether kidney transplantation is an appropriate treatment in non-Stx-HUS patients who have progressed to ESKD is still a matter of debate. Actually, around 50% of the patients who had a renal transplant had a recurrence of the disease in the grafted organ [47]. There is no effective treatment for recurrences, and graft failure occurs in more than 90% of patients. Screening for mutations may help to define graft prognosis, and genotyping for *CFH, MCP*, and *CFI* should be performed in all patients with ESRD secondary to non-Stx-HUS being considered for a transplant. In patients with *CFH* mutations, the graft outcome is poor, the recurrence rate ranges from 30% to 100% according to different surveys, and it is significantly higher than in patients without *CFH* mutations [5, 45, 47]. As CFH is mainly produced by the liver, a kidney transplant will not correct the *CFH* genetic defect in these patients. Simultaneous kidney and liver transplant has been performed in two young children with non-Stx-HUS and *CFH* mutations, with the objective of correcting the genetic defect and prevent disease recurrences [47]. However, both cases treated with this procedure were complicated by premature irreversible liver failure. The reasons for this may include increase susceptibility of the transplanted liver to ischemic or immune injury related to uncontrolled complement activation.

Four more cases of combined kidney and liver transplant in patients with *CFH* mutations have been subsequently reported [33, 62]. In all cases posttransplant outcome was favorable with good renal and liver function recorded at follow-up after several years. Extensive plasma exchange was given prior to surgery to provide patients with enough normal CFH to prevent liver graft damage. Thus, in this setting, combined liver and kidney transplant may be an effective way to gain independence from chronic dialysis and may be life-saving in those infants who, on dialysis, have a poor life expectancy.

As CFI and CFB are plasma proteins, one could speculate that HUS recurrence may take place on the transplanted kidney, and patients may experience graft failure. The few data available are in line with this hypothesis, as graft failures for recurrence occurred in most patients with *CFI* and *CFB* mutations [8, 26]. On the other hand, kidney graft outcome is favorable in patients with *MCP* mutations, as found in four patients who have been successfully transplanted with no disease recurrence [46]. There is a strong theoretical rationale for this: MCP is a transmembrane protein highly expressed in the kidney. Transplantation of a kidney expressing normal MCP not surprisingly corrects the defects in these patients.

6.9.3.2 TTP Associated with Congenital Deficiency of ADAMTS13

This rare form of TMA is associated with a congenital defect of a plasma metalloprotease, ADAMTS13, that cleaves ULVWF multimers into smaller multimers. The defect was originally described in TTP [20, 21], however emerging data indicate that also patients with HUS [51, 72] may have a complete lack of ADAMTS13 activity, albeit less frequently. Thus on clinical grounds, a possible congenital defect of ADAMTS13 can not be excluded only on the basis of the predominant renal localization of disease manifestation. TTP associated with congenital ADAMTS13 deficiency presented either in families, or in patients with no familial history of the disease [20, 21, 38, 72]. In both cases, the disease is inherited as an autosomal recessive trait, as documented by ADAMTS13 levels in healthy relatives of patients that fell into bimodal distribution with a group with half normal values, consistent with carriers, and the other with normal values [38].

Recurrences are very frequent and may occur even after symptom-free periods of months or years. Although they are more frequent in adults, relapsing forms of TMA have also been reported in children with congenital ADAMTS13 deficiency in whom renal symptoms are predominant [57].

To date, more than 50 *ADAMTS13* mutations have been identified in patients with the familial form of TTP [19, 38]. Affected individuals within families were either homozygous for the same mutation or compound heterozygous for two different mutations, confirming that the disease was inherited as a recessive trait.

The mutations have been found along the entire *ADAMTS13* gene and no clustering is evident, although more than 70% of them are located from the metalloprotease through the Tsp-1-2 domains [24]. Studies on secretion and activity of the mutated forms of the protease showed that most of these mutations led to an impaired secretion from the cells, and, when the mutated protein is secreted, the proteolytic activity is greatly reduced [13].

6.9.3.2.1 Therapy

At the moment, therapy of ADAMTS13-associated TMA involves plasma infusion or exchange to replenish the active protease. Actually, providing just a 5% normal enzymatic activity may be sufficient to degrade large VWF multimers – which may be relevant to induce remission of the microangiopathic process – and this effect is sustained over time due to the relatively long half-life (2–4 days) of the protease. In two brothers with complete deficiency of the protease and relapsing TTP, disease remission was achieved by plasmapheresis and was concurrent with an almost full recovery of the ADAMTS13 activity. Both patients achieved a long-lasting remission, although protease activity decreased to less than 20% over 20 days after plasma therapy withdrawal [22]. Although individual attacks usually respond to treatment, long-term prognosis is invariably poor if therapy fails to achieve lasting remission.

6.9.3.3 HUS Associated with Inborn Abnormal Cobalamin Metabolism

This is a rare autosomal recessive form of HUS associated with an inborn abnormality of cobalamin metabolism [3]. The disease manifests in the first days or months of life. Children fail to thrive, have poor feeding, suffer from vomiting, and may present neurologic symptoms of fatigue, delirium, psychosis, seizures. In cases with early onset, the disease has a fulminant evolution and occasionally involves the pulmonary vasculature, but when it ensues later in childhood it may follow a more chronic course. The hallmarks of defective cobalamin metabolism are hyperhomocysteinemia and methylmalonic aciduria, and the extremely high homocysteine levels have been suggested to have a role in the pathogenesis of the vascular lesions. Without treatment, the disease is fatal, and it is likely that some children die undiagnosed.

6.9.3.3.1 Therapy

Treatment is finalized to correct the metabolic disorder as effectively as possible [71]. Daily intramuscular administrations of hydroxycobalamin may reduce both homocysteine levels and methylmalonic aciduria, while oral hydroxycobalamin and cyanocobalamin are ineffective. Oral betaine contributes to further reduce serum homocysteine levels by activating betaine-homocysteine methyltransferase. Supplementation of folic acid to avoid folate deficiency induced by methyltetrahydrofolate trapping, and of L-carnitine to increase propionyl carnitine excretion have been suggested, but their role in improving disease outcome is unclear.

Despite treatment, the majority of children with early onset disease die or have severe neurologic sequelae. Intensified treatment in older children with less acute disease may achieve remission of the microangiopathic process and amelioration of the other clinical manifestations of the metabolic disorder. Whether plasma therapy has a role in improving disease outcome is unknown.

6.9.3.4 Other Genetic Forms

Conceivably, the mutations described above account for around 50% of genetic forms of TMA. Patients with decreased C3 but no evidence of CFH, MCP, CFI, or CFB abnormalities have been described. In these cases, uncontrolled activation of the alternative complement pathway may be due to genetic defects in other complement proteins, including C3, DAF, CR1, CR2, and C4 binding protein. Other cases may be associated with still unrecognized genetic defects.

6.9.3.4.1 Therapy

Plasma infusion or exchange is the only therapy that may have some effect. Regardless of treatment, however, disease outcome is usually poor.

6.9.4 Idiopathic

These are forms of unknown etiology with progressive renal function deterioration and neurologic involvement that may resemble TTP. They may follow a progressive course to end-stage renal failure or death, and very likely constitute a disease closer to TTP that requires more specific therapies to stop the progression of the microangiopathic process. These cases recur more often after kidney transplantation [52].

6.9.4.1 Therapy

Plasma infusion and exchange have been retrospectively found to limit residual renal insufficiency or the risk of end-stage renal failure in children. Uncontrolled studies suggest that plasma infusion or exchange may markedly lower the mortality rate and risk of end-stage renal failure in adults [27, 59]. Intravenous immunoglobulins have been suggested, to limit neurologic involvement, but their effectiveness too is still unproved. Bilateral nephrectomy (see above) may be attempted as rescue therapy in patients with severe renal involvement, refractory hypertension/thrombocytopenia, and hypertensive encephalopathy.

6.9.5 Treatment Guidelines

6.9.5.1 Plasma Manipulation

The infusion is intended to deliver the equivalent of one plasma volume (about 30 ml/kg of body weight) over the first 24 h and about 20 ml/kg of body weight daily thereafter. To avoid fluid overload, diuretics or ultrafiltration may be employed. The exchange procedure is usually intended to replace one to two plasma volumes every day.

Two procedures are available for plasma separation in the setting of plasma exchange: filtration and centrifugation. The total extracorporeal volume of the plasma circuit affects the choice of the procedure. It is estimated that the total extracorporeal volume should not exceed 8–10% of total blood volume of the patient (taken as 100 ml/kg in infants < 10 kg, and 80 ml/kg in children > 10 kg). Thus, the filtration system, which has an extracorporeal volume of less than 100 ml, is preferred for small children and in patients with cardiovascular instability. Plasma centrifugation is the standard procedure for all other cases.

Plasma exchange procedure may carry the risk of major complications and death. Severe complications include systemic infections, venous thrombosis, and hypotension requiring dopamine [29]. However, the benefits outweigh the risks because of the poor prognosis of untreated TMA.

6.9.5.2 Other Specific Treatments

In a large series of TTP patients [55], 200 mg of oral prednisone (or 200 mg of intravenous prednisolone in patients with evidence of hepatic dysfunction) were given per day until complete normalization of the markers of hemolysis, when corticosteroids were rapidly tapered to 60 mg per day and then more slowly by 5 mg per week. In the HELLP syndrome, dexamethasone was given, 10 mg intravenously every 12 h until delivery and for 36 h thereafter.

The recommended initial dose of vincristine is 1.4 mg/m^2 (not to exceed 2 mg) by intravenous injection, followed by 1 mg intravenously every 4 days until complete remission is achieved. On account of its severe neurotoxicity, the drug should be used with caution.

6.9.5.3 Rescue Treatments

Bilateral nephrectomy and splenectomy are irreversible procedure and should be considered only for patients at imminent risk of death or with disabling disease. In patients at increased risk of bleeding because of severe refractory thrombocytopenia, platelet transfusion may be indicated before surgery.

6.9.6 Future Directions

Acquired forms – Several agents aimed to interrupt the pathogenic cascade starting with the ingestion of Stx-producing *E. coli* strains and eventually culminating in full-blown HUS are currently under investigation [59]. Molecular decoys such as orally administered harmless recombinant bacteria that display a Stx receptor on the surface [48, 50, 65] have been successfully used to bind and inactivate the toxin in the mice intestine. In another study, a plant-based oral vaccination with *Nicotiana tabacum* cells transfected with the gene encoding inactivated Stx2, fully protected mice from challenge with a lethal dose of the toxin [74]. Another approach is to use Stx inhibitors, among them is "STARFISH," an oligobivalent, water-soluble carbohydrate ligand that can simultaneously engage all five B subunits of the toxin, which might help to prevent toxin that has already entered the circulation from binding to specific receptors [44]. Others have ameliorated disease in pigs by injection of toxin-neutralizing antibodies [42]. Although natural infection with *E. coli* O157 does not confer immunity and no human vaccine is currently available, Shiga toxoid vaccines have been shown effective in preventing related diseases in animals.

Genetic forms – New information derived from recent genetic studies will hopefully open the perspective of new specific treatments for patients with genetic forms of HUS and TTP. Specific replacement therapies with recombinant CFH and ADAMTS13 or with complement inhibitor compounds, could become a viable alternative to plasma treatment. This is reasonably feasible for patients with *ADAMTS13* gene mutations, since even a small (5% of normal) VWF cleaving protease activity may be sufficient to degrade large VWF multimers. Finally, the full definition of the *CFH* and *ADAMTS13* gene sequence will soon render gene therapy a realistic option for patients with inherited HUS or TTP.

6.9.7 Take Home Pearls

- Conservative therapy alone is the intervention of choice in most cases of childhood Stx-associated HUS, which usually recover spontaneously, and, probably, a waiting attitude before considering plasma therapy is the best strategy in cases associated with *MCP* mutations, since these forms appear to have a high rate of spontaneous remissions that does not appear to be appreciably increased by plasma therapy.
- Patients with immune mediated deficiency of factor H or ADAMTS13 may benefit the most from the

exchange procedure that, in addition to supplying an extra amount of these two plasma components that may saturate the autoantibody activity, may also remove the autoantibody from the circulation.

- Similarly in immune forms, steroids, vincristine, immunoglobulins, immunosuppressants, and splenectomy may help to inhibit the production of the autoantibody and, combined with plasma exchange, may result in an effective clearance of the autoantibody from the circulation. On the contrary, they have definitely no room in the treatment of genetic forms. Trials considering the two forms together, invariably diluted the potential benefits of steroids or immunosuppressive therapy in subjects with immune mediated disease. This may explain the inconclusive results of previsous studies in HUS and TTP. Novel studies should likely focus on the role of steroids as first line therapy for immune–mediated forms, and on vincristine, high dose immunoglobulins or other immunosuppressants as second line therapy, being splenectomy to be considered as resuc therapy for those patients with tefractory disease and life–threatening thrompocytopenia or neurological involvement.
- Patients with genetically determined deficiency of plasma components, CFH, CFI, and ADAMTS13, may benefit from both plasma infusion and exchange, since both the procedures may replace the defective activity, with the exchange procedure offering the possibility of supplying larger amounts of plasma without the risk of fluid overload.
- The role of plasma therapy, either as infusion or exchange, in forms associated with abnormalities of membrane bound regulatory proteins such as MCP is unknown.
- Whenever indicated, specific therapy should be started as soon as diagnosis is established in order to speed up disease recovery and minimize morbidity and mortality. Treatment should be continued until complete disease remission is achieved.
- Platelet count and serum lactate dehydrogenase are the most sensitive markers for monitoring the response to therapy. In conditions associated with decreased platelet production (cancer- or AIDS-associated TMA), serum lactate dehydrogenase concentration is a more reliable indicator of disease activity than platelet count. In pregnancy-associated TMA, monitoring serum transaminases may be helpful.

References

1. Ake, J.A., Jelacic, S., Ciol, M.A., Watkins, S.L., Murray, K.F., Christie, D.L., Klein, E.J. & Tarr, P.I. (2005). Relative nephroprotection during *Escherichia coli* O157:H7 infections: association with intravenous volume expansion. *Pediatrics*, **115**, e673–80.
2. Artz, M.A., Steenbergen, E.J., Hoitsma, A.J., Monnens, L.A. & Wetzels, J.F. (2003). Renal transplantation in patients with hemolytic uremic syndrome: high rate of recurrence and increased incidence of acute rejections. *Transplantation*, **76**, 821–6.
3. Baumgartner, E.R., Wick, H., Maurer, R., Egli, N. & Steinmann, B. (1979). Congenital defect in intracellular cobalamin metabolism resulting in homocysteinuria and methylmalonic aciduria. I. Case report and histopathology. *Helv Paediatr Acta*, **34**, 465–82.
4. Bell, W.R., Braine, H.G., Ness, P.M. & Kickler, T.S. (1991). Improved survival in thrombotic thrombocytopenic purpura-hemolytic uremic syndrome. Clinical experience in 108 patients. *N Engl J Med*, **325**, 398–403.
5. Bresin, E., Daina, E., Noris, M., Castelleti, F., Stefanov, R., Hill, P., Goodship, T.M., Remuzzi, G. & HUS/TTP, f.t.I.R.o.R.a.F. (2006). Outcome of renal transplantation in patients with non-Shiga Toxin-associated haemolytic uremic syndrome: prognostic significance of genetic background. *Clin J Am Soc Nephrol*, **1**, 88–99.
6. Caletti, M.G., Lejarraga, H., Kelmansky, D. & Missoni, M. (2004). Two different therapeutic regimes in patients with sequelae of hemolytic-uremic syndrome. *Pediatr Nephrol*, **19**, 1148–52.
7. Caprioli, J., Castelletti, F., Bucchioni, S., Bettinaglio, P., Bresin, E., Pianetti, G., Gamba, S., Brioschi, S., Daina, E., Remuzzi, G. & Noris, M. (2003). Complement factor H mutations and gene polymorphisms in haemolytic uraemic syndrome: the C-257T, the A2089G and the G2881T polymorphisms are strongly associated with the disease. *Hum Mol Genet*, **12**, 3385–95.
8. Caprioli, J., Noris, M., Brioschi, S., Pianetti, G., Castelletti, F., Bettinaglio, P., Mele, C., Bresin, E., Cassis, L., Gamba, S., Porrati, F., Bucchioni, S., Monteferrante, G., Fang, C.J., Liszewski, M.K., Kavanagh, D., Atkinson, J.P. & Remuzzi, G. (2006). Genetics of HUS: the impact of MCP, CFH, and IF mutations on clinical presentation, response to treatment, and outcome. *Blood*, **108**, 1267–79.
9. Carter, A.O., Borczyk, A.A., Carlson, J.A., Harvey, B., Hockin, J.C., Karmali, M.A., Krishnan, C., Korn, D.A. & Lior, H. (1987). A severe outbreak of Escherichia coli O157:H7 – associated hemorrhagic colitis in a nursing home. *N Engl J Med*, **317**, 1496–500.
10. Chiurchiu, C., Firrincieli, A., Santostefano, M., Fusaroli, M., Remuzzi, G. & Ruggenenti, P. (2003). Adult nondiarrhea hemolytic uremic syndrome associated with Shiga toxin *Escherichia coli* O157:H7 bacteremia and urinary tract infection. *Am J Kidney Dis*, **41**, E4.
11. Cho, H.Y., Lee, B.S., Moon, K.C., Ha, I.S., Cheong, H.I. & Choi, Y. (2007). Complete factor H deficiency-associated atypical hemolytic uremic syndrome in a neonate. *Pediatr Nephrol*, **22**, 874–80.
12. Cuttner, J. (1980). Thrombotic thrombocytopenic purpura: a ten-year experience. *Blood*, **56**, 302–6.

13. Donadelli, R., Banterla, F., Galbusera, M., Capoferri, C., Bucchioni, S., Gastoldi, S., Nosari, S., Monteferrante, G., Ruggeri, Z.M., Bresin, E., Scheiflinger, F., Rossi, E., Martinez, C., Coppo, R., Remuzzi, G. & Noris, M. (2006). In-vitro and in-vivo consequences of mutations in the von Willebrand factor cleaving protease ADAMTS13 in thrombotic thrombocytopenic purpura. *Thromb Haemost*, **96**, 454–64.
14. Dragon-Durey, M.A., Loirat, C., Cloarec, S., Macher, M.A., Blouin, J., Nivet, H., Weiss, L., Fridman, W.H. & Fremeaux-Bacchi, V. (2005). Anti-Factor H autoantibodies associated with atypical hemolytic uremic syndrome. *J Am Soc Nephrol*, **16**, 555–63.
15. Dundas, S., Murphy, J., Soutar, R.L., Jones, G.A., Hutchinson, S.J. & Todd, W.T. (1999). Effectiveness of therapeutic plasma exchange in the 1996 Lanarkshire Escherichia coli O157:H7 outbreak. *Lancet*, **354**, 1327–30.
16. Ferrari, S., Scheiflinger, F., Rieger, M., Mudde, G., Wolf, M., Coppo, P., Girma, J.P., Azoulay, E., Brun-Buisson, C., Fakhouri, F., Mira, J.P., Oksenhendler, E., Poullin, P., Rondeau, E., Schleinitz, N., Schlemmer, B., Teboul, J.L., Vanhille, P., Vernant, J.P., Meyer, D. & Veyradier, A. (2007). Prognostic value of anti-ADAMTS 13 antibody features (Ig isotype, titer, and inhibitory effect) in a cohort of 35 adult French patients undergoing a first episode of thrombotic microangiopathy with undetectable ADAMTS 13 activity. *Blood*, **109**, 2815–22.
17. Ferraris, J.R., Ramirez, J.A., Ruiz, S., Caletti, M.G., Vallejo, G., Piantanida, J.J., Araujo, J.L. & Sojo, E.T. (2002). Shiga toxin-associated hemolytic uremic syndrome: absence of recurrence after renal transplantation. *Pediatr Nephrol*, **17**, 809–14.
18. Fremeaux-Bacchi, V., Dragon-Durey, M.A., Blouin, J., Vigneau, C., Kuypers, D., Boudailliez, B., Loirat, C., Rondeau, E. & Fridman, W.H. (2004). Complement factor I: a susceptibility gene for atypical haemolytic uraemic syndrome. *J Med Genet*, **41**, e84.
19. Fujikawa, K., Suzuki, H., McMullen, B. & Chung, D. (2001). Purification of human von Willebrand factor-cleaving protease and its identification as a new member of the metalloproteinase family. *Blood*, **98**, 1662–6.
20. Furlan, M., Robles, R., Galbusera, M., Remuzzi, G., Kyrle, P.A., Brenner, B., Krause, M., Scharrer, I., Aumann, V., Mittler, U., Solenthaler, M. & Lammle, B. (1998a). von Willebrand factor-cleaving protease in thrombotic thrombocytopenic purpura and the hemolytic-uremic syndrome. *N Engl J Med*, **339**, 1578–84.
21. Furlan, M., Robles, R. & Lamie, B. (1996). Partial purification and characterization of a protease from human plasma cleaving von Willebrand factor to fragments produced by in vivo proteolysis. *Blood*, **87**, 4223–34.
22. Furlan, M., Robles, R., Morselli, B., Sandoz, P. & Lammle, B. (1999). Recovery and half-life of von Willebrand factor-cleaving protease after plasma therapy in patients with thrombotic thrombocytopenic purpura. *Thromb Haemost*, **81**, 8–13.
23. Furlan, M., Robles, R., Solenthaler, M. & Lammle, B. (1998b). Acquired deficiency of von Willebrand factor-cleaving protease in a patient with thrombotic thrombocytopenic purpura. *Blood*, **91**, 2839–46.
24. Galbusera, M., Noris, M. & Remuzzi, G. (2006). Thrombotic thrombocytopenic purpura – then and now. *Semin Thromb Hemost*, **32**, 81–9.
25. Garg, A.X., Suri, R.S., Barrowman, N., Rehman, F., Matsell, D., Rosas-Arellano, M.P., Salvadori, M., Haynes, R.B. & Clark, W.F. (2003). Long-term renal prognosis of diarrhea-associated hemolytic uremic syndrome: a systematic review, meta-analysis, and meta-regression. *JAMA*, **290**, 1360–70.
26. Geelen, J., van den Dries, K., Roos, A., van de Kar, N., de Kat Angelino, C., Klasen, I., Monnens, L. & van den Heuvel, L. (2007). A missense mutation in factor I (IF) predisposes to atypical haemolytic uraemic syndrome. *Pediatr Nephrol*, **22**, 371–5.
27. George, J.N. (2000). How I treat patients with thrombotic thrombocytopenic purpura-hemolytic uremic syndrome. *Blood*, **96**, 1223–9.
28. George, J.N. (2003). The association of pregnancy with thrombotic thrombocytopenic purpura-hemolytic uremic syndrome. *Curr Opin Hematol*, **10**, 339–44.
29. George, J.N. (2007). Evaluation and management of patients with thrombotic thrombocytopenic purpura. *J Intensive Care Med*, **22**, 82–91.
30. Goicoechea de Jorge, E., Harris, C.L., Esparza-Gordillo, J., Carreras, L., Arranz, E.A., Garrido, C.A., Lopez-Trascasa, M., Sanchez-Corral, P., Morgan, B.P. & Rodriguez de Cordoba, S. (2007). Gain-of-function mutations in complement factor B are associated with atypical hemolytic uremic syndrome. *Proc Natl Acad Sci USA*, **104**, 240–5.
31. Goodship, T.H., Liszewski, M.K., Kemp, E.J., Richards, A. & Atkinson, J.P. (2004). Mutations in CD46, a complement regulatory protein, predispose to atypical HUS. *Trends Mol Med*, **10**, 226–31.
32. Hayward, C.P., Sutton, D.M., Carter, W.H., Jr., Campbell, E.D., Scott, J.G., Francombe, W.H., Shumak, K.H. & Baker, M.A. (1994). Treatment outcomes in patients with adult thrombotic thrombocytopenic purpura-hemolytic uremic syndrome. *Arch Intern Med*, **154**, 982–7.
33. Jalanko, H., Peltonen, S., Koskinen, A., Puntila, J., Isoniemi, H., Holmberg, C., Pinomaki, A., Armstrong, E., Koivusalo, A., Tukiainen, E., Makisalo, H., Saland, J., Remuzzi, G., de Cordoba, S., Lassila, R., Meri, S. & Jokiranta, T.S. (2008). Successful liver-kidney transplantation in two children with aHUS caused by a mutation in complement factor H. *Am J Transplant*, **8**, 216–21.
34. Jozsi, M., Manuelian, T., Heinen, S., Oppermann, M. & Zipfel, P.F. (2004). Attachment of the soluble complement regulator factor H to cell and tissue surfaces: relevance for pathology. *Histol Histopathol*, **19**, 251–8.
35. Jozsi, M., Strobel, S., Dahse, H.M., Liu, W.S., Hoyer, P.F., Oppermann, M., Skerka, C. & Zipfel, P.F. (2007). Anti-factor H autoantibodies block C-terminal recognition function of factor H in hemolytic uremic syndrome. *Blood* 110, 1516–8.
36. Kavanagh, D., Kemp, E.J., Mayland, E., Winney, R.J., Duffield, J.S., Warwick, G., Richards, A., Ward, R., Goodship, J.A. & Goodship, T.H. (2005). Mutations in complement factor I predispose to development of atypical hemolytic uremic syndrome. *J Am Soc Nephrol*, **16**, 2150–5.
37. Landau, D., Shalev, H., Levy-Finer, G., Polonsky, A., Segev, Y. & Katchko, L. (2001). Familial hemolytic uremic syndrome associated with complement factor H deficiency. *J Pediatr*, **138**, 412–7.
38. Levy, G.G., Nichols, W.C., Lian, E.C., Foroud, T., McClintick, J.N., McGee, B.M., Yang, A.Y., Siemieniak, D.R.,

Stark, K.R., Gruppo, R., Sarode, R., Shurin, S.B., Chandrasekaran, V., Stabler, S.P., Sabio, H., Bouhassira, E.E., Upshaw, J.D., Jr., Ginsburg, D. & Tsai, H.M. (2001). Mutations in a member of the ADAMTS gene family cause thrombotic thrombocytopenic purpura. *Nature*, **413**, 488–94.

39. Loirat, C. & Niaudet, P. (2003). The risk of recurrence of hemolytic uremic syndrome after renal transplantation in children. *Pediatr Nephrol*, **18**, 1095–101.
40. Loirat, C., Veyradier, A., Foulard, M., et al. (2001). von Willebrand factor (vWF)-cleaving protease activity in pediatric hemolytic uremic syndrome (HUS). Abs. Twelth Congress of the International pediateic Nepheology Association; September 1–5, 2005 Seattle, WA.
41. Mannucci, P.M. & Peyvandi, F. (2007). TTP and ADAMTS13: When Is Testing Appropriate? *Hematology Am Soc Hematol Educ Program*, **2007**, 121–6.
42. Matise, I., Cornick, N.A., Booher, S.L., Samuel, J.E., Bosworth, B.T. & Moon, H.W. (2001). Intervention with Shiga toxin (Stx) antibody after infection by Stx-producing *Escherichia coli*. *J Infect Dis*, **183**, 347–350.
43. McGraw, M.E., Lendon, M., Stevens, R.F., Postlethwaite, R.J. & Taylor, C.M. (1989). Haemolytic uraemic syndrome and the Thomsen Friedenreich antigen. *Pediatr Nephrol*, **3**, 135–9.
44. Mulvey, G.L., Marcato, P., Kitov, P.I., Sadowska, J., Bundle, D.R. & Armstrong, G.D. (2003). Assessment in mice of the therapeutic potential of tailored, multivalent Shiga toxin carbohydrate ligands. *J Infect Dis*, **187**, 640–9.
45. Neumann, H.P., Salzmann, M., Bohnert-Iwan, B., Mannuelian, T., Skerka, C., Lenk, D., Bender, B.U., Cybulla, M., Riegler, P., Konigsrainer, A., Neyer, U., Bock, A., Widmer, U., Male, D.A., Franke, G. & Zipfel, P.F. (2003). Haemolytic uraemic syndrome and mutations of the factor H gene: a registry-based study of German speaking countries. *J Med Genet*, **40**, 676–81.
46. Noris, M., Brioschi, S., Caprioli, J., Todeschini, M., Bresin, E., Porrati, F., Gamba, S. & Remuzzi, G. (2003). Familial haemolytic uraemic syndrome and an MCP mutation. *Lancet*, **362**, 1542–7.
47. Noris, M., Bucchioni, S., Galbusera, M., Donadelli, R., Bresin, E., Castelletti, F., Caprioli, J., Brioschi, S., Scheiflinger, F. & Remuzzi, G. (2005). Complement factor H mutation in familial thrombotic thrombocytopenic purpura with ADAMTS13 deficiency and renal involvement. *J Am Soc Nephrol*, **16**, 1177–83.
48. Paton, A.W., Morona, R. & Paton, J.C. (2000). A new biological agent for treatment of Shiga toxigenic Escherichia coli infections and dysentery in humans. *Nat Med*, **6**, 265–70.
49. Perez-Caballero, D., Gonzalez-Rubio, C., Gallardo, M.E., Vera, M., Lopez-Trascasa, M., Rodriguez de Cordoba, S. & Sanchez-Corral, P. (2001). Clustering of missense mutations in the C-terminal region of factor H in atypical hemolytic uremic syndrome. *Am J Hum Genet*, **68**, 478–84.
50. Pinyon, R.A., Paton, J.C., Paton, A.W., Botten, J.A. & Morona, R. (2004). Refinement of a therapeutic Shiga toxin-binding probiotic for human trials. *J Infect Dis*, **189**, 1547–55.
51. Remuzzi, G., Galbusera, M., Noris, M., Canciani, M.T., Daina, E., Bresin, E., Contaretti, S., Caprioli, J., Gamba, S., Ruggenenti, P., Perico, N. & Mannucci, P.M. (2002a). von Willebrand factor cleaving protease (ADAMTS13) is deficient in recurrent and familial thrombotic thrombocytopenic purpura and hemolytic uremic syndrome. *Blood*, **100**, 778–85.
52. Remuzzi, G., Ruggenenti, P., Codazzi, D., Noris, M., Caprioli, J., Locatelli, G. & Gridelli, B. (2002b). Combined kidney and liver transplantation for familial haemolytic uraemic syndrome. *Lancet*, **359**, 1671–2.
53. Richards, A., Kemp, E.J., Liszewski, M.K., Goodship, J.A., Lampe, A.K., Decorte, R., Muslumanoglu, M.H., Kavukcu, S., Filler, G., Pirson, Y., Wen, L.S., Atkinson, J.P. & Goodship, T.H. (2003). Mutations in human complement regulator, membrane cofactor protein (CD46), predispose to development of familial hemolytic uremic syndrome. *Proc Natl Acad Sci USA*, **100**, 12966–71.
54. Rizzoni, G., Claris-Appiani, A., Edefonti, A., Facchin, P., Franchini, F., Gusmano, R., Imbasciati, E., Pavanello, L., Perfumo, F. & Remuzzi, G. (1988). Plasma infusion for hemolytic-uremic syndrome in children: results of a multicenter controlled trial. *J Pediatr*, **112**, 284–90.
55. Rock, G.A., Shumak, K.H., Buskard, N.A., Blanchette, V.S., Kelton, J.G., Nair, R.C. & Spasoff, R.A. (1991). Comparison of plasma exchange with plasma infusion in the treatment of thrombotic thrombocytopenic purpura. Canadian Apheresis Study Group. *N Engl J Med*, **325**, 393–7.
56. Rodriguez de Cordoba, S., Esparza-Gordillo, J., Goicoechea de Jorge, E., Lopez-Trascasa, M. & Sanchez-Corral, P. (2004). The human complement factor H: functional roles, genetic variations and disease associations. *Mol Immunol*, **41**, 355–67.
57. Ruggenenti, P., Galbusera, M., Cornejo, R.P., Bellavita, P. & Remuzzi, G. (1993). Thrombotic thrombocytopenic purpura: evidence that infusion rather than removal of plasma induces remission of the disease. *Am J Kidney Dis*, **21**, 314–8.
58. Ruggenenti, P., Galli, M. & Remuzzi, G. (2001a). Hemolytic uremic syndrome, thrombotic thrombocytopenic purpura, and antiphospholipid antibody syndromes. In *Immunologic Renal Diseases*, E.G., N. & Couser, W.G. (eds), 2nd ed. pp. 1179–1208. Lippincott Williams & Wilkins: Philadelphia.
59. Ruggenenti, P., Noris, M. & Remuzzi, G. (2001b). Thrombotic microangiopathy, hemolytic uremic syndrome, and thrombotic thrombocytopenic purpura. *Kidney Int*, **60**, 831–46.
60. Ruggenenti, P. & Remuzzi, G. (1996). The pathophysiology and management of thrombotic thrombocytopenic purpura. *Eur J Haematol*, **56**, 191–207.
61. Safdar, N., Said, A., Gangnon, R.E. & Maki, D.G. (2002). Risk of hemolytic uremic syndrome after antibiotic treatment of *Escherichia coli* O157:H7 enteritis: a meta-analysis. *JAMA*, **288**, 996–1001.
62. Saland, J.M., Emre, S.H., Shneider, B.L., Benchimol, C., Ames, S., Bromberg, J.S., Remuzzi, G., Strain, L. & Goodship, T.H. (2006). Favorable long-term outcome after liver-kidney transplant for recurrent hemolytic uremic syndrome associated with a factor H mutation. *Am J Transplant*, **6**, 1948–52.
63. Saunders, R.E., Abarrategui-Garrido, C., Fremeaux-Bacchi, V., Goicoechea de Jorge, E., Goodship, T.H., Lopez Trascasa, M., Noris, M., Ponce Castro, I.M., Remuzzi, G., Rodriguez de Cordoba, S., Sanchez-Corral, P., Skerka, C., Zipfel, P.F. & Perkins, S.J. (2007). The interactive Factor H-atypical hemolytic uremic syndrome mutation database and website: update and integration of membrane cofactor protein and Factor I mutations with structural models. *Hum Mutat*, **28**, 222–34.

64. Stratton, J.D. & Warwicker, P. (2002). Successful treatment of factor H-related haemolytic uraemic syndrome. *Nephrol Dial Transplant*, **17**, 684–5.
65. Takahashi, M., Taguchi, H., Yamaguchi, H., Osaki, T., Komatsu, A. & Kamiya, S. (2004). The effect of probiotic treatment with *Clostridium butyricum* on enterohemorrhagic Escherichia coli O157:H7 infection in mice. *FEMS Immunol Med Microbiol*, **41**, 219–26.
66. Taylor, C.M. (2001). Complement factor H and the haemolytic uraemic syndrome. *Lancet*, **358**, 1200–2.
67. Trachtman, H., Cnaan, A., Christen, E., Gibbs, K., Zhao, S., Acheson, D.W., Weiss, R., Kaskel, F.J., Spitzer, A. & Hirschman, G.H. (2003). Effect of an oral Shiga toxin-binding agent on diarrhea-associated hemolytic uremic syndrome in children: a randomized controlled trial. *JAMA*, **290**, 1337–44.
68. Tsai, H.M. & Lian, E.C. (1998). Antibodies to von Willebrand factor-cleaving protease in acute thrombotic thrombocytopenic purpura. *N Engl J Med*, **339**, 1585–94.
69. Tsai, H.M., Rice, L., Sarode, R., Chow, T.W. & Moake, J.L. (2000). Antibody inhibitors to von Willebrand factor metalloproteinase and increased binding of von Willebrand factor to platelets in ticlopidine-associated thrombotic thrombocytopenic purpura. *Ann Intern Med*, **132**, 794–9.
70. Van Dyck, M. & Proesmans, W. (2004). Renoprotection by ACE inhibitors after severe hemolytic uremic syndrome. *Pediatr Nephrol*, **19**, 688–90.
71. Van Hove, J.L., Van Damme-Lombaerts, R., Grunewald, S., Peters, H., Van Damme, B., Fryns, J.P., Arnout, J., Wevers, R., Baumgartner, E.R. & Fowler, B. (2002). Cobalamin disorder Cbl-C presenting with late-onset thrombotic microangiopathy. *Am J Med Genet*, **111**, 195–201.
72. Veyradier, A., Obert, B., Houllier, A., Meyer, D. & Girma, J.P. (2001). Specific von Willebrand factor-cleaving protease in thrombotic microangiopathies: a study of 111 cases. *Blood*, **98**, 1765–72.
73. Weiner, C.P. (1987). Thrombotic microangiopathy in pregnancy and the postpartum period. *Semin Hematol*, **24**, 119–29.
74. Wen, S.X., Teel, L.D., Judge, N.A. & O'Brien, A.D. (2006). A plant-based oral vaccine to protect against systemic intoxication by Shiga toxin type 2. *Proc Natl Acad Sci USA*, **103**, 7082–7.
75. Wong, C.S., Jelacic, S., Habeeb, R.L., Watkins, S.L. & Tarr, P.I. (2000). The risk of the hemolytic-uremic syndrome after antibiotic treatment of *Escherichia coli* O157:H7 infections. *N Engl J Med*, **342**, 1930–6.

Acute Tubulointerstitial Nephritis

6.10

David J. Border and Richard J. Baker

Core Messages

- Acute tubulointerstitial nephritis (ATIN) is a cause of acute kidney injury (AKI) which is characterized by the presence of inflammatory cells within the renal tubules and interstitium.
- The etiology of ATIN is diverse but is most frequently associated to a drug reaction, infection, or autoimmune pathology.
- Diagnostic clues can be found from the patient's history, examination, and laboratory investigation results, but a renal biopsy is recommended to confirm the diagnosis and facilitate early treatment.
- Drug-induced ATIN should be treated by stopping any causative agent and starting oral steroids.
- Infection-related and autoimmune ATIN should be managed by treating the underlying cause.

6.10.1 Background

Acute tubulointerstitial nephritis (ATIN) is an often reversible cause of acute kidney injury (AKI) characterized by the presence of inflammatory cells within the renal tubules and interstitium. The etiology of ATIN is diverse but is most frequently associated to a drug reaction, infection, or autoimmune condition. The clinical features are often nonspecific and the "classical" description of a triad of fever, rash, and eosinophilia are now uncommon. ATIN should be considered in cases of AKI, especially when there is no obvious precipitant. A prompt renal biopsy is recommended for diagnosis since early administration of steroids has been associated with a more rapid and complete recovery of renal function. The renal outcome will usually be good but in a small proportion, particularly the elderly, significant renal impairment can persist.

6.10.2 Historical

ATIN was first described by Councilman in 1898 [1]. Describing a series of 42 autopsies of victims of diphtheria and scarlet fever, he noted that the kidneys displayed "cellular and fluid exudation in the interstitial tissue …." This exudate was not purulent and the kidneys were themselves sterile, suggesting that the tissue damage was not due to direct microbial invasion but due to an allergic-type phenomenon. In 1946, a further series was described in which all patients had been treated with sulfonamides [2], but it was not clear whether the inciting agent was the drug itself or the underlying infection. Subsequently cases of ATIN associated with phenindione and methicillin were described, establishing it as a form of drug allergy [3, 4]. Widespread adoption of percutaneous biopsy techniques has led to ATIN becoming increasingly recognized as a cause of AKI. Today an ever increasing numbers of drugs and infections have been associated with ATIN, highlighting the need for ongoing vigilance when patients present with acute renal impairment [5–9].

R. J. Baker (✉)
Department of Renal Medicine, St James's University Hospital, Beckett Street, Leeds, LS9 7TF, UK
e-mail: richard.baker@leedsth.nhs.uk

A. Jörres, et al. (eds.), *Management of Acute Kidney Problems*,
DOI: 10.1007/978-3-540-69441-0_6.10, © Springer-Verlag Berlin Heidelberg 2010

6.10.3 Epidemiology

Amongst asymptomatic Finnish army recruits, biopsied for either hematuria or proteinuria, the incidence of ATIN was 0.7 per 100,000 [10]. Other series have found ATIN in only 2–3% of renal biopsy series [11, 12], but in up to 25% of those biopsied for drug-induced renal failure [13]. In a series of 109 patients from a large center, biopsied for unexplained renal impairment with normal sized kidneys, ATIN accounted for 27% of cases [14].

There is an equal sex distribution at presentation which occurs across a wide age range [15]. Studies have suggested ATIN is more common in the elderly [16) with a series showing an incidence of 18.6% amongst 259 patients aged over 60 years biopsied for acute renal insufficiency [17].

6.10.4 Clinical Features

ATIN should be suspected in any unexplained case of AKI, particularly when there is no obvious precipitant. Most cases of ATIN present with non-specific symptoms of acute renal dysfunction, or no symptoms at all. Usually individuals are normotensive without peripheral edema and serum creatinine will be acutely raised. Evidence of tubular dysfunction may be present with renal tubular acidosis, fanconi syndrome, or abnormalities of sodium and potassium handling. Renal impairment is severe enough to require dialysis in approximately one third of patients.

Eosinophilia is present in 23–36% of individuals, rash in 15–21%, and fever in 27–30%. Together the characteristic "classic" triad of signs is rare and seen in less than 10% of ATIN cases [15, 18], and typically is absent in those related to nonsteroidal anti-inflammatory drugs (NSAIDs) [19, 20]. Older series consist largely of cases caused by beta lactam antibiotics (such as methcillinam) and sulfonamides, and feature a high incidence of the "allergic-type" elements of rash, fever, arthralgia, and eosinophilia [21–26]. It is thought the incidence of "classic" symptoms is less due to the reduced use of these antibiotics.

Urinalysis usually reveals proteinuria although normally less than 2 g/24 h is excreted. Nephrotic range proteinuria (more than 3 g/24 h excreted) can occur but should arouse suspicion of coincident minimal change disease secondary to NSAID usage. Mild hematuria on urinalysis is common but macroscopic hematuria and red cell casts on microscopy are rarely found.

White cells and white cell casts may also be present in the urine and examination for eosinophiluria (eosinophils > 1% total urine white cells) with Hansel's stain is often positive. This test is not routinely performed and has a low sensitivity and positive predictive value (38%) [27, 28].

Enlarged renal bipolar length is a non-specific finding in ATIN but associated distension of the renal capsule can cause patients to present with flank pain.

6.10.5 Etiology

There are an ever increasing number of associations with ATIN so constant vigilance is required. Historically, prior to the widespread use of antibiotics, exposure to infective agents was the most frequent cause of ATIN, but now drugs predominate. Based on a number of contemporary series causes include [15]:

- Drugs 71%
- Infections 15%
- Idiopathic 8%
- Tubulointerstitial Nephritis and Uveitis (TINU) syndrome 5%
- Sarcoidosis 1%

Recent examples of drug associations include celecoxib, etanercept, sorafenib, linazolid, and several antiretroviral agents [29–35]. ATIN associated with infections such as BK virus, adenovirus, and histoplasmosis has also been described [31, 33, 36].

6.10.5.1 Drug-Induced ATIN

There are numerous agents associated with drug-induced ATIN (DI-ATIN) (see Table 6.10.1). Eighty percent of cases develop within 3 weeks of stating the precipitant drug, but the time following exposure to developing ATIN ranges from 1 day to over 12 months. The development of DI-ATIN is not dose dependent and can reoccur on rechallenging with the same or related drug, usually rapidly within 2–3 days. Historically methicillin was a significant cause of DI-ATIN, which is reflected in the literature, and has subsequently been withdrawn

Table 6.10.1 Common causes of drug-induced-ATIN

NSAIDs (diclofenac, ibuprofen, naproxen, indomethacin, COX2 inhibitors)
Antibiotics (beta-lactams [penicillins and cephalosporins], rifampin, sulfonamides, Tetracyclines, Quinolones)
Proton pump inhibitors (omeprazole and lansoprazole)
Diuretics (loop and thiazide types)
Phenytoin
Salicylates (Aspirin, 5-aminosalicylates)
H2 antagonists (cimetidine)
Allopurinol
Phenindione

from clinical use. The clinical signs found with methicillin induced ATIN included a high frequency of abnormal urinalysis and extrarenal symptoms and good preservation of renal function.

6.10.5.1.1 NSAID-Associated DI-ATIN

Nonsteroidal anti-inflammatory drug (NSAID) associated DI-ATIN differs in its behavior from other causes as it presents later (median 3 months) can be associated with significant proteinuria or nephrotic syndrome secondary to minimal change disease [37, 38]. Most cases occur in patients aged over 50 years, reflecting the cohort exposed to the drug, and it has even been described after application of topical NSAID preparations [39]. Extrarenal signs (fever, rash) and hematuria are rare with NSAID ATIN. Some authors have stated that NSAID-related ATIN has a poor outlook and is often irreversible though this finding has not been universal [18, 40].

6.10.5.2 Infection-Related ATIN (IR-ATIN)

The advent of antibiotics is believed to have reduced the frequency of ATIN cases caused by infections. However direct microbial infection causing a similar histological picture (e.g., pyelonephritis) must be distinguished from sterile "allergic-type" ATIN as described originally by Councilman in diphtheria and scarlet fever. Histologically identical to DI-ATIN the clinical presentation will depend upon the underlying infection. A number of pathogens are associated with IR-ATIN (see Table 6.10.2). The infecting agents are thought to cause ATIN by stimulating the release of chemokines leading to leukocyte infiltration of the interstitium [41].

Table 6.10.2 Causes of infection-related ATIN

Bacterial	Streptococci	Staphylococcae
	Legionella	*Cornybacterium diptheriae*
	Brucella	*Campylobacter jejuni*
	Escherichiacoli	Tuberculosis
	Salmonella	Leptospirosis
	Syphilis	
Viral	Epstein Barr virus	Cytomegalovirus
	Polyomavirus	BK virus
	Hantavirus	Hepatitis B virus
	Herpes simples virus	HIV
	Measles	
Others	Mycoplasma	Toxoplasma
	Leishmania donovani	Chlamydia

Table 6.10.3 Causes of Autoimmune Related ATIN

Sjogren's syndrome
Systemic lupus erythematosus
Sarcoidosis
Behcet's disease
Glomerulonephritis
Wegner's granulomatosis
Necrotising vasculitis
Primary biliary cirrhosis
Essential cryoglobulinaemia
Acute graft (renal transplant) rejection

6.10.5.3 Autoimmune ATIN

Most autoimmune conditions associated with an interstitial infiltrate cause a chronic interstitial nephritis. Several of these may also be associated with a more acute presentation (see Table 6.10.3). Sarcoidosis is a cause of granulomatous ATIN. It is associated with extrarenal symptoms in approximately 90% of cases. Hilar lymphadenopathy and pulmonary infiltrates are found in around half the patients [42].

6.10.5.4 Idiopathic ATIN

Idiopathic ATIN is a heterogeneous entity where a causes of interstitial nephritis is not clear. Management of these cases is discussed in Section 6.10.9.

6.10.5.5 Tubulointerstitial Nephritis and Uveitis Syndrome

TINU syndrome was first reported in 1975 as an association between ATIN and anterior uveitis, sometimes associated with bone marrow granulomas [43]. It is a rare disease and despite a number (>150) of such patients having now been described [44] it remains poorly understood. Although associations with chlamydia, mycoplasma, and Epstein Barr infections have been suggested, the etiology remains obscure [45]. Exposure to some drugs, such as cephalosporins and NSAIDs have also been associated with the development of TINU syndrome, as well as some autoimmune conditions (e.g., hypoparathyroidism and thyroiditis). Uveitis is often bilateral and ocular symptoms may proceed (21%) be concurrent (15%) or occur after (25%) the ATIN [62]. Cases can sometimes be difficult to distinguish from sarcoidosis and Sjogren syndrome. Amongst adults, females usually predominate (3:1). They may suffer from weight loss and anemia, and have a raised ESR alongside renal impairment, but presentation is often nonspecific [62]. Renal biopsy findings include granulomas (13%), interstitial eosinophils (33%), and neutrophils (25%). Treatment is discussed in Section 6.10.9.

6.10.5.6 Renal Transplant ATIN

ATIN can be problematic in the renal allograft as the histological appearance is similar to acute interstitial cellular rejection. Interestingly DI-ATIN can still occur despite ongoing immunosuppression. Similar histological appearances may also be found in association with viral allograft infections such as BK or CMV nephropathy, although in these cases the tissue damage is thought to be mediated by direct viral cytotoxicity [36].

6.10.6 Pathogenesis

The majority of cases of ATIN are thought secondary to an immune reaction against an extra-renal antigen (Ag), produced by drugs or infectious agents, which subsequently induces an inflammatory response through T-cell-mediated delayed hypersensitivity reaction or direct T-cell cytotoxicity.

The features that suggest ATIN being an immunologically induced hypersensitivity reaction include:

- Its occurrence in a small proportion of patients exposed to the agent.
- Its incidence is not dose dependent.
- The time course is typical of a delayed type hypersensitivity reaction.
- Inadvertent rechallenge can cause recurrence [24, 47, 48].
- Drug specific T-cell responses have been demonstrated in vitro to share many features with cutaneous hypersensitivity reactions [49].
- A demonstrable association with extrarenal manifestations of hypersensitivity.
- There is sterile interstitial tissue with a paucity of neutrophils.

This reaction may occur by a number of different mechanisms:

- Direct Ag binding to kidney structures, modifying the immunogenicity of native renal proteins
- A molecular mimicry of renal Ags
- Precipitation of immune complexes within the interstitium

Cell-mediated immunity is believed to play the major role in ATIN, with T-cells and occasionally granulomas found in the interstitium. Antibody-mediated immunity also has a role as well however, as immune complexes are sometimes found in biopsy tissue. Immune complex deposition is often found in autoimmune ATIN, especially lupus nephritis (50%) and less frequently in Sjogrens and mixed cryoglobulinemia. Both forms of immune reaction will result in inflammation through activation of the complement cascade and the release of cytokines which can lead ultimately to interstitial fibrosis and renal failure.

6.10.7 Histology

The typical histological findings on renal biopsy are interstitial edema and cellular infiltrates largely composed of T-lymphocytes with some macrophages, eosinophils, and plasma cells. Often patchy in the deep cortex and outer medulla, the infiltrates can become diffuse in severe forms of ATIN. Occasionally, usually in the distal tubule, tubulitis can be found with

T-lymphocytes crossing the tubule-basement membrane to sit between tubular cells. The interstitial edema is often seen to separate the tubules. Infiltrative changes are also associated with focal tubular damage but spare the vascular structures and glomeruli, which appear normal on light microscopy. Interstitial granulomata can be found in any form of ATIN [50], but in DI-ATIN certain drugs are more commonly associated than others (e.g., NSAIDs). Immune deposits are rarely found but occasionally granular or linear IgG deposits are seen on immunofluorescence staining of the tubular or capsular basement membrane.

Signs of chronic renal damage with interstitial scarring and fibrosis may develop over time to be present on biopsy. This can provide prognostic information for renal recovery (see Section 6.10.10).

Interstitial infiltration by malignant cells may be seen in leukemia or lymphoma and can mimic the typical ATIN biopsy findings.

6.10.8 Diagnosis

The patients history, including recent drug use, infection, and immune conditions alongside a physical examination, looking for fever, rash, or signs of inflammatory disease as well as urinalysis and the laboratory investigations highlighted previously will provide clues to the diagnosis.

Imaging techniques are of minimal help in the diagnosis of ATIN. The kidneys may appear enlarged on ultrasound scan (USS) but this is a non-specific finding. Gallium scanning has been used to diagnose DI-ATIN, typically revealing bilateral renal parenchymal uptake consistent with an interstitial infiltrative process. False negative diagnoses have been described as well as false positives in patients with pyelonephritis, cancer, or glomerular disease [53–55]. Given the varying sensitivities this test is rarely used.

A renal biopsy is recommended for a confirmation of diagnosis to facilitate early treatment [51]. In addition the histology, as discussed previously, can provide useful prognostic information [23, 40, 52]. The clinical diagnosis sometimes has to be made without kidney tissue in those where the risks of biopsy are significant.

Identifying the causative drug when there is more than one potential suspect can be difficult. In vitro lymphocyte stimulation assays are not widely available or validated [49]. In practice one or more potential offending drugs have to be stopped at the same time, leading to uncertainty over the actual inciting agent.

6.10.9 Treatment

In suspected cases of DI-ATIN the mainstay of treatment is stopping the causative agent and steroid therapy. Unfortunately there have been no significant prospective randomized studies investigating the treatment of ATIN and so therapeutic guidance must be drawn from retrospective uncontrolled case series. There is increasing evidence that treating with steroids is superior to conservative therapy alone [11, 22–24]. A retrospective study of 20 patients with ATIN demonstrated that the seven patients who were treated with steroids had a significantly better renal outcome than those who were not [23]. Other reports have also described benefits from steroids in small series of patients [22, 24]. In another study of 27 patients with ATIN, 17 improved spontaneously with conservative measures and drug discontinuation [11]. The remaining ten showed further deterioration of renal function in the 2 weeks following admission, and were then treated with steroids. In all these patients renal function then improved, returning to normal in six.

Other studies however have come to opposing conclusions regarding steroid therapy. One described 61 patients in multiple centers all of whom were diagnosed with DI-ATIN on the basis of renal biopsy and clinical history [51]. Fifty-two were treated with steroids and enjoyed a better clinical outcome than those who remained untreated. Moreover those who were treated within 2 weeks of drug withdrawal had a more complete recovery. In the other single center retrospective study no effect of steroid treatment could be demonstrated, although the patients in this particular series were treated later after diagnosis and tended to have worse renal function than those who were not treated [18].

In summary in the absence of prospective randomized controlled trial data we recommend that a short course of steroid is administered and this should begin as soon as possible after diagnosis. In cases where there are potential significant steroid side effects it is not unreasonable to withhold treatment to assess first for renal recovery on inciting drug withdrawal. A period of 3–7 days without the causal drug is usually enough time to see whether improvement of kidney function without steroid will occur.

The optimal steroid dose regimen is also unknown. Short courses of pulsed methylprednisolone (e.g., 500 mg i/v for 3 days consecutively) have been used as well as relatively short tapered courses of oral steroids (0.5–1 mg/kg/day tapered over 4–12 weeks). We recommend the latter as the preferred treatment option.

Ideally steroid use should be based on a biopsy findings demonstrating ATIN. Sometimes, as discussed, a renal biopsy is not technically possible and in such cases an empirical "trial" of steroids is justified.

Second line agents are poorly defined with only limited case reports. A recent report of eight cases of ATIN suggested that mycophenolate mofetil might be beneficial in patients who are unresponsive to or intolerant of steroid therapy [56]. Cyclosporine and cyclophosphamide have also been used as alternative agents, mainly in steroid resistant cases, and should only be considered in this situation.

Ideopathic ATIN cases are treated in a similar fashion to DI-ATIN with steroids. Some cases respond well to steroids and others will recover normal renal function without any specific treatment.

In cases of TINU syndrome prolonged steroid therapy (1 mg/kg oral prednisolone slowly tapered over 3–6 months) usually leads to improvement in both renal function and uveitis, though the latter may relapse [46]. The nephritis however usually resolves spontaneously [62].

The treatment of Autoimmune ATIN is of the underlying immune condition. This will usually involve immunosuppression with steroids or stronger immunomodulatory agents.

6.10.10 Prognosis

The following factors have been identified with a poor renal prognosis:

- Increasing patient age [52, 61]
- The degree of interstitial fibrosis on renal biopsy [57, 58]
- Granulomas and tubular atrophy on biopsy [15]
- An association with NSAID use
- Duration of renal failure more than 3 weeks [23, 61]

Attempts have been made to gain prognostic information from the renal biopsy, with variable outcomes. The degree of tubular atrophy predicted renal outcome in one series [15], whereas some authors have reported that patchy cellular infiltration predicts a better outcome than diffuse disease [23, 52]. Other studies showed that there was no correlation between the degree of cellular infiltration or tubulitis and outcome [11, 57]. The degree of interstitial fibrosis has been correlated to outcome [57, 58] and is known to reflect background chronic renal damage. No such relationship was found in another study which may be due to the patchy nature of the disease and the random sampling on renal biopsy [59]. The infiltrate is generally most prominent at the corticomedullary boundary, and the medulla is relatively spared. This was recognized over 100 years ago by Councilman, who commented on the localized nature of the histological changes [1].

Historical data demonstrated that renal function improved in the majority of methicillin induced ATIN patients with either discontinuation of the drug or steroid treatment, but that a lower proportion recovered renal function from ATIN secondary to other drugs [22, 40]. Acute dialysis is sometimes required but only a few patients (<10%) become dialysis dependent [60]. Renal function does not return to baseline in up to 40% of patients with ATIN, but the final creatinine does not correlate with the peak value [9] or a poorer renal prognosis [22].

6.10.11 Take Home Pearls

- ATIN is a common cause of unexplained ARF.
- Most ATIN cases are probably allergic-type responses to drugs.
- ATIN usually occurs within 3 weeks of starting medication.
- Early clinical suspicion and renal biopsy are essential.
- "Offending" drug withdrawal is essential.
- Early steroid treatment is beneficial and probably hastens recovery.
- Mycophenolate Mofetil may offer an effective second-line therapy.
- Recovery may be incomplete, especially those over 60 years of age.

References

1. Councilman W (1898) Acute interstitial nephritis. J Exp Med 3:393–418
2. More R, McMillan, G, Duff, G (1946) The pathology of sulphonamide allergy in man. Am J Pathol 22:703–725
3. McMenamin RA, Davies, LM, Craswell, PW (1976) Drug induced interstitial nephritis, hepatitis and exfoliative dermatitis. Aust N Z J Med 6:583–587
4. Hewitt W, Finegold, S, Monzon, O (1961) Untoward side effects associated with methicillin therapy. Antimicrob Agents Chemother 765–769
5. Droz D, Kleinknecht, D (1997) Acute interstitial nephritis. In Cameron J, Davison, A (eds) Oxford Textbook of Clinical Nephrology. Oxford University Press, Oxford, pp 1634–1646
6. Michel DM, Kelly, CJ (1998) Acute interstitial nephritis. J Am Soc Nephrol 9:506–515
7. Neilson EG (1989) Pathogenesis and therapy of interstitial nephritis. Kidney Int 35:1257–1270
8. Rastegar A, Kashgarian, M (1998) The clinical spectrum of tubulointerstitial nephritis. Kidney Int 54:313–327
9. Rossert J (2001) Drug-induced acute interstitial nephritis. Kidney Int 60:804–817
10. Pettersson E, von Bonsdorff, M, Tornroth, T, Lindholm, H (1984) Nephritis among young Finnish men. Clin Nephrol 22:217–222
11. Buysen JG, Houthoff, HJ, Krediet, RT, Arisz, L (1990) Acute interstitial nephritis: a clinical and morphological study in 27 patients. Nephrol Dial Transplant 5:94–99
12. Cameron JS (1988) Allergic interstitial nephritis: clinical features and pathogenesis. Q J Med 66:97–115
13. Landais P, Goldfarb, B, Kleinknecht, D (1987) Eosinophiluria and drug-induced acute interstitial nephritis. N Engl J Med 316:1664
14. Farrington K, Levison, DA, Greenwood, RN, Cattell, WR, Baker, LR (1989) Renal biopsy in patients with unexplained renal impairment and normal kidney size. Quart J Med 70:221–233
15. Baker RJ, Pusey, CD (2004) The changing profile of acute tubulointerstitial nephritis. Nephrol Dial Transplant 19:8–11
16. Davison AM (1998) Renal disease in the elderly. Nephron 80:6–16
17. Haas M, Spargo, BH, Wit, EJ, Meehan, SM (2000) Etiologies and outcome of acute renal insufficiency in older adults: a renal biopsy study of 259 cases. Am J Kidney Dis 35:433–447
18. Clarkson MR, Giblin, L, O'Connell, FP, O'Kelly, P, Walshe, JJ, Conlon, P, O'Meara, Y, Dormon, A, Campbell, E, Donohoe, J (2004) Acute interstitial nephritis: clinical features and response to corticosteroid therapy. Nephrol Dial Transplant 19:2778–2783
19. Clive DM, Stoff, JS (1984) Renal syndromes associated with nonsteroidal antiinflammatory drugs. N Engl J Med 310:563–572
20. Pirani CL, Valeri, A, D'Agati, V, Appel, GB (1987) Renal toxicity of nonsteroidal anti-inflammatory drugs. Contrib Nephrol 55:159–175
21. Shibasaki T, Ishimoto, F, Sakai, O, Joh, K, Aizawa, S (1991) Clinical characterization of drug-induced allergic nephritis. Am J Nephrol 11:174–180
22. Galpin JE, Shinaberger, JH, Stanley, TM, Blumenkrantz, MJ, Bayer, AS, Friedman, GS, Montgomerie, JZ, Guze, LB, Coburn, JW, Glassock, RJ (1978) Acute interstitial nephritis due to methicillin. Am J Med 65:756–765
23. Laberke HG (1980) Treatment of acute interstitial nephritis. Klin Wochenschr 58:531–532
24. Pusey CD, Saltissi, D, Bloodworth, L, Rainford, DJ, Christie, JL (1983) Drug associated acute interstitial nephritis: clinical and pathological features and the response to high dose steroid therapy. Quart J Med 52:194–211
25. Linton AL, Clark, WF, Driedger, AA, Turnbull, DI, Lindsay, RM (1980) Acute interstitial nephritis due to drugs: Review of the literature with a report of nine cases. Ann Intern Med 93:735–741
26. Nolan CM, Abernathy, RS (1977) Nephropathy associated with methicillin therapy. Prevalence and determinants in patients with staphylococcal bacteremia. Arch Intern Med 137:997–1000
27. Nolan CR, 3rd, Anger, MS, Kelleher, SP (1986) Eosinophiluria – a new method of detection and definition of the clinical spectrum. N Engl J Med 315:1516–1519
28. Ruffing KA, Hoppes, P, Blend, D, Cugino, A, Jarjoura, D, Whittier, FC (1994) Eosinophils in urine revisited. Clin Nephrol 41:163–166
29. Esposito L, Kamar, N, Guilbeau-Frugier, C, Mehrenberger, M, Modesto, A, Rostaing, L (2007) Linezolid-induced interstitial nephritis in a kidney-transplant patient. Clin Nephrol 68:327–329
30. Fine DM, Perazella, MA, Lucas, GM, Atta, MG (2008) Kidney biopsy in HIV: beyond HIV-associated nephropathy. Am J Kidney Dis 51:504–514
31. Henao J, Hisamuddin, I, Nzerue, CM, Vasandani, G, Hewan-Lowe, K (2002) Celecoxib-induced acute interstitial nephritis. Am J Kidney Dis 39:1313–1317
32. Izzedine H, Brocheriou, I, Rixe, O, Deray, G (2007) Interstitial nephritis in a patient taking sorafenib. Nephrol Dial Transplant 22:2411
33. Kopp JB, Falloon, J, Filie, A, Abati, A, King, C, Hortin, GL, Mican, JM, Vaughan, E, Miller, KD (2002) Indinavir-associated interstitial nephritis and urothelial inflammation: clinical and cytologic findings. Clin Infect Dis 34:1122–1128
34. Schmid S, Opravil, M, Moddel, M, Huber, M, Pfammatter, R, Keusch, G, Ambuhl, P, Wuthrich, RP, Moch, H, Varga, Z (2007) Acute interstitial nephritis of HIV-positive patients under atazanavir and tenofovir therapy in a retrospective analysis of kidney biopsies. Virchows Arch 450:665–670
35. Sugimoto T, Yasuda, M, Sakaguchi, M, Koyama, T, Uzu, T, Nishioka, J, Kashiwagi, A (2008) Acute interstitial nephritis associated with etanercept. Rheumatol Int 28(12): 1283–1284
36. Randhawa PS, Finkelstein, S, Scantlebury, V, Shapiro, R, Vivas, C, Jordan, M, Picken, MM, Demetris, AJ (1999) Human polyoma virus-associated interstitial nephritis in the allograft kidney. Transplantation 67:103–109
37. Kleinknecht D (1995) Interstitial nephritis, the nephrotic syndrome, and chronic renal failure secondary to nonsteroidal anti-inflammatory drugs. Semin Nephrol 15:228–235
38. Porile JL, Bakris, GL, Garella, S (1990) Acute interstitial nephritis with glomerulopathy due to nonsteroidal anti-inflammatory agents: a review of its clinical spectrum and effects of steroid therapy. J Clin Pharmacol 30:468–475

39. O'Callaghan CA, Andrews, PA, Ogg, CS (1994) Renal disease and use of topical non-steroidal anti-inflammatory drugs. BMJ 308:110–111
40. Schwarz A, Krause, PH, Kunzendorf, U, Keller, F, Distler, A (2000) The outcome of acute interstitial nephritis: risk factors for the transition from acute to chronic interstitial nephritis. Clin Nephrol 54:179–190
41. Hung CC, Chang, CT, Chen, KH, Tian, YC, Wu, MS, Pan, MJ, Vandewalle, A, Yang, CW (2006) Upregulation of chemokine CXCL1/KC by leptospiral membrane lipoprotein preparation in renal tubule epithelial cells. Kidney Int 69:1814–1822
42. Hannedouche T, Grateau, G, Noel, LH, Godin, M, Fillastre, JP, Grunfeld, JP, Jungers, P (1990) Renal granulomatous sarcoidosis: report of six cases. Nephrol Dial Transplant 5:18–24
43. Dobrin RS, Vernier, RL, Fish, AL (1975) Acute eosinophilic interstitial nephritis and renal failure with bone marrow-lymph node granulomas and anterior uveitis. A new syndrome. Am J Med 59:325–333
44. Mandeville JT, Levinson, RD, Holland, GN (2001) The tubulointerstitial nephritis and uveitis syndrome. Surv Ophthalmol 46:195–208
45. Stupp R, Mihatsch, MJ, Matter, L, Streuli, RA (1990) Acute tubulo-interstitial nephritis with uveitis (TINU syndrome) in a patient with serologic evidence for Chlamydia infection. Klin Wochenschr 68:971–975
46. Rodriguez-Perez JC, Cruz-Alamo, M, Perez-Aciego, P, Macia-Heras, M, Naranjo-Hernandez, A, Plaza-Toledano, C, Hortal-Cascon, L, Fernandez-Rodriguez, A (1995) Clinical and immune aspects of idiopathic acute tubulointerstitial nephritis and uveitis syndrome. Am J Nephrol 15:386–391
47. Saltissi D, Pusey, CD, Rainford, DJ (1979) Recurrent acute renal failure due to antibiotic-induced interstitial nephritis. Br Med J 1:1182–1183
48. Sloth K, Thomsen, AC (1971) Acute renal insufficiency during treatment with azathioprine. Acta Med Scand 189: 145–148
49. Spanou Z, Keller, M, Britschgi, M, Yawalkar, N, Fehr, T, Neuweiler, J, Gugger, M, Mohaupt, M, Pichler, WJ (2006) Involvement of drug-specific T cells in acute drug-induced interstitial nephritis. J Am Soc Nephrol 17:2919–2927
50. Joss N, Morris, S, Young, B, Geddes, C (2007) Granulomatous interstitial nephritis. Clin J Am Soc Nephrol 2:222–230
51. Gonzalez E, Gutierrez, E, Galeano, C, Chevia, C, de Sequera, P, Bernis, C, Parra, EG, Delgado, R, Sanz, M, Ortiz, M, Goicoechea, M, Quereda, C, Olea, T, Bouarich, H, Hernandez, Y, Segovia, B, Praga, M (2008) Early steroid treatment improves the recovery of renal function in patients with drug-induced acute interstitial nephritis. Kidney Int 73:940–946
52. Kida H, Abe, T, Tomosugi, N, Koshino, Y, Yokoyama, H, Hattori, N (1984) Prediction of the long-term outcome in acute interstitial nephritis. Clin Nephrol 22:55–60
53. Graham GD, Lundy, MM, Moreno, AJ (1983) Failure of Gallium-67 scintigraphy to identify reliably noninfectious interstitial nephritis: concise communication. J Nucl Med 24:568–570
54. Linton AL, Richmond, JM, Clark, WF, Lindsay, RM, Driedger, AA, Lamki, LM (1985) Gallium67 scintigraphy in the diagnosis of acute renal disease. Clin Nephrol 24:84–87
55. Wood BC, Sharma, JN, Germann, DR, Wood, WG, Crouch, TT (1978) Gallium citrate Ga 67 imaging in noninfectious interstitial nephritis. Arch Intern Med 138:1665–1666
56. Preddie DC, Markowitz, GS, Radhakrishnan, J, Nickolas, TL, D'Agati, VD, Schwimmer, JA, Gardenswartz, M, Rosen, R, Appel, GB (2006) Mycophenolate mofetil for the treatment of interstitial nephritis. Clin J Am Soc Nephrol 1:718–722
57. Ivanyi B, Hamilton-Dutoit, SJ, Hansen, HE, Olsen, S (1996) Acute tubulointerstitial nephritis: phenotype of infiltrating cells and prognostic impact of tubulitis. Virchows Arch 428:5–12
58. Bhaumik SK, Kher, V, Arora, P, Rai, PK, Singhal, M, Gupta, A, Pandey, R, Sharma, RK (1996) Evaluation of clinical and histological prognostic markers in drug-induced acute interstitial nephritis. Ren Fail 18:97–104
59. Cheng HF, Nolasco, F, Cameron, JS, Hildreth, G, Neild, GH, Hartley, B (1989) HLA-DR display by renal tubular epithelium and phenotype of infiltrate in interstitial nephritis. Nephrol Dial Transplant 4:205–215
60. Laberke HG, Bohle, A (1980) Acute interstitial nephritis: correlations between clinical and morphological findings. Clin Nephrol 14:263–273
61. Ditlove J, Weidmann, P, Bernstein, M, Massry, SG (1977) Methicillin nephritis. Medicine (Baltimore) 56:483–491
62. Herlitz LC, Chun, MJ, Stokes, MB, Markowitz, GS (2007) Uveitis and acute renal failure. Kidney Int 72:1554

Myoglobinuric Acute Kidney Failure 6.11

Mehmet Sükrü Sever and Raymond Vanholder

Core Messages

- Myoglobinuric acute kidney failure (AKF) is a variant of acute kidney dysfunction due to rhabdomyolysis, while rhabdomyolysis is the disintegration of striated muscles resulting in the release of muscular cell contents into the extracellular fluid.
- Rhabdomyolysis may result from nontraumatic and traumatic etiologies; its clinical spectrum varies from asymptomatic elevations in serum creatine kinase, to AKF and multiorgan failure, i.e., the crush syndrome.
- Most important laboratory findings include myoglobinuria, increased serum levels of myoglobin, creatine kinase, and hyperkalemia.
- Vigorous hydration by isotonic saline followed by alkaline solutions and mannitol are useful in the prophylaxis of myoglobinuric AKF.
- Usually, dialysis is required in patients with established kidney failure; intermittent hemodialysis is the preferred renal replacement therapy.

M. S. Sever (✉)
Department of Internal Medicine/Nephrology, Istanbul School of Medicine, Millet caddesi, Çapa Topkapi TR 34390, Istanbul, Turkey
e-mail: severm@hotmail.com

6.11.1 Introduction

Myoglobinuria is presence of myoglobin in the urine.

Myoglobin is the oxygen-carrier protein of the muscle and serves to store the oxygen required for oxidative metabolism that is used by the mitochondria during muscle contraction. Its molecular weight is 17,800 Da and accounts for 1–3% of the dry weight of the skeletal muscle [67], where each gram of wet muscle contains 4 mg of myoglobin [17]. Normal serum level of myoglobin ranges from 0 to 0.003 mg/dl; half-life is about 3 h, but lengthens in renal failure. It disappears from the plasma within 6 h to be converted to bilirubin [14, 17]. Normally, 50–85% of myoglobin binds weakly to certain plasma globulins (haptoglobulin and α2-globulin) and is excreted in the urine in minimal amounts (less than 5 ng/ml) [55]. The renal threshold value for myoglobinuria is 1.5 mg/dl; approximately 100 g of muscle tissue should be damaged for serum myoglobin to exceed this critical level [19]. Therefore, lack of myoglobinuria does not exclude rhabdomyolysis; however, positive myoglobinuria indicates that the dimensions of muscle tissue necrosis is extensive.

Rhabdomyolysis is disintegration of striated muscles, which results in the release of myoglobin and other muscular cell contents into the extracellular fluid and the circulation. The manifestations range from asymptomatic elevations of serum muscle enzymes to life-threatening electrolyte imbalances, acute kidney failure (AKF), and multiorgan failure.

Myoglobinuric AKF is kidney dysfunction due to rhabdomyolysis. Twenty to 50% of rhabdomyolysis cases are complicated by AKF; the wide variation is related to timing of the analysis and inconsistent definitions of rhabdomyolysis and AKF in the literature [51, 64]. On the other hand, rhabdomyolysis is responsible for 5–20% of all cases of AKF [34].

A. Jörres et al. (eds.), *Management of Acute Kidney Problems*,
DOI: 10.1007/978-3-540-69441-0_6.11, © Springer-Verlag Berlin Heidelberg 2010

6.11.1.1 Structure of the Muscles

Muscles are the largest organ in the body accounting for approximately 40% of total body mass; they are located in compartments, which are spaces restricted by rigid, noncompliant fascias surrounding the muscles. Normally, the pressure in these compartments is very low; increased pressure is referred to as *compartment syndrome,* which can disrupt the perfusion and hinder the function of the muscles.

Anatomically, muscles are comprised of innumerable, elongated, multinucleated cells (*muscle fibers* or *myocytes*). Each myocyte contains thousands of thin, longitudinal fibers, i.e., *myofibrils*. Each myofibril contains nearly 1,500 thick (myosin) and 3,000 thin (actin) filaments, lying side by side.

The cell membrane of myocytes (*sarcolemma*) is impermeable to extracellular fluid and electrolytes. The cytoplasm of myocytes containing intracellular organelles is called *sarcoplasm*; it holds large amounts of potassium, magnesium, phosphate, proteolytic enzymes, and mitochondria; the latter forms adenosine triphosphate (ATP) which supplies energy to the muscle during contraction. As compared with the extracellular fluid, the sarcoplasm is hyperoncotic and electronegative; it contains significantly lower calcium and sodium, but markedly higher potassium concentrations [16, 67]. *Sarcoplasmic reticulum* is the endoplasmic reticulum of the muscle fiber and contains plenty of calcium ions.

6.11.2 Etiology and Pathogenesis

6.11.2.1 Etiology of Rhabdomyolysis

Nonphysical and physical causes play a role in the etiology of rhabdomyolysis (Table 6.11.1); the incidence of the listed causes varies according to the geographical region. Drug abuse is a major cause in the Western countries, while traumatic events are more common in developing countries. Etiology may also differ according to timing of analysis; nontraumatic causes are approximately five times more frequent than traumatic ones in daily practice [63]; during wars and natural disasters, however, traumatic etiology becomes the leading cause.

Table 6.11.1 Etiology of rhabdomyolysis [13, 60, 63]

Nonphysical causes	Physical causes
Electrolyte abnormalities	**Trauma and/or compression of the muscles**
Hypokalemia, hypocalcemia, hypophosphatemia	Natural and man-made disasters
Hyponatremia, hypernatremia	Traffic or working accidents
Alcohol, drugs, and toxins	Torture, beating
Regular and illegal drugs	Long-term confinement to the same position
Toxins	**Occlusion or hypoperfusion of the muscular vessels**
Snake and insect venoms	Thrombosis
Fish toxins	Embolism
Infections and infestations	Vessel clamping
Infections localized to muscles (pyomyositis)	Shock
Metastatic infections (sepsis)	**Strainful exercise of muscles**
Systemic effects	Strenuous exercising
Toxic shock syndrome, *Legionella* spp., *Streptococcus* spp., *Staphylococcus* spp., *Clostridium perfringes, Salmonella* spp., *Plasmodium falciparum,* HIV, Influenza, Herpes and Coxsackie virus infections	Epilepsy Delirium tremens Tetanus Status asthmaticus
Metabolic myopathies	**Electrical current**
Myophosphorylase deficiency (Mc Ardle disease)	High-voltage electrical injury
Carnitine palmitoyl transferase deficiency	Cardioversion
Phosphofructokinase deficiency	**Hyperthermia**
Endocrine disorders	High ambient temperatures
Hypothyroidism, diabetic coma and resulting electrolyte imbalances	Neuroleptic malignant syndrome
Disseminated intravascular coagulation	Malignant hyperthermia
Polymyositis, dermatomyositis	Sepsis
	Exercise

HIV: Human Immudeficiency Virus

Overall, the vast majority of etiologic factors are related to alcohol consumption, drug use, and compression of muscles resulting from prolonged immobility.

6.11.2.2 Pathogenesis of Rhabdomyolysis

Two features predispose muscles to be readily damaged. First, they are not protected by bony structures; hence the risk of being traumatized is very high. Second, their metabolism is highly variable; although blood flow, oxygen consumption, and energy needs are limited at rest, they increase drastically, even up to 25 times, during strenuous exercise [16].

Overall, rhabdomyolysis develops due to an imbalance between muscle energy production and consumption. Factors resulting in an insufficient supply of substrates and/or oxygen required for energy production (e.g., crush injury, ischemia), impaired cellular energy production (e.g., hereditary enzymatic defects) and/or increased calcium influx into the cell (e.g., malignant hyperthermia) may cause rhabdomyolysis. On the other hand, when the cell consumes excessive energy (e.g., strenuous exercise) and when the sources delivering this energy cannot be replaced in an adequate manner, again rhabdomyolysis can develop. Sometimes the definite cause cannot be determined; whereas, in most cases, multiple factors play a role [13].

In what follows, the pathogenesis of pressure-induced rhabdomyolysis will be described as an example.

When muscles are compressed, sarcolemmal permeability increases and substances that are highly concentrated in the muscle cells (i.e., myoglobin, potassium, and phosphate) flow out to the extracellular environment, whereas substances abundant in the extracellular environment such as water, sodium, and calcium move into the intracellular milieu [6]. Once a critical calcium concentration is reached, the following events are observed: (1) sustained muscle contraction depletes ATP stores, (2) mitochondrial damage results in oxidant stress, and (3) activation of proteases, phospholipases, and other enzymes, causes myofibril and membrane phospholipid damage [67].

Local accumulation of intracellular elements in the extracellular milieu cause microvascular damage producing capillary leak, and subsequently compartmental syndrome. This syndrome, in turn, increases pressure on the capillaries triggering occlusion of the microcirculation and depleting myoglobin oxygen content. However, most of these pathologic events occur after flow into the injured muscles is restored. At that moment, leukocytes migrate into the damaged tissue, release cytokines and proteolytic enzymes and contribute to free radical production (reperfusion injury) [60]. Typically, this scenario occurs at the moment of rescue of the entrapped crush victims, who initially appear well, then suddenly deteriorate and even die shortly after successful extrication (rescue death) [36]. It has been hypothesized that when the patient is under the rubble, perfusion of the extremity is prevented by existing pressure on the muscles. When this pressure is removed by extrication, however, huge amounts of plasma fluid leak into the injured extremity, leading to compartment syndrome, hypovolemia, and shock. Also, extensive amounts of muscle breakdown products, cytokines, proteolytic enzymes, and free radicals enter the circulation, exposing the rest of the body to their adverse effects [6, 36, 65].

6.11.2.3 Pathogenesis of Myoglobinuric AKF

AKF due to crush injury is prerenal in the first phase; if not treated in this early period, however, parenchymal AKF, which is almost always due to acute tubular necrosis (ATN), develops. Mechanisms contributing to AKF in this setting are (Fig. 6.11.1):

1. Intravascular volume depletion, renal hypoperfusion, and ischemia due to fluid third spacing in necrotic muscles,
2. Intratubular myoglobin and uric acid cast formation,
3. Scavenging of nitric oxide (NO) by myoglobin,
4. Renal vasoconstriction due to cytokines released from damaged muscles,
5. Release of free iron from intratubular myoglobin, which catalyzes free radical production, enhancing ischemic damage,
6. Hypocalcemia-induced cardiac output depression potentiating renal hypoperfusion,
7. Induction of inflammation of the kidney tissue by precipitation of $CaPO_4$ salts, secondary to hyperphosphatemia,
8. Disseminated intravascular coagulation due to release of tissue thromboplastin from the damaged muscles [60, 67].

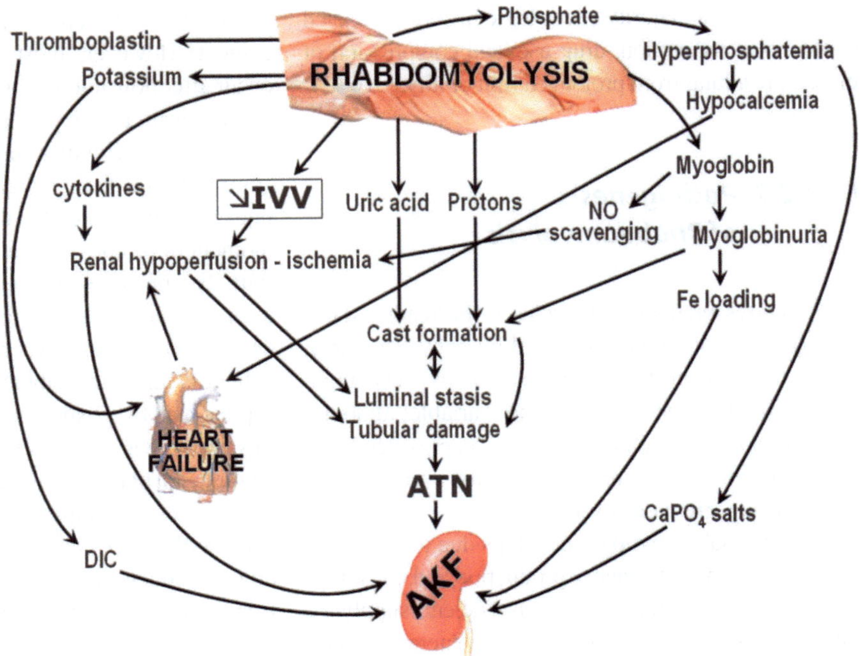

Fig. 6.11.1 Pathophysiology of rhabdomyolysis-related acute kidney failure (Please see the text for description of the figure) IVV: intravascular volume, NO: nitric oxide, ATN: acute tubular necrosis, Fe: iron, DIC: disseminated intravascular coagulation, AKF: acute kidney failure

6.11.3 Clinical Findings

Clinical findings of myoglobinuric AKF include local findings of rhabdomyolysis and systemic findings (or findings of crush syndrome) [45, 61].

The most typical local finding is *compartment syndrome* due to swollen muscles. Patients suffer from severe pain, weakness, paresthesia, paresis, or paralysis and pallor in the affected extremities. Distal pulses may be absent when intracompartmental pressure is very high. In traumatic rhabdomyolysis, signs of blunt or penetrating trauma are present as well.

Crush syndrome develops in 30–50% of cases; symptoms include hypovolemic shock, sepsis, electrolyte disturbances (most importantly hyperkalemia), heart failure, arrhythmias, acute respiratory distress syndrome, disseminated intravascular coagulation, bleeding, psychological trauma, and most importantly AKF [45, 50, 54].

Myoglobinuric AKF is usually characterized by an initial oliguric period that is followed by polyuria, which usually starts within 1–3 weeks after the primary event, while some cases may present with a nonoliguric course from the beginning.

6.11.4 Laboratory Findings

6.11.4.1 Urinary Findings

Dirty-brownish discoloration of the urine as a result of myoglobinuria is typical [20]. However, normal color can be noted as well when filtered myoglobin load is low, myoglobinuria resolves before the patient seeks medical attention, or pigment excretion is limited because of kidney dysfunction. In practice, myoglobinuria is most often detected by dipstick testing; a positive test can indicate hematuria, myoglobinuria, or hemoglobinuria, which is not helpful in leading to a final diagnosis. Very few erythrocytes in the urine sediment in spite of a strong blood reaction by dipstick testing and detection of dark-pigmented casts at microscopic investigation of the urine rule out hematuria.

Other urinary findings are related to the extent of renal involvement. In the early course, when the patients are usually hypovolemic, urinary indices are consistent with prerenal AKF (high specific gravity and osmolality, low urinary sodium concentration, and lower than 1% fractional sodium excretion [FENa]). On the other hand, proteinuria, isostenuria, and necrotic tubular epithelial cells in the urinary sediment can be detected in the later course, all of which suggest development of ATN. Interestingly, FENa may continue to be low at this stage as well, a finding that may reflect the primacy of tubular obstruction rather than tubular necrosis [11].

6.11.4.2 Biochemical Features

Increased serum levels of substances – myoglobin, urea, creatinine, uric acid, potassium, phosphate, protons, and muscle enzymes (creatine kinase [CK], aspartate aminotransferase [AST], alanine aminotransferase [ALT], and lactic dehydrogenase [LDH]) – released from the injured muscles, together with a decrease of serum calcium due to shift into the muscles, form the basis for biochemical abnormalities. Among these, serum myoglobin, CK, potassium, calcium, and creatinine deserve special mention.

Serum myoglobin: The most reliable laboratory finding of rhabdomyolysis is increased serum myoglobin. However, it has no practical diagnostic value because the half-life of myoglobin is very short (about 1–3 h), so that it is completely removed from the plasma within approximately 6 h [17]. Except for patients who reach the hospital within a very short time period after initiation of rhabdomyolysis, myoglobin level is usually found within normal limits at admission to hospital.

Serum CK: This enzyme is abundant in the striated muscles; it catalyzes the formation of ATP from ADP by using the high-energy phosphate bond in creatine phosphate, and passes to the circulation in case of muscle injury. Subtypes of CK exist; they are specific for the striated muscle (CK-MM), the myocardium (CK-MB), and the brain (CK-BB). Normal serum CK levels vary between 45 and 260 U/l [55]. An increased level is the most typical indicator of muscle damage, although a specific cutoff value allowing a definite diagnosis is not available. Levels higher than 500, 1,000, or even 3,000 U/l [14, 58, 64] have been suggested; mostly serum CK-MM levels are much higher than these values, and occasionally exceed 10,000 or even 100,000 U/l. This enzyme reaches peak levels usually within the first 12–24 h after muscle injury and half-life is normally 48 h [22]; serum level does not differ in the patients with or without renal failure [38]. Contradictory opinions exist regarding the prognostic value of serum CK; increased levels may point to an increased risk of subsequent AKF and/or dialysis needs [18, 38, 46, 62] or not [14].

Serum potassium: Muscular cell potassium content is about 100 mmol/kg; rapid and total necrosis of only about 150 g of muscle releases more than 15 mmol potassium, which is sufficient to acutely elevate the serum and extracellular fluid potassium concentration by 1.0 mmol/l [14]. Many other factors play a role in the development of hyperkalemia following rhabdomyolysis: (1) failure to excrete potassium load due to renal failure, (2) efflux of intracellular potassium to the extracellular environment due to acidosis resulting from either rhabdomyolysis and/or coexisting renal failure, (3) increased catabolism, and (4) medical interventions (i.e., blood transfusions, administration of potassium-containing drugs or surgery).

The daily rise in the plasma potassium concentration may exceed 1.0 mEq/l in patients with rhabdomyolysis or other hypercatabolic states [27], which is much larger than with renal failure in patients who are not hypercatabolic (usual daily rise of 0.3 mEq/l) [57]. Hyperkalemia-related cardiac arrhythmia is a frequent cause of sudden death in patients with myoglobinuric AKF.

Serum calcium: Hypocalcemia is common in patients with rhabdomyolysis and can lead to tetany, seizures, and potentiate cardiotoxic effects of hyperkalemia [1, 22, 60]. Controversy exist on the incidence of hypocalcemia with reported figures ranging from 20% to 100% [3, 13]. Various factors may be involved in the pathogenesis [17, 22, 25, 60], such as: (1) direct effects of hyperphosphatemia, (2) suppression of calcitriol synthesis by hyperphosphatemia, (3) influx of plasma calcium into the injured muscle cells, (4) precipitation of calcium salts into the damaged tissues (metastatic calcification), and (5) resistance of bones to the calcium releasing effects of parathyroid hormone (PTH) during renal failure. On the other hand, hypercalcemia may also develop (in 20–30% of cases) both at the early and late stages of rhabdomyolysis. An early rise may be due to increased serum protein due to severe dehydration [17]. Late hypercalcemia can be secondary to (1) mobilization of the calcium salts previously precipitated into the muscles, (2) improvement of skeletal response to the calcium-releasing actions of PTH, and (3) increased vitamin D synthesis in the recovering kidneys, resulting in increased absorption of calcium from the guts [13, 24, 25, 63].

Hypercalcemia is more common in the patients who had been initially treated with calcium salts during the hypocalcemic stage; hence calcium supplementation is suggested only for symptomatic hypocalcemia or severe hyperkalemia.

Serum creatinine: Intracellular energy production largely depends upon presence of creatine, which is abundant in the muscles. It is released in large quantities from the damaged muscle cells and is converted into creatinine in the circulation. Therefore, a higher ratio of serum creatinine to blood urea nitrogen (BUN) has been suggested in patients with myoglobinuric AKF [6, 15, 17, 21]. However, not all authors confirm this hypothesis [14, 39, 46, 60]. In the Marmara earthquake database, mean serum creatinine to BUN ratio was (3.9/55.1 = 1/14.1), which fits into the presumed physiologic ratio of 1/10–15 [42]. Therefore, the possibility should be considered that creatinine generation is not always increased in rhabdomyolysis. Alternatively, besides a high production rate of creatinine, increased urea generation by the liver in seriously traumatized and highly catabolic patients [42] may contribute to the maintenance of this physiologic ratio.

6.11.5 Prognosis

Overall, mortality rate in patients with AKF ranges between 7% and 80% in various series [59]. Many factors such as the primary cause, the demography of the patients, the need for various therapeutic interventions, and especially the presence of comorbid factors may affect the mortality rates [9, 10, 23, 37]. Myoglobinuric AKF is most often linked to multiple surgical and medical comorbidities; therefore, a worse prognosis can be expected as compared with patients with AKF due to other etiologies. In accordance with this hypothesis, mortality rates reaching up to 40% have been reported [4, 38, 64]. Following the Marmara earthquake, however, overall mortality rate of the patients with AKF was only 15.2%; this rate was 9.3% in the patients who did not require dialysis support and 17.2% in the dialyzed victims [12], suggesting a more favorable prognosis than had been described before.

6.11.6 Prophylaxis

Volume resuscitation: The goals of volume repletion are enhancing renal perfusion to minimize ischemic injury and increasing the urine flow rate to wash out obstructing casts. A urine output of 200–300 ml/h is desirable while myoglobinuria (discolored urine) persists. Fluids should be given at the earliest occasion to interfere with release of the heme pigment into the circulation and before hypovolemia (due to sequestration of plasma water in the injured muscle) develops [49]. For crush casualties, volume resuscitation should be considered even when the patient is entrapped under the rubble [6]. Isotonic saline (at a rate of 1 l/h or 10–15 ml/kg of body weight/h) is the preferred solution at the first stage; fluids should be hypotonic saline later on overall, 10-12 l/day. Adding sodium bicarbonate ampoules of 50 mEq to each second or third liter of this solution keeps urinary pH above 6.5 and is useful not only for preventing myoglobin and uric acid casts, but also copes with acidosis and hyperkalemia and minimizes the release of free iron from myoglobin [32, 67]. The usual requirement for bicarbonate is 200–300 mEq for the first day. If the urine pH does not rise above 6.5 after 3–4 h of the alkaline solution or if symptomatic hypocalcemia develops, alkaline administration should be discontinued.

If urinary output is more than 20 ml/h, 50 ml of 20% mannitol (1–2 g/kg/day [total, 120 g], given at a rate of 5 g/h) may be added to each liter of this solution (mannitol-alkaline solution). Mannitol may be beneficial by: (1) generating osmotic diuresis, which minimizes intratubular myoglobin deposition and cast formation, (2) acting as a free radical scavenger, thereby minimizing cell injury, and (3) extracting sequestered water from the injured muscles, thus preventing compartment syndrome [8]. However, mannitol may cause various adverse effects, such as volume depletion, hypernatremia, hyperosmolality, volume expansion, and even AKF, especially when administered in high doses. Mannitol is contraindicated in oliguric patients.

Since large amounts of fluid accumulate in the damaged muscles of crush cases, it is useful to administer 4–5 l more fluids than all visible losses. However, administering extensive volumes to oligoanuric patients carries the risk of hypervolemia, hypertension, and heart failure as well. Therefore, if the patients cannot be monitored closely due to specific circumstances, mannitol-alkaline solution should be applied less aggressively (i.e., 4–6 l/day) to avoid inadvertent volume overload, especially in the elderly victims [60]. Placing a central venous pressure (CVP) catheter at the earliest occasion, and adjusting the volume of fluids according to CVP measurements is useful [49].

This protocol should be continued until myoglobinuria disappears (practically until normalization of the urinary color), which usually occurs within 2–3 days following the initial insult. Subsequently, mannitol-alkaline infusion can be tapered and then discontinued.

By no means should potassium-containing solutions be used empirically in crush patients; this intervention may result in death of many already hyperkalemic casualties, who could not be diagnosed due to specific circumstances [48].

Other interventions: Elimination of myoglobin by plasma exchange or special hemofilters, which can permit passage of molecules even up to 30,000 Da, has been proposed since myoglobin cannot be cleared by standard hemodialysis membranes. However, there is controversy about the beneficial effects of this intervention [5, 22, 67]. On the other hand, the induction of myoglobin excretion through the kidneys by intravenous fluids is certainly useful and safe.

Loop diuretics may be beneficial by increasing urine volume [20]. However, they may worsen hypocalcemia by inducing calciuria and increase the risk of cast formation by inhibiting the sodium/hydrogen pump in the distal tubule, thus acidifying the urine [6, 55]. Despite these concerns, however, in elderly patients, especially if volume overloaded, use of loop diuretics may be justified.

Among other controversial interventions interfering with uric acid production by allopurinol [22], increasing capillary blood flow and decreasing neutrophil adhesion/cytokine release by pentoxifylline [28], preventing oxidant injury by glutathione [2, 63], interfering with lipid peroxidation at the cell membrane level by aminosteroids [35, 43], removing iron by deferoxamine [40, 66], and decreasing intracellular calcium by dantrolene [26] can be cited.

An important controversy in myoglobinuric AKF is performing routine fasciotomies to patients with compartment syndrome (Fig. 6.11.2). Fasciotomy may effectively lower intracompartmental pressure, thus decreasing the extent of rhabdomyolysis, and in turn, preventing AKF. Also, it may prevent irreversible neurologic damage by restoring circulation [52, 53, 68]. However, it has many drawbacks as well; a closed injury turns into an open wound with a high risk of infection, which may increase the risk of amputation; fasciotomy wounds are prone to leakage of plasma and bleeding, and, also, fasciotomies may cause severe disabilities in the long-term [7, 30, 41, 45]. However, even the authors who favor a more conservative approach suggest emergent fasciotomy in the case of certain indications, such as an open crush injury, absence of distal pulses, and overall perfusion failure of the extremity [8, 31, 41].

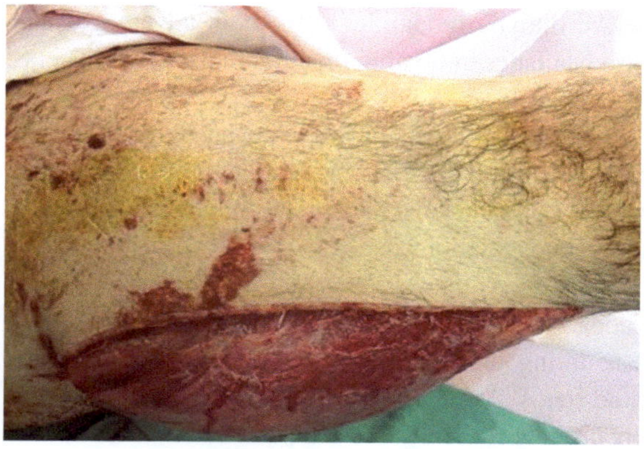

Fig. 6.11.2 Fasciotomy operation for treating compartment syndrome in one of the crush casualties of the Marmara earthquake. Please note the protruded muscle due to high pressure in the compartment

Measurement of intracompartmental pressure is the best method for defining an objective criterion for fasciotomies. Clinically significant ischemia occurs if intracompartmental pressure is higher than 30–50 mm Hg [29, 33], especially if it lasts longer than 6 h [60] or the difference between compartmental pressure and diastolic blood pressure is less than 30 mm Hg [6, 52].

6.11.7 Treatment

There is no specific therapy of myoglobinuric AKF once overt kidney failure develops. Dialysis is initiated in response to the usual indications, including volume overload, hyperkalemia, severe acidemia and uremia. More frequent (twice or even thrice daily) hemodialysis may be indicated since the risk of fatal hyperkalemia is considerably higher compared with other etiologies of AKF [44].

All dialytic modalities carry both advantages and disadvantages in treating myoglobinuric AKF patients [47, 56, 60]:

Intermittent hemodialysis is the preferred modality, because of the high clearance rate of uremic solutes as well as potassium and the possibility of dialyzing without anticoagulation.

Continuous dialysis strategies may be used in these patients as well; they do not adversely affect blood pressure during fluid removal, hence allow a better control of fluid status. Avoiding disequilibrium syndrome and the opportunity to freely feed the patients are other advantages. However, they are contraindicated in subjects with bleeding tendency and major surgical interventions, due to the continuous need for anticoagulation.

In cases with traumatic rhabdomyolysis, peritoneal dialysis (PD) might be difficult to perform because of abdominal and/or thoracic trauma and the inability of the patients to lie down due to hypervolemia-related heart failure and/or respiratory failure. Also, PD may not cope with the metabolic and electrolyte derangements of rhabdomyolysis, especially in heavily traumatized patients.

6.11.8 Take Home Pearls

- Rhabdomyolysis may result from both physical and nonphysical causes; 20–50% of rhabdomyolysis cases are complicated by myoglobinuric AKF, while this pathology is responsible for 5–20% of overall cases of AKF.
- Rhabdomyolysis is a frequent cause of AKF following earthquakes; surgical and medical complications, especially hyperkalemia, are more frequent in these patients as compared with AKF due to other etiologies.
- Early fluid resuscitation by isotonic saline at a rate of 1 l/h, followed by mannitol-alkaline solution in cases with adequate urine response are useful to prevent myoglobinuric AKF.
- Empirical administration of potassium-containing solutions are contraindicated in these patients.
- Dimensions of metabolic derangements are extensive; thus, intermittent hemodialysis is the preferred renal replacement therapy in patients with myoglobinuric AKF.

References

1. Abassi ZA, Hoffman A, Better OS (1998) Acute renal failure complicating muscle crush injury. Semin Nephrol 8: 558–565.
2. Abul-Ezz SR, Walker PD, Shah SV (1991) Role of glutathione in an animal model of myoglobinuric acute renal failure. Proc Natl Acad Sci USA 88:9833–9837.
3. Akmal M, Bishop JE, Telfer N, et al. (1986) Hypocalcemia and hypercalcemia in patients with rhabdomyolysis with and without acute renal failure. J Clin Endocrinol Metab 63: 137–142.
4. Atef MR, Nadjatfi I, Boroumand B, Rastegar A (1994) Acute renal failure in earthquake victims in Iran: epidemiology and management. Quart J Med 87:35–40.
5. Berns JS, Cohen RM, Rudnick MR (1991) Removal of myoglobin by CAVH-D in traumatic rhabdomyolysis. Am J Nephrol 11:73.
6. Better OS, Stein JH (1990) Early management of shock and prophylaxis of acute renal failure in traumatic rhabdomyolysis. N Engl J Med 322:825–829.
7. Better OS, Rubinstein I, Reis D (2003) Muscle crush compartment syndrome: Fulminant local edema with threatening systemic effects. Kidney Int 63:1155–1157.
8. Better OS, Rubinstein I, Winaver JM, Knochel JP (1997) Mannitol therapy revisited (1940–1997). Kidney Int 52:886–894.
9. Bullock ML, Umen AJ, Finkelstein M, Keane WF (1985) The assessment of risk factors in 462 patients with acute renal failure. Am J Kidney Dis 5:97–103.
10. Chertow GM, Christiansen CL, Cleary PD, et al. (1995) Prognostic stratification in critically ill patients with acute renal failure requiring dialysis. Arch Intern Med 155:1505–1511.
11. Corwin HL, Schreiber MJ, Fang LS (1984). Low fractional excretion of sodium. Occurrence with hemoglobinuric- and myoglobinuric-induced acute renal failure. Arch Intern Med 144:981.
12. Erek E, Sever M, Serdengecti K, et al. (2002) An overview of morbidity and mortality in the patients with acute renal failure due to crush syndrome. Nephrol Dial Transplant 17: 33–40.
13. Frisoni A, Jacob F, Voltz C, Bollaert P (1998). Rhabdomyolysis in acute renal failure. In: Progress in Acute Renal Failure, Cantarovich F, Rangoonwala B, Verho M (eds). New Jersey: Bridgewater, pp 139–152.
14. Gabow PA, Kaehny WD, Kelleher SP (1982) The spectrum of rhabdomyolysis. Medicine 61:141–152.
15. Grossman RA, Hamilton RW, Morse BM, et al. (1974) Non-traumatic rhabdomyolysis and acute renal failure. N Engl J Med 291:807–811.
16. Guyton AC, Hall JE (1996) Contraction of skeletal muscle. In: Textbook of Medical Physiology, 9th edn. Philadelphia: Saunders, pp 73–85.
17. Honda N (1983) Acute renal failure and rhabdomyolysis. Kidney Int 23:888–898.
18. Hwang S, Shu K, Lain J, Yang W (2001) Renal replacement therapy at the time of the Taiwan Chi-Chi earthquake. Nephrol Dial Transplant 16 (Suppl 5) 78–82.

19. Knochel JP (1981) Serum calcium derangements in rhabdomyolysis (editorial). N Engl J Med 305:161–162.
20. Knochel, JP (1982) Rhabdomyolysis and myoglobinuria. Annu Rev Med 33:435.
21. Knochel JP (1990) Catastrophic medical events with exhaustive exercise "White collar rhabdomyolysis." Kidney Int 38:709–719.
22. Knochel JP (1998) Rhabdomyolysis and acute renal failure. In: Current Therapy in Nephrology and Hypertension, Glassock RJ (ed), 4th edn. St. Louis: Mosby, pp 262–265.
23. Lameire N, Matthys E, Vanholder R, et al. (1987) Causes and prognosis of acute renal failure in elderly patients. Nephrol Dial Transplant 2:316–322.
24. Lane JT, Boudreau RJ, Kinlaw WB (1990) Disappearance of muscular calcium deposits during resolution of prolonged rhabdomyolysis-induced hypercalcemia. Am J Med 89: 523–525.
25. Llach F, Felsenfeld AJ, Haussler MR (1981) The pathophysiology of altered calcium metabolism in rhabdomyolysis-induced acute renal failure N Engl J Med 305:117–123.
26. Lopez JR, Rojas B, Gonzales MA, Terzic A (1995) Myoplasmic Ca^{2+} concentration during exertional rhabdomyolysis. Lancet 345:424–425.
27. Lordon, RE, Burton, JR (1972) Post-traumatic renal failure in military personnel in Southeast Asia. Experience at Clark USAF hospital, Republic of the Philippines. Am J Med 53:137.
28. Mandell GL (1988) ARDS, neutrophils, and pentoxifylline. Am Rev Respir Dis 138:1103–1105.
29. Matsen FA, Mayo KA, Sheridan GW (1976) Monitoring of intramuscular pressure. Surgery 79:702–709.
30. Matsuoka T, Yoshioka T, Tanaka H, et al. (2002) Long-term physical outcome of patients who suffered crush syndrome after the 1995 Hanshin-Awaji earthquake: Prognostic indicators in retrospect. J Trauma 52:33–39.
31. Michaelson M, Taitelman U, Bshouty Z, et al. (1984) Crush syndrome: experience from the Lebanon war, 1982. Isr J Med Sci 20:305–307.
32. Moore KP, Holt SG, Patel RP, et al. (1998) A causative role for redox cycling of myoglobin and its inhibition by alkalinization in the pathogenesis and treatment of rhabdomyolysis-induced renal failure. J Biol Chem 273:31731–31737.
33. Mubarak SJ, Owen CA, Hargens AR, et al. (1978) Acute compartment syndromes: diagnosis and treatment with the aid of the wick catheter. J Bone Joint Surg Am 60:1091–1095.
34. Murali NS, Nath KA (2005) Myoglobinuric and hemoglobinuric acute renal failure. In: A Primer on Kidney Diseases (National Kidney foundation), Greenberg A (Ed), 4th edn. China: Elsevier Saunders, pp 308–314.
35. Nath KA, Balla J, Croatt AJ, Vercellotti GM (1995) Heme protein-mediated renal injury: a protective role for 21-aminosteroids in vitro and in vivo. Kidney Int 47:592–602.
36. Noji EK (1992) Acute renal failure in natural disasters. Ren Fail 14:245–249.
37. Obialo CI, Okonofura EC, Nzerue M, et al. (1999) Role of hypoalbuminemia and hypercholesterolemia as co-predictors of mortality in acute renal failure. Kidney Int 56:1058–1063.
38. Oda J, Tanaka H, Yoshioka T, et al., (1997) Analysis of 372 patients with crush syndrome caused by the Hanshin-Awaji earthquake. J Trauma 42:470–476.
39. Oh MS (1993) Does serum creatinine rise faster in rhabdomyolysis? Nephron 63:255–257.
40. Paller MS (1988) Hemoglobin- and myoglobin-induced acute renal failure in rats: role of iron in nephrotoxicity. Am J Physiol 255:F539–F544.
41. Reis ND, Michaelson M (1986) Crush injury to the lower limbs. J Bone Joint Surg 68A:414–418.
42. Rose BD (2001) Clinical Physiology of Acid-Base and Electrolyte Disorders, 5th edn. New York: McGraw-Hill.
43. Salahudeen AK, Wang C, Bigler SA, et al. (1996) Synergistic renal protection by combining alkaline-diuresis with lipid peroxidation inhibitors in rhabdomyolysis: possible interaction between oxidant and non-oxidant mechanisms. Nephrol Dial Transplant 11:635–642.
44. Sever MS (2005) The Crush Syndrome (and Lessons from the Marmara Earthquake). Basel: Karger AG.
45. Sever MS, Erek E, Vanholder R, et al. (2002) Clinical findings in the renal victims of a catastrophic disaster: the Marmara earthquake. Nephrol Dial Transplant 17:1942–1949.
46. Sever MS, Erek E, Vanholder R, et al. (2002) The Marmara earthquake: admission laboratory features of the patients with nephrological problems. Nephrol Dial Transplant 17: 1025–1031.
47. Sever MS, Erek E, Vanholder R, et al. (2002) Renal replacement therapies in the aftermath of the catastrophic Marmara earthquake. Kidney Int 62:2264–2271.
48. Sever MS, Erek E, Vanholder R, et al., (2003) Serum potassium in the crush victims of the Marmara disaster.Clin Nephrol 59:326–333.
49. Sever MS, Vanholder R, Lameire N (2006) Management of crush-related injuries after disasters. N Engl J Med 354: 1052–1063.
50. Sharma R (2002) Gujarat earthquake causes major mental health problems. BMJ 324:259..
51. Sharp, LS, Rozycki, GS, Feliciano, DV (2004) Rhabdomyolysis and secondary renal failure in critically ill surgical patients. Am J Surg 188:801.
52. Shaw AD, Sjolin SU, McQueen MM (1994) Crush syndrome following unconsciousness. Need for urgent orthopedic referral. Br Med J 309:857–859.
53. Sheridan GW, Matsen FAIII (1976) Fasciotomy in the treatment of acute compartment syndrome. J Bone Joint Surg Am 58:112–115.
54. Shoaf KI, Sareen HR, Nguyen LH, Bourque LB (1998) Injuries as a result of California earthquakes in the past decade. Disasters 22:218–35.
55. Slater MS, Mullins RJ (1998) Rhabdomyolysis and myoglobinuric renal failure in trauma and surgical patients: a review. J Am Coll Surg 186:693–716.
56. Solez K, Bihari D, Collins AJ, et al., (1993) International dialysis aid in earthquakes and other disasters. Kidney Int 44:479–483.
57. Strauss, M (1948) Acute renal insufficiency due to lower-nephron nephrosis. N Engl J Med 239:693.
58. Tanaka H, Oda J, Iwai A, et al. (1999) Morbidity and mortality of hospitalized patients after the 1995 Hanshin-Awaji earthquake. Am J Emerg Med 17:186–191.

59. Thadhani R, Pascual M, Bonventre JV (1996) Acute renal failure. N Engl J Med 334:1448–1460.
60. Vanholder R, Sever MS, Erek E, Lameire N (2000) Rhabdomyolysis. J Am Soc Nephrol 11:1553–61.
61. Vanholder R, Sever MS, Erek E, Lameire N (2000) Acute renal failure related to crush syndrome: Towards an era of seismo-nephrology? Nephrol Dial Transplant 15: 517–521.
62. Veenstra J, Smit WM, Krediet RT, Arisz L (1994) Relationship between elevated creatine phosphokinase and the clinical spectrum of rhabdomyolysis. Nephrol Dial Transplant 9:637–641.
63. Visweswaran P, Guntupalli J (1999) Rhabdomyolysis. Crit Care Clin 15:415–428.
64. Ward MM (1988) Factors predictive of acute renal failure in rhabdomyolysis. Arch Intern Med 148:1553.
65. Zager RA, Burkhart KM, Conrad DS, Gmur DJ (1995) Iron, heme oxygenase, and glutathione: Effects on myohemoglobinuric proximal tubular injury. Kidney Int 48:1624–1634.
66. Zager RA (1992) Combined mannitol and deferoxamine therapy for myohemoglobinuric renal injury and oxidant tubular stress: Mechanistic and therapeutic implications. J Clin Invest 90:711–719.
67. Zager RA (1996) Rhabdomyolysis and myohemoglobinuric acute renal failure. Kidney Int 49: 314–326.
68. Zhi-Yong S (1987) Medical support in Tangshan earthquake: a review of the management of mass casualties and certain major injuries. J Trauma 27:1130–1136.

Tropical Infections and Acute Kidney Injury

6.12

Rashad S. Barsoum

Core Messages

- Infections are responsible for about 50% of cases with acute kidney injury (AKI) in the tropics.
- Many tropical infections can cause AKI by direct invasion of the renal parenchyma, inducing a systemic inflammatory response, critically altering the renal hemodynamics and/or provoking a morbid immune response.
- Genetic, environmental, and socioeconomic factors interact in increasing morbidity from tropical infections, including AKI. Drug nephrotoxicity may confer additional damage.
- The clinical syndrome of tropical AKI is confounded by the associated primary disease, multiorgan affection, rhabdomyolysis, hemolysis, disseminated intravascular coagulation, preexisting morbidities, malnutrition, multiple infections, and late referral.
- The typical laboratory features reflect the catabolic state of infection, the associated humoral response, and the manifestations of tissue hypoxia.
- In most patients, AKI is reversible by adequate treatment of infection, hydration, and supportive treatment.
- Unfortunately the lack of equipment and experience with continuous renal replacement therapy limit its use in endemic areas. Intermittent dialysis is the only available alternative. Plasmapheresis or blood exchange may be useful in a few infections.

R. S. Barsoum
Cairo University, Cairo Kidney Center, 3 Hussein El-Memar Street, Antique Khana, P.O. Box 91, Bab El-Louk, Cairo 11513, Egypt
e-mail: rashad.barsoum@gmail.com

6.12.1 Introduction

The tropical zone is classically defined as that lying 10° north and south of the Equator. However, since the medical profile in this region is very similar to that in the "subtropical" zone, extending to the Tropic of Cancer and Tropic of Capricorn at 23.5°N and 23.5°S, respectively, the term "tropical infections" applies to the extended definition.

This zone is inhabited by several ethnic groups with known genetic characteristics relevant to susceptibility to infection [44] or its complications, particularly in the kidneys [45]. Relevant examples include the high prevalence G6PD deficiency [37] or gene mutation [47] which may lead to intravascular hemolysis, and subsequently acute kidney injury (AKI), in several tropical infections as typhoid, typhus, and hepatitis A viral infection [46]. Another genetic factor attracting considerable interest is polymorphism of proinflammatory and antiinflammatory cytokines [45] or of the regulators of oxidative stress [48], which may be responsible for significant differences in the renal response to infection.

Besides the effect of a typically warm and humid environment on the prevalence of infectious disease and its rapid spread [2], it also confounds the pathogenesis by superadding the impact of pyrexia and excessive fluid

A. Jörres et al. (eds.), *Management of Acute Kidney Problems*,
DOI: 10.1007/978-3-540-69441-0_6.12, © Springer-Verlag Berlin Heidelberg 2010

Table 6.12.1 Main tropical infections causing acute kidney injury

Agent	Disease	High-prevalence regions	Pathogenetic mechanism(s)	
			Tissue invasion	*SIR*[a]
Bacterial				
Bacillus anthracic (cereus)	Intestinal anthrax	Sub-Sahelian Africa and Asia, Latin America, Australia		+++
b-Hemolytic streptococci	Infected scabies	Brazil, Senegal, South Africa		
Burkholderia pseudomallei	Whitmore's disease; septicemic melioidosis	Southeast Asia, northern Australia	+++	+++
Corynebacterium diphtheriae	Diphtheria	Throughout tropical zone	+	
Leptospira icterohemorrhagica	Weil's disease; leptospirosis	Throughout tropical zone	+++	+++
Mycobacterium leprae	Lepromatous leprosy	Brazil, India, Madagascar, Mozambique, Nepal	++	
Mycobacterium tuberculosis		Southeast Asia, sub-Saharan Africa		
Orientia (*Rickettsia*) tsutsugamushi	Tsutsugamushi fever; scrub typhus	China, Indian subcontinent	++	++
Salmonella paratyphi A	Salmonellosis	Throughout tropical zone		++
Salmonella typhi	Typhoid	Asia, Africa, Latin America	++	++
Shigella dysenteriae	D+ hemolytic uremic syndrome	Indian subcontinent		
Treponema pallidum	Secondary syphilis	Sub-Saharan Africa		
Vibrio cholera		Indian subcontinent, Southeast Asia		
Viral				
Dengue virus	Dengue hemorrhagic fever (DHF)	Southeast Asia, western Pacific, India	++	++
Hantaan virus	Korean hemorrhagic fever; hemorrhagic fever with renal syndrome (HFRS)	Korea, Southeast Asia	++	
Hepatitis A virus (HAV)	Acute viral hepatitis	Throughout tropical zone	+	
Hepatitis B virus (HBV)	ANCA vasculitis	India, China, Taiwan, Southeast Asia, sub-Saharan Africa	+	
Hepatitis C virus (HCV)	ANCA vasculitis, acute graft dysfunction (?)	Africa, Southeast Asia, western Pacific	±	
Human Immunodeficiency Virus (HIV)	Acute HIV nephropathy	Sub-Saharan Africa	+	
Parasitic				
Leishmania donovani	Kala-azar; visceral leishmaniasis	Bangladesh, India, Nepal	++	
Plasmodium falciparum	Malignant malaria	Sub-Saharan Africa, Southeast Asia, India, Latin America		+++
Wuchereria bancrofti	Filariasis	India, Southeast Asia, sub-Saharan Africa, west Pacific		

[a]SIR = Systemic inflammatory response
[b]ATN = Acute tubular necrosis
[c]CIC = Circulating immune complexes

loss in sweat and perspiration. Increased body temperature may be an independent risk factor in rhabdomyolysis associated with infection. Dehydration may accelerate the development of AKI in many tropical infections particularly those associated with gastrointestinal fluid loss, systemic inflammatory response (SIR), or peripheral circulatory pooling.

Acute tropical infection is often superimposed on a background of chronic endemic disorders such as malnutrition, parasitic infections, chronic liver disease,

Pathology			Reference
Hemodynamic	*Immune-mediated*		
Gastrointestinal fluid losses		ATN[b]	[3]
	CIC[c]	Acute glomerulonephritis	[4]
		Diffuse interstitial nephritis with microabscess formation	[5]
		Acute interstitial nephritis	[6]
		Acute interstitial nephritis, hemorrhages, ATN[b]	[7]
	Cryoglobulins, ANCA	ATN[b], crescentic glomerulonephritis	[8, 9, 43]
Hypercalcemia	Vasculitis, ANCA	Necrotizing glomerulitis, ATN[b]	[10, 11, 43]
		Acute interstitial nephritis	[12]
	CIC[c]	Exudative glomerulonephritis, ATN[b]	[13, 14]
	CIC[c]	Acute interstitial nephritis with solitary abscesses, acute glomerulonephritis	[15, 16]
+	Shigatoxin	Thrombotic microangiopathy	[17]
	Cryoglobulins	Crescentic glomerulonephritis	[18]
Gastrointestinal fluid losses		ATN[b], hypokalemic tubulopathy	[19]
		Interstitial edema, hemorrhages, ATN	[20]
		Interstitial edema, hemorrhages, ATN	[21]
		ATN[b]	[22]
	Cryoglobulins	Necrotizing glomerulopathy	[23, 24]
		Necrotizing glomerulopathy, acute transplant glomerulopathy	[25, 26]
Gastrointestinal fluid losses		ATN[b]	[27, 28]
		Acute posttransplant interstitial nephritis	[29, 30]
Peripheral pooling	CIC[c] ANCA	Exudative glomerulonephritis	[31, 43]
	CIC[c]	Exudative glomerulonephritis	[32]

malignancy, which modify the clinical impact, suppress host immunity leading to persistence or dissemination and augment the chances of complications.

Because of the same background and of the biologically polluted environment, the chances of acquiring multiple infections are quite high, with a morbidity impact that often exceeds simple algebraic summation of individual effects. This is attributed to a positive agent–agent interaction such as that in-between lymphotropic viruses as HIV, HCV, or EBV, and other infections as malaria or typhoid [2]. On the other hand, there is experimental [49] and epidemiologic [50] evidence that certain tropical infections may attenuate the replication of concomitant HIV infection.

In addition to the above-mentioned bioecological factors, the tropical zone encompasses the lowest economic level countries, while being inhabited by over 85% of the world population [1]. This discrepancy drastically reflects on poor primary health care and subsequently the incidence of communicable diseases.

Tropical infection is responsible for a large proportion of AKI (Table 6.12.1). While accurate statistics are lacking, sporadic reports and regional surveys hold it responsible for 45–50% of acute renal failure cases in the tropics [2].

6.12.2 Pathogenetic Mechanisms

6.12.2.1 Direct Invasion

The kidneys are exposed to pathogens during their intravascular circulation as a part of their life cycle in humans. However, only a few are able to settle in the renal parenchyma (Fig. 6.12.1), subject to the availability of respective ligands. These are able to cause acute kidney injury by direct cytopathic effect (e.g., viral infections) or by inducing a local inflammatory reaction (e.g., bacterial infections). When multiple nephropathic mechanisms are involved, direct tissue injury is suggested by detection of the causative organism at the site of injury regardless of the extent of systemic reaction [22, 25, 27, 33], or its ability to induce similar lesions by direct inoculation in experimental models [34].

6.12.2.2 Systemic Inflammatory Response

Systemic inflammatory response is often the major pathogenetic factor in AKI. The peripheral resistance may be critically reduced and renal vascular resistance increased leading to diminished perfusion [35]. The latter may be further amplified by the outrageous release of catecholamines in neuropathic organisms or their toxins, such as with tetanus [41]. In addition, tropical infection is typically associated with overt [35] or subclinical [36] rhabdomyolysis, hemolysis particularly in G6PD-deficient subjects [2, 31], or disseminated intravascular coagulation (DIC) [14].

6.12.2.3 Hemodynamic Perturbation

Pyrexial illness in the warm tropical climate leads to excessive fluid depletion through perspiration and sweating. This may be amplified by associated gastrointestinal and electrolyte fluid loss (e.g., cholera) or excessive diuresis as a consequence of hypercalcemia (e.g., tuberculosis), or diabetes insipidus (e.g., encephalopathic viral infections).

Peripheral circulatory pooling may result from specific tropical infections in the absence of SIR. The typical example is falciparum malaria, where there is increased “stickiness” of parasitized red cells. The erythrocyte membrane anchoring points are morphologically distinct as knobs, which acquire ligands to the red cell complement receptor CR1 and to adhesion molecules on the platelets and endothelial cells. Parasitized red cells thus aggregate with each other, and with nonparasitized erythrocytes, platelets, and capillary endothelium, thereby leading to large thrombi which clog the peripheral capillaries.

6.12.2.4 Immune-Mediated Renal Lesions

The offending antigen in *Escherichia coli* O157:H7, which causes the hemolytic uremic syndrome (HUS) is a verocytotoxin known as Shigatoxin. This has a specific affinity to a glycolipid receptor, Gb3, which is constitutively expressed on eukaryotic cells, activation of which triggers a cascade of reactions ending in capillary wall damage and lumenal thrombosis. As its name implies, Shigatoxin is the principal toxin produced by *Shigella* species, the cause of bacillary dysentery in many tropical countries. This infection is a notorious cause of HUS in Argentinean [42] and Indian [17] children.

Immune complexes are responsible for AKI in postinfectious proliferative, exudative, or crescentic glomerulonephritis (Table 6.12.1). The extent and type of glomerular response in different tropical infections are influenced by their specific cytokine or chemokine profile, and the associated local release of free oxygen radicals.

Infections associated with cryoglobulinemia may lead to AKI by inducing renal vasculitis and subsequent glomerular necrosis. There is evidence that massive complement activation via the classical and

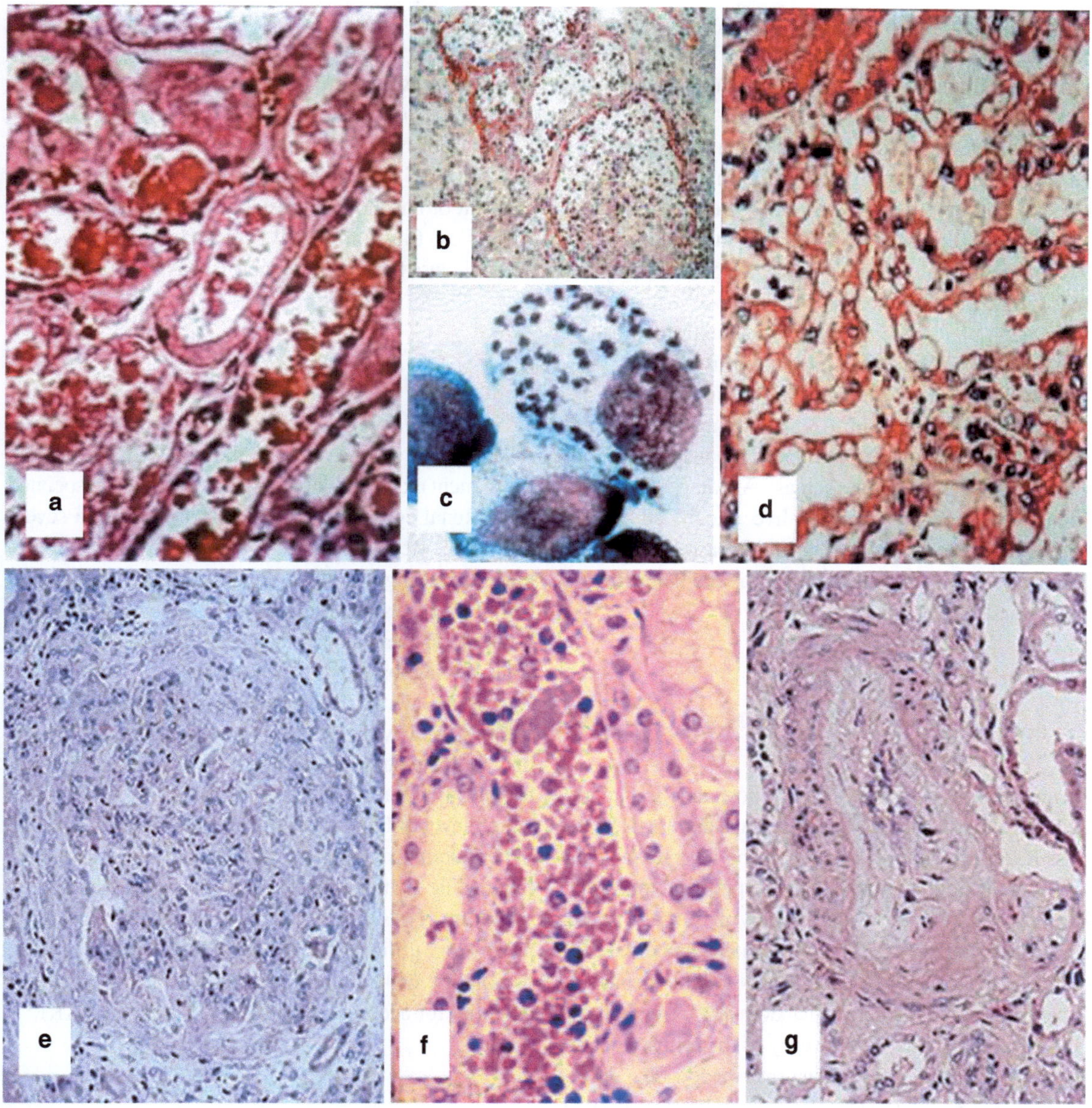

Fig. 6.12.1 Main histopathologic lesions in tropical infections causing AKI. (**a**) Acute tubular necrosis with intralumenal red cell debris and interstitial hemorrhage in leptospirosis. (**b**) Acute interstitial nephritis with abscess formation in typhoid. (**c**) Amastigotes of *Leishmania donovani* (Leishman-Donovan bodies) in an interstitial renal macrophage in kala-azar. (**d**) Proximal tubular vacuolation associated with hypokalemia in cholera. (**e**) Crescentic glomerulonephritis in scabies. (**f**) Clumps of aggregated blood cells in a renal venule in falciparum malaria. (**g**) Salmonella-associated acute vascular rejection of a renal allograft

mannose-binding pathways is responsible for the endothelial damage.

Tuberculosis, leprosy, and less commonly malaria [43] may be associated with the formation of anti-neutrophil cytoplasmic antibodies (ANCA), which may lead to renal vasculitis by their own right.

6.12.2.5 Iatrogenic Renal Injury

Amphotericin B, aminoglycosides, cephalosporins, and, to a lesser extent, vancomycin are the main nephrotoxic antibiotics commonly used in the treatment of tropical infections. Their nephrotoxicity is considerably augmented when these agents are used in combination, and when diuretics or nonsteroidal antiinflammatory agents are added.

Other notoriously nephrotoxic agents used in specific tropical infections include rifampicin in tuberculosis or leprosy, dapsone in the latter [51], topical carbon tetrachloride in scabies [52], and others.

Antimalarial drugs are the prototype of drugs that cause intravascular hemolysis in those with G6PD deficiency; blackwater fever being an extreme form in malaria with an extremely high mortality [2].

Interferon treatment for HCV infection may be associated with vasculitic AKI [53]. Anaphylactic and serum-sickness types of immune response have been described with several vaccines. An alarming report from Brazil incriminates the live attenuated yellow fever vaccine for transmitting the disease to immunocompromised individuals, leading to fatal hemorrhagic acute renal failure [54].

6.12.3 Clinical Characteristics

Fortunately, AKI usually stops short at Risk-Injury-Failure-Loss of Function-End stage renal disease (RIFLE) class R (Risk) or class I (Injury), being reversed by control of infection, hydration, and supportive treatment. RIFLE class F (Failure) occurs only in severe disease, usually neglected or resistant to treatment, and often confounded by collateral factors such as volume depletion, hepatic or pulmonary injury, rhabdomyolysis, hemolysis, DIC, or drug toxicity. The severity of the primary condition and its complications often overshadows the development of AKI, which tends to remain underdiagnosed until too late. Indeed, the ultimate survival, in malaria for example, depends on the extent of extrarenal complications rather than the AKI itself, although the latter remains as an independent risk factor for death [31].

The uremic syndrome in the tropics is often far advanced compared with that is usually encountered in the industrialized world, owing to late diagnosis and referral, high catabolic rate, and lack of specialized treatment facilities. Clinical signs as the "urea frost," acute polyneuritis, and extensive pericarditis are fairly common. Similarly, extreme laboratory abnormalities are often observed, such as severe metabolic acidosis (partly due to associated lactic acidosis), low serum sodium (due to SIADH or the "sick-cell syndrome" attributed to microbial toxins and tissue hypoxia), and severe hyperkalemia (augmented by hemolysis, rhabdomyolysis, and acidosis).

Since the eventual patient survival largely depends on the control of the primary infection and adequate management of nutrition and metabolic derangement, living with "Lost function" (RIFLE class L) or "End stage" (RIFLE class E) as a consequence of AKI is unusual.

6.12.4 Diagnosis

Awareness is the key issue in the timely diagnosis and subsequent management of tropical infection–associated AKI. Renal complications usually occur with a severe infection, often associated with multiple organ involvement including the liver, lungs, muscles, brain, and hemopoietic system. Monitoring of urine output and relevant blood chemistry in such cases should avoid undue delay in diagnosis and management.

Confusion may result from the overlap of the parameters of AKI with those of infection per se. Oliguria may indicate dehydration due to fluid losses in the gastro intestinal tract (GIT) or skin. In the absence of AKI, a high level of blood urea nitrogen (BUN), acidosis, or hyperkalemia may be attributed to the high catabolic rate, while a high serum creatinine may occur with rhabdomyolysis. Accordingly, standard laboratory parameters utilizing the urinary/plasma ratios of urea, osmolality, or sodium (Chapters 3.1 and 3.2) may be essential for accurate diagnosis and staging of AKI.

6.12.5 Management

Adequate management of AKI requires a triad of (a) proper diagnosis and management of the primary infection; (b) timely diagnosis of AKI; and (c) appropriate staging of renal injury.

Treatment of the primary infection is obviously the most important single measure, without which AKI will progress and add an independent risk factor for death. This should include specific therapy – avoiding as much as possible the use of nephrotoxic antimicrobials – and supportive treatment including hydration and maintenance of electrolyte and acid–base balance.

The use of symptomatic measures such as antipyretics should consider drug–drug interactions and nephrotoxicity particularly in a dehydrated patient.

The timely diagnosis and staging of AKI is essential in all stages. The main focus in RIFLE class R and I should be the maintenance of adequate hydration as guided by circulatory parameters and urine volume. Unfortunately, sophisticated facilities for circulatory monitoring may be lacking, hence the need for expert clinical judgment taking into consideration the skin turgor, mucous membrane wetness, and jugular venous pressure.

There is no evidence that the use of diuretics (including mannitol), dopamine, or other vasoactive drugs have any beneficial effect. An old study has shown some benefit from the intra-arterial installation of the calcium-channel blocker gallopamil into the renal artery of patients with malarial acute renal failure [55], but this has not been subsequently confirmed, and the logistics for its implementation on a large scale are difficult.

The challenge in RIFLE class F is to provide adequate nutrition and proper replacement therapy. It is important to take into consideration that the catabolic state associated with severe infection is augmented by the uremic state, and that food and drink intake is largely deficient because of loss of consciousness, poor appetite, or vomiting. Therefore, adequate enteral or parenteral nutrition should be secured as a fundamental component of treatment at this stage, even more importantly than in the earlier stages.

There are several ways of providing renal replacement therapy as detailed in Part VII. Ideally, continuous renal replacement therapy would provide many advantages including removal of uremic and possibly microbial toxins and injurious cytokines, and permitting adequate fluid balance. However, the facilities and experience with the respective modalities are often deficient in most tropical medical facilities.

Conventional intermittent hemodialysis or peritoneal dialysis is the second best option, if used early enough and with adequate dosing and frequency. Plasmapheresis has been used as an adjuvant to hemodialysis for the removal of microbial toxins with good results [56]. Where this was not possible, blood exchange was used in the hopes of reducing parasitemia in malarial acute renal failure with some success [57].

As explained earlier, only a few patients reach RIFLE class L or E, since the patient's outcome is usually decided during the first three stages. When permanent loss of function occurs, the supervening regional policies apply.

6.12.6 Take Home Pearls

- Infections are a frequent reason for AKI in the tropical zone.
- In most patients, AKI is reversible, however, it constitutes an independent risk factor for mortality.
- Extracorporeal therapies should be seen as a supplement to a comprehensive treatment plan including the control of infection, fluid balance, maintenance of adequate nutrition, and care of extrarenal complications.

References

1. The World Bank Data & Statistics. http://web.worldbank.org/WBSITE/EXTERNAL/DATASTATISTICS. Viewed 26 Feb 2008.
2. Barsoum R, Sitprija V. Tropical nephrology. In: Schrier RW (ed) Schrier's Diseases of the Kidney and Urinary Tract, 8 th ed. (2006). Lippincott Williams & Wilkins, Philadelphia, PA, pp 2013–2055.
3. Tomiyama J, Hasegawa Y, Nagasawa T, et al. (1989) Bacillus cereus septicemia associated with rhabdomyolysis and myoglobinuric renal failure.1. Jpn J Med 28(2):247–50.
4. Heukelbach J, Feldmeier H (2006) Scabies Lancet 367(9524):1767–74.
5. Chou DW, Chung KM, Chen CH, et al. (2007) Bacteremic melioidosis in southern Taiwan: clinical characteristics and outcome. J Formos Med Assoc 106(12):1013–22.
6. Futrakul P, Sitprija V, Teranaparin C, et al. (1984): Diphtheria with renal failure. Abstracts of the 4th Collequium in Nephrology Hongkong p 44.
7. Visith S, Kearkiat P (2005) Nephropathy in leptospirosis. J Postgrad Med 51(3):184–8.
8. Jayalakshmi P, Looi LM, Lim KJ, et al. (1987) Autopsy findings in 35 cases of leprosy in Malaysia. Int J Lepr Other Mycobact Dis 55:510–4.
9. Madiwale CV, Mittal BV, Dixit M, et al. (1994) Acute renal failure due to crescentic glomerulonephritis complicating leprosy. Nephrol Dial Transplant 9(2):178–9.
10. Simon A, Chalumeau M, Mougenot B, et al. (2006) Severe hypercalcaemia and acute renal failure: atypical complications of generalized tuberculosis. Acta Paediatr 95(11):1517–8.
11. Singarayar J, Umerah B (1978) Tropical vasculitis and tuberculosis. Med J Zambia 12:74–6.
12. Tsay RW, Chang FY (1998) Serious complications in scrub typhus. J Microbiol Immunol Infect 31:240–4.
13. Bassily S, Farid Z, Barsoum RS, et al. (1976) Renal biopsy in schistosoma-salmonella associated nephrotic syndrome. J Trop Med Hyg 79:256–9.
14. Glover SC, Smith CC, Porter IA (1982) Fatal salmonella septicaemia with disseminated intravascular coagulation and renal failure. J Med Microbiol 15:117–21.
15. Lwanga D, Wing AJ (1970) Renal complications associated with typhoid fever. East Afr Med J 47:146–9.

16. Dhawan A, Marwaha RK (1992) Acute glomerulonephritis in multi-drug resistant Salmonella typhi infection. Indian Pediatr 29:1039–41.
17. Srivastava RN, Moudgil A, Bagga A, et al. (1991) Hemolytic uremic syndrome in children in northern India. Pediatr Nephrol 5:284–8.
18. Eknoyan G, Dillman RO (1978) Renal complications of infectious diseases. Med Clin North Am 62(5):979–1003.
19. Benyajati C, Keoplug M, Beisel WR, et al. (1960) Acute renal failure in Asiatic cholera: clinicopathologic correlations with acute tubular necrosis and hypokalemic nephropathy. Ann Intern Med 52:960–75.
20. Tkachenko EA, Lee HW (1991) Etiology and epidemiology of hemorrhagic fever with renal syndrome. Kidney Int [Suppl] 35:S54–61.
21. Kim YK, Lee SC, Kim C, et al. (2007) Clinical and laboratory predictors of oliguric renal failure in haemorrhagic fever with renal syndrome caused by Hantaan virus. J Infect 54(4):381–6.
22. Faust RL, Pimstone N (1996) Acute renal failure associated with nonfulminant hepatitis A viral infection. Am J Gastroenterol 91:369.
23. Guilpain P, Servettaz A, Tamby MC, et al. (2005) Pathogenesis of primary systemic vasculitides (II): ANCA-negative vasculitides. Presse Med 34(14):1023–33.
24. Li PK, Lai FM, Ho SS, et al. (1992) Acute renal failure in hepatitis B virus-related membranous nephropathy with mesangiocapillary transition and crescentic transformation. Am J Kidney Dis 9(1):76–80.
25. Barsoum R (2007) Hepatitis C virus: from entry to renal injury – facts and potentials. Nephrol Dial Transplant 22(7): 1840–8.
26. D'Amico G (1998) Renal involvement in hepatitis C infection: cryoglobulinemic glomerulonephritis. Kidney Int 54:650–71.
27. Izzedine H, Baumelou A, Deray G (2007) Acute renal failure in HIV patients. Nephrol Dial Transplant 22(10): 2757–62.
28. Praditpornsilpa K, Napathorn S, Yenrudi S, et al. (1999) Renal pathology and HIV infection in Thailand. Am J Kidney Dis 33(2):282–6.
29. Duarte MIS, Silva MRR, Goto H, et al. (1983) Interstitial nephritis in human kala-azar. Trans R Soc Trop Med Hyg 77:531–7.
30. Caravaca F, Munoz A, Pizarro, et al. (1991) Acute renal failure in visceral leishmaniasis. Am J Nephrol 11:350–2.
31. Barsoum RS (2000) Malarial acute renal failure. J Am Soc Nephrol 11:2147–54.
32. Langhammer J, Birk HW, Zahner H (1997) Renal disease in lymphatic filariasis: evidence for tubular and glomerular disorders at various stages of the infection. Trop Med Int Health 2:875–84.
33. Lima EQ, Gorayeb FS, Zanon JR, et al. (2007) Dengue haemorrhagic fever-induced acute kidney injury without hypotension, haemolysis or rhabdomyolysis. Nephrol Dial Transplant 22(11):3322–6.
34. Boonpucknavig S, Vuttiviroj O, Boonpucknavig V (1981) Infection of young adult mice with dengue virus type 2. Trans Roy Soc Trop Med Hyg 75:647–53.
35. Sitprija V (2008) Altered fluid, electrolyte and mineral status in tropical disease, with an emphasis on malaria and leptospirosis. Nat Clin Pract Nephrol 4(2):91–101.
36. Chusil S, Kasantikul V, Sitprija V. (1986): Subclinical rhabdomyolysis in tropical acute renal failure. Abstracts, 3rd Asian Pacific Congr Nephrol Singapore, p 60.
37. Knox-Macaulay HHM (1995). Blood diseases in the tropics. In: Ashworth G (ed) Tropical Pathology, 2nd ed. Springer, Hamburg, pp 1131–1134.
38. Sabeti PC, Reich DE, Higgins JM, et al. (2002) Detecting recent positive selection in the human genome from haplotype structure. Nature 419:832–7.
40. Dosquet C, Wautier JL (1992) Contact factors in severe sepsis. Presse Med 21(5):210–5.
41. Daher EF, Abdulkader RC, Motti E, et al. (1997) Prospective study of tetanus-induced acute renal dysfunction: role of adrenergic overactivity. Am J Trop Med Hyg 57:610–4.
42. Lopez EL, Diaz M, Grinstein S, et al. (1989) Hemolytic uremic syndrome and diarrhea in Argentine children: the role of Shiga-like toxins. J Infect Dis 160(3):469–75.
43. Ghosh K, Pradhan V, Ghosh K (2008) Background noise of infection for using ANCA as a diagnostic tool for vasculitis in tropical and developing countries. Parasitol Res 102(5): 1093–5.
44. Jaber BL, Pereira BJ, Bonventre JV, et al. (2005) Polymorphism of host response genes: implications in the pathogenesis and treatment of acute renal failure. Kidney Int 67(1):14–33.
45. Jaber BL, Liangos O, Pereira BJ, et al. (2004) Polymorphism of immunomodulatory cytokine genes: implications in acute renal failure. Blood Purif 22(1):101–11.
46. Agarwal RK, Moudgil A, Kishore K, et al. (1985) Acute viral hepatitis, intravascular hemolysis, severe hyperbilirubinemia and renal failure in glucose.6.phosphate dehydrogenase deficient patients. Postgrad Med J 61:971.
47. Beutler E, Vulliamy TJ (2002) Hematologically important mutations: glucose-6-phosphate dehydrogenase. Blood Cells Mol Dis 28:93–103.
48. Perianayagam MC, Liangos O, Kolyada AY, et al. (2007) NADPH oxidase p22phox and catalase gene variants are associated with biomarkers of oxidative stress and adverse outcomes in acute renal failure. J Am Soc Nephrol 18(1): 255–63.
49. Kannangara S, DeSimone JA, Pomerantz RJ (2005) Attenuation of HIV-1 infection by other microbial agents. J Infect Dis 192(6):1003–9.
50. Goyal S, Kannangai R, Abraham AM, et al. (2007) Lack of increased frequency of human immunodeficiency virus infection in individuals with dengue-like illness in South India. Indian J Med Microbiol 25(3):300–1.
51. Nishioka Sde A (1997) Acute renal failure and multidrug therapy for leprosy. Int J Lepr Other Mycobact Dis 65(2): 259–60.
52. Javier Perez A, Courel M, Sobrado J, et al. (1987) Acute renal failure after topical application of carbon tetrachloride. Lancet 1(8531):515–6.
53. Dimitrov Y, Heibel F, Marcellin L, et al. (1997) Acute renal failure and nephrotic syndrome with alpha interferon therapy. Nephrol Dial Transplant 12:200–3.
54. Vasconcelos PF, Luna EJ, Galler R, et al. (2001) Serious adverse events associated with yellow fever 17DD vaccine in Brazil: a report of two cases. Lancet 358:91–7.
55. Lumlertgul D, Wongmekiat O, Sirivanichai C, et al. (1991) Intrarenal infusion of gallopamil in acute renal failure. A preliminary report. Drugs 42(Suppl 1):44–50.

56. Lercari G, Paganini G, Malfanti L, et al. (1992) Apheresis for severe malaria complicated by cerebral malaria, acute respiratory distress syndrome, acute renal failure, and disseminated intravascular coagulation. J Clin Apheresis 7: 93–96.

57. Hoontrakoon S, Suputtamongkol Y (1998) Exchange transfusion as an adjunct to the treatment of severe falciparum malaria. Trop Med Int Health 3:156–61.

AIDS and Acute Kidney Failure

6.13

Hassane Izzedine

Core Messages

- HIV-infected patients may present with a variety of patterns of renal involvement
- Acute kidney failure (AKF) is common and is often the result of acute tubular necrosis (ATN), acute interstitial nephritis, and thrombotic microangiopathy
- The most common precipitating factors of ATN include medications and dehydration superimposed on sepsis, hypotension, and respiratory failure
- It is potentially avoidable, and support through the period of renal failure may lead to resolution of the renal dysfunction
- Although it is potentially reversible with dialysis support, AKF nonetheless carries a high mortality

Acute kidney failure (AKF) incidence rates vary from 0.9% to 20% and mortality rates between 25% to 80% [1]. The mortality rate in AKF depends on the type of AKF and comorbidities of the patient. Indeed, in the Madrid study [2], patients with acute tubular necrosis (ATN) had a mortality rate of 60%, while those with prerenal or postrenal disease had a 35% mortality rate. Most deaths are not due to the AKF itself but rather to underlying disease (such as acquired immunodeficiency syndrome [AIDS] status) or complications.

Renal disease is an increasingly prevalent entity in -infected patients. In contrast to AKF due to prerenal and postrenal causes, renal forms of AKF in HIV-infected patients are often related to HIV-mediated viral or immunologic disease, or to treatment-related toxicity, both of which have changed since the introduction of highly active antiretroviral therapy (HAART) [3–5]. The AIDS Clinical Trials Group has accepted the diagnosis of AKF in HIV1-seropositive patients as a creatinine level greater than 1.5 mg/dl or a 1.3-fold increase above laboratory baseline that resolves within 3 months. This definition has been included in recent guidelines from the HIV Medicine Association of the Infectious Diseases Society of America (HIVMA-IDSA) [6]. Because consensus on defining AKF does not exist, these findings need to be interpreted with caution.

6.13.1 Epidemiology: Incidence and Risk Factors

HIV-positive individuals have an increased risk of developing AKF while hospitalized, and AKF is associated with increased mortality [7]. Rao and Friedman [8] estimated mortality to be 60% in HIV-infected patients diagnosed with ARF, and Lopes et al. [9] found a 43% overall mortality for HIV-infected patients who developed acute kidney injury (AKI) as defined by the RIFLE criteria. The adjusted odds ratio for AKF in HIV-positive individuals was elevated in both the pre-HAART [10, 11] and post-HAART [3, 12] eras.

Wyatt et al. examined the incidence and predictors of AKF in acute care hospitals in New York State during

H. Izzedine
Department of Nephrology, La Pitié-Salpêtrière Hospital, 47-80 Boulevard de l'Hôpital, Assistance Publique-Hopitaux de Paris, Pierre et Marie Curie University, 75013 Paris, France
e-mail: hassan.izzedine@psl.aphp.fr

A. Jörres et al. (eds.), *Management of Acute Kidney Problems*,
DOI: 10.1007/978-3-540-69441-0_6.13,

1995 (pre-HAART) or 2003 (post-HAART) and the impact of AKF on in-hospital mortality in the post-HAART era from the state Planning and Research Cooperative System database. The presence of AKF was determined based on the clinical judgment of the treating physician. There were 52,580 adult HIV-infected patients discharged from hospital in 1995 and 25,114 in 2003. Compared with uninfected patients, HIV-infected patients had an increased incidence of AKF in both the pre-HAART (2.9 vs 1.0%, adjusted odds ratio [OR], 4.62; 95% confidence interval [95% CI], 4.30–4.95) and post-HAART eras (6.0% vs 2.7%, adjusted OR, 2.82; 95% CI, 2.66–2.99). AKF was associated with mortality among HIV-infected patients in the post-HAART era (OR, 5.83; 95% CI, 5.11–6.65). Renal replacement therapy was prescribed in only 1% of discharges among patients with HIV in 2003 and in <1% in 1995. Hospitalizations of HIV-infected patients that were complicated by AKF were also complicated by much higher in-hospital mortality (27%) than seen in admissions of HIV-infected patients without AKF (4.5%). After adjusting for confounding factors, AKF was associated with a nearly sixfold increase in in-hospital mortality among HIV-infected patients in 2003 (OR, 5.83; 95% CI, 5.11–6.65) [7]. Franceschini et al. conducted an observational study of 754 HIV-infected patients recruited from a university-based infectious diseases clinic to assess the effect of low CD4 cell counts on the incidence of AKF in ambulatory HIV-positive patients HAART treated. AKF incidence was 5.9 per 100 person-years (PY) [13]. AKF was defined as increases in serum creatinine level lasting at least 2 days: 0.5 mg/dl for patients with a baseline level less than 2.0 mg/dl; 1.0 mg/dl for patients with a baseline level between 2.0–5.0 mg/dl; 1.5 mg/dl for patients with a baseline level of 5.0 mg/dl or higher. Renal failure was most common during the first year on HAART (19 cases per 100 PY). Given that, the authors recommended that kidney function should be carefully monitored during this period. In a retrospective study, including 36 HIV-infected adults developing AKF after intensive care unit (ICU) admission, Spichler et al. reported that AKF was oliguric in 55.6%. Peritoneal dialysis was performed in 47% of them. AKF mortality in the ICU is very high and occurs most frequently in patients with a mean 75 months of HIV infection. Surviving patients presented lower levels of urea and creatinine and lower CD4 cells count at admission than did nonsurvivors [14]. Another retrospective analysis of 2,274 HIV-infected patients in London from January 1998 to December 2005 found a 5.7% prevalence of ARF [15].

Several acute kidney injury and/or mortality risk factors have been identified. In the study by Franceschini et al, risk factors for AKF included male sex, CD4 cell count less than 200/μl (15 cases per 100 PY for CD4 counts below 100 cells/mm^3 vs 1 case per 100 PY for CD4 count of 500 cells/mm^3 or higher, $p < 0.001$), HIV RNA level greater than 10,000 copies/ml, number of years of previous antiretroviral therapy ($p < 0.001$), and hepatitis C coinfection ($p = 0.02$) [13]. HCV coinfection occurs in 15–30% of all HIV-infected patients in the United States [13]. Among HIV/HCV-coinfected patients, an estimated 30% of AKF events are caused by underlying liver disease [16]. Furthermore, liver failure has been associated with a higher risk of renal toxicity for a number of drugs, e.g., antivirals [17], and increased in-hospital death in patients with AKF in the ICU (OR, 3.1; 95% CI, 1.9–4.9) [18]. The highest incidence was observed in HIV/HCV coinfected patients who also had low CD4 cell counts (25 cases per 100 PY for those with CD4 counts below 100 cells/mm^3) [13]. This risk factor remained an independent predictor of experiencing AKF [13] and the most important predictor of HIV-1-related morbidity and mortality. Furthermore, Wyatt et al. reported that AKF was significantly associated with age, diabetes mellitus, and chronic kidney disease, as well as acute or chronic liver failure or hepatitis coinfection in the post-HAART cohort [7]. Finally, most AKF episodes (52%) in the study by Franceschini et al. were due to infections or antibiotic and antifungal drug toxicity [13].

6.13.2 Causes

6.13.2.1 Prerenal and/or ATN

Although pre-HAART AKF was associated with younger age, severe immunosuppression, opportunistic infections, and septicemia [19] and their treatments, earlier data during the AIDS epidemic showed that ATN and thrombotic microangiopathies were the most common etiologies of AKF in immunosuppressed patients [5, 20]. A study from South Africa [21] found ATN and thrombotic microangiopathies (TMA) to be the most common causes of AKI in HIV-infected patients. Significantly, HIV-infected patients who developed AKI had a sixfold higher inpatient mortality compared with those HIV-infected patients whose renal function remained normal throughout hospitalization. However, these studies have only considered AKF identified through hospital records or biopsy databases [20, 22–24], biasing these findings toward severe clinical conditions associated with ATN. In the study by Franceschini et al, the most common mechanisms of AKF were prerenal in 38% of cases (most frequently due to dehydration, sepsis, or liver disease) and most AKF episodes (52%) were due to infections or antibiotic and antifungal drug toxicity, with fewer than 10% of events directly related to antiretroviral reversible nephrotoxicity (including indinavir, tenofovir, and nevirapine) [13]. Less common causes included obstructive nephropathy and interstitial nephritis.

HIV infection has also been associated with states of decreased effective circulatory volume and intravascular volume depletion related to capillary leak or endotoxin-mediated arteriolar vasoconstriction in states of severe sepsis, congestive heart failure, or cirrhosis post HBV or HCV, which can lead to AKI [25]. Both ischemic and nephrotoxic ATN is a common cause of ARF, particularly among hospitalized HIV-infected patients [25, 26]. HIV-infected patients may also be at risk for contrast nephropathy due to their often volume-depleted state or preexisting renal insufficiency [25–27]. Prophylaxis should be considered for any patient with classic risk factors for contrast-induced nephropathy [28]. Although it is potentially reversible with dialytic support, AKF nonetheless carries a high mortality.

6.13.2.2 Postrenal AKF

Obstructive uropathy in HIV-infected patients includes nephrolithiasis, which can occur during states of volume depletion, following use of indinavir, acyclovir, and sulfadiazine [25, 29], retroperitoneal lymphadenopathy in the setting of aggressive high-grade B cell lymphomas [26], and/or radiation used to treat such lymphomas. Noncontrast computerized tomography of the abdomen is necessary if retroperitoneal fibrosis diagnosis is suspected. Other etiologies include lower urinary tract obstruction from a neuropathic bladder and benign prostatic hypertrophy [25, 30], and obstructing fungus balls [25, 30].

6.13.3 Intrinsic Renal Failure

6.13.3.1 Acute Interstitial Nephritis

Acute interstitial nephritis (AIN) in the setting of HIV infection may be related to an allergic idiosyncratic drug reaction (classic allergic interstitial nephritis), direct cytotoxic effects of the HIV infection, or to associated opportunistic infections, which can promote tubulointerstitial injury, including tuberculosis, cytomegalovirus, candidiasis, polyomavirus, and histoplasmosis [26]. If a drug-induced allergic interstitial nephritis is suspected based on history including fever, drug rash, and peripheral eosinophilia, prompt discontinuation of the suspected agent is appropriate. A kidney biopsy is often necessary to evaluate for other associated renal diseases, particularly before treatment with immunosuppressive agents, such as steroids, is considered [26].

Two recently identified diseases (the immune restoration syndrome or immune reconstitution inflammatory syndrome [IRIS] and the diffuse infiltrative lymphocytosis syndrome [DILS]) should be considered as a cause of AKF and acute interstitial nephritis in HIV-infected patients.

IRIS is a result of an exuberant inflammatory response towards previously diagnosed or incubating opportunistic pathogens, as well as responses towards other as yet undefined antigens. The frequency of IRIS has not been reported conclusively, but it may be estimated to occur in 10–25% of patients who receive HAART. IRIS was documented by the increase in the CD4 cell count within the first months of HAART, and supported by the presence of granulomatous reaction. The clinical profile bears some resemblance to sarcoidosis hence its name "sarcoidosis-like disease." The interval between the start of HAART and the onset of IRIS is highly variable, ranging from <1 week to several months, but the majority of events occur within the first 8 weeks after HAART initiation. To date, only three cases of AKF related to IRIS has been reported [31–33].

DILS is a disorder that is characterized by salivary and lacrimal glandular swelling and sicca symptoms of varying intensity, frequently accompanied by persistent circulating and visceral CD8-positive lymphocytic infiltration [34]. It is also sometimes called "Sjögren-like disease." The frequency appears to be diminishing remarkably with HAART therapy. In a recent review, Basu et al. [35] reported that the mean duration from

HIV diagnosis to DILS diagnosis was 59.55 ± 43.8 months, and the mean duration of DILS-related symptoms was 9.05 ± 2.3 months. In this cohort, 12.9% of 129 patients developed renal involvement, of which 3 had lymphocytic interstitial nephritis without glomerular involvement on renal biopsies leading to renal insufficiency. Three patients had type IV renal tubular acidosis [35]. A few other cases of acute interstitial nephritis related to DILS have also been reported [36, 37].

6.13.3.2 Thrombotic Microangiopathy

HIV-associated TMA includes hemolytic uremic syndrome and thrombotic thrombocytopenic purpura [3]. Microangiopathic anemia and renal impairment predominate in hemolytic uremic syndrome, whereas in thrombotic thrombocytopenic purpura a pentad of microangiopathic anemia, thrombocytopenia, renal impairment, fever, and neurologic features occurs. Proteinuria can be in the nephrotic range but is usually less marked than in human immunodeficiency virus-associated nephropathy (HIVAN) [38]. Pathologic findings are similar in both forms, with fibrin-rich thrombi and platelets deposited in the glomerular capillaries and arterial microvessels [27]. The incidence of TMA in HIV-infected patients has ranged from 0% to 7% in prospective and retrospective analyses [26]. HIV-associated TMA predominantly affects children and young white male populations [38, 39]. In a series of 71 HIV-infected patients with ARF from North Carolina, United States, TMA was the cause of 2 of the 111 cases of ARF reported [13]. In a single-center study from Paris, Peraldi et al. [5] found TMA to be the cause of approximately 50% of their biopsy-proven cases of AKI (32 out of 60 cases) in HIV-infected patients.

Compared with HIVAN, TMA is rare, but HIV-related TMA may account for up to 35% of all TMA cases [5, 40]. Endothelial CMV inclusion has been incriminated in a subset of HIV-associated TMA, but whether CMV contributes to pathogenesis remains unclear [41]. Down-regulation of von Willebrand factor cleaving protease (ADAMTS13), a metalloproteinase that cleaves multimers of von Willebrand factor on platelets, is a key feature of TMA, and a case report illustrated that antibodies against this protease can be a feature of HIV-associated TMA [42]. However, one study did not show a relationship between the presence of inhibitors of ADAMTS13 and the development of HIV-associated TMA [43]. Treatment included plasma infusion and/or plasmapheresis [42]. The role of adjunct immune modulating therapies, such as steroids or rituximab, is still unclear. These drugs must be used with caution in this immunosuppressed group of patients in the absence of evidence-based recommendations [26]. HIV1-infected patients seem to be more responsive to plasma infusion with fresh frozen plasma than HIV-negative patients and less likely to require plasma exchange [39]. Furthermore, the time for platelet counts and lactate dehydrogenase to normalize was shorter. Responses to antiretroviral therapy, antiplatelet agents, corticosteroids, and vincristine have been reported [42]. Mortality exceeds 60% in HIV-associated TMA [27].

6.13.3.3 Acute Glomerulopathies

Micropathologic studies have expanded the spectrum of AKF related to glomerular lesions in HIV-infected patients including HIVAN, HIV-immune complex kidney diseases (HIVICK), crescentic immunoglobulin A nephropathy, membranoproliferative glomerulonephritis (MPGN), cryoglobulinic vasculitis especially in HCV coinfected patients, fibrillary and immunotactoid glomerulopathies, AA amyloidosis, and lupus-like immune complex glomerulonephritis.

HIVAN is a distinct clinicopathologic entity that is characterized by a proteinuria in the nephrotic range and, in the absence of antiretroviral therapy, rapid progression to end-stage renal disease. Its most common renal manifestation is the collapsing variant of focal segmental glomerular sclerosis.

Most such cases are among young, African-American men. MPGN may be the most common of the immune complex-mediated glomerulonephritides seen in white HIV-infected patients (mostly among intravenous drug abusers coinfected with HIV and hepatitis C virus).

Crescentic glomerulonephritis is not common in HIV-positive patients and false-positive antibodies to antineutrophil cytoplasmic antibodies and anti-glomerular basement membrane antibodies are a feature of HIV infection and must be interpreted cautiously during HIV-associated AKF [44, 45]. Optimal therapy for the treatment of acute glomerulonephritis in the setting of HIV infection is unclear [26, 46].

6.13.3.4 Drug Related AKF

Many drugs used in the treatment or prophylaxis of opportunistic infections in HIV infection may cause acute nephrotoxicity (Table 6.13.1). Acute tubular necrosis, crescentic glomerulonephritis, and acute interstitial nephritis can occur, and the last may respond to corticosteroid therapy. Of note, trimethoprim can increase serum creatinine levels by altering normal elimination pathways, with no evidence of deterioration in glomerular filtration rate (GFR) [47, 48].

Amid the many antiretroviral drugs available nowadays, clinicians should differentiate between the agents, which were classically known to be nephrotoxic in the doses in which they were prescribed such as indinavir and ritonavir, and the more modern agents notorious for their toxicity even in the usual therapeutic doses as tenofovir. Finally, anecdotical acute nephrotoxicity cases have been reported related to didanosine, atazanavir, abacavir, and lamivudine-stavudine treatment [49].

Table 6.13.1 Drug induced acute kidney failure (AKF) in HIV-infected patients

Type of renal injury	Drug
Prerenal	IEC, amphotericin B, COX-2 inhibiters
	Diuretics, interferon, AINS
Acute tubular necrosis	Acyclovir, abacavir, adefovir, aminoglycosides
	Amphotericin B, cidofovir, cocaine, foscarnet
Intratubular obstruction secondary to crystal precipitation	Indinavir, pentamidine, rifampicin, ritonavir, sulfonamides
	Indinavir, sulfadiazine, foscarnet, acyclovir, atazanavir, efavirens, sulfonamides
Interstitial nephritis	β-Lactam antibiotics, quinolones, trimethorpim-sulfamethoxazole
	Rifampicin, acyclovir, abacavir, indinavir, rifampicin
Crescentic glomerulonephritis	Foscarnet, rifampicin
Thrombotic microangiopathy	Interferons, valaciclovir

NSAID (nonsteroidal anti-inflammatory drug), *ACEI* (angiotensin converting enzyme inhibitor)

6.13.3.5 Drug-Induced Acute Crystal Nephropathy

Commonly prescribed medications given to HIV-infected patients, which may promote crystal nephropathy including indinavir, acyclovir, atazanavir, and sulfadiazine [50, 51]. Other drugs may induced crystal nephropathy in the setting of an acid urine or volume depletion (e.g., ganciclovir and sulfadiazine) [50, 52].

6.13.3.6 Rhabdomyolysis

Rhabdomyolysis should also be considered when HIV-infected patients present with AKI. In one renal biopsy series of HIV-infected patients in Europe, approximately 10% of the ARF cases were attributed to myoglobinuric pigment nephropathy [5]. Myoglobinuric AKI among HIV-infected patients may be related to direct cytoxic effect of HIV on muscle cells, the adverse myotoxic effects of HAART, substance abuse (cocaine and alcohol use both are associated with myotoxicity), and electrolyte derangements that can promote muscle injury (hypokalemia and hypophosphatemia) [26].

Zidovudine and didanosine have been associated with rhabdomyolysis. Zidovudine affects mitochondrial DNA by promoting deletional mutations or by inhibiting mitochondrial DNA polymerase activity [53, 54]. There have been multiple reports of rhabdomyolysis in HIV-infected patients taking both HAART and statin therapy by interaction through the cytochrome P450 system [26, 55, 56].

The potential renal effects of indinavir are worth mentioning. An increase in the serum creatinine level has been observed with indinavir treatment in 14–33% of patients [57]. Most elevations in serum creatinine levels normalize within weeks after the discontinuation of indinavir. Presentations of indinavir nephrotoxicity include AKF, symptomatic (flank pain and dysuria), or asymptomatic crystalluria, nephrolithiasis, and chronic renal impairment with tubulointerstitial injury [58, 59]. Insidious renal impairment develops with tubular crystals, tubule necrosis, and dilation, with diffuse eosinophilic interstitial infiltrates and scarring [59]. Leukocyturia is common and persistent in 32% of individuals taking indinavir [60]. Fluid deprivation, unadjusted of indinavir dose to creatinine clearance, acyclovir or trimethoprim-sulfamethoxazole coadministration, low baseline body mass index, and the presence of chronic viral hepatitis are cofactors in indinavir nephrotoxicity [61, 62]. The HIVMA-IDSA guidelines recommend that individuals receiving indinavir should drink at least 1.5 L of water per day and that periodic creatinine and urinalysis monitoring should be performed in the first 6 months of treatment [6]. Case reports have linked ritonavir use to reversible renal failure [49]. All reported patients who showed an increase in the serum creatinine level received ritonavir at a dose of 800–1,200 mg/day. Withdrawing the drug leads to a full regression of the renal dysfunction within few days making an underlying hemodynamic mechanism possible. There were no reports of ritonavir or indinavir nephrotoxicity when used at the dose of 100 mg twice a day or 400 mg twice a day, respectively.

The drug that is the most problematic in this context is undoubtedly tenofovir (TDF). Presentations of TDF nephrotoxicity include AKF, Fanconi syndrome, and progressive increase serum creatinine levels. Pivotal controlled clinical studies in humans found tenofovir DF (TDF) to be safe, with the incidence of TDF-associated renal impairment (elevated serum creatinine or hypophosphatemia) being 1–3% and with minimal differences from comparative non-TDF arms [62, 63]. Further studies have shown only minimal decreases in the GFR of individuals taking TDF and a low incidence (0.3%) of AKF [64, 65]. However, during postmarketing surveillance, several cases of Fanconi syndrome and/or AKF have been observed in patients receiving TDF in combination with other antiretroviral agents, raising concerns about the risk of renal toxicity using this drug. Recent reports have linked HAART regimens that contain TDF to a mild, time-dependant elevation in the serum creatinine level and a decrease in the glomerular filtration rate. One study of 174 patients found a lower mean GFR, as calculated by creatinine clearance (97 ml/min/1.73 m^2 vs 107 ml/min/1.73 m^2), with 38% of patients showing an impaired GFR in the TDF arm compared with 29% in the control group [64]. The decrease in GFR in those on a TDF-containing regimen remained well within the normal range of GFR and did not lead to discontinuation of TDF. However, in the prospective HIV Outpatient Study (HOPS) Cohort, despite more advanced HIV disease at baseline that could predispose to incident renal insufficiency, patients on TDF-containing HAART with either ritonavir/lopinavir or ritonavir/atazanavir did not experience greater decrements in renal function during the first year of observation than patients on TDF-containing HAART regimens without these agents or other protease inhibitors [66]. At contrary, there was recent support for the theory from a clinical trial which showed that a regimen of tenofovir combined with protease inhibitors had a greater decline in creatinine clearance compared with a regimen of tenofovir combined with non-nucleoside-reverse-transcriptase inhibitors [67]. The estimated decline in GFR as measured by the Modification of Diet in Renal Disease (MDRD) equation was approximately 15 ml/min in the tenofovir-protease inhibitor group compared with a decline of 4.5 ml/min in the tenofovir-NNRTI group ($p < 0.02$) [67]. There was no significant difference in GFR decline in the tenofovir-NNRTI group compared with the group of HIV-infected patients who did not receive any tenofovir as part of their HAART regimen [67]. The reasons for the disparate results between these two studies are not clear but may reflect the limitations of using estimating equations for GFR which have not been validated in HIV-infected patients. Actually, the incidence and significance of nephrotoxicity associated with the use of TDF in clinical practice remains unanswered, and more safety data are needed. Predisposing factors for the development of acute renal failure with the use of TDF remain obscure.

6.13.4 Underlying Mechanisms

Over the past few years, considerable progress has been made in the molecular identification and characterization of organic anion and cation transporters in the kidney. The process of secreting organic anions (OA) and cations (OC) through the proximal tubular cells is achieved via unidirectional transcellular transport, involving the uptake of OA and OC into the cells from the blood across the basolateral membrane, followed by extrusion across the brush-border membrane into urine. Drug accumulation in renal proximal tubule cells is classically a function of both uptake at the basolateral membrane and efflux at the luminal membrane. Alterations of this equilibrium between blood-into-cell and cell-into-lumen transports may result in intracellular accumulation of the drug that may result in local toxicity. Treatments that block efflux, like those that enhance uptake, may thus increase both accumulation and toxicity [68]. The observation that 93% of cases of TDF-associated renal impairment occurred in individuals taking protease inhibitors has led to speculation that ritonavir-mediated inhibition of the multidrug resistance protein 2, which secretes TDF into the urine, might lead to intracellular accumulation of the drug [69]. Others have argued that multidrug resistance protein 4, not multidrug resistance protein 2, mediates TDF efflux and is not inhibited by ritonavir [70, 71]. A population-based pharmacokinetic study demonstrated that the combination of lopinavir and ritonavir decreases TDF clearance [72]. Furthermore, Kiser et al. identified an interaction between lopinavir/ritonavir and tenofovir that manifests as a decrease in the renal clearance of tenofovir. Tenofovir renal clearance was 17.5% lower in subjects on lopinavir/ritonavir compared with those on TDF without a protease inhibitor, after controlling for differences in GFR [73]. However, the impact of this potential interaction between boosted PIs and tenofovir was not confirmed in the prospective HOPS cohort [66]. Prospective studies are needed to definitively identify those patients at risk.

A renal biopsy series suggested that the mitochondrial to nuclear DNA ratio was unchanged in HIV-positive individuals who received TDF compared with those who did not, although the combination of TDF with didanosine was associated with a reduced ratio [74]. Competition between TDF and didanosine for active uptake into proximal renal tubular cells, a process controlled by the human organic anion transporter 1[75] could facilitate greater didanosine serum concentrations and therefore mitochondrial damage and nephrotoxicity during coadministration without dose adjustment of didanosine [69]. We hypothesized that polymorphisms in the renal tubular drug transporter genes *MRP2* or *MRP4* would influence the disposition of TDF and could therefore affect the risk of renal toxicity [56]. We showed that renal tubular dysfunction related to TDF therapy outcome was significantly associated with a single nonsynonymous G-A substitution at position 1249 of *ABCC2* (also called *MRP2*, which encodes multidrug resistance protein 2 [MRP2]) and with an *ABCC2* haplotype comprising four polymorphisms, including 1249 G-A (unadjusted OR, 4.25; lower bound of 95% confidence interval, 1.25). Additionally, a T-A substitution at position 3563 and a haplotype including this polymorphism were significantly associated with the absence of renal toxicity (none of the case patients had these variants). A synonymous polymorphism in *ABCC4* (also called *MRP4*, which encodes MRP4) was also associated with the outcome ($p = 0.04$) but did not alter the amino acid sequence of the encoded protein. We provided the first report of a possible association between a human genetic variant and TDF-associated renal dysfunction [76]. In their human transporter genotype and tenofovir pharmacokinetics association study, Kiser et al. found that tenofovir renal clearance was 15% lower in ABCC4 3463G SNP variants compared with wild-type and that ABCC2-24T carriers excreted 19% more tenofovir in urine than wild-type. This decreased renal clearance translated into a 32% increased area under the concentration-time curve (AUC) in the ABCC4 3463G SNP variants [77]. Candidates for a nephrotoxic antiretroviral therapy should be considered in the future for renal tubular pharmacogenetic testing before starting treatment. Prevention of nephrotoxicity should be directed towards early detection of proximal-tubular injury, adjustment of tenofovir dose for level of renal function, and avoidance of drugs that may inhibit tenofovir's renal elimination, such as ritonavir [50].

6.13.5 Conclusion

HIV-infected patients have multiple risk factors for the development of AKI. The incidence of AKF (defined on RIFLE criteria) and of AKF as a predictor of mortality in HIV-infected patients in the HAART era will be confirmed in future prospective clinical studies. Future pharmacogenetic studies are awaited to determine patients susceptible to develop renal side effects and to personalize our approach to each.

6.13.6 Take Home Pearls

- Acute kidney failure is a common complication in HIV-infected patients
- Typical causes are acute tubular necrosis, acute interstitial nephritis, and thrombotic microangiopathy
- The most common precipitating factors include medications and dehydration superimposed on sepsis, hypotension, and respiratory failure

References

1. Lameire N, Van BW, Vanholder R: Acute renal failure. *Lancet* 2005; 365: 417 –430.
2. Liano F, Pascual J. Epidemiology of acute renal failure: a prospective, multicenter, community-based study. Madrid Acute Renal Failure Study Group. *Kidney Int* 1996; 50: 811–818.
3. Kimmel PL, Barisoni L, Kopp JB. Pathogenesis and treatment of HIV-associated renal diseases: lessons from clinical and animal studies, molecular pathologic correlations, and genetic investigations. *Ann Intern Med* 2003; 139:214–226.
4. Perazella MA. Acute renal failure in HIV-infected patients: a brief review of common causes. *Am J Med Sci* 2000; 319:385–391.
5. Peraldi MN, Maslo C, Akposso K, Mougenot B, Rondeau E, Sraer JD. Acute renal failure in the course of HIV infection: a single institution retrospective study of ninety-two patients and sixty renal biopsies. *Nephrol Dial Transplant* 1999; 14:1578–1585.
6. Gupta SK, Eustace JA, Winston JA, Boydstun II, Ahuja TS, Rodriguez RA, Tashima KT, Roland M, Franceschini N, Palella FJ, Lennox JL, Klotman PE, Nachman SA, Hall SD, Szczech LA. Guidelines for the management of chronic kidney disease in HIV-infected patients: recommendations of the HIV Medicine Association of the Infectious Diseases Society of America. *Clin Infect Dis* 2005;40:559–1585.
7. Wyatt CM, Arons RR, Klotman PE, Klotman ME. Acute renal failure in hospitalized patients with HIV: risk factors and impact on in-hospital mortality. *AIDS* 2006; 20:561–565.
8. Rao TKS, Friedman EA. Outcome of severe acute renal failure in patients with acquired immunodeficiency syndrome. *Am J Kidney Dis* 1995; 25:390–398.
9. Lopes JA, Fernandes J, Jorge S, Neves J, Antunes F, Prata MM. An assessment of the RIFLE criteria for acute renal failure in critically ill HIV-infected patients. *Crit Care* 2007; 11:401.
10. Pardo V, Aldana M, Colton RM, Fischl MA, Jaffe D, Moskowitz L, Hensley GT, Bourgoignie JJ. Glomerular lesions in the acquired immunodeficiency syndrome. *Ann Intern Med* 1984; 101:429–434.
11. Schwartz EJ, Szczech LA, Ross MJ, Klotman ME, Winston JA, Klotman PE. Highly active antiretroviral therapy and the epidemic of HIV+ end-stage renal disease. *J Am Soc Nephrol* 2005; 16:2412–2420.
12. Selik RM, Byers RH Jr, Dworkin MS. Trends in diseases reported on U.S. death certificates that mentioned HIV infection, 1987–1999. *J Acquir Immune Defic Syndr* 2002; 29: 378–387.
13. Franceschini N, Napravnik S, Eron JJ Jr, Szczech LA, Finn WF. Incidence and etiology of acute renal failure among ambulatory HIVinfected patients. *Kidney Int* 2005; 67: 1526–1531.
14. Spichler A., Andrade L., Seguro A.C. Acute renal failure in HIV patients in intensive care. 9th European AIDS Conference (EACS) 1st EACS Resistance & Pharmacology Workshop. October 25–29, 2003 Warsaw, Poland.
15. Roe J, Campbell LJ, Ibrahim F, Hendry BM, Post FA. HIV care and the incidence of acute renal failure. *Clin Infect Dis* 2008; 47:242–249.
16. Sherman KE, Rouster SD, Chung RT, Rajicic N: Hepatitis C virus prevalence among patients infected with human immunodeficiency virus: A cross-sectional analysis of the US adult AIDS Clinical Trials Group. *Clin Infect Dis* 2002; 34: 831–837.
17. Blaas S, Schneidewind A, Gluck T, Salzberger B. Acute renal failure in HIV patients with liver cirrhosis receiving tenofovir: a report of two cases. *AIDS* 2006; 20: 1786–1787.
18. Mehta RL, Pascual MT, Gruta CG, Zhuang S, Chertow GM. Refining predictive models in critically ill patients with acute renal failure. *J Am Soc Nephrol* 2002; 13:1350–1357.
19. Rao TK, Friedman EA. Outcome of severe acute renal failure in patients with acquired immunodeficiency syndrome. *Am J Kidney Dis* 1995; 25:390–398.
20. Bourgoignie JJ, Meneses R, Ortiz C, Jaffe D, Pardo V. The clinical spectrum of renal disease associated with human immunodeficiency virus. *Am J Kidney Dis* 1988; 12: 131–137.
21. Naicker S, Aboud O, Gharbi MB. Epidemiology of acute kidney injury in Africa. *Semin Nephrol* 2008; 28:348–353.
22. Rao TK, Friedman EA, Nicastri AD. The types of renal disease in the acquired immunodeficiency syndrome. *N Engl J Med* 1987; 316:1062–1068.
23. Valeri A, Neusy AJ. Acute and chronic renal disease in hospitalized AIDS patients. *Clin Nephrol* 1991; 35:110–118.
24. Williams DI, Williams DJ, Williams IG, Unwin RJ, Griffiths MH, Miller RF. Presentation, pathology, and outcome of HIV associated renal disease in a specialist centre for HIV/AIDS. *Sex Transm Infect* 1998; 74:179–184.
25. Perazella MA. Acute renal failure in HIV-infected patients: a brief review of common causes. *Am J Med Sci* 2000; 319:385–391.
26. Cohen SD, Chawla LS, Kimmel PL. Acute kidney injury in patients with human immunodeficiency virus infection. *Curr Opin Crit Care* 2008; 14:647–653.
27. Weiner NJ, Goodman JW, Kimmel PL. The HIV-associated renal diseases: current insight into pathogenesis and treatment. *Kidney Int* 2003; 63:1618–1631.
28. Pannu N, Wiebe NM, Tonelli M. Prophylaxis strategies for contrast-induced nephropathy. *JAMA* 2006; 295:2765–2779.
29. Moriyama Y, Minamidate Y, Yasuda M, Ehara H, Kikuchi M, Tsuchiya T, Deguchi T, Tsurumi H. Acute renal failure due to bilateral ureteral stone impaction in an HIV-positive patient. *Urol Res* 2008; 36:275–277.
30. Kennedy WA II, Benson MC, Kaplan SA. Urologic manifestations of HIV infection. In: Kimmel PL, Berns JS, J Stein, eds. Renal and urologic complications of HIV infection. Contemporary issues in nephrology. New York: Churchill Livingstone; 1995. pp. 181–193.
31. Jehle AW, Khanna N, Sigle JP, Glatz-Krieger K, Battegay M, Steiger J, Dickenmann M, Hirsch HH. Acute renal failure on immune reconstitution in an HIV-positive patient with miliary tuberculosis. *Clin Infect Dis* 2004; 38: 32–35.
32. Daugas E, Plaisier E, Boffa JJ, Guiard-Schmid JB, Pacanowski J, Mougenot B, Ronco P. Acute renal failure associated with immune restoration inflammatory syndrome. *Nat Clin Pract Nephrol* 2006; 2: 594–598;
33. Izzedine H, Brocheriou I, Martinez V, Deray G. IRIS and acute granulomatous interstitial nephritis. *AIDS* 2007; 21:534–535.
34. Itescu S, Brancato LJ, Buxbaum J, Gregersen PK, Rizk CC, Croxson TS, Solomon GE, Winchester R. A diffuse infiltrative CD8 lymphocytosis syndrome in human immunodeficiency virus (HIV) infection: a host immune response

associated with HLA-DR5. *Ann Intern Med* 1990; 112:3–10.
35. Basu D, Williams FM, Ahn CW, Reveille JD. Changing spectrum of the diffuse infiltrative lymphocytosis syndrome. *Arthritis Rheum* 2006; 55: 466–472.
36. Zafrani L, Coppo P, Dettwiler S, Molinier-Frenkel V, Agbalika F, Guiard-Schmid JB, Pialoux G, Xu-Dubois YC, Rondeau E, Hertig A.Nephropathy associated with the diffuse infiltrative lymphocytosis syndrome. *Kidney Int* 2007; 72:219–224.
37. Izzedine H, Brocheriou I, Valantin MA, Camous L, Bourry E, Baumelou A, Deray G, Katlama C. A case of acute renal failure associated with diffuse infiltrative lymphocytosis syndrome. *Nat Clin Pract Nephrol* 2008; 4:110–114.
38. Meisenberg BR, Robinson WL, Mosley CA, Duke MS, Rabetoy GM, Kosty MP. Thrombotic thrombocytopenic purpura in human immunodeficiency (HIV)-seropositive males. *Am J Hematol* 1988; 27:212–215.
39. Novitzky N, Thomson J, Abrahams L, du Toit C, McDonald A. Thrombotic thrombocytopenic purpura in patients with retroviral infection is highly responsive to plasma infusion therapy. *Br J Haematol* 2005; 128:373–129.
40. Thompson CE, Damon LE, Ries CA, Linker CA. Thrombotic microangiopathies in the 1980s: clinical features, response to treatment, and the impact of the human immunodeficiency virus epidemic. *Blood* 1992; 80:1890–1895.
41. Maslo C, Buré-Rossier A, Girard PM, Gholizadeh Y, Lebrette MG, Rozenbaum W. Clinical and bacteriologic impact of rifabutin prophylaxis for Mycobacterium avium complex infection in patients with human immunodeficiency virus infection. *Clin Infect Dis* 1997; 24:344–349.
42. Sahud MA, Claster S, Liu L, Ero M, Harris K, Furlan M. von Willebrand factor-cleaving protease inhibitor in a patient with human immunodeficiency syndrome-associated thrombotic thrombocytopenic purpura. *Br J Haematol* 2002; 116:909–911.
43. Gunther K, Garizio D, Nesara P. ADAMTS13 activity and the presence of acquired inhibitors in human immunodeficiency virus-related thrombotic thrombocytopenic purpura. *Transfusion* 2007; 47:1710–1716.
44. Savige JA, Chang L, Horn S, Crowe SM. Anti-nuclear, anti-neutrophil cytoplasmic and anti-glomerular basement membrane antibodies in HIV-infected individuals. *Autoimmunity* 1994; 18:205–211.
45. Szczech LA, Anderson A, Ramers C, Engeman J, Ellis M, Butterly D, Howell DN. The uncertain significance of anti-glomerular basement membrane antibody among HIV-infected persons with kidney disease. *Am J Kidney Dis* 2006; 48:e55–59.
46. Szczech LA, Gupta SK, Habash R, Guasch A, Kalayjian R, Appel R, Fields TA, Svetkey LP, Flanagan KH, Klotman PE, Winston JA. The clinical epidemiology and course of the spectrum of renal diseases associated with HIV infection. *Kidney Int* 2004; 66:1145–1152.
47. Andreev E, Koopman M, Arisz L. A rise in plasma creatinine that is not a sign of renal failure: which drugs can be responsible? *J Intern Med* 1999;246:247–252.
48. Ducharme MP, Smythe M, Strohs G. Drug-induced alterations in serum creatinine concentrations. *Ann Pharmacother* 1993; 27:622–633.
49. Roling J, Schmid H, Fischereder M, Draenert R, Goebel FD. HIV-associated renal diseases and highly active antiretroviral therapy-induced nephropathy. *Clin Infect Dis* 2006; 42:1488–1495.
50. Izzedine H, Launay-Vacher V, Deray G. Antiviral drug-induced nephrotoxicity. *Am J Kidney Dis* 2005; 45:804–817.
51. Izzedine H, Isnard-Bagnis C, Hulot JS, Vittecoq D, Cheng A, Jais CK, Launay-Vacher V, Deray G. Renal safety of tenofovir in HIV treatment-experienced patients. *AIDS* 2004; 18:1074–1076.
52. Perazella M. Drug-induced renal failure: update on new medications and unique mechanisms of nephrotoxicity. *Am J Med Sci* 2003; 325:349–362.
53. Chariot P, Ruet E, Authier FJ, Lévy Y, Gherardi R. Acute rhabdomyolysis in patients infected by human immunodeficiency virus. *Neurology* 1994; 44:1692–1696.
54. Mhiri C, Baudrimont M, Bonne G, Geny C, Degoul F, Marsac C, Roullet E, Gherardi R. Zidovudine myopathy: a distinctive disorder associated with mitochondrial dysfunction. *Ann Neurol* 1991; 29:606–614.
55. Chuck SK, Penzak SR. Risk-benefit of HMG-CoA reductase inhibitors in the treatment of HIV protease inhibitor-related hyperlipidemia. *Expert Opin Drug Saf* 2002; 1:5–17.
56. Fontaine C, Guaird-Schmid JB, Slama L, et al. Severe rhabdomyolysis during a hypersensitivity reaction to abacavir in a patient treated with ciprofibrate. *AIDS* 2005; 19:1927–1928.
57. Kopp JB, Miller KD, Mican JA, Feuerstein IM, Vaughan E, Baker C, Pannell LK, Falloon J. Crystalluria and urinary tract abnormalities associated with indinavir. *Ann Intern Med* 1997; 127:119–125.
58. Reilly RF, Tray K, Perazella MA. Indinavir nephropathy revisited: a pattern of insidious renal failure with identifiable risk factors. *Am J Kidney Dis* 2001; 38:E23.
59. Dieleman JP, van Rossum AM, Stricker BC, Sturkenboom MC, de Groot R, Telgt D, Blok WL, Burger DM, Blijenberg BG, Zietse R, Gyssens IC. Persistent leukocyturia and loss of renal function in a prospectively monitored cohort of HIV-infected patients treated with indinavir. *J Acquir Immune Defic Syndr* 2003; 32:135–142.
60. Brodie SB, Keller MJ, Ewenstein BM, Sax PE. Variation in incidence of indinavir-associated nephrolithiasis among HIV-positive patients. *AIDS* 1998; 12:2433–2437.
61. Malavaud B, Dinh B, Bonnet E, Izopet J, Payen JL, Marchou B. Increased incidence of indinavir nephrolithiasis in patients with hepatitis B or C virus infection. *Antivir Ther* 2000; 5:3–5.
62. Squires K, Pozniak AL, Pierone G Jr, et al. Tenofovir disoproxil fumarate in nucleoside-resistant HIV-1 infection: a randomized trial. *Ann Intern Med* 2003; 139:313–320.
63. Izzedine H, Hulot JS, Vittecoq D, Gallant JE, Staszewski S, Launay-Vacher V, Cheng A, Deray G; Study 903 Team. Long-term renal safety of tenofovir disoproxil fumarate in antiretroviral-naive HIV-1-infected patients. Data from a double-blind randomized active-controlled multicentre study. *Nephrol Dial Transplant* 2005; 20: 743–746.
64. Mauss S, Berger F, Schmutz G. Antiretroviral therapy with ténofovir is associated with mild renal dysfunction. *AIDS* 2005; 19:93–95.
65. Gallant JE, Parish MA, Keruly JC, Moore RD. Changes in renal function associated with tenofovir disoproxil fumarate treatment, compared with nucleoside reverse-transcriptase inhibitor treatment. *Clin Infect Dis* 2005;40: 1194–1198.

66. Buchacz K, Young B, Baker RK, Moorman A, Chmiel JS, Wood KC, Brooks JT; the HIV Outpatient Study (HOPS) Investigators. Renal function in patients receiving Tenofovir with Ritonavir/Lopinavir or Ritonavir/Atazanavir in the HIV Outpatient Study (HOPS) Cohort. *J Acquir Immune Defic Syndr* 2006; 43: 626–628.
67. Goicoechea M, Liu S, Best B, et al. Greater tenofovir-associated renal function decline with protease inhibitor-based versus non nucleoside reverse-transcriptase inhibitor-based therapy. *J Infect Dis* 2008; 197:102–108.
68. Izzedine H, Launay-Vacher V, Deray G. Renal tubular transporters and antiviral drugs: an update. *AIDS* 2005; 19: 455–462.
69. Zimmermann AE, Pizzoferrato T, Bedford J, Morris A, Hoffman R, Braden G. Tenofovir-associated acute and chronic kidney disease: a case of multiple drug interactions. *Clin Infect Dis* 2006; 42:283–290.
70. Winston A, Amin J, Mallon P, Marriott D, Carr A, Cooper DA, Emery S. Minor changes in calculated creatinine clearance and anion-gap are associated with tenofovir disoproxil fumarate-containing highly active antiretroviral therapy. *HIV Med.* 2006; 7:105–111.
71. Ray AS, Cihlar T, Robinson KL, Tong L, Vela JE, Fuller MD, Wieman LM, Eisenberg EJ, Rhodes GR. Mechanism of active renal tubular efflux of tenofovir. *Antimicrob Agents Chemother* 2006; 50:3297–304.
72. Jullien V, Tréluyer JM, Rey E, Jaffray P, Krivine A, Moachon L, Lillo-Le Louet A, Lescoat A, Dupin N, Salmon D, Pons G, Urien S. Population pharmacokinetics of tenofovir in human immunodeficiency virus-infected patients taking highly active antiretroviral therapy. *Antimicrob Agents Chemother* 2005; 49:3361–3366.
73. Kiser JJ, Carten ML, Aquilante CL, Anderson PL, Wolfe P, King TM, Delahunty T, Bushman LR, Fletcher CV. The effect of lopinavir/ritonavir on the renal clearance of tenofovir in HIV-infected patients. *Clin Pharmacol Ther* 2008; 83:265–272.
74. Côté HC, Magil AB, Harris M, Scarth BJ, Gadawski I, Wang N, Yu E, Yip B, Zalunardo N, Werb R, Hogg R, Harrigan PR, Montaner JS. Exploring mitochondrial nephrotoxicity as a potential mechanism of kidney dysfunction among HIV-infected patients on highly active antiretroviral therapy. *Antivir Ther* 2006; 11:79–86.
75. Izzedine H, Hulot JS, Vittecoq D, Gallant JE, Staszewski S, Launay-Vacher V, Cheng A, Deray G; Study 903 Team. Long-term renal safety of tenofovir disoproxil fumarate in antiretroviral-naive HIV-1-infected patients. Data from a double-blind randomized active-controlled multicentre study. *Nephrol Dial Transplant* 2005; 20:743–746.
76. Izzedine H, Hulot JS, Villard E, Goyenvalle C, Dominguez S, Ghosn J, Valantin MA, Lechat P, Deray AG. Association between ABCC2 gene haplotypes and tenofovir-induced proximal tubulopathy. *J Infect Dis* 2006; 194: 1481–1491.
77. Kiser JJ, Aquilante CL, Anderson PL, King TM, Carten ML, Fletcher CV. Clinical and genetic determinants of intracellular tenofovir diphosphate concentrations in HIV-infected patients. *J Acquir Immune Defic Syndr* 2008; 47: 298–303.

Acute Kidney Injury in Oncological Disorders and Tumor Lysis Syndrome

6.14

Claudio Ronco

Core Messages

- Acute kidney injury (AKI) is a serious complication in cancer patients
- Multiple causes such as metabolic disturbances, tumor lysis syndrome, renal infiltration by malignant cells, sepsis, or drug-induced toxicity may lead to AKI in cancer patients
- In some cases, cancer treatment is the main cause of AKI

6.14.1 Introduction

Acute kidney injury (AKI) is a serious complication of cancer and constitutes a major source of morbidity and mortality. Moreover, AKI may preclude optimal cancer treatment by requiring a decrease in chemotherapy dosage or by contraindicating potentially curative treatment.

In general, the initial pathways leading to AKI in cancer patients are common to the development of AKI in other conditions. However, in cancer patients, AKI may also develop due to additional etiologies arising from treatment of cancer or the disease itself. Multiple causes leading to AKI in critically ill cancer patients are often present in combination (Table 6.14.1). Although some of these causes are common to the general intensive care unit (ICU) population (e.g., sepsis, shock, and aminoglycosides), some are related to the malignancy itself or to its treatment. A better knowledge of organ failure related to malignant disease may potentially lead to an improvement in these patients' outcomes.

6.14.2 Negative Impact of AKI on Prognosis for Cancer Patients

Although AKI is a frequent occurrence, little is known about its impact on morbidity and mortality in this population. Nevertheless, currently available data on AKI and its consequences suggest that AKI has the potential to substantially alter the outcome of patients with cancer and jeopardize their chances of receiving optimal cancer treatment and a potential cure. Data are scarce about global AKI related mortality rates in patients with cancer, and physicians have no choice but to rely on data generally extrapolated from studies on the general ICU population. The risk for AKI seems higher in critically ill cancer patients than in other critically ill patients. Among critically ill cancer patients, 12–49% experience AKI and 9–32% require renal replacement therapy during their ICU stay. In critically ill patients with cancer, acute renal dysfunction usually occurs in the context of multiple organ dysfunctions and is associated with mortality rates ranging from 72–85% when renal replacement therapy is needed [1–3].

Managing chemotherapy is delicate since the pharmacokinetics of most cytotoxic agents have not been adequately studied in patients with altered renal function. The necessary dose adjustments may therefore

C. Ronco
Department of Nephrology, Dialysis and Transplantation, S. Bortolo Hospital, Viale Rodolfi 37, 36100 Vicenza, Italy
e-mail; claudio.ronco@vlssvicenza.it

A. Jörres et al. (eds.), *Management of Acute Kidney Problems*,
DOI: 10.1007/978-3-540-69441-0_6.14, © Springer-Verlag Berlin Heidelberg 2010

Table 6.14.1 Causes of acute kidney injury in cancer patients

Prerenal failure
• Sepsis
• Extracellular dehydration (diarrhea, mucitis, vomiting)
• Sinusoidal obstruction syndrome (formerly called hepatic veno-occlusive disease)
• Drugs (e.g., calcineurin inhibitors, angiotensin-converting enzyme inhibitors, nonsteroidal antiinflammatory agents)
• Capillary-leak syndrome (IL-2)
Intrinsic failure
• Acute tubular necrosis
– Ischemia (shock, severe sepsis)
– Nephrotoxic agents (contrast agents, aminoglycosides, amphotericin, ifosfamide, cisplatin)
– Disseminated intravascular coagulation
– Intravascular hemolysis
• Acute interstitial nephritis
– Immunoallergic nephritis
– Pyelonephritis
– Cancer infiltration (e.g., lymphoma, metastasis)
– Nephrocalcinosis
• Vascular nephritis
– Thrombotic microangiopathy
– Vascular obstruction
• Glomerulonephritis
– Amyloidosis (AL, myeloma; AA, renal carcinoma, or Hodgkin's disease)
– Immunotactoid glomerulopathy
– Membranous glomerulonephritis (pulmonary, breast, or gastric carcinoma)
– IgA glomerulonephritis, focal glomerulosclerosis
Postrenal failure
• Intrarenal obstruction (e.g., urate crystals, light chain, acyclovir, methotrexate)
• Extrarenal obstruction (retroperitoneal fibrosis, ureteral, or bladder outlet obstruction)

be approximate, inappropriate, or even omitted. Consequently, patients may be underdosed, with a decreased chance of remission, or overdosed with an increased risk of systemic toxicity leading to potentially severe and unexpected complications in the course of chemotherapy. Furthermore, physicians will have to repeatedly adjust doses of supportive therapies, which carries some additional risk of treatment-related toxicity to the patient with potentially dramatic consequences. Underdosing drugs is also unacceptable; pain may not be relieved, immunosuppression becomes insufficient or anti-infective treatment ineffective especially in neutropenic patients, with the risk of emergence of antibiotic-resistant organisms.

6.14.3 Causes of AKI in Cancer Patients

6.14.3.1 Nephrotoxic Chemotherapy Agents

Currently, the five primary agents most commonly responsible for chemotherapy-induced nephrotoxicity are mitomycin C, gemcitabine, platinum compounds, methotrexate, and ifosfamide. These agents produce subacute or chronic renal insufficiency, except for cisplatin and methotrexate (when given in high doses), which can cause AKI. In addition, patients receiving repeated, high doses of bisphosphonates, such as pamidronate, can develop nephrotic syndrome and a form of collapsing glomerulopathy [4]. Most recently, zoledronate has been reported to produce acute tubular necrosis. Interferons also have the potential to cause nephrotoxicity, including the development of thrombotic microangiopathy. Pentostatin, a drug used to treat some hematological malignancies, can also produce AKI when used at doses higher than 4 mg/m^2. The nitrosoureas, semustine, carmustine, and lomustine, can lead to chronic renal insufficiency after prolonged use. Streptozotocin causes proximal tubular toxicity and in rare cases can lead to AKI [5–7].

6.14.3.1.1 Mitomycin C

Mitomycin C–induced nephrotoxicity has a significant mortality rate, with associated pulmonary and neurological manifestations being the most common signs of poor prognosis. Long-term treatment with mitomycin C can lead to progressive renal insufficiency and subacute kidney injury. Most cases of mitomycin C nephrotoxicity present as hemolytic uremic syndrome (HUS) caused by thrombotic microangiopathy. This is due to the direct toxic effects of mitomycin C on the endothelium. Patients experience gradual onset of anemia and thrombocytopenia, with high lactate dehydrogenase levels and undetectable haptoglobin levels. Progressive renal insufficiency is accompanied by increasing blood urea nitrogen (BUN) and creatinine levels, as well as severe hypertension. The urinalysis shows microhematuria and proteinuria. A clear-cut relationship exists between the cumulative dose of mitomycin C and risk of HUS: the incidence of nephrotoxicity rises markedly after total doses above 40–60 mg/m^2 are given over several months. Current practice therefore restricts mitomycin C treatment to 2–3 months. However, some patients are still seen who have received mitomycin C for 4 or 5 months, and these usually present with a slow rise in BUN and creatinine levels, hypertension, thrombocytopenia, and anemia [8–9].

6.14.3.1.2 Gemcitabine

HUS induced by gemcitabine is an increasingly common scenario [10]. Gemcitabine-induced HUS follows the same pathogenesis as that caused by mitomycin-C, and is accompanied by anemia, thrombocytopenia, hypertension, and raised BUN and creatinine levels. In these cases, the urinalysis also shows blood and protein. Unlike mitomycin C, there is no clear-cut relationship between the cumulative dose of gemcitabine and risk of HUS. However, most patients had received gemcitabine for at least 3–5 months before the onset of HUS. The hematological abnormalities often improve spontaneously, and renal function may also improve with time.

6.14.3.1.3 Platinum Compounds

Cisplatin is probably the most extensively studied nephrotoxic anticancer agent. Although direct tubular toxicity may cause AKI, cisplatin has also been associated with chronic dose-dependent reduction of the glomerular filtration rate (GFR) [11]. Cisplatin usually induces only mild renal failure that does not require dialysis, and patients usually recover renal function. Patients are usually nonoliguric and hyponatremia may be observed, which is probably related to a salt-losing nephropathy. Hypomagnesemia, which can be long-lasting, is much more common than AKI and is related to urinary magnesium losses. The maximum dose should not exceed 120 mg/m^2 body surface area, and renal dysfunction may require a dosage reduction. Repeated administration up to a cumulative dose of 850 mg was associated with a 9% reduction in GFR over a 5-year period, compared with a 40% reduction in patients given more than 850 mg [11]. The most widely used protective measure is saline infusion to induce solute diuresis. Amifostine (inorganic thiophosphate) has been found to be effective in preventing renal failure, even after repeated exposure. Therefore, the American Society of Clinical Oncology stated that amifostine (910 mg/m^2) may be considered for the prevention of nephrotoxicity in patients receiving cisplatin-based chemotherapy (grade of recommendation A) [12]. Stevens-Johnson syndrome and toxic epidermic necrolysis have been reported in patients given amifostine.

6.14.3.1.4 Methotrexate

Methotrexate is a widely used anticancer drug. High doses of methotrexate (w0 g/m^2) are used to treat osteosarcoma, Burkitt's lymphoma, and to facilitate brain penetration in central nervous lymphoma. These high doses are associated with a high risk of AKI due to precipitation of methotrexate or its metabolite, 7-OH methotrexate, within the renal tubules. When AKI occurs, the resulting decrease in methotrexate clearance leads to extrarenal toxicity (neutropenia, hepatitis, orointestinal mucositis, and/or neurological impairment). Thus, methotrexate toxicity may manifest as multiple organ failure [13]. Prevention of nephrotoxicity, together with methotrexate level monitoring, is crucial to prevent extrarenal methotrexate toxicity. During methotrexate infusion and elimination, fluids should be given to maintain a high urinary output and urinary alkalization should be performed to keep the urinary pH above 7.5. Rescue with folinic acid (50 mg four times a day) should be started 24 h after each high-dose methotrexate infusion, and serum methotrexate concentrations should be measured every day. Patients are considered at high risk for methotrexate toxicity when serum levels are greater than 15 µM/l at 24 h, 1.5 µM/l at 48 h, or 0. µM/l at 72 h. Unless absolutely necessary, patients should not be given medications that inhibit folate metabolism 5 (e.g., trimethoprim-sulfamethoxazole), exhibit intrinsic renal toxicity (e.g., nonsteroidal anti-inflammatory agents and contrast agents), or decrease the fraction of methotrexate bound to albumin (e.g., aspirin). When all these measures were taken, the incidence of AKI was 1.8% in patients with sarcoma [14]. Because methotrexate is highly protein bound, regular dialysis will not clear the drug efficiently and high doses of leucovorin are needed to prevent systemic toxicity. Hemoperfusion and daily high-flux hemodialysis have also been used to remove methotrexate [15–16]

Carboxypeptidase-G2 is a bacterial enzyme that converts methotrexate into an inactive metabolite (2,4-diamino-N10-methylpteroic acid), thus providing an alternative route of elimination. Its use lowered plasma methotrexate concentrations to nontoxic levels (by 98% in 15 min), although rebounds (with an increase no greater than 10% in plasma methotrexate concentrations) occurred in 60% of patients. Carboxypeptidase-G2 and high-dose leucovorin have been tested in patients with methotrexate intoxication and AKI, with similar results [17]. Therefore, no recommendations can be made concerning renal replacement therapy or carboxypeptidase-G2 in this population.

6.14.3.1.5 Alkylating Agents

The main anticancer agents responsible for hemorrhagic cystitis are alkylating agents, such as cyclophosphamide and ifosfamide. Maintaining a high urinary output and concomitantly administering the bladder epithelium protectant mesna virtually eliminated hemorrhagic cystitis related to the toxicity of anticancer agents. However, several other toxic effects of these drugs have been described, including emesis, alopecia, myelosuppression, and neurotoxicity. Moreover, ifosfamide has been associated with AKI or acute tubular dysfunction. Ifosfamide causes proximal tubular defects (Fanconi syndrome) and chronic renal insufficiency but rarely AKI [18]. Hypokalemia, hyperchloremic metabolic acidosis, hypophosphatemia (despite concomitant renal insufficiency), and renal glucosuria are characteristic of ifosfamide-induced nephrotoxicity. Fanconi syndrome should therefore be considered if a patient receiving ifosfamide develops phosphaturia, glucosuria with normal glucose levels, aminoaciduria, and a proximal tubular metabolic acidosis.

6.14.3.2 Urinary Tract Obstruction or Infiltration of The Kidney By Tumors

Cancer can damage the kidneys in a variety of ways. Renal compression or urinary tract obstruction by a tumor close to the kidney, such as an ovarian or bladder tumor, is frequently seen in cancer patients. Metastatic disease is also observed in the kidneys, but it is rare for lung, breast, or colon cancer metastases to cause AKI. Metastatic solid tumors usually result in AKI through involvement of.the lymph nodes, causing ureteric obstruction and vascular occlusion. Lymphomas, particularly high-grade lymphomas, and acute lymphoblastic leukemia often infiltrate the kidneys and, although usually clinically silent, can lead to AKI. Chemotherapy, however, usually produces a prompt improvement in tumor mass and infiltration. Unfortunately, a rapid decrease in tumor size can induce tumor lysis syndrome, which in turn increases the risk of AKI.

6.14.3.3 Tumor Lysis Syndrome

Tumor lysis syndrome (TLS) is a potentially life-threatening condition that frequently occurs following the rapid degradation of tumors. It is particularly common in patients with a high tumor burden and cellular turnover following cytotoxic therapy (including steroids in steroid-sensitive hematological malignancies), but can also occur spontaneously, especially in patients with lymphoid malignancies, due to rapid cell turnover and an increased rate of purine metabolism. The release of large volumes of intracellular contents into the systemic circulation leads to the accumulation of purine-derived metabolites such as uric acid, and of cytoplasmic ionic content (mainly phosphorous and potassium), overwhelming the renal excretion capacity. Renal dysfunction in TLS results principally from acute uric acid accumulation, hyperkalemia, hyperphosphatemia, and hypocalcemia. TLS-related AKI is believed to be the consequence of tubular obstruction through intratubular precipitation of several compounds, such as uric acid and xanthine, whose concentrations in urine exceed their solubility threshold. Although still not completely understood, the exact pathophysiology of TLS is probably more complex, resulting from the combination of several phenomena, including acute urate nephropathy and acute nephrocalcinosis, with one aggravating the other. Animal models have shown that hyperuricemia leads to urate nephropathy through both intratubular and parenchymatous uric acid precipitations, with further renal injury being caused by a granulomatous reaction and necrosis of the distal tubule epithelium. In addition to urate nephropathy, acute nephrocalcinosis caused by hyperphosphatemia can play a pivotal role in TLS-related AKI, with diffuse parenchymatous depositions of calcium–phosphate complexes, explaining why some patients will develop AKI despite adequate treatment of hyperuricemia. Finally, TLS-related AKI is frequently precipitated by volume depletion, which has repeatedly been observed as a major aggravating factor over the past 3 decades [18,]. TLS primarily occurs in patients with hematological malignancies, those with a high tumor burden and rapidly proliferating diseases being particularly at risk. The incidence of TLS varies between 20% and 50% in high-risk groups (Burkitt's lymphoma, aggressive non-Hodgkin's lymphoma, acute lymphoid leukemia, acute myeloid leukemia [mainly type 4 and 5], and chronic lymphocytic leukemia, mainly aggressive lymphoma and childhood acute lymphoid leukemia). With the exception of small cell lung cancer, neuroblastoma, and breast cancer, occurrence of AKI in patients with solid malignancies is rare. Prevention of TLS-related AKI is a cornerstone in the care of patients with hematological malignancies since the introduction of allopurinol, a xanthine oxidase inhibitor, and urate oxidase more than 25 years ago (in France and Italy). Allopurinol specifically inhibits xanthine oxidase which catalyzes the metabolism of xanthine to uric acid, thus preventing uric acid formation. Uric acid formation is therefore stopped, and the existing uric acid is slowly excreted over 2–3 days. However the uric acid load may not be eliminated in patients with impaired renal function, and allopurinol may also lead to accumulation of poorly soluble xanthine in the kidney, which is less soluble than uric acid, and occasional cases of xanthine nephropathy and calculi have been reported. In most mammals, uric acid is oxidized to allantoin via the urate oxidase enzymatic pathway. However, urate oxidase is not present in humans because of a nonsense mutation of the encoding gene [19]. Nonrecombinant urate oxidase can be extracted from *Aspergillus flavus* although the yield is low. Injection of urate oxidase reduces plasma uric acid levels by catalyzing the breakdown of uric acid to allantoin, which is a readily excreted metabolite that is 5–10 times more soluble than uric acid [20]. Nonrecombinant urate oxidase has been shown to reduce the risk of AKI from TLS when compared with allopurinol, and can reduce the need for dialysis in patients with aggressive lymphoma at high risk of TLS [19]. Less than 2% of patients who received urate oxidase-based therapy in France and Italy required dialysis, whereas 16–20% of patients who had allopurinol-based therapy in England and the United States needed dialysis. Nevertheless, approximately 4.5% of patients experience allergic reactions to this preparation, with serious events such as bronchospasm and hypoxemia being rare. Recently rasburicase, a recombinant form of urate oxide has been engineered [20]. Clinical studies have demonstrated that rasburicase is a highly effective drug for the prevention and treatment of TLS-related hyperuricemia [21].

Vigorous hydration increases elimination of uric acid and urinary alkalinization increases the solubility of uric acid in urine. However, the widespread use of urinary alkalinization is now a controversial practice as an alkaline urine pH favors calcium phosphate crystal precipitation. Sodium bicarbonate administration therefore increases the risk of acute nephrocalcinosis, which may contribute to rapid alteration of renal function. Rasburicase lowers uric acid levels so quickly that the need for urinary alkalization no longer exists, thereby reducing the risk of acute nephrocalcinosis.

6.14.3.4 Uric Acid

Uric acid can be considered a new potential factor in the pathogenesis of AKI. Uric acid can cause both mechanical obstruction due to intratubular precipitation of urate crystals, and direct glomerular and tubular cell toxicity as a result of endothelial dysfunction, oxidant stress, cell disruption, and platelet activation. Uric acid is also a mediator in the local inflammatory response and the progression to systemic inflammation, by stimulating production of cytokines (interleukin-1b

Table 6.14.2 Uric acid: a new pathogenetic factor in AKI

Tubular obstruction	Tissue damage	Acute inflammation
Uric acid crystals	Endothelial dysfunction (Nitric oxide (NO) mediated)	Correlates with circulating cytokines
Mechanical obstruction	Platelet activation	Stimulates synthesis of MCP1 (monocyte chemoattractant protein 1)
Tubular nephropathy	Oxidant stress and cell disruption	Stimulates monocyte production of interleukin-1b and tumor necrosis factor-α

and tumor necrosis factor-α) and chemoattractants (Table 6.14.2). Hyperuricemia is commonly associated with hypertension and elevated uric acid levels may be a risk factor for cardiovascular and renal disease [22]. Preclinical studies in the rat have shown that reducing uric acid levels prevented the development of hypertension, vascular disease, and renal disease. These findings raise the possibility that lowering uric acid levels may be similarly beneficial in reducing the incidence of cardiovascular disease in man [22].

6.14.3.5 AKI in Patients with Multiple Myeloma

Multiple myeloma is the hematological neoplasia most frequently associated with acute or chronic renal failure. Renal failure predates the diagnosis of myeloma in half of patients in whom renal dysfunction will occur, and develops in most of the remainder within 1 month of the diagnosis of myeloma. Of the 50% of multiple myeloma patients who experience renal impairment, 10% will require dialysis. Patients with multiple myeloma and renal failure have a significantly worse survival compared with all patients with multiple myeloma. Myeloma is characterized by the uncontrolled proliferation of a B cell clone. The aberrant B lymphocyte population secretes a paraprotein: either an intact monoclonal immunoglobulin, or a derived fragment (usually a light chain fragment). Production of this nephrotoxic paraprotein by the abnormal B cells is primarily responsible for AKI in multiple myeloma. The light chains are normally found together with heavy chains in the immunoglobulin molecule and detected by urine protein electrophoresis and immunofixation. Renally excreted light chains cause nephrotoxicity by two main mechanisms. Free light chains are directly nephrotoxic and they contribute also to the formation of casts in the distal tubules. Myeloma casts are composed principally of monoclonal light chains and Tamm-Horsfall glycoprotein (THP), a major constituent of normal urine synthesized exclusively by cells of the thick ascending limb of the loop of Henle. THP is able to form high-molecular-weight aggregates at high (but physiological) concentrations of sodium and calcium, and at low urinary pH. It is thus understandable why precipitating factors leading to an acute fall in GFR increase the intratubular factors of light chains and thus their precipitation. Renal dysfunction may develop in patients with multiple myeloma for a number of reasons. Specific mechanisms of renal injury include myeloma cast nephropathy, amyloid depositions, and glomerular infiltration with light chains. Frequently AKI is triggered by an event such as treatment with nonsteroidal antiinflammatory agents for pain control, use of intravenous contrast agents, development of hypercalcemia, volume depletion (diuretic treatment, septicemia), or cryoglobulinemia ssociated renal failure. Furthermore, many patients with myeloma have water, electrolyte, and acid–base disturbances, which may impact on renal load. In addition to the avoidance of precipitating factors, including the treatment of hyperuricemia, active management of AKI associated with multiple myeloma includes maintaining sufficient urine flow by volume expansion and administration of loop diuretics, and at times alkalinizing the urine. Reports also describe the benefits of plasma exchange with myeloma and renal failure. Furthermore, although response to chemotherapy is the major factor determining overall survival, recovery of renal function is also associated with improved survival. Specific treatment for multiple myeloma may improve renal function, and for those on chronic dialysis, improvement can be sufficient to allow discontinuation of dialysis. Nevertheless, chronic renal failure is common in many of the patients who present with severe alteration of renal function. Therefore, prevention of further renal damage is imperative and particular attention must be paid to the avoidance of nephrotoxic drugs and hypovolemia. The prognosis for patients with multiple myeloma with chronic renal failure has improved considerably over the past 2 decades, with more than 50% of patients recovering normal function with appropriate treatment. Renal failure alone should therefore no longer be considered to be an absolute contraindication to intensive treatment of myeloma if appropriate dose reduction is applied [23,24].

6.14.3.6 AKI in Patients Given Hematopoietic Progenitor Cell Transplants

AKI in patients receiving hematopoietic progenitor cell transplants (HPCTs) is extremely common, with studies reporting incidences ranging from 6.5% in some autologous HPCT series, 26–64% in most series, and up to 81% in allogeneic transplant settings [25]. Identified risk factors include allogeneic stem cell donor, veno-occlusive disease, and age greater than 25 years. AKI in patients undergoing HPCT is associated with severe prognosis. Mortality rates are primarily dependent on the severity of renal failure, the need for dialysis, and the type of transplant (autologous versus allogeneic).

Patients given HPCT are exposed to a number of factors that contribute to their worsening renal function. In the conditioning phase of transplantation, two rare conditions can cause rapidly progressive AKI. Firstly, acute TLS is a rare occurrence in patients undergoing a transplant, since candidates for HPCT are given routine prophylaxis for this syndrome. Secondly, marrow infusion toxicity is another complication that is now rare. AKI is caused by massive hemoglobinuria due to both intravascular hemolysis caused by dimethyl sulfoxide (DMSO) used as a cryoprotectant and free hemoglobin released by red cells disrupted during the thawing of the graft [25]. This complication has become infrequent since lower DMSO concentrations are now used, and marrow grafts are "rinsed" after thawing and prior to infusion.

During the month after transplant, patients are at risk of developing AKI from acute tubular necrosis of various etiologies discussed above. The most frequent of these is sepsis, followed by exposure to nephrotoxic drugs, especially antimicrobials, volume depletion caused by vomiting and diarrhea, and more rarely, hemorrhage. The role of cyclosporin A in the pathogenesis of AKI after allogeneic transplantation has been the subject of debate. The major dose-limiting toxicity of cyclosporin A is nephrotoxicity, while the AKI it induces usually responds to dose reduction and is reversible on drug discontinuation. The risk of acute cyclosporin A–related renal dysfunction, generally correlates with plasma concentrations, but above all, is markedly increased by concomitant administration of other nephrotoxic drugs, especially amphotericin B [26].

Most importantly in this time frame, most patients with severe forms of AKI have developed a complication known as veno-occlusive disease of the liver. Liver damage is a common complication of cytoreductive therapy and develops in 20–40% of bone marrow transplant (BMT) recipients [27].

The main site of liver damage in this setting is the hepatic sinusoid, and the resulting clinical syndrome is called SOS. Most cases of SOS are clinically obvious, with jaundice, liver pain, edema, and ascites. These clinical manifestations may be associated with AKI mimicking hepatorenal syndrome, with normal kidney histology. SOS can be classified as mild (clinically obvious, requires no treatment, and resolves completely), moderate (signs and symptoms require treatment but resolve completely), or severe (requires treatment but does not resolve before death or day 100). Severe SOS carries a bleak prognosis, with 98% mortality in a cohort study [28]. AKI, similar to any other organ failure, influences the prognosis of SOS. In patients with moderate SOS, diuretic therapy and/or analgesics are usually sufficient. In patients with severe SOS, the treatment rests on supportive care. No satisfactory specific treatments are available. Defibrotide (a polydeoxyribonucleotide with anti-ischemic, antithrombotic, and thrombolytic properties) produced promising results in an open-label study but has not yet been investigated in randomized studies. Thrombolytic therapy is of uncertain efficacy and carries a risk of fatal bleeding.

6.14.3.7 Viral Infections

Viral infections are an emergent cause of AKI in BMT patients. Several studies confirm that AKI is associated with adenovirus, polyomavirus (BK virus or JC virus), and simian polyomavirus. The well-documented association between the BK virus and hemorrhagic cystitis may explain not only the high incidence of hemorrhagic cystitis after BMT (20–25%), but also the occurrence of nephropathy. The simian 40 virus was recently found in association with AKI and hemorrhagic cystitis [29]. Finally, adenovirus is associated with disseminated infections, encephalitis, pneumonitis, and AKI. To allow either a prompt reduction in immunosuppression or the initiation of antiviral therapy, the diagnosis of adenoviral disease must be made early. Polymerase chain reaction testing or enzyme-linked immunosorbent assay may help to achieve this goal [29].

6.14.4 Conclusions

AKI is a serious complication in cancer patients that causes additional morbidity and mortality. It results from various causes, including metabolic disturbances, renal infiltration by malignant cells, sepsis, and drug-induced toxicity. Prevention of AKI is mandatory in critically ill cancer patients. Protecting against AKI involves identifying those patients most at risk and, where applicable, timely intervention with preventive strategies. AKI from a number of etiologies, particularly contrast-agent nephropathy and TLS, can be avoided. Fluid expansion and uricolytic treatment in patients with a high risk of acute TLS, prevention of contrast nephropathy, elimination of nephrotoxic drugs in high-risk patients, and monitoring of serum methotrexate concentrations are among the measures that may reduce the risk of AKI. Further studies are needed to improve the prognosis of these patients, to determine optimal treatments, and to identify additional causative factors. In conclusion, a multidisciplinary approach is needed to ensure adequate assessment, appropriate preventive measures, and early intervention to reduce the incidence of life-threatening AKI in cancer patients

6.14.5 Take Home Pearls

- Acute kidney injury in cancer patients may result from metabolic disturbances, tumor lysis syndrome, renal infiltration by malignant cells, sepsis, or drug-induced toxicity.
- In patients with a high risk of acute tumor lysis syndrome, fluid expansion and uricolytic treatment are among the key measures for prevention of AKI.
- A multidisciplinary approach is required to ensure adequate assessment, appropriate preventive measures, and early interventions to reduce the incidence of AKI in cancer patients.

References

1. Benoit DD, Depuydt PO, Vandewoude KH, Offner FC, Boterberg T, De Cock CA, Noens LA, Janssens AM, Decruyenaere JM: Outcome in critically ill medical patients treated with renal replacement therapy for Acute Kidney Injury: comparison between patients with and those without haematological malignancies. *Nephrol Dial Transplant* 2005; 20:552–558.
2. Darmon M, Thiery G, Ciroldi M, de Miranda S, Galicier L, Raffoux E, Le Gall JR, Schlemmer B, Azoulay E: Intensive care in patients with newly diagnosed malignancies and a need for cancer chemotherapy. *Crit Care Med* 2005; 33:2488–2493.
3. Bagshaw SM, Laupland KB, Doig CJ, Mortis G, Fick GH, Mucenski M, Godinez-Luna T, Svenson LW, Rosenal T: Prognosis for long-term survival and renal recovery in critically ill patients with severe Acute Kidney Injury: a population-based study. *Crit Care* 2005; 9:R700–R709.
4. Markowitz GS, Appel GB, Fine PL, Fenves AZ, Loon NR, Jagannath S, et al. Collapsing focal segmental glomerulosclerosis following treatment with high-dose pamidronate. *J Am Soc Nephrol*. 2001; 12:1164–1172.
5. Markowitz GS, Fine PL, Stack JI, Kunis CL, Radhakrishnan J, Palecki W, et al. Toxic acute tubular necrosis following treatment with zoledronate (Zometa). *Kidney Int*. 2003; 64:281–289.
6. Quesada JR, Talpaz M, Rios A, Kurzrock R, Gutterman JU. Clinical toxicity of interferons in cancer patients: a review. *J Clin Oncol*. 1986; 4:234–243.
7. Zuber J, Martinez F, Droz D, Oksenhendler E, Legendre C. Alpha-interferon-associated thrombotic microangiopathy: a clinicopathologic study of 8 patients and review of the literature. *Medicine (Baltimore)*. 2002; 81:321–331.
8. Cantrell JE, Jr., Phillips TM, Schein PS. Carcinomaassociated hemolytic-uremic syndrome: a complication of mitomycin C chemotherapy. *J Clin Oncol*. 1985; 3:723–734.
9. Valavaara R, Nordman E. Renal complications of mitomycin C therapy with special reference to the total dose. *Cancer*. 1985; 55:47–50.
10. Fung MC, Storniolo AM, Nguyen B, Arning M, Brookfield W, Vigil J. A review of hemolytic uremic syndrome in patients treated with gemcitabine therapy. *Cancer*. 1999; 85:2023–2032.
11. Arany I, Safirstein RL: Cisplatin nephrotoxicity. *Semin Nephrol* 2003; 23:460–464.
12. Schuchter LM, Hensley ML, Meropol NJ, Winer EP, American Society of Clinical Oncology Chemotherapy and Radiotherapy Expert Panel: 2002 update of recommendations for the use of chemotherapy and radiotherapy protectants: clinical practice guidelines of the American Society of Clinical Oncology. *J Clin Oncol* 2002; 20:2895–2903.
13. Arany I, Safirstein RL: Cisplatin nephrotoxicity. *Semin Nephrol* 2003; 23:460–464.
14. Widemann BC, Balis FM, Kempf-Bielack B, Bielack S, Pratt CB, Ferrari S, Bacci G, Craft AW, Adamson PC: High-dose methotrexate- induced nephrotoxicity in patients with osteosarcoma. *Cancer* 2004; 100:2222–2232.
15. Relling MV, Stapleton FB, Ochs J, Jones DP, Meyer W, Wainer IW, et al. Removal of methotrexate, leucovorin, and their metabolites by combined hemodialysis and hemoperfusion. *Cancer*. 1988; 62:884–888.
16. Wall SM, Johansen MJ, Molony DA, DuBose TD, Jr., Jaffe N, Madden T. Effective clearance of methotrexate using high-flux hemodialysis membranes. *Am J Kidney Dis*. 1996; 28: 846–854.
17. Buchen S, Ngampolo D, Melton RG, Hasan C, Zoubek A, Henze G, Bode U, Fleischhack G: Carboxypeptidase G2 rescue in patients with methotrexate intoxication and renal failure. *Br J Cancer* 2005; 92:480–487.

18. Suarez A, McDowell H, Niaudet P, Comoy E, Flamant F: Longterm follow-up of ifosfamide renal toxicity in children treated for malignant mesenchymal tumors: an International Society of Pediatric Oncology report. *J Clin Oncol* 1991; 9:2177–2182.
19. Andreoli SP, Clark JH, Mcguire WA, Bergstein JM. Purine excretion during tumour lysis in children with acute lymphocytic leukaemia receiving allopurinol: relationship to Acute Kidney Injury. *J Pediatr*. 1986; 109:292–298.
20. Brogard JM, Coumaros D, Franckhauser J, Stahl A, Stahl J. Enzymatic uricolysis: a study of the effect of a fungal urate-oxydase. *Rev Eur Etud Clin Biol*. 1972; 17:890–895.
21. Mahmoud HH, Leverger G, Patte C, Harvey E, Lascombes F. Advances in the management of malignancy-associated hyperuricaemia. *Br J Cancer*. 1998; 77:18–20.
22. Verdecchia P, Schillaci G, Reboldi GP, Santeusanio F, Porcellati C, Brunetti P. Relation between serum uric acid and risk of cardiovascular disease in essential hypertension: the PIUMA Study. *Hypertension*. 2000; 36:1072–1078.
23. Johnson WJ, Kyle RA, Pineda AA, O'Brien PC, Holley KE. Treatment of renal failure associated with multiple myeloma. Plasmapheresis, hemodialysis, and chemotherapy. *Arch Intern Med*. 1990; 150:863–869.
24. Alexanian R, Barlogie B, Dixon D. Renal failure in multiple myeloma. *Arch Intern Med*. 1990; 150:1693–1695.
25. Reiter E, Kalhs P, Keil F, Rabitsch W, Gisslinger H, Mayer G, et al. Effect of high-dose melphalan and peripheral blood stem cell transplantation on renal function in patients with multiple myeloma and renal insufficiency: a case report and review of the literature. *Ann Hematol*. 1999; 78:189–191.
26. Smith DM, Weisenburger DD, Bierman P, Kessinger A, Vaughan WP, Armitage JO. Acute Kidney Injury associated with autologous bone marrow transplantation. *Bone Marrow Transplant*. 1987; 2:195–210.
27. Kennedy MS, Deeg HJ, Siegel M, Crowley JJ, Storb R, Thomas ED. Acute renal toxicity with combined use of amphotericin B and cyclosporine after marrow transplantation. *Transplantation*. 1983; 35:211–215.
28. McDonald GB, Hinds MS, Fisher LD, Schoch HG, Wolford JL, Banaji M, Hardin BJ, Shulman HM, Clift RA: Veno-occlusive disease of the liver and multiorgan failure after bone marrow transplantation: a cohort study of 355 patients. *Ann Intern Med* 1993; 118:255–267.
29. Mori K, Yoshihara T, Nishimura Y, Uchida M, Katsura K, Kawase Y, Hatano I, Ishida H, Chiyonobu T, Kasubuchi Y, et al.: AKI due to adenovirus-associated obstructive uropathy and necrotizing tubulointerstitial nephritis in a bone marrow transplant recipient. *Bone Marrow Transplant* 2003; 31: 1173–1176.

Kidney Failure Following Cardiovascular Surgery

6.15

Michael Haase and Anja Haase-Fielitz

Core Messages

- Acute kidney injury (AKI) following cardiovascular surgery is a common and serious condition with substantial morbidity and mortality.
- Several patient- and procedure-related risk factors for the development of AKI have been identified.
- The use of conventional renal markers, such as serum creatinine, delays the diagnosis of postoperative AKI, however, novel early and specific renal biomarkers are emerging.
- The perioperative avoidance of nephrotoxic agents (e.g., contrast media, nonsteroidal antiinflammatory drugs, aprotinin) and hypovolemia, and the cautious use of packed red blood cells are of importance.
- To date, there is no internationally acknowledged consensus with regard to any specific pharmacologic intervention to prevent AKI after cardiovascular surgery using cardiopulmonary bypass (CPB).
- Treatment of established AKI after CPB attempts to prevent further damage to the kidney and remains largely supportive until renal function recovers.

M. Haase (✉)
Department of Nephrology and Intensive Care Medicine, Charité Campus Virchow-Klinikum, 13343 Berlin, Germany
e-mail: michael.haase@charite.de

6.15.1 Introduction

Cardiovascular surgery with the use of cardiopulmonary bypass (CPB) is a common and life-saving procedure. It is the most frequent major surgical procedure performed in hospitals worldwide, with well over one million operations undertaken each year [1]. Surgical revascularization is associated with improved long-term outcomes compared with percutaneous stenting in most subgroups of patients with multivessel coronary artery disease [2]. During the last few years, a rising number of cardiac surgical procedures has been reported by the American Heart Association (about 600,000 in 2005), mostly due to increasing numbers of older patients who are considered "high risk" secondary to substantial comorbidities [3]. Overall, despite advances in cardiovascular surgical techniques, intensive care, and renal replacement therapy (RRT), mortality and morbidity associated with kidney failure have not markedly changed in the last decade [3]. After cardiovascular surgery, major morbidities known to be primary contributors to perioperative mortality are cardiac failure, respiratory failure, the need for mediastinal (re)exploration, and kidney failure [4].

6.15.2 Epidemiology and Outcome

Acute kidney injury (AKI), previously referred to as acute renal failure or kidney failure, is a frequent and serious complication encountered in 1–5% of patients [5, 6] requiring RRT, or 20–50% of patients [7–11] developing acute increases in serum creatinine after CPB, depending on the definition used, premorbidities of the populations investigated, and procedures performed. Development of RRT-dependent AKI was

A. Jörres et al. (eds.), *Management of Acute Kidney Problems*,
DOI: 10.1007/978-3-540-69441-0_6.15, © Springer-Verlag Berlin Heidelberg 2010

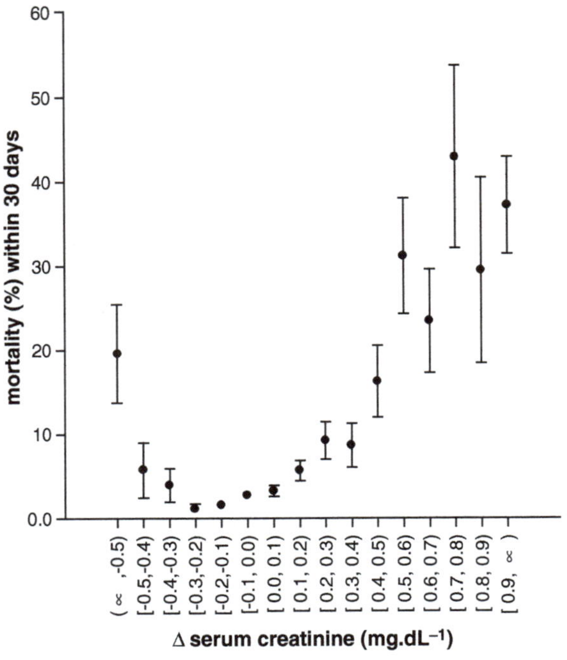

Fig. 6.15.1 Distribution of mortality rates according to delta creatinine intervals (From [15])

identified as the strongest risk factor for death with an odds ratio of 7.9 in this setting [12]. Mortality associated with the development of AKI is as high as 50–80% in some studies [12, 13] but likely averages 15–30% [14] depending on postoperative period studied. Even minimal postoperative changes in serum creatinine are associated with a substantial and progressive decrease in hospital (Fig. 6.15.1) [14–17] and long-term [18–20] survival. In a prospective cohort study of 4,118 cardiac surgical patients, every 8.8 μmol/l (0.1mg/dl) increase in plasma creatinine was associated with an increase in mortality from about 3% to 4.5%, then 9%, 12% and 16% [15]. AKI after CPB is associated with numerous adverse outcomes including prolonged length of stay in the intensive care unit and in hospital. In addition, patients developing AKI experience higher readmission rates to the hospital and lower quality of life [6, 18, 21].

Simultaneously to the number of procedures performed, the incidence of AKI after cardiac surgery has increased over time. In two recent retrospective analyses, the proportion of patients developing AKI or RRT-dependent AKI decreased and mortality rates declined significantly over time [13, 22]. However, this might be explained, at least in part, by a shift in case mix including patients with less severe AKI, in more sensitive diagnostic criteria for AKI, and the earlier timing of commencing RRT [23].

Overall, the onset of AKI portends a poor prognosis, not only from the loss of kidney function, but also from associated life-threatening complications including sepsis, gastrointestinal hemorrhage, and central nervous system dysfunction [24, 25].

6.15.3 Risk Factors

Multiple risk factors for AKI after CPB have been identified, mostly in multicenter retrospective observational trials. The majority of studies defined risk factors for development of RRT-dependent AKI [26]. Several patient- and procedure-related factors have been repeatedly associated with an increased risk for AKI [3] (Table 6.15.1).

6.15.3.1 Patient-Related Risk Factors

Impaired preoperative renal function is one of the most important predictors of postoperative AKI. A progressive relationship between preoperative serum creatinine concentration and risk of postoperative AKI has

Table 6.15.1 Important risk factors associated with acute kidney injury (AKI) after cardiovascular surgery

Patient-related risk factors for AKI	Procedure-related risk factors for AKI
Preoperative chronic renal impairment	Type of cardiovascular surgery
Age	Duration of cardiopulmonary bypass/cross-clamp
Female sex	Number and age of red blood cells transfused
Chronic obstructive pulmonary disease	
Peripheral vascular disease	
Reduced left ventricular function	
Cardiogenic shock	
Emergency surgery	
Radiocontrast exposure	
Body mass index	
Genetic risk	

Source: Adapted from [3]

been found [5, 27–30]. The risk for postoperative RRT may be increased by up to ten times if preoperative glomerular filtration rate (GFR) is less than 30 ml/min [31]. Other important risk factors include age, chronic obstructive pulmonary disease, peripheral vascular disease, reduced left ventricular function, diabetes mellitus, particularly when insulin-dependent, cardiogenic shock, and need for emergency cardiac surgery [3, 30, 31]. Reoperation carries a higher risk than primary cardiovascular surgery [44]. Female sex is an independent risk factor for adverse renal outcomes after open heart surgery, particularly in women at younger age (< 60 years) [27, 32, 33]. The risk of female sex risk is not explained by illness severity, presurgery health status, and smaller coronary artery diameter [34], or by longer delays for the procedure [35]. The influence of race is less clear [27, 31].

Beside established risk factors, pulse pressure is independently associated with adverse renal outcome. Patients with pulse pressure hypertension > 80 mm Hg were three times more likely to die a renal-related death compared with those without [30]. Extreme obese and malnourished patients have an independently higher incidence of AKI and mortality [36, 37]. Cardiac catheterization performed within five days before operation is a significant risk factor for AKI after CPB [38].

Clinical predictors and biochemical markers identified for the development of AKI only explain a part of this individual risk. There is evidence that several genetic polymorphisms accounting for CPB-associated AKI involve genes, which participate in the control of inflammatory or vasomotor processes [7, 39–43].

6.15.3.2 *Procedure-Related Risk Factors*

In addition, there are several factors specifically related to the surgical procedure itself such as type of surgery, use and duration of CPB and aortic cross-clamp, and blood transfusion (Table 6.15.1). Valve replacement and simultaneous valve surgery and coronary artery revascularization involve a greater risk for AKI than coronary artery revascularization or valve repair alone [28, 31, 44]. This might be, at least in part, related to the duration of CPB, as there is evidence that a longer duration of CPB is associated with an increased likelihood of AKI [5, 45–47]. Moreover, correction of anemia in cardiovascular surgical patients by red blood cell transfusion may be associated with incrementally increased risk for AKI [48]. An independent association between duration of red blood cell storage and AKI and in-hospital mortality was observed [49, 50].

Clinical scoring systems to predict the risk for RRT-dependent AKI weighting the most important patient- and procedure-related risk factors described have been developed [31, 44, 45]. Patients identified at increased risk, may be suitable for renal protection strategies. The risk score developed by Thakar et al. includes preoperative variables thereby making it preoperatively readily available and appears to be of good predictive value [44].

6.15.4 Pathomechanisms

Several general mechanisms have been implicated in the pathogenesis of cardiovascular surgery–associated AKI. Available evidence suggests that they are likely to involve the following mechanisms, processes, factors, and pathways [52]:

1. Toxins
2. Metabolic factors
3. Ischemia-reperfusion
4. Neurohormonal activation
5. Inflammation
6. Oxidative stress

Such major causes may amplify their pathophysiologic renal effects and are typically classified according to their timely occurrence (Table 6.15.2).

6.15.4.1 *Preoperative Events*

Radiocontrast-induced nephropathy represents a common type of *toxin-induced AKI*. Mechanisms may act in concert in causing radiocontrast-induced nephropathy, such as hypoxia, apoptosis, oxidative stress perturbed renal medullary hemodynamics, and direct toxic effects of contrast media on renal cells [51]. The use of nonsteroidal antiinflammatory drugs (NSAIDs), angiotensin-converting enzyme (ACE) inhibitors and angiotensin II receptor 1 blockers (ARBs) can impair the autoregulation of renal blood flow and such cause preoperative sublethal renal injury in selected patients at risk [52]. Antimicrobials such as aminoglycoside and

Table 6.15.2 Important pathomechanisms contributing to acute kidney injury (AKI) after cardiovascular surgery

Preoperative events	Intraoperative events	Postoperative events
AKI prior to cardiovascular surgery	Nephrotoxins	Nephrotoxins
Nephrotoxins	Free hemoglobin	Myoglobin
Radiocontrast media	Aprotinin	NSAID
NSAID	Aminoglycosides, e.g., gentamicin	ACE-inhibitors/ARB
ACE inhibitors / ARBs	Ischemia-reperfusion	Ischemia-reperfusion
Ischemia-reperfusion	Hypotension	Hypovolemia
Cardiogenic shock	Vasopressors	SIRS
Noncardiogenic hypotension	Duration of CPB	Packed red blood cells
SIRS	Emboli	Hyperglycemia
Activated sympathetic nervous system, e.g., chronic heart failure	Packed red blood cells	
	CPB-induced inflammation	

AKI, acute kidney injury; NSAID, nonsteroidal antiinflammatory drugs; angiotensin converting enzyme (ACE); ARB, angiotensin II receptor1 blockers; CPB, cardiopulmonary bypass; SIRS, systemic inflammatory response syndrome

amphotericin can cause interstitial nephropathy or direct injury [53].

Causes of *renal ischemia* are renal arterial embolism as a complication of cardiac catheterization or spontaneously released emboli from infected valve, cardiogenic shock, or noncardiogenic hypotension as in hypovolemia, overdose of antihypertensive medication, septic endocarditis, or allergic reaction to preoperatively given drugs [52].

Preoperatively, *neurohormonal activation* occurs most commonly in the setting of chronic heart failure. Low cardiac output syndrome leads to elevated sympathetic nervous system activation, activated renin-angiotensin-aldosterone system and increased levels of plasma catecholamines and vasopressin contributing to vasoconstriction, reduced glomerular filtration, and increased sodium and water retention [52], and further promotes tubular ischemia and injury.

Inflammation is relevant in patients undergoing cardiovascular surgery presenting with atherosclerotic heart disease and impaired endothelial function and in patients with infection, e.g., endocarditis.

Oxidative stress can harm the renal tubular cell and is caused by nephrotoxic medication (e.g. gentamicin) and radiocontrast agents.

6.15.4.2 Intraoperative Events

The intraoperative period is a critical time when patients are exposed to anesthesia and CPB [3].

Major potential mechanisms of *ischemic renal injury* are related to hemodynamic instability caused by hypotension or reduced cardiac output due to the induction of anesthesia, the initiation of mechanical ventilation, blood loss, especially for reoperations, release of emboli from atherosclerotic plaques of the aorta or from atrial or ventricular thrombi or air embolism after puncture of the great vessels for CPB and potential aortic dissection occluding renal artery exits. Cardiopulmonary bypass itself is associated with substantial hemodynamic changes – particularly, its initiation and its weaning are periods of hemodynamic instability and renal hypoperfusion. Cardioplegia is applied to provide the best operative conditions possible for the surgeon while the CPB machine takes over circulation and oxygenation. If flow from the pump is maintained at the normal level of cardiac output (2.2–2.4 L min/m^2), mean arterial pressure may be lower than normal due to substantial CPB-induced vasodilatation. Recent studies in cardiac surgical patients who had normal preoperative renal function found that lower CPB flows and longer periods of CPB at mean arterial pressures less than 60 mmHg were associated with postoperative AKI [46, 54]. In addition, the duration of CPB is associated with AKI [5, 45–47]. This may relate to the generation of *inflammatory and oxidative mediators* due to contact of leukocytes with foreign body material of the oxygenation membrane, ischemia-reperfusion injury, operative trauma, and the release of free hemoglobin. Subsequently, a systemic inflammatory response syndrome and multiorgan injury including AKI may develop. During CPB, neutrophils, platelets, and vascular endothelial cells are activated with up-regulation of adhesion molecules such as CD11b and CD41 [55]. These events lead to amplification of renal cytotoxic oxygen-derived free radicals, proteases, cytokines, and chemokines [3].

In regard to hypoperfusion, in almost all centers, CPB is accomplished using nonpulsatile pumps. No clear advantage was found for the use of more elaborate technique of pulsatile CPB [56]. Most centers employ mild to moderate hypothermia (26–34°C) during CPB to provide protection against hypoperfusion-related ischemia. If severe hypotension in previously normotensive patients occurs or renal atherosclerotic disease is recognized, arterial perfusion pressure can be elevated using vasopressors.

Free hemoglobin in the serum scavenges endothelium-derived nitric oxide, and after glomerular filtration free urine hemoglobin releases iron, which is involved in the generation of *radical oxygen species*. Free urine hemoglobin may cause occlusion of renal tubules with hemoglobin casts contributing to necrosis of tubular cells [57]. However, no studies have clearly linked free hemoglobin or free iron directly to AKI in humans.

Prothrombotic drugs such as aprotinin are potential renal *toxins*. Unlike amino caproic and tranexamic acid, aprotinin – after free glomerular passage – binds selectively to the brush border of the proximal tubule membrane, inhibiting prostaglandin and renin synthesis, prostasin secretion, and bradykinin release and focal tubular necrosis ensues [58]. Aprotinin also may instigate macrovascular or microvascular thrombosis [59].

Neurohormonal factors such as elevated plasma levels of catecholamines and vasopressin may contribute to a reduction in renal blood flow and further promote renal injury during CPB.

6.15.4.3 Postoperative Events

In addition to *toxins* mentioned above, myoglobin released through surgical muscle injury can significantly contribute to the development of AKI in the postoperative period [60]. *Metabolic factors* such as increased blood glucose level may contribute to renal injury [61]. During Intensive Care stay, cardiogenic shock and noncardiogenic hypotension, e.g., from sepsis, typically sternal wound infection, and on the normal ward of care arrhythmia, e.g., atrial fibrillation, may be associated with *ischemia-reperfusion* and *inflammatory response* causing AKI.

6.15.4.4 Diagnosis

In clinical practice, the diagnosis of AKI is based on an increase in serum creatinine and decrease in urine output, with the latter being highly variable due to the use of fluid infusion and loop diuretics [62, 63]. Serum creatinine is affected by several non-renal factors and is considered a late indicator of AKI as it typically increases only when the GFR has decreased to < 50% of normal [64]. Substantial rises in serum creatinine often occur as late as 48–72 h after the initial injurious event to the kidney [65]. Early diagnosis of AKI may however contribute to timely intervention aimed at improving patient outcome [66]. In response to this problem, several biomarkers have been recently investigated as possible tools for the early detection of AKI. Among these biomarkers particularly promising results have been reported for neutrophil gelatinase-associated lipocalin (NGAL), urine interleukin 18 (IL-18), and cystatin C [64, 67–71]. Serum and urine NGAL and urine IL-18 measured immediately after surgery have been found to be of good predictive value for AKI in children undergoing cardiac surgery [67, 68]. Adult patients differ from pediatric patients in many ways including diminished renal reserve and the presence of age-related comorbidities. Therefore, observations made in children may not apply to adult patients. In a recent prospective cohort study of 100 adult cardiac surgical patients, serum NGAL and serum cystatin C measured on arrival in the intensive care unit were of good value in the prediction of AKI [69]. For urine IL-18, however, its initial value in children undergoing cardiac surgery for congenital heart disease could not be confirmed in an adult cohort of cardiac surgical patients [72]. In adults, urine IL-18 may rather be a nonspecific marker of CPB-associated inflammation and not a specific marker for AKI [72].

Future studies are supposed to confirm or refute preliminary results on renal biomarkers and to investigate a combination of serum and urine markers to further improve the early diagnosis of CPB-associated AKI.

6.15.5 Prevention

Multiple causes of CPB-associated AKI have been proposed, including ischemia-reperfusion, generation of reactive oxygen species, hemolysis, and activation of inflammatory pathways. In addition, the identification of several patient- and procedure-related risk factors of AKI after cardiovascular surgery has led to the evaluation of numerous preventive strategies [73]. Most of these strategies aim at avoidance of renal vasoconstriction or improvement of renal blood flow. Others target the inflammatory reaction or generation of reactive oxygen species. Such strategies include variation in hemodynamic management of patients, pharmacologic, and nonpharmacologic measures. Patients enrolled into such trials include those at low, intermediate, and high risk for AKI. Regenerative strategies remain to be investigated.

6.15.5.1 Hemodynamic Strategies

Hemodynamic management is of importance in cardiovascular surgery patients – with the majority of patients developing hemodynamic instability at some stage – and includes perioperative assessment and maintenance of adequate cardiac output, perfusion pressure, and oxygen delivery. To date, monitoring techniques used in clinical practice are pulmonary artery catheter and transesophageal echocardiography.

The avoidance of hypovolemia is of significance. Particularly, in cardiovascular surgery patients presenting with preoperative chronic renal impairment, prehydration during the 12 h prior to surgery, may reduce AKI and the need for RRT [74]. This remains, however, to be confirmed in larger trials. Intraoperatively and postoperatively, the hemodynamic response (stroke volume, cardiac output) to volume challenge may guide fluid therapy. If a positive response results directly after a fluid challenge, more fluid substitution appears to be required as long as cardiac output increases. If cardiac output fails to increase after fluid challenge further application of fluids may not be beneficial. A fall in cardiac output suggests that cardiac efficiency is decreasing [73].

A grossly positive fluid balance can be harmful and is associated with adverse outcomes [75]. In general, early and appropriate goal-directed fluid therapy aiming at improved hemodynamics contributes to a degree of fluid overload in most patients. In patients with AKI and/or oliguria, a positive fluid balance is almost universal. No study has examined the impact of postoperative fluid balance on clinical outcomes in cardiovascular surgery patients with AKI. However, a secondary analysis of the SOAP (Sepsis Occurrence in Acutely Ill Patients) study shows that there is an independent association between mortality and positive fluid balance in a cohort of critically ill patients with AKI [76]. Therefore, a positive fluid balance has recently been suggested as biomarker of critical illness [77]. If fluid substitution alone is not sufficient, different approaches including inotrope agents (e.g., dobutamine, milrinone), vasopressors (e.g., norepinephrine, vasopressin), or a combination of both have been suggested to maximize oxygen delivery [78, 79]. These issues need to be addressed in future studies in cardiovascular patients where hemodynamic monitoring is critical and where grossly positive fluid balances of several liters up to many days after surgery may occur.

6.15.5.2 Pharmacologic Strategies

Pharmacologic renoprotective strategies in the setting of cardiovascular surgery include the avoidance or cautious dosing of red blood cells, particularly when priorly stored for long-term [48–50]. Medications such as NSAIDs and other nephrotoxic agents should be discontinued. Whether ACE inhibitors and ARBs should be ceased before cardiovascular surgery and also the timing of their restart after surgery is a matter of controversy [80]. However, the controversy regarding the safety of aprotinin [81–84] has recently come to an end after an early termination of a large randomized controlled trial (RCT) which showed increased all-cause mortality in the aprotinin group compared with tranexamic acid or amino caproic acid [85]. The marketing of aprotinin has been suspended by the pharmaceutical company.

Increased blood glucose level may contribute to renal injury and its control appears to reduce the incidence of AKI and the need for RRT, as shown in a cohort of critically ill patients with predominantly postcardiac surgery patients [61].

In addition, numerous pharmacologic interventions have been tested in RCTs of their nephroprotective effect in cardiovascular surgery patients [86–119]. There are no known drugs that have demonstrated renal protection conclusively. Table 6.15.3 summarizes results of RCTs using pharmacologic interventions to prevent AKI after cardiovascular surgery during the last 2 decades. Such drugs might exert multiple actions and aim at increasing natriuresis (e.g., furosemide, atrial, and brain natriuretic peptide), increasing renal blood flow, (e.g., dopamine, fenoldopam, pentoxifylline, and theophylline – a phosphodiesterase inhibitor that blocks neutrophils), inhibiting inflammatory or oxidative stress, (e.g., dexamethasone, sodium bicarbonate [11], N-acetylcysteine [10] – a thiol group containing antioxidant and vasodilator) and inhibiting renal vasoconstriction induced for example by sympathetic nervous system activation, (e.g., clonidine). The failure of many of these interventions to reliably prevent AKI after CPB may be related in part to its more complex pathophysiology than originally considered with only single pathways targeted unlikely to succeed, uncertain timing to commence and end the intervention, no clear evidence for dosing of specific drugs and due to the fact that most RCTs to date in this setting were underpowered.

Despite an increasing number of reports of renal protective properties from fenoldopam, two RCTs found this drug to be associated with significant hypotension [9, 95] and one with hemolysis [9]. Nevertheless, a recent meta-analysis provides evidence that fenoldopam may confer significant benefits in preventing renal replacement therapy and reducing mortality in patients undergoing cardiovascular surgery despite increased incidence of hypotension [120].

In two recent RCTs, the perioperative use of nesiritide was associated with less renal injury [115, 116] and in one of them with reduced mortality [116]. On the other hand, nesiritide, investigated in the setting of congestive heart failure, was repeatedly found not to improve renal function [121, 122] and in a meta-analysis of >850 patients, it was associated with increased short-term risk of death [123].

Basing on renal protective effect and safety, some of the preventive interventions described deserve further investigation in large multicenter studies sufficiently powered for important patient outcomes such as need for renal replacement therapy, length of stay in hospital, and mortality. Until then, there is no internationally acknowledged consensus with regard to any pharmacologic intervention to prevent AKI after CPB.

6.15.5.3 Nonpharmacologic Strategies

Nonpharmacologic renoprotective strategies in the setting of cardiovascular surgery include measures associated with the procedure of CPB and preemptive RRT. Cardiac catheterization performed during the immediate preoperative period is a significant risk factor for AKI after CPB [38] and should therefore be avoided, whenever possible.

First of all, given the putative role of CPB in the development of AKI, it has been postulated that off-pump coronary artery bypass surgery reduces the risk of renal injury. Several studies demonstrated a significant reduction of AKI with the use of off-pump surgery on the beating heart [124–128]. Independent from the number of coronary artery grafts, off-pump surgery appears to be associated with reduced adjusted risk of AKI compared with on-pump cardiac surgery [129]. Nonetheless, infrequent studies in low-risk patients report no renal effects [130] with no reduction in hemodialysis [131]. In a recent meta-analysis of 37 small randomized controlled trials encompassing 3,499 subjects and 22 risk-adjusted observational studies encompassing 293,617 subjects, conflicting results regarding the impact of off-pump surgery on the development of AKI were reported [132]. Although there was a trend toward reduction in AKI in the pooled analyses of the five randomized trials, only the analysis of the eight observational studies reached statistical significance [133]. Thus, ultimate assessment of the benefits of off-pump cardiac surgery must await the results of well-designed, adequately powered, prospective, randomized, multiple-center trials. The results of ongoing larger RCTs on off-pump cardiovascular surgery including a US Department of Veterans Affairs cooperative study of approximately 2,200 patients, which is due to be completed in 2009 (ClinicalTrials.gov Identifier NCT00032630) are therefore awaited.

Numerous small trials have evaluated different aspects of CPB management including flow, perfusion pressure, pulsatile versus non-pulsatile CPB, leukocyte depletion, temperature, and degree of hemodilution [46, 134, 135]. The results were mostly negative or inconclusive with no recommendations to be made for clinical practice. For example, in a recent study, low pressure or flow during CPB were not predictors of adverse renal outcome [135]. Also, the use of pulsatile compared with nonpulsatile perfusion did not show renal benefit in a recent RCT in children undergoing CPB [134]. Finally, leukocyte depletion using filters decreases mediators of tubular and glomerular injury but the effect on postoperative serum creatinine is inconsistent [136]. Needle-puncture of the aorta for the initiation of CPB should be guided by echocardiography to avoid plaque rupture and embolism, particularly in patients with severe atherosclerotic disease.

Table 6.15.3 Results of randomized controlled trials using pharmacologic interventions to prevent acute kidney injury after

Intervention	No. (drug/total)	Risk for postoperative AKI	Timing of intervention
Furosemide			
Lassnigg et al. [86]	41/123	Low	Beginning of surgery – 24 h
Lim et al. [87]	35/70	Low	After CPB – up to 5 days postoperation
Mannitol			
Carcoana et al. [88]	26/100	Low	Induction of anesthesia – 1 h after CPB
Yallop et al. [89]	20/40	Low	Induction of CPB – end of CPB
Smith et al. [90]	23/47	High	Induction of CPB – end of CPB
Dopamine			
Lassnigg et al. [86]	42/123	Low	Beginning of surgery – 24 h
Gatot et al. [91]	41/81	Low	After surgery – 48 h
Bove et al. [9]	40/80	High	Induction of anesthesia – 24 h
Piper et al. [92]	20/60	Low	Arrival in ICU
Woo et al. [93]	20/42	Intermediate	Induction of anesthesia – 48 h postoperation
Dopamine + diltiazem			
Yavuz et al. [94]	15/60	Low	Form 24 h prior to surgery to 48 h postoperation
Fenoldopam			
Barr et al. [95]	19/79	High	From surgical induction – 48 h Postoperation
Bove et al. [9]	40/80	High	Induction of anesthesia – 24 h Postoperation
Halpenny et al. [96]	16/31	Low	After end of CPB
Caimmi et al. [97]	80/160	High	Commencement of CPB – 24 h postoperation
Theophylline			
Krämer et al. [98]	28/56	Low	Induction of anesthesia – 96 h post-op
Pentoxyfylline			
Hoffmann et al. [99]	15/37	High	Postoperative day 1– Postoperative day 7
Boldt et al. [100]	20/40	High	Before surgery – morning of the second postoperative day
Diltiazem			
Piper et al. [92]	20/60	Low	Arrival in ICU
Bergman et al. [101]	12/25	High	Induction of anesthesia – 24 h postoperation
Amano et al. [102]	13/23	Low	Pericardiotomy – 24 h postoperation
Zanardo et al. [103]	23/35	Low	Sternotomy – 24 h postoperation
Clonidine			
Kulka et al. [104]	23/48	Low	Bolus 1 h before induction of anesthesia
Myles et al. [105]	78/156	Low	During the first 24 h
Dexamethasone			
Morariu et al. [106]	10/20	Low	Induction of anesthesia – 8 h postoperation
Loef et al. [107]	10/20	Low	Induction of anesthesia – 8 h postoperation
NAC			
Haase et al. [10]	31/61	High	Induction of anesthesia up to 24 h postoperation
Barr et al. [95]	20/79	High	4 h prior to surgery up to day 1 postoperation
Adabag et al. [108]	50/102	High	Day prior to surgery – day 6 postoperation
Sisillo et al. [109]	125/256	High	Induction of anesthesia – 48 h postoperation
Wijeysundera et al. [110]	88/175	High	Induction of anesthesia – 4 h after CPB
Ristikankare et al. [111]	38/77	Intermediate	Induction of anesthesia – 20 h postoperation
NAC + fenoldopam			
Barr et al. [95]	21/79	High	From surgical induction until 48 h postoperation

cardiovascular surgery

Nephroprotection	Outcomes (compared with placebo if not stated otherwise)
No	Deleterious effect on kidney function, no effect on LOS in ICU or in hospital
No	No effect on LOS in ICU or in hospital
No	No effect on urine markers and creatinine clearance 24 h post-op, no further outcomes reported
No	No renal effect (on course of serum creatinine or urine markers), no further outcomes reported
No	No renal effect (on course of serum creatinine or need for renal replacement therapy), no further outcomes reported
No	No effect on LOS in ICU or in hospital
No	No effect on LOS in ICU or in hospital
No	Compared with fenoldopam no renal effect no effect on LOS in ICU or in hospital
No	No effect on urine markers, no further outcomes reported
No	No renal effect, no tubular protection as measured by urine markers, no further outcomes reported
Yes	Improvement in urine markers and in free-water clearance
Yes	Reduced loss of eGFR, caused hypotension, no effect on RRT, LOS in ICU or in hospital
No	Compared to dopamine no renal effect, caused hypotension and hemolysis, no effect on LOS in ICU or in hospital
Yes	Less reduced eGFR, within 14 h postoperation, no further outcomes reported
Yes	Less reduced creatinine clearance, shorter stay in ICU
No	No renal effect, no further outcomes reported
Yes	Less hemofiltration needed, shorter stay in ICU
Yes	Less renal injury by urine markers, no difference in mortality
Yes	Less injury by urine markers, no other outcomes reported
Yes	Less reduced GFR, no effect on dialysis, LOS in ICU or in hospital
No	No renal effect at 24 h, no other outcomes reported
Yes	Less reduced GFR during CPB but not at 24 h, no effect on dialysis, LOS in ICU or in hospital
Yes	Less reduced GFR at 24 h but not at 72 h postoperation, no effect on dialysis, LOS in ICU or in hospital
Yes	Less reduced creatinine clearance, improved quality of life
No	No effect on renal function, stay in ICU or in hospital, prolonged intubation
No	No effect on renal function, stay in ICU or in hospital, prolonged intubation
No	No renal effect, no effect on LOS in ICU or in hospital
Yes	Reduced loss of eGFR, no effect on RRT, LOS in ICU or in hospital
No	No renal effect, no effect on LOS in ICU or in hospital
No	No clear renal effect, shorter LOS in ICU, no difference in mortality
No	No clear renal effect, no effect on LOS in ICU or in hospital
No	No renal effect, no effect on LOS in ICU or in hospital
Yes	Reduced loss of eGFR, caused hypotension, no effect on RRT, LOS in ICU or in hospital

(*continued*)

Table 6.15.3 (continued)

Intervention	No. (drug/total)	Risk for postoperative AKI	Timing of intervention
Atrial natriuretic peptide (Anaritide)			
Hayashida et al. [112]	9/18	High	After commencement of CPB – for 6 h
Bergman et al. [113]	15/30	Low	Chest closure – for 3 h
Swärd et al. [114]	10/19	Low	6 h after end of CPB – for 1 h
Brain natriuretic Peptide (Nesiritide)			
Chen et al. [115]	17/36	High	Induction of anesthesia – 24 h postoperation
Mentzer et al. [116]	141/279	High	Induction of anesthesia – at least 24 h up to 96 postoperation
Nitroprusside sodium			
Kaya et al. [117]	124/250	Intermediate	Rewarming on CPB – end of CPB
Statins			
Christenson et al. [118]	37/77	Low	4 weeks prior to surgery – day of surgery
Chello et al. [119]	20/40	Low	3 weeks prior to surgery – day of surgery
Sodium bicarbonate			
Haase et al. [11]	50/100	High	Induction of anesthesia – 24 h postoperation

[a]AKI = Acute kidney injury (according to study-specific definition used); No., number
[b]CPB = Cardiopulmonary bypass
[c]LOS = Length of stay
[d]ICU = Intensive care unit
[e]GFR = Estimated glomerular filtration rate
[f]RRT = Renal replacement therapy
[g]NAC = N-Acetylcysteine

Preemptive RRT may have a significant effect on postoperative morbidity and mortality [137, 138]. Recently, new technologies of extracorporeal blood purification achieving removal of circulating proinflammatory and antiinflammatory mediators have also been developed; however, these remain to be tested in this setting [139–141].

In summary, observational or small controlled trials of off-pump surgery and avoidance of aortic manipulation and preemptive RRT show some efficacy in preventing AKI following cardiovascular surgery [73]. Pending results of ongoing large RCTs, the avoidance of CPB should be considered, particularly in high-risk patients. Finally, there is insufficient evidence to recommend preemptive RRT.

6.15.6 Treatment

The prevention of further damage to the kidney directed at its underlying cause is the cornerstone in the management of established AKI after CPB. Early diagnosis of AKI using novel renal biomarkers may facilitate specific measures particularly in the setting of cardiovascular surgery using CPB where the timing of the injurious event to the kidney is known [67–72]. By then, treatment of AKI remains largely supportive until renal function recovers. In the following, specific therapeutic principles in AKI are discussed.

Basic treatment of AKI after CPB includes avoidance of nephrotoxins such as radiocontrast agents, NSAID, or aminoglycoside antibiotics; the switch to drugs preferably metabolized in the liver; or adjustment of drug dosing according to renal function.

Drugs that increase renal blood flow, promote natriuresis, and block inflammation have been investigated for treatment of AKI in cardiovascular surgery patients [142]. In general, few RCTs have been performed to investigate such strategies and therefore the evidence to date is very limited. In an uncontrolled, small trial in post cardiac surgical patients, "renal-dose" dopamine improved creatinine clearance in patients with established AKI [143]. On the other hand, renal-dose dopamine worsened renal perfusion in critically ill patients with AKI, which adds to questioning the routine use of renal-dose dopamine as a treatment option [144]. In the only multicenter international RCT on renal-dose dopamine, it could not improve renal function or any other outcome of critically ill patients, with however only 7.5% of patients admitted after cardiac surgery [145]. In a meta-analysis, Friedrich et al. concluded

Nephroprotection	Outcomes (compared with placebo if not stated otherwise)
No	No renal effect
(Yes)	Increased diuresis and natriuresis immediately postoperation
Yes	Compared to baseline increased GFR and diuresis
Yes	Reduced loss of creatinine Clearance at 48 h but not at 72 h, no effect on LOS in ICU
Yes	Less renal injury by creatinine increase and less mortality, no reduction in RRT
Yes	Less reduced GFR, no effect on dialysis, LOS in ICU or in hospital
Yes	Reduced incidence of AKI, no effect on LOS in ICU or in hospital
No	No renal effect, no effect on LOS in ICU or in hospital
Yes	Less injury by creatinine increase and urine markers, no effect on RRT, LOS in ICU or in hospital

that renal-dose dopamine offers transient improvements in renal physiology, but there is no good evidence that it offers important clinical benefits to patients with AKI [146].

Fenoldopam mesylate, a selective dopamine receptor 1 agonist, has been shown to reduce systemic vascular resistance in a dose-dependent manner. It is able to augment renal blood flow in patients with normal renal function and chronic renal failure. Clinicians use fenoldopam in the belief that improving renal blood flow and oxygen delivery will disrupt the progression toward dialysis-dependent ARF. Despite early success in the prevention of AKI [95–97], there is no convincing evidence for the treatment of established AKI after CPB using fenoldopam, yet.

In a pharmacologic dose effect study, atrial natriuretic peptide increased GFR in a cohort of patients with established AKI after cardiac surgery [147]. A small RCT demonstrated that low-dose atrial natriuretic peptide, administered after development of postoperative AKI, improved dialysis-free survival in patients with AKI after cardiac surgery [148]. In a larger RCT in critically ill patients with AKI, the administration of atrial natriuretic peptide did not improve the overall rate of dialysis-free survival [149]. However, atrial natriuretic peptide may improve dialysis-free survival in those patients with oliguria and may worsen it in patients without oliguria who have developed AKI [149].

In another RCT enrolling patients with oliguric AKI after cardiac surgery, the combined use of furosemide, mannitol, and dopamine improved renal function after cardiac surgery compared with intermittent use of furosemide alone [150]. Such results remain to be confirmed prior to routine administration of this solution in the early postoperative period for oliguric AKI.

Various other therapeutic agents such as insulin-like growth factor and erythropoietin [151] have shown promising results in other settings than cardiovascular surgery [152].

Renal replacement therapy is initiated for uremic symptoms, or when volume overload, electrolyte abnormalities or acidosis are refractory to medical management. Current data suggests the modality of RRT used does not impact survival or renal recovery. There is no consensus as to timing of initiation or dose of RRT in AKI following cardiovascular surgery.

The acute dialysis quality initiative working group concludes that routine use of diuretics cannot be supported, other than to maintain fluid balance in oliguric patients [142]. Iatrogenic hypovolemia should be avoided. No pharmacologic interventions to revert established AKI have consistently resulted in improved outcomes. Several methods of RRT have been utilized with no differences in outcome. No recommendations can be made on mode and timing of beginning and ending of RRT in AKI after cardiovascular surgery [142].

6.15.7 Summary

AKI following cardiovascular surgery can develop through multiple pathophysiologic events including ischemia-reperfusion, inflammatory and oxidative stress, sympathetic nervous system activation, and nephrotoxins. Nephrotoxic agents should be discontinued and hypovolemia needs to be avoided. As timing of the injurious event to kidney is known in this setting, specific preventive strategies appear conceivable; however, they need further investigation. Preliminary successful use of off-pump cardiovascular surgery in patients at increased risk of AKI needs confirmation in large randomized controlled trials before general recommendations can be made. Increased understanding of pathomechanisms contributing to AKI and individualized prevention or treatment strategies might be the key to improve outcomes of kidney failure following cardiovascular surgery.

6.15.8 Take Home Pearls

- AKI following cardiovascular surgery is a common and serious condition with substantial morbidity and mortality.
- Key measures to reduce the perioperative incidence of AKI are to avoid nephrotoxic drugs and contrast agents whenever possible, to maintain euvolemia, and to carefully restrict the use of packed red blood cell transfusions.
- There are no specific pharmacologic interventions to prevent AKI after cardiovascular surgery that could be generally recommended.

Acknowledgments We thank Dr Andrea Lassnigg, Department of Cardiothoracic and Vascular Anesthesia and Intensive Care Medicine, University Hospital of Vienna, A-1090 Vienna, Austria for providing us with Fig. 6.15.1.

References

1. Albert MA, Antman EM: Preoperative evaluation for cardiac surgery. In Cohn LH, Edmunds LH jr. (eds.): Cardiac surgery in the adult, New York, MacGraw-Hill, 2003, pp 235–248
2. Bair TL, Muhlestein JB, May HT, et al. (2007) Surgical revascularization is associated with improved long-term outcomes compared with percutaneous stenting in most subgroups of patients with multivessel coronary artery disease: results from the Intermountain Heart Registry. Circulation 116(11 Suppl):I226–231
3. Rosner M, Okusa M (2006) Acute kidney injury associated with cardiac surgery. Clin J Am Soc Nephrol 1:19–32
4. Hein OV, Birnbaum J, Wernecke KD, et al. (2006) Three-year survival after four major post-cardiac operative complications. Crit Care Med 34:2729–2737
5. Conlon PJ, Stafford-Smith M, White WD, et al. (1999) Acute renal failure following cardiac surgery. Nephrol Dial Transplant 14:1158–1162
6. Mangano CM, Diamondstone LS, Ramsay JG, et al. (1998) Renal dysfunction after myocardial revascularization: risk factors, adverse outcomes, and hospital resource utilization. The Multicenter Study of Perioperative Ischemia Research Group. Ann Intern Med 128:194–203
7. Stafford-Smith M, Podgoreanu M, Swaminathan M, et al. (2005) Association of genetic polymorphisms with risk of renal injury after coronary bypass graft surgery. Am J Kidney Dis 45:519–530
8. Wagener G, Gubitosa G, Wang S, et al. (2008) Urinary Neutrophil Gelatinase-Associated Lipocalin and Acute Kidney Injury After Cardiac Surgery. Am J Kidney Dis Jul 21. [Epub ahead of print]
9. Bove T, Landoni G, Calabro MG et al. (2005) Renoprotective action of fenoldopam in high-risk patients undergoing cardiac surgery: a prospective, double-blind, randomized clinical trial. Circulation 111:3230–3235
10. Haase M, Haase-Fielitz A, Bagshaw SM, et al. (2007) Phase II, randomized, controlled trial of high-dose N-acetylcysteine in high-risk cardiac surgery patients. Crit Care Med 35:1324–1331
11. Haase M, Haase-Fielitz A, Bellomo R, et al. (2008) Sodium bicarbonate to prevent Increases in serum creatinine after cardiac surgery: A pilot double-blind, randomized controlled trial. Crit Care Med 37:39–47
12. Chertow GM, Levy EM, Hammermeister KE, et al. (1998) Independent association between acute renal failure and mortality following cardiac surgery. Am J Med 104: 343–348
13. Thakar CV, Worley S, Arrigain S, et al. (2007) Improved survival in acute kidney injury after cardiac surgery. Am J Kidney Dis 50:703–711
14. Lassnigg A, Schmid ER, Hiesmayr M, et al. (2008) Impact of minimal increases in serum creatinine on outcome in patients after cardiothoracic surgery: do we have to revise current definitions of acute renal failure? Crit Care Med 36: 1129–1137
15. Lassnigg A, Schmmidlin D, Mouhieddine M, et al. (2004) Minimal changes of serum creatinine predict prognosis in patients after cardiothoracic surgery: a prospective cohort study. J Am Soc Nephrol 15:1597–1605
16. Zanardo G, Michielon P, Paccagnella A et al. (1994) Acute renal failure in the patient undergoing cardiac operation. Prevalence, mortality rate, and main risk factors. J Thorac Cardiovasc Surg 107:1489–1495
17. Arnaoutakis GJ, Bihorac A, Martin TD, et al. (2007) RIFLE criteria for acute kidney injury in aortic arch surgery. J Thorac Cardiovasc Surg 134:1554–1561
18. Loef BG, Epema AH, Smilde TD, et al. (2005) Immediate postoperative renal function deterioration in cardiac surgical patients predicts in-hospital mortality and long-term survival. J Am Soc Nephrol 16:195–200
19. Khoynezhad A, Donayre CE, Smith J, et al. (2008) Risk factors for early and late mortality after thoracic endovascular aortic repair. J Thorac Cardiovasc Surg 135:1103–1114

20. Brown JR, Cochran RP, MacKenzie TA, et al. (2008) Long-term survival after cardiac surgery is predicted by estimated glomerular filtration rate. Ann Thorac Surg 86:4–11
21. Lok CE, Austin PC, Wang H, et al. (2004) Impact of renal insufficiency on short- and long-term outcomes after cardiac surgery. Am Heart J 148:430–438
22. Swaminathan M, Shaw AD, Phillips-Bute BG, et al. (2007) Trends in acute renal failure associated with coronary artery bypass graft surgery in the United States. Crit Care Med 35: 2286–2291
23. Blot SI, Vandijck DM, Hoste EA (2008) Trends in mortality in coronary artery bypass graft patients with acute renal failure. Crit Care Med 36:656
24. Thakar CV, Yared JP, Worley S, et al. (2003) Renal dysfunction and serious infections after open-heart surgery. Kidney Int 64:239–246
25. Levy EM, Viscoli CM, Horwitz RI (1996) The effect of acute renal failure on mortality. A cohort analysis. JAMA 275:1489–1494
26. Hoste EA, Cruz DN, Davenport A, et al. (2008) The epidemiology of cardiac surgery-associated acute kidney injury. Int J Artif Organs 31:158–165
27. Thakar CV, Liangos O, Yared JP, et al. (2003) ARF after open-heart surgery: Influence of gender and race. Am J Kidney Dis 41:742–751
28. Chertow GM, Lazarus JM, Christiansen CL, et al. (1997) Preoperative renal risk stratification. Circulation 95:878–884
29. Macedo E, Castro I, Yu L, et al. (2008) Impact of mild acute kidney injury (AKI) on outcome after open repair of aortic aneurysms. Ren Fail 30:287–296
30. Aronson S, Fontes ML, Miao Y, et al. (2007) Risk index for perioperative renal dysfunction/failure: critical dependence on pulse pressure hypertension. Circulation 115:733–742
31. Mehta RH, Grab JD, O'Brien SM, et al. (2006) Bedside tool for predicting the risk of postoperative dialysis in patients undergoing cardiac surgery. Circulation 114:2208–2216
32. Brown JR, Cochran RP, Leavitt BJ, et al. (2007) Multivariable prediction of renal insufficiency developing after cardiac surgery. Circulation 116(11 Suppl):I139–143
33. Vaccarino V, Abramson JL, Veledar E, et al. (2002) Sex differences in hospital mortality after coronary artery bypass surgery: evidence for a higher mortality in younger women. Circulation 105:1176–1181
34. Vaccarino V, Lin ZQ, Kasl SV, et al. (2003) Gender differences in recovery after coronary artery bypass surgery. J Am Coll Cardiol 41:307–314
35. Levy AR, Sobolev BG, Kuramoto L, et al. (2007) Do women spend longer on wait lists for coronary bypass surgery? Analysis of a population-based registry in British Columbia, Canada. BMC Cardiovasc Disord 7:24
36. Tyson GH 3rd, Rodriguez E, Elci OC, et al. (2007) Cardiac procedures in patients with a body mass index exceeding 45: outcomes and long-term results. Ann Thorac Surg 84:3–9
37. Engelman DT, Adams DH, Byrne JG, et al. (1999) Impact of body mass index and albumin on morbidity and mortality after cardiac surgery. J Thorac Cardiovasc Surg 118: 866–873
38. Del Duca D, Iqbal S, Rahme E, et al. (2007) Renal failure after cardiac surgery: timing of cardiac catheterization and other perioperative risk factors. Ann Thorac Surg 84: 1264–1271
39. Haase-Fielitz A, Haase M, Bellomo R, et al. (2007) Genetic polymorphisms in sepsis- and cardiopulmonary bypass-associated acute kidney injury. Contrib Nephrol 156: 75–91
40. Gaudino M, Di Castelnuovo A, Zamparelli R, et al. (2003) Genetic control of postoperative systemic inflammatory reaction and pulmonary and renal complications after coronary artery surgery. J Thorac Cardiovasc Surg 126:1107–1112
41. Chew ST, Newman MF, White WD, et al. (2000) Preliminary report on the association of apolipoprotein E polymorphisms, with postoperative peak serum creatinine concentrations in cardiac surgical patients. Anesthesiology 93: 325–331
42. MacKensen GB, Swaminathan M, Ti LK, et al. (2004) Preliminary report on the interaction of apolipoprotein E polymorphism with aortic atherosclerosis and acute nephropathy after CABG. Ann Thorac Surg 78:520–526
43. Isbir SC, Tekeli A, Ergen A, et al. (2007) Genetic polymorphisms contribute to acute kidney injury after coronary artery bypass grafting. Heart Surg Forum 10:E439–444
44. Thakar CV, Arrigain S, Worley S, et al. (2005) A clinical score to predict acute renal failure after cardiac surgery. J Am Soc Nephrol 16:162–168
45. Palomba H, de Castro I, Neto AL et al. (2007) Acute kidney injury prediction following elective cardiac surgery: AKICS Score. Kidney Int 72:624–631
46. Fischer UM, Weissenberger WK, Warters RD, et al. (2002) Impact of cardiopulmonary bypass management on post-cardiac surgery renal function. Perfusion 17:401–406
47. Boldt J, Brenner T, Lehmann A et al. (2003) Is kidney function altered by the duration of cardiopulmonary bypass? Ann Thorac Surg 75:906–912
48. Koch CG, Li L, Duncan AI, et al. (2006) Morbidity and mortality risk associated with red blood cell and blood-component transfusion in isolated coronary artery bypass grafting. Crit Care Med 34:1608–1616
49. Basran S, Frumento RJ, Cohen A, et al. (2006) The association between duration of storage of transfused red blood cells and morbidity and mortality after reoperative cardiac surgery. Anesth Analg 103:15–20
50. Koch CG, Li L, Sessler DI, Figueroa P, Hoeltge GA, Mihaljevic T, Blackstone EH. Duration of red-cell storage and complications after cardiac surgery. N Engl J Med. 2008 Mar 20;358(12):1229–1239.
51. Seeliger E, Flemming B, Wronski T, et al. (2007) Viscosity of contrast media perturbs renal hemodynamics. J Am Soc Nephrol 18:2912–2920
52. Bellomo R, Auriemma S, Fabbri A, et al. (2008) The pathophysiology of cardiac surgery-associated acute kidney injury (CSA-AKI). Int J Artif Organs 31:166–178
53. Taber SS, Mueller BA (2006) Drug-associated renal dysfunction. Crit Care Clin 22:357–374
54. Gold JP, Charlson ME, Williams-Russo P, et al. (1995) Improvement of outcomes after coronary artery bypass. A randomized trial comparing intraoperative high versus low meanarterial pressure. J Thorac Cardiovasc Surg 110: 1302–1311
55. Galinanes M, Watson C, Trivedi U, et al. (1996) Differential patterns of neutrophil adhesion molecules during cardiopulmonary bypass in humans. Circulation 94(9 Suppl): II364–369

56. Alghamdi AA, Latter DA (2006) Pulsatile versus nonpulsatile cardiopulmonary bypass flow: an evidence-based approach. J Card Surg 21:347–354
57. Haase M, Haase-Fielitz A, Bagshaw SM, et al. (2007) Cardiopulmonary bypass-associated acute kidney injury: a pigment nephropathy? Contrib Nephrol 156:340–353
58. Seto S, Kher V, Scicli AG, et al. (1983) The effect of aprotinin (a serine protease inhibitor) on renal function and renin release. Hypertension 5:893–899
59. Samama CM, Mazoyer E, Bruneval P, et al. (1994) Aprotinin could promote arterial thrombosis in pigs: a prospective randomized, blind study. Thromb Haemost 71:663–669
60. Maccario M, Fumagalli C, Dottori V, et al. (1996) The association between rhabdomyolysis and acute renal failure in patients undergoing cardiopulmonary bypass. J Cardiovasc Surg 37:153–159
61. van den Berghe G, Wouters P, Weekers F, et al. (2001) Intensive insulin therapy in the critically ill patients. N Engl J Med 345:1359–1367
62. Bellomo R, Kellum JA, Ronco C (2007) Defining and classifying acute renal failure: from advocacy to consensus and validation of the RIFLE criteria. Intensive Care Med 33: 409–413
63. Mehta RL, Kellum JA, Shah SV et al. (2007) Acute kidney injury Network: report of an initiative to improve outcomes in acute kidney injury. Crit Care 11:R31
64. Herget-Rosenthal S, Marggraf G, Hüsing J, et al. (2004) Early detection of acute renal failure by serum cystatin C. Kidney Int 66:1115–1122
65. Mehta RL, Chertow GM (2003) Acute renal failure definitions and classification: time for change? J Am Soc Nephrol 14:2178–2187
66. Bennett M, Dent CL, Ma Q, et al. (2008) Urine NGAL predicts severity of acute kidney injury after cardiac surgery: a prospective study. Clin J Am Soc Nephrol 3:665–673
67. Mishra J, Dent C, Tarabishi R, et al. (2005) Neutrophil gelatinase-associated lipocalin (NGAL) as a biomarker for acute renal injury after cardiac surgery. Lancet 365: 1231–1238
68. Parikh CR, Mishra J, Thiessen-Philbrook H, et al. (2006) Urinary IL-18 is an early predictive biomarker of acute kidney injury after cardiac surgery. Kidney Int 70:199–203
69. Haase-Fielitz A, Bellomo R, Devarajan P, et al. (2008) Novel and conventional serum biomarkers predicting acute kidney injury in adult cardiac surgery – A prospective cohort study. Crit Care Med 37:553-560
70. Abu-Omar Y, Mussa S, Naik MJ, et al. (2005) Evaluation of Cystatin C as a marker of renal injury following on-pump and off-pump coronary surgery. Eur J Cardiothorac Surg 27:893–898
71. Zhu J, Yin R, Wu H, et al. (2006) Cystatin C as a reliable marker of renal function following heart valve replacement surgery with cardiopulmonary bypass. Clin Chim Acta 374:116–121
72. Haase M, Bellomo R, Story D, et al. (2008) Urinary interleukin-18 does not predict acute kidney injury after adult cardiac surgery – A prospective observational cohort study. Crit Care 12:R96. Epub 2008 Aug 1
73. Schetz M, Bove T, Morelli A, et al. (2008) Prevention of cardiac surgery-associated acute kidney injury. Int J Artif Organs 31:179–189
74. Marathias KP, Vassili M, Robola A, et al. (2006) Preoperative intravenous hydration confers renoprotection in patients with chronic kidney disease undergoing cardiac surgery. Artif Organs 30:615–621
75. McArdle GT, Price G, Lewis A, et al. (2007) Positive fluid balance is associated with complications after elective open infrarenal abdominal aortic aneurysm repair. Eur J Vasc Endovasc Surg 34:522–527
76. Payen D, de Pont AC, Sakr Y, et al. (2008) A positive fluid balance is associated with a worse outcome in patients with acute renal failure. Crit Care 12:R74. Epub 2008 Jun 4
77. Bagshaw S, Brophy P, Cruz D, et al. (2008) Fluid balance as a biomarker: impact of fluid overload on outcome in critically ill patients with acute kidney injury. Critical Care 12:R169 Epub 2008 July 24
78. Kern JW, Shoemaker WC (2002) Meta-analysis of hemodynamic optimization in high-risk patients. Crit Care Med 30:1686–1692
79. Egi M, Bellomo R, Langenberg C, et al. (2007) Selecting a vasopressor drug for vasoplegic shock after adult cardiac surgery: a systematic literature review. Ann Thorac Surg 83:715–723
80. Devbhandari MP, Balasubramanian SK, Codispoti M, et al. (2004) Preoperative angiotensin-converting enzyme inhibition can cause severe post CPB vasodilation – current UK opinion. Asian Cardiovasc Thorac Ann 12:346–349
81. Mangano DT, Tudor IC, Dietzel C, (2006) Multicenter Study of Perioperative Ischemia Research Group; Ischemia Research and Education Foundation. The risk associated with aprotinin in cardiac surgery. N Engl J Med 354: 353–365
82. Hausenloy DJ, Pagano D, Keogh B (2008). Aprotinin – still courting controversy Lancet 371: 449–450
83. Furnary AP, Wu Y, Hiratzka LF, et al. (2007) Aprotinin does not increase the risk of renal failure in cardiac surgery patients. Circulation 116(11 Suppl):I127–133
84. Levy JH, Pifarre R, Schaff HV, et al. (1995) A multicenter, double-blind, placebo-controlled trial of aprotinin for reducing blood loss and the requirement for donor-blood transfusion in patients undergoing repeat coronary artery bypass grafting. Circulation 92:2236–2244
85. Fergusson DA, Hébert PC, Mazer CD, et al. (2008) A comparison of aprotinin and lysine analogues in high-risk cardiac surgery. N Engl J Med 358:2319–2331
86. Lassnigg A, Donner E, Grubhofer G, et al. (2000) Lack of renoprotective effects of dopamine and furosemide during cardiac surgery. J Am Soc Nephrol 11:97–104
87. Lim E, Ali ZA, Attaran R, et al. (2002) Evaluating routine diuretics after coronary surgery: a prospective randomized controlled trial. Ann Thorac Surg 73:153–155
88. Carcoana OV, Mathew JP, Davis E, et al. (2003). Mannitol and dopamine in patients undergoing cardiopulmonary bypass: a randomized clinical trial. Anesth Analg 97: 1222–1229
89. Yallop KG, Sheppard SV, Smith DC (2008) The effect of mannitol on renal function following cardio-pulmonary

bypass in patients with normal pre-operative creatinine. Anaesthesia 63:576–582
90. Smith MN, Best D, Sheppard SV, et al. (2008) The effect of mannitol on renal function after cardiopulmonary bypass in patients with established renal dysfunction. Anaesthesia 63:701–704
91. Gatot I, Abramov D, Tsodikov V, et al. (2004) Should we give prophylactic renal-dose dopamine after coronary artery bypass surgery? J Card Surg 19:128–133
92. Piper SN, Kumle B, Maleck WH, et al. (2003) Diltiazem may preserve renal tubular integrity after cardiac surgery. Can J Anaesth 50:285–292
93. Woo EB, Tang AT, el-Gamel A, et al. (2002) Dopamine therapy for patients at risk of renal dysfunction following cardiac surgery: science or fiction? Eur J Cardiothorac Surg 22:106–11
94. Yavuz S, Ayabakan N, Goncu MT, et al. (2002) Effect of combined dopamine and diltiazem on renal function after cardiac surgery. Med Sci Monit 8:PI45–50
95. Barr LF, Kolodner K (2008) N-acetylcysteine and fenoldopam protect the renal function of patients with chronic renal insufficiency undergoing cardiac surgery. Crit Care Med 36:1427–1435
96. Halpenny M, Lakshmi S, O'Donnell A, et al. (2001) Fenoldopam: renal and splanchnic effects in patients undergoing coronary artery bypass grafting. Anaesthesia 56: 953–960
97. Caimmi PP, Pagani L, Micalizzi E, et al. (2003) Fenoldopam for renal protection in patients undergoing cardiopulmonary bypass. J Cardiothorac Vasc Anesth 17:491–494
98. Krämer BK, Preuner J, Ebenburger A, et al. (2002) Lack of renoprotective effect of theophylline during aortocoronary bypass surgery. Nephrol Dial Transplant 17:910–915
99. Hoffmann H, Markewitz A, Kreuzer E, et al. (1998) Pentoxifylline decreases the incidence of multiple organ failure in patients after major cardio-thoracic surgery. Shock 9:235–240
100. Boldt J, Brosch C, Piper SN, et al. (2001) Influence of prophylactic use of pentoxifylline on postoperative organ function in elderly cardiac surgery patients. Crit Care Med 29:952–958
101. Bergman AS, Odar-Cederlöf I, Westman L, et al. (2002) Diltiazem infusion for renal protection in cardiac surgical patients with preexisting renal dysfunction. J Cardiothorac Vasc Anesth 16:294–299
102. Amano J, Suzuki A, Sunamori M, et al. (1995) Effect of calcium antagonist diltiazem on renal function in open heart surgery. Chest 107:1260–1265
103. Zanardo G, Michielon P, Rosi P, et al. (1993) Effects of a continuous diltiazem infusion on renal function during cardiac surgery. J Cardiothorac Vasc Anesth 7:711–716
104. Kulka PJ, Tryba M, Zenz M et al. (1996) Preoperative alpha2-adrenergic receptor agonists prevent the deterioration of renal function after cardiac surgery: results of a randomized, controlled trial. Crit Care Med 24: 947–952
105. Myles PS, Buckland MR, Schenk NJ, et al. (1993) Effect of "renal-dose" dopamine on renal function following cardiac surgery. Anaesth Intensive Care. 21:56–61
106. Morariu AM, Loef BG, Aarts LP, et al. (2005) Dexamethasone: benefit and prejudice for patients undergoing on-pump coronary artery bypass grafting: a study on myocardial, pulmonary, renal, intestinal, and hepatic injury. Chest 128:2677–2687
107. Loef BG, Henning RH, Epema AH, et al. (2004) Effect of dexamethasone on perioperative renal function impairment during cardiac surgery with cardiopulmonary bypass. Br J Anaesth 93:793–798
108. Adabag AS, Ishani A, Koneswaran S, et al. (2008) Utility of N-acetylcysteine to prevent acute kidney injury after cardiac surgery: a randomized controlled trial. Am Heart J 155:1143–1149
109. Sisillo E, Ceriani R, Bortone F, et al. (2008) N-acetylcysteine for prevention of acute renal failure in patients with chronic renal insufficiency undergoing cardiac surgery: a prospective, randomized, clinical trial. Crit Care Med 36:81–86
110. Wijeysundera DN, Beattie WS, Rao V, et al. (2007) N-acetylcysteine for preventing acute kidney injury in cardiac surgery patients with pre-existing moderate renal insufficiency. Can J Anaesth 54:872–881
111. Ristikankare A, Kuitunen T, Kuitunen A, et al. (2006) Lack of renoprotective effect of i.v. N-acetylcysteine in patients with chronic renal failure undergoing cardiac surgery. Br J Anaesth 97:611–616
112. Hayashida N, Chihara S, Kashikie H, et al. (2000) Effects of intraoperative administration of atrial natriuretic peptide. Ann Thorac Surg 70:1319–1326
113. Bergman A, Odar-Cederlöf I, Westman L, et al. (1996) Effects of human atrial natriuretic peptide in patients after coronary artery bypass surgery. J Cardiothorac Vasc Anesth 10:490–496
114. Swärd K, Valsson F, Sellgren J, et al. (2005) Differential effects of human atrial natriuretic peptide and furosemide on glomerular filtration rate and renal oxygen consumption in humans. Intensive Care Med 31:79–85
115. Chen HH, Sundt TM, Cook DJ, et al. (2007) Low dose nesiritide and the preservation of renal function in patients with renal dysfunction undergoing cardiopulmonary-bypass surgery: a double-blind placebo-controlled pilot study. Circulation. 116(11 Suppl):I134–138
116. Mentzer RM Jr, Oz MC, Sladen RN, et al. (2007) Effects of perioperative nesiritide in patients with left ventricular dysfunction undergoing cardiac surgery: the NAPA Trial. J Am Coll Cardiol 49:716–726
117. Kaya K, O uz M, Akar AR, et al. (2007) The effect of sodium nitroprusside infusion on renal function during reperfusion period in patients undergoing coronary artery bypass grafting: a prospective randomized clinical trial. Eur J Cardiothorac Surg 31:290–297
118. Christenson JT (1999) Preoperative lipid-control with simvastatin reduces the risk of postoperative thrombocytosis and thrombotic complications following CABG. Eur J Cardiothorac Surg 15:394–399
119. Chello M, Patti G, Candura D, et al. (2006) Effects of atorvastatin on systemic inflammatory response after coronary bypass surgery. Crit Care Med 34:660–667
120. Landoni G, Biondi-Zoccai GG, Marino G, et al. (2008) Fenoldopam reduces the need for renal replacement therapy

and in-hospital death in cardiovascular surgery: a meta-analysis. J Cardiothorac Vasc Anesth 22:27–33
121. Sackner-Bernstein JD, Skopicki HA, Aaronson KD (2005) Risk of worsening renal function with nesiritide in patients with acutely decompensated heart failure. Circulation 111:1487–1491
122. Wang DJ, Dowling TC, Meadows D, et al. (2004) Nesiritide does not improve renal function in patients with chronic heart failure and worsening serum creatinine. Circulation 110:1620–1625
123. Sackner-Bernstein JD, Kowalski M, Fox M, et al. (2005) Short-term risk of death after treatment with nesiritide for decompensated heart failure. JAMA 293:1900–1905
124. Sabik JF, Gillinov AM, Blackstone EH, et al. (2002) Does off-pump coronary surgery reduce morbidity and mortality? J Thorac Cardiovasc Surg 124:698–707
125. Mack MJ, Pfister A, Bachand D, et al. (2004) Comparison of coronary bypass surgery with and without cardiopulmonary bypass in patients with multivessel disease. J Thorac Cardiovasc Surg 127:167–173
126. Haase M, Sharma A, Fielitz A, et al. (2003) On-pump coronary artery surgery versus off-pump exclusive arterial coronary grafting: a matched cohort comparison. Ann Thorac Surg 75:62–67
127. Hix JK, Thakar CV, Katz EM, et al. (2006) Effect of off-pump coronary artery bypass graft surgery on postoperative acute kidney injury and mortality. Crit Care Med 34: 2979–2983
128. Di Mauro M, Gagliardi M, Lacò AL, et al. (2007) Does off-pump coronary surgery reduce postoperative acute renal failure? The importance of preoperative renal function. Ann Thorac Surg 84:1496–1502
129. Lattouf OM, Puskas JD, Thourani VH, et al. (2007) Does the number of grafts influence surgeon choice and patient benefit of off-pump over conventional on-pump coronary artery revascularization in multivessel coronary artery disease? Ann Thorac Surg 84:1485–1495
130. Tang AT, Knott J, Nanson J, et al. (2002) A prospective randomized study to evaluate the renoprotective action of beating heart coronary surgery in low risk patients. Eur J Cardiothorac Surg 22:118–123
131. Straka Z, Widimsky P, Jirasek K, Stros P, et al. (2004) Off-pump versus on-pump coronary surgery: final results from a prospective randomized study PRAGUE-4. Ann Thorac Surg 77:789–793
132. Wijeysundera DN, Beattie WS, Djaiani G, et al. (2005) Off-pump coronary artery surgery for reducing mortality and morbidity: meta-analysis of randomized and observational studies. J Am Coll Cardiol 46:872–882
133. Palevsky PM (2006) Off-pump cardiac surgery and acute kidney injury. Crit Care Med 34:3052–3053
134. Alkan T, Akçevin A, Undar A, et al. (2006) Effects of pulsatile and nonpulsatile perfusion on vital organ recovery in pediatric heart surgery: a pilot clinical study. ASAIO J 52:530–535
135. Slogoff S, Reul GJ, Keats AS, et al. (1990) Role of perfusion pressure and flow in major organ dysfunction after cardiopulmonary bypass. Ann Thorac Surg 50: 911–918
136. Bolcal C, Akay HT, Bingol H, et al. (2007) Leukodepletion improves renal function in patients with renal dysfunction undergoing on-pump coronary bypass surgery: a prospective randomized study. Thorac Cardiovasc Surg 55: 89–93
137. Durmaz I, Yagdi T, Calkavur T, et al. (2003) Prophylactic dialysis in patients with renal dysfunction undergoing on-pump coronary artery bypass surgery. Ann Thorac Surg 75:859–864
138. Bingol H, Akay HT, Iyem H, et al. (2007) Prophylactic dialysis in elderly patients undergoing coronary bypass surgery. Ther Apher Dial 11:30–35
139. Haase M, Silvester W, Uchino S, et al. (2007) A pilot study of high-adsorption hemofiltration in human septic shock. Int J Artif Organs 30:108–117
140. Haase M, Bellomo R, Baldwin I, et al. (2007) Hemodialysis membrane with a high-molecular-weight cutoff and cytokine levels in sepsis complicated by acute renal failure: a phase 1 randomized trial. Am J Kidney Dis 50: 296–304
141. Haase M, Bellomo R, Baldwin I, et al. (2008) The effect of three different miniaturized blood purification devices on plasma cytokine concentration in an ex-vivo model of endotoxinemia. Int J Artif Organs 31:722-729
142. Tolwani A, Paganini E, Joannidis M, et al. (2008) Treatment of patients with cardiac surgery associated-acute kidney injury. Int J Artif Organs 31:190–196
143. Davis RF, Lappas DG, Kirklin JK, et al. (1982) Acute oliguria after cardiopulmonary bypass: renal functional improvement with low-dose dopamine infusion. Crit Care Med 10:852–856
144. Lauschke A, Teichgräber UK, Frei U, et al. (2006) 'Low-dose' dopamine worsens renal perfusion in patients with acute renal failure. Kidney Int 69:1669–1674
145. Bellomo R, Chapman M, Finfer S, et al. (2000) Low-dose dopamine in patients with early renal dysfunction: a placebo-controlled randomised trial. Australian and New Zealand Intensive Care Society (ANZICS) Clinical Trials Group. Lancet 356:2139–2143
146. Friedrich JO, Adhikari N, Herridge MS, et al. (2005) Meta-analysis: low-dose dopamine increases urine output but does not prevent renal dysfunction or death. Ann Intern Med 142:510–524
147. Valsson F, Ricksten SE, Hedner T, et al. (1996) Effects of atrial natriuretic peptide on acute renal impairment in patients with heart failure after cardiac surgery. Intensive Care Med 22:230–236
148. Swärd K, Valsson F, Odencrants P, et al. (2004) Recombinant human atrial natriuretic peptide in ischemic acute renal failure: a randomized placebo-controlled trial. Crit Care Med 32:1310–1315
149. Allgren RL, Marbury TC, Rahman SN, et al. (1997) Anaritide in acute tubular necrosis. N Engl J Med 20 336: 828–834
150. Sirivella S, Gielchinsky I, Parsonnet V (2000) Mannitol, furosemide, and dopamine infusion in postoperative renal failure complicating cardiac surgery. Ann Thorac Surg 69: 501–506
151. Vesey DA, Cheung C, Pat B, et al. (2004) Erythropoietin protects against ischaemic acute renal injury. Nephrol Dial Transplant 19:348–355
152. Hirschberg R, Kopple J, Lipsett P, et al. (1999) Multicenter clinical trial of recombinant human insulin-like growth factor I in patients with acute renal failure. Kidney Int 55: 2423–2432

Burns and Acute Kidney Failure

6.16

Filippo Mariano, Ezio Nicola Gangemi,
Daniela Bergamo, Zsuzsanna Hollo,
Maurizio Stella, and Giorgio Triolo

Core Messages

- Renal alterations such as proteinuria, hematuria, and electrolyte disturbances are common in patients with severe burns.
- Two distinct pictures with an early and a late form of acute kidney failure (ARF) have been described: The early form occurs in the immediate postburns period and can in most cases be effectively prevented by early aggressive fluid resuscitation. The late form develops after 2–3 weeks from initial injury and is usually due to sepsis and multiorgan dysfunction syndrome.
- In the last 20 years, onset and outcome of acute kidney failure in these patients has been improved by early aggressive burn wound excision, new powerful antibiotics, and early enteral nutrition for maintaining gastrointestinal trophism.
- In patients with established ARF, early intensive extracorporeal treatment is effective in reaching a mean survival rate of 20–50% of treated patients.

6.16.1 Introduction

A severe burn is a skin injury accompanied by a serious systemic illness with aftermaths in several distant organs leading to high mortality rates. The main risk factors for burn patient outcome are age, percentage of total burn surface area (TBSA), the presence of inhalation injury or other traumatic lesions, and comorbidities. Taking into consideration a patient over 60 years of age, with more than 40% TBSA, and inhalation injury, probability of death is estimated to be higher than 90% [33]. Fortunately, in the last 20 years, burn-related mortality has decreased in Western countries thanks to a systematic primary prevention of burns and specific treatment protocols for burn shock, including early fluid resuscitation and immediate admission to highly specialized burn centers with skilled medical personnel.

However, the major fatal complication is the multiorgan dysfunction syndrome (MODS) which is prevalently a consequence of sepsis in that lungs are among the organs invariably affected (100%) followed by the intestine and kidneys (68%) [38].

6.16.2 Pathophysiology of Burns

6.16.2.1 Thermal Injury

Thermal injuries cause coagulative necrosis of the skin and underlying soft tissue. As soft tissue temperature increases, capillary permeability increases and fluid loss occurs leading to hypovolemia and shock proportionally to burn extension and thickness. After a few hours from the burn injury, the body elicits a systemic release of inflammatory mediators and changes into hormonal and immunologic responses that increase vasodilation and extravascular fluid loss phenomena. Increased mesenteric vascular resistance and decreased intestinal perfusion can be observed in the gut, leading to bacterial translocation and endotoxemia. Circulating

F. Mariano (✉)
Department of Internal Medicine, Division of Nephrology and Dialysis, CTO Hospital, Via G. Zurreti 29, 10126 Turin, Italy
e-mail: filippo.mariano@cto.to.it

A. Jörres et al. (eds.), *Management of Acute Kidney Problems*,
DOI: 10.1007/978-3-540-69441-0_6.16, © Springer-Verlag Berlin Heidelberg 2010

and local mediators include cytokines (interleukin-1 [IL-1], IL-2, IL-6, IL-8, IL-12, and tumor necrosis factor [TNF]), growth factors, activation products of coagulation and contact phase cascades, complement factors, nitric oxide, platelet-activating factor (PAF), prostaglandins (PGs), and leukotrienes. Endocrine rearrangement includes increased levels of cortisol and prolactin, a state of insulin resistance and peripheral inactivation of thyroid hormones that may jointly affect the metabolic response to burns leading to nitrogen and calcium negative balance, lipolysis, and massive peripheral muscle catabolism (the so-called wasting syndrome).

6.16.2.2 Chemical Injury

Potentially dangerous chemicals are ubiquitous in modern life. Noxious agents include alkalis, acids, or organic compounds. Prolonged contact with gasoline, kerosene, or diesel fuel may produce a chemical burn that is a full-thickness injury. Systemic absorption may cause organ dysfunction and death if exposure to the aforementioned substances is prolonged and the surface area involved is large. This may be evident within 6–24 h after injury with pulmonary insufficiency and/or hepatic and renal failure.

6.16.2.3 Electrical Injury

Most tissue damage in electrical injury is caused by heat generated by current flow which causes tissue destruction at the contact site and along the current pathway. Electrical current injury may be fatal or cause arrhythmia, direct cardiac damage, respiratory arrest, and neurological complications. Acute renal failure (AFR) arising from myoglobinemia and myoglobinuria due to massive rhabdomyolysis can complicate clinical picture.

6.16.2.4 Inhalation-Associated Injury

Carbon monoxide inhalation, direct thermal injury to the upper aerodigestive tract, and inhalation of products of combustion are the mechanisms of inhalation injury. This associated lesion may increase mortality from 30% to 40% owing to acute lung injury or acute respiratory distress syndrome (ARDS) which are likely to occur during the course of the burn patients.

6.16.2.5 Fluid Management and Prevention of Septic Complications

Fluid resuscitation and circulating blood volume monitoring are of primary importance in the acute treatment of the burn patient. In the first 24 h postburn, the goal is to restore and maintain adequate tissue perfusion and oxygenation, avoid organ ischemia, and preserve heat-injured but viable soft tissue. Thus, both exogenous contribution to edema and infection risk in compromised tissue are minimized. Many resuscitation formulas based on crystalloids (lactated Ringer's solution) or colloids (frozen plasma and albumin) have been proposed by Parkland, Evans, Brooke, and Slater [7, 31]. All these formulas have to be considered as guidelines only, with careful precise monitoring of the patient's status in order to adjust the amount of fluid resuscitation given accurately to decrease the incidence of shock-related complications such as early ARF [5, 16]. Colloid use has decreased because controlled trials have shown no clear advantage: during administration of albumin after 24 h of clinically satisfactory crystalloid resuscitation, an increased rate of pulmonary complications [10] and a decrease in the glomerular filtration rate have been observed [11].

Presence of a concomitant inhalation injury needs even larger volumes of infusion. In 51 burn patients with TBSA > 25% and inhalation injury, after an initial fluid resuscitation according to the Parkland formula, an infusion was performed to provide a urine output of 30–50 ml/h. For successful resuscitation, patients with inhalation injuries required a mean infusion rate of 5.76 ml/kg/%TBSA and sodium replacement of 0.94 mEq/kg/%TBSA. Furthermore, the infusion rate and sodium requirement were significantly higher than those observed in the group without inhalation injury (3.98 ml/kg/%TBSA and 0.68 mEq/kg/%TBSA, respectively, $p < 0.05$) [30].

To obtain urine alkalinization when patients present rhabdomyolysis with myoglobinuria, useful treatments for preventing toxic renal failure include elicited infusion rate, forced diuresis by mannitol or furosemide (higher than 300 ml/h) and the administration of sodium bicarbonate.

Renal damage can arise even from hemoglobinuria in burn patients with associated hemolysis, and the administration of haptoglobin may prevent hemoglobinuria-induced renal failure. In fact, in a controlled study in ten extensively burned patients with overt hemoglobinuria, five received fluid resuscitation (control group) and the other five patients also received haptoglobin in addition to fluid resuscitation. In the therapy group, free serum hemoglobin dropped rapidly, whereas its levels in the control group remained unchanged for at least 12 h. The time required for macroscopic hemoglobinuria to clear showed a statistically significant difference between the haptoglobin-treated patients and the control patients [45].

Sepsis is still currently the most important cause of burn death and is closely associated with the development of late renal damage in the context of MODS. However, in the last few decades, early and aggressive burn wound excision, better use of topical antimicrobial agents to limit local bacterial colonization, new powerful antibiotics, and early nutritional enteric support for the gastrointestinal trophism have been decisive in improving infection control and burn patient survival.

6.16.3 Renal and Electrolyte Abnormalities

In severe burn patients, the kidney is invariably affected, with a wide range of morphologic and functional alterations. Several pathogenic mechanisms such as, filtered breakdown products, antibiotic toxicity, and sepsis are thought to be involved in these alterations. Renal alterations often include a transitory contraction of renal function and, more rarely, severe forms of ARF requiring renal replacement therapy (RRT) (see Table 6.16.1).

Table 6.16.1 Renal alterations in patients with burns

Changes in renal blood flow and glomerular filtration rate
Increased mean kidney mass and renal blood flow
Increased/decreased glomerular filtration rate
Proximal renal tubular abnormalities
Glycosuria, excessive loss of Na^+, K^+, Ca^{++}, Mg^{++}, and phosphate
Na^+ and water retention, hyponatremia, and hypokalemia
Proteinuria and hematuria
Acute renal failure
End-stage renal failure

6.16.3.1 Renal Blood Flow and Glomerular Filtration Rate Changes

In convalescent burn patients, renal blood flow was increased [9], while glomerular filtration rate (GFR) was found to be decreased or increased [36]. Autopsy findings showed mean kidney weight was usually increased [9]. In ordinary clinical evaluation, estimated GFR by creatinine clearance could lead to unreliable results, because hyperhydration and reduced muscle mass overestimate renal function.

6.16.3.2 Tubular and Electrolyte Alterations

In burn patients, electrolyte abnormalities such as hypernatremia, hyponatremia, hypokalemia, and decreased calcium and magnesium blood levels were commonly observed [3]. Losses through the burn wound exudates not completely replaced and abnormal urinary output contributed to fluid impairment and electrolyte abnormalities. Other alterations involved increased fractional sodium excretion, high uric acid clearance, a low phosphate adsorption threshold, glycosuria, and aminoaciduria. Rare cases of hypercalcemia likewise due to prolonged immobilization have also been described [18, 20, 35, 36].

6.16.3.3 Hematuria and Proteinuria

Microscopic hematuria is a common finding in burn patient with an indwelling bladder catheter. Frank hematuria was described in about 5% of children with burns. In most cases, underlying causes were urinary tract infections (50%), followed by renal stones (15%), catheter-related trauma, and renal vein thrombosis. When hematuria was associated with acute tubular necrosis (ATN), it was seen as a negative prognostic factor [41].

Proteinuria is usually present in severe burn patients, starting in the first few days after admission and increasing over time. Proteinuria is of a mixed type, reflecting both increased glomerular permeability and decreased tubular reabsorption of filtered proteins such as lysozyme, β2-microglobulin, and amylase [32, 35]. Proteinuria, which was in the nephrotic range, lasted several weeks and peaked in the second to third week when all patients showed full clinical signs of severe sepsis [22]. The extent of proteinuria was correlated in a significantly positive manner with indices of renal function, such as blood creatinine and urea. Proteinuria also correlated with indices of systemic inflammation (positively with white blood cells and negatively with platelet count) and negatively with outcome [25]. In addition, the plasma of severe burn septic patients with ARF contain factors that functionally affect glomerular and tubular epithelial cells. These plasmas were able to promote cell polarity alteration and a dose-dependent proapoptotic effect on both podocytes and tubular cells that correlated with the extent of proteinuria. Proteinuria could be considered as a hallmark of renal involvement in systemic inflammatory reaction due to burns and sepsis, and it is a negative prognostic factor [22].

6.16.4 Acute Renal Failure

ARF in burn patients is not common. Two distinct pictures of ARF can be observed: early ARF, occurring either few hours after injury or in the first few days, and late ARF developing approximately 1 or more weeks after burn injury. Early ARF may be due to hypovolemia and hypoperfusion of the kidneys, whereas late ARF is a consequence of infection, endotoxemia, and MODS. In the last 20 years, ARF clinical presentation has changed from early to late findings in accordance with the evolution in burn care.

6.16.4.1 *Incidence and Prognosis*

Data as to ARF incidence in burn patients varies widely from 0.5% to 30%, and the mortality rate has been described to be between 50% and 100%. Different definitions of ARF and the nonhomogeneous population studied justify the observed high variation of these reported data [27–29,35,37].

However, in previous reports regarding the period before the 1980s (when RRT was not always available or feasible), the survival rate of patients with ARF was very low or zero. On the basis of published data between 1953 and 1979, 119 patients out of 7,126 developed ARF, and only eight of these survived [6].

As an impressive experience, in 1984 Sawada et al. published a case report of ARF survival in a severe burn patient who had been anuric for 20 days and was treated by RRT for 35 days. On reviewing the literature, they found only 20 cases of oliguric ARF survival prior to 1984 [34].

Since then, ARF incidence has fallen and survival rate in ARF burn patients has improved considerably. By analyzing data of about 5,000 children with burns admitted from 1966 to 1997 at the Shriners Burns Institute (Galveston, TX, USA), Jeschke et al. found 60 children who had developed ARF. ARF onset was bimodal with one peak occurring in the first week and another at 19–23 days after the burn. By dividing the patients into two periods (one period before 1984 and the other after 1984), they found that the mortality rate of children with ARF decreased from 100% before 1984 and to 56% thereafter. Factors involved in survival improvement were a significantly shorter time delay for fluid resuscitation, early wound excision, and reduced incidence of sepsis (19% vs 60%, $p < 0.05$) [16].

In a study from the same group on 1,404 acute burn adults, ARF incidence was 5.4% (76 patients with burns >30% TBSA). Diagnosis was made on the basis of oliguria, creatinine >2 mg/dl, blood urea nitrogen to serum creatinine ratio >20, and dialysis requirement (diagnosis if present three out of four criteria). Dividing the patients with ARF into survivors and nonsurvivors, the independent risk factors for mortality were found to be age (age <40 years in 67% of survivors and 25% of nonsurvivors, $p < 0.02$), sepsis (44% in survivors and 96% in nonsurvivors $p < 0.05$), ARF as part of MODS (11% in survivors and 96% in nonsurvivors, $p < 0.001$), and time between burn injury and fluid resuscitation initiation (1.7 ± 1.0 h in survivors vs 4.4 ± 2.1 in nonsurvivors, $p < 0.001$). In the multivariate analysis, no significant differences between survivors and nonsurvivors were found for TBSA, third-degree burns (%), and presence of inhalation injury. On comparing ARF patients admitted from 1981 to 1989 (n = 35) with those admitted from 1990 to 1998 ($n = 41$), no significant differences between the two periods could be seen in the ARF incidence (5.4% vs 5.1%) or mortality (88% vs 87%) [5]. From these data they conclude that "the aggressive early fluid resuscitation and the prevention of sepsis may reduce the incidence of ARF in burned adults. This, in turn, may decrease the mortality associated with ARF" [5].

In another series of 147 severely burned patients (mean TBSA 60 ± 21.8%), Gheun-Ho et al. found an ARF incidence of 19% (28 patients). Mortality rate of these patients was 100%, in comparison with 29.4% of those without ARF. In addition, patients with had a significantly larger TBSA (79.5 ± 15.4% vs 55.3 ± 20.5%) and lower serum albumin concentration on admission (1.92 ± 0.66 vs. 2.48 ± 0.82 g/dl). In a multivariate analysis, TBSA >65% was associated with an ARF risk 9.9 times higher than that for patients with burn size <65% [8]. However, in most studies, no data were provided on timing of dialysis initiation or on dialysis dose.

Apart from specific causes of mortality relating to burns, the acute uremic state could be per se an important negative factor for outcome, as was demonstrated in a wide survey of Austrian intensive care units [26].

6.16.4.2 Early Acute Renal Failure

During the first few days after burn injury, alterations in renal functions and urinary abnormalities are common. Many factors affect renal homeostasis, such as acute change in volemia, electrolyte disturbances, hormones, presence of a plethora of inflammatory mediators, and elevated levels of toxic breakdown products such as myoglobin and hemoglobin in blood.

Acute change in volemia is prolonged by excessive fluid loss from the burn wound and movement of large quantities of fluid from the intravascular compartment to the interstitial space due to a massive capillary leakage. Because depletion of circulating volume and both local and generalized edema are fully manifested in a few hours after injury, any delay in fluid resuscitation may exacerbate volume depletion and decreased renal blood flow. Sodium retention in the interstitial space and sodium-potassium pump impairment also contribute to generalized edema.

Burn stress stimulates the production and release of hormones such as catecholamines, aldosterone, angiotensin II, and vasopressin, which can lead to vasoconstriction and changes in renal blood flow. On the other hand, plasma atrial natriuretic polypeptide (ANP) levels elevated after burns counterbalance the action of the stress-related hormones through vasodilatation and natriuresis. Excessively high levels of stress-related hormones and/or impairment of ANP secretion may participate in reduced renal function.

Moreover, many inflammatory mediators including cytokines (TNF, IL-1, IL-6), eicosanoids (PGs, thromboxane, and leukotrienes), and PAF can affect the kidney in the early postburn period, because they variably increase microvascular permeability as well as activate circulating inflammatory cells. Inflammatory mediators promote adhesion and migration of activated neutrophils in burned tissue. As a specific PG in the kidney, the vasodilator PG-E_2 counteracts the above vasoconstrictor substances, but its production is inhibited in the early phase of a burn. In addition, acute burns cause immediate depression of cardiac inotropism before any detectable reduction in plasma volume. This effect is due to an apoptotic mechanism induced by circulating endotoxin. Bacterial translocation and gut derived-factors are likely to be involved in this depression of myocardial function [4].

As a result of muscular damage, massive rhabdomyolysis and/or hemolysis due to extensive full-thickness burns or electric injury burns, massive amounts of myoglobin and hemoglobin, often in excess of haptoglobin-binding capability, are released in the blood compartment. Hemoglobin and myoglobin are freely filtered, absorbed by tubular epithelium, and degraded into globin and heme. The latter is directly toxic on tubular cells by generating oxygen free radicals via iron ions. When combined with dehydration, acidosis, shock, or endotoxemia, toxic effects of myoglobin or hemoglobin affect the kidney, with occlusion of tubules, formation of hemoglobin casts, and acute loss of kidney function [5].

6.16.4.3 Late Acute Renal Failure

Sepsis and MODS, the main late complications arising from 1 to 2 weeks after burn injury, are usually responsible for late acute renal dysfunction [5, 16, 33, 35]. Sepsis as a life-threatening complication mainly originates from the burn wound infection.

However, impaired gastrointestinal barrier function is another potential cause of MODS. Increasing evidence suggests that bacterial translocation occurring through the damaged intestinal mucosa may lead to repetitive episodes of endotoxemia and sepsis. These episodes which can last several weeks impact on distant organs including the kidney. The lipopolysaccharide component of gram-negative bacterial cell wall endotoxin, as well as lipoteichoic acid and other bacterial wall components are capable of inducing ARF either directly or by synthesis of secondary mediators [17, 21, 43]. Microcirculatory derangement due to sepsis leads to inadequate delivery of oxygen to peripheral tissues and lactic acidosis, perpetuating the vicious cycle of renal ischemia and tubular injury.

ARF may also be due to antibiotic drugs administered to control sepsis. Some antibiotics, such as aminoglycosides and certain cephalosporins, are known to be nephrotoxic. Drug nephrotoxicity is highlighted by the concomitant presence of septic shock and fever [46].

Acute or chronic intoxication with alcohol, barbiturates, chlorpromazine, toluene, and paint thinner have been reported as possible associated agents inducing renal failure in burn patients, but early resuscitation therapy was delayed in some of these patients [33].

6.16.5 Renal Replacement Therapy in Burn Patients

6.16.5.1 *Early Experiences of Dialysis*

Even though RRT in burn patients has been reported since the 1950s, the first survivor from ARF secondary to burns was indicated in literature only in 1965 [44].

Until the mid-1980s, the standard intermittent hemodialysis was the only option of treatment. This was usually performed daily to achieve a low-level azotemia maintenance and a wide fluid removal which was necessary to balance the massive amounts of liquid infused for hemodynamic stabilization, parenteral nutrition, and drug administration. However, burn patients were often suffering from septic shock, with low tolerance to high-rate fluid removal, and their survival rate was very low. In 1986, continuous arteriovenous hemofiltration (CAVH) was first proven to be an effective tool in removing fluid in severe burn patients with anasarca and ARF, allowing the maintenance of a nutritional support and other fluid intake [15].

6.16.5.2 *Dialysis Data in the Last 20 Years*

Despite the use of dialytic support in this kind of patient being popular, there are few data available in literature, patients groups are insufficient, and trials are lacking. During the last 2 decades, continuous RRT has reached a good standard quality, and different therapy modalities (hemodialysis, hemodiafiltration, and hemofiltration) have been reported for burn adults with an overall mortality rate of 70% (on about 200 patients altogether) [1, 6, 12–15, 19, 23, 39–41, 44].

Currently, early dialysis initiation is always recommended in burn patients when signs of renal failure appear, both in early and late ARF [2].

In 1999, Holm et al. reported a 15% survival in a large population of 48 patients with ARF following burns and requiring RRT (corresponding to 15% of the total burn population cared for in his unit) [14]. The mean burned TBSA was 48% (ranging from 13% to 95%), and 79% of patients had an inhalation injury. Patients were all treated with continuous arteriovenous hemofiltration for a mean of 10.5 days (from 1 to 47 days). Complications relating to vascular catheter were observed in 10%, with two patients experiencing thromboembolic complications in the lower leg, and three patients had significant bleeding from the catheter insertion site in the femoral artery. The percentage of burned surface area and the presence of inhalation injury significantly correlated with ARF development, whereas the degree of burns, age, and electric injury showed no correlation. The need for RRT was frequently associated with the development of multiple organ failure (MOF), and 83% of patients with ARF died because of MOF. Neither age, day of ARF onset, dialysis support duration, nor TBSA proved predictive for patient survival.

Since the mid-1990s, a blood pump has become available for continuous venovenous techniques.

Leblanc et al. reported their experience with continuous RRT in 16 and in 12 burn patients treated, respectively, from 1987 to 1994 and from 1995 to 1998, and corresponding to 1.6% of the total population admitted to the burn unit in the related periods [19, 39]. In patients requiring RRT, the burned TBSA was respectively 58 ± 5.7% and 48 ± 16%, the APACHE II score was 18.4 ± 2% and 19.7 ± 3%, and 11/16 and 12/12 patients were septic. Leblanc et al. made use of different techniques of continuous treatment, such as, continuous arteriovenous hemofiltration and hemodiafiltration (CAVH and CAVHDF), only used in the first period of time, while continuous venovenous hemofiltration and venovenous hemodiafiltration (CVVH and CVVHDF) were preferred in the second period. Overall mortality rate was 67.8% (19 out of 28), but survival improved from 18% to 50% from 1987–1994 to 1995–1998.

By comparing the burn population to a group of critically ill patients admitted to the intensive care unit in the same period of time and requiring dialytic support, Leblanc et al. observed that in burn patients the mean duration of replacement treatment was longer (24.2 ± 9.4 vs 5.3 ± 0.8 days, $p < 0.006$), the mean fluid intake was higher (8.2 ± 0.7 vs 3.3 ± 0.2 l/day, $p < 0.0001$) while total weight loss during the whole therapy was lower (12.6 ± 3.6 kg vs 6.8 ± 1.0 kg, $p < 0.03$). Moreover, the authors indicated a higher incidence of hemorrhagic complications in burn patients (56% vs 15%), mostly related to wound bleeding [1]. When platelet count was lower than 50,000/ml, no heparin was used [39].

The anticoagulation modality of the extracorporeal circuit was one of the critical problems for the application of the continuous treatments. In fact, the long therapy duration required the use of a large amount of anticoagulant drugs to maintain blood circulation patency. The critically ill population in general, and burn patients in particular, often have a high bleeding risk because of possible ongoing hemorrhage, frequent associated injuries, or extensive open surfaces or surgery. Heparin may be considered as an invasive procedure that can expose these patients to an unbearable hemorrhagic risk [23]. Regional anticoagulation with citrate may be an effective alternative especially for continuous dialysis, which is useful even when sorbent technology is applied [23–25].

In critically ill patients, citrate anticoagulation is reported to be related to an increased filter survival and to a reduced incidence of bleeding complications when compared with heparin. In severe burn patients with septic shock, associated ARF citrate, applied as sole anticoagulant, appeared to be effective and safe during coupled plasma filtration absorption (CPFA)-continuous venovenous hemofiltration treatment [23]. By comparing 58 CPFA sessions using systemic anticoagulation with heparin (mean heparin 741 U/h) with 28 sessions using citrate regional anticoagulation (citrate-containing replacement solutions), no differences in number of used cartridges were observed, while the number of lost cartridges was significantly lower in the citrate patients. In these conditions, citratemia mean level in the extracorporeal circuit was 4 mmol/l, and no accumulation of citrate in systemic blood was reported (systemic citratemia remained below 0.5 mmol/l). A citrate peak serum level of 2.68 mmol/l was observed after 7 h of treatment only in one patient with acute kidney and liver failure, nevertheless the reduction of blood flow rate and citrate infusion proved to be promptly effective at lowering citratemia [23].

Some experiences of peritoneal dialysis in burn patients with ARF are reported in the literature, especially in children [30]. This treatment modality offers the advantages of better hemodynamic tolerance and no need for anticoagulation therapy. However, it only allows limited fluid removal, besides not providing the clearance required in the severe hypercatabolic status of burn patients and the risk of peritonitis is particularly high in septic patients. In addition, intact abdomen skin has to be preserved for future skin grafts. For all this reasons, extracorporeal treatment has been preferred to peritoneal dialysis for some time.

6.16.6 Take Home Pearls

- Proteinuria, hematuria, and electrolyte disturbances are common in patients with severe burns. True ARF is a rare and life-threatening complication.
- Two distinct pictures of ARF can be observed: early ARF, due to hypovolemia, and late ARF arising from sepsis and MODS.
- Early ARF occurring in the immediate postburn period is nowadays effectively prevented by aggressive fluid resuscitation. Late ARF develops after 2–3 weeks from initial injury and is usually associated with microcirculatory derangement of sepsis and MODS.

References

1. Abdel-Rahman EM, Moorthy AV, Helgerson RB, et al. (1997) ARF requiring dialysis in patients with burns: 16 years' experience in one center. J Am Soc Nephrol 8:121A
2. Bellomo R, Ronco C, Kellum JA, et al. (2004) Acute renal failure – definition, outcome measures, animal models, fluid therapy and information technology needs: the Second International Consensus Conference of the Acute Dialysis Quality Initiative (ADQI) Group. Critical Care 8:R204–12

3. Berger MM, Rothen C, Cavadini C, et al. (1997) Exudative mineral losses after serious burns: a clue to the alterations of magnesium and phosphate metabolism. Am J Clin Nutr 65:1 473–81
4. Carlson DL, Lightfoot E Jr, Bryant DD, et al. (2002)Burn plasma mediates cardiac myocyte apoptosis via endotoxin. Am J Physiol Heart Circ Physiol 282:H1907–14
5. Chrysopoulo MT, Jeschke MG, Dziewulski P, et al. (1999) Acute renal dysfunction in severely burned adults. J Trauma 46:141–4
6. Davies MP, Evans J, McGonigle RJS (1994) The dialysis debate: acute renal failure in dialysis patients. Burns 20: 71–3
7. Dries DJ (2009) Management of burn injuries – recent developments in resuscitation, infection control and outcomes research. Scand J Trauma Resusc Emerg Med 17:14–27
8. Gheun-Ho K, Kook Hwan O, Ja-Ryong K, et al. (2003) Impact of burn size and initial serum albumin level on acute renal failure occurring in major burn. Am J Nephrol 23: 55–60
9. Goodwin CW, Aulick LH, Becker RA, et al. (1980) Increased renal perfusion and kidney size in convalescent burn patients. JAMA 244:1588–90
10. Goodwin CW, Dorethy J, Lam V, et al. (1983) Randomized trial of efficacy of crystalloid and colloid resuscitation on hemodynamic response and lung water following thermal injury. Ann Surg 197:520–31
11. Gore DC, Dalton JM, Gehr TW (1996) Colloid infusions reduce glomerular filtration in resuscitated burn victims. J Trauma 40:356–60
12. Gueugniaud PY (1993) Apport de l'hemodiafiltration continue au traitement des bruleès graves. In: Journois D (ed) Hemofiltration continue. Elsevier, Paris, pp 209–19
13. Hladlik M, Tymonova J, Zaoral T, et al. (2001) Treatment by continuous renal replacement therapy in patients with burns injuries. Acta Chir Plast 43:21–5
14. Holm C, Horbrand F, von Donnersmarck GH, Muhlbauer W (1999) Acute renal failure in severely burned patients. Burns 25:171–8
15. Hubsher J, Olshan AR, Schwartz AB, et al. (1986) Continuous arteriovenous hemofiltration for the treatment of anasarca and acute renal failure in severely burned patients. ASAIO Trans 32:401–4
16. Jeschke MG, Barrow RE, Wolf SE, et al. (1998) Mortality in burned children with acute renal failure. Arch Surg 133: 752–6
17. Kellum JA, Leblanc M, Gibney RT, et al. (2005) Primary prevention of acute renal failure in the critically ill. Curr Opin Crit Care 11:537–41
18. Klein GL, Nicolai M, Langman CB, et al. (1997) Dysregulation of calcium homeostasis after severe burn injury in children: possible role of magnesium depletion. J Pediatr 131:246–51
19. Leblanc M, Thibeault Y, Querin S (1997) Continuous hemofiltration and hemodiafiltration for acute renal failure in severely burned patients. Burns 23:160–5
20. Lindquist J, Drueck C, Simon NM, et al. (1984) Proximal renal tubular dysfunction in severe burns. Am J Kidney Dis 4:44–7
21. Mariano F, Guida G, Donati D, et al. (1999) Production of platelet-activating factor in patients with sepsis-associated acute renal failure. Nephrol Dial Transplant 14:1150–7
22. Mariano F, Stella M, Pezzuto C, et al. (2000) Role of sepsis in inducing renal injury in severe burns patients with acute renal failure. Nephrol Dial Transpl 15:A81
23. Mariano F, Tetta C, Stella M, et al. (2004) Regional citrate anticoagulation in critically ill patients treated with plasma filtration and adsorption. Blood Purif 22:313–9
24. Mariano F, Tetta C, Ronco C, et al. (2006) Is there a real alternative anticoagulant to heparin in continuous treatments? Expert Rev Med Devices. 3:5–8
25. Mariano F, Cantaluppi V, Mauriello G, et al. (2008) Plasma of burn septic patients induced functional glomerular and tubular epithelial cell alterations that may account for proteinuria and acute renal failure. Crit Care 12: R42–R54
26. Metnitz PG, Krenn CG, Steltzer H, et al. (2002) Effect of acute renal failure requiring renal replacement therapy on outcome in critically ill patients. Crit Care Med 30: 2051–8
27. Monafo WW (1996) Initial management of burns. N Engl J Med 21:1581–86
28. Mustonen KM, Vuola J (2008) Acute renal failure in intensive care burn patients (ARF in burn patients). J Burn Care Res 29:227–37
29. Navar PD, Saffle JR, Warden GD (1985) Effect of inhalation injury on fluid resuscitation requirements after thermal injury. Am J Surg 150:716–20
30. Pomeranz A, Reichenberg Y, Schurr D, et al. (1985) Acute renal failure in a burn patient: the advantages of continuous peritoneal dialysis. Burns Incl Therm Inj 11:367–70
31. Prelack K, Dylewski M, Sheridan RL(2007) Practical guidelines for nutritional management of burn injury and recovery. Burns 33:14–24
32. Richmond JM, Sibbald WJ, Linton AM, et al. (1982) Patterns of urinary protein excretion in patients with sepsis. Nephron 31:219–23
33. Ryan CM, Schoenfeld DA, Thorpe WP, et al. (1999) Objective estimates of the probability of death from burn injuries. N Engl J Med 338:362–6
34. Sawada Y, Momma S, Takamizawa A, et al. (1984) Survival from acute renal failure after severe burns. Burns 11: 143–7
35. Schiavon M, Di Landro D, Baldo M, et al. (1988) A study of renal damage in seriously burned patients. Burns Incl Therm Inj 14:107–12
36. Sevitt S (1965) Renal function after burning. J Clin Pathol 18:572–8
37. Sevitt S (1979) A review of the complications of burns, their origin and importance for illness and death. J Trauma 19:358–69
38. Sheridan RL, Ryan CM, Yin LM, et al. (1998) Death in the burn unit: sterile multiple organ failure. Burns 24:307–11
39. Tremblay R, Ethier J, Querin S, et al. (2000) Veno-venous continuous renal replacement therapy for burned patients with acute renal failure. Burns 26:638–43
40. Triolo G, Mariano F, Stella M, et al. (2002) Dialytic therapy in severely burnt patients with acute renal failure. G Ital Nefrol 19:155–9
41. Tweddell JS, Waymack JP, Warden GD, et al. (1987) Haematuria in the burned child. J Pediatr Surg 22:899–903ù
42. Vertel RM, Knochel JP (1967) Nonoliguric acute renal failure. JAMA 15:200:598–602

43. Wan L, Bellomo R, Di Giantomasso D, et al. (2002) The pathogenesis of septic acute renal failure. Curr Opin Crit Care 9:496–502
44. Weksler N, Chorni I, Gurman G, et al. (1997) Improved survival with continuous veno-venous hemofiltration in nonoliguric burned septic patients. Blood Purif 15:137
45. Yoshioka T, Sugimoto T, Ukai T, et al. (1985) Haptoglobin therapy for possible prevention of renal failure following thermal injury: a clinical study. J Trauma 25:281–7
46. Zager RA (1992) Endotoxemia, renal hypoperfusion, and fever: interactive risk factors for aminoglycoside and sepsis-associated acute renal failure. Am J Kidney Dis 20: 223–30

6.17 Acute Kidney Transplant Failure

Ralf Schindler

Core Messages

- The glomerular filtration rate (GFR) of the renal transplant usually averages around 40–50 ml/min. Thus, even slight decreases in GFR that may remain undetected in a healthy patient will cause a rapid increase in serum creatinine in the transplanted patient.
- Calcineurin inhibitors as part of immunosuppressive protocols may cause renal vasoconstriction and also interact with a variety of other drugs, thus potentially increasing their nephrotoxic potential.
- Acute allograft failure may occur in the context of severe infections, secondary to diarrhea and fluid loss, or as a consequence of disturbed (arterial of venous) graft perfusion. If these potential reasons have been investigated and excluded, a renal biopsy must be performed to establish the diagnosis of rejection.

6.17.1 Introduction

Basically, acute failure in a renal transplant follows the same rules as in native kidneys (Table 6.17.1). Every event causing deterioration of native kidney function such as severe infection or hypotension will certainly also affect the renal transplant. There are, however, several issues specific for allograft recipients. The function of the renal transplant is usually not "normal," but glomerular filtration rate (GFR) averages around 40–50 ml/min. Thus, even slight decreases in GFR that remain undetected in a patient with normal baseline renal function of the native kidneys will cause rapid increases in serum creatinine in the transplanted patient due to the hyperbolic relation between GFR and creatinine. This may give the impression that the allograft is particularly vulnerable to any noxious event. In addition, most immunosuppressive protocols include calcineurin inhibitors such as cyclosporin A or tacrolimus. These substances cause vasoconstriction especially at high doses, and vasoconstriction renders the allograft susceptible to ischemia, for instance, during volume depletion or after contrast media.

Another important issue specific for transplant patients is the interaction between immunosuppressive drugs and other medications. For instance, the metabolism of tacrolimus and cyclosporin A is strongly influenced by antibiotics (fluconazol, erythromycin, azithromycin, rifampicin, etc.), calcium channel blockers (diltiazem, verapamil, nifedipine), anticonvulsive drugs (phenytoin), and others. Another example is the synergistic bone marrow toxicity of azathioprine and allopurinol. Other drugs may be especially toxic only because of their retention in chronic renal failure, such as cotrimoxazole. Thus, in transplant patients as in other patients with decreased GFR, great care must be taken to adjust drug doses and drug combinations. One of the best sources for drug adjustments in renal failure is the Renal Drug Book (available online at http://www.kdp-baptist.louisville.edu/renalbook/adult/1/).

R. Schindler
Department of Nephrology and Intensive Care Medicine,
Charité, Campus Virchow-Klinikum,
Augustenburger Platz 1, 13353 Berlin, Germany
e-mail: ralf.schindler@charite.de

A. Jörres et al. (eds.), *Management of Acute Kidney Problems*,
DOI: 10.1007/978-3-540-69441-0_6.17, © Springer-Verlag Berlin Heidelberg 2010

Table 6.17.1 Possible causes of acute allograft failure

	Possible cause	Diagnostic procedure	Treatment
Prerenal	Hypotension	Clinical observation	Volume repletion, catecholamines
	Volume depletion, diarrhea	CMV diagnosis, endoscopy	Antibiotics
	Renal artery stenosis	Doppler ultrasound, MRI	PTA, surgical revision
	Renal vein thrombosis		Intra-arterial thrombolysis
Intrarenal	Drug toxicity	Drug-monitoring	Drug level adjustment
	Rejection	Biopsy	Steroids, antibodies
Postrenal	Ureteral obstruction	Ultrasound	Double J-catheter
	Postvesical obstruction		Nephrostomy
			Bladder catheter
			Supravesical catheter

CMV cytomegalovirus, *MRI* magnetic resonance imaging, *PTA* percutaneous transluminal angioplasty

6.17.2 Clinical Approach and Diagnostic Procedures

6.17.2.1 History

A thorough history must be taken for the patient with acute allograft failure. Charts must be reviewed for nephrotoxic substances such as aminoglycosides, cotrimoxazole, contrast media, and reverse-transcriptase inhibitors. Nonsteroidal antiinflammatory drugs may lead to renal vasoconstriction, especially in the presence of volume depletion. A history of rejection episodes and a "bad" match of the allograft with several HLA-antigen mismatches make the recurrence of rejection more likely. Nonadherence with medication, especially immunosuppressive drugs, is seldom admitted by the patient and must be carefully evaluated. The time after transplant may also give clues to the diagnosis. Within the first days after the transplant, surgical complications involving the renal artery (thrombosis, bleeding, or kinking) or the renal vein (thrombosis) are to be considered. Routine monitoring by Doppler ultrasound, especially in the case of initial nonfunction of the allograft is mandatory. Although severe acute rejection may occur at any time, it is more likely to be early (weeks) after transplant. In contrast, recurrence of the underlying disease usually occurs later (months to years) after transplant and typically leads not to acute but slow deterioration of allograft function or proteinuria. The same is true for polyomavirus infection of the allograft [1].

6.17.2.2 The Patient with Fever or Inflammation

Acute allograft failure may occur in the context of severe infections. Infections are very common after a renal transplant. In a recent large study comparing four different immunosuppressive regimens, the incidence of infections within the first year was approximately 75%, including approximately 20% opportunistic infections [2]. Again, the time after transplant may give clues to the type of infection.

Within the first month, postsurgical infections similar to those in nonimmunocompromised individuals are common. These include urinary tract infections, wound infections, pneumonia, and catheter sepsis, and are mostly caused by bacteria and fungal species [3]. Common viral infections that reactivate in the first month are herpes virus types 1 and 2. Other infections that occur in the first month are untreated infections in the recipient that may be exacerbated by immunosuppression. The most common entity, however, is urinary tract infection, which is not difficult to diagnose. Fever and a urine dipstick positive for leukocytes indicate infection even in the absence of symptoms. While mild symptoms may be treated with quinolones, the patient with high fever and acute allograft failure should be administered a broad-spectrum combination therapy covering gram-negative bacteria, enterobacter, and enterococci.

The second to the sixth month posttransplant is the period where opportunistic infections are most common such as those resulting from cytomegalovirus (CMV), *Pneumocystis, Nocardia, Listeria, Legionella,* and others. Also, latent infections that were present in the recipient or transmitted from the donor may be reactivated or become clinically apparent in this period. Examples include tuberculosis and viral hepatitis.

Beyond the sixth month, the type of infection is mostly related to the degree of immunosuppression, with increased risk of opportunistic infections in patients with poor allograft function and those with repeated episodes of acute rejection requiring increased immunosuppressive therapy. One possible explanation for late infections with allograft dysfunction is unrecognized increased immunosuppression. Up to now, there is no good and clinically established test for the degree of immunosuppression, and most patients are treated by the maxim "one size fits all" instead of receiving tailored immunosuppression. A viral infection commonly seen during this period is reactivated varicella-zoster virus infection manifesting as herpes zoster. Chronic viral infections such as those from hepatitis B virus, hepatitis C virus, Epstein-Barr virus, and CMV are apparent in 10–15% of patients in this time period. It is very unusual for viral infections to cause direct allograft failure by infecting the graft. CMV and herpes rather cause infection of extrarenal tissues (lung, gut) and only secondarily lead to renal failure. In contrast, polyomavirus infects the allograft directly but does not cause acute but rather chronic allograft dysfunction.

6.17.2.3 Diarrhea

Diarrhea is very common in transplanted patients. Possible causes are side effects of drugs, infections with *Clostridium difficile* or CMV. Maes et al. suggested a diagnostic workup including seven different steps [4]. They concluded that in most patients a cause could be identified and successfully treated (Table 6.17.2). Although mycophenolate mofetil (CellCept or Myfortic) is often accused as the main culprit, these drugs were responsible for diarrhea in only 25% of cases. Very common is infection with clostridia after generous treatment of urinary or respiratory tract infections with antibiotics or CMV infections. The latter is especially common in the constellation of donor-positive/recipient-negative CMV status before transplant. Tissue-invasive CMV infection of the gut often can only be diagnosed in biopsy specimens, while the CMV tests (APAAP, PCR) in peripheral blood remain negative.

Diarrhea may provoke prerenal renal failure that causes typical urine findings. These include low urinary sodium concentration and high urine osmolarity. However, since treatment with diuretics is very common, the measurement of fractional urea excretion is more reliable. The fractional excretion of urea can be easily determined by dividing (U-urea × P-creat) by (P-urea × U-creat) × 100. If the result is lower than 35%, prerenal failure is likely. Improvement of renal function after volume repletion also makes prerenal causes plausible.

6.17.2.4 Ultrasound

Immediate ultrasound and Doppler examination by an experienced investigator is mandatory in acute allograft failure [5]. Simple postvesical obstruction must be

Table 6.17.2 Diagnostic work-up for diarrhea in transplanted patients (Derived from Maes et al. [4])

Step	Patients treated	Patients cured
1. Stop superfluous medication: antiarrhythmics, antidiabetics, diuretics, laxantives, proton pump blockers, antihypertensives	14	7
2. Stool cultures for shigella, salmonella, vibrio, aeromonas, mykobacteria, fungi, and clostridial toxins	22	17
3. Virus-screening for CMV, adenovirus, rotavirus	8	5
4. Breath test, D-xylose, 14C-glycocholic acid	39	13
5. Changes of immunosuppression	65	25
6. Coloscopy, biopsies for CMV, parasites, fungi	19	13
7. Symptomatic treatment: lactobacilli, lactose-free diet	28	11
Total		91

CMV cytomegalovirus

excluded. Dilation of the renal pelvis and ureter may indicate urine outflow obstruction due to uereteral stenosis at the bladder anastomosis or due to postvesical obstruction. The functional significance of obstruction, however, is not easily diagnosed. Grade I dilatation of the pelvis is rather common and is caused by the absence of renal innervation. When grade II or III dilatation and a simultaneous creatinine increase are present, urinary obstruction must be excluded by insertion of a double-J catheter and a bladder catheter. Subsequent improvement in renal function makes the functional significance of the dilatation most likely.

Renal perfusion and resistance indices must be examined by Doppler ultrasound. Increased renal resistance may be caused by vasoconstriction (hypovolemia, toxic levels of calcineurin inhibitors) or venous outflow obstruction. In these cases, resistive index is high (above 0.9) and there is little or no diastolic flow. Venous obstruction may be caused by thrombosis of the femoral and renal vein (Fig. 6.17.1). In this patient, postoperative thrombosis of the femoral and iliac veins included partially the allograft vein and could be treated by intra-arterial lysis with t-plasminogen activator.

In contrast, decreases in allograft resistance (resistive index below 0.6 and increased diastolic flow as shown in Fig. 6.17.2), may indicate renal artery stenosis. In addition, high blood flows (above 200 cm/s) and turbulent flow may be detected within the stenosis. Because many patients are older and bear significant atherosclerotic disease, stenosis may also occur at more proximal sites, for instance the main iliac artery (Fig. 6.17.3). Thus, Doppler examination is a valuable tool and must be performed in all cases of acute allograft failure.

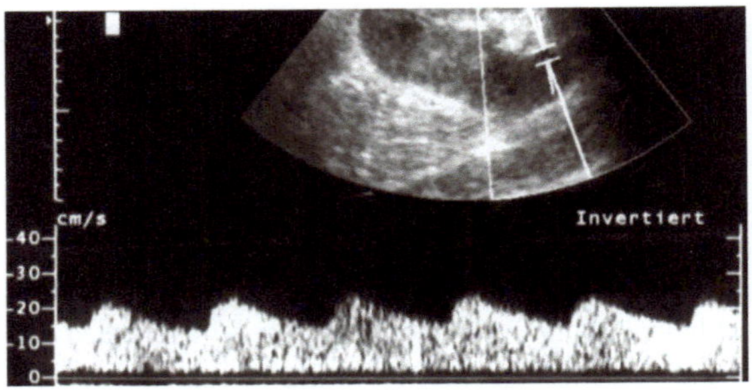

Fig. 6.17.2 Doppler profile in an allograft distal to a renal artery stenosis. Note the high diastolic flow, RI was 0.5

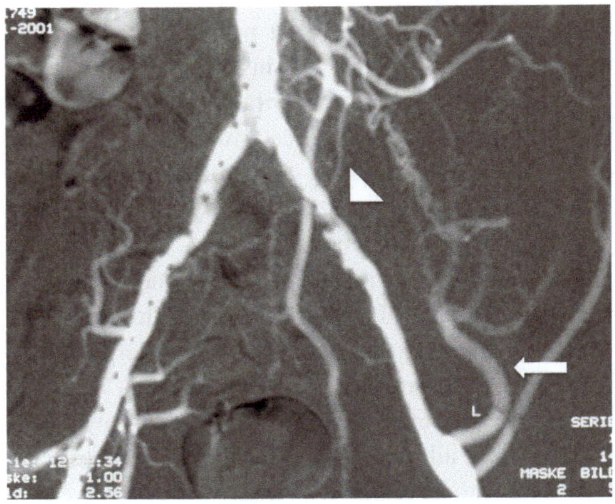

Fig. 6.17.3 Stenosis of the left iliac artery (*arrowhead*) proximal to a renal transplant artery (*solid arrow*)

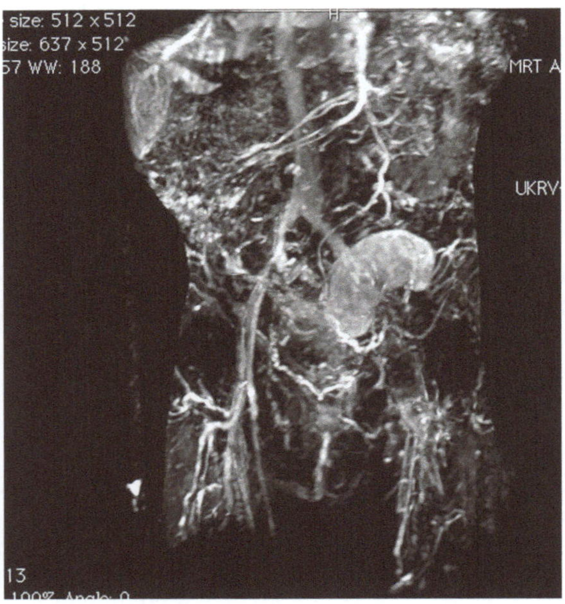

Fig. 6.17.1 Thrombosis of the femoral and iliac common vein including the renal transplant vein (magnetic resonance imaging). The patient presented with oliguria and pain in the left groin

6.17.2.5 Allograft Biopsy

If all of the above reasons for acute allograft failure have been excluded, a renal biopsy must be performed without delay. In most cases, light microscopy is sufficient to establish the diagnosis of rejection. It is important to obtain enough material, at least ten glomeruli and two small arteries to differentiate between grade I and grade II rejection. Staining for C4d is helpful for establishing the diagnosis of vascular rejection. An experienced pathologist must evaluate biopsy specimens. Differential diagnoses include calcineurin inhibitor toxicity, interstitial nephritis (bacterial or viral infections), and ischemic tubular lesions. If rejection is the most likely clinical cause in the absence of other possible causes, treatment with steroid pulses (usually 500 mg/day i.v.) may be initiated before pathologic confirmation. Rejection can also be histologically diagnosed in a biopsy obtained after one or two steroid pulses.

6.17.3 Take Home Pearls

- In patients with suspected acute allograft failure, infections must be searched for and treated, fluid status must be evaluated and corrected if necessary, and (arterial and venous) graft perfusion needs to be evaluated.
- As soon as the above potential reasons for acute allograft failure have been excluded, a renal biopsy must be performed to establish the diagnosis of rejection.

References

1. Weikert BC, Blumberg EA: Viral infection after renal transplantation: surveillance and management. *Clin J Am Soc Nephrol* 3 (Suppl 2):S76–86, 2008
2. Ekberg H, Tedesco-Silva H, Demirbas A, Vitko S, Nashan B, Gurkan A, Margreiter R, Hugo C, Grinyo JM, Frei U, Vanrenterghem Y, Daloze P, Halloran PF: Reduced exposure to calcineurin inhibitors in renal transplantation. *N Engl J Med* 357:2562–2575, 2007
3. Khoury JA, Brennan DC: Infectious complications in kidney transplant recipients: review of the literature. *Saudi J Kidney Dis Transplant* 16:453–497, 2005
4. Maes B, Hadaya K, de Moor B, Cambier P, Peeters P, de Meester J, Donck J, Sennesael J, Squifflet JP: Severe diarrhea in renal transplant patients: results of the DIDACT study. *Am J Transplant* 6:1466–1472, 2006

Acute Kidney Failure During Pregnancy and Postpartum

6.18

Duska Dragun and Michael Haase

Core Messages

- A multidisciplinary, experienced team including nephrologists, gynecologists, and obstetricians should be formed for optimal care in pregnancy-related acute kidney injury (PR-AKI) for both mother and child.
- Management of blood pressure, choice of drugs, and adjustment for drug dosing according to renal function are of great importance. Likewise, correction of anemia and the replacement of water-soluble vitamins, trace elements, and phosphate are mandatory.
- If renal replacement therapy is required, daily intermittent hemodialysis may be the preferred treatment option as it provides intensive solute clearance and better hemodynamic stability compared with alternate-day treatment.
- Measurement of Doppler flow velocity waveform and fetal heart trace should be routinely established as part of the surveillance of pregnancy in patients requiring hemodialysis.

6.18.1 Introduction and Scope

The uniqueness of medical care in pregnancy lies in (1) the body's dramatic adaptation caused by gestation and (2) the need to treat two individuals endangered simultaneously with, however, only one directly accessible [1]. Pregnancy-related acute kidney injury (PR-AKI) is rare and requires the care of an interdisciplinary team of experienced physicians. PR-AKI usually occurs in women with previously healthy kidneys. Known risk factors include (pre)-eclampsia, infection, and autoimmune diseases such as systemic lupus erythematodes.

Despite converging trends, there are still huge differences in the incidence, causes, and outcome of PR-AKI in developed countries compared with developing countries [76]. This is closely linked to environmental and socioeconomic conditions. With the liberalization of abortion laws and improved obstetric care resulting in a decrease in septic abortion and the improvement of prenatal care in developed countries, PR-AKI is now an uncommon occurrence [2, 3]. Since the 1960s, the incidence of PR-AKI has decreased from 1/3,000 to 1/15,000–1/20,000 with respect to the total number of pregnancies. Similarly, the proportion of PR-AKI from total cases of acute kidney injury (AKI) has fallen from 20–40% in the 1960s to 0–1% in the last decade [2].

In developing countries such as India, PR-AKI despite a decrease in renal cortical necrosis following obstetrical complication [4] still accounts for 5–20% of total AKI [4–6]. Simultaneously, mortality decreased from 70% in 1984–1994 to 10–35% in 1995–2005 [4, 7].

In developing countries the most common contributing factors to PR-AKI are abruptio placentae, puerperal sepsis, septic abortion, and postpartum hemorrhage [4], whereas in developed countries the most common causes of PR-AKI are (pre)-eclampsia, microangiopathic thrombocytopenia, sepsis, and hemorrhage by abruptio placentae [2] (Table 6.18.3). Despite decreasing incidence, PR-AKI remains a serious complication with 10–30% [2, 4] of patients progressing to end-stage renal disease.

D. Dragun (✉)
Department of Nephrology and Intensive Care Medicine, Charité Campus Virchow-Klinikum, 13343 Berlin, Germany
dragun@charite.de

A. Jörres et al. (eds.), *Management of Acute Kidney Problems*,
DOI: 10.1007/978-3-540-69441-0_6.18, © Springer-Verlag Berlin Heidelberg 2010

6.18.1.1 Physiology of Maternal Renal Adaptation During Pregnancy

Normal pregnancy is associated with marked hemodynamic alterations within maternal circulation, including increases in cardiac output and plasma volume and reductions in vascular resistance and arterial pressure. Significant alterations in the activity of various neurohormonal systems and in vascular and endothelial function are associated with this adaptational process. Pregnancy requires a salt-conserving state for a period of several months to allow the accumulation of approximately 8 l of fluid. However, sodium waste tends to be facilitated by the increase in glomerular filtration, the high circulating levels of progesterone, and the decrease in plasma albumin observed during the pregnancy [8].

Rising glomerular filtration rate (GFR) and renal plasma flow contribute to increased creatinine clearance with reestablishment of a steady state in serum creatinine concentration with lower values ranging from 45 to 55 μmol/l [9] (Tables 6.18.1 and 6.18.2). In terms of substrate handling, mild proteinuria (<300 mg/day) occurs and does not indicate renal injury. During pregnancy, increased minute ventilation with hypocapnia is compensated by renal acidosis with reduced plasma bicarbonate concentrations (18–20 mmol/l) [10].

Plasma progesterone levels tend to increase more than 20-fold over the nonpregnant average exerting a natriuretic effect via its mineralocorticoid action as well as direct effects on distal tubular reabsorption. Increased levels of aldosterone and the increased rennin activity counterbalance actions of progesterone. The reduction in the arterial pressure in the face of marked increase in cardiac output during pregnancy is due to a considerable decrease in vascular tone. An increase in nitric oxide (NO) during normal pregnancy has been suggested to mediate decreases in vascular resistance by direct actions and by blunting the vascular responsiveness to vasoconstrictors. The renal circulation is among other vascular beds particularly affected already during normal pregnancy. Both renal plasma flow and GFR increase over 50% above in normal pregnant women, averaging 149 ± 34 ml/min/1.73 m² [11, 12]. Although numerous factors, including vasodilatory hormone relaxin, may be involved in this marked renal vasodilatation, NO has been implicated as an important mediator of the renal hyperfiltration during pregnancy. Pregnancy is associated with enhanced renal expression and activation of NO synthase isoforms.

Table 6.18.1 Laboratory values in healthy pregnancies

Variable	Normal value during pregnancy
Glomerular filtration rate	↑ Approx. 40% over baseline
Creatinine clearance	↑ Approx. 25% over baseline
Blood urea nitrogen	↓ 9.0 mg/dl
pCO_2	↓ 10 mmHg below baseline
Bicarbonate	↓ 18–20 mmol/l
Urinary protein	Max. 300 mg/24 h

Source: Adapted from [1]

6.18.2 Diagnosis

During recent decades, there was a paucity of AKI definitions, and these mainly relied on arbitrary cutoff values of increases in serum creatinine within various periods of time. Recently, there are suggestions for consensus definitions of AKI, previously referred to as acute renal failure [13, 14]. Nevertheless, these

Table 6.18.2 Mean plasma concentration of renal function markers and albumin during pregnancy

	Controls (*n* = 58)	6–13 weeks (*n* = 94)	22–27 weeks (*n* = 107)	34–36 weeks (*n* = 88)	37–42 weeks (*n* = 109)
	65.2	52.9**	50.8**	52.7**	54.9*
Creatinine (μmol/l)	48–82 (100%)	36–70 (–19%)	37–64) (–22%)	(39–66) (–20%)	37–73 (–16%)
	236	173**	204*	241	295**
Urate (μmol/l)	121–351 (100%)	107–239 (–27%)	127–281 (–13%)	146–336 (+2%)	162–428 (+25%)
	0.84	0.820	0.84	1.08**	1.16***
Cystatin C (mg/l)	0.66–1.02 (100%)	66–1.00 (–2%)	0.64–1.04 (±0%)	0.79–1.37 (+29%)	0.79–1.53 (+39%)
	1.45	1.48	1.64	1.83**	2.10***

Reference interval (mean ± 1.96 SD) and percentage (%) relationship to the nonpregnant group for each trimester group
Source: Adapted from [10]
* Significant differences
** Significant differences
*** Significant differences

definitions are also partly serum creatinine-based with creatinine being a surrogate parameter of renal function that is affected by several nonrenal factors such as muscle mass, age, sex, and drugs [15]. Serum creatinine is considered a late indicator of AKI as it typically increases only when the GFR has decreased to <50% of its normal value [15]. During pregnancy, diagnosis of AKI might be further delayed due to serum creatinine concentrations reestablished at lower levels caused by increased GFR and hemodilution. Novel renal biomarkers independent from serum creatinine such as neutrophil gelatinase-associated lipocalin [16] are needed for early and specific diagnosis of PR-AKI at a time when it might still be amenable to therapeutic interventions to protect mother and child from morbidity and mortality. However, such markers have not yet been investigated in pregnancy.

6.18.3 Preeclampsia/Eclampsia/HELLP Syndrome

6.18.3.1 Preeclampsia

Preeclampsia is defined as hypertension associated with proteinuria occurring after 20 weeks of gestation. Hypertension is defined as a blood pressure of at least 140 mm Hg (systolic) or at least 90 mm Hg (diastolic) on at least two occasions and at least 4–6 h apart after the 20 weeks of gestation in women known to be previously normotensive [17]. Proteinuria is defined as excretion of 300 mg or more of protein every 24 h. Preeclampsia is regarded as serious if severe hypertension is associated with proteinuria or if hypertension is associated with severe proteinuria (>5 g/day) [17]. Presence of multiorgan involvement such as pulmonary edema, oliguria (<500 ml/day), thrombocytopenia (platelet count <100,000/μl), are also characteristic features of severe preeclampsia [17]. Preeclampsia is a major cause of maternal and neonatal mortality worldwide and a major contributor to premature births and intrauterine growth restriction [18]. Frequency of preeclampsia ranges between 2% and 7% in healthy nulliparous women and increases substantially in women with multifetal gestation, chronic hypertension, previous preeclampsia, pregestational diabetes mellitus, and preexisting thrombophilias [19].

Although many of the clinical and physiologic manifestations associated with preeclampsia resolve after delivery, in some women the disease process can worsen during the first 48 h after delivery. Such women might be at risk for pulmonary edema, renal failure, postpartum eclampsia, HELLP syndrome, and stroke [17]. Impact of preeclampsia also persists in the late postpartum period. Epidemiologic studies provide evidence that women with history of preeclampsia are more likely to develop hypertension compared with women who had normal pregnancies, and women who experience recurrent preeclamptic pregnancies are at even greater risk. History of preeclampsia is also associated with greater risk of cardiovascular disease (CVD), including myocardial infarction, ischemic heart disease, and stroke. The underlying mechanism that places women with a history of preeclampsia at risk for CVD remains speculative. This is a clinically important area of investigation because maternal-fetal stress is a major factor for poor obstetric and infant outcomes, including prematurity and intrauterine growth restriction as well as susceptibility to CVD and metabolic disease throughout life.

The predominant reason for the hypofiltration in preeclampsia is impaired hydraulic permeability of glomerular capillary walls, owing mainly to reductions in size and density of endothelial cell fenestrae, to the accumulation of subendothelial fibrinoid deposits, and to the interposition of mesangial cells. Glomerular capillary endotheliosis is a characteristic glomerular lesion of preeclampsia. Kidneys of women with preeclampsia also develop prominent swelling of endocapillary cells (mesangial and endothelial cells) [12, 20]. Podocytes also usually appear swollen. Preeclampsia is the leading cause of nephrotic syndrome during pregnancy [21]. Glomerular enlargement and endothelial swelling usually disappear within 8 weeks of delivery, coinciding with resolution of the hypertension and proteinuria. Focal segmental glomerulosclerosis can accompany the generalized glomerular endotheliosis of preeclampsia in 50% of cases [22].

The edema in preeclampsia is unlike the "underfill edema" of congestive heart failure, hepatic cirrhosis, and nephrotic syndrome, where low effective circulating volume leads to high plasma renin and aldosterone concentrations with secondary renal sodium retention [23]. In contrast, the edema of preeclampsia resembles "overfill edema" of acute glomerulonephritis or acute ischemic renal failure in which glomerular-tubular imbalance has been invoked as a cause of salt retention [24]. Hypoalbuminemia is common and may contribute to edema, although the correction of hypoalbuminemia with albumin infusions in preeclamptic patients usually does not increase a diuresis.

Coincident with glomerular endotheliosis, there is an overall decrease in GFR and effective renal plasma flow to approximately 24–34% [25]. In addition to the primary effects of preeclampsia on renal function, preeclampsia can also predispose to acute renal failure through secondary effects of relative intravascular volume depletion, vasoconstriction, and activation of the inflammatory and coagulation cascades. In this setting, the superimposed insult of hemorrhage (e.g., abruption placentae or postpartum hemorrhage) can substantially impair renal perfusion, thus increasing risks of renal deterioration. Indeed, patients with pregnancy complication superimposed on preeclampsia are at increased risk for development of acute renal failure [26]. In preeclampsia-related acute renal failure, the structural injury is acute tubular necrosis, with the most severe cases at risk for renal cortical necrosis, yet they occur rather rare.

Trials aimed at prevention or at reduction of the rate or severity of preeclampsia showed a minimum to no benefit. Women with a low baseline dietary calcium intake and at high risk for preeclampsia may benefit from calcium supplementation, as they had lower blood pressure levels and reduced incidence of disease [27]. Low-dose aspirin had small to moderate benefits in prevention of preeclampsia and was noted to be safe [28].

Antihypertensive treatment is aimed at prevention of potential cerebrovascular and cardiovascular complications [29]. Although the use of antihypertensives has been shown to prevent cerebrovascular problems, they do not prevent or alter the natural course of the disease in women with mild preeclampsia. In preeclampsia, the gestational age as well as the level of blood pressure influences the use of antihypertensives. At term, women with preeclampsia are likely to be delivered, treatment of hypertension (unless severe) can be delayed, and blood pressure can be reevaluated postpartum. If preeclampsia develops remote from term, and expectant management is undertaken, treatment of hypertension is initiated, and blood pressure can usually be safely lowered to 140/90 mm Hg with oral agents nifedipine or labetalol. Antihypertensive treatment is also recommended for sustained values of systolic blood pressure of at least 160 mm Hg and for sustained diastolic values of at least 110 mm Hg [17]. Parenteral hydralazine, labetalol, and short-acting oral nifedipine are the most commonly used drugs to control acute severe hypertension in women with preeclampsia. When antihypertensives are used, fetal monitoring is mandatory to recognize any signs of fetal distress that might be attributable to reduced placental perfusion. Control of severe hypertension has been studied in a recent meta-analysis, and this suggested that intravenous labetalol or oral nifedipine is as effective as intravenous hydralazine, with fewer adverse effects [30].

Adequate prenatal care is most important in the management of preeclampsia [19, 31]. Maternal antenatal monitoring includes identification of women at high risk, early detection by the recognition of clinical symptoms, and increase in the severity of the condition [29]. Subsequent treatment depends on results of the initial maternal and fetal assessment. The main objective of management of preeclampsia is the safety of the mother. Although delivery is always appropriate for the mother, it poses a difficulty for a very premature fetus. Fetal gestational age, fetal status, and severity of maternal condition should be considered in the decision-making process. In cases of severe preeclampsia characterized by progressive deterioration of both maternal and fetal conditions, delivery is clearly indicated if the disease develops after 34 weeks of gestation. The same recommendations apply when there is imminent eclampsia, multiorgan dysfunction, severe intrauterine growth restriction, suspected abruption placentae, or non-reassuring fetal testing before 34 weeks of gestation [19]. There is no consensus as to whether to pursue interventionist or expectant care [32]. Short-term morbidity for the baby might be reduced by a policy of expectant care [33].

Choice of antihypertensive treatment in the postpartum period is often influenced by breast feeding [29], but in general, agents commonly used in the antepartum period can be used postpartum. Patients with hypertension accompanied by symptomatic pulmonary or peripheral edema benefit from a brief course of furosemide treatment in the days postpartum [34].

6.18.3.2 Eclampsia

Eclampsia is defined as the occurrence of generalized seizures during pregnancy or postpartum period, without an apparent neurologic etiology, in a woman who has or subsequently develops preeclampsia. Preeclampsia may evolve from mild to severe disease and then to eclampsia, yet only about 2% of women with preeclampsia will have seizures. However, the old paradigm implicating the transition from the mild to more severe disease manifestations has been challenged, as it has been reported that 60% of seizures were the first sign of preeclampsia, before hypertension occurred, and only 13% women had had severe preeclampsia prior to seizures [35]. Seizures may occur as late as after 1 week after delivery, without preceding hypertension. Many of the neurologic abnormalities of eclampsia are similar to hypertensive encephalopathy, including abnormalities localized to regions of posterior circulation, and may represent focal areas of cerebral edema, as detected on computed tomography scan and magnetic resonance imaging [36].

Magnesium-sulfate prophylaxis in women with preeclampsia may prevent or reduce the rate of eclampsia and its complications [31]. Secondary benefits also include reduced maternal and perinatal morbidities in women with severe preeclampsia and lower rate of progression to severe disease in those with mild preeclampsia [31]. On the other hand, magnesium sulfate showed no benefit on perinatal outcome in women with mild preeclampsia [31].

Women with hypertensive encephalopathy, hemorrhage, or eclampsia require treatment with parenteral antihypertensives to lower 2/3 diastolic plus 1/3 systolic blood pressure by 25% over minutes to hours and then to further lower blood pressure to 160/100 mm Hg over subsequent hours [17].

6.18.3.3 HELLP Syndrome

HELLP syndrome develops in approximately 10–20% of women with severe preeclampsia. HELLP syndrome is considered to be severe preeclampsia with the additional prominent features of (a) microangiopathic hemolytic anemia with fragmented erythrocytes and polychromasia on the peripheral blood smear, and increased lactate dehydrogenase (LDH), (b) liver function abnormalities (increased serum aspartate aminotransferase [AST] and alanine aminotransferase [ALT]). HELLP syndrome is described as severe when the platelet count is less than 50,000/μl [37]. The incidence of acute renal failure in HELLP syndrome is much higher than in preeclampsia, affecting almost 10% of the patients [38]. Management is similar to severe preeclampsia, and delivery is the only cure.

There has been uncertainty regarding the safety and efficacy of corticosteroids in women with severe preeclampsia with or without HELLP syndrome. The available data support the effectiveness and safety of corticosteroids to reduce neonatal complications in women with severe preeclampsia at 34 weeks of gestation or less [39].

6.18.4 Thrombotic Microangiopathies

Thrombotic thrombocytopenic purpura (TTP) and hemolytic uremic syndrome (HUS) are rather rare during pregnancy and postpartum. Most cases develop antepartum with average gestational age at diagnosis of 26 weeks. Increasing concentrations of procoagulant factors, decreased fibrinolytic activity, loss of endothelial cell thrombomodulin, and decreasing activity of ADAMTS13 may contribute to development of TTP-HUS in susceptible individuals. The critical diagnostic difficulty in pregnant and postpartum women is that thrombocytopenia and microangiopathic hemolytic anemia are also characteristic clinical features of preeclampsia/HELLP syndrome, where neurologic and renal abnormalities may also occur. Similar to nonpregnant patients, plasma exchange is the essential therapy for TTP-HUS [40, 41]. There is no benefit from delivery, and anticoagulation with heparin is potentially harmful. TTP-HUS is often diagnosed postpartum, especially in patients with an initial diagnosis of severe preeclampsia who have worsening renal function, further hematologic deterioration, or multisystemic ischemia despite delivery [42]. Women who develop TTP-HUS should be aware of the potential for relapse as well as of the risk of relapse in subsequent pregnancies [43].

6.18.5 SLE and Antiphospholipid Syndrome

Patients with systemic lupus erythematosus (SLE) and associated antiphospholipid antibodies are at risk for tissue ischemia secondary to thromboembolic events and thrombotic microangiopathy resembling HELLP syndrome, and TTP-HUS [44]. Patients with renal involvement, hypertension, and proteinuria, have identical pictures as patients with preeclampsia. However, the management of the SLE flare will differ from the management of preeclampsia. Prednisone is used in patients with lupus nephritis, whereas combined regimens of prednisone and low-dose aspirin are recommended in patients with antiphospholipid antibodies. The catastrophic antiphospholipid syndrome occurs in less than 1% of patients with associated antiphospholipid antibody syndrome. Acute thrombotic microangiopathy may affect at least three organs, among which the kidneys, cardiorespiratory system, and central nervous system are most common. Patients with catastrophic antiphospholipid syndrome should be treated with full anticoagulation with heparin and steroids plus plasma exchange.

6.18.6 Sepsis

Sepsis is an infrequent, yet important cause of morbidity and possible death in gravitas. Most cases occur during late pregnancy and the postpartum period. It is frequently associated with severe hypotension, inflammation, disseminated intravascular coagulopathy, and AKI endangering mother and child. Early recognition and treatment of sepsis-associated PR-AKI may prevent complications.

In a European retrospective study, over an 11-year period, of 1,321 women, about 1% of all pregnancies required intensive care unit admission, and 52 of them (4%) had severe sepsis or septic shock [45]. The most common infection was chorioamnionitis in about 40%, and endomyometritis in about 20% [45]. Other common infections were septic abortion, pneumonia, pyelonephritis, and postpartum fever [45, 46]. The factors that contribute to a decreased rate of severe sepsis, septic shock, and death in pregnant women are young age and few comorbid conditions. The organisms responsible for infections in pregnant women presenting with sepsis are mostly gram-negative followed by gram-positive bacteria, both usually responsive to common broad-spectrum antimicrobial agents [45].

The incidence of sepsis-associated PR-AKI in developed countries is not well described in the literature. However, in a recent Indian study, postpartum sepsis (40%) was the most common cause of PR-AKI [5, 6]. Dialysis was needed in 50% of these patients, with 60% of them recovering [5]. Sepsis accounts for the majority of maternal mortality (60%) in developing countries [6].

Extracorporeal blood purification directed at elimination of inflammatory and antiinflammatory agents might be an option in therapy-refractory multiorgan failure; however, this is of an experimental nature [47–49].

6.18.7 Therapeutic Principles

The prevention of further damage to the kidney directed at its underlying cause is the cornerstone in the management of established PR-AKI. It remains largely supportive until the renal function recovers. Basic treatment of AKI includes avoidance of nephrotoxins such as radiocontrast agents or aminoglycoside antibiotics, adjustment of drug dosing, fluid management, application of antibiotics, and surgical treatment of a septic focus where possible, which also applies to PR-AKI. In the following, specific therapeutic principles in PR-AKI are discussed.

6.18.7.1 Drug Choice and Drug Dosing

Serious problems with drug choice and drug dose adjustment may arise in pregnant women with renal impairment.

In PR-AKI, antihypertensives, anticoagulants, and antibiotics are essential drugs where dosing is dependent on renal function. Also, the dosages of magnesium, lithium, and morphine must be reduced in AKI. The drug-related risk must be weighed against the disease-related risk for mother and child [50].

6.18.7.1.1 Antihypertensives

Many patients who develop PR-AKI present with hypertension. The target blood pressure in PR-AKI should not be too low to maintain sufficient placental perfusion for optimal fetal growth [51]. Angiotensin-converting enzyme inhibitors and angiotensin II receptor-1 antagonists are contraindicated during pregnancy due to fetopathy including vascular malformation, pulmonary hypoplasia, and neonatal anuria [52, 53]. During pregnancy, methyldopa and hydralazine are antihypertensives of choice. Increase of methyldopa dose should be blood pressure adjusted and administered slowly in patients with PR-AKI. If PR-AKI does not resolve within 4 weeks, 50% of maximal dose in patients with normal renal function should not be exceeded. Dosing of hydralazine is not restricted in PR-AKI. However, frequent blood monitoring is encouraged. Longer use of hydralazine more than 3 months should be avoided as a lupus erythematosus-like disorder may develop.

Selective beta-blockers, particularly metoprolol, are increasingly used for blood pressure control if a combination of methyldopa and hydralazine is not sufficient. However, there are reports describing intrauterine growth retardation and postpartum hypotension in the newborn.

6.18.7.1.2 Antibiotics

Penicillins and other beta-lactams are antibiotics of choice during pregnancy and no adjustment according to renal function is needed. However, dose adjustment to renal function is essential for several antiinfective agents such as cephalosporins (e.g., ceftazidime). Tetracyclines, quinolones, and gentamicin are associated with adverse fetal outcome and should be avoided.

6.18.7.1.3 Erythropoietin

Anemia in PR-AKI may occur in the setting of HELLP syndrome or due to uremia-associated red blood cell membrane fragility and decreased synthesis of erythropoietin. Recombinant human erythropoietin appears to be tolerated during pregnancy [54], however an increased dose is necessary because of pregnancy-related lower drug potency or erythropoietin resistance due to enhanced cytokine production [55] (Table 6.18.3). Care must be taken when higher doses are needed to correct anemia above target levels recommended (hematocrit > 33%, [56]) because erythropoietin-related hypertension may develop [57].

Table 6.18.3 Pregnancy-related causes of acute kidney injury

Variable	Normal value during pregnancy
Sepsis	Urinary tract infection
	Septic abortion
	Puerperal sepsis
(Pre)-eclampsia	Microangiopathic thrombocytopenia
Hemorrhage	Abruptio placentae
Ureteric obstruction	Renal stones
	Surgical ligation
Urethral obstruction	Blood clots
	Kinked urinary bladder catheter

Source: Adapted from Mantel Best Practice & Research Clinical Obstetrics and Gynaecology 2001

6.18.7.1.4 Anticoagulants

Pregnant women are at increased risk of thromboembolism [58]. Oral anticoagulation such as warfarin or dicumarol should be discouraged because of fetal bleeding, stillbirth, and embryopathy [59]. In PR-AKI, anticoagulation must be achieved with reduced dose of parenteral heparin – fractionated (low-molecular-weight) or unfractionated – and monitored by laboratory.

6.18.7.1.5 Loop Diuretics

Loop diuretics are frequently used in the treatment of oliguric renal failure with fluid overload after exclusion of postrenal causes. Specific fetal risks of loop diuretics such as frusemide have not been reported; however, any agent that alters maternal hemodynamics and has the potential to affect uteroplacental perfusion should be used with caution in pregnancy.

6.18.7.2 Renal Replacement Therapy

If conservative therapy of PR-AKI fails to control fluid overload, symptomatic uremia (pericarditis, vomiting and diarrhea, and mental status changes), and hyperkalemia using resins (polystyrene sulfonate) or glucose and insulin, renal replacement therapy (RRT) needs to be commenced. Bicarbonate should be used cautiously if the correction of severe renal acidosis appears to be necessary.

AKI requiring RRT occurs in <1 in 10,000–15,000 pregnancies [3, 60]. Such a condition predicts a significant increase in mortality in different patient populations [61, 62] without being investigated specifically in PR-AKI.

To date, there is little evidence to guide the management of patients requiring RRT during pregnancy. No multicenter international studies have been performed to clarify the questions regarding, when in the setting of RRT-dependent PR-AKI such therapy is best begun, whether continuous or intermittent application would be most beneficial for mother and child, and which dose of dialysis, hemofiltration, or hemodiafiltration in combination with which simultaneous gynecologic and prenatal care should be used. The vast majority of these data are from patients with chronic renal disease. Our ability to translate medical evidence to the bedside of pregnant patient care is, therefore, primarily extrapolative [1]. In short, innumerable case reports and case series over the past decades suggest high rates of preterm birth, low weight birth, and refractory hypertension in pregnancies on maintenance dialysis [63–65]. There has been substantial improvement in successful pregnancy rates in the chronic renal failure patients over the past 3 decades [63–69]. In two larger surveys, longer duration of dialysis time during pregnancy resulted in a reduced prematurity rate and an increased number of viable pregnancies [67, 70]. By lowering the urea level and water load, the incidence of polyhydramnios and dialysis-induced hypotension may be reduced [71, 72], thereby improving fetal outcome.

A joint systematic nephrologic, gynecologic, prenatal, and obstetric treatment protocol for optimal outcome of mother and child was investigated in two uncontrolled case series with prospective data collection from a total of 12 pregnant women on maintenance hemodialysis who delivered 11 live newborns (in one the mother electively terminated her conception because of the suggestion of a molar pregnancy) [63, 64]. Such protocol was of some success as in both studies all newborns left the hospital alive and in good health [63, 64]. In the following, these and other studies serve as a basis for the cautious recommendations made for the use of RRT in PR-AKI.

Polyhydramnios develops due to fetal solute diuresis caused by high placental blood urea nitrogen (BUN) concentration. This disorder and maternal hypertension and premature rupture of the fetal membranes are suspected of causing premature delivery [73].

In this regard, there is evidence that, particularly in PR-AKI, earlier rather than later commencement might be beneficial to the fetus.

6.18.7.2.1 Beginning of Renal Replacement Therapy

The first decision to make is when to begin RRT in severe PR-AKI. The Kidney Disease Outcomes Quality Initiative (KDOQI) guidelines recommend evaluating the benefits and risks of starting RRT when patients reach stage 5 (estimated GFR <15 ml/min/1.73 m^2), although the ideal time for RRT initiation remains a matter of debate, and the results of prospective clinical trials are awaited to resolve this issue [74].

However, particularly the developing fetus appears to be susceptible to uremia. Retrospective data have suggested that maintaining a predialysis BUN value <50 mg/dl leads to a longer gestation, and increased likelihood of successful pregnancy [75]. On the other hand each session of intensified RRT also represents a psychological and physical burden for the mother. Much empathy from the treating clinician is needed to get her informed consent for early initiation of intensified RRT.

6.18.7.2.2 Choice of Modality of Renal Replacement Therapy

Acute shifts in fluid volume, electrolyte imbalance, and hypotension could constitute major RRT-related complications that impair the uteroplacental circulation. The choice of RRT modality in PR-AKI should not only take into account hemodynamic stability, degree of uremia and electrolyte derangements, and access to RRT, but should also address individual circumstances and severity of disease of mother and child.

Most of the literature suggests that the largest body of experience exists for the use of intermittent hemodialysis in PR-AKI [7, 64, 67–69]. In a case series, the use of frequent and extended intermittent hemodiafiltration in pregnant women on maintenance dialysis has been reported [63]. Hemodiafiltration was chosen to further increase the effectiveness and safety of the dialysis prescription. In critically ill patients, daily hemodiafiltration was used with excellent cardiovascular stability [77]. In some patients, hemodiafiltration might be also advantageous due to substantially improved elimination of larger solutes such as phosphate, while preserving a high clearance for small solutes such as urea and creatinine.

Nocturnal home hemodialysis appears to be another treatment option for kidney failure with favorable fertility and fetal and maternal outcomes described for pregnant women on maintenance dialysis [64, 78]. This may however not be transferable to PR-AKI where kidney failure may be associated with sepsis and hypotension or shock. Whether nocturnal dialysis may be applied in PR-AKI in hemodynamically stable pregnancies warrants further investigation.

Peritoneal dialysis has also been used as a modality of RRT in pregnant dialysis-dependent women. In a large case series of 87 patients, fetal survival was similar in pregnancies treated with peritoneal hemodialysis compared with intermittent hemodialysis [65, 78]. However, peritoneal dialysis may itself be associated with specific risks, such as peritonitis and catheter-related mechanical hazards to the fetus.

Continuous RRT, such as venovenous hemodialysis, hemofiltration, or hemodiafiltration appears to be the modality of choice for AKI in critically ill, hemodynamically instable pregnancies with septic or cardiogenic shock and multiorgan failure treated in the intensive care unit [79].

The decision for this modality of RRT should be made cautiously, and the pregnancies should be monitored for the risks associated.

6.18.7.2.3 Dose of Renal Replacement Therapy

To date, there are no guidelines basing on good-quality evidence on the dose of RRT in severe PR-AKI. However, evidence is growing that with increasing dose of RRT, fetal outcomes can be improved [63, 67]. In successful pregnancies, a correlation between birth weight and dose of dialysis was found [70]. Greater attention to a high intake of protein (>1.5 g/kg) and higher dose of RRT, achieved by longer, daily RRT, may be the optimal approach to pregnant patients developing RRT-dependent PR-AKI [63, 64, 78]. Fetal survival was positively influenced by lower serum creatinine level, lower BUN to serum creatinine ratio and increased hours of dialysis [78].

In the setting of high-caloric, high-protein diet, increased dose of RRT appears to achieve improved control of blood concentrations of waste products, preventing potential negative effects on the fetus [63, 64]. Dialysis efficacy expressed as Kt/V (double-pool) >10/week and urea reduction rate of >50% have been reported in two series of successful pregnancies in women treated with about 30–50 h of hemodialysis per week (6×5 h daily or 7×7 h nocturnal using nonreusable high-flux membranes) [63, 64]. The weight gain achieved is closely related to ultrafiltration rate during each session of RRT. By maintaining a lower targeted ultrafiltration goal per treatment, daily RRT allows improved fluid management – with less hypotension, decreased fluid restrictions, and decreased interdialytic weight gain known to be associated with increased workload for the heart. It also allows maintaining stable arterial blood pressures with a reduction of antihypertensive medication [80]. Mean weight gain during RRT in five pregnant women has been reported at about 1,000 g during the first trimester, about 5,000 g during the second and about 5,000 g during the third trimester [64].

6.18.7.2.4 Practical Problems of Renal Replacement Therapy

Extensive dialysis regimen previously described may result in a decrease in the serum levels of water-soluble vitamins, trace elements, and inorganic phosphorus, with possible detrimental effects to the health of the mother and the unborn child. Such effects after initiation of intensive hemodialysis need to be compensated for by substituting and monitoring of water-soluble vitamins such as folate, trace elements, and sodium phosphate [81, 82]. Hazardous effects such as alkalemia, hypokalemia, hypocalcemia, or hypercalcemia need also to be avoided. Bicarbonate content of the dialysate may be reduced in alkalemic patients [63]. Strict precautions should be taken to avoid maternal hypotension, including maintaining left lateral tilt, limiting average maternal dry weight gain to 500 g every 10 days, and avoiding large fluid shifts by limiting net fluid removal to <500 ml per session [83]. Blood pressure should be monitored every 15 min. Anemia needs to be corrected using increasing doses of erythropoietin or, if refractory, transfusion of red blood cells to achieve recommended hematocrit levels >33% in kidney failure [56].

Finally, postpartum dose of RRT may be decreased and anticoagulation may be switched from heparin to regional anticoagulation using citrate due to increased risk of bleeding [84, 85].

6.18.7.2.5 Nonrenal Indications for Extracorporeal Treatment in Peripartum Patients

There are also nonrenal indications for extracorporeal treatment in critically ill peripartum patients such as severe fluid retention in cardiomyopathy [86, 87]. This has been repeatedly successfully performed using hemofiltration to achieve stabilization of cardiac function before cesarean section [87].

6.18.8 Prenatal and Obstetric Management

Although there are no randomized prospective trials in patients who become pregnant while on maintenance dialysis, more intensive and more frequent treatment have been advocated to increase gestation time, raise infant birth weight, produce more viable pregnancies, and improve fetal outcome [67, 70, 88]. The improvement in outcomes of pregnant women on maintenance dialysis during the last decades is likely the result of successful multidisciplinary management by nephrologists, gynecologists, and obstetricians, with intensified dialysis, better anemia management, and improved perinatal monitoring. This is particularly important as this subgroup of patients has a high or even higher risk of prematurity than any other group. It is tempting to speculate that improvements in hemodynamics during prolonged daily or nocturnal RRT are attributable to less extreme fluctuations of solutes and fluid and may help to minimize shifts in maternal and fetal intravascular volume. The incidence of maternal complications that lead to indicated preterm delivery, such as preeclampsia or severe hypertension, seems to be reduced, potentially because a higher frequency of dialysis minimizes shifts in maternal intravascular volume [89].

However, acute shifts in fluid volume, electrolyte imbalance, and hypotension still constitute dialysis-related complications that can lead to impairment of uteroplacental circulation and fetal distress. This emphasizes the need for close maternal and fetal surveillance by frequent Doppler ultrasound and fetal heart rate tracings.

6.18.8.1 Monitoring of Mother and Child

Preterm delivery, usually before 32 weeks' gestation [75, 81], and fetal distress are still the primary perinatal complications for pregnant women on dialysis. In this setting, intensive maternal and fetal monitoring may reduce perinatal morbidity and mortality for pregnant women on maintenance dialysis [89]. Obstetric surveillance should consist of careful monitoring of maternal blood pressure, Doppler flow velocity waveforms of fetal and maternal vessels, and continuous fetal heart rate tracing immediately before, half-way through, and immediately after each hemodialysis session [83]. This surveillance may commence at the time of fetal viability (25 weeks) and should be continued until delivery or RRT-dependent PR-AKI resolves.

6.18.8.2 Doppler Velocimetry and Fetal Heart Tracings

Doppler velocimetry is used to assess right-sided uterine artery and umbilical artery systolic to diastolic ratios as an assessment of uteroplacental perfusion, while umbilical artery systolic to diastolic ratio and continuous fetal heart tracings are used as an assessment of fetal perfusion. It is recommended that all Doppler evaluations and fetal heart rate tracing interpretations are performed by a single observer [83].

During the past decade, serial assessments of such techniques have been performed in several cases and case series where increased dose of intermittent RRT at gentle ultrafiltration and urea reduction rates was achieved [83, 89–91]. In a case series of five pregnancies and a single report, relatively stable umbilical artery flow velocities were reported [89, 91]. Regular fetal ultrasound examinations contribute to more exact estimation of ultrafiltration goals for each RRT session as well as determine the optimal timing of semielective deliveries in these high-risk pregnancies.

Regular sonographic measurement of cervical length may be used to detect pregnancies with threatened preterm delivery and need for interventions, such as hospitalization, cervical cerclage, administration of tocolysis by infusion of magnesium and β2-mimetics, as well as application of corticosteroids to improve lung maturity [92].

6.18.8.3 Decision for Timing and Mode of Delivery

Close monitoring of fetal distress, maturity, and growth may be extremely important for some of the patients with PR-AKI. It may allow better control of cervix cerclage and tocolysis, and most importantly it may allow an early decision for planned delivery by cesarean section, which may have contributed to the favorable outcomes reported [63]. In eight cases, ultrasound-indicated cervical cerclage [63, 93] combined with short-term tocolysis and corticosteroid administration was performed. This management likely improves perinatal outcome. Intrauterine growth restriction is a frequent complication of pregnancies of women on maintenance dialysis. Fetuses affected by this condition are at increased risk for acidemia and hypoxemia [94] and significant mortality and morbidity, not only during the perinatal period [95, 96] but likely also during adult life [97]. Measurement of the Doppler flow velocity waveform in numerous maternal and fetal vessels can be used to diagnose fetuses at risk, and improve fetal outcome (Fig. 6.18.1) [96, 98]. In none of the five cases reported, were significant Doppler changes observed comparing before to after hemodialysis measurements [89]. Intrauterine growth restriction was diagnosed in four of five cases, one of them associated with severely abnormal arterial and venous Doppler flow patterns which led to indicated preterm delivery by cesarean section. In another case, formerly normal arterial Doppler patterns became abnormal, followed by a severely abnormal fetal heart trace (late decelerations) and emergency cesarean section. The authors speculated that intensive monitoring saved these babies from intrauterine damage [89].

6.18.9 Take Home Pearls

- Pregnancy-related AKI is a rare, yet serious condition for mother and child and requires the care of an interdisciplinary team of experienced physicians. It can develop through multiple pathophysiologic events including sepsis and eclampsia.
- Normal pregnancy is characterized by increased renal perfusion and glomerular filtration rate, making it a state of augmented renal clearance. What constitutes adequate renal replacement therapy in the nonpregnancy setting is thus likely inadequate in pregnancy.
- Experience from treatment of pregnant women with end-stage renal disease on maintenance hemodialysis provides evidence that an azotemic intrauterine environment has deleterious fetal effects. It suggests that increased uremic clearance leads to an increase in successful pregnancies and better fetal outcomes which has been confirmed in several case series.
- Intensified hemodialysis and frequent maternal and fetal surveillance might be the key to further improving outcomes of mother and child.

Acknowledgment We thank Dr. Bamberg, Charité University Medicine, Berlin, Germany, for providing us with the Doppler ultrasound figures.

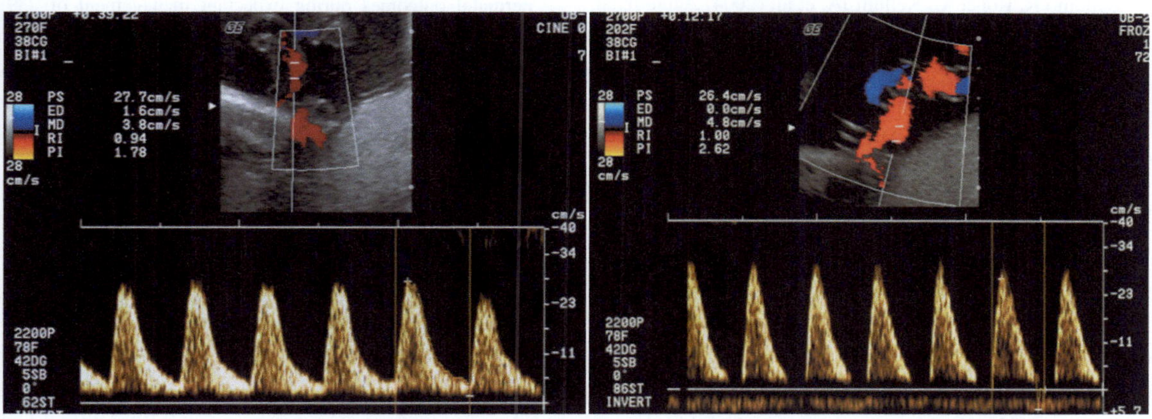

Fig. 6.18.1 Normal umbilical artery Doppler velocity after a hemodialysis session (*left picture*), absent diastolic flow in the umbilical artery (*right picture*)

References

1. Gammill HS, Jeyabalan A (2005) Acute renal failure in pregnancy. CCM 33 (Suppl.):372–384.
2. Stratta P, Besso L, Canavese C, et al. (1996) Is pregnancy-related acute renal failure a disappearing clinical entity? Ren Fail 18:575–584.
3. Mantel GD (2001) Care of the critically ill parturient: oliguria and renal failure. Best Pract Res Clin Obstet Gynaecol 15:563–581.
4. Prakash J, Vohra R, Wani IA, et al. (2007) Decreasing incidence of renal cortical necrosis in patients with acute renal failure in developing countries: a single-centre experience of 22 years from Eastern India. Nephrol Dial Transplant 22:1213–1217.
5. Kumar KS, Krishna CR, Kumar VS (2006) Pregnancy related acute renal failure. J Obstet Gynecol India 56:308–310.
6. Goplani KR, Shah PR, Gera DN, et al. (2008) Pregnancy-related acute renal failure: a single-center experience. Indian J Nephrol 18:17–21.
7. Jayakumar M, Prabahar MR, Fernando EM, et al. (2006) Epidemiologic trend changes in acute renal failure – a tertiary center experience from South India. Ren Fail 28:405–410.
8. Krutzén E, Olofsson P, Bäck SE, et al. (1992) Glomerular filtration rate in pregnancy: a study in normal subjects and in patients with hypertension, preeclampsia and diabetes. Scand J Clin Lab Invest 52:387–392.
9. Kristensen K, Lindström V, Schmidt C, et al. (2007) Temporal changes of the plasma levels of cystatin C, beta-trace protein, beta2-microglobulin, urate and creatinine during pregnancy indicate continuous alterations in the renal filtration process. Scand J Clin Lab Invest 67:612–618.
10. Greenhill A, Gruskin AB (1976) Laboratory evaluation of renal function. Pediatr Clin North Am 23:661–679.
11. Sims EAH, Krantz KE (1958) Serial studies of renal function and the puerperium in normal women. J Clin Invest 37:1764–1774.
12. Lafayette RA, Druzin M, Sibley R, et al. (1998) Nature of glomerular dysfunction in pre-eclampsia. Kidney Int 54:1240–1249.
13. Bellomo R, Ronco C, Kellum JA, et al. (2004) Acute renal failure – definition, outcome measures, animal models, fluid therapy and information technology needs: the Second International Consensus Conference of the Acute Dialysis Quality Initiative (ADQI) Group. Crit Care 8:R204–212.
14. Mehta RL, Kellum JA, Shah SV, et al. (2007) Acute kidney injury network: report of an initiative to improve outcomes in acute kidney injury. Crit Care 11:R31.
15. Bellomo R, Kellum JA, Ronco C (2004) Defining acute renal failure: physiological principles. Intensive Care Med 30:33–37.
16. Haase-Fielitz A, Bellomo R, Devarajan P, et al. (2008) Novel and conventional serum biomarkers predicting acute kidney injury in adult cardiac surgery – a prospective cohort study. Crit Care Med 34(4):592–594.
17. Report of the National High Blood Pressure Education Program (2000) Working group report on high blood pressure in pregnancy. Am J Obstet Gynecol 183:1–22.
18. Eskenazi B, Fenster L, Sidney S, et al. (1993) Fetal growth retardation in infants of multiparous and nulliparous women with preeclampsia. Am J Obstet Gynecol 169: 1112–1118.
19. Sibai B, Dekker G, Kupferminc M (2005) Pre-eclampsia. Lancet 365:785–99.
20. Kincaid-Smith PS (1991) The renal lesion of pre-eclampsia revisited. Am J Kid Dis 17:144–148.
21. Moran P, Baylis PH, Lindheimer MD, et al. (2003) Glomerular ultrafiltration in normal and pre-eclamptic pregnancy. J Am Soc Nephrol 14:648–652.
22. Gaber LW, Spargo BH (1987) Pregnancy induced nephropathy. Am J Kid Dis 9:317–323.
23. Schrier RW (1988) Pathogenesis of sodium and water retention in high-output and low-output cardiac failure, nephrotic syndrome, cirrhosis, and pregnancy. N Engl J Med 319:1127–1134.
24. Karumanchi SA, Maynard SE, Stillman IE, et al. (2005) Preeclampsia: a renal perspective. Kidney Int 67:2101–2113.
25. Lafayette RA (2005) The kidney in preeclampsia. Kidney Int 67:1194–1203.
26. Drakeley AJ, Le Roux PA, Anthony J, et al. (2002) Acute renal failure complicating severe preeclampsia requiring admission to an obstetric intensive care unit. Am J Obstet Gynecol 186:253–256.
27. Attalah AN, Hofmayr GJ, Duley L (2002) Calcium supplementation during pregnancy for preventing hypertensive disorders and related problems. Cochrane Database Syst Rev3: CD001059.
28. Knight M, Duley L, Henderson-Smart DJ, et al. (2000) Antiplatelet agents for preventing and treating pre-eclampsia. Cochrane Database Syst Rev 2:CD000492.
29. Podymow T, August P (2008) Update on the use of antihypertensive drugs in pregnancy. Hypertension 51:960–969.
30. Magee LA, Cham C, Waterman EJ, et al. (2003) Hydralazine for treatment of severe hypertension in pregnancy: meta-analysis. BMJ 327:955–960.
31. Sibai BM (2004) Magnesium sulfate prophylaxis in preeclampsia. Lessons learned from recent trials. Am J Obstet Gynecol 190:1520–1526.
32. Churchill D, Duley L (2002) Interventionist versus expectant care for severe pre-eclampsia before term. Cochrane Database Syst Rev 3: CD003106.
33. Haddad D, Deis S, Goffinet T, et al. (2004) Maternal and perinatal outcomes during expectant management of 239 severe preeclamptic women between 24 and 33 weeks gestation. Am J Obstet Gynecol 190:1590–1595.
34. Ascarelli MH, Johnson V, McCreary H, et al. (2005) Postpartum preeclampsia management with furosemide: a randomized controlled trial. Obstet Gynecol 105:29–33.
35. Katz VL, Farmer R, Kuller JA (2000) Preeclampsia into eclampsia: toward a new paradign. Am J Obstet Gynecol 182:1389–1394.
36. Thomas SV (1998) Neurological aspect of eclampsia. J Neurol Sci 155:37–43.
37. Martin JN, Rinehart BK, May WL, et al. (1999) The spectrum of severe pre-eclampsia: comparative analysis by HELLP (hemolysis, elevated liver enzymes, and low platelet count) syndrome classification. Am J Obstet Gynecol 180:1373–1382.
38. Sibai BM, Ramadan MK (1993) Acute renal failure in pregnancies complicated by hemolysis, elevated liver enzymes, and low platelets. Am J Obstet Gynecol 168: 1682–1690

39. Matchaba P, Moodley J (2002) Corticosteroids for HELLP syndrome in pregnancy. Cochrane Database Syst Rev 4:CD002076.
40. Hayward CP, Sutton DM, Carter WH Jr, et al. (1994) Treatment outcomes in patients with adult thrombotic thrombocytopenic purpura-hemolytic uremic syndrome. Arch Intern Med 154:982–987.
41. Roberts G, Gordon MM, Porter D, et al. (2003) Acute renal failure complicating HELLP syndrome, SLE and antiphospholipid syndrome: successful outcome using plasma exchange therapy. Lupus 12:251–257.
42. Egerman RS, Witlin AG, Friedman SA, et al. (1996) Thrombotic thrombocytopenic purpura and hemolytic uremic syndrome in pregnancy. Am J Obstet Gynecol 175:950–956.
43. George JN (2003) The association of pregnancy with thrombotic thrombocytopenic purpura-hemolytic uremic syndrome. Curr Opin Hematol 10: 339–344.
44. Lockshin MD, Erkan D (2003) Treatment of the antiphospholipid syndrome. N Engl J Med 349:1177–1779.
45. Pactitis S, Koutra G, Charalambidis C, et al. (2007) Severe sepsis and septic shock in pregnancy and puerperium: an 11-year review in a maternity intensive care unit. Crit Care 11(Suppl. 4):P39.
46. Medve L, Csitári IK, Molnár Z (2005) Recombinant human activated protein C treatment of septic shock syndrome in a patient at 18th week of gestation: a case report. Am J Obstet Gynecol 193:864–865.
47. Haase M, Silvester W, Uchino S, et al. (2007) A pilot study of high-adsorption hemofiltration in human septic shock. Int J Artif Organs 30:108–117.
48. Haase M, Bellomo R, Baldwin I, et al. (2007) Hemodialysis membrane with a high-molecular-weight cutoff and cytokine levels in sepsis complicated by acute renal failure: a phase 1 randomized trial. Am J Kidney Dis 50:296–304.
49. Haase M, Bellomo R, Baldwin I, et al. (2008) The effect of three different miniaturized blood purification devices on plasma cytokine concentration in an ex-vivo model of endotoxinemia. IJAO Int J Artif Organs 31(8):722–729
50. Keller F, Griesshammer M, Häussler U, et al. (2001) Pregnancy and renal failure: the case for application of dosage guidelines. Drugs 61:1901–1920.
51. Von Dadelszen P, Ornstein MP, Bull SB, et al. (2000) Fall in mean pressure and fetal growth restriction in pregnancy hypertension: a meta-analysis. Lancet 355:87–92.
52. Saji H, Yamanaka M, Hagiware A, et al. (2001) Losartan and fetal toxic effects. Lancet 357: 363.
53. Anonymus (1997) Postmarketing surveillance for angiotensin-converting enzyme inhibitor use during the first trimester of pregnancy – United States, Canada, and Israel, 1987–1995. MMWR Morb Mortal Wkly Rep 46: 240–242.
54. Thorp M, Pulliam J (1998) Use of recombinant erythropoietin in a pregnant renal transplant recipient. Am J Nephrol 18:448–451.
55. Al Shohaib S (1999) Erythropoietin therapy in a pregnant post-renal transplant patient. Nephron 81: 81–83.
56. Hou S, Orlowski J, Pahl M, et al. (1993) Pregnancy in women with end-stage renal disease: treatment of anaemia and premature labor. Am J Kidney Dis 21:16–22.
57. Morgera S, Scholle C, Voss G, et al. (2004) Metabolic complications during regional citrate anticoagulation in continuous venovenous hemodialysis: single-center experience. Nephron Clin Pract 97:c131–136.
58. Hunt BJ, Doughty HA, Majumdar G, et al. (1997) Thromboprophylaxis with low molecular weight heparin (fragmin) in high risk pregnancies. Thromb Haemost 77:39–43.
59. Vitale N, DeSanto LS, Pollice A, et al. (1999) Dose-dependent fetal complications of warfarin in pregnant women with mechanical heart valves. J Am Coll Cardiol 33:1637–1641.
60. Agraharkar M (2006) Renal disease and pregnancy. E-medicine May 17.
61. Lassnigg A, Schmid ER, Hiesmayr M (2008) Impact of minimal increases in serum creatinine on outcome in patients after cardiothoracic surgery: do we have to revise current definitions of acute renal failure? Crit Care Med 36:1129–1137.
62. Uchino S, Kellum JA, Bellomo R, et al. (2005) Beginning and ending supportive therapy for the kidney (BEST kidney) investigators. Acute renal failure in critically ill patients: a multinational, multicenter study. JAMA 294:813–818.
63. Haase M, Morgera S, Bamberg C, et al. (2005) A systematic approach to managing pregnant dialysis patients – the importance of an intensified haemodiafiltration protocol. Nephrol Dial Transplant 20:2537–2542.
64. Barua M, Hladunewich M, Keunen J, et al. (2008) Successful pregnancies on nocturnal home hemodialysis. Clin J Am Soc Nephrol 3:392–396.
65. Chou CY, Ting IW, Lin TH, et al. (2008) Pregnancy in patients on chronic dialysis: a single center experience and combined analysis of reported results. Eur J Obstet Gynecol Reprod Biol 136:165–170.
66. Confortini P, Galanti G, Ancona G, et al. (1971) Full term pregnancy and successful delivery in a patient on chronic haemodialysis. Proc Eur Dial Transplant Assoc 8:74–78.
67. Okundaye I, Abrinko P, Hou S (1998) Registry of pregnancy in dialysis patients. Am J Kidney Dis 31:766–773.
68. Hou SH (1994) Frequency and outcome of pregnancy in women on dialysis. Am J Kidney Dis 23:60–63.
69. Ero lu D, Lembet A, Ozdemir FN, et al. (2004) Pregnancy during hemodialysis: perinatal outcome in our cases. Transplant Proc 36:53–55.
70. Bagon JA, Vernaeve H, De Muylder X, Lafontaine JJ, Martens J, Van Roost G. (1998) Pregnancy and dialysis. Am J Kidney Dis 31(5):756–765.
71. Maruyama H, Shimada H, Obayashi H, et al. (1998) Requiring higher doses of erythropoietin suggests pregnancy in hemodialysis patients. Nephron 79:413–419.
72. Hou SH (1994) Pregnancy in women on haemodialysis and peritoneal dialysis. Baillieres Clin Obstet Gynaecol 8: 481–500.
73. Levy DP, Giatras I, Jungers P (1998) Pregnancy and end-stage renal disease – past experience and new insights. Nephrol Dial Transplant 13:3005–3007.
74. Triolo G, Savoldi S (2008) When to start dialysis. The predialysis patient. G Ital Nefrol 25(Suppl. 41):9–20.
75. Holley JL, Reddy SS (2003) Pregnancy in dialysis patients: a review of outcomes, complications, and management. Semin Dial 16:384–388.
76. Jayakumar M, Prabahar MR, Fernando EM (2006) Epidemiologic trend changes in acute renal failure - a tertiary center experience from South India. Ren Fail 28: 405–410.
77. Marshall MR, Ma T, Galler D, et al. (2004) Sustained low-efficiency daily diafiltration (SLEDD-f) for critically ill patients requiring renal replacement therapy: towards an adequate therapy. Nephrol Dial Transplant 19:877–884.

78. Chan WS, Okun N, Kjellstrand CM (1998) Pregnancy in chronic dialysis: a review and analysis of the literature. Int J Artif Organs 21:259–268.
79. Batashki I, Milchev N, Uchikova E, et al. (2006) Hyperlipidemic pancreatitis during pregnancy - a case report. Akush Ginekol (Sofiia) 45 Suppl 1:41–43.
80. Ting GO, Kjellstrand C, Freitas T, et al. (2003) Long-term study of high-comorbidity ESRD patients converted from conventional to short daily hemodialysis. Am J Kidney Dis 42:1020–1035.
81. Hou S (1999) Pregnancy in chronic renal insufficiency an end-stage renal disease. Am J Kidney Dis 33:235–252.
82. Hussain S, Savin V, Piering W (2005) Phosphorus-enriched hemodialysis during pregnancy: two case reports. Hemodial Int 9:147–152.
83. Giatras I, Levy DP, Malone FD, et al. (1998) Pregnancy during dialysis: case report and management guidelines. Nephrol Dial Transplant 13:3266–3272.
84. Morgera S, Scholle C, Melzer C, et al. (2004) A simple, safe and effective citrate anticoagulation protocol for the genius dialysis system in acute renal failure. Nephron Clin Pract 98:c35–40.
85. Haase M, Morgera S, Bamberg C, et al. (2006) Successful pregnancies in dialysis patients including those suffering from cystinosis and familial Mediterranean fever. J Nephrol 19:677–681.
86. Beards SC, Freebairn RC, Lipman J (1993) Successful use of continuous veno-venous haemofiltration to treat profound fluid retention in severe peripartum cardiomyopathy. Anaesthesia 48:1065–1067.
87. Fall LH, Young WW, Power JA, et al. (1990) Severe congestive heart failure and cardiomyopathy as a complication of myotonic dystrophy in pregnancy. Obstet Gynecol 76: 481–485.
88. Rizzoni G, Ehrich JH, Broyer M, et al. (1992) Successful pregnancies in women on renal replacement therapy: report from the EDTA registry. Nephrol Dial Transplant 7: 279–287.
89. Bamberg C, Diekmann F, Haase M, et al. (2007) Pregnancy on intensified hemodialysis: fetal surveillance and perinatal outcome. Fetal Diagn Ther 22:289–293.
90. Nakai Y, Nishio J, Nishimura S, et al. (1998) Umbilical arterial flow change during hemodialysis. Perinat Med 26: 54–55.
91. Malone FD, Craigo SD, Giatras I, et al. (1998) Suggested ultrasound parameters for the assessment of fetal well-being during chronic hemodialysis. Ultrasound Obstet Gynecol 11:450–452.
92. Tsoi E, Fuchs IB, Rane S, et al. (2005) Sonographic measurement of cervical length in threatened preterm labor in singleton pregnancies with intact membranes. Ultrasound Obstet Gynecol 25:353–356.
93. To MS, Palaniappan V, Skentou C, et al. (2002) Elective cerclage vs. ultrasound-indicated cerclage in high-risk pregnancies. Ultrasound Obstet Gynecol 19:475–477.
94. Soothill PW, Nicolaides KH, Campbell S (1987) Prenatal asphyxia, hyperlacticaemia, hypoglycaemia, and erythroblastosis in growth retarded fetuses. Br Med J 294: 1051–1053.
95. Kurkinen-Räty M, Kivelä A, Jouppila P (1997) The clinical significance of an absent end-diastolic velocity in the umbilical artery detected before the 34th week of pregnancy. Acta Obstet Gynecol Scand 76:398–404.
96. Hartung J, Kalache KD, Heyna C, et al. (2005) Outcome of 60 neonates who had ARED flow prenatally compared with a matched control group of appropriate-for-gestational age preterm neonates. Ultrasound Obstet Gynecol 25:566–572.
97. Barker DJ (1997) The long-term outcome of retarded fetal growth. Clin Obstet Gynecol 40:853–863.
98. Hecher K, Bilardo CM, Stigter RH, et al. (2001) Monitoring of fetuses with intrauterine growth restriction: a longitudinal study. Ultrasound Obstet Gynecol 18:564–570.

Acute Kidney Failure in Children

6.19

Michael Zappitelli and Stuart L. Goldstein

Core Messages

- Until recently, most pediatric acute kidney failure (AKF) resulted from primary renal diseases (such as glomerulonephritis or hemolytic uremic syndrome), whereas current pediatric AKF results more often from secondary renal injury such as sepsis, nephrotoxic medications, and renal ischemia.
- The prevention and treatment of metabolic derangements comprise the primary goals of pharmacologic therapy in children with AKF. Preservation or restoration of renal perfusion with appropriate inotropic agents is essential and the first pharmacologic measure to maintain urine output in critically ill children unresponsive to volume repletion.
- In patients requiring renal replacement therapy, modern technology enables the choice for intermittent hemodialysis, peritoneal dialysis, or a continuous renal replacement therapy even for small children and infants.

6.19.1 Introduction

Acute kidney failure (AKF) management in children requires special considerations not commonly encountered in the care of adult patients. Pediatric patients with AKF may range in weight from a 1.5-kg neonate to a 200-kg young adult. In addition, disease states that may require acute renal replacement therapy (RRT) in the absence of significant renal dysfunction, such as inborn errors of metabolism or postoperative care of an infant with congenital cardiac defects, are more prevalent in the pediatric setting. Optimal care for the pediatric patient requiring RRT requires an understanding of the causes and patterns of pediatric AKF and multiorgan dysfunction syndrome (MODS) and recognition of the local expertise with respect to the personnel and equipment resources. The aim of this chapter is to review pediatric AKF epidemiology, etiology, and management, with an emphasis on emerging practice patterns with respect to modality and the timing of treatment.

6.19.2 Epidemiology

Pediatric AKF incidence is generally less than 1% when defined by need for RRT [6, 60]. Other studies have used a wide variety of definitions, ranging from mild to large changes in serum creatinine (SCr) and/or urine output which has led to variable reports of AKF incidence [3, 4, 6, 62]. Two pediatric AKF studies in critically ill children highlight the impact of AKF definition and patient characteristics on epidemiology description. In the first, almost all patients admitted to a pediatric intensive care unit (PICU) were eligible for

S. L. Goldstein (✉)
Baylor College of Medicine, Medical Director, Renal Dialysis Unit and Pheresis Service, Texas Children's Hospital,
6621 Fannin Street, MC 3-2482, Houston, Texas 77054, USA
e-mail: stuartg@bcm.tmc.edu

A. Jörres et al. (eds.), *Management of Acute Kidney Problems*,
DOI: 10.1007/978-3-540-69441-0_6.19, © Springer-Verlag Berlin Heidelberg 2010

enrollment, and AKF was defined as SCr doubling [6]. In the second, only patients receiving invasive mechanical ventilation and vasopressors (therefore with very high illness severity) were included, and AKF was defined as a ≥1.5 times SCr increase (a less "strict" AKF definition) [3]. Both population and definition characteristics in the latter study led to a higher estimate of AKI incidence (82 vs 4.5%) than in the former. However, the *actual* occurrence of AKI in each intensive care unit (ICU) may not have truly differed – AKI ascertainment merely differed in relation to the study population and AKI definition.

The Acute Dialysis Quality Initiative recently proposed the RIFLE criteria (Risk, Injury, Failure, Loss, End-Stage Renal Disease) for defining AKF [9], which stratify AKF from mild (RIFLE class R, "risk": ≥50% SCr increase from baseline) to severe (RIFLE class F, "failure": ≥3 × baseline SCr). We defined AKF in a cohort of critically ill children using a pediatric-modified (pRIFLE) criteria, and found that AKF occurred in 82% of patients and was an independent risk factor for mortality and longer hospital stay [3]. A recent modification of the RIFLE criteria was proposed by the Acute Kidney Injury Network (the AKIN criteria staging system) [39], however, this definition has not been evaluated in children. Further epidemiologic research utilizing these definitions in children will contribute to understanding the true incidence of mild to severe AKF in a wide range of geographic and diagnostic patient populations.

6.19.3 Etiology and Diagnosis

The most common causes of pediatric AKF have changed over the last 10–20 years. Until recently, most AKF resulted from primary renal diseases (such as glomerulonephritis or hemolytic uremic syndrome), whereas current AKF results more often from secondary renal injury, such as sepsis, nephrotoxic medications, and ischemia due to several disease states [3, 6, 30, 60, 62]. While each of these conditions causes AKF via different mechanisms, they lead to a final common pathway of acute tubular necrosis (ATN), characterized by renal tubular cell death, as discussed in other chapters. Common clinical pediatric conditions leading to these mechanisms are multiple organ dysfunction syndrome, stem cell transplantation, and cardiopulmonary bypass (CPB) surgery, as discussed below (Section 6.19.5). Infants with AKF after corrective congenital heart surgery comprise a well-studied cohort. The incidence of dialysis requirement after infant CPB ranges from 2.7% to 5.3% with survival rates ranging from 21% to 70% [12, 43, 44], and the incidence of serum creatinine doubling ranges from approximately 6% to 30%, depending on the specific patient and surgical characteristics [41, 54]. Stem cell transplant recipients are also an important specific patient group at risk for AKF from a number of causes including nephrotoxic medications, radiation-induced nephropathy, and a hepatorenal-like syndrome associated with vaso-occlusive disease [32]. Because of the large amounts of fluid received during their treatment, these patients are also at particularly high risk of developing substantial fluid overload.

Diagnostic evaluation of AKF revolves around determining the causes and extent of AKF severity. Because the diagnostic evaluation of AKF is detailed in other chapters, and does not differ substantially in children, only certain salient points will be discussed.

When evaluating a child for the presence and severity of AKF, it is important to know the baseline serum creatinine, since serum creatinine concentrations depend upon the child's muscle mass, age, and sex and are highly variable between individuals. When baseline serum creatinine is unknown, it can be estimated by assuming the child has normal published values for age and sex or by assuming a normal glomerular filtration rate (120 ml/min/1.73 m^2) and back-calculating serum creatinine using the pediatric-specific Schwartz formula (glomerular filtration rate = k × height/serum creatinine, where $k = 0.43$ in infants, 0.7 in adolescent boys and 0.55 in all other children) [51].

Many children with significant kidney injury will not be oliguric. A detailed fluid balance history is necessary to evaluate whether a positive fluid balance is occurring. Urine output assessment alone without considering the contemporaneous fluid administration is not useful in the evaluation of children with AKF. A perceived mildly positive fluid balance may actually represent a substantial amount of fluid overload, especially in smaller children. One suggested formula derived in children to assess fluid overload status, is to express the difference in fluid output from fluid intake since PICU admission, as a percentage of the patient's estimated dry weight, using the following formula:

Fluid overload = (fluid in liters − fluid out liters)/weight in kg × 100% [25].

Children with stem cell transplants and greater than 10% fluid overload during AKF may exhibit a higher mortality than children with less than 10% fluid overload [40]. Increased fluid overload is associated with mortality in patients receiving continuous RRT [23, 25]. Fluid overload management options are discussed in Section 6.19.4.

Hyponatremia and hyperkalemia are frequent findings in patients with AKF. However, some specific pediatric conditions may lead to severe hypernatremia with AKF (such as Bartter syndrome) or hypokalemia and hypophosphatemia (as seen with congenital tubulopathies or a Fanconi syndrome). It is also important to obtain renal ultrasound imaging to assure that renal anatomy is normal and that there is no underlying congenital chronic kidney disease (such as dysplasia or obstructive uropathy), particularly if the degree of AKF severity is out of proportion to prior events.

6.19.4 Treatment

6.19.4.1 Fluid and Electrolyte Considerations

Careful attention to fluid and electrolyte management in pediatric AKF is critical to prevent or mitigate associated comorbidities, and is dependent on an accurate assessment of the underlying cause of AKF. For example, patients with prerenal azotemia most often have reversible AKF, which is responsive to fluid resuscitation, whereas patients with acute tubular necrosis should be treated with volume, sodium, and potassium restriction, to prevent development of worsening fluid overload and hyperkalemia. Finally, patients with AKF secondary to nephrotoxic medications or interstitial nephritis often demonstrate polyuria.

The standard practice of providing "maintenance fluids" based on patient size or caloric requirement (e.g., the Holliday-Seger method [29] or 400 ml/m^2 of body surface area) was derived from patients with normal renal function and the amount of urine volume needed to excrete a normal daily solute load. Such maintenance fluid algorithms are not appropriate and can be dangerous for children with AKF. The fluid prescription for children with AKF should be directed by the individual clinical situation. A safe starting point in most cases is insensible losses plus replacement of ongoing losses. A daily volume of 400 ml/m^2 of body surface area to replace insensible fluid losses should be prescribed for patients with a normal basal metabolic rate, whereas higher volumes may be required for febrile patients. Lower insensible loss volume replacement may be appropriate for patients receiving invasive mechanical ventilation who have decreased respiratory insensible fluid loss. Patients with oligoanuric kidney failure should not receive potassium or phosphorus unless they exhibit hypokalemia or hypophosphatemia. Sodium administration should be restricted to 2–3 mEq/kg body weight per day to prevent fluid retention and hypertension in children with oligoanuric AKF.

Depending on the clinical situation, replacement of all or only part of a patient's ongoing losses may be warranted. For example, patients with fluid overload might be managed appropriately with a fluid rate that contains insensible losses plus half of ongoing losses to provide sufficient glucose and electrolytes, but to allow the patient to attain negative fluid balance. Patient weight and serum electrolyte concentrations should be measured at least daily to modify the fluid and electrolyte prescription appropriately.

Optimal fluid repletion strategies for patients with intravascular volume contraction also require a rationale approach. Clinical signs and symptoms including tachycardia, degree of skin turgor, mucus membrane hydration, and mental status can be used to estimate patient fluid deficits. Aggressive rehydration is warranted for patients with significant circulatory compromise to restore organ perfusion. For patients with less severe dehydration, the fluid deficit can be replaced over 24–48 h while continuing to replace insensible and ongoing fluid losses.

Significant clinical research has been conducted recently to assess various fluid repletion strategies based on physiologic directed end points in patients with shock. Recent data from adult patients with septic shock demonstrate that goal-directed fluid therapy using physiologic end points could significantly improve patient survival [45, 57]. Adult patients who received early goal-directed fluid therapy in the emergency center received more fluid in the emergency center, but received less fluid and had better survival in the ICU compared with patients who received standard therapy. Fluid resuscitation in critically ill children is essential for patients with acute hypovolemia and septic shock [21]. The subacute effects of fluid overload, however, are more uncertain. Several studies have suggested an association between excessive fluid retention and negative patient outcome. Adult surgical ICU patients who develop fluid retention have increased morbidity, increased requirements for blood products, prolonged dependency on pressors, and a twofold increase in death [53]. Fluid overload has also been associated with decreased survival in adult patients with ARDS [31, 50].

6.19.4.2 Pharmacologic Therapy

AKF management should begin prior to consultation of a nephrologist and provision of RRT. Maintenance of adequate urine volumes and prevention/treatment of metabolic derangements comprise the goals of pharmacologic therapy in children with AKF. Preservation or restoration of renal perfusion with appropriate inotropic agents is essential and the first pharmacologic measure to maintain urine output in critically ill patients unresponsive to volume repletion [34].

6.19.4.2.1 Vasopressors

The effects of dopamine are varied and complex, leading to controversy with respect to its utility in the setting of AKF. At low or so-called renal doses of 0.5–2 μg/kg/min, dopamine increases renal plasma flow and sodium excretion. At 2–5 μg/kg/min, dopamine binds β-adrenergic receptors and at doses above 5 μg/kg/min, dopamine's α-adrenergic receptor binding becomes activated. These complex actions render it difficult to ascertain whether any observed renal benefit from dopamine occurs as a result its dopaminergic or intropic effect. However, well-designed prospective randomized studies of adult patients at risk for acute tubular necrosis have called into question the utility of renal-dose dopamine in reversing oliguria [7, 35], and many centers have abandoned its use in the setting of ATN [36, 48].

Dobutamine does not exhibit a direct effect on the kidney, but rather acts primarily on the β1-adrenergic receptors. The benefit of dobutamine for patients with AKF resides in its ability to increase cardiac output, leading to an increase in renal blood flow.

Norepinephrine also exerts complex systemic and renal actions [49], which have the contradictory effects of decreasing renal blood flow in healthy individuals but improving systemic pressure and leading to renal vasodilatation. Norepinephrine appears to be the most beneficial vasopressor in euvolemic patients with hypotension, such as those with septic shock, leading to improved glomerular filtration rate.

Vasopressin increases systemic vascular resistance by direct action on the vascular smooth muscle cells. Vasopressin has been shown to be especially effective in maintaining renal perfusion in patients with septic shock who were unresponsive to catecholamines [58].

Prospective randomized studies of adult patients at risk for ATN have called into question the utility of intravenous furosemide in reversing oliguria [33, 52]. However, the practice of providing furosemide, either as an intermittent bolus or as a continuous infusion (0.1–0.3 mg/kg/h) in combination with a thiazide diuretic has potential to maintain urine output in patients at risk of developing anuria.

Another recent study supports the use of fenoldopam, a dopamine α-1 agonist to prevent AKF in certain critically ill adult populations [47, 59]. No published pediatric study exists with respect to the effect of fenoldopam in pediatric AKF.

Many other agents, which are still considered to be experimental, have shown inconsistent results with respect to preventing or ameliorating a course of AKF. *N*-Acetylcysteine has been studied most extensively in the setting of contrast-induced nephropathy prevention. Results from an early successful trial [46], in which only 2% of patients who received *N*-acetylcysteine versus 21% who received placebo demonstrated increased serum creatinine, have not been reproduced [10, 13]. Less well-studied agents, including insulin-like growth factor I [28] and thyroxine [2] have not been effective in improving an AKF course.

6.19.4.3 Renal Replacement Therapy

Provision of RRT as intermittent hemodialysis, peritoneal dialysis (PD), or a continuous renal replacement therapy (CRRT) is now a mainstay of treatment for the child with AKF. Technological advances aimed at providing accurate ultrafiltration with volumetric control incorporated into hemodialysis and CRRT equipment and disposable lines, circuits, and dialyzers sized for the entire pediatric weight spectrum have made RRT safer in the pediatric setting [19]. Transition from the use of adaptive CRRT equipment, to production of hemofiltration machines with volumetric control allowing for accurate ultrafiltration (UF) flows has likewise led to a change in pediatric RRT modality prevalence patterns. Accurate UF and blood flow rates are crucial for pediatric RRT since the extracorporeal circuit volume can comprise more than 15% of a small pediatric patients' total blood volume and small UF inaccuracies may represent a large percentage of a small pediatric patient's total body water. Polls of US pediatric nephrologists demonstrate increased CRRT use over PD as the preferred modality for treating pediatric AKF. In 1995, 45% of pediatric centers ranked PD and 18 percent ranked CRRT as the most common modality used for initial AKF treatment. In 1999, 31% of centers chose PD versus 36% of centers reporting CRRT as their primary initial modality for AKF treatment [61].

In the last decade, survival rates stratified by RRT modality have been stable; survival rates for patients receiving hemodialysis (73–89%) are higher than those receiving PD (49–64%) or CRRT (34–42%) [20, 25]. Better survival in patients who receive hemodialysis likely results from improved hemodynamic stability, but no prospective pediatric study that controls for patients' illness severity has compared survival across modalities exists.

Acute drug intoxications and hyperammonemia secondary to inborn errors of metabolism are often best treated with hemodialysis since rapid drug removal is important to prevent morbidity, and hemodialysis is the most efficient RRT modality [16, 38]. However, recent studies demonstrate CRRT to be very effective in protein-bound drug removal and hyperammonemia [5, 42].

6.19.4.4 Vascular Access

Provision of intermittent hemodialysis and CRRT requires vascular access. In the acute setting, the most common sites for catheter placement are the internal jugular, subclavian, and femoral veins. Avoidance of the subclavian vein is preferable in order to prevent subclavian vein stenosis in patients who may not recover renal function and who would need permanent vascular access in the ipsilateral upper extremity. A study of adult patients reported increased recirculation and worse performance in catheters placed in the femoral vein versus subclavian or jugular veins [37], but these data have not been reproduced in children. Catheter size should also be matched to patient size. Table 6.19.1 lists catheter configurations and patient size combinations.

Table 6.19.1 Acute catheter configuration and patient size combination

Patient size	Catheter size and source	Site of insertion
Neonate	Single-lumen 5 French (Cook)	Femoral artery or vein
	Dual-lumen 7F (Cook/Medcomp)	Femoral vein
3–6 kg	Dual-lumen 7F (Cook/Medcomp)	Internal/external-jugular, subclavian, or femoral vein
	Triple-Lumen 7F (Medcomp)	Internal/external-jugular, subclavian, or femoral vein
6–30 kg	Dual-lumen 8F (Kendall, Arrow)	Internal/external-jugular, subclavian, or femoral vein
>15 kg	Dual-lumen 9F (Medcomp)	Internal/external-jugular, subclavian, or femoral vein
>30 kg	Dual-lumen 10F (Arrow, Kendall)	Internal/external-jugular, subclavian, or femoral vein
>30 kg	Triple-lumen 12.5F (Arrow, Kendall)	Internal/external-jugular, subclavian, or femoral vein

6.19.4.5 Patient Factors

In general, factors that determine the optimal modality for a clinical situation include patient size, hemodynamic stability, and institutional expertise. PD and CRRT are better suited for patients with hemodynamic instability, because daily total ultrafiltration goals can be achieved over a 24-h period instead of a 3–4 h intermittent hemodialysis treatment. Table 6.19.2 outlines various advantages and disadvantages of the different acute renal replacement therapy modalities.

Acute PD requires much less technical expertise, expense, and equipment compared with intermittent hemodialysis and CRRT. PD catheters can be placed quickly and easily. Initial dwell volumes should be limited to 10 ml/kg of patient body weight to minimize intra-abdominal pressure and potential for fluid leakage along the catheter tunnel. Although PD may deliver less efficient solute removal than hemodialysis or CRRT, its relative simplicity and minimal associated side effects allow for RRT provision in settings lacking pediatric dialysis specific support and personnel.

Table 6.19.2 Advantages and disadvantages of different acute renal replacement therapy modalities

Modality	Advantages	Disadvantages
Intermittent hemodialysis	Short treatment times Accurate UF	Vascular access necessary Hemodynamic instability Heparin anticoagulation
Peritoneal dialysis	No need for vascular access Minimal equipment needs Minimal training needs Feasible in small infants Continuous treatment	Less efficient than hemodialysis/CRRT Variable UF dependent on BP
CRRT	Accurate UF that can be altered to account for changes in intake/patient BP Smaller circuit volumes Citrate anticoagulation	Vascular access necessary

BP blood pressure, *CRRT* continuous renal replacement therapy, *UF* ultrafiltration

6.19.4.6 CRRT

Various CRRT aspects including dose, dialysis/hemofiltration fluid composition, and anticoagulation methods have been studied in recent years. Until recently, most CRRT hemofiltration fluid or dialysis fluid used lactate as a buffer. A crossover study in adult patients receiving CRRT revealed that lactate-based solutions could lead to a rising serum lactate level in patients [63], a phenomenon that could lead to unnecessary investigation for tissue ischemia. Bicarbonate-buffered solutions can be made by hospital pharmacies, but are also now available from industry sources [17]. A recent pediatric study has highlighted the potential patient safety implications with pharmacy-prepared solutions, that can arise from compounding errors [8]. Thus, a solution composition validation program should exist in centers that opt to use pharmacy-made solutions for CRRT.

Anticoagulation of the CRRT circuit is essential to provide the therapy. Heparin and citrate are the two most common forms of anticoagulation. The adverse effects of heparin include systemic anticoagulation and the rare occurrence of induction of heparin-induced thrombocytopenia. Citrate anticoagulation occurs by decreasing the ionized calcium in the blood. CRRT circuits can undergo regional anticoagulation, where citrate is infused into the access line of the CRRT circuit and calcium is infused into a separate systemic central venous line or at the return line to maintain physiologic ionized calcium in the patient. The potential complications of regional citrate anticoagulation include metabolic alkalosis (especially if used in combination with bicarbonate-buffered CRRT replacement/dialysis solutions) and citrate lock. Citrate lock is a phenomenon where the delivery of citrate exceeds the patient's hepatic clearance. As a result, citrate concentrations increase in the blood and act as a buffer to bind calcium. Citrate lock is identified by a decreasing serum ionized calcium in the presence of a rising total calcium. The treatment for citrate lock is to discontinue citrate for 4 h and then restart at a lower citrate delivery rate. Recent pediatric studies have reported practical and safe citrate anticoagulation protocols [15, 17, 18].

6.19.5 Specific Patient Populations

6.19.5.1 Infants

Infants and neonates with AKF present unique problems for RRT provision. As noted earlier, delivery of hemodialysis or CRRT to these small patients entails a significant portion of their blood volume to be pumped through the extracorporeal circuit. Therefore, extracorporeal circuit volumes that comprise more than 10–15% of patient blood volume should be primed with whole blood to prevent hypotension and anemia. Since the prime volume is not discarded, it is important to not reinfuse the blood into the patient at the end of the treatment, to prevent volume overload and hypertension. Patients who receive CRRT with an AN-69 membrane are at risk for the bradykinin release syndrome when circuits require blood priming. The bradykinin release syndrome leads to hypotension and can be mitigated by normalizing the blood pH and giving a calcium bolus to the patient to counter the citrate in the blood unit [14].

6.19.5.2 Congenital Heart Disease

A recent trend toward providing PD therapy earlier in the post-CPB course has been reported, with one study of 20 patients demonstrating 80% patient survival [55]. While improved survival with early PD initiation may result from prevention of fluid overload, some posit that improved survival with early PD initiation results from increased clearance of CPB-induced proinflammatory cytokines, although further study is required to support this hypothesis [11].

6.19.5.3 Multiorgan Dysfunction Syndrome

The most critically ill patient population with multiorgan dysfunction syndrome has been a focus of significant outcome study in recent years. The concept that worsening fluid overload is associated with worse outcome in critically ill pediatric patients with multiorgan dysfunction syndrome who require RRT has been the focus of recent pediatric study. Both single-center data [23–26] and a multicenter effort [27], the Prospective Pediatric Continuous Renal Replacement Therapy Registry Group, demonstrate that worsening fluid overload is an independent risk factor for mortality, irrespective of severity of illness, in patients who receive CRRT. These data, coupled with the predilection for early multiorgan system failure and death in critically ill children with AKF, may argue for early and aggressive initiation of RRT in association with a goal-directed fluid repletion strategy in patients with multiorgan dysfunction syndrome.

6.19.5.4 Stem Cell Transplantation

Early recognition of AKF and prevention of fluid overload in patients with a recent stem cell transplant is critical because the need for mechanical ventilation in these patients is associated with increased mortality. A recent pediatric study has demonstrated that aggressive fluid control with early initiation of diuretics and CRRT can lead to improved survival in children with stem cell transplant and AKF [1].

6.19.6 Outcome

Depending on the definition used and the population studied, mortality in children with AKF ranges from 10 to 69% [20, 22, 40]. Children receiving CRRT with nonrenal organ disease or MODS have a higher mortality rate (>50%) compared with other diagnoses (<30%) [30]. Infants demonstrate even higher mortality when compared with older children [56]. Few data exist to describe the long-term outcome of children with PICU-acquired AKF. About 30% of children with hospital-acquired AKF had incomplete recovery of renal function or some element of chronic kidney disease by hospital discharge, and 5% required RRT at discharge [56]. The same group performed a 3–5 year follow-up of patients who suffered from AKF during PICU admission. Patient survival was 80%, and 60% of patients had some renal abnormality at follow-up (low GFR, hypertension, microalbuminuria, hematuria) [62]. In summary, hospital mortality of patients with AKF is related to the level of illness severity. In those who survive, there appears to be a definite risk of long-term negative effects on renal function and potentially increased risk for chronic kidney disease.

6.19.7 Take Home Pearls

- Acute kidney failure (AKF) in children may result from primary renal diseases or from secondary renal injury, such as sepsis, nephrotoxic medications, and renal ischemia.
- AKF management in children requires special considerations, as pediatric patients with AKF may range in weight from a 1.5-kg neonate to a 200-kg young adult.
- The primary goals of pharmacologic therapy are the preservation/restoration of renal perfusion and the prevention/treatment of metabolic derangements.
- For pediatric patients requiring renal replacement therapy, adequately sized therapy systems are available to enable the choice for intermittent hemodialysis, peritoneal dialysis, or continuous renal replacement therapy.

References

1. Michael, M., Kuehnle, I., Goldstein, S. L. (2004). Fluid overload and acute renal failure in pediatric stem cell transplant patients. Pediatr Nephrol. 19:91–5
2. Acker, C. G., Singh, A. R., Flick, R. P., et al. (2000) A trial of thyroxine in acute renal failure. Kidney Int 57:293–8
3. Akcan-Arikan, A., Zappitelli, M., Loftis, L. L., et al. (2007) Modified RIFLE criteria in critically ill children with acute kidney injury. Kidney Int 71:1028–35
4. Arora, P., Kher, V., Rai, P. K., et al. (1997) Prognosis of acute renal failure in children: a multivariate analysis. Pediatr Nephrol 11:153–5
5. Askenazi, D. J., Goldstein, S. L., Chang, I. F., et al. (2004) Management of a severe carbamazepine overdose using albumin-enhanced continuous venovenous hemodialysis. Pediatrics 113:406–9
6. Bailey, D., Phan, V., Litalien, C., et al. (2007) Risk factors of acute renal failure in critically ill children: A prospective descriptive epidemiological study. Pediatr Crit Care Med 8:29–35
7. Baldwin, L., Henderson, A., Hickman, P. (1994) Effect of postoperative low-dose dopamine on renal function after elective major vascular surgery. Ann Intern Med 120:744–7
8. Barletta, J. F., Barletta, G. M., Brophy, P. D., et al. (2006) Medication errors and patient complications with continuous renal replacement therapy. Pediatr Nephrol 21:842–5
9. Bellomo, R., Ronco, C., Kellum, J. A., et al. (2004) Acute renal failure – definition, outcome measures, animal models, fluid therapy and information technology needs: the Second International Consensus Conference of the Acute Dialysis Quality Initiative (ADQI) Group. Crit Care 8:R204–12
10. Boccalandro, F., Amhad, M., Smalling, R. W., et al. (2003) Oral acetylcysteine does not protect renal function from moderate to high doses of intravenous radiographic contrast. Catheter Cardiovasc Interv 58:336–41
11. Bokesch, P. M., Kapural, M. B., Mossad, E. B., et al. (2000) Do peritoneal catheters remove pro-inflammatory cytokines after cardiopulmonary bypass in neonates? Ann Thorac Surg 70:639–43
12. Book, K., Ohqvist, G., Bjork, V. O., et al. (1982) Peritoneal dialysis in infants and children after open heart surgery. Scand J Thorac Cardiovasc Surg 16:229–33
13. Briguori, C., Manganelli, F., Scarpato, P., et al. (2002) Acetylcysteine and contrast agent-associated nephrotoxicity. J Am Coll Cardiol 40:298–303
14. Brophy, P. D., Mottes, T. A., Kudelka, T. L., et al. (2001) AN-69 membrane reactions are pH-dependent and preventable. Am J Kidney Dis 38:173–8
15. Brophy, P. D., Somers, M. J., Baum, M. A., et al. (2005) Multi-centre evaluation of anticoagulation in patients receiving continuous renal replacement therapy (CRRT). Nephrol Dial Transplant 20:1416–21
16. Brusilow, S. W., Danney, M., Waber, L. J., et al. (1984) Treatment of episodic hyperammonemia in children with inborn errors of urea synthesis. N Engl J Med 310:1630–4
17. Bunchman, T. E., Maxvold, N. J., Barnett, J., et al. (2002) Pediatric hemofiltration: Normocarb dialysate solution with citrate anticoagulation. Pediatr Nephrol 17:150–4
18. Bunchman, T. E., Maxvold, N. J., Brophy, P. D. (2003) Pediatric convective hemofiltration: Normocarb replacement fluid and citrate anticoagulation. Am J Kidney Dis 42:1248–52
19. Bunchman, T. E., Maxvold, N. J., Kershaw, D. B., et al. (1995) Continuous venovenous hemodiafiltration in infants and children. Am J Kidney Dis 25:17–21
20. Bunchman, T. E., McBryde, K. D., Mottes, T. E., et al. (2001) Pediatric acute renal failure: outcome by modality and disease. Pediatr Nephrol 16:1067–71
21. Carcillo, J. A., Fields, A. I. (2002) Clinical practice parameters for hemodynamic support of pediatric and neonatal patients in septic shock. Crit Care Med 30:1365–78
22. DiCarlo, J. V., Alexander, S. R., Agarwal, R., et al. (2003) Continuous veno-venous hemofiltration may improve survival from acute respiratory distress syndrome after bone marrow transplantation or chemotherapy. J Pediatr Hematol Oncol 25:801–5
23. Foland, J. A., Fortenberry, J. D., Warshaw, B. L., et al. (2004) Fluid overload before continuous hemofiltration and survival in critically ill children: a retrospective analysis. Crit Care Med 32:1771–6
24. Gillespie, R. S., Seidel, K., Symons, J. M. (2004) Effect of fluid overload and dose of replacement fluid on survival in hemofiltration. Pediatr Nephrol 19:1394–9
25. Goldstein, S. L., Currier, H., Graf, C., et al. (2001) Outcome in children receiving continuous venovenous hemofiltration. Pediatrics 107:1309–12
26. Goldstein, S. L., Somers, M. J., Baum, M. A., et al. (2005) Pediatric patients with multi-organ dysfunction syndrome

receiving continuous renal replacement therapy. Kidney Int 67:653–8
27. Goldstein, S. L., Somers, M. J., Brophy, P. D., et al. (2004) The rospective pediatric continuous renal replacement therapy (ppCRRT) registry: design, development and data assessed. Int J Artif Organs 27:9–14
28. Hladunewich, M. A., Corrigan, G., Derby, G. C., et al. (2003) A randomized, placebo-controlled trial of IGF-1 for delayed graft function: a human model to study postischemic ARF. Kidney Int 64:593–602
29. Holliday, M. A., Segar, W. E. (1957) The maintenance need for water in parenteral fluid therapy. Pediatrics 19:823–32
30. Hui-Stickle, S., Brewer, E. D., Goldstein, S. L. (2005) Pediatric ARF epidemiology at a tertiary care center from 1999 to 2001. Am J Kidney Dis 45:96–101
31. Humphrey, H., Hall, J., Sznajder, I., et al. (1990) Improved survival in ARDS patients associated with a reduction in pulmonary capillary wedge pressure. Chest 97:1176–80
32. Kist-van Holthe, J. E., Goedvolk, C. A., Brand, R., et al. (2002) Prospective study of renal insufficiency after bone marrow transplantation. Pediatr Nephrol 17:1032–7
33. Klinge, J. (2001) Intermittent administration of furosemide or continuous infusion in critically ill infants and children: does it make a difference? Intensive Care Med 27:623–4
34. Lameire, N. H., De Vriese, A. S., Vanholder, R. (2003) Prevention and nondialytic treatment of acute renal failure. Curr Opin Crit Care 9:481–90
35. Lassnigg, A., Donner, E., Grubhofer, G., et al. (2000) Lack of renoprotective effects of dopamine and furosemide during cardiac surgery. J Am Soc Nephrol 11:97–104
36. Lauschke, A., Teichgraber, U. K., Frei, U., et al. (2006) "Low-dose" dopamine worsens renal perfusion in patients with acute renal failure. Kidney Int 69:1669–74
37. Little, M. A., Conlon, P. J., Walshe, J. J. (2000) Access recirculation in temporary hemodialysis catheters as measured by the saline dilution technique. Am J Kidney Dis 36:1135–9
38. McBryde, K. D., Kudelka, T. L., Kershaw, D. B., et al. (2004) Clearance of amino acids by hemodialysis in argininosuccinate synthetase deficiency. J Pediatr 144:536–40
39. Mehta, R. L., Kellum, J. A., Shah, S. V., et al. (2007) Acute kidney injury network: report of an initiative to improve outcomes in acute kidney injury. Crit Care 11:R31
40. Michael, M., Kuehnle, I., Goldstein, S. L. (2004) Fluid overload and acute renal failure in pediatric stem cell transplant patients. Pediatr Nephrol 19:91–5
41. Mishra, J., Dent, C., Tarabishi, R., et al. (2005) Neutrophil gelatinase-associated lipocalin (NGAL) as a biomarker for acute renal injury after cardiac surgery. Lancet 365:1231–8
42. Picca, S., Dionisi-Vici, C., Abeni, D., et al. (2001) Extracorporeal dialysis in neonatal hyperammonemia: modalities and prognostic indicators. Pediatr Nephrol 16:862–7
43. Picca, S., Principato, F., Mazzera, E., et al. (1995) Risks of acute renal failure after cardiopulmonary bypass surgery in children: a retrospective 10-year case-control study. Nephrol Dial Transplant 10:630–6
44. Rigden, S. P., Barratt, T. M., Dillon, M. J., et al. (1982) Acute renal failure complicating cardiopulmonary bypass surgery. Arch Dis Child 57:425–30
45. Rivers, E., Nguyen, B., Havstad, S., et al. (2001) Early goal-directed therapy in the treatment of severe sepsis and septic shock. N Engl J Med 345:1368–77
46. Safirstein, R., Andrade, L., Vieira, J. M. (2000) Acetylcysteine and nephrotoxic effects of radiographic contrast agents – a new use for an old drug. N Engl J Med 343:210–2
47. Samuels, J., Finkel, K., Gubert, M., et al. (2005) Effect of fenoldopam mesylate in critically ill patients at risk for acute renal failure is dose dependent. Ren Fail 27:101–5
48. Schenarts, P. J., Sagraves, S. G., Bard, M. R., et al. (2006) Low-dose dopamine: a physiologically based review. Curr Surg 63:219–25
49. Schetz, M. (2002) Vasopressors and the kidney. Blood Purif 20:243–51
50. Schuller, D., Mitchell, J. P., Calandrino, F. S., et al. (1991) Fluid balance during pulmonary edema. Is fluid gain a marker or a cause of poor outcome? Chest 100:1068–75
51. Schwartz, G. J., Haycock, G. B., Edelmann, C. M., Jr., et al. (1976) A simple estimate of glomerular filtration rate in children derived from body length and plasma creatinine. Pediatrics 58:259–63
52. Shilliday, I. R., Quinn, K. J., Allison, M. E. (1997) Loop diuretics in the management of acute renal failure: a prospective, double-blind, placebo-controlled, randomized study. Nephrol Dial Transplant 12:2592–6
53. Simmons, R. S., Berdine, G. G., Seidenfeld, J. J., et al. (1987) Fluid balance and the adult respiratory distress syndrome. Am Rev Respir Dis 135:924–9
54. Skippen, P. W., Krahn, G. E. (2005) Acute renal failure in children undergoing cardiopulmonary bypass. Crit Care Resusc 7:286–91
55. Sorof, J. M., Stromberg, D., Brewer, E. D., et al. (1999) Early initiation of peritoneal dialysis after surgical repair of congenital heart disease. Pediatr Nephrol 13:641–5
56. Symons, J. M., Chua, A. N., Somers, M. J., et al. (2007) Demographic characteristics of pediatric continuous renal replacement therapy: a report of the prospective pediatric continuous renal replacement therapy registry. Clin J Am Soc Nephrol 2:732–8
57. Trzeciak, S., Dellinger, R. P., Abate, N. L., et al. (2006) Translating research to clinical practice: a 1-year experience with implementing early goal-directed therapy for septic shock in the emergency department. Chest 129:225–32
58. Tsuneyoshi, I., Yamada, H., Kakihana, Y., et al. (2001) Hemodynamic and metabolic effects of low-dose vasopressin infusions in vasodilatory septic shock. Crit Care Med 29:487–93
59. Tumlin, J. A., Finkel, K. W., Murray, P. T., et al. (2005) Fenoldopam mesylate in early acute tubular necrosis: a randomized, double-blind, placebo-controlled clinical trial. Am J Kidney Dis 46:26–34
60. Vachvanichsanong, P., Dissaneewate, P., Lim, A., et al. (2006) Childhood acute renal failure: 22-year experience in a university hospital in southern Thailand. Pediatrics 118:e786–91
61. Warady, B. A., Bunchman, T. (2000) Dialysis therapy for children with acute renal failure: survey results. Pediatr Nephrol 15:11–3
62. Williams, D. M., Sreedhar, S. S., Mickell, J. J., et al. (2002) Acute kidney failure: a pediatric experience over 20 years. Arch Pediatr Adolesc Med 156:893–900
63. Zimmerman, D., Cotman, P., Ting, R., et al. (1999) Continuous veno-venous haemodialysis with a novel bicarbonate dialysis solution: prospective cross-over comparison with a lactate buffered solution. Nephrol Dial Transplant 14:2387–91

Part VII

Temporary Replacement of Kidney Function

Indications to Start Kidney Replacement Therapy

7.1

Nathalie Neirynck and An S. De Vriese

Core Messages

- In the absence of high-quality trials, no evidence-based criteria for the initiation of dialysis can be provided.
- A serum potassium > 6.5 mEq/l and/or ECG changes is a generally accepted threshold to initiate dialysis.
- Pulmonary edema and overt fluid overload are definite indications for kidney replacement therapy (KRT).
- Oliguria (diuresis < 200 ml/12 h) or anuria (diuresis < 50 ml/12 h) after optimization of volume status are generally accepted indications to start KRT. It remains unclear whether an earlier start of KRT, triggered by a less pronounced or less prolonged decline of diuresis, is beneficial.
- A trial of loop diuretics (furosemide 20 mg/h or bumetanide 1 mg/h) can be considered in volume-overloaded patients. Failure to increase diuresis to 0.5–1 ml/kg/h within a few hours should lead to prompt withdrawal of the diuretic and institution of dialytic support.
- A serum urea concentration of 190–215 mg/dl (32–36 mmol/l) is a commonly accepted threshold to initiate KRT. Whether earlier dialysis provides a survival advantage is unknown.
- The value of urea cutoff levels to initiate dialysis has been questioned. The use of biomarkers appears promising to predict the necessity of KRT, but still requires validation.

7.1.1 Introduction

Once acute kidney failure (AKF) has developed, 50–75% of patients require kidney replacement therapy (KRT) [1, 20, 41, 62]. This chapter will focus on the indications to start KRT and the studies that evaluated timing of KRT in relation to outcome. Traditionally accepted "definite" indications to start KRT are electrolyte disorders, acid–base disorders, fluid overload, oligoanuria, the requirement to administer large volumes of fluid and nutrition, uremic complications, and progressive uremia [5, 20, 21, 28, 45, 58]. Unfortunately, no consensus exists on the precise cutoff values triggering initiation of KRT. Consequently, clinicians have adopted individual practice patterns that vary substantially. In a survey by Ricci et al., 90 different criteria to start KRT are described [50]. With 27%, oligoanuria was the most frequently reported motivation [50]. Since most indications for KRT have not been the subject of randomized controlled trials (RCTs), we have chosen a pragmatic approach and will integrate the evidence – when available – with generally accepted clinical management strategies. Nonrenal indications for KRT, including hyperthermia, intoxications with a dialyzable toxin, congestive heart failure, and elimination of inflammatory mediators will be discussed elsewhere in this book.

A. S. De Vriese (✉)
The Renal Unit, AZ Sint-Jan AV, Ruddershove, 10, 8000 Brugge, Belgium
e-mail: an.devriese@azbrugge.be

A. Jörres et al. (eds.), *Management of Acute Kidney Problems*,
DOI: 10.1007/978-3-540-69441-0_7.1, © Springer-Verlag Berlin Heidelberg 2010

7.1.2 Electrolyte Disorders

7.1.2.1 Hyperkalemia

Because of the well-known cardiac toxicity, hyperkalemia has been one of the first indications to start dialysis [45]. A generally accepted threshold, albeit purely opinion-based, is a serum potassium >6.5 mEq/l and/or electrocardiogram (ECG) changes [5, 20, 21, 33, 45]. The expectation that AKF will persist, the presence of muscle or other tissue injury or gastrointestinal ischemia, and the requirement for blood transfusion, all will influence the decision to start dialysis immediately, rather than to await the effect of conservative measures [5]. Hemodialysis is more effective in removing potassium than hemofiltration or peritoneal dialysis. The removal rate depends on the initial serum potassium concentration, the potassium concentration of the dialysate, the type of dialyzer used, and the blood and dialysate flow rates. Using a potassium-free dialysate, a decrease of serum potassium up to 1.2–1.5 mEq/l/h can be achieved. Two strategies can be used to avoid a rapid decrease of the serum potassium, which by itself has been associated with the induction of cardiac arrythmias. Either dialysis is begun with a 3 mEq/l potassium dialysate, with a decrease of the dialysate potassium concentration each subsequent hour. Alternatively, dialysis is initiated at a 0–1 mEq/l dialysate potassium, to be substituted by a higher concentration once the serum potassium is no longer life-threatening [27].

7.1.2.2 Hypo- and Hypernatremia

Aggressive correction of hyponatremia or hypernatremia in the absence of AKF by means of KRT will rarely, if ever, be indicated. Severe hyponatremia and hypernatremia in patients with AKF can be corrected by continuous KRT, when respectively fluid restriction or administration of free water is not possible [5]. Different thresholds have been proposed: <115 mEq/l and >160 mEq/l [5], or < 120 mEq/l and >155 mEq/l [33]. Rapid changes of the sodium concentration should evidently be avoided, for fear of osmotic demyelination [45]. In a case of hypernatremia associated with a hyperglycemic nonketotic coma and AKF, custom-made dialysate was used and the sodium concentration was adapted every 6 h [35]. In other case reports of hypernatremia, hypertonic fluid replacement was used to prevent rapid correction [43, 65].

7.1.2.3 Hypercalcemia

Severe hypercalcemia can be an indication to start KRT, although no specific thresholds are proposed [45]. Dialysis should be considered as a last resort treatment in patients with severe hypercalcemia and mental alterations in whom aggressive hydration cannot be accomplished. An efficient reduction can be achieved using a calcium-free dialysate [32]. Another strategy to correct severe hypercalcemia is continuous KRT with regional citrate anticoagulation [29].

7.1.3 Acid–Base Disorders

Severe metabolic acidosis is an accepted indication for KRT. Opinion-based thresholds are a pH < 7.1 [5] or pH < 7.0 [33]. Both intermittent hemodialysis (IHD) and continuous venovenous hemodiafiltration (CVVHDF) can be used to correct metabolic acidosis, with a preference for CVVHDF [44, 60].

7.1.4 Fluid Management

7.1.4.1 Volume Overload and Oligoanuria

Volume overload is generally recognized as an indication for KRT in AKF. Subjective criteria for the initiation of therapy include the impairment of cardiopulmonary function by pulmonary vascular congestion and the compromise of cutaneous integrity or wound healing by peripheral edema [45]. Objective and reproducible measurements, such as oxygen saturation, central venous pressure, pulmonary artery occlusion pressure, end-diastolic ventricular volume, or bioimpedance measurements, all have limitations in assessing volume status [38, 49]. More reliable parameters to determine volume status and volume responsiveness are dynamic measures such as inspiratory decrease in right atrial pressure, expiratory decrease in atrial systolic pressure, respiratory changes in pulse pressure, and respiratory changes in aortic blood velocity [49]. Unfortunately, what constitutes "optimal volume status" in a critically ill patient with AKF remains largely undefined. In addition, none of these measures has been studied rigorously as a parameter to guide the initiation of KRT.

The presence of oliguria or anuria despite an "optimal" volume status is an accepted indication to start KRT [20, 33]. Oliguria is defined as a diuresis < 200 ml/12 h and anuria as a diuresis < 50 ml/12 h [5]. In the perioperative period and intensive care unit (ICU) population, oliguria is often defined as an urinary flow rate of < 0.5 ml/kg/h [56]. The RIFLE criteria for urine output are a diuresis of < 0.5 ml/kg/h for 6 h, < 0.5 ml/kg/h for12 h, and < 0.3 ml/kg/h for 24 h or anuria to define class R (risk), class I (injury), and class F (failure) AKF, respectively [7]. Oligoanuria was the most common indication for KRT reported by clinicians in a questionnaire [50]. The presence of oligoanuria is generally associated with a subjective appreciation of more severe AKF. Some studies indeed found that the mortality rate of oliguric AKF was higher than that of nonoliguric AKF [2, 55], but patients with preserved diuresis had a lower APACHE II score and a higher creatinine clearance at inclusion [55]. In contrast, larger urine output and lower serum creatinine was counterintuitively associated with higher mortality in ICU patients with AKF in an observational study [39]. Another small retrospective analysis of nonoliguric AKF requiring dialysis reported a higher diuresis in nonsurvivors versus survivors [34].

7.1.4.2 Loop Diuretics

Before starting KRT in patients with fluid overload or oligoanuria, a trial of loop diuretics is generally given. Loop diuretics convert oliguria to diuresis in a subset of patients with AKF. While the mortality rate of nonoliguric AKF was found to be lower than that of oliguric AKF, there were no significant differences in the clinical characteristics, the severity of renal failure, and the mortality rate between spontaneously nonoliguric patients and patients becoming nonoliguric after furosemide [2, 54]. These observations imply that patients responding to loop diuretics are characterized by a less severe form of renal failure, rather than a beneficial effect of therapy [16]. In a retrospective multicenter study of 522 critically ill patients with AKF [40], diuretic use was evaluated in relation to timing of dialysis, recovery of renal function, and mortality. At the time of the first nephrology consultation, 59% of the patients received diuretics. An additional 12% were started on diuretics later on. Diuretic use was associated with a 68% increase in mortality and a 77% increase in the odds of death or nonrecovery of renal function. The time from consultation to dialysis was 1–2 days longer in patients receiving diuretics. The authors suggested that the adverse outcome was due either to direct deleterious effects of diuretics or to a delay in the recognition of the severity of AKF and subsequent institution of dialytic support when urine output is sustained. Alternatively, diuretics may have been preferentially used in patients with an intrinsically more severe course of disease [16]. These results are at variance with those of another multicenter observational study in 1,743 critically ill patients with AKF [61]. At study inclusion, 70% of the patients were treated with diuretics. The use of diuretics was not associated with mortality [61]. A few smaller retrospective studies found no effect of loop diuretics on the course of established AKF [9, 11, 42]. Loop diuretics did not accelerate renal recovery, reduce the need for dialysis or affect mortality. Three RCTs comparing a bolus of a loop diuretic with no drug found no difference in renal recovery or mortality [12, 31, 55]. Most of these studies were, however, relatively small and lacked statistical power to entirely rule out an effect of diuretics. In an attempt to resolve the controversy generated by the lack of high-quality trials, three meta-analysis pooled the results of the available RCTs on the use of loop diuretics in the prevention and treatment of AKF [3, 26, 54]. None found a beneficial effect on mortality or renal recovery, although two reported the requirement of a reduced number of dialysis treatments [3, 54].

A recent international survey revealed diverse practice patterns in the use of diuretics for the management of acute kidney injury (AKI) [4]. Only 5.3% of the respondents reported the use of a protocol to guide therapy. Diuretics were more frequently given in bolus than as a continuous infusion. There is, however, evidence that a greater overall natriuresis can be achieved with a continuous infusion than with repeated bolus injections [52]. In addition, the high peak plasma levels attending bolus administration are associated with an enhanced risk of ototoxicity [10, 22]. Continuous infusions are therefore the preferred mode of administration [37, 53]. The most studied loop diuretic is furosemide, which is usually given in a single intravenous dose from 40 mg up to 160–200 mg two or three times daily or as a continuous infusion at 20 mg/h. Although extremely high doses (up to 2,400 mg/day) have increased urine output in selected cases, they should be avoided for fear of ototoxicity. Bumetanide is given at a dose of 2 mg up to 8–10 mg in bolus or as a continuous infusion at 1 mg/h. The dose should be titrated to achieve a diuresis of 0.5–1 ml/kg/h and avoid volume depletion. Since the onset of action starts within a few minutes after intravenous administration with a maximum effect after 30–40 min, continuation of the drug in the absence of an increase in diuresis within a few hours appears futile.

In conclusion, the judicious use of loop diuretics in AKF remains more in the realm of art than of science. Large and rigorously designed RCTs on the position of loop diuretics in the management of AKF are therefore urgently required. Pending data from such studies, a trial of diuretic therapy in volume-overloaded patients can be considered, but should have as its sole objective the increase of diuresis. Failure to achieve this goal within a few hours should lead to prompt withdrawal of the diuretic and institution of dialytic support.

7.1.4.3 Trials on Timing of Dialysis

Early start of dialysis triggered by the onset of oligoanuria has been evaluated in three retrospective studies [15, 18, 34] and two RCTs [8, 57] (Table 7.1.1). Two retrospective studies performed in patients with AKF after cardiac surgery [15, 18] compared early start of KRT triggered by the development of oliguria with a more delayed start based on metabolic derangement. Both studies found a shorter length of stay in both ICU and hospital and a lower mortality when KRT was initiated early. One study [15] used a historical control group, making unmeasured confounding very likely. Another retrospective study analyzed the initiation of KRT in survivors versus nonsurvivors [34]. Survivors underwent KRT 9 days earlier than nonsurvivors and had a lower diuresis at initiation of dialysis. However, they also had a significantly lower MOF score, which appears a more probable explanation for their ultimate survival. The RCT by Bouman et al. [8] examined the effect of timing and intensity of KRT in 106 patients with circulatory and respiratory insufficiency and oliguric AKI, the majority of which were post-cardiac surgery. Patients were randomized into an early start, high-volume hemofiltration group (n = 35), an early start, low-volume hemofiltration group (n = 35), or a late start, low-volume hemofiltration group (n = 36). In the last group, six patients ultimately did not require KRT. Survival was not different among the groups. Time from inclusion to initiation of KRT differed by only 36 h between the early and late starters, which is perhaps too short to be of pathophysiologic significance. Another small RCT included 36 patients post-cardiac surgery when diuresis was < 30 ml/h for 3 h and creatinine increased by 0.5 mg/dl/day [57]. Patients were randomized to start dialysis immediately or when diuresis decreased further. Eight patients were excluded because they never met the criteria to start dialysis. Survival at 14 days was remarkably higher in the early start group. Surprisingly, there was no difference in time to initiation of dialysis expressed as days after surgery, nor in serum creatinine at the start of dialysis.

7.1.4.4 Summary

Pulmonary edema and overt fluid overload are definite indications to start KRT. Oliguria (diuresis < 200 ml/12 h) or anuria (diuresis < 50 ml/12 h) after optimization of volume status are generally used criteria to start KRT. Before the initiation of KRT, a trial of loop diuretics is defendable, provided volume depletion is avoided and the restoration of diuresis does not delay the institution of dialysis when required by other indicators. Whether loop diuretics ultimately affect mortality remains equivocal. The available evidence does not allow us to conclude whether an earlier start of KRT, triggered by a less pronounced or less prolonged decline of diuresis, is beneficial. All nonrandomized trials on this subject are burdened by an inherent bias that rules out any reliable conclusions. The "early" groups will always include patients who may never have required dialysis had they been observed longer and who therefore intrinsically have a better prognosis. Only two small RCT have been performed, unfortunately with conflicting results.

Table 7.1.1 Retrospective studies of early versus late kidney replacement therapy in acute kidney failure

Reference	Timing	Patient number and type	Initiation of dialysis: A = "early"; B = "late"	Mean urea (mg/dl) Time to initiation of dialysis (days)	End points (p value)
[23]	1989–1997	$n = 100$ Polytrauma	**A**: urea < 129 mg/dl **B**: urea > 129 mg/dl	**A**: 98; **B**: 203 **A**: 10.5; **B**: 19.4 (from hospital admission)	Survival: **A**: 39%; **B**: 20.3% ($p = 0.041$) Hospital LOS: **A**: 46.5 d; **B**: 53.0 d ($p = 0.459$) Duration KRT: **A**: 17.7 d; **B**: 20.2 d ($p = 0.448$)
[15]	**A**: 1996–2001 **B**: 1992–1996	$n = 61$ Post-cardiac surgery	**A**: urine output < 100 ml within 8 h after surgery despite furosemide **B**: SCreat > 5 mg/dl or potassium > 5.5 mEq/l regardless of urine output	No data **A**: 0.78; **B**: 2.55 (from surgery)	Hospital mortality: **A**: 23.5%; **B**: 55.5% ($p = 0.016$) ICU mortality: **A**: 17.6%; **B**: 48.1% ($p = 0.014$) Hospital LOS: **A**: 15.4 d; **B**: 20.9 d ($p = 0.016$) ICU LOS: **A**: 7.8 d; **B**: 12.4 d ($p = 0.0001$)
[36]	1999–2001	$n = 243$ PICARD, heterogeneous ICU population	**A**: urea < 163 mg/dl **B**: urea > 163 mg/dl	**A**: 102; **B**: 246 No data	14-day survival: **A**: 80%; **B**: 75% ($p = 0.09$) 28-day survival: **A**: 65%; **B**: 59% ($p = 0.09$)
[18]	2002–2003	$n = 64$ Post-cardiac surgery	**A**: urine output < 100 ml within 8 h after surgery despite furosemide **B**: urea ≥ 180 mg/dl or SCreat ≥ 2.8 mg/dl or potassium > 6.0 mEq/l regardless of urine output	**A**: 143; **B**: 160 **A**: 0.78; **B**: 2.55	Hospital mortality: **A**: 22%; **B**: 43% ($p < 0.05$) Hospital LOS: **A**: 15.4 d; **B**: 20.9 d ($p < 0.05$) -ICU LOS: **A**: 8.5 d; **B**: 12.5 d ($p < 0.05$)
[48]	**A**: 1999–2004 **B**: 1996–1999	$n = 80$ Septic AKF	**A**: SCreat > 1.35 mg/dl, urea >48 mg/dl, urine output <800 ml/24 h despite furosemide **B**: SCreat > 2.7 mg/dl, urea > 96 mg/dl, urine output < 400 ml/24 h or < 100 ml/6 h	**A**: 235; **B**: 257 **A**: < 12 h after ICU admission; **B**: no data	28-day survival: **A**: 55%; **B**: 27.5% ($p = 0.005$) ICU survival: **A**: 70%; **B**: 40% ($p = 0.003$) Hospital stay: **A**: 19 d; **B**: 34 d ($p < 0.001$) Duration of mechanical ventilation: **A**: 11 d; **B**: 20 d ($p < 0.001$)
[34]	? published in 2005	$n = 43$ Nonoliguric AKF	**A**: survivors **B**: nonsurvivors	**A**: 163; **B**: 90 **A**: 7; **B**: 16	Urine output at start of dialysis: **A**: 0.7 l/d; B: 1.5 l/d ($p = 0.02$) MOF score at start of dialysis: **A**: 1.7; **B**: 2.7 ($p < 0.01$)

LOS: length of stay; IHF: isovolemic hemofiltration; AKF: acute kidney failure; CVVH: continuous venovenous hemofiltration; SCreat: serum creatinine; MOF: multiple organ failure

7.1.5 Azotemia

Uremic complications such as uremic encephalopathy, neuropathy, myopathy, and pericarditis require urgent initiation of KRT. Although traditionally mentioned as indications to start KRT, this extent of uremia is no longer seen in the current setting of AKI in ICU patients. Uremic symptoms, such as anorexia, nausea, vomiting, and pruritus are difficult to distinguish in critically ill patients, and therefore serum urea is used as a surrogate marker. Unfortunately, the optimal threshold for serum urea to initiate KRT is not known.

Based on historical trials [13, 17, 19, 20, 30, 47, 59], a threshold of 190 – 215 mg/dl (32–36 mmol/l) is commonly advised [21, 45, 46, 51].

During the 1960s and 1970s, several retrospective studies supported "early" start of KRT, and the concept of prophylactic dialysis was introduced. In 1960, Teschan et al. reported an all-cause mortality of 30% in 15 oliguric patients who were dialyzed when urea reached 200 mg/dl (36 mmol/l), to keep it below 150 mg/dl (25 mmol/l) [59]. There was no control group, but the authors reported that the results were better than their own earlier experience. In 1964, Easterling et al. reported a similar overall mortality of 36% in 45 patients dialyzed to keep urea below 322 mg/dl (54 mmol/l) [17]. Three further retrospective studies reported dramatically lower mortality rates when dialysis was started earlier than in more traditional practices [19, 30, 47]. In the study by Parson et al., initiation of dialysis when urea was 257–320 mg/dl (42–54 mmol/l) resulted in a mortality of 25%, while 88% of patients died when dialysis was started when urea was > 428 mg/dl (77 mmol/l) [47]. Fischer reported mortality rates of 57% and 74% in early (urea 320 mg/dl or 54 mmol/l) versus late (urea 428 mg/dl or 77 mmol/l) starters, respectively [19]. Kleinknecht et al. found a mortality of 29% when dialysis was started to maintain urea < 200 mg/dl (33 mmol/l), and a mortality of 42% when dialysis was initiated when urea was > 350 mg/dl (58 mmol/l) or when severe electrolyte disturbances were present [30]. The survival benefit was borne largely by lower rates of fatal gastrointestinal hemorrhage (5% vs 14%, $p < 0.02$) and sepsis (12% vs 24%, $p < 0.01$) [30]. These studies evidently have only historical significance, since the thresholds used to define "late" dialysis are no longer applicable.

A subsequent prospective case control study of 18 Vietnam war casualties introduced a lower threshold of urea to define "early" dialysis [13, Table 7.1.2]. In the early group predialysis urea was kept at < 150 mg/dl (25 mmol/l) and creatinine < 5 mg/dl (446 μmol/l), while in the late group, dialysis was not initiated until urea reached 320 mg/dl (54 mmol/l), creatinine reached 10 mg/dl (893 μmol/l), or other indications to start treatment, such as hyperkalemia, fluid overload, or

Table 7.1.2 Prospective studies of early versus late kidney replacement therapy in acute kidney failure

Reference	Timing	Patient number and type	Initiation of dialysis: A = "early"; B = "late"	Mean urea (mg/dl) Time to initiation of dialysis	End points (*p* value)
Prospective case-control study					
13	1970	*n* = 18 trauma	**A**: maintain predialysis urea < 150 mg/dl and SCreat < 5 mg/dl **B**: urea > 322 mg/dl, SCreat > 10 mg/dl or clinical indication for earlier dialysis	**A**: 107; **B**: 257 No data	Survival: **A**: 64%; **B**: 20% ($p < 0.1$)
Randomized controlled trials					
57	1995–1997	*n* = 36 Post-cardiac surgery	**A**: diuresis < 30 ml/min for 3 h **B**: diuresis < 20 ml/min for 2 h	No data **A**: 1.8 d; **B**: 1.7 d (from surgery)	14-day survival: **A**: 85%; **B**: 14% ($p < 0.01$)
8	1998–2000	*n* = 106 Oliguric AKF, ventilated	**A**: urine output < 30 ml/h for > 6 h and creatinine clearance < 20 ml/min and < 12 h after inclusion; **A1**: EHVH; **A2**: ELVH **B**: LLVH: oliguria and creatinine clearance < 20 ml/min and urea > 240 mg/dl (40 mmol/l), severe pulmonary edema	**A**: 101; **B**: 226 **A**: 6-7 h; **B**: 42 h	28-day survival: **A1**: 74.3%; **A2**: 68.8%; **B**: 75% ($p = 0.80$) Hospital survival: **A1**: 62.9%; **A2**: 48.6%; **B**: 61.1% ($p = 0.42$)

AKF: acute kidney failure; EHVH: early high-volume hemofiltration with blood flow rate 200 ml/min and ultrafiltration rate 72 l/day; ELVH: early low-volume hemofiltration with blood flow rate 100–150 ml/min and ultrafiltration rate 24–36 l/day; LLVH: late low-volume hemofiltration with blood flow rate 100–150 ml/min and ultrafiltration rate 24–36 l/day uremic encephalopathy were present. There was a marked difference in mortality, sepsis, and bleeding in favor of the early group [13]. The difference in mortality was not significant, however, owing to the small number of patients studied. Gettings et al. [23], [Table 7.1.1] retrospectively analyzed data of 100 posttraumatic patients with AKF, in whom continuous renal replacement therapy (CRRT) was initiated at the discretion of the attending physician. The patients were divided in an early or late group, if urea at initiation of dialysis was less than or greater than 129 mg/dl (21.5 mmol/l). While no differences in the duration of CRRT, length of hospital stay, or recovery of renal function were noted, mortality was lower in the early group. However, the study stretched over a 9-year period, during which general intensive care and dialysis techniques improved significantly and overall survival tended to improve over the study period. The findings could therefore be attributed to a systematic bias, if physicians were more likely to start "early" dialysis during the most recent period covered by the study. In addition, AKF due to rhabdomyolysis was more prevalent in the early starters, whereas the proportion of patients with multiorgan failure was lower in the early starters, both of which may have beneficially affected their survival. The PICARD study is an observational multicenter study of AKF in the ICU [41]. Liu et al. retrospectively analyzed a subpopulation of patients who required KRT, as determined by the attending physician [36], [Table 7.1.1]. The 243 patients whose urea on the day of start of dialysis was known were divided into an early or late group, if urea was ≤ 163 mg/dl (27 mmol/l) or > 163 mg/dl (27 mmol/l), respectively. Mean urinary output or occurrence of oliguria was comparable between the groups. Survival rates were not different, but the number of failing organs was higher in the early start group. Piccini et al. studied 80 patients with septic shock, acute lung injury, and oliguric acute kidney injury, defined as serum creatinine >1.35 mg/dl (120 µmol/l), serum urea > 48 mg/dl (8 mmol/l) [5, 6], and diuresis < 800 ml/24 h despite fluid resuscitation and furosemide administration in the previous 24 h [48], [Table 7.1.1]. Isovolemic hemofiltration at 45 m/kg/h of plasma–water exchange over 6 h within 12 h after admission to the ICU, followed by continuous venovenous hemofiltration (CVVH) at 20 ml/min/h during the remaining 18 h, was compared with initiation of CVVH at 20 ml/min/h when "classical criteria" [5, 6] to start KRT were fulfilled, i.e., serum creatinine >2.7 mg/dl (240 µmol/l), serum urea >96 mg/dl (16 mmol/l), and/or a urine output <400 ml/24 h or <100 ml/6 h. In the early group, every patient received extracorporeal treatment, whereas in the late group only 30% developed AKF of which 75% (n = 9) were treated with KRT. Both ICU and 28-day survival were better in the early CVVH group. The early group was, however, treated in a later period and could therefore have profited from improvements in general critical care medicine and dialysis techniques.

Serum urea concentration is the oldest surrogate marker for renal function. Although its limitations as a biomarker to estimate kidney function have long been recognized, more recently the use of urea cutoff levels to initiate dialysis has been questioned [63]. Serum urea may be too unspecific for kidney injury, since it is also influenced by tissue protein catabolism and subclinical gastrointestinal hemorrhage. A new series of biomarkers for AKI, such as the urinary tubular enzymes, neutrophil gelatinase-associated lipocalin (NGAL), kidney injury molecule-1 (KIM-1), interleukin 18 (IL-18), and Na^+/H^+ exchanger isoform 3 (NHE3), are promising tools for early detection, grading of severity, differential diagnosis, and time course of kidney injury, as well as for monitoring the response to therapy [14, 24, 64]. Urinary cystatine C and a1-microglobulin may predict the requirement for KRT in nonoliguric AKF [25]. Most of these tests still want validation, however. Hopefully, the initiation of KRT may in the future be more reliably triggered by a combination of biomarkers than by serum urea [14].

7.1.6 Conclusion

Half a century ago it was hypothesized that early dialysis could prevent the development of the uremic syndrome and the associated adverse outcome [59]. Although the decision to initiate dialysis in AKF is made on a daily basis by most practicing nephrologists, the optimal timing to improve survival presently remains moot. There are no reliable predictors of the time course of AKF. Clinicians therefore often intuitively have to assess the potential that renal function will recover without the requirement for KRT. They must weigh the importance of early correction of uremia and fluid overload against the potential adverse consequences and logistic and economic burden of

KRT. Most trials have been performed several decades ago and may no longer be applicable today. The availability of regional anticoagulation, biocompatible membranes, bicarbonate buffer, and other sophistications in dialysis delivery may have decreased the adverse effects of dialysis in patients with AKI, and thus may have tipped the balance in favor of early dialysis. It is our hope that a new generation of clinical trials will be designed and prove illuminating in this important matter. This information may than pave the way for a standardized approach to dialysis in the ICU.

References

1. Abosaif NY, Tolba YA, Heap M, et al. (2005) The outcome of acute renal failure in the intensive care unit according to RIFLE: model application, sensitivity and predictability. Am J Kidney Dis 46: 1038–1048
2. Anderson RJ, Linas SL, Berns AS, et al. (1977) Non oliguric acute renal failure. N Engl J Med 296: 1134–1138
3. Baghsaw SM, Delaney A, Haase M, et al. (2007) Loop diuretics in the management of acute renal failure: a systematic review and meta-analysis. Crit Care Rescusc 9: 60–68
4. Bagshaw SM, Delaney A, Jones D, et al. (2007) Diuretics in the management of acute renal injury: a multinational survey. Contrib Nephrol 156: 236–249
5. Bellomo R, Ronco C (1998) Indications and criteria for initiating renal replacement therapy in intensive care unit. Kidney Int 53 (Suppl 66): S106–109
6. Bellomo R, Kellum J, Ronco C (2001) Acute renal failure: time for consensus. Intensive Care Med 27: 1585–1588
7. Bellomo R, Ronco C, Kellum JA, et al. (2004) Acute renal failure: definition, outcome measures, animal models, fluid therapy and information technology needs. The second international consensus conference of Acute Dialysis Quality Initiative (ADQI) group. Crit Care 8: R204–R2012
8. Bouman CSC, Oudemans-van Straaten H, Tijssen JGP, et al. (2002) Effects of early high volume CVVH on survival and recovery of renal function in intensive care patients with acute renal failure; a prospective randomised trial. Crit Care Med 30: 2205–2211
9. Borirakchanyavat V, Vongsthongsri M, Sitprija V (1978) Furosemide and acute renal failure. Postgrad Med J 54: 30–2
10. Brown CB, Ogg CS, Cameron JS (1981) High dose frusemide in acute renal failure: a controlled trial. Clin Nephrol 15: 90–96
11. Cantarovich F, Galli C, Benedetti L, et al. (1973) High dose frusemide in established acute renal failure. Br Med J 4: 449–450
12. Cantarovich F, Rangoonwala B, Lorenz H, et al. (2004) High dose furosemide for established ARF: a prospective randomised double-blind placebo controlled multicenter trial. Am J Kidney Dis 44: 402–409
13. Conger JD (1975) A controlled evaluation of prophylactic dialysis in post-traumatic acute renal failure. J Trauma 15:1056–1063
14. Dennen P, Parikh CR (2007) Biomarkers of acute kidney injury: can we replace serum creatinine? Clin Nephrol 68: 269–278
15. Demirkiliç U, Kurulay E, Yenicesu M, et al. (2004) Timing of replacement therapy for acute renal failure after cardiac surgery. J Card Surg 19: 17–20
16. De Vriese AS (2003) Prevention and treatment of acute renal failure in sepsis. J Am Soc Nephrol 14: 792–805
17. Easterling RE. Forland M. (1964) A five year experience with prophylactic dialysis for acute renal failure. Trans Am Soc Artif Intern Organs 10: 200–208.
18. Elahi M, Lim MY, Joseph RN, et al., (2004) Early hemofiltration improves survival in post-cardiotomy patients with acute renal failure. Eur J Cardiothorc Surg 26: 1027–1031
19. Fisher RP, Griffen WO Jr, Reiser M, et al. (1966) Early dialysis in the treatment of acute renal failure. Surg Gynecol Obstet 123: 1019–1023
20. Formica M, Inguaggiato P, Bainotti S, et al. (2007) Acute renal failure in critically ill patients: indications for and choice of extracorporeal treatment. J Nephrol 20: 15–20
21. Fry AC, Farrington K (2006) Management of acute renal failure. Postgrad Med J 82: 106–116
22. Gallagher KL, Jones JK (1979) Furosemide-induced ototoxicity. Ann Int Med 91: 744–745
23. Gettings LG, Reynolds HN, Scalea T (1999) Outcome in posttraumatic acute renal failure when continuous renal replacement is applied early vs late. Intensive Care Med 25: 805–813
24. Han WK, Bonventre JV (2004) Biological markers for the early detection of acute kidney injury. Curr Opin Crit Care 10: 476–482
25. Herget-Rosenthal S, Poppen D, Marggraf G, et al. (2004) Prognostic value of tubular proteinuria and enzymuria in nonoliguric acute tubular necrosis. Clin Chem 50: 552–58
26. Ho KM, Sheridan DJ (2006) Meta-analysis of frusemide to prevent or treat acute renal failure. BMJ 333: 420–425
27. Hou S, McElroy PA, Nootens J, et al. (1989) Safety and efficacy of low-potassium dialysate. Am J Kidney Dis 13:137–143
28. John S, Eckardt KU (2006) Renal replacement therapy in the treatment of acute renal failure- Intermittent and continuous. Semin Dial 19: 455–464
29. Kindgen-Milles D, Kram R, Kleinefort W, et al. (2008) Treatment of severe hypercalcemia using continuous renal replacement therapy with regional citrate anticoagulation. ASAIO 54: 442–444
30. Kleinknecht D, Jungers P, Chanard J, Barbanel C, et al. (1972) Uremic and non-uremic complications in acute renal failure: Evaluation of early and frequent dialysis on prognosis. Kidney Int 1: 190–196
31. Kleinknecht D, Ganeval D, Gonzalez- Duque LA, et al., (1976) Furosemide in acute renal failure. A controlled trial. Nephron 17: 51–58
32. Koo WS, Jeon DS, Ahn SJ, et al., (1996) Calcium-free hemodialysis for the management of hypercalcemia. Nephron 72: 424–428
33. Lameire N, Van Biesen W, Vanholder R (2005) Acute renal failure. Lancet 365: 417–430

34. Liangos O, Rao M, Balakrishnan VS, et al. (2005) Relationship of urine output to dialysis initiation and mortality in acute renal failure. Nephron Clin Pract 99: c56–60
35. Lin JJ, McKenney DW, Price C, et al., (2002) Continuous venovenous hemodiafiltration in hypernatremic hyperglycemic nonketotic coma. Pedriatr Nephrol 17: 969–973
36. Liu KD, Himmelfarb J, Paganini E, et al. (2006) Timing of initiation of dialysis in critically ill patient with acute kidney injury. Clin J Am Soc Nephrol 1: 915–919
37. Martin SJ, Danziger LH (1994) Continuous infusion of loop diuretics in the critically ill: A review of the literature. Crit Care Med 22: 1323–1329
38. Mehta RL, Clark WC, Schetz M (2002) Techniques for assessing and achieving fluid balance in acute renal failure. Curr Opin Crit Care 8: 535–543
39. Mehta RL, McDonald B, Gabbai F, et al. (2002) Nephrology consultation in acute renal failure: does timing matter? Am J Med 113: 456–461.
40. Mehta RL, Pascual MT, Soroko S, et al. (2002) Diuretics, mortality and non-recovery of renal function and acute renal failure. JAMA 288: 2547–2553
41. Mehta RL, Pascual MT, Soroko S, et al. (2004) Spectrum of acute renal failure in the intensive care unit: the PICARD experience. Kidney Int 66: 613–21
42. Minuth AN, Terrel JB, Suki WN (1976) A study of the course and prognosis of 104 patients and the role of furosemide. Am J Med Sci 271: 317–324
43. Moss GD, Primavesi RJ, McGraw ME (1990) Correction of hypernatraemia with continuous arteriovenous haemodiafiltration. Arch Dis Child 65: 628–630
44. Naka T, Bellomo R (2004) Bench-to-bedside review: treating acid base abnormalities in the ICU- the role of renal replacement therapy. Crit Care 8: 108–114
45. Palevsky PM (2005) Renal replacement therapy I: indication and timing. Crit Care Clin 21: 347–356
46. Palevsky PM (2006) Dialysis modality and dosing strategy in acute renal failure. Semin Dial 19: 165–170
47. Parson FM, Hobson SM, Blagg CR, et al. (1961) Optimum of dialysis in acute reversible renal failure. Desciption and value of an improved dialyser with large surface area. Lancet 1: 129–134
48. Piccinni P, Maurizio D, Barbacini S, et al. (2006) Early isovolaemic haemofiltration in oliguric patients with septic shock. Intensive Care Med 32: 80–86
49. Pinsky MR, Brophy P, Padilla J, et al. (2008) Fluid and volume monitoring. Int J Artif Organs 31: 111–126
50. Ricci Z, Ronco C, D'amico G, et al. (2006) Practice patterns in the management of acute renal failure in the critically ill patient: an international survey. Nephrol Dial Transplant 21: 690–696
51. Rondon- Berrios H, Palevsky PM (2007) Treatment of acute kidney injury: an update in the management of renal replacement therapy. Curr Opin Nephrol Hypertens 16: 64–70
52. Rudy DW, Voelker JR, Greene PK, et al. (1991) Loop diuretics for chronic renal insufficiency: a continuous infusion is more efficacious than bolus therapy. Ann Int Med 115: 360–366
53. Salvador DR, Rey NR, Ramos GC, et al. (2005) Continuous infusion versus bolus injection of loop diuretics in congestive heart failure. Cochrane Database Syst Rev 20: CD003178
54. Sampath S, Moran JL, Graham PL, et al. (2007) The efficacy of loop diuretics in acute renal failure: assessment using Bayesian evidence synthesis techniques. Crit Care Med 35: 2516–2524
55. Shilladay IR, Quin KJ, Allison ME (1997) Loop diuretics in the managment of acute renal failure: A prospective, double-blind, placebo-controlled, randomized study. Nephrol Dial Transplant 12: 2592–2596
56. Sladen RN (2000) Oliguria in the ICU: systematic approach to diagnosis and treatment. Anesthesiol Clin North America 18: 739–752
57. Sugahara S, Suzuki H (2004) Early start on continuous dialysis improves survival rate in patients with acute renal failure following coronary bypass surgery. Hemodial Int 8: 320–325
58. Star RA (1998) Treatment of acute renal failure. Kidney Int 54: 1817–1831
59. Teschan PE, Baxter CR, O'Brien TF, et al. (1960) Prophylactic hemodialysis in the treatment of acute renal failure. Ann Intern Med 53: 992–1016
60. Uchino S, Bellomo R, Ronco C (2001) Intermittent versus continuous renal replacement therapy in the ICU: impact on electrolyte and acid-base-balance. Intensive Care Med 27: 1037–1043
61. Uchino S, Doig GS, Bellomo R, et al. (2004) Diuretics and mortality in acute renal failure. Crit Care Med 32: 1669–1677
62. Uchino S, Kellum JA, Bellomo R, et al. (2005) Acute renal failure in critically ill patients. JAMA 294: 813–818
63. Waikar SS, Bonventre JV (2006) Can we rely on blood urea nitrogen as a biomarker to determine when to initiate dialysis. Clin J Am Soc Nephrol 1: 903–904
64. Waikar SS, Bonventre JV (2007) Biomarkers for diagnosis of acute kidney injury. Curr Opin Nephrol Hyperten 16: 557–564
65. Yang YF, Wu V, Huang C (2005) Successful management of extreme hypernatraemia by haemofiltration in a patient with severe metabolic acidosis and renal failure. Nephrol Dial Transplant 20:2013–2014

Principles of Extracorporeal Therapy: Haemodialysis, Haemofiltration and Haemodiafiltration

7.2

Mathavakkannan Suresh and Ken Farrington

Core Messages

- Dialysis allows separation of the components of a complex solution by diffusive solute exchange across a semipermeable membrane.
- Convective movement of water from blood across the membrane is driven by the transmembrane pressure and also involves the bulk movement of dissolved solute across the membrane (solute drag).
- Diffusion is the underlying physicochemical principle of haemodialysis, whilst solute transport in haemofiltration is purely convective. The two principles are combined in haemodiafiltration.
- Early dialysers were manufactured from cellulose membranes. Modern dialysers are made of synthetic materials such as polysulfone, polycarbonate, polyamide, polyacrylonitrile or polymethylmethacrylate and are constructed in a hollow fibre configuration. Blood traverses through each individual capillary, whilst dialysis fluid flows in between the capillaries in a countercurrent fashion, thus maximising concentration gradients.
- Modern dialysis machines are designed to control and monitor the production of dialysis fluid at the prescribed flow rate, temperature and chemical composition, to control ultrafiltration, and to monitor and control the extracorporeal circuit.

K. Farrington (✉)
Renal Unit, Lister Hospital, Corey Mill Lane, Stevenage, SG 14AB, UK
e-mail: ken.farrington@nbs.net

7.2.1 Introduction

Dialysis plays a vital role in the management of acute kidney failure (AKF). It has the capacity to reverse metabolic derangements resulting from the rapid loss of kidney function, and to facilitate the achievement and maintenance of optimal fluid balance. A range of techniques is available, the choice of which depends on a number of factors including the haemodynamic stability of the patient and the presence or absence of other mitigating factors such as the impairment of function of other organs in multiorgan failure, the presence of bleeding or bleeding diatheses and the characteristics of ingested substances in the management of drug overdoses. Haemodialysis (HD) remains the most widely used modality when patients are haemodynamically stable, while haemofiltration is favoured in labile blood pressure situations. Variations of both and the introduction of hybrid therapies have improved the management of AKF though it remains to be seen whether these new techniques confer a survival benefit compared with the standard therapies.

7.2.2 A Brief History of Dialysis

The evolution of HD therapy has passed through three distinct phases: a pioneering phase ending in the application of the treatment in cases of AKF, a phase of standardisation and expansion as a maintenance treatment for patients with chronic kidney failure, and the current phase in which, in the developed world, there is almost universal access to the treatment for patients with acute and chronic renal failure, and individualisation of treatment is possible, though still largely aspirational.

A. Jörres et al. (eds.), *Management of Acute Kidney Problems*,
DOI: 10.1007/978-3-540-69441-0_7.2, © Springer-Verlag Berlin Heidelberg 2010

The pioneers. The term 'dialysis' was first coined by Thomas Graham, a professor of chemistry in Glasgow, Scotland, in 1861. He was able to separate urea from urine using a vegetable parchment coated with albumin. In 1913, Abel, Rowntree and Turner invented a vivi-diffusion device for use in experimental animals, consisting of celloidin tubes enclosed in a glass jacket through which blood could be passed. Hirudin, obtained from leeches, was the anticoagulant. They suggested that their 'artificial kidney' could be used to remove toxins from circulating blood which might help to tide a patient over a chemical emergency, such as might occur with acute kidney damage. Subsequently, the first human dialysis was performed by George Haas in Germany in 1924, though the treatment time was only 15 min. The first device used successfully in AKF in humans was invented by W. J. Kolff and H. Berk in the Netherlands in 1943. It consisted of a cellophane tube (30 m × 2.5 mm) wound helically around a cylinder that rotated slowly while immersed in a dialysate bath of 70–100 l. Blood from the radial artery was fed through a rotating coupling device into the tube and returned through a cannula in an antecubital vein. Heparin was used as the anticoagulant. There was no control over ultrafiltration (UF), though a later development by Nils Alwall allowed the application of hydrostatic pressure to control UF. Further modifications by Merrill and his coworkers (Kolff-Brigham kidney) led to the first widespread use of dialysis for the treatment of AKF and suggested that the treatment was reasonably safe, repeatable, and that it removed toxins other than nitrogen metabolites, could control sodium, potassium and calcium imbalances and remove excess water.

Expansion and standardisation. Further developments of dialyser technology included the 'twin coil' dialysis delivery system, the parallel plate dialyser in which the cellophane membrane was configured into flat sheets with countercurrent flow of blood and dialysate to improve diffusion characteristics, and the Kiil dialyser, which utilised a sandwich system of flat membranes and plastic (epoxy resin) boards, and required assembly before each dialysis. These developments in dialyser technology, coupled with parallel developments including the use of the Scribner silastic shunt and the Brescia-Cimino arteriovenous fistula to facilitate safe and reliable long-term venous access, as well as the use of single-pass flow of acetate-buffered dialysis fluid from a central delivery system, permitted the expansion of programmes for the maintenance treatment of patients with chronic kidney failure [1].

Universal access and individualisation. The advent of the disposable hollow fibre dialysers around 1970, and concurrent technical advances allowing the development of volumetric control of UF, heralded entry into the modern era. These and other advances in membrane technology have allowed the evolution of high-volume convection as an adjunct to diffusion and to the blood purification techniques of haemofiltration (HF) and haemodiafiltration (HDF). In addition, machine technology has also advanced, with modern dialysis delivery systems incorporating complex circuitry to control dialysate composition, flow, conductance, and temperature and to monitor and to control the extracorporeal circuit. Many machines also offer the capacity for online HDF, blood volume monitoring, blood temperature monitoring and online clearance estimates. The capacity to individualise treatments is at the operator's finger tips. In addition the dialysis population has expanded hugely, and currently there are well-over half a million people worldwide receiving regular HD for chronic kidney disease.

7.2.3 Physiological Principles

Dialysis is physicochemical process which allows separation of the components of a complex solution by diffusive solute exchange across a semipermeable membrane. These membranes act as molecular size–selective filters, the size threshold of which varies depending on the composition of the membrane. In HD the membrane is interposed between the patient's bloodstream and a rinsing solution – the dialysis fluid (Fig. 7.2.1).

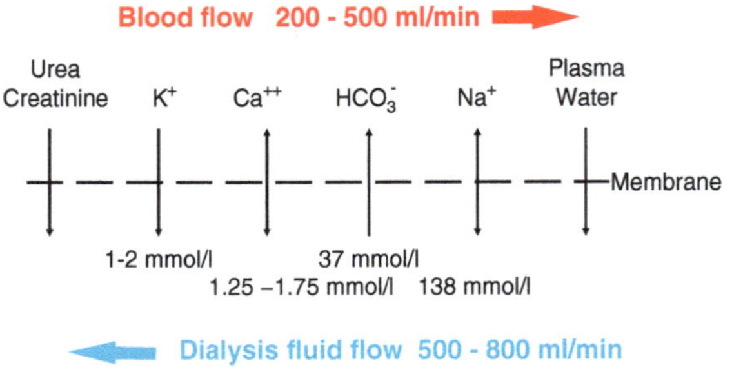

Fig. 7.2.1 Schema of diffusive processes across haemodialysis membrane

In addition to diffusion, convective transfer also takes place across the membrane, driven by the pressure drop across the membrane – the transmembrane pressure (TMP). Changes in the composition of body fluid compartments during HD and HDF are produced by the combined effects of diffusion and convection.

7.2.3.1 Diffusion

Diffusion is a passive process by which solute moves from an area of high concentration to an area of low concentration down a concentration gradient, the solute flux (J) being given by:

$J = -D^* \Delta C/\Delta x$, where D is the diffusivity of the solute which is a constant depending on the molecular size and charge of the particular solute, ΔC is the concentration gradient and Δx is the distance diffused. The negative sign indicates the direction of solute flux toward the lower solute concentration.

In dialysis, diffusion takes place across a semipermeable membrane and solute flux (J) depends on the diffusivity of the solute, the blood-dialysis fluid concentration gradient (ΔC), and the composition, area (A) and thickness (Δx) of the membrane.

Hence $J = -D^* \Delta C^* A/\Delta x$

$= -K_0{}^*A^*\Delta C$, where $K_0 = D/\Delta x$ = the mass transfer coefficient for a particular solute

$= -K_0A^* \Delta C$, where K_0A = the mass transfer area coefficient for that solute.

K_0A reflects the intrinsic capacity of a specific dialyser to remove a specific solute. It can be conceived as the theoretical maximum clearance of that solute, i.e. its clearance at infinite blood and dialysis fluid flow rates.

7.2.3.2 Osmosis

Osmosis is the process by which solvent (water) moves passively across a semipermeable membrane from a dilute solution (high water concentration) to a more concentrated solution (low water concentration). In early HD systems (and currently in peritoneal dialysis), glucose was deployed as an osmotic agent to achieve UF, but in modern haemodialysis, UF is achieved by regulation of the transmembrane hydrostatic pressure gradient.

7.2.3.3 Convection

Convective movement of water from blood across the membrane (UF), is driven by the TMP. This is adjusted by application of variable negative pressure to the dialysate side of the membrane. The UF rate depends on the TMP and the membrane's permeability to water as indicated by its UF coefficient (K_{uf}). Convection also involves the bulk movement of dissolved solute across the membrane (solute drag). In general, convection contributes little to the clearance of rapidly diffusible small solutes such as urea, but can add significantly to the diffusive clearance of middle molecules by high-flux membranes.

7.2.3.4 Combining Diffusion and Convection

During dialysis, there are interactions between convective and diffusive modes of solute transport. Along the length of the dialyser, solute concentration reduces due to diffusion, thus limiting convective transport. Likewise, the UF-driven intradialyser fall in blood flow rate limits diffusive transport. The total clearance (diffusive plus convective – K_{total}) can be represented as [2]:

$$K_{total} = K_{d0} + T_r Q_u$$

where K_{d0} = diffusive clearance in the absence of UF; Q_u = UF rate; T_r = transmittance coefficient, which is related to K_{d0}, the dialyser inlet blood flow, and the sieving coefficient.

7.2.4 Membrane and Dialysers

Early dialysis delivery systems used cellulose membranes, which were bioincompatible and caused frequent dialyser reactions. Subsequent developments resulted in thinner cuprophane membranes, in substituted cellulose membranes with higher diffusion coefficients, and later in cellulosynthetic membranes produced by the addition of a synthetic material to liquefied cellulose. Now, most dialysis membranes are synthetic, made of materials such as polysulfone, polycarbonate, polyamide, polyacrylonitrile and

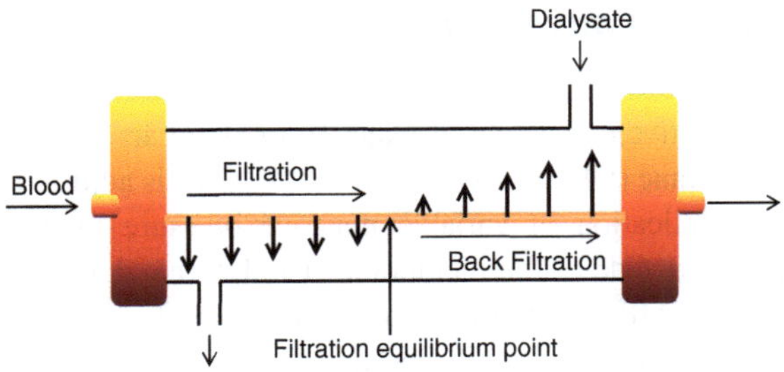

Fig. 7.2.2 The phenomena of obligate backfiltration in a high-flux hollow-fibre dialyser

polymethylmethacrylate. The modern dialyser is constructed in a hollow fibre configuration, consisting of thousands of tightly bound capillaries in a cylindrical shell. Blood traverses through each individual capillary, whilst dialysis fluid flows in between the capillaries in a countercurrent fashion, thus maximising concentration gradients.

The performance of a dialyser is defined by its K_{uf} (ml/h of ultrafiltrate per mm Hg of TMP) and its dialyser clearance (K_d) for a range of solutes (including urea, creatinine, Vitamin B_{12}, inulin and β_2-microglobulin), at various blood and dialysate flow rates. K_0A for urea is also often quoted. Modern synthetic dialysers have high K_d and K_{uf} (high flux) achieving better clearances of β_2-microglobulin and other middle molecules compared to conventional (cuprophane) dialysers. The synthetic membranes are also more 'biocompatible', reducing complement activation and inflammatory reactions during dialysis. High-flux membranes permit high-volume UF, which can be utilised in the techniques of HF, and in combination with the diffusive clearance offered by HD in the technique of HDF. A consequence of the high blood and dialysis fluid flow rates and the countercurrent configuration, is an unavoidable movement of dialysis fluid into blood ('obligatory back-filtration', Fig. 7.2.2). This provides some useful convective clearance (internal HDF) and underlines the requirement for ultrapure water in the preparation of dialysis fluids.

7.2.5 Dialysis Fluid

Patients on HD are intimately exposed to huge quantities of water. The potential for poisoning by waterborne impurities, both chemical and microbiological, is significant. Aluminium and chloramines are examples of proven chemical toxins. Bacterial and endotoxin contamination is potentially harmful, causing problems such as intradialytic pyrexias and hypotension, and adding to the inflammatory milieu. Use of ultrapure water is imperative, especially in high-flux HD and on-line HDF. Water is purified by a combination of techniques, including softening and deionisation, carbon adsorption, reverse osmosis, ultraviolet irradiation and microfiltration. Regular monitoring of water quality standards, both chemical and microbiological, is mandatory. For ultrapure dialysate, the guidelines of many bodies including the UK Renal Association, specify a bacterial count limit of less than 0.1 colony forming units (CFU)/ml and an endotoxin level of less than 0.03 EU/ml [3].

To produce dialysis fluid of the desired composition, acid and bicarbonate concentrates are mixed with treated water in a single-patient proportionating system within the dialysis machine (Table 7.2.1 and Fig. 7.2.3). Dialysis fluid composition (Table 7.2.1) is the major means of maintaining normal electrolyte, and mineral and acid–base balance, concentrations being set to achieve various goals including net loss (e.g. potassium), net gain (e.g. bicarbonate) and net zero balance (e.g. calcium). Sodium concentrations are generally set to achieve net zero diffusive balance with the required sodium removal being attained by UF.

In addition to contributing to the achievement of optimal mineral and electrolyte balance, the composition of the dialysis fluid may also have a role in the maintenance of haemodynamic stability during the dialysis session. Low dialysate sodium levels by augmenting diffusive loss, may improve blood pressure control between sessions, at the risk of increased intradialytic hypotension. A patient prone to this problem may benefit from an increased dialysis fluid sodium level, yet risk fluid retention, interdialytic hypertension and their cardiovascular sequelae. Varying the sodium level – from a higher level initially to lower levels at the end of the session (sodium

Table 7.2.1 Typical dialysis fluid concentrate composition (many dialysis fluid concentrates also contain low concentrations of acetate)

	Acid	Base
Na^+	99–110	27–40
K^+	0–3	0
Ca^{++}	1.25–2.0	0
Mg^{++}	0.75	0
Cl^-	99–110	0
CH_3COO^-	0	0
HCO_3^-	0	27–40
$C_6H_{12}O_6$	0–5.5	0

Fig. 7.2.3 The basic dialysis fluid pathway through the dialyser. A = acid concentrate, B = bicarbonate concentrate, UF Pump = ultrafiltration pump

modelling), may be of benefit in some situations. Increased dialysis fluid potassium levels may reduce the propensity for dysrhythmias, but reduce potassium removal. Increased dialysis fluid calcium levels may also be helpful in patients prone to intradialytic hypotension. These examples illustrate the great potential for tailoring dialysis fluids to suit the prevailing needs of individual patients, and point to the practical limitations [4].

7.2.6 The Dialysis Machine

The dialysis machine is designed to control and monitor the production of dialysis fluid at the prescribed flow rate, temperature and chemical composition, to control UF, and to monitor and control the extracorporeal circuit. The machines operate in fail-safe mode, such that a deviation of a monitored variable outside its control limits, or a fault in the monitoring equipment itself, will automatically trigger the return of the system to a safe configuration, in which the patient is isolated from the malfunction and its effects.

7.2.6.1 The Dialysis Fluid Pathway

The basic elements of the dialysis fluid pathway through the dialysis machine are shown in Fig. 7.2.3.

Fluid enters the machine passing through a heat exchanger and is then warmed to the desired temperature (usually 35–37°C) by a heater immersed in the flow-through heater vessel. The fluid is then degassed under negative pressure, since gas bubbles forming in the dialyser and downstream venous lines may reduce both dialysis efficiency and the efficiency of volumetric balancing devices. Metered quantities of acid (A) and bicarbonate concentrates, powders or granules (B) are then mixed with appropriate volumes of water by a proportionating device to produce dialysis fluid of the appropriate chemical composition. A volumetric balancing chamber or flow cell placed in the fluid pathway ensures equal dialysis fluid flow rates to and from the dialyser. Precise control of UF is achieved by varying TMP by use of a UF pump which removes fluid from the return limb from the dialyser, causing an equal volume to be drawn from the blood across the dialysis membrane into the dialysis fluid, in order to maintain balance. The fluid composition is checked by conductivity monitoring. Other safety monitors include a blood leak detector in the return limb from the dialyser (not shown). Dialysis fluid flow rates are typically 500–800 ml/min).

7.2.6.2 The Extracorporeal Circuit

The basic elements of the extracorporeal circuit are shown in Fig. 7.2.4.

In maintenance HD, blood is withdrawn from the patient via an arterial (A) needle placed in the fistula, and circulated by a peristaltic pump through the dialyser, returning to the patient through the venous (V)

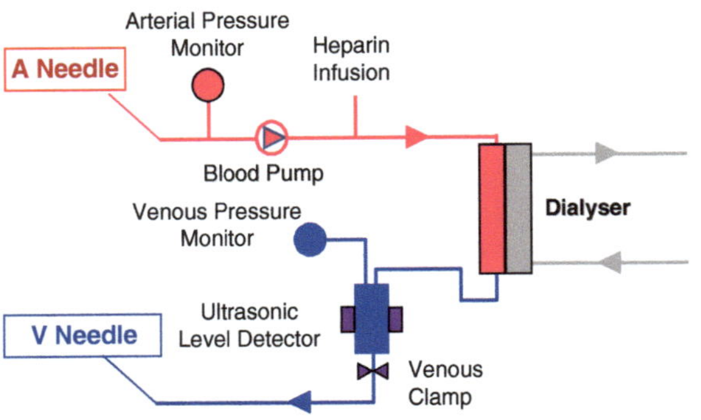

Fig. 7.2.4 Standard extracorporeal circuit. A needle = arterial needle; V needle = venous needle

needle. A double-lumen HD catheter inserted into a central vein is the usual mode of access for acute treatments. For maintenance treatments, blood pump speeds are usually in the range 200–450 ml/min. The circuit is anticoagulated, normally with heparin, which is infused on the positive pressure side of the blood pump, to prevent the in-drawing of air. An arterial pressure monitor is placed on the negative pressure side of the blood pump. Its purpose is to protect the access; low arterial pressures (high negative pressures) indicate high shear rates and turbulence at the arterial cannula/catheter ostium. The venous pressure monitor was originally introduced to detect accidental disconnection of circuit from the V needle, falling venous pressures reflect blood loss to the environment, though under modern operating conditions, it is of limited efficacy [5]. Increased venous pressures suggest downstream obstruction, which undetected may lead to line rupture and haemolysis. Newer machines also monitor the dialyser inlet pressure, which, if raised, could indicate clotting within the dialyser. The bubble trap level-detector protects against air embolus. A falling level activates the venous clamp and stops the blood pump.

7.2.6.3 Other Features of HD Machines

Most modern machines also incorporate additional devices allowing single-needle dialysis and online HDF. Many also offer other capabilities. Online monitoring of relative blood volume utilising ultrasonic devices, which follow changes in blood density throughout the dialysis, may help to optimise UF strategies and maintain intradialytic haemodynamic stability. Blood temperature monitoring may also contribute to the maintenance of haemodynamic stability by allowing heat gain to be limited, thus preventing vasodilatation. Technologies such as ionic dialysance allow estimates of online clearance, and may contribute to achievement of adequacy standards. These last methods can also be used to estimate access flow and assess the degree of access recirculation.

7.2.7 Anticoagulation

Unfractionated heparin (UFH) remains the standard anticoagulant for maintenance HD, monitored with whole-blood activated clotting times. Low-molecular-weight heparins (LMWH) are increasingly used, their major advantage being that continuous infusion is not required. Different LMWHs have different half-lives and differing propensities for reversal by protamine, and monitoring is difficult. Heparin-free dialysis, deploying frequent saline flushes, can be used when bleeding risks are high. Heparin is also standard for continuous treatments in the acute setting. The long half-life and difficulties in measuring the anticoagulation effect preclude use of LMWH in these settings. The synthetic analog of prostacyclin I_2 (PGI_2) can be used in patients with bleeding diatheses. Regional citrate anticoagulation, a strategy in which infusion of calcium and magnesium at the dialyser outlet neutralises citrate administered at the inlet, can avoid systemic anticoagulation. The technique however, requires custom-made continuous venovenous hemofiltration (CVVH) replacement solutions and careful monitoring.

7.2.8 Haemodialysis/Filtration Techniques

7.2.8.1 Conventional Haemodialysis

Conventional HD classically deployed cuprophane (low-flux, bioincompatible) membranes in standard circuits for long hours. There was diffusive but little convective solute removal. Smaller molecules such as urea were cleared efficiently but middle molecule clearance was poor. The definition of conventional HD would also have included the use of acetate as buffer. However, our notions of what constitutes conventional HD have changed dramatically and continue to evolve. Cuprophane is no longer available in Europe, short hours are the norm, and acetate has long been superseded by bicarbonate. Use of biocompatible synthetic membranes is almost standard, and use of the high-flux variety is growing rapidly. It is now difficult to define 'conventional HD'.

7.2.8.2 Haemofiltration

Haemofiltration is a purely convective treatment. Although convection enhances middle molecule clearance, small molecule clearance is much less efficient than in diffusive mode, and this the limits applicability of the technique as a maintenance intermittent treatment for chronic kidney failure. However, the technique has a major role as a continuous treatment in the management of haemodynamically unstable patients with AKF, avoiding the rapid swings in solute concentrations and volume status which characterise intermittent treatments. Highly permeable membranes are used in haemofilters, permitting high-volume ultrafiltration. Haemofiltrate volumes of 25–50 l/day are readily achievable. Dissolved solutes are removed by solvent drag. High volumes of substitution fluid are required. Substitution fluid, from commercially prepared bags, is delivered either on the arterial side of the filter (predilution) or into the venous bubble-trap (postdilution). The postdilution technique commands better solute clearance, whilst predilution tends to reduce clotting within the filter, prolonging its life span. There are number of variants. Continuous arteriovenous haemofiltration (CAVH), which required femoral artery cannulation, has given way to CVVH (Fig. 7.2.5), which requires a pumped venous supply. Continuous venovenous haemodialysis (CVVHD) is a further variant, which combines convective and diffusive clearances. Dialysis fluid is infused through the dialyser inlet and the effluent is collected at the dialyser outlet, and pumped to adjust UF rates. In CVVHDF, both dialysis fluid and substitution fluid are deployed.

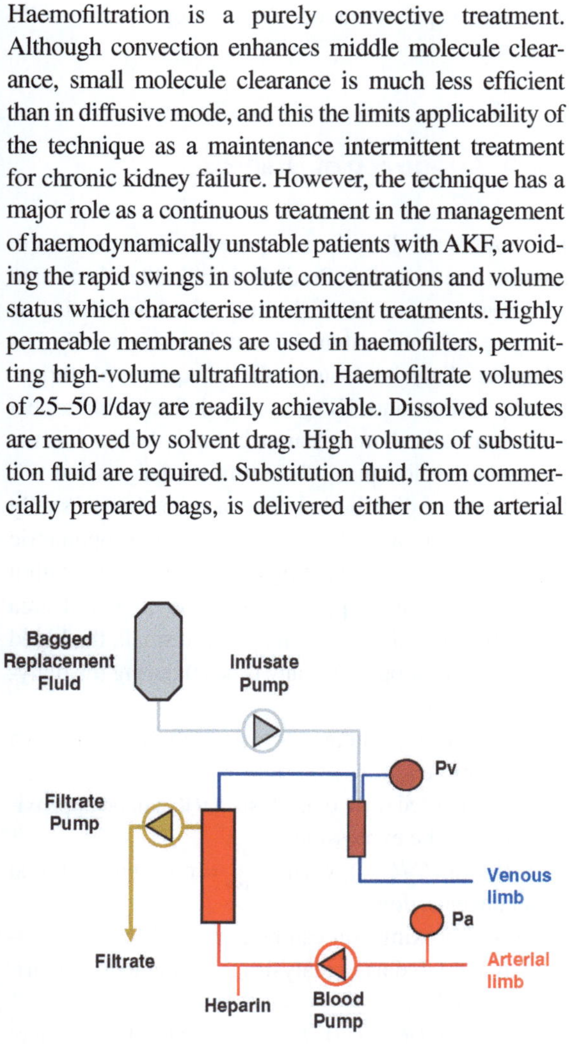

Fig. 7.2.5 Basic circuit for continuous venovenous haemofiltration

7.2.8.3 High-flux Haemodialysis

Poor clearance of middle molecules, notably β_2-microglobulin, fuelled the increasing use of high-flux membranes. High-flux HD uses highly permeable, biocompatible membranes, which provide good diffusive clearance of small solutes combined with much better diffusive removal of middle molecules than low-flux techniques. This is augmented by a convective contribution to middle molecule clearance resulting from obligate back-filtration (internal HDF) within the dialyser.

7.2.8.4 Haemodiafiltration

HDF describes the addition of a prescribed convective component (haemofiltration) to the technique of high-flux HD, allowing the benefits of both these modalities to be maximised. The major benefit is enhanced removal of middle molecules. The postdilution mode also offers a small increment in small solute clearance. During each high-flux session, up to 25 l of haemofiltrate is removed and replaced by substitution fluid. Initially the substitution fluid was only available in the form of commercially prepared bags, as used in continuous treatments, which made HDF an expensive option. The advent of cheap ultrapure substitution fluid produced online from dialysis fluid by the dialysis machine has allowed online HDF to become established as a viable maintenance therapy for patients

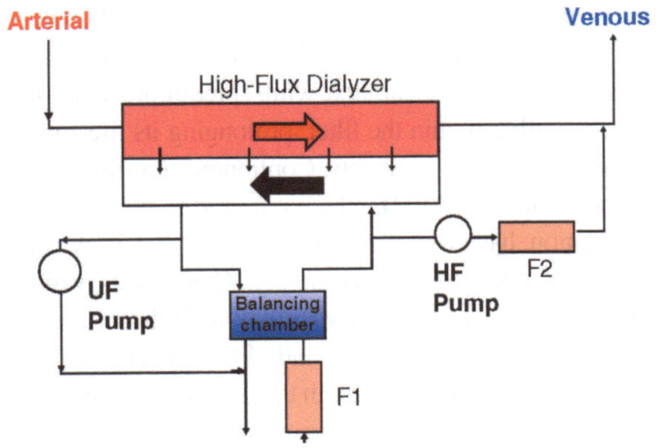

Fig. 7.2.6 Blood and fluid pathways in online haemodiafiltration. UF Pump = ultrafiltration pump, HF Pump = haemodiafiltrate pump, F1 = ultrafilter 1, F2 = ultrafilter 2

with chronic kidney failure. Figure 7.2.6 shows the basic modifications of the dialysis machine, which allow online production of HDF fluid. Fluid is removed from the dialysis fluid pathway supplying the dialyser by a haemofiltration pump (HF pump), passed through an ultrafilter (F2), and infused in to the 'V' line (postdilution) or the 'A' line (predilution [not shown]). To maintain volumetric balance in the fixed-volume loop between the balance chamber and the dialyser, an equal volume of fluid is drawn from the blood across the dialysis membrane.

7.2.8.5 Other Haemodialysis Techniques Applicable to AKF

7.2.8.5.1 Sustained Low-Efficiency Dialysis

Sustained low-efficiency dialysis (SLED) is a hybrid technique combining the theoretical advantages of intermittent haemodialysis (IHD) and CVVH [6]. Dialysis flow rates are reduced to 300 ml/min with blood-pump speeds of around 200 ml/min. The treatment is carried out daily, typically for 6–12 h per session. Solute clearances are comparable to IHD and haemodynamic stability to CVVH.

7.2.8.5.2 HVHF and PHVHF

Increasing the UF rates to > 35 ml/kg/h in an otherwise conventional CVVH set-up is called high-volume haemofiltration (HVHF) [7]. The theoretical benefits include removal of larger inflammatory mediators, though there is insufficient data to justify its routine use. Pulse high-volume haemofiltration (PVHF) is a further modification with UF rates of 85 ml/kg/h for 4–6 h followed by conventional CVVH.

7.2.8.5.3 Renal Assist Device

This experimental device consists of a hollow-fibre dialyser coated with cultured proximal tubular epithelial cells, arranged in series with a conventional haemofilter, allowing the blood to pass from the dialyser outlet into the renal assist device. Phase II trials in sepsis-induced ARF suggest improved outcomes.

7.2.9 Adequacy of Dialysis

Just how much dialysis is required to maintain health remains controversial. Predialysis blood levels of urea and creatinine can be misleading, low levels being as likely to indicate malnutrition and muscle wasting as adequate dialysis. Instead the adequacy of thrice-weekly maintenance HD is usually defined with respect to the normalised urea clearance, Kt/V – where K is the dialyser urea clearance, 't' the time on dialysis and 'V', the volume of distribution of urea in the body usually calculated as total body water using an anthropometric formula (Watson). Assuming urea is distributed within the body in a single pool and that the effects of urea generation and UF during dialysis are small, the blood urea concentration (C_t) at any time (t) during the dialysis is given by:

$C_t = C_0 e^{-Kt/V}$, where C_0 = predialysis blood urea concentration.

The delivered dose of dialysis Kt/V, can be approximated from the expression:

$Kt/V = \ln(C_0/C_{post})$, where C_{post} = postdialysis blood urea concentration.

This approximation can be corrected for urea generation and UF during dialysis according to an empirical formula [8]:

$Kt/V = -\ln(R - 0.008T) + (4 - 3.5R)\Delta W/W$, where $R = C_{post}/C_0$, T = treatment time (hours), ΔW = interdialytic weight gain, W = post-dialysis weight.

A further correction for two-pool effects allows the calculation of equilibrated Kt/V (eKt/V), using either of the formulas given below:

eKt/V = spKt/V – 0.6(spKt/V)/T + 0.03 [9], where spKt/V = single pool Kt/V, T = treatment time in hours.

eKt/V = spKt/V ($t/(t + 38)$) [10], where t = treatment time in minutes.

An eKt/V in excess of 1.2 is established as the target for thrice-weekly maintenance dialysis. It is calculated from predialysis and postdialysis blood urea concentrations, treatment time, ultrafiltration volume (interdialytic weight gain) and postdialysis weight, using the equation from [8] and the equations from [9] or [10], as set out above. The HEMO study [11] suggested that outcomes of thrice-weekly HD regimens are not improved by achievement of higher dialysis doses. Neither was there a significant benefit of high-flux over low-flux membranes. These findings have refocused attention on the contribution to adequacy of the duration and particularly, the frequency of HD sessions. There are suggestions of improved outcomes from more frequent treatments (quotidian dialysis), either daily short-hours treatments, or long-hours nocturnal treatments, though little of the data is controlled [12].

Targets for the treatment of AKF have been intensely debated in terms of frequency and duration of treatments, solute clearances, and in continuous treatments, exchange volumes and UF rates. However, the outcome of the recent VA/NIH Acute Renal Failure Trial Network Study [13] suggests that adequacy criteria similar to those outlined above in relation to maintenance treatment, also apply in the acute setting. Outcomes were not improved by providing IHD more frequently than thrice-weekly, with an achieved Kt/V of 1.2–1.4, or by providing continuous renal replacement therapy at an effluent flow rate of >20 ml/h. In addition, the optimal timing of dialysis initiation remains uncertain in both acute and chronic settings, and a pragmatic approach is required.

7.2.10 Take Home Pearls

- Dialysis is the physicochemical process which allows separation of the components of a complex solution by diffusive solute exchange across a semipermeable membrane.
- In addition to diffusion, convective transfer also takes place across the membrane, driven by the pressure drop across the membrane.
- Hemofiltration is a purely convective treatment during which the passage of solutes across a membrane is carried by water flux.

References

1. Scribner BH: Lasker Clinical Medicine Research Award. Medical dilemmas: the old is new. Nat Med 2002;8: 1066–1067.
2. Villarroel F, Klein E, Holland F: Solute flux in hemodialysis and hemofiltration membranes. Trans Am Soc Artif Intern Organs 1977;23:225–233.
3. Renal Association. Clinical Practice Guidelines for Haemodialysis. 2007.
4. Hoenich N, Thijssen S, Kitzler T, Levin R, Ronco C: Impact of water quality and dialysis fluid composition on dialysis practice. Blood Purif 2008;26:6–11.
5. Ahlmen J, Gydell KH, Hadimeri H, Hernandez I, Rogland B, Strombom U: A new safety device for hemodialysis. Hemodial Int 2008;12:264–267.
6. O'Reilly P, Tolwani A: Renal replacement therapy III: IHD, CRRT, SLED. Crit Care Clin 2005;21:367–378.
7. House AA, Ronco C: Extracorporeal blood purification in sepsis and sepsis-related acute kidney injury. Blood Purif 2008;26:30–35.
8. Daugirdas JT: Second generation logarithmic estimates of single-pool variable volume Kt/V: an analysis of error. J Am Soc Nephrol 1993;4:1205–1213.
9. Daugirdas JT, Schneditz D: Overestimation of hemodialysis dose depends on dialysis efficiency by regional blood flow but not by conventional two pool urea kinetic analysis. ASAIO J 1995;41:M719-M724.
10. Tattersall JE, DeTakats D, Chamney P, Greenwood RN, Farrington K: The post-hemodialysis rebound: predicting and quantifying its effect on Kt/V. Kidney Int 1996;50: 2094–2102.
11. Eknoyan G, Beck GJ, Cheung AK, Daugirdas JT, Greene T, Kusek JW, Allon M, Bailey J, Delmez JA, Depner TA, Dwyer JT, Levey AS, Levin NW, Milford E, Ornt DB, Rocco MV, Schulman G, Schwab SJ, Teehan BP, Toto R: Effect of dialysis dose and membrane flux in maintenance hemodialysis. N Engl J Med 2002;347: 2010–2019.
12. Suri RS, Nesrallah GE, Mainra R, Garg AX, Lindsay RM, Greene T, Daugirdas JT: Daily hemodialysis: a systematic review. Clin J Am Soc Nephrol 2006;1:33–42.
13. Palevsky PM, Zhang JH, O'Connor TZ, Chertow GM, Crowley ST, Choudhury D, Finkel K, Kellum JA, Paganini E, Schein RM, Smith MW, Swanson KM, Thompson BT, Vijayan A, Watnick S, Star RA, Peduzzi P: Intensity of renal support in critically ill patients with acute kidney injury. N Engl J Med 2008;359:7–20.

Membranes for Dialysis and Hemofiltration

7.3

Detlef H. Krieter and Christoph Wanner

Core Messages

- Materials for dialyzers and hemofilters are either based on cellulose or modified cellulosic membranes or made from synthetic polymers such as polysulfone, polyethersulfone, polyamide, polyacrylonitrile, or polymethylmethacrylate.
- Membranes can be classified according to permeability (water flux and permeability for larger molecules) and biocompatibility characteristics. The latter may include properties such as:
  - *Complement system activation*
  - *Cell activation*
  - *Reactive oxygen species production*
  - *Cell aggregate formation*
  - *Premature cellular senescence*
  - *Coagulation system activation*
  - *Increased apoptosis*
  - *Contact phase system activation*
- Requirements for modern dialysis membrane include:
  - *High diffusive clearance*
  - *High permeability for uremic middle molecules*
  - *Adequate hydraulic permeability*
  - *Pyrogen retention capability*
  - *High biocompatibility*

7.3.1 Introduction

For the first successful dialysis treatment in a patient with acute renal failure in 1945, Kolff and Berk used a simple cellophane tube as dialysis membrane for their dialysis apparatus, the "rotating drum" [35]. In principle, nothing has changed since that breakthrough, but tremendous progress has been achieved to develop dialysis membranes into today's highly biocompatible and efficient medical product suitable for the long-term replacement of the excretory renal function.

Dialysis membranes serve as a semipermeable barrier, which selectively allow smaller solutes to diffuse through their pore structure from blood into dialysate and vice versa along a concentration gradient. Larger solutes are retained and, if their steric structure does not exclude a passage, they preferably permeate the dialysis membrane by convection, together with plasma water, as a consequence of solvent drag generated by a hydrostatic transmembrane pressure. The mass transfer by diffusion and convection is not solely determined by the tertiary structures of the membrane, i.e., the pore sizes and pore distribution and the membrane wall thickness, which correlates with the diffusive resistance. Depending on the membrane material and formation, also physicochemical interactions may promote the adsorption of proteins and cells onto the surface. Adsorption is a third, but saturable mechanism involved in the removal of solutes and also in hemocompatibility. It alters the sieving properties of a dialysis membrane over time.

Two different dialysis membrane forms have been adopted for current large-scale production of dialyzers: flat plate and particularly hollow fiber membranes. First presented by Stewart during the mid-1960s [74], hollow fiber or capillary membranes have the advantage of

D. H. Krieter (✉)
University Hospital Würzburg, Department of Medicine,
Division of Nephrology, Josef-Schneider-Strasse 2,
97080 Würzburg, Germany
e-mail: krieter_d@medizin.uni-wuerzburg.de

A. Jörres et al. (eds.), *Management of Acute Kidney Problems*,
DOI: 10.1007/978-3-540-69441-0_7.3, © Springer-Verlag Berlin Heidelberg 2010

Table 7.3.1 Classification of dialyzers based on dialysis membrane permeability.

	Low-flux	Mid-flux	High-flux	Super-flux (Protein-leaking)
Ultrafiltration coefficient (K_{UF}) (ml/h/mm Hg)	<10	10–20	>20	>20
Instantaneous β_2-microglobulin plasma clearance (ml/min)	<10	10–20	>20	>20
Albumin loss per 4 h treatment (g)	0	0	<2	>2
Suitable treatment modality	HD	HD (HDF)	HD, HF, HDF	HD

HD, hemodialysis; HF, hemofiltration; HDF, hemodiafiltration

serving as their own support, thus, avoiding costly flow channels, which are essential for the parallel plate design of flat membrane dialyzers. This difference in device manufacturing has led to the almost complete elimination of parallel plate filters from the market.

7.3.2 Classification of Dialysis Membranes

From a clinical perspective, it is appropriate to classify dialysis membranes according to permeability and biocompatibility characteristics. Several classifications focusing on membrane permeability and dialyzer performance have been proposed in the past. Table 7.3.1 is a simplified approach based on water flux and permeability for larger proteins indicated by β_2-microglobulin clearance and albumin loss. This classification reflects the relevant information on a dialyzer to decide about the suitability for the different treatment modes of current renal replacement therapy. Water flux or water permeability is usually derived from in vitro tests and expressed as the ultrafiltration coefficient K_{UF} measured in milliliters per hour per mm Hg transmembrane pressure. The ultrafiltration rate (UFR) describes the water permeability of a dialysis membrane per square meter, while the K_{UF} is a parameter for a given dialyzer. The K_{UF} for a certain dialysis membrane correlates with the surface area. K_{UF} and permeability for larger proteins are associated, but, depending on the pore morphology of the membrane, do not necessarily correlate.

Due to historical reasons, "biocompatibility" refers to the effects of the membrane on the two classical parameters: complement system activation and induction of transient leukopenia in blood during dialysis treatment. Not reflecting small differences within each class, three classes of biocompatibility can be defined according to the chemical composition of the dialysis membranes: bioincompatible unsubstituted cellulose, more biocompatible substituted cellulosic, and biocompatible synthetic dialysis membranes (see Table 7.3.2). Several reports suggest that with increasing biocompatibility, patient outcome improves, while others did not find differences in morbidity and mortality. Many of these studies were confounded by differences in membrane permeabilities, which were always low-flux in bioincompatible, but not in biocompatible dialyzers (refer to Chapters 2.4 and 2.5). However, even if convincing prospective studies are lacking, this issue seems to be no longer relevant, because the production of bioincompatible unsubstituted cellulose dialysis membranes is approaching an end, and the same may be imminent for substituted cellulose.

7.3.3 Dialysis Membrane Materials

7.3.3.1 Cellulose Membranes

From the beginning of chronic hemodialysis until the 1990s, unsubstituted cellulose has been the most frequently used polymer for dialysis membranes. Cellulose is a natural hydrophilic polysaccharide forming tight crystalline regions, which lead to homogenous membranes with high mechanical strength, regardless whether they are produced as flat or capillary types. This property allows the production of very thin dialysis membranes, which, together with its quality to form a hydrogel after moistening, results in excellent diffusive small solute clearances. In contrast, unsubstituted cellulose membranes are almost impermeable for larger substances. Only small middle molecules, such as vitamin B_{12} (1,355 Da), pass the membrane, and to a very limited extent. Unsubstituted cellulose is only available

Table 7.3.2 Classification of dialysis membranes based on biocompatibility. The different permeabilities are highlighted

Unsubstituted cellulose *bioincompatible*	Substituted/modified cellulose *more biocompatible*	Synthetic membranes *biocompatible*
Cuprophan® *LF*	Cellulose (di-)acetate *LF*, triacetate *LF, HF, SF*	AN69® *HF*, AN69® ST *HF*
Cuprammonium-rayon *LF*	Hemophan® *LF*	Polysulfone
Saponified cellulose ester (SCE) *LF*	SMC® *LF*	Fresenius Polysulfon® PS400/600 *LF/HF,*
	Cuprammonium-rayon polyethylene glycol *LF, MF, HF*	Helixone® *HF,*
	Excebrane® LF	α-Polysulfone *LF, HF,*
		APS HF, SF,
		VitabranE® *HF,*
		Toraysulfone *HF, SF*
		Polyethersulfone
		DIAPES® *LF, MF, HF, SF*
		PUREMA® *LF, HF, SF,*
		Polyamix® *LF, HF,*
		Arylane® *HF,*
		Polyester–Polymer–Alloy (PEPA) *HF, SF,*
		PES alpha *HF*
		Polymethylmethacrylate *LF, MF, HF, SF*
		Ethylene vinyl-alcohol (EVAL) *LF*

LF, low-flux; *MF*, mid-flux; *HF*, high-flux; *SF*, super-flux

as low-flux dialysis membrane. Due to relative bioincompatibility (refer to Chapter 2.4), the use of unsubstituted cellulose membranes has become unpopular, and production will most likely be ceased completely within the near future.

7.3.3.2 Modified Cellulosic Membranes

From a clinical perspective, modified or substituted cellulose (synonymous with semisynthetic) dialysis membranes must be distinguished from unsubstituted cellulose. They differ in that a certain portion of the free hydroxyl groups of cellulose are substituted by defined hydrophobic substances with the effect of improved biocompatibility while retaining the favorable diffusive capacity and mechanical strength of unsubstituted cellulose membranes. In Hemophan®, about 5% of the hydroxyl groups are modified by binding of the positively charged tertiary amino group diethyl-amino-ethyl (DEAE). Due to the resulting positive charge, negatively charged substances such as heparin, but also blood cells, tend to bind to the membrane, giving it a typical reddish color after use. In SMC®, a similar amount of electroneutral hydrophobic aromatic benzyl groups are substituted, making the membrane more biocompatible, particularly with respect to reduced thrombogenicity.

While both Hemophan® and SMC® are typical low-flux membranes, the substitution of the hydroxyl groups with polyethylene glycol (PEG) is performed to not only improve biocompatibility, but also to create a larger pore membrane. PEG avoids the formation of a tight skin layer, whereby the molecular weight of the covalently bonded PEG seems to be crucial for the membrane's permeability.

Excebrane® has been introduced in an attempt to reduce oxidative stress during dialysis [73]. It is a multilayer, cellulose-based (cuprammonium rayon) membrane with an acrylic copolymer coating on the internal phase. The liposoluble physiological antioxidant vitamin E is covalently bound to the copolymer and serves as a scavenger for free radicals [62].

Cellulose acetate membranes are the most widely used substituted cellulose membranes to date. According to the degree of acetylation, they are labeled as cellulose (di-)acetate or triacetate. In cellulose triacetate, almost 100% of the cellulosic hydroxyl groups are substituted with acetate, while in cellulose acetate the portion is about 50%. Cellulose triacetate is available in the complete range of permeabilities, from low-flux to protein-leaking super-flux membranes. The membrane wall thickness is rather thin compared with synthetic membranes, favoring diffusive solute transfer. It is important to note that cellulose acetate is sensitive to pH changes [82]. An increase in pH leads to deacetylation of the membrane, while pH reduction causes hydrolyzation of the polymer. Cellulose acetate membrane degradation in the form of deacetylation and polymer scission due to very long storage and aging of dialyzers (>10 years) has been responsible for severe patient injury, such as persistently decreased vision and hearing [27].

7.3.3.3 Synthetic Membranes

Synthetic membranes represent the by far most frequently used dialysis membranes, with still increasing market share. In general, they are regarded as the most hemocompatible membranes. This quality is the reason synthetic membranes have displaced cellulose filters since the mid-1990s. Most probably, synthetic membranes will also eliminate modified cellulosic membranes in the foreseeable future.

Most synthetic membranes are a blend of rather hydrophobic base polymers (e.g., polysulfone and polyethersulfone), which favorably determines biocompatibility, and hydrophilic copolymers, often polyvinylpyrrolidone, to improve transmembrane solute passage. Some membranes consist of hydrophilized (e.g., AN69® and polymethyl-methacrylate) or hydrophilic (ethylene vinyl-alcohol) copolymers. The chemical composition, i.e., the base polymer and the ratio of base polymer to copolymer, is particularly important for the pore morphology and pore size distribution of a membrane, but also the sophisticated spinning process determines the sieving characteristics of the end product. Therefore, in clinical practice, synthetic membranes can deliver widely varying treatment results due to differences in their selectivity, despite a virtually similar or even identical chemical structure and the assignment to the same flux class. Depending on specific polymer properties, some types of membrane eliminate considerable amounts of toxins by adsorption, which is a saturable process, while in other membranes this mechanism is an only negligible feature. Since the development of the first synthetic dialysis membrane in 1970, named the RP69 (Rhône-Poulenc) and later AN69®, which reflected the desire for more permeable membranes as a consequence of the "middle molecule hypothesis" stated by Babb et al. [4], a variety of different synthetic dialysis membranes have emerged, particularly within the last 10 years (Table 7.3.2). The "middle molecule hypothesis" suspected larger solutes as a cause of the uremic neuropathy seen in maintenance dialysis patients. Optimized synthetic membranes with improved permselectivity have been engineered recently to ideally combine best biocompatibility with excellent toxin removal characteristics. They fully cover the whole range of requirements of current extracorporeal renal replacement therapies.

The oldest synthetic membrane, AN69®, is composed of the copolymers acrylonitrile and metallyl-Na-sulfonate. It is a symmetric and homogenous membrane only available as a high-flux type, which eliminates proteins efficiently by adsorption due to an intensely negatively charged surface resulting from the sulfonate groups. The electronegativity of AN69® has been made also responsible for several fatal anaphylactoid reactions in patients taking angiotensin-converting enzyme (ACE) inhibitors, since it induces the activation of the contact phase system with generation of bradykinin (refer to Chapter 2.4) [37, 77, 81]. Therefore, AN69® is strictly contraindicated in patients on ACE inhibitor therapy. To eliminate contact activation while keeping the favorable adsorbent properties, a surface-modified version of the membrane, AN69® ST, was developed. In this membrane, the negative charges are neutralized by coating with polyethyleneimine during membrane processing [53]. As an additional effect, heparin binds to the surface of AN69® ST if added to the extracorporeal circuit during pre-rinsing. This allows a significant reduction of heparin for anticoagulation during dialysis, which may be beneficial in patients at bleeding risk [6].

Polysulfone and several polyethersulfone (synonymous with polyarylethersulfone) derivatives are the most widely used, highly biocompatible dialysis membranes. The first polysulfone membrane was initially developed in the 1970s as an appropriate filter for the emerging convective therapy forms, particularly hemofiltration. A first low-flux version was introduced much later during the 1980s. The original polysulfone membrane (Fresenius Polysulfon®) has an asymmetric, microreticular structure, which is different from many polyethersulfone derivates. Despite chemical similarities, other membranes feature symmetric, microreticular, and three-layer (DIAPES®) or asymmetric, anisotrop, and macroreticular (Polyamix®) structures (see Fig. 7.3.1). Both polysulfone and polyethersulfone are rather hydrophobic polymers, which need a hydrophilic copolymer to

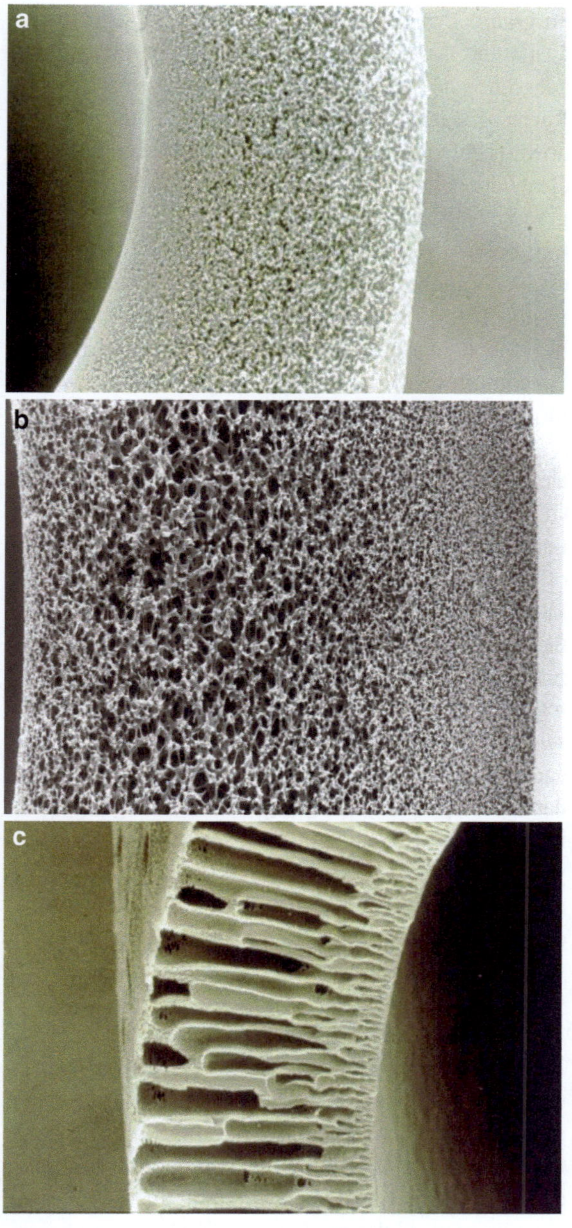

Fig. 7.3.1 Electron microscopic cross-section view of three different synthetic high-flux dialysis membranes. (**a**) Polysulfone membrane (Fresenius Polysulfon® PS600). Asymmetric, microreticular structure. Wall thickness 40 µm. (**b**) Polyethersulfone membrane (DIAPES® HF800). Symmetric, microreticular, three-layer structure. Wall thickness 35 µm. (**c**) Polyethersulfone/polyamid blended membrane (Polyamix®). Asymmetric, anisotrop, macroreticular structure. Wall thickness 50 µm (Photographs are courtesy of Membrana GmbH, Germany)

provide the excellent diffusive performances delivered with these membranes. Except for the polyester–polymer alloy (PEPA) membrane, in which polyethersulfone is amalgamated with polyacrylate, this is achieved by blending with polyvinylpyrrolidone. In this respect, Polyamix® is not different, even if it is often distinguished as a polyamide membrane, because small quantities of this polymer are added to the polyethersulfone/polyvinylpyrrolidone blend. VitabranE™ is a polysulfone/polyvinylpyrrolidone high-flux membrane coated with vitamin E, for which a first report has recently shown a beneficial effect on oxidative stress in maintenance dialysis patients [47]. Adsorption is a minor mechanism of toxin removal with polysulfone and polyethersulfone. Solutes are preferably eliminated by transmembrane passage. Polysulfone and polyethersulfone dialysis membranes are available in the whole range of permeabilities for all current clinical applications (Table 7.3.2).

Several further developments of existing high-flux polysulfone/polyethersulfone membranes have been introduced. These membranes possess a very similar water flux compared to their original membrane and, hence, belong to the same class of permeability. Due to a more homogenous and dense pore size distribution, they have a significantly steeper sieving curve for low-molecular-weight proteins, i.e., an improved middle molecule removal at low albumin loss. Current examples are Helixone® and the even more efficient PUREMA® H. Helixone® is based on the PS600 polysulfone membrane, but has a smaller inner fiber diameter for enhanced internal filtration (185 vs 200 µm) [55]. PUREMA® H is the result of a modified spinning process of its polyethersulfone precursor DIAPES® HF800 [38].

Polymethylmethacrylate (PMMA) is an asymmetric, hydrophobic dialysis membrane produced since 1977 by fusion of isotactic polymethylacrylate and dimethylsulfoxide. This relatively biocompatible membrane is available in the whole range of water fluxes (Table 7.3.2). Differences in membrane permeability are obtained by variation of the polymer composition and the water content during production. PMMA membranes have a considerable adsorptive capacity for low-molecular-weight proteins [3].

Ethylene vinyl-alcohol (EVAL) is a copolymer made of ethylene and vinyl acetate. It forms a relatively hydrophilic, symmetric low-flux dialysis membrane. Based on low activation of the coagulation system, it has been used for heparin-free dialysis. Regarding cell and complement activation, EVAL demonstrates a less favorable biocompatibility profile, which is similar to that of modified cellulosic membranes [85].

7.3.4 Dialysis Membrane Biocompatibility

- *Complement system activation*

The contact of blood with the dialysis membrane induces biological responses involving circulating cells and plasma components. During the 1970s, the apparent relative bioincompatibility of unsubstituted cellulose membranes was already suggested as the cause for acute pulmonary dysfunction during hemodialysis due to complement-mediated leukostasis [9]. The magnitude of leukocyte and complement system activation has since been established as classical parameters of biocompatibility. The relative bioincompatibility of unsubstituted cellulose membranes has been linked to free hydroxyl groups on the surface, which trigger intense complement system activation via the alternative pathway with the cleavage of several complement products, such as C3a, C5a, and the membrane attack complex C5b-9. These and other complement products serve as marker substances and can be detected with a maximum at 5–10 min after the start of dialysis. Substituted cellulose membranes with less, and particularly synthetic membranes without, free hydroxyl groups lead to much lower complement and cell activation. It must be noted that not only the dialysis membrane material itself, but also the removal of generated complement fragments by adsorption or transmembrane transport may interfere with the blood–membrane response.

- *Cell activation*

The complement system is a potent mechanism for the initiation and amplification of inflammation. Notably the anaphylatoxins C3a and C5a stimulate chemotaxis and activation of leukocytes. Complement-induced activation of leukocytes, but also direct cell–dialysis membrane contact causes a transient leukopenia with a nadir during the first 10–15 min of dialysis. Activated neutrophils sequestrate specifically in the pulmonary capillary bed where they are thought to be involved in the multifactorial mechanisms compromising gas exchange, which lead to dialysis-associated hypoxemia [48]. Pulmonary neutrophil sequestration is related to the expression of C5a receptors specifically within the lungs [80]. Also other factors, such as an increased expression of adhesion molecules localized on granulocytes (L-selectin, the integrins CD11b and CD61, etc.), which play a role in cell aggregation and adherence to endothelium, are involved [32, 61]. Reversal of leukopenia has been linked to the selective down-regulation of C5a receptors on polymorphonuclear leukocytes, internalization of C5a receptors on granulocytes, and reduction of plasma C5a concentration below the critical threshold needed for granulocyte–endothelial adhesion [22]. Leukocyte rebound results from sequestrated neutrophils returning into blood and recruitment from the marginated pool or bone marrow stores leading to granulocytosis after more than 1 h of dialysis.

Activated peripheral blood mononuclear cells generate proinflammatory cytokines, such as interleukin-1β (IL-1β) and tumor necrosis factor α (TNF-α) [22], particularly in the presence of endotoxin [18]. The secretion of IL-1β and TNF-α precedes the generation of interleukin-6 (IL-6) and subsequently acute-phase protein synthesis, which is equivalent to inflammation, a frequent finding in maintenance dialysis patients. Inflammation is regarded as a main cause for malnutrition and atherosclerosis in this patient population. The presence of endotoxins and other bacterial fragments in blood originating from contaminated dialysate is a strong trigger for inflammation. Retention of these substances by the dialysis membrane from passing into blood via backdiffusion or backfiltration may also be regarded in the context of biocompatibility (see Chapter 2.6).

- *Reactive oxygen species production*

Increased production of reactive oxygen species (ROS) during hemodialysis contributes to oxidative stress in uremia, which has been implicated in long-term complications including anemia, amyloidosis, accelerated atherosclerosis, and malnutrition. A transient increase in the production of ROS during hemodialysis is observed particularly with cellulose membranes, which seem to both stimulate and prime neutrophil oxidative burst activity, but these effects are partially obscured by neutropenia [84]. Both synthetic and cellulose membranes cause ROS production by neutrophils, but with cellulose it is significantly higher compared with, e.g., polysulfone [21, 60]. In addition, endotoxin from dialysate crossing the dialysis membranes may also prime the production of ROS by activated neutrophils. Not only dialysis membrane material, also membrane permeability seems to influence oxidative stress. Compared with low-flux synthetic and high-flux cellulosic membrane materials, high-flux synthetic membranes have demonstrated a beneficial long-term effect on lipid oxidation as evidenced by lower plasma levels of oxidatively modified low-density lipoprotein [83]. ROS production during dialysis with different high-flux synthetic membranes seems to be similar [38]. Reducing oxidative stress in hemodialysis should comprise the improvement of the hemocompatibility of the dialysis system including dialysis membranes and the supplementation of deficient patients with antioxidants. One approach in this direction has been made by coating cellulosic and synthetic dialysis membrane materials with vitamin E. Long-term treatment with vitamin-coated cellulose membranes was demonstrated to improve parameters of oxidative stress, such as malondialdehyde, advanced glycation end products, and 8-hydroxydeoxyguanosine plasma levels [63]. However, this effect was similar to that of noncoated synthetic membranes and seemed to be associated with higher plasma levels of vitamin E [75]. When vitamin E-coated synthetic polysulfone was tested in a long-term study, plasma levels of parameters of oxidative stress were lower compared with a similar membrane without coating [47]. Whether the beneficial effects of vitamin E-coating exceed those of a simple supplementation therapy with vitamin E is currently not clear.

- *Cell aggregate formation*

The formation of circulating platelet-leukocyte and platelet-erythrocyte aggregates as a consequence of cell activation by dialysis membranes has been observed during hemodialysis, but whether these phenomena are of potential relevance in biological processes including inflammation, atherogenesis, and hemostasis remains speculative [70]. However, differences between the membranes are present and not necessarily to the disadvantage of bioincompatible cellulosic membranes. As an example, the expression of P-selectin (CD62P) as a measure of platelet activation and the formation of platelet-neutrophil and platelet-erythrocyte aggregates is similar between cellulose diacetate and polysulfone [69]. Platelet activation in the form of CD62P, CD63, and PAC-1 expression appears to be even lower in cuprammonium than in polysulfone dialysis membranes [76]. Platelets also directly adsorb to the dialysis membrane without forming aggregates with other cells. As a consequence, the number of platelets in blood can decrease by 10–15% during dialysis.

- *Premature cellular senescence*

Dialysis membrane bioincompatibility is discussed as being also involved in the stress-induced premature senescence (SIPS) of mononuclear cells, which has been linked to the selective activation of these cells by cellulosic membranes. In contrast to patients on maintenance dialysis with biocompatible membranes, those treated with cellulosic membranes had a subset of mononuclear cells with decreased telomere length and a predominant CD14dim/CD16bright phenotype, which are typical features of SIPS [52]. The percentage of SIPS mononuclear cells seems to be associated with chronic inflammation because it correlates with C-reactive protein [29].

- *Increased apoptosis*

Increased cell apoptosis has been linked to uremia per se, but also to differences in dialysis membrane biocompatibility. A higher proportion of apoptotic cells has been demonstrated in maintenance dialysis patients on cellulosic membranes as compared with synthetic membranes [44]. However, the permeability of tested dialysis membranes may have confounded the results because it also impacts on apoptosis. Patients on high-flux synthetic membranes were found to have a significantly lower percentage of apoptotic lymphocytes than patients on low-flux membranes made of the same material [72]. Although of interest, all previous studies on both SIPS of mononuclear cells and cellular apoptosis must be interpreted with caution because the chosen study designs were inappropriate to allow definite conclusions.

- *Coagulation system activation*

The contact of blood with the dialysis membrane leads to activation of the coagulation system and platelets. Thrombin generation and thrombus formation is largely prevented by anticoagulation, if not, fouling of the membrane and ultimately clotting of fibers would result. The procoagulatory activity of dialysis membranes, which can be characterized by measuring the generation of coagulation products, such as thrombin–anti-thrombin III complexes, or of fibrinolytic activity, such as D-dimers, can be very different. Generally, cellulosic and most synthetic membranes have a low thrombogenicity. In contrast, the synthetic AN69® membrane has an enhanced thrombogenic activity [15]. A strong induction of the coagulation cascade is triggered by intense contact activation via factor XII (Hageman factor) due to the negative charge of this membrane. In dialysis membranes without negative charge and contact activation, thrombin formation is reduced and not induced via factor XII [15].

- *Contact phase system activation*

During contact activation by the AN69® membrane, factor XIIa also generates kallikrein from prekallikrein. Plasma kallikrein, in turn, cleaves high-molecular-weight kininogen under release of bradykinin. This activation of the kallikrein-kinin system, occurring during each dialysis with the AN69® membrane, has been clinically insignificant until ACE (synonymous with kininase II) inhibitors were introduced for clinical routine use. Inhibition of kininase II, the major enzyme of kinin degradation, which is localized in the pulmonary vasculature, allows high concentrations of bradykinin passing into the arterial system and, thus, causing potentially severe anaphylactoid reactions [37, 77, 81]. Neutralizing the membrane electronegativity of AN69® by coating with polyethyleneimine (AN69® ST membrane) dramatically decreases kinin formation [10]. However, a recent study suggested that the absolute value of the zeta potential, as a measure of electronegativity, does not correlate with contact phase activation. Rather other parameters, particularly the quantity of highly charged functional groups on the membrane surface, were assumed to be involved in this phenomenon [38].

7.3.5 Dialysis Membrane Biocompatibility and Clinical Outcome

Observational data in maintenance dialysis patients from the US Renal Data System published in 1996 suggested that unsubstituted cellulose membranes were associated with 20% greater mortality compared with biocompatible substituted cellulose and synthetic membranes [20]. This observation was attributed to differences in complement activation, but the membranes also differed with respect to water flux and larger molecule clearance. A post hoc analysis of a large prospective study population of maintenance dialysis patients with type 2 diabetes mellitus basically confirmed these results without confounding for permeability differences [36]. Unsubstituted cellulose was identified as the dialysis membrane with the highest relative overall mortality risk. Additionally, patients on substituted cellulose had a worse outcome than patients on synthetic membranes. To date, the effect of dialysis membrane biocompatibility on the mortality of long-term hemodialysis patients has never been evaluated in a prospective study of sufficient biostatistical power.

In contrast to maintenance dialysis patients, patients with acute renal failure who require dialysis are often critically ill and have sepsis. This important difference makes it more difficult to perceive the consequences of the biological responses resulting from membrane bioincompatibility. Two initial prospective clinical studies published in 1994 have shifted the use of dialysis membranes in intermittent hemodialysis in patients with acute renal failure toward synthetic membranes [19, 64]. One trial compared unsubstituted cellulose to polymethylmethacrylate [19] and the other to polyacrylonitrile [64]. Both studies reported a significantly better recovery of renal function and a trend toward superior survival among patients dialyzed with biocompatible synthetic dialysis membranes. However, numerous shortcomings in the study designs led to a controversial debate about the validity of these results. Several subsequently performed prospective trials, some of them thoroughly designed, failed to demonstrate a difference between synthetic and unsubstituted cellulose membranes [31, 40] and between synthetic and substituted cellulose membranes in the outcome of patients with acute renal failure being treated with intermittent hemodialysis [1, 16].

Two recent meta-analyses focusing on membrane biocompatibility and outcome of patients with acute renal failure came to the same inconclusive results [2, 28]. In summary, the use of biocompatible synthetic membranes in the often complex patients with acute renal failure requiring renal replacement therapy is certainly safe, but a general recommendation to prefer synthetic over cellulosic dialysis membranes is not justified by convincing evidence.

7.3.6 Dialysis Membrane Permeability and Clinical Outcome

In contrast to low-flux dialysis membranes, which almost completely retain substances with a molecular weight of more than about 1,000 Da, the removal of larger molecules including putative uremic toxins by more permeable, i.e., high-flux membranes is an acknowledged concept to deliver more adequate dialysis therapy. Particularly with regard to complex cases, where acute renal failure is one symptom of multiorgan failure and sepsis, extracorporeal renal replacement with highly permeable membranes provides the opportunity to target humoral mediators of disease, such as proinflammatory cytokines. Many of these substances are larger than 20,000 Da and their removal may potentially modulate the course of disease.

In chronic hemodialysis, several mainly observational studies showed better outcomes for patients treated with high-flux membranes [7, 34, 36, 41, 51, 87], but the only published randomized controlled trial in this respect, the Hemodialysis (HEMO) Study, which enrolled in total 1,846 patients on maintenance hemodialysis, did not find a difference between low- and high-flux membranes [8, 12]. Primary data analysis of the HEMO Study, which had a two-by-two factorial design comparing also standard with high-dose dialysis, only proved a benefit of high-flux versus low-flux membranes regarding cardiac death [12]. In a secondary analysis, an additional 32% lower relative mortality risk was found for patients on high-flux dialysis membranes with a mean duration of dialysis for longer than 3.7 years before randomization [8]. The overall inconclusive results of the HEMO Study led to intense criticisms of the study design, which excluded overweight patients and allowed widespread dialyzer reuse. Some reuse practices significantly change the characteristics of dialysis membranes. Therefore, it may be conceivable that a possible survival advantage of high-flux versus low-flux dialyzers is attenuated if high-flux dialyzers are reused.

Very recently, the results of the European membrane Permeability Outcome (MPO) Study on 738 incident chronic hemodialysis patients treated with high-flux compared with low-flux membranes were presented. The MPO Study demonstrated that patients with an elevated risk as characterized by the presence of diabetes mellitus and/or low serum albumin levels </= 4 g/dl, which is associated with protein energy wasting (malnutrition, inflammation, and atherosclerosis) and increased morbidity and mortality risk, show a favorable outcome on high-flux dialysis [42]. In the population overall, no significant survival benefit with either high-flux or low-flux membranes was detected [42].

In patients presenting acute renal failure, only two, rather small prospective studies investigating intermittent hemodialysis are suited to draw conclusions on the effects of different dialysis membrane permeabilities on outcome [16, 50]. All other available trials confounded for biocompatibility by comparing high-flux synthetic with low-flux cellulosic membranes. However, except for the study by Schiffl et al., who observed in their patients that, compared with low-flux cellulose, intermittent hemodialysis with a high-flux synthetic membrane had beneficial effects on the outcome (mortality, death from sepsis, and renal function) [64], no study was able to demonstrate differences in survival between low- and high-flux membranes [1, 16, 40, 50]. It is only with respect to the recovery of renal function that a possible advantage of high- over low-flux membranes cannot be excluded [1, 2].

Based on the insufficient existent body of evidence, a recommendation for the use of either low- or high-flux membranes in the intermittent hemodialysis treatment of acute renal failure patients is not justified. Furthermore, it is still unclear whether an intermittent renal replacement therapy is inferior to a continuous treatment, the latter always requires the use of a high-flux membrane. The severity of the often fatal underlying disease, in which acute renal failure is only part of multiorgan dysfunction, seems to be more crucial for the patient outcome than differences in dialysis membrane permeability.

7.3.7 Dialysis Membrane Requirements in Acute Renal Failure

Basically, the specifications of dialysis membranes for the treatment of patients presenting acute renal failure do not differ from those for maintenance dialysis. They must be defined rather by virtue of theoretical and practical considerations than on the basis of conclusive clinical data. The ideal dialysis membrane should allow constant high diffusive and convective clearances for the removal of a wide range of toxins. It should have the best biocompatibility to avoid undesirable interactions with blood components, adequate hydraulic permeability for use in intermittent or continuous renal replacement therapy modes, and high pyrogen retention capability when used with non-ultrapure dialysate. These demands are best met by the latest generation of synthetic high-flux membranes.

- *High diffusive clearance*

The small solute clearance of a dialyzer is not only determined by the dialysis membrane, i.e., its porosity and wall thickness. Modern synthetic high-flux membranes no longer form a significant diffusive barrier. With a wall thickness between only 20–60 μm, their morphology differs considerably from the first high-flux membranes, which originally were designed for hemofiltration and had a wall thickness of more than 100 μm. Modification of the dialysate flow distribution is able to enhance the diffusive clearance of a modern dialyzer. This has been achieved by changes of the dialysate path of the dialyzer housing [57], by ondulation/microondulation of the dialysis membrane hollow fibers [59], by modifying the packing density of the fiber bundle [57], or by adding spacer yarns to the fiber bundle [49].

- *High permeability for middle molecules*

Observational trials indicate that an efficient removal of middle molecules and also larger substances by convective treatment procedures may be associated with improved outcome in patients on maintenance renal replacement therapy [5]. Compared with those undergoing low-flux dialysis, chronic patients on high-efficiency hemodiafiltration had a 35% lower mortality [5]. In patients with acute renal failure, the plasma level of cytokines predicts mortality [68], and the reduction of high levels of cytokines and other proinflammatory mediators, which are often larger than 20,000 Da, may have beneficial effects on the outcome of these often critically ill patients [58]. In continuous venovenous hemofiltration, the ultrafiltration rate, which is equivalent to the dose of convection and which correlates with the removal of middle molecules and larger solutes, impacts on the mortality in acute renal failure. It is recommended to be at least at 35 ml/h per /kg body weight [56]. For the efficient removal of cytokines, highly permeable dialysis membranes are a prerequisite, irrespective of continuous or intermittent dialysis mode. Basically, all available high-flux dialysis membranes are suited for convective therapy modes, but they differ considerably in terms of hydraulic permeability and solute permselectivity. While the permeability for middle molecules should be as high as possible, essential proteins, such as albumin or immunoglobulins, should be retained. However, it is currently unclear, and even more so in acute renal failure, how much albumin permeability is tolerable. Recently developed high-flux membranes have much enhanced middle molecule permeability without important albumin loss. This has been obtained by increasing internal filtration (i.e., forward filtration of plasma water followed by backward filtration of dialysate) in the dialysis membrane fiber either due to reduction of the inner fiber diameter [55], which leads to a higher pressure gradient along the fiber, or by improving the pore morphology [38]. When used in simple hemodialysis, such a dialysis membrane is able to match the efficacy of high-efficiency hemodiafiltration with a conventional high-flux membrane [39]. Protein-leaking or super-flux dialysis membranes are also highly permeable for middle molecules, but, at least in maintenance dialysis therapy, they are not suited for convective treatment forms due to the loss of essential proteins. In critically ill, septic patients with acute renal failure, the employment of these (what are also called high-cutoff dialysis membranes) in continuous mode is regarded differently despite the necessity of substituting significant amounts of albumin. Small-scale studies have indicated that high-permeability continuous venovenous hemofiltration is able to modulate the inflammatory response and to improve peripheral blood mononuclear cell functions [45, 46], but larger prospective randomized trials on patient outcome are lacking.

- *Constant clearances*

Ideally, a dialysis membrane should deliver a constant performance during the whole treatment time, provided that treatment parameters are not changed and no clotting has taken place. The ability of dialysis membranes to adsorb protein and cells alters their permeability and, hence, solute clearances. Adsorption is particularly intense early during blood–membrane contact, i.e., at the beginning of the renal replacement treatment, and becomes saturated with time. The degree of adsorption is different from membrane to membrane. In some membranes, it is even the most important mode of solute removal [11]. To give an example, for polysulfone, the adsorptive removal of β_2-microglobulin during a 4-h hemodialysis session is only 17% of the total removed amount, while for AN69 it is much higher at 60% [33]. Clogging due to adsorption or saturation of adsorption of the dialysis membranes may significantly decrease treatment efficiency [11, 17]. Therefore, the practice of changing the dialyzer in continuous treatment forms at fixed time intervals has been established in many centers to guarantee adequate treatment delivery even without any evidence for impaired patency of the extracorporeal circuit. Dialysis membranes with only marginal adsorption permit changing the hemofilter less frequently.

- *Adequate hydraulic permeability*

For hemodialysis, as a mainly diffusive therapy form, technically either low-flux dialysis membranes or those with any higher fluxes are appropriate. Current dialysis machines are equipped with an ultrafiltration control. This essential technical feature allows using large-pore dialysis membranes in hemodialysis mode without uncontrolled fluid removal from the patient. Without ultrafiltration control, the use of low-flux dialysis membranes was necessary to avoid accidental fluid loss. For intermittent or continuous convective treatment forms, i.e., hemofiltration and hemodiafiltration, high-flux membranes must be used, allowing the ultrafiltration of adequate amounts of plasma water without unacceptably high transmembrane pressure increase. Filters with large surface area (>1.6 m^2) should be chosen for intermittent renal replacement to assure treatment efficiency and practicability. In continuous convective treatments, much lower fluid rates are ultrafiltered, and, hence, filters with smaller surface areas (around 1.0 m^2) are usually adequate.

- *High biocompatibility*

Convincing evidence for a significant role of dialysis membrane biocompatibility in the outcome of patients with acute renal failure is lacking (refer to Chapter 2.5). However, due to the complexity of underlying disease with often fatal outcome particularly in critically ill septic patients, the use of highly biocompatible dialysis membranes should be considered to avoid putatively undesirable interactions with the patients' blood components. Neither a further induction of the systemic inflammatory response by activation of the complement system and peripheral blood cells, nor an activation of the coagulation system can be regarded as beneficial. Routinely, coagulation is avoided by systemic anticoagulation with heparin. In patients at bleeding risk, a heparin-coated dialysis membrane (AN69® ST) with reduced procoagulatory effects [6] has been successfully used without systemic heparin injection, but regional anticoagulation with citrate appears to be much superior in preventing clotting of the extracorporeal system [13]. Contact system-activating dialysis membranes have the potential to aggravate blood pressure instability and should be used with caution, although a comparison between such a membrane and polysulfone did not reveal differences with respect to their effects on the hemodynamic response [30].

- *Pyrogen retention capability*

Bacterial endotoxin and other cytokine-inducing bacterial substances from contaminated standard dialysate have the potential to pass through dialysis membranes into blood by backdiffusion and backfiltration. In vitro experiments have demonstrated that the composition and flux property of the membrane affects the permeability for bacterial material. In principle, all dialysis membranes are permeable for pyrogens. On the one hand, low-flux membranes are regarded to be somewhat safer because of smaller pores and minimal backfiltration of dialysate. On the other hand, some synthetic larger pore high-flux dialysis membranes have the capacity to adsorb bacterial substances, which also may prevent the pyrogen passage. These characteristics together with the quality and quantity of the bacterial challenge and other significant differences in the experimental settings have led to in part contradictory results in the same membranes [43, 67, 78, 86]. However, despite lacking controlled clinical studies on patient morbidity and mortality, we can say that the passage of endotoxins from dialysate through the dialysis membrane may induce the activation of proinflammatory cytokines and represents a potential hazard for the patient [65, 66, 71]. Therefore, the use of ultrapure dialysate in hemodialysis is generally suggested.

7.3.8 Future Trends in Dialysis Membranes: The Bioartificial Kidney

Despite some progress in renal replacement treatment delivery, the outcomes in acute renal failure are still poor. Therefore, the concept of current renal replacement therapies needs to be reconsidered, particularly in patients presenting sepsis and multiorgan dysfunction. Compared with the human kidney, the rather unselective replacement of renal function in critically ill patients with traditional dialysis membranes is not equivalent. All studies investigating conventional intermittent or continuous therapy forms in these patients demonstrated low survival. Future concepts, such as microfluidics and membraneless systems, nanofabricated membranes with synthetic channels, or silicon membranes with slit pores [26] are still far from clinical application. Whether they will improve mortality rates is uncertain.

Encouraging results have been demonstrated by first clinical trials on a bioartificial kidney. The bioartificial kidney consists of a conventional continuous venovenous hemofiltration in series with a renal tubule assist device (RAD) containing approximately 10^9 functional renal proximal tubule cells. This setting replaces not only excretory, but also transport, metabolic, and endocrine functions of the kidney [23]. Renal tubule cells seem to play critical roles in immunoregulation. In acute renal failure associated with sepsis, they potentially alter the detrimental multiple-organ consequences of sepsis. The results of animal studies and recent phase I/II and phase II clinical trials have shown that the RAD is able to modify the sepsis condition and to improve survival in acute renal failure [14, 24, 25]. The first clinical trial demonstrated the safety, durability, viability, and functionality of this biologic therapy for up to 24 h. Six of ten critically ill patients with a mean predicted hospital mortality rate above 85% survived for at least 30 days after the treatment [25]. In a subsequent multicenter randomized controlled study involving 58 patients with acute renal failure, a 72-h treatment with the bioartificial kidney reduced the relative mortality risk by approximately 50% and was associated with more rapid recovery of kidney function compared with conventional continuous renal replacement therapy alone. At day 28, the mortality rate was only 33% in the bioartificial kidney group and 61% in the control group [79]. These intriguing data indicate that the novel renal tubular cell therapy has the potential to add significant benefit to current renal replacement strategies in the outcome of critically ill patients with acute renal failure.

7.3.9 Take Home Pearls

- The dialysis membrane represents the critical component for toxin and fluid removal by extracorporeal renal replacement therapy.
- Dialysis membranes should have (1) high diffusive and convective clearances for the removal of a wide range of toxins, (2) the best possible biocompatibility to avoid undesirable interactions with blood components, (3) adequate hydraulic permeability for use in intermittent or continuous renal replacement therapy modes, and (4) the highest pyrogen retention capability for the use with non-ultrapure dialysate.
- Outcome studies in patients with acute renal failure, focusing on dialysis membrane characteristics did not yield conclusive clinical data, indicating that the severity of the underlying disease is crucial.
- Overall, the trend is toward the use of biocompatible synthetic high-flux membranes in both acute and maintenance dialysis therapy forms.

References

1. Albright RC Jr, Smelser JM, McCarthy JT, Homburger HA, Bergstralh EJ, Larson TS (2000) Patient survival and renal recovery in acute renal failure: randomized comparison of cellulose acetate and polysulfone membrane dialyzers. Mayo Clin Proc 75:1141–1147.
2. Alonso A, Lau J, Jaber BL (2008) Biocompatible hemodialysis membranes for acute renal failure. Cochrane Database Syst Rev 23:CD005283
3. Aoike I (2007) Clinical significance of protein adsorbable membranes – Long-term clinical effects and analysis using a proteomic technique. Nephrol Dial Transplant 22(Suppl. 5):v13–v19.
4. Babb AL, Popovich RP, Christopher TG, Scribner BH (1971) The genesis of the square meter-hour hypothesis. Trans Am Soc Artif Intern Organs 17:81–91.
5. Canaud B, Bragg-Gresham JL, Marshall M, Desmeules S, Gillespie BW, Depner T, Klassen P, Port FK (2006) Mortality risk for patients receiving hemodiafiltration versus hemodialysis: European results from the DOPPS. Kidney Int 69:2087–2093.
6. Chanard J, Lavaud S, Maheut H, Kazes I, Vitry F, Rieu P (2007) The clinical evaluation of low-dose heparin in haemo-

dialysis: A prospective study using the heparin-coated AN69 ST membrane. Nephrol Dial Transplant Dec 21 [Epub ahead of print]
7. Chauveau P, Nguyen H, Combe C, et al. for the French Study Group for Nutrition in Dialysis (2005) Dialyzer membrane permeability and survival in hemodialysis patients. Am J Kidney Dis 45:565–571.
8. Cheung AK, Levin NW, Greene T, Agodoa L, Bailey J, Beck G, Clark W, Levey AS, Leypoldt JK, Ornt DB, Rocco MV, Schulman G, Schwab S, Teehan B, Eknoyan G (2003) Effects of high-flux hemodialysis on clinical outcomes: Results of the HEMO Study. J Am Soc Nephrol 14:3251–3263.
9. Craddock PR, Fehr J, Brigham KL, Kronenberg RS, Jacob HS (1977) Complement and leukocyte-mediated pulmonary dysfunction in hemodialysis. N Engl J Med 296:769–774.
10. Désormeaux A, Moreau ME, Lepage Y, Chanard J, Adam A (2008) The effect of electronegativity and angiotensin-converting enzyme inhibition on the kinin-forming capacity of polyacrylonitrile dialysis membranes. Biomaterials 29:1139–1146.
11. De Vriese AS, Colardyn FA, Philippé JJ, Vanholder RC, De Sutter JH, Lameire NH (1999) Cytokine removal during continuous hemofiltration in septic patients. J Am Soc Nephrol 10:846–853.
12. Eknoyan G, Beck GJ, Cheung AK, et al. (2002) Effect of dialysis dose and membrane flux in maintenance hemodialysis. N Engl J Med 347:2010–2019.
13. Evenepoel P, Dejagere T, Verhamme P, Claes K, Kuypers D, Bammens B, Vanrenterghem Y (2007) Heparin-coated polyacrylonitrile membrane versus regional citrate anticoagulation: a prospective randomized study of 2 anticoagulation strategies in patients at risk of bleeding. Am J Kidney Dis 49:642–649.
14. Fissell WH, Lou L, Abrishami S, Buffington DA, Humes HD (2003) Bioartificial kidney ameliorates gram-negative bacteria-induced septic shock in uremic animals. J Am Soc Nephrol 14:454–461.
15. Frank RD, Weber J, Dresbach H, Thelen H, Weiss C, Floege J (2001) Role of contact system activation in hemodialyzer-induced thrombogenicity. Kidney Int 60:1972–1981.
16. Gastaldello K, Melot C, Kahn RJ, Vanherweghem JL, Vincent JL, Tielemans C (2000) Comparison of cellulose diacetate and polysulfone membranes in the outcome of acute renal failure. A prospective randomized study. Nephrol Dial Transplant 15:224–230.
17. Haase M, Silvester W, Uchino S, Goldsmith D, Davenport P, Tipping P, Boyce N, Bellomo R (2007) A pilot study of high-adsorption hemofiltration in human septic shock. Int J Artif Organs 30:108–117.
18. Haeffner CN, Cavaillon JM, Laude M, Kazatchkine MD (1987) C3a (C3adesArg) induces production and release of interleukin 1 by cultured human monocytes. J Immunol 139:794–799.
19. Hakim RM, Wingard RL, Parker RA (1994) Effect of the dialysis membrane in the treatment of patients with acute renal failure. New Engl J Med 331:1338–1342.
20. Hakim RM, Held PJ, Stannard DC, Wolfe RA, Port FK, Daugirdas JT, Agodoa L (1996) Effect of the dialysis membrane on mortality of chronic hemodialysis patients. Kidney Int 50:566–570.
21. Himmelfarb J, Ault KA, Holbrook D, Leeber DA, Hakim RM (1993) Intradialytic granulocyte reactive oxygen species production: a prospective, crossover trial. J Am Soc Nephrol 4:178–186.
22. Hörl WH (2002) Hemodialysis membranes: Interleukins, biocompatibility, and middle molecules. J Am Soc Nephrol 13:S62–S71.
23. Humes HD, Buffington DA, MacKay SM, Funke AJ, Weitzel WF (1999) Replacement of renal function in uremic animals with a tissue-engineered kidney. Nat Biotechnol 17:451–455.
24. Humes HD, Buffington DA, Lou L, Abrishami S, Wang M, Xia J, Fissell WH (2003) Cell therapy with a tissue-engineered kidney reduces the multiple-organ consequences of septic shock. Crit Care Med 31:2421–2428.
25. Humes HD, Weitzel WF, Bartlett RH, Swaniker FC, Paganini EP, Luderer JR, Sobota J (2004) Initial clinical results of the bioartificial kidney containing human cells in ICU patients with acute renal failure. Kidney Int 66:1578–1588.
26. Humes HD, Fissell WH, Tiranathanagul K (2006) The future of hemodialysis membranes. Kidney Intl 69:1115–1119.
27. Hutter JC, Kuehnert MJ, Wallis RR, Lucas AD, Sen S, Jarvis WR (2000) Acute onset of decreased vision and hearing traced to hemodialysis treatment with aged dialyzers. JAMA. 283:2128–2134.
28. Jaber BL, Lau J, Schmid CH, Karsou SA, Levey AS, Pereira BJ (2002) Effect of biocompatibility of hemodialysis membranes on mortality in acute renal failure: A meta-analysis. Clin Nephrol 57:274–282.
29. Jimenez R, Carracedo J, Santamaría R, Soriano S, Madueño JA, Ramírez R, Rodríguez M, Martín-Malo A, Aljama P (2005) Replicative senescence in patients with chronic kidney failure. Kidney Int Suppl 99:S11–S15.
30. Jones CH, Goutcher E, Newstead CG, Will EJ, Dean SG, Davison AM (1998) Hemodynamics and survival of patients with acute renal failure treated by continuous dialysis with two synthetic membranes. Artif Organs 22:638–643.
31. Jörres A, Gahl GM, Dobis C, Polenakovic MH, Cakalaroski K, Rutkowski B, Kisielnicka E, Krieter DH, Rumpf KW, Guenther C, Gaus W, Hoegel J (1999) Haemodialysis-membrane biocompatibility and mortality of patients with dialysis-dependent acute renal failure: a prospective randomised multicentre trial. International Multicentre Study Group. Lancet 354:1337–1341.
32. Kawabata K, Nagake Y, Shikata K, Makino H, Ota Z (1996) The changes of Mac-1 and L-selectin expression on granulocytes and soluble L-selectin level during hemodialysis. Nephron 73:573–579.
33. Klinke B, Röckel A, Abdelhamid S, Fiegel P, Walb D (1989) Transmembranous transport and adsorption of beta-2-microglobulin during hemodialysis using polysulfone, polyacrylonitrile, polymethylmethacrylate and cuprammonium rayon membranes. Int J Artif Organs 12:697–702.
34. Koda Y, Nishi S, Miyazaki S, Haginoshita S, Sakurabayashi T, Suzuki M, Sakai S, Yuasa Y, Hirasawa Y, Nishi T (1997) Switch from conventional to high-flux membrane reduces the risk of carpal tunnel syndrome and mortality of hemodialysis patients. Kidney Int 52:1096–1101.
35. Kolff WJ (1965) First clinical experience with the artificial kidney. Ann Intern Med 62:608–619.
36. Krane V, Krieter DH, Olschewski M, März W, Mann JFE, Ritz E, Wanner C, for the German Diabetes and Dialysis

Study Investigators (2007) Dialyzer membrane characteristics and outcome of patients with type 2 diabetes on maintenance hemodialysis. Am J Kidney Dis 49:267–275.
37. Krieter DH, Grude M, Lemke HD, Fink E, Bönner G, Schölkens BA, Schulz E, Müller GA (1998) Anaphylactoid reactions during hemodialysis in sheep are ACE inhibitor dose-dependent and mediated by bradykinin. Kidney Int 53:1026–1035.
38. Krieter DH, Morgenroth A, Barasinski A, Lemke HD, Schuster O, von Harten B, Wanner C (2007) Effects of a polyelectrolyte additive on the selective dialysis membrane permeability for low-molecular-weight proteins.Nephrol Dial Transplant 22:491–499.
39. Krieter DH, Hunn E, Morgenroth A, Lemke HD, Wanner C (2008) Matching efficacy of online hemodiafiltration in simple hemodialysis mode. Artif Organs 32:903–909
40. Kurtal H, von Herrath D, Schaefer K (1995) Is the choice of membrane important for patients with acute renal failure requiring hemodialysis? Artif Organs 19:391–394.
41. Locatelli F, Marcelli D, Conte F, Limido A, Malberti F, Spotti D (1999) Comparison of mortality in ESRD patients on convective and diffusive extracorporeal treatments. The Registro Lombardo Dialisi E Trapianto. Kidney Int 55:286–293.
42. Locatelli F, Martin-Malo A, Hannedouche T, Loureiro A, Papadimitriou M, Wizemann V, Jacobson SH, Czekalski S, Ronco C, Vanholder R; Membrane Permeability Outcome (MPO) Study Group (2009) Effect of membrane permeability on survival of hemodialysis patients. J Am Soc Nephrol 20:645–654
43. Lonnemann G, Sereni L, Lemke HD, Tetta C (2001) Pyrogen retention by highly permeable synthetic membranes during in vitro dialysis. Artif Organs 25:951–960.
44. Martín-Malo A, Carracedo J, Ramírez R, Rodriguez-Benot A, Soriano S, Rodriguez M, Aljama P (2000) Effect of uremia and dialysis modality on mononuclear cell apoptosis. J Am Soc Nephrol 11:936–942.
45. Morgera S, Haase M, Rocktäschel J, Böhler T, von Heymann C, Vargas-Hein O, Krausch D, Zuckermann-Becker H, Müller JM, Kox WJ, Neumayer HH (2003) High permeability haemofiltration improves peripheral blood mononuclear cell proliferation in septic patients with acute renal failure. Nephrol Dial Transplant 18:2570–2576.
46. Morgera S, Haase M, Kuss T, Vargas-Hein O, Zuckermann-Becker H, Melzer C, Krieg H, Wegner B, Bellomo R, Neumayer HH (2006) Pilot study on the effects of high cutoff hemofiltration on the need for norepinephrine in septic patients with acute renal failure. Crit Care Med 34:2099–2104.
47. Morimoto H, Nakao K, Fukuoka K, Sarai A, Yano A, Kihara T, Fukuda S, Wada J, Makino H (2005) Long-term use of vitamin E-coated polysulfone membrane reduces oxidative stress markers in haemodialysis patients. Nephrol Dial Transplant 20:2775–2782.
48. Munger MA, Ateshkadi A, Cheung AK, Flaharty KK, Stoddard GJ, Marshall EH (2000) Cardiopulmonary events during hemodialysis: effects of dialysis membranes and dialysate buffers. Am J Kidney Dis 36:130–139.
49. Poh CK, Hardy PA, Liao Z, Huang Z, Clark WR, Gao D (2003) Effect of spacer yarns on the dialysate flow distribution of hemodialyzers: a magnetic resonance imaging study. ASAIO J 49:440–448.
50. Ponikvar JB, Rus RR, Kenda RB, Bren AF, Ponikvar RR (2001) Low-flux versus high-flux synthetic dialysis membrane in acute renal failure: prospective randomized study. Artif Organs 25:946–950.
51. Port FK, Wolfe RA, Hulbert-Shearon TE, Daugirdas JT, Agodoa LY, Jones C, Orzol SM, Held PJ (2001) Mortality risk by hemodialyzer reuse practice and dialyzer membrane characteristics: Results from the USRDS Dialysis Morbidity and Mortality Study. Am J Kidney Dis 37:276–286.
52. Ramírez R, Carracedo J, Soriano S, Jiménez R, Martín-Malo A, Rodríguez M, Blasco M, Aljama P (2005) Stress-induced premature senescence in mononuclear cells from patients on long-term hemodialysis. Am J Kidney Dis 45:353–359.
53. Randoux C, Gillery P, Georges N, Lavaud S, Chanard J (2001) Filtration of native and glycated beta2-microglobulin by charged and neutral dialysis membranes. Kidney Int 60:1571–1577.
54. Ronco C, Bowry S (2001) Nanoscale modulation of the pore dimensions, size distribution and structure of a new polysulfone-based high-flux dialysis membrane. Int J Artif Organs 24:726–735.
55. Ronco C, Bellomo R, Homel P, Brendolan A, Dan M, Piccinni P, La Greca G (2000) Effects of different doses in continuous veno-venous haemofiltration on outcomes of acute renal failure: a prospective randomised trial. Lancet 356:26–30.
56. Ronco C, Brendolan A, Lupi A, Metry G, Levin NW (2000) Effects of a reduced inner diameter of hollow fibers in hemodialyzers. Kidney Int 58:809–817.
57. Ronco C, Bowry SK, Brendolan A, Crepaldi C, Soffiati G, Fortunato A, Bordoni V, Granziero A, Torsello G, La Greca G (2002) Hemodialyzer: from macro-design to membrane nanostructure; the case of the FX-class of hemodialyzers. Kidney Int Suppl. 80:126–142.
58. Ronco C, Bonello M, Bordoni V, Ricci Z, D'Intini V, Bellomo R, Levin NW (2004) Extracorporeal therapies in non-renal disease: treatment of sepsis and the peak concentration hypothesis. Blood Purif 22:164–174.
59. Ronco C, Levin N, Brendolan A, Nalesso F, Cruz D, Ocampo C, Kuang D, Bonello M, De Cal M, Corradi V, Ricci Z (2006) Flow distribution analysis by helical scanning in polysulfone hemodialyzers: effects of fiber structure and design on flow patterns and solute clearances. Hemodial Int 10:380–388.
60. Rosenkranz AR, Templ E, Traindl O, Heinzl H, Zlabinger GJ (1994) Reactive oxygen product formation by human neutrophils as an early marker for biocompatibility of dialysis membranes. Clin Exp Immunol 98:300–330.
61. Rousseau Y, Carreno MP, Poignet JL, Kazatchkine MD, Haeffner-Cavaillon N (1999) Dissociation between complement activation, integrin expression and neutropenia during hemodialysis. Biomaterials 20:1959–1967.
62. Sasaki M, Hosoya N, Saruhashi M (1999) Development of vitamin E-modified membrane. Contrib Nephrol 127: 49–70.
63. Satoh M, Yamasaki Y, Nagake Y, Kasahara J, Hashimoto M, Nakanishi N, Makino H (2001) Oxidative stress is reduced by the long-term use of vitamin E-coated dialysis filters. Kidney Int 59:1943–195.

64. Schiffl H, Lang SM, Konig A, Strasser T, Haider MC, Held E (1994) Biocompatible membranes in acute renal failure: prospective case-controlled study. Lancet 344:570–572.
65. Schiffl H, Lang SM, Stratakis D, Fischer R (2001) Effects of ultrapure dialysis fluid on nutritional status and inflammatory parameters. Nephrol Dial Transplant 16:1863–1869.
66. Schindler R, Lonnemann G, Schäffer J, Shaldon S, Koch KM, Krautzig S (1994) The effect of ultrafiltered dialysate on the cellular content of interleukin-1 receptor antagonist in patients on chronic hemodialysis. Nephron 68:229–233.
67. Schindler R, Christ-Kohlrausch F, Frei U, Shaldon S (2003) Differences in the permeability of high-flux dialyzer membranes for bacterial pyrogens.Clin Nephrol 59:447–454.
68. Simmons EM, Himmelfarb J, Sezer MT, Chertow GM, Mehta RL, Paganini EP, Soroko S, Freedman S, Becker K, Spratt D, Shyr Y, Ikizler TA; PICARD Study Group (2004) Plasma cytokine levels predict mortality in patients with acute renal failure. Kidney Int 65:1357–1365.
69. Sirolli V, Ballone E, Di Stante S, Amoroso L, Bonomini M (2002) Cell activation and cellular-cellular interactions during hemodialysis: effect of dialyzer membrane. Int J Artif Organs 25:529–537.
70. Sirolli V, Amoroso L, Pietropaolo M, Grandaliano G, Pertosa G, Bonomini M (2006) Platelet-leukocyte interactions in hemodialysis patients: culprit or bystander? Int J Immunopathol Pharmacol 19:461–470.
71. Sitter T, Bergner A, Schiffl H (2000) Dialysate related cytokine induction and response to recombinant human erythropoietin in haemodialysis patients. Nephrol Dial Transplant 15:1207–1211.
72. Soriano S, Martín-Malo A, Carracedo J, Ramírez R, Rodríguez M, Aljama P (2005) Lymphocyte apoptosis: role of uremia and permeability of dialysis membrane. Nephron Clin Pract 100:c71–c77.
73. Sosa MA, Balk EM, Lau J, Liangos O, Balakrishnan VS, Madias NE, Pereira BJG, Jaber BL (2006) A systematic review of the effect of the Excebrane dialyser on biomarkers of lipid peroxidation. Nephrol Dial Transplant 21:2825–2833.
74. Stewart RD, Cerny JC, Mahon HI (1964) The capillary "kidney": Preliminary report. Med Bull (Ann Arbor) 30:116–118.
75. Tarng DC, Huang TP, Liu TY, Chen HW, Sung YJ, Wei YH (2000) Effect of vitamin E-bonded membrane on the 8-hydroxy 2'-deoxyguanosine level in leukocyte DNA of hemodialysis patients. Kidney Int 58:790–799.
76. Thijs A, Grooteman MP, Zweegman S, Nubé MJ, Huijgens PC, Stehouwer CD (2007) Platelet activation during haemodialysis: comparison of cuprammonium rayon and polysulfone membranes. Blood Purif 25:389–394.
77. Tielemans C, Madhoun P, Lenaers M, Schandene L, Goldman M, Vanherweghem JL (1990) Anaphylactoid reactions during hemodialysis on AN69 membranes in patients receiving ACE inhibitors. Kidney Int 38:982–984.
78. Tielemans C, Husson C, Schurmans T, Gastaldello K, Madhoun P, Delville JP, Marchant A, Goldman M, Vanherweghem JL (1996) Effects of ultrapure and non-sterile dialysate on the inflammatory response during in vitro hemodialysis. Kidney Int 49:236–243.
79. Tumlin J, Wali R, Williams W, Murray P, Tolwani AJ, Vinnikova AK, Szerlip HM, Ye J, Paganini EP, Dworkin L, Finkel KW, Kraus MA, Humes HD (2008) Efficacy and safety of renal tubule cell therapy for acute renal failure. J Am Soc Nephrol 2008 Feb 13 [Epub ahead of print]
80. van Teijlingen ME, Nubé MJ, ter Wee PM, van Wijhe MH, Borgdorff P, Tangelder GJ (2003) Haemodialysis-induced pulmonary granulocyte sequestration in rabbits is organ specific. Nephrol Dial Transplant 18:2589–2595.
81. Verresen L, Waer M, Vanrenterghem Y, Michielsen P (1990) Angiotensin-converting-enzyme inhibitors and anaphylactoid reactions to high-flux membrane dialysis. Lancet 336:1360–1362.
82. Vos KD, Burris FO, Riley RL (1966) Kinetic study of the hydrolysis of cellulose acetate in the pH range of 2–10. J Appl Polymer Sci 10:825–832.
83. Wanner C, Bahner U, Mattern R, Lang D, Passlick-Deetjen J (2004) Effect of dialysis flux and membrane material on dyslipidaemia and inflammation in haemodialysis patients. Nephrol Dial Transplant 19:2570–2575.
84. Ward RA, McLeish KR (1995) Hemodialysis with cellulose membranes primes the neutrophil oxidative burst. Artif Organs 9:801–807.
85. Ward RA, Schaefer RM, Falkenhagen D, Joshua MS, Heidland A, Klinkmann H, Gurland HJ (1993) Biocompatibility of a new high-permeability modified cellulose membrane for haemodialysis. Nephrol Dial Transplant 8:47–53.
86. Weber V, Linsberger I, Rossmanith E, Weber C, Falkenhagen D (2004) Pyrogen transfer across high- and low-flux hemodialysis membranes. Artif Organs 28:210–217.
87. Woods HF, Nandakumar M (2000) Improved outcome for haemodialysis patients treated with high-flux membranes. Nephrol Dial Transplant 15 (Suppl 1):S36–S42.

Dialysates and Substitution Fluids

7.4

Isabelle Plamondon and Martine Leblanc

Core Messages

- The goal of renal replacement therapies is to maintain acid–base balance and physiologic electrolyte concentrations, to control azotemia, to resolve fluid overload, and to allow optimal nutrition.
- Dialysates and substitution fluids must be composed to suit the patients' requirements especially regarding acid–base status and electrolyte concentrations.
- To this end, bicarbonate-based fluids are routinely used for intermittent hemodialysis whilst dialysates and substitution fluids for continuous therapies can be either bicarbonate-based or lactate-buffered.
- Dialysate and substitution fluid may also serve as the source of the anticoagulant, e.g., in regional citrate anticoagulation.
- The temperature of dialysates and substitution fluids needs to be adequately controlled as it will impact on patients' body temperature.

7.4.1 Introduction

Acid–base status of critically ill patients certainly largely depends on their underlying condition; however, for patients on continuous renal replacement therapy (CRRT), the composition of the dialysate and substitution fluids used, as well as the operational characteristics of the therapy are the major determinants of the acid–base equilibrium and influence correction of any underlying imbalance.

The Stewart-Figge approach provides an explanation of the physiology of electrolytes and acid–base imbalance in critical illness [1]. Strong ions are considered almost completely dissociated in solutions; therefore, strong cations and anions in blood plasma are sodium $[(Na^+ + K^+ + Ca^{2+} + Mg^{2+}) - (Cl^- + \text{lactate})]$. Since the "normal" apparent strong ion difference of human blood plasma is 40–42 mmol/l, it can be concluded that unmeasured anions are normally present [2]. However, in critical illness, the apparent strong ion difference is often found to be lower, in the 30–35 mmol/l range, as a consequence of an underlying metabolic acidosis with excessive unmeasured anions, and also as the consequence of the low serum albumin usually found in such patients.

During critical illness, catabolism is greater and both nonvolatile acid production and volatile acid burden may be enhanced. Nonvolatile acid elimination is reduced in renal failure, and a normal strong ion difference can not be restored by the failing kidneys [3].

In renal failure, a mixed type of metabolic acidosis (both hyperchloremic and high-anion gap) is commonly found [4]; the apparent strong ion difference of renal failure patients is usually reduced. Chloride and unmeasured anions in blood plasma (phosphates, sulfates, various organic acids not completely oxidized, and other unknown molecules) just accumulate, being not eliminated by the kidneys. Hyperkalemia and hyperphosphatemia are common features in acute renal failure. Natremia can be variable but can be found low in cases of fluid overload, hypotonic enteral or parenteral nutrition and when drugs are administrated in dextrose solutions.

M. Leblanc (✉)
University of Montreal, Nephrology and Critical Care, Maisonneuve-Rosemont Hospital, 5415 boulevard de l'Assomption, Montreal, QC H1T 2M4, Canada
e-mail: martine.leblanc@sympatico.ca

A. Jörres et al. (eds.), *Management of Acute Kidney Problems*,
DOI: 10.1007/978-3-540-69441-0_7.4, © Springer-Verlag Berlin Heidelberg 2010

A high anion gap acidosis in critical illness may indicate hyperlactatemia but the latter may exist without acidemia. Moreover, the strong ion difference of fluid given to patients has an impact on their acid–base balance, and the effect can be marked when a patient has received massive amounts of fluid for resuscitation.

Patients on CRRT often have abnormal respiratory function with either respiratory acidosis or alkalosis. The respiratory component of the acid–base disturbance should be taken into account, even for patients in acute renal failure (ARF); efforts should be directed at normalizing the pH rather than only the bicarbonate level.

7.4.2 Fluids for CRRT

The goals of renal support in ARF are to restore acid–base balance and physiologic electrolyte concentrations, control azotemia, resolve fluid overload, and allow optimal nutrition.

Both the composition of fluids used for CRRT and the operational conditions of the CRRT system will be determinant in the achievement of such goals. Fluids used for CRRT include dialysate and replacement/substitution solutions with electrolytes in concentrations similar to those in normal blood plasma, except for electrolytes that are protein-bound. Preexisting deficits or excesses in water and/or electrolytes, as well as all inputs and losses should be taken into account to assess the impact of the CRRT treatment.

Supraphysiologic sodium concentration in the dialysate is a recognized tool to improve hemodynamic stability during intermittent hemodialysis. To our knowledge, in CRRT, there is no study that has evaluated whether the use of supraphysiologic concentrations of sodium help maintain hemodynamics or improve the outcome after head injury.

When initiating CRRT, a solution containing no potassium is often needed since hyperkalemia is frequent in ARF. If treatment is prolonged, a commercial solution containing potassium has to be used, or potassium supplement should be added to the replacement fluid and/or dialysate. Commercial solutions exist with different potassium concentrations (Table 7.4.1).

Hyperphosphatemia is a typical disturbance in ARF; nonetheless, the majority of patients on CRRT will require phosphate supplementation shortly after CRRT initiation, despite nutritional support. Commercial replacement solutions and dialysates contain no phosphate. Phosphate salts can be added to the dialysate and replacement fluid to achieve final phosphate concentration within the normal range [5]. However, oral or parenteral supplementation is the preferred option in most centers.

The magnesium concentration in the different solutions is at the lower limit of the normal serum range, while the calcium concentration is usually higher than the normal blood plasma ionized calcium concentration. Using a calcium content in dialysate/replacement fluid higher than in blood plasma results in a net calcium influx, especially when considering that most patients are hypoalbuminemic. A slightly higher calcium concentration in CRRT solutions may help

Table 7.4.1 Composition of some of the commercially available fluids of CRRT (ion concentrations in mmol/l)

	Plasma	Accusol (Baxter)	Prism0cal (Gambro)	Prismasol (Gambro)	Premixed dialysate (Baxter)	PrismaSate dialysate (Gambro)	Normocarb HF (Dialysis solutions)
Na^+	135–145	140	140	140	140	0–3.5	140
K^+	3.3–5.0	0–4	0	0–4	2	0–4	0
Cl^-	100–108	109.5–116.3	106	106.5–111.5	117	108.0–120.5	106.5–116.5
Ca^{2+}	1.15–1.30	0–1.75	0	0–1.75	1.75	0–3.5	0
Mg^{2+}	0.7–1.0	0.5–0.75	0.5	0.5–0.75	0.75	1.0–1.5	0.75
Phosphate	1.0	0	0	0	0	0	0
HCO_3	22–26	30–35	32	32	0	22–32	25–35
Lactate	0.5–2.0	0	3	3	30	3	0
pH	7.4	7.4		7.0–8.5			8.55 ± 0.25
Dextrose anhydrous (mg/dl)	70–110	0–100	0	0–100	100	0–110	0

improve hemodynamic stability, as shown for intermittent hemodialysis in an acute care setting.

Several of the commercially available solutions and their content are presented in Table 7.4.1. Despite slight differences, it may not be convenient to have several solutions in stock, in a single institution. Most of the time, two different solutions are selected, providing suitable options for the metabolic needs of most patients, also knowing that adjustments can be achieved with enteral or parenteral supplements. Shelf-life of commercial substitution fluids is usually 1 year. Some centers prefer to customize their fluids to avoid storage and for financial reasons. Errors are more frequent with customized solutions.

Because a loss of glucose (and thus calories) occurs through the effluent, a physiologic glucose concentration (near 5 mmol/l) in dialysate and replacement fluid may be preferred. On the other hand, if glucose losses are accounted for in the nutritional regimen, solutions without dextrose can also be used. Solutions with supraphysiologic glucose or dextrose content should be avoided, since they may induce hyperglycemia which is associated with poor outcomes. Moreover, dextrose-containing solutions may enhance lactate production, possibly detrimental in presence of brain injury [6]. We currently ignore the effect of glucose degradation products resulting from heat sterilization of hyperglycemic solutions (such as the peritoneal dialysate previously used at the beginning of the technique and still used in some countries).

Since the replacement or substitution fluid is directly infused into the circulation, the solutions should preferably be sterile. Commercial solutions are heat-sterilized. Backdiffusion and/or backfiltration of cytokine-inducing substances can theoretically occur during CRRT. Membrane hydraulic permeability and transmembrane pressure are the main factors influencing backfiltration. Membranes with high adsorptive capabilities could reduce the risk in theory. The literature on CRRT does not stipulate if the dialysate fluid should be sterile or not. We may see in the near future more sophisticated CRRT solutions, for example containing nutrients or antioxidants. More research is definitely required in that area. Whatever solution is used, electrolytes and acid–base balance should be assessed frequently during CRRT, especially if high-volume exchanges are performed.

7.4.3 Choice of Buffer

The strong ion difference (SID) of CRRT solutions has a significant impact on the patient's acid–base balance, especially when high rates or massive amounts are delivered. It can be appreciated that strong ion differences of commercially available solutions for CRRT are relatively close to the strong ion difference of normal human blood plasma, compared with normal saline (with a SID of 0) and to Ringer's lactate (with a SID of 28). Buffer anion in CRRT fluids is usually in a concentration above 25–30 mmol/l [7].

One of the major objectives of CRRT is to restore and maintain acid–base homeostasis. Acidemia has deleterious effects on cardiovascular hemodynamics. A loss of buffer base occurs during CRRT, whether pure hemofiltration, dialysis, or hemodiafiltration mode is chosen. Replacement of forced bicarbonate loss and correction of systemic acidemia require buffer replacement either through replacement fluid or from dialysate. As the main alkalinazing anion, citrate and bicarbonate are the most frequently used in CRRT solutions.

The availability of commercial bicarbonate-based fluids for CRRT is relatively recent due to manufacturing and storage difficulties. Indeed, a higher pH increases the risk of bacterial contamination and precipitation of divalent cations (Ca and Mg) [8]. Moreover, during storage, bicarbonate dissociates into carbonate and CO_2, requiring the storage of the solution in a CO_2 impermeable container. Some bicarbonate-based solutions currently available (Accusol and Prismasol) are packaged in two-compartment bags, one containing electrolytes and the other the buffer. The solution is reconstituted prior to use. There is also on the market an electrolyte concentrate (Normocarb HF) containing no lactate, no calcium with a reconstituted concentration of bicarbonate of 25–35 mEq/l.

Another option is to use a dialysate containing no buffer concomitantly with the administration of $NaHCO_3$ given distally in the renal replacement circuit or via a distant venous access.

Lactate solutions are usually well tolerated because the human body can rapidly metabolize large amounts of lactate (at a rate of 100 mmol/h for as much as 2,000 mmol/day). It is converted by the liver into bicarbonate in a 1:1 ratio and usually does not remain in circulation as a strong ion for a long time. The sieving coefficient of lactate in continuous venovenous hemofiltration (CVVH) or continuous venovenous hemodiafiltration (CVVHDF) is close to 1; therefore, lactate filter clearance is similar to the ultrafiltration (or ultradiafiltration) flow rate. The filter lactate clearance during CVVHDF when using bicarbonate-buffered fluids is negligible compared with the total systemic lactate clearance, and the blood plasma lactate concentration remains a reliable marker of systemic hypoperfusion [9]. Controlled trials have demonstrated that lactate or bicarbonate-buffered solutions for CRRT have a similar efficacy to correct metabolic acidosis [10–12]. However, serum lactate was found to be slightly higher with use of lactate solutions, without clear evidence of detrimental impact on outcome. Nonetheless, this may complicate the clinical interpretation of blood lactate levels.

Generally, the use of bicarbonate-buffered fluids has been associated with an improved control of metabolic acidosis [13]. Although lactate solutions are well tolerated during CRRT when infused at moderate flows of 2–3 l/h, the infusion of large amounts of D,L-lactate could possible increase catabolism and induce cerebral dysfunction [14]. In addition, in patients who are limited in their capacity to convert lactate (liver failure or severe shock), lactate solutions should be avoided. In such circumstances, the infused lactate anion remains in circulation as a strong anion, while the endogenous bicarbonate is lost through the effluent, both contributing to a metabolic acidosis. Replacement fluid used during CRRT for critically ill patients with severe hepatic failure and acute renal failure are generally bicarbonate-based solutions. Despite that choice, blood plasma lactate concentration often remains abnormally high with persistent lactic acidosis and low bicarbonate levels [15]. Lactate and unmeasured anions uptake is altered in severe hepatic failure and has a significant impact on acid–base balance, even during CRRT.

Acetate has also been proposed as the alkalinizing anion, since it is metabolized into bicarbonate by the liver and the muscle in a 1:1 ratio. However, acetate has not been frequently used in CRRT fluids, probably because of uneventful effects of hyperacetatemia observed previously with intermittent hemodialysis. The impact of acetate-based fluids in CRRT are poorly defined. In 84 critically ill patients with acute renal failure treated with continuous venovenous hemofiltration (CVVH), substitution with lactate was associated with a significant increase in serum bicarbonate and in blood pH after 48 h when compared with acetate [16].

7.4.4 Citrate Anticoagulation

Lactate has fallen out of favor, and citrate has gained in popularity in recent years. Citrate is a chelator of calcium, an essential cofactor in the coagulation cascade. It is used for regional anticoagulation of the extracorporeal circuit during CRRT. Citrate is infused in the arterial line of the circuit and anticoagulates the blood in the extracorporeal circuit only. A calcium infusion at the end of the venous line or in the periphery reverses anticoagulation. Thus, this approach does not confer systemic anticoagulation. Even for critically ill patients at low risk of bleeding, the risk of a bleeding event and the need for red blood cell transfusion have been shown to be lower during CVVH with citrate anticoagulation compared with unfractionated heparin anticoagulation [17].

Beside its anticoagulant role, citrate also serves as the main alkalinizing anion being converted into bicarbonate by the tricarboxylic pathway in the liver and by the muscle in a 1:3 ratio. If sodium tricitrate is administered without taking into account the sodium load, hypernatremia may occur. Hypocalcemia and hypomagnesemia are also predictable if appropriate substitution is not provided. Hypercalcemia is also possible if too much calcium is infused. This technique is particularly appealing for patients at risk for bleeding and with thrombocytopenia [18]. It should be used very cautiously in patients with liver impairment, shock, and high anion gap metabolic acidosis. Indeed, in patients with severe liver failure, citrate can accumulate and induce a progressive metabolic acidosis and a fall in systemic ionized calcium level. Regional citrate anticoagulation may prolong circuit survival compared with systemic heparin anticoagulation, but the results are inconsistent in the literature [17,19].

Several regional citrate anticoagulation regimens for CRRT have been proposed. Cointault et al. [20] suggested a protocol where citrate (3.22%; 112.9 mmol/l) is delivered prefilter by an independent pump. The replacement solution and the dialysate are calcium-containing standard commercial isotonic solution (Hemosol®; Hospal, Lyon, France). The dialysate composition was adapted according to the patient's acid–base status by adding different quantity of bicarbonate to the Hemosol® B0 solution. To compensate for the loss of calcium through the filter, a calcium chloride solution was infused in the venous line of the circuit.

Tolwani et al. published a protocol using a non-concentrated citrate solution (0.50% or 18 mmol/l trisodium citrate solution) as replacement fluid with a bicarbonate-based dialysate [21]. They achieved effluent rates of 35 ml/kg/h. Calcium gluconate was administered through a separate line. A similar protocol was published by Gabutti et al. [22], but they used the same diluted citrate solution (13.30 mmol/l) as substitution and dialysate fluids.

We suggested a protocol using Hemocitrasol-20 (Na 145 mmol/l, Cl 100 mmol/l, citrate 20 mmol/l, and glucose 10 mmol/l), a manufactured solution (by Biosol, Sondalo, Italy) for Hospal-Gambro as substitution fluid in predilution [23]. Blood flow rate was 125 ml/min with an initial flow rate of the replacement fluid of 1,250 ml/h and adjusted subsequently according to a scale of the activated coagulation time measured posthemofilter. When a diffusive component of clearance was added, the dialysate solution was normal saline 0.9% at a rate of 1 l/h. A calcium plus magnesium-containing solution was infused using a separate intravenous pump in the venous blood line return.

Most studies on citrate CRRT show correction of the metabolic acidosis [12]. However, since one molecule of citrate provides three molecules of bicarbonate, metabolic alkalosis may ensue. [24]. Citrate delivery is titrated according to its anticoagulation properties and not according to its effect on the plasmatic pH. When citrate metabolism is not impaired, the quantity of citrate administrated will determine its effect on acid–base status.

7.4.5 Influence of CRRT Prescription

Diffusion, the main exchange mechanism in continuous venovenous hemodialysis (CVVHD), is excellent for removing small molecules but is much more limited for middle-sized solutes. Cations and anions involved in the strong ion difference are available to be exchanged by diffusive fluxes. Convection is the exchange mechanism used during CVVH. Most ions considered in the strong ion difference equation pass easily through the membrane with convective fluxes and have sieving coefficients near one. Thus, diffusion and convection are both efficient processes to restore electrolytes and acid–base balance. However, there are differences in biochemical outcomes between the different approaches. CVVHDF and CVVH have a different effect on electrolytes and acid–base homeostasis despite obtaining comparable blood and dialysate/replacement fluid flow rate [25].

During convection, large amounts of bicarbonate can be lost in the ultrafiltration, inducing potentially rapidly a metabolic acidosis if not replaced appropriately by the substitution fluid. For example, during CVVH at an ultrafiltration rate of 3 l/h, as much as 50 mmol of HCO^{-}_{3} can be lost hourly. The amount of bicarbonate lost in the effluent can be easily assessed since both the sieving coefficient and ultrafiltration rate are known. If the replacement consists in normal saline, a hyperchloremic acidosis would rapidly occur. Since the composition of replacement fluids can be flexible, the alkalinizing performance of CVVH may be superior to CVVHD and may be more versatile.

Continuous renal replacement therapies provide a constant restoration of electrolytes and acid–base balance, avoiding large fluctuations. However, since flow rates during CRRT are lower than during intermittent modalities, acid–base balance restoration is progressive and usually occurs over 36–48 h in most cases. As well, at usual CRRT rates in average-size patients, a metabolic steady state is expected to occur after 3 or 4 days; this may apply to several electrolytes [26].

When applying higher flows, for example to reach an ultrafiltration rate of 35 ml/kg/h, as recommended by Ronco et al. [27], acid–base correction and metabolic steady state may both occur sooner. In high-volume CVVH, because of the potential massive influx of lactate anions, bicarbonate fluids are recommended. On the other hand, a metabolic alkalosis may be induced by high-volume CVVH if using replacement fluids containing too much bicarbonate, and its concentration may have to be reduced under certain circumstances.

Replacement solution can be infused before or after the hemofilter. In the prefilter mode, the solution dilutes the blood cellular component improving blood rheology and thus, enhancing filter patency and/or diminishing anticoagulation needs. Higher ultrafiltration rate could be obtained with predilution, but for the same ultrafiltration rate, solute clearance is smaller compared with postdilution. To obtain similar clearances, more ultrafiltration volume and replacement fluid are required as well as more porous membranes with a larger surface area for high-volume CVVH [13]. Postdilutional treatments are limited by filter clotting if the filtration fraction is too high. The maximal blood flow delivered by the catheter is also a limitation. The sieving coefficient of cations and anions is also affected as whether the predilutional or the postdilutional mode is chosen [28].

As a general statement, it can be said that the net effect on acid—base status induced by the different CCRT approaches depends on the buffer concentration in the substitution/dialysate fluids, the metabolic conversion rate of the buffers, the total ultradiafiltration (or effluent) rate, the predilution or postdilution modes, in addition to the initial blood plasma acid–base balance [29].

7.4.6 Temperature

Renal support with CRRT has an impact on body temperature; energy is lost within the circuit, but patient body weight and presence or absence of intact thermal autoregulatory mechanisms have an influence [30]. A low blood flow and a high dialysate or replacement solution infusion rate both increase the heat loss from blood in the extracorporeal circuit. The cooling effect of CRRT could contribute to the better hemodynamic stability after CRRT initiation. It has been suggested that patients treated by hemofiltration have less symptomatic hypotension than patients on hemodiafiltration. Cooling the dialysate could decrease the disparity in vascular reactivity between the two modalities of treatment since the difference in arterial blood pressure appears related to variations in the extracorporeal blood temperature [31]. Hypothermia is also beneficial for cerebral protection by reducing oxygen consumption. However, it may have a negative impact on the heat shock response and decrease time to clotting of the circuit. Moreover, nutritional calorific balance is affected by extracorporeal heat loss, but also by reduction of the metabolic rate induced by hypothermia. Hypothermia may be avoided or controlled by using a heating device.

7.4.7 High Volume Hemofiltration

High-volume hemofiltration (6–8 l/h exchange rate) has been advocated to improve patient outcomes. However, the risk of acid–base and electrolyte imbalances is high, and this technique requires well-balanced fluids. As the current substitution fluids are not designed for high volume CVVH, electrolytes and acid–base balance should be assessed frequently during CRRT, or else, customized solutions may be required. An approach limiting high volume CVVH to short periods of time may be a reasonable alternative [28].

7.4.8 Take Home Pearls

- Dialysates and substitution fluids need to be composed in a suitable fashion to enable the correction of metabolic acidosis and to maintain physiologic electrolyte concentrations
- Bicarbonate-based fluids are routinely used for intermittent hemodialysis; dialysates and substitution fluids for continuous therapies can be bicarbonate-based or lactate-buffered
- Substitution fluids administered in predilution fashion can also be used as the source of the anticoagulant such as in regional citrate anticoagulation
- Controlling the temperature of dialysates and substitution fluids is important as this will impact on body temperature of patients

References

1. Kellum JA. Metabolic acidosis in the critically ill: Lessons from physical chemistry. Kidney Int 1997;53(Suppl 66): S81–S86.
2. Leblanc M, Kellum JA. Biochemical and biophysical principles of hydrogen ion regulation. In Ronco C, Bellomo R (eds). Critical Care Nephrology, 1 edn. Dordrecht, Kluwer, 1998, pp 261–277.
3. Warnock DG. Uremic acidosis. Kidney Int 1988;34: 278–287.
4. Wallia R, Greenberg A, Piraino B, Mitrio R, Puschett JB. Serum electrolytes in end-stage renal disease. Am J Kidney Dis 1986;8:98–104.
5. Troyanov S, Geadah D, Ghannoum M, Cardinal J, Leblanc M. Phosphate addition to hemodiafiltration solutions during continuous renal replacement therapy. Intensive Care Med 2004; 30:1662–1665.
6. Sieber FE, Traystman RJ. Special issues: Glucose and the brain. Critical Care Med 1992;20:104–114.
7. Macias WL, Clark WR. Acid-base balance in continuous renal replacement therapy. Seminars in Dialysis 1996;9: 145–151.

8. Maccariello E, Rocha E, Dalboni MA, Ferreira AT, Draibe S, Cendoroglo M. Customized bicarbonate buffered dialysate and replacement solutions for continuous renal replacement therapies: Effect of crystallization on the measured levels of electrolytes and buffer. Artif Organs 2001; 25:870–875.
9. Levraut, J, Ciebiera, J-P, Jambou, P, Ichai, C, Labib Y, Grimaud D. Effect of continuous venovenous hemofiltration with dialysis on lactate clearance in critically ill patients. Critical Care Med 1997 25:58–62.
10. Thomas AN, Guy JM, Kishen R, Geraghty IF, Bowles BJ, Vadgama P. Comparison of lactate and bicarbonate buffered haemofiltration fluids: Use in critically ill patients. Nephrol Dial Transplant 1997;12:1212–1217.
11. Heering P, Ivens K, Thumer OM, Grabensee B. Acid-base balance and substitution fluid during continuous hemofiltration. Kidney Int 1999;56(Suppl 72):S37–S40.
12. Zimmerman D, Cotman P, Ting R, Karanicolas S, Tobe SW. Continuous veno-venous haemodialysis with a novel bicarbonate dialysis solution: Prospective cross-over comparison with a lactate buffered solution. Nephrol Dial Transplantation 1999;14:2387–2391.
13. Schetz M, Leblanc M, Murrray P. The Acute Dialysis Quality Initiative VII: Fluid composition and management in CRRT. Adv Renal Replace Ther 2002;9:282–289.
14. Veech RL. The untoward effects of the anions of dialysis fluid. Kidney Int 1988;34:587–597.
15. Naka T, Bellomo R, Morimatsu H, Rocktaschel J, Wan L, Gow P, Angus P. Acid-base balance during continuous venovenous hemofiltration: the impact of severe hepatic failure. Int J Artif Organs 2006;29:668–674.
16. Morgera S, Heering P, Szentandrasi T, Manassa E, Heintzen M, Willers R, Passklick-Deetjen J, Grabensee B. Comparison of a lactate-versus acetate-based hemofiltration replacement fluid in patients with acute renal failure. Renal Failure 1997;19:155–164.
17. Betjes MG, van Oosterom D, van Agteren M, van de Wetering J. Regional citrate versus heparin anticoagulation during venovenous hemofiltration in patients at low risk for bleeding: similar hemofilter survival but significantly less bleeding. J Nephrol 2007;20:602–608.
18. Palsson R, Laliberte KA, Niles JL. Choice of replacement solution and anticoagulant in continuous venovenous hemofiltration. Clin Nephrol 2006 Jan;65:34–42.
19. Monchi M, Berghmans D, Ledoux D, Canivet JL, Dubois B, Damas P. Citrate vs. heparin for anticoagulation in continuous venovenous hemofiltration: A prospective randomized study. Intensive Care Med 2004;30:260–265. Epub 2003 Nov 5
20. Cointault O, Kamar N, Bories P, Lavayssiere L, Angles O, Rostaing L, Genestal M, Durand D. Regional citrate anticoagulation in continuous venovenous haemodiafiltration using commercial solutions. Nephrol Dial Transplantation 2004;19:171–178.
21. Tolwani AJ, Prendergast MB, Speer RR, Stofan BS, Wille KM. A practical citrate anticoagulation continuous venovenous hemodiafiltration protocol for metabolic control and high solute clearance. Clin J Am Soc Nephrol. 2006;1: 79–87. Epub 2005 Nov 23
22. Gabutti L, Marone C, Colucci G, Duchini F. Citrate anticoagulation in continuous venovenous hemodiafiltration: a metabolic challenge. Intensive Care Med 2002;28:1419–1425. Epub 2002 Sep 6
23. Dorval M, Madore F, Courteau S, Leblanc M. A novel citrate anticoagulation regimen for continuous venovenous hemodiafiltration. Intensive Care Med 2003;29:1186–1189. Epub 2003 May 22.
24. Morgera S, Scholle C, Voss G, Haase M, Vargas-Hein O, Krausch D, Melzer C, Rosseau S, Zuckermann-Becker H, Neumayer HH. Metabolic complications during regional citrate anticoagulation in continuous venovenous hemodialysis: single-center experience. Nephron Clin Pract. 2004; 97(4):c131–136.
25. Morimatsu H, Uchino S, Bellomo R, Ronco C. Continuous renal replacement therapy: does technique influence electrolyte and bicarbonate control? Int J Artif Organs. 2003 Apr;26 (4):289–296.
26. Clark WR, Mueller BA, Kraus MA, Macias WL. Extracorporeal therapy requirements for patients with acute renal failure. J Am Soc Nephrol 1997;8:804–812.
27. Ronco C, Bellomo R, Homel P, Brendolan A, Dan M, Piccinni P, La Greca G. Effects of different doses in continuous venovenous haemofiltration on outcomes of acute renal failure: A prospective randomized trial. Lancet 2000;356: 26–30.
28. Davenport A. Potential adverse effects of replacing high volume hemofiltration exchanges on electrolyte balance and acid-base status using the current commercially available replacement solutions in patients with acute renal failure. Int J Artif Organs. 2008;31(1):3–5.
29. Bouchard J, Mehta RL. Acid-base disturbances in the intensive care unit: Current issues and the use of continuous renal replacement therapy as a customized treatment tool. Int J Artif Organs. 2008;31:6–14.
30. Yagi N, Leblanc M, Sakai K, Wright EJ, Paganini EP. Cooling effect of continuous renal replacement therapy in critically ill patients. Am J Kidney Dis. 1998;32:1023–30.
31. van Kuijk WH, Hillion D, Savoiu C, Leunissen KM. Critical role of the extracorporeal blood temperature in the hemodynamic response during hemofiltration. J Am Soc Nephrol. 1997;8:949–55.

7.5 Intermittent Hemodialysis

Christophe Vinsonneau and Mourad Benyamina

Core Messages

- Intermittent hemodialysis (IHD) is not only the preferred treatment option for patients with isolated kidney failure, but also the most powerful method to quickly control life-threatening situations associated with acute kidney failure, such as severe hyperkalemia, severe metabolic acidosis, and pulmonary edema with fluid overload in oliguric patients without severe hemodynamic impairment.
- As intermittent hemodialysis can often be performed without anticoagulation it may also have advantages in patients at risk of bleeding complications.
- Intermittent hemodialysis can be used in various modalities, combining diffusion and convection with different session frequency or duration:
  - Conventional IHD
  - Sequential IHD
  - Sustained low-efficiency dialysis (SLED)

7.5.1 Introduction

Until the early 1980s, intermittent hemodialysis (IHD) was the only available method to treat patients with acute renal failure (ARF) in intensive care units (ICUs). IHD was first developed for chronic renal failure patients and was implemented in nephrology. This is why nephrologists became the specialists who administered IHD to ARF patients in ICUs. However, the implementation of IHD derived from nephrology practices raised some concerns, especially as regards hemodynamic tolerance. The description of a new mode of renal replacement therapy (RRT), continuous arteriovenous hemofiltration (CAVH), by Kramer et al. in 1977 [1] offered a new way to treat ARF. Given the arteriovenous access, the treatment was directly controlled by the arterial pressure, which led to improved hemodynamic tolerance. In the absence of well-conducted comparative studies, continuous hemofiltration (usually called continuous renal replacement therapy [CRRT]) gained wide acceptance in ICUs [2] to treat ARF because of its supposedly better hemodynamic tolerance and its easy bedside use. Meanwhile IHD improved, in particular for the treatment of ARF. Based on clinical studies, IHD standards for ICU patients became quite different from the ones of chronic renal failure patients. Hemodynamic tolerance and therefore efficiency were improved by the use of synthetic membranes, bicarbonate-based buffers, and specific settings [3].

Despite an abundant literature comparing IHD with CRRT in critically ill patients, no significant differences in terms of mortality or renal recovery have ever been shown [4–7] – even in the most recent prospective randomized studies [8–9]. Therefore, it appears that both methods can be used in critically ill

C. Vinsonneau (✉)
Department of Intensive Care, Cochin Port-Royal, University Hospital, René Descartes University, 75014 Paris, France
e-mail: christophe.vinsonneau@cch.aphp.fr

A. Jörres et al. (eds.), *Management of Acute Kidney Problems*,
DOI: 10.1007/978-3-540-69441-0_7.5, © Springer-Verlag Berlin Heidelberg 2010

patients and that almost all patients can be treated with IHD [9]. The two methods appear complementary and can be used for specific indications, given their own advantages and limitations.

7.5.2 Operational Characteristics of IHD

7.5.2.1 Physical Principles

In IHD, molecule removal is driven by a concentration gradient between the vascular and dialysate side of the membrane, using a diffusive mechanism of exchange. This method favors small molecule removal given their high diffusibility across the membrane and provides a high efficiency (clearance around 200 ml/min). In a standard way, this method is based on a high dialysate flow (500 ml/min) but needs, however, a high blood flow (250–300 ml/min).

In contrast to IHD, CRRT refers to all extrarenal therapies using convection as solute or water removal mechanism. Therefore, solute and water removals are driven by a pressure gradient between blood and the ultrafiltrate side of the membrane. In IHD a certain amount of convection is used during each session to remove excess fluids, which is called "net ultrafiltration." Its effect on metabolic control or solute removal is however nonsignificant.

7.5.2.2 Technical Aspects

The implementation of IHD needs some specific equipment: a dialysis machine, a water treatment system, and electrolyte concentrates. Some other aspects may be quite different from CRRT: i.e., vascular access, dialysis membrane, and anticoagulation.

7.5.2.2.1 Dialysis Machine

The machine is devoted to the production of the dialysate using the online-prepared pure water and the electrolyte concentrates, as well as the extracorporeal blood circulation, to control the ultrafiltration and for monitoring of the treatment. Different safety alarms are available especially to monitor the circuit pressure, and the presence of air or blood leakage across the membrane. Recent improvements have been implemented in some machines, such as the online monitoring of the ionic dialysance (delivered dialysis dose) or the blood volume.

The machine used in ICU must be robust, compact, and easy to use for the ICU team.

7.5.2.2.2 Pure Water

The microbiologic quality of the prepared water is essential to achieve the best tolerance, including the absence of endotoxin which may pass through the membrane from the dialysate to the vascular side. From the water supply, inorganic and organic substances are removed to obtain pure water. The water treatment system is composed of filters, charcoal cartridge, and a reverse osmosis system. The water delivery may use three different approaches: a central distribution from a specific water treatment system as in a chronic hemodialysis unit, a mobile water treatment incorporated in the dialysis machine, or more recently a batch-delivered system [10]. Each system presents some limitations.

7.5.2.2.3 Dialysate

The electrolytic composition of the dialysate should achieve a good electrolytic equilibrium and a good uremic control at the end of the session. The choice of the electrolytic concentrate is of paramount importance. The standard buffer is now bicarbonate based, given the hemodynamic effects provided by the old acetate-based buffer. For the electrolytic solution, particular attention has to be paid to the potassium concentration (from 2 to 3 mmol/l) and the calcium concentration (from 1.25 to 1.75 mmol/l), the final concentrations of which are defined by the solution used. The final sodium concentration (from 140 to 150 mmol/l) and bicarbonate concentration (from 30 to 36 mmol/l), however, may be selected on the dialysis machine and may be modified during treatment. The dialysate flow may be modified in almost all machines (from 500 to 1,000 ml/min). The reduction of the dialysate flow is one of the ways to decrease the solute removal when hemodynamic instability is present or when a prolongation of the dialysis session is considered (see Section 7.5.4.3 SLED).

7.5.2.2.4 Vascular Access

For the treatment of ARF in the ICU, double-lumen catheters are used instead of single-lumen catheters. The latter needs a dialysis machine able to deliver dialysis using the mode "single-needle" but is associated with higher recirculation, decreasing the delivered dialysis dose. The best insertion site providing the higher blood flow is the right jugular vein, but femoral access still remain the emergency site and is associated with a lower rate of acute complications during insertion. Concerning the rate of nosocomial infection between jugular and femoral access, recent data seem to challenge the usually reported higher rate of infection with femoral access [11].The subclavian access should be avoided due to the high rate of venous stenosis following dialysis catheter insertion. Usually the use of an arteriovenous fistula in chronic renal failure patients is discouraged in the ICU because of the risk of infection, the risk of low cardiac output, and the low levels of experience of many ICU nurses. The use of a long-term cuffed catheter may be considered after the acute phase in a stable patient, but the occurrence of systemic infection leads usually to catheter removal. The diameter of the catheter is important to consider, to obtain a good blood flow with acceptable pressures. In this setting, 12F seems to be the minimum acceptable inner diameter.

7.5.2.2.5 Dialysis Membrane

Two different membrane families are available: cellulosic (unmodified or modified) and synthetic membranes (polysulfone, polyacrylonitrile, polymethylmethacrylate, and polyamide). Unmodified cellulosic membranes have a low molecular permeability and a low ultrafiltration coefficient. In addition, they are well known to activate inflammation (complement and leukocyte activation) which is described as a "bioincompatibility" property. This induces hemodynamic impairment and may induce pulmonary and kidney damage. In ARF patients, modified cellulosic or synthetic membranes are preferred. Several studies have shown that these latter, when compared with unmodified cellulosic membrane, could be able to improve the survival and the renal recovery of patients treated for ARF, which was barely significant in a recent meta-analysis [12]. In contrast, no study has reported any significant difference for major outcomes between modified cellulosic or synthetic membranes, or between different synthetic membranes. Concerning the molecular permeability or the ultrafiltration coefficient, no study has demonstrated that high permeability or high-flux membranes are needed to treat ARF. The surface of the membrane is usually between 1.3 and 1.6 m^2. Larger surfaces need to be used with caution to avoid retrofiltration.

7.5.2.2.6 Anticoagulation

One of the major advantages of IHD however is the lower need for anticoagulation compared with CRRT. Some authors have reported that IHD may be used without any anticoagulation, but usually for short-duration sessions [13]. New membranes (heparin-coated) can be used without anticoagulation after a priming with heparin and may offer a longer duration. Unfractionated heparin remains, however, the conventional anticoagulant in IHD. Several other options may be used including low-molecular-weight heparin, regional citrate anticoagulation, heparinoids, hirudin, or prostacyclin. Regional heparinization with protamine infusion is no longer recommended given the systemic anticoagulation usually observed. Heparinoids and hirudin may be used for heparin-induced thrombocytopenia. Regional citrate anticoagulation may also be used when heparin is contraindicated, or for patients at high risk of bleeding.

7.5.3 Advantages and Limits

The high efficiency achieved with IHD is responsible for a rapid decrease of the concentration gradient, leading to a decrease in the removal rate that limits the amount of solute removed. This explains why IHD is used discontinuously, usually for 4–6 h every day or every other day. This high efficiency and the short

Table 7.5.1 Advantages and limitations of intermittent hemodialysis

Advantage	Limitation
High clearance for small molecules	Hemodynamic tolerance
Patient's mobility	Abrupt osmolality variation
Several patients treated a day with one machine	Fluid management
Low or no anticoagulation, low bleeding risk	Unpredictable dialysis dose
Low cost	Microbiologic safety
	Nurse training

duration of each session explain some important differences between IHD and CRRT (Table 7.5.1):

- The refilling of urea from the interstitial space to the vascular compartment is limited during the session and occurs soon after the end of the treatment. Given the high extravascular volume of urea distribution, we observe a significant increase of serum urea after each session that is called urea rebound. This phenomenon limits IHD efficiency.
- The rapid exchange of solute induces high and fast osmolality variations during the treatment. These variations involve the vascular compartment and may induce hemodynamic instability as well as cellular edema, which is particularly deleterious for the brain.
- The fluid balance control needs high ultrafiltrate rates considering the short session duration which may be involved in hemodynamic impairment.

These characteristics offer, however, some advantages (Table 7.5.1). The nurse's workload is diminished, the patient's mobility is preserved, and the bleeding risk is decreased because of low exposure to anticoagulants. On top of that, from a practical point of view, one machine can treat several patients a day, whereas continuous therapies require one monitor for each patient-day. Yet IHD presents some technical limitations in the ICU: it demands a specific water production unit, more complex care provider training, and, in many countries, the intervention of a nephrology team.

7.5.4 Different Modalities

Several modalities can be used combining diffusion and convection with different session frequency or duration.

7.5.4.1 Conventional IHD

This modality is directly derived from the use in chronic dialysis units. The sessions are performed on a daily or alternate-day basis. In the ICU, short daily dialysis has become very popular to improve hemodynamic tolerance, fluid balance control, and metabolic control, as reported by Schiffl et al. [14].

7.5.4.2 Sequential IHD

Ultrafiltration and diffusion are not performed simultaneously during the same session. Usually, ultrafiltration is performed alone using convection to manage the fluid balance, and thereafter, diffusion is used alone. In hemodynamically unstable patients, this modality has been reported to improve the hemodynamic tolerance.

7.5.4.3 Sustained Low-Efficiency Dialysis

The principle behind sustained low-efficiency dialysis (SLED) is to decrease the solute clearance and to maintain the treatment over prolonged periods of time. The dialysate and the blood flow rate are decreased (100 and 200 ml/min, respectively) and the session duration is increased (8–10 h). The lower clearance induces a lower solute removal rate and a lower decrease of the concentration gradient. Therefore, the refilling from the interstitium to the vascular bed is enhanced, and given the prolonged duration of the treatment, the effective solute removal (i.e., efficiency) is increased. The hemodynamic tolerance of SLED has been reported to be equivalent to that of CRRT. The Genius system from Fresenius (Fresenius Medical Care Germany, Bad Homburg, Germany) is dedicated to SLED, even if the machine may provide standard IHD [10].

7.5.5 Specificity of IHD Use in ICU

Many pathophysiologic differences are obvious between chronic renal failure and ARF. In addition, ARF is usually part of a multiple-organ failure syndrome with hemodynamic instability in the ICU patient. Therefore, specific settings are needed to treat ICU patients with IHD. In this population, the main objectives are metabolic control and good hemodynamic tolerance to avoid any further damage to the kidney and other organs.

7.5.5.1 Metabolic Control and Dialysis Dose

Dialysis adequacy has been recognized as a strong prognostic factor in chronic IHD for at least the past 2 decades. Its role in the treatment of ARF has been suspected when old studies reported a lower mortality with an early initiation of IHD in ARF [15]. More recently a retrospective study in almost 1,500 patients provided strong data to support the relation between the dialysis adequacy and outcomes [16]. Nowadays, there is accumulating evidence to support the link between dialysis efficacy and outcomes for treatment of ARF in the ICU. One major unresolved issue is the target dose able to provide the better outcome. Using CRRT, two prospective randomized studies reported a significant relation between higher delivered dose and survival [17, 18]. Based on a study from Ronco et al. [17], many experts recommended that patients treated with CRRT for ARF should receive at least 35 ml/kg/h. However recently, two other studies have been unable to support these previous results [19, 20]. In IHD, the study by Schiffl et al. [14] showed that daily dialysis (six sessions a week, mean session duration 3 h 20 min) improved significantly the patient's survival compared with alternate-day sessions (three sessions a week, same mean duration). This study presents several shortcomings, especially in the alternate-day group. In this group, the fluid balance had to be managed during 3 h 20 min every 2 days. The net ultrafiltration was around 1 l/h during IHD sessions compared with around 400 ml/h in the other group. Unsurprisingly, the alternate-day group experienced more frequent hypotensive episodes (25 ± 5% vs 5 ± 2%), more frequent oliguria (73% vs 21%), and a worsening of organ failure score. Therefore, it is difficult to conclude from the study whether the higher delivered dose provided a better outcome or if the characteristics of the alternate-day treatment worsened the prognosis. A recent prospective randomized multicenter study challenges the role of high delivered dialysis dose in ARF [21]. The authors randomized 1,124 patients with ARF and at least one nonrenal organ failure or sepsis, to receive intensive or less intensive RRT. Patients were assigned to IHD if hemodynamically stable, or CRRT or SLED if hemodynamic impairment was present. Intensive treatment was IHD or SLED six times per week or 35 ml/kg/h for CRRT; while the less intensive treatment was IHD or SLED three times per week or CRRT 20 ml/kg/h. In the less intensive group assigned to IHD, sequential dialysis could be used to control the fluid balance (ultrafiltration alone the other day). In IHD the prescribed dose based on formal urea kinetic modeling (Kt/V) derived from chronic hemodialysis patients was 1.2–1.4, which is the target recommended to improve outcome in chronic renal failure patients. They found no differences between the two groups regarding 60-day survival, renal recovery, duration of renal support, or rate of organ failure. No definitive comparison can be drawn between this study and the other because the control group (less intensive treatment) received a treatment definitively more intensive than the control group in the study by Schiffl et al. [14]. We can, however, conclude that the most important way to improve the outcome may be the adequacy of the treatment to avoid hemodynamic worsening and severe electrolytic disorders. Nevertheless, these data underline the lack of consensus regarding the target dose.

Another major issue concerns the method of measurement. Traditionally, nephrologists evaluate dialysis adequacy by measurement of urea concentration. Several indices are well accepted in chronic renal failure patients: urea reduction ration (URR), Kt/V (K: urea clearance; t: session duration; V: urea distribution volume), and Kt. None of these parameters have been validated in the treatment of ARF. Moreover, they are not expected to evaluate correctly the delivered dose. The URR is influenced by the ultrafiltration rate and does not account for the urea rebound usually markedly increased in ICU patients. The assumption needed to use the Kt/V index is a stable urea generation rate over time, and a predictable urea distribution volume. The urea generation ratio in ICU patients differs over time in response to the inflammatory process as well as urea distribution volume affected by edema and third space. The near future may provide a new powerful method to monitor online the delivered dose using the ionic dialysance. A recent study in ICU patients showed that the correlation between the Kt measured with ionic dialysance and the Kt measured with dialysate sampling was very good [22].

7.5.5.2 Hemodynamic Tolerance

Hypotension during IHD still remains a serious problem in ICU patients, occurring in around 30% of all sessions in cases of multiple organ dysfunction syndrome. This complication is of multiple origin, mainly hypovolemia (fluid removal during the priming and during treatment), sodium and water loss (osmolality variation), and vascular vasodilation. Most of the studies published in ICU patients, reporting a high incidence of hypotension, used settings directly derived from chronic renal failure patients. Taking into account the particular characteristics of ICU patients, particular settings may dramatically improve the hemodynamic tolerance of IHD. It has been reported that high dialysate sodium concentration may reduce sodium loss at the initiation of, and osmolality variation during, treatment. Mild dialysate hypothermia may also contribute to better tolerance by the preservation of vascular tone. These positive effects have been reported by Schortgen et al. [3] showing that specific settings decreased significantly the hypotension rate during treatment and the rate of any intervention to maintain arterial pressure. These aforementioned settings were saline priming with isovolemic connection, application of a high dialysate sodium concentration, mild hypothermic dialysate, and low ultrafiltration rate. Recent prospective randomized studies using optimized settings in IHD illustrate the tolerance improvement [8, 9]. No differences in hypotension rate were found between IHD and CRRT groups, whereas CRRT is usually advocated to provide better hemodynamic tolerance. New technological developments are available to monitor blood volume with online hematocrit or hemoglobin measurement. The could be useful in ICU patients but still remains to be evaluated in this population.

7.5.5.3 Outcome Improvement or Renal Recovery

Whether or not CRRT improves outcome or renal recovery as compared with IHD remained controversial until recent publications. Several studies compared both methods, but most of them were nonrandomized retrospective trials. Many methodologic biases preclude conclusive recommendations based on these studies. The membranes used were not standardized (biocompatible in CRRT, cuprophane in IHD), different therapies were pooled in CRRT (arteriovenous and venovenous methods) and in IHD (peritoneal dialysis and IHD). Probably the most important limitation was the lack of standardization for efficiency and hemodynamic tolerance in IHD. Indeed, nowadays, we know that hemodynamic tolerance can be significantly improved using specific settings in IHD for the critically ill [3] and that dialysis dose may play a role. Nevertheless, these retrospective studies reported conflicting results with a significantly higher mortality, a lack of significant difference, or a lower mortality with CRRT. Four meta-analyses report the absence of significant differences in terms of hospital mortality between the two methods [4–7], but study heterogeneity and their poor methodologic quality preclude any definitive conclusions. To date, six prospective randomized studies have been published [8, 9, 23–26]. The study from Mehta et al. [23] found a significant higher mortality in the continuous treatment group, whereas the five remaining studies found no significant difference in terms of mortality [8, 9, 24–26]. In the study from Mehta et al. [23], however, despite randomization, the two groups were not comparable for several covariates (number of organ failures, severity score, etc.), but the multivariate analysis showed no relation between mode of RRT and mortality. It is important to note that most of these studies have included a small number of patients (from 30 to 166 patients), and some major weaknesses can be outlined (randomization failure [23], modifications of therapeutic protocol during the study period [25], combination of different types of CRRTs [23], and small number of heterogeneous groups of patients enrolled [9, 24–26]). However the last published study from Vinsonneau et al. [9] enrolled 360 patients and found no significant difference in survival between the two groups (60-day survival 32% vs 33% for IHD vs CRRT). In this study, both techniques were standardized for polymer membranes and dialysis buffers, factors known to affect the ability of patients to tolerate RRTs. In addition, guidelines were provided to improve hemodynamic tolerance in IHD based on the study from Schortgen et al. [3]. Regarding renal recovery, no convincing data exist to support the conclusion that CRRT could be able to decrease renal replacement duration or patient's dialysis dependency in the ICU or at hospital discharge. Except for a few studies reporting a significant benefit with CRRT or a trend toward a benefit, all other studies did not find any effect. Especially, the most recently published prospective randomized studies [8, 9] have found no significant difference in terms of RRT duration or rate of dialysis dependency.

7.5.6 Preferential Indication for IHD

Best indications are acute metabolic or toxic situations in acutely ill patients without uncontrolled hemodynamic instability. The need to treat patients without anticoagulation or the possibility of the patients moving are other good indications. Finally, inefficient CRRT for repeated filter clotting despite adequate anticoagulation or insufficient metabolic control can be good indications as well.

7.5.6.1 ARF Complications

IHD is certainly the most powerful method to easily and quickly control life-threatening situations associated with ARF. This is the case for severe hyperkalemia and severe metabolic acidosis, but also for pulmonary edema with fluid overload in oliguric patients without severe hemodynamic impairment. These situations require rapid disorder control and are usually associated with a noncompromised hemodynamic situation.

7.5.6.2 Hyperkalemia

The advantage of IHD for small molecule removal is more evident for transient disorders (hyperkalemia complicating the acute phase of ARF), but its value could be questioned in cases of persistent abnormalities such as tumor lysis syndrome or severe hyperphosphatemia. These situations can justify a combination of IHD early in the course of treatment, followed by the use of a continuous modality, given that sufficient initial control is achieved.

7.5.6.3 Metabolic Acidosis

Severe uncontrolled metabolic acidosis in shock remains a classical indication for RRT, despite the lack of consensus. Lactic acidosis related to tissue hypoperfusion accounts for the main etiology, and bicarbonate infusion is usually insufficient. Using CRRT in a standard way may lead to insufficient control, especially when liver dysfunction is present.

7.5.6.4 Azotemia

For azotemia control, IHD is also a good method, but its efficiency can be limited by the urea rebound. In some hypercatabolic patients, IHD may be the best method to control azotemia given the inability to deliver target dialysis doses in some patients with CRRT. In fact, the mean duration of CRRT reported in clinical studies is between 16 and 20 h, which leads to a decrease of efficiency with no steady-state situation.

7.5.6.5 Poisoning

Many toxins can be removed from the blood by extrarenal therapies. Some poisonings need rapid toxin removal because they are life-threatening. How efficient the extrarenal therapy is to remove the toxin is determined by the toxin's characteristics. The toxin has to be of low molecular weight (<500 Da), with high water solubility, low protein bound fraction, and low volume of distribution (<1.5 l/kg). Besides these characteristics, the clearance offered by the extrarenal technique is of paramount importance, because one of the main prognostic factors is the rapidity of toxin elimination. Therefore, IHD is the best method in these situations because the rapid removal of the toxic leads to a prompt efficacy compared with CRRT. In practice, CRRT can be considered in poisoning with a high volume of distribution and low refilling rate, such as in prolonged-release lithium intoxication, for example, but it must be performed with high performance and only following initial management with IHD to rapidly improve the symptoms.

7.5.6.6 Hemorrhage Risk and Contraindications to Anticoagulant

Filter and line patency are major determinants of filter life span and therefore of delivered dialysis dose. IHD can be performed with the use of a low dose or no dose of anticoagulant, which represents a major advantage in patients at high risk of bleeding or with any anticoagulation contraindication. In addition, it seems easier to treat patients with IHD in cases of heparin-induced thrombocytopenia and for alternative treatments to heparin (heparinoid), given the pharmacologic properties of these molecules and the difficult management of these treatments in continuous methods.

7.5.6.7 Other Indications

After primary care of patients treated with CRRT, when the hemodynamic situation improves, IHD makes ICU care and the comfort of the patient better. Moreover patients' increased mobility makes investigations outside the ICU easier (computed tomography, MRI, etc.), helps to prevent decubitus-related complications (decubitus ulcer, venous thrombosis, atelectasis, etc.), and helps to start rehabilitation. Indeed, IHD can be an alternative for some patients for whom CRRT is not suitable, because of iterative surgical procedures and frequent treatment interruptions that lead to low delivered dialysis dose.

7.5.7 Take Home Pearls

- The best indications for intermittent hemodialysis in acute patients are acute metabolic or toxic derangements in the absence of uncontrolled hemodynamic instability.
- Intermittent hemodialysis can often be performed without anticoagulation and thus has advantages in patients at risk of bleeding complications.
- It is the preferred treatment option for patients with isolated kidney failure, as it preserves patient mobility.

References

1. Kramer P, Wigger W, Rieger J, Matthaei D, Scheler F. Arteriovenous hemofiltration: a new and simple method for treatment of over-hydrated patients resistant to diuretics. Wien Klin Wochenschr 1977;55:1121–22.
2. Uchino S, Kellum JA, Bellomo R, et al. Acute renal failure in critically ill patients: a multinational multicenter study. JAMA, 2005;294:813–8.
3. Schortgen F, Soubrier N, Delclaux C, et al. Hemodynamic tolerance of intermittent hemodialysis in ICU: usefulness of practice guidelines. Am J Respir Crit Care Med, 2000; 162:197–20.
4. Kellum JA, Angus DC, Johnson JP, et al. Continuous versus intermittent renal replacement therapy: a meta-analysis. Intensive Care Med 2002;28:29–37.
5. Tonelli M, Manns B, Feller-Kopman D. Acute renal failure in the intensive care unit: a systematic review of the impact of dialytic modality on mortality and renal recovery. Am J Kidney Dis 2002;40:875–85.
6. Rabindranath K, Adams J, Macleod AM, Muirhead N. Intermittent versus continuous renal replacement therapy for acute renal failure in adults. Cochrane Database Syst Rev. 2007 July 18;(3):CD003773.
7. Bagshaw SM, Berthiaume LR, Delaney A, Bellomo R. Continuous versus intermittent renal replacement therapy for critically ill patients with acute kidney injury: a meta-analysis. Crit Care Med. 2008;36:610–7.
8. Uehlinger DE, Jakob SM, Ferrari P, et al. Comparison of continuous and intermittent renal replacement therapy for acute renal failure. Nephrol Dial Transplant 2005;20:1630–7.
9. Vinsonneau C, Camus C, Combes A, et al. Continuous venovenous haemodiafiltration versus intermittent haemodialysis for acute renal failure in patients with multiple-organ dysfunction syndrome: a multicentre randomised trial. Lancet 2006;368:379–85.
10. Fliser D, Kielstein JT. A single-pass batch dialysis system: an ideal dialysis method for the patient in intensive care with acute renal failure. Curr Opin Crit Care 2004;10:483–8.
11. Parienti JJ, Thirion M, Mégarbane B, et al. Femoral vs jugular venous catheterization and risk of nosocomial events in adults requiring acute renal replacement therapy: a randomized controlled trial. JAMA 2008;299:2413–22.
12. Alonso A, Lau J, Jaber BL. Biocompatible hemodialysis membranes for acute renal failure. Cochrane Database Syst Rev 2008 Jan 23;(1):CD005283.
13. McGill RL, Blas A, Bialkin S, Sandroni SE, Marcus JR. Clinical consequences of heparin-free hemodialysis. Hemodial Int 2005;9:393–8.
14. Schiffl H, Lang SM, Fischer R. Daily hemodialysis and the outcome of acute renal failure. N Engl J Med, 2002;346: 305–10.
15. Kleinknecht D, Jungers P, Chanard J, Barbanel C, Ganeval D. Uremic and non-uremic complications in acute renal failure: Evaluation of early and frequent dialysis on prognosis. Kidney Int 1972;1:190–6.
16. Paganini EP, Tapolyai M, Goormastic M, et al. Establishing a dialysis therapy/patient outcome link in intensive care unit dialysis for patients with acute renal failure. Am J Kidney Dis. 1996;28:S81–S89.
17. Ronco C, Bellomo R, Homel P, et al. Effects of different doses in continuous veno-venous haemofiltration on outcomes of acute renal failure: a prospective randomised trial. Lancet 2000;356:26–30.
18. Saudan P, Niederberger M, De Seigneux S, et al. Adding a dialysis dose to continuous hemofiltration increases survival in patients with acute renal failure. Kidney Int. 2006;70:1312–7.

19. Bouman CS, Oudemans-Van Straaten HM, Tijssen JG, Zandstra DF, Kesecioglu J. Effects of early high-volume continuous venovenous hemofiltration on survival and recovery of renal function in intensive care patients with acute renal failure: a prospective, randomized trial. Crit Care Med 2002;30:2205–11.
20. Tolwani AJ, Campbell RC, Stofan BS, Lai KR, Oster RA, Wille KM. Standard versus high-dose CVVHDF for ICU-related acute renal failure. J Am Soc Nephrol. 2008;19: 1233–8.
21. VA/NIH Acute Renal Failure Trial Network, Palevsky PM, Zhang JH, O'Connor TZ et al. Intensity of renal support in critically ill patients with acute kidney injury. N Engl J Med. 2008;359:7–20.
22. Ridel C, Osman D, Mercadal L, Anguel N, Petitclerc T, Richard C, Vinsonneau C. Ionic dialysance: a new valid parameter for quantification of dialysis efficiency in acute renal failure? Intensive Care Med 2007;33:460–5.
23. Mehta RL, McDonald B, Gabbai FB, et al. A randomized clinical trial of continuous versus intermittent dialysis for acute renal failure. Kidney Int 2001;60:1154–63.
24. John S, Griesbach D, Baumgärtel M, Weihprecht H, Schmieder RE, Geiger H. Effects of continuous haemofiltration vs intermittent heamodialysis on systemic heamodynamics and splanchnic regional perfusion in septic shock patients: a prospective, randomized clinical trial. Nephrol Dial Transplant 2001;16:320–7.
25. Gasparovic V, Filipovic-Greie I, Merkler M, Pisl Z. Continuous renal replacement therapy (CRRT) or intermittent hemodialysis (IHD) – what is the procedure of choice in critically ill patients? *Ren Fail* 2003;25:855–62.
26. Augustine JJ, Sandy D, Seifert TH, Paganini EP. A randomized controlled trial comparing intermittent with continuous dialysis in patients with ARF. *Am J Kidney Dis* 2004;44:1000–7.

Continuous Renal Replacement Therapies 7.6

Shigehiko Uchino and Claudio Ronco

Core Messages

- Continuous renal replacement therapy (CRRT) can provide improved hemodynamic stability and better solute control; thus it is often viewed as being the preferred choice for the treatment of critically ill patients.
- Modern CRRT systems are based on pump-driven venovenous circuits (V-V circuits), however, if a CRRT machine is not available, the procedures may also be performed in arteriovenous fashion with blood flow driven by the arteriovenous blood pressure gradient.
- CRRT can be performed as continuous hemofiltration, hemodialysis, or hemodiafiltration. Hemofiltration and hemodiafiltration circuits are further classified based on the infusion site of replacement fluids relative to the hemofilter (predilution vs postdilution). Predilution reinfusion reduces hemoconcentration within the hemofilter and may thus have the advantage of longer filter patency. However, this must be weighed against the reduced efficacy that is predictable based on the dilution-induced reduction in plasma solute concentrations.

S. Uchino (✉)
Intensive Care Unit, Department of Anesthesiology, Jikei University School of Medicine, 3-19-18, Nishi-Shinbashi, Minato-ku, Tokyo 105-8471, Japan
e-mail: s.uchino@jikei.ac.jp

7.6.1 Introduction

Acute kidney injury (AKI) is a common condition in the ICU. Approximately 6% of critically ill patients develop AKI, and 4% require renal replacement therapy (RRT) [1]. Continuous renal replacement therapy (CRRT) is often the preferred choice over intermittent renal replacement therapy (IRRT) and peritoneal dialysis in the ICU. This is because AKI occurring in the ICU is often different from the syndrome observed in renal wards. Patients are critically ill and several organ systems are involved in the syndrome. Under such circumstances, standard hemodialysis or peritoneal dialysis has displayed significant limitations in these patients, while CRRT is rapidly gaining consensus and displaying interesting clinical advantages. The critically ill patient presents a severe hemodynamic instability, sepsis, and septic shock, and may require mechanical ventilation, cardiac mechanical support, and other types of vital supports. In these conditions, CRRT can provide improved hemodynamic stability and better solute control compared with IRRT and peritoneal dialysis [2–4].

In this chapter, an overview of CRRT (including history, nomenclature, operational characteristics, indications, and complications) will be discussed. More thorough information for some of these subjects can be obtained in other chapters. To describe the current practice of CRRT, data from the Beginning and Ending Supportive Therapy for the Kidney (BEST Kidney) study will be presented [1, 5]. The BEST Kidney study is a prospective epidemiologic study conducted at 54 centers in 23 countries, mainly in 2001. Such information should help readers to understand how CRRT is actually conducted in ICUs worldwide.

A. Jörres et al. (eds.), *Management of Acute Kidney Problems*,
DOI: 10.1007/978-3-540-69441-0_7.6, © Springer-Verlag Berlin Heidelberg 2010

7.6.2 Historical Review

In 1977, Peter Kramer described a new technique called continuous arteriovenous hemofiltration (CAVH) [6]. The system originated from an accidental puncture of the femoral artery instead of the femoral vein. Kramer's intuition was to connect a highly permeable filter to the arterial access and to return the blood into another venous access thus creating an arteriovenous circuit (A-V circuit) without need of a pump. The arteriovenous pressure gradient was adequate to move the blood throughout the circuit and to create sufficient hydrostatic pressure in the filter to produce a certain amount of ultrafiltration. The transmembrane pressure gradient was further increased by lowering the position of the ultrafiltrate collection bag to create a negative pressure in the ultrafiltrate compartment. Blood purification was exclusively obtained by convection, and the ultrafiltrate produced was totally or partially replaced with fresh solutions. Anticoagulation was achieved by infusion of heparin in the arterial line.

The low efficiency of CAVH stimulated the use of countercurrent dialysate flow in low permeable dialyzers (CAVHD) or in highly permeable hemodiafilters (CAVHDF) [7, 8]. The newer membranes applied in the field allowed the combination of diffusion and convection to remove molecules in a wider spectrum of molecular weights. The arteriovenous circulation was progressively substituted with a venovenous circulation thanks to the application of peristaltic pumps. Special techniques to reduce the risk of bleeding were developed including the use of predilution, or the utilization of alternative agents such as citrate, low-molecular-weight heparin (LMWH) and prostacyclin [9]. Special filters were designed for particular patients such as neonates or small infants [10], and heparin-coated membranes were made available for special treatment conditions. The same technology was applied to catheters and lines to achieve a completely anti-thrombogenic surface in the whole circuit. Finally, a series of machines specifically designed to perform CRRT have been developed, and the new technology spurred new interest in the use of CRRT not only as blood purification techniques but also as possible treatments for multiple organ dysfunction syndromes and septic shock [11].

7.6.3 CRRT Techniques and Nomenclature

Several techniques are today available in the family of CRRT. Techniques may differ in terms of vascular access, extracorporeal circuit design, infusion sites of replacement fluid, anticoagulation, intensity of treatment, and type of membrane.

7.6.3.1 Arteriovenous and Venovenous Circuits

In the arteriovenous circuit (A-V circuit), blood is taken from an artery through an arterial indwelling catheter and returns to a vein through a venous indwelling catheter. Blood flow is regulated by the arteriovenous pressure gradient, and the circuit must be designed to prevent any unnecessary resistance to the circulation. When used in hemofiltration, the rate of ultrafiltration may vary, and it may be increased by lowering the position of the ultrafiltrate collecting bag. The A-V circuit requires arterial puncture and an indwelling arterial catheter, which can be the cause of bleeding, especially when anticoagulation is used. In the venovenous circuit (V-V circuit), blood is taken from a vein and returns to a vein, usually with a double-lumen catheter. Blood flow is regulated by a pump and therefore does not depend on blood pressure. Because of the bleeding issue and blood pressure-dependent blood flow, the A-V form is rarely used today. For example, in the BEST Kidney study, only one among 1,006 patients treated with CRRT had the A-V circuit [5].

7.6.3.2 Hemofiltration, Hemodialysis, and Hemodiafiltration

The most important mechanisms of solute and water transport across semipermeable membranes are diffusion and convection. Diffusion is the process of transport in which molecules that are present in a solvent and can freely go through a semipermeable membrane tend to move from the region of higher concentration into the region of lower concentration. Convection is the mass transfer mechanism associated with ultrafiltration of plasma water. If a solute is small enough to pass through the pore structure of the membrane, it is driven ("dragged") across the membrane in association with the ultrafiltrated plasma water. This movement of plasma water is a consequence of a transmembrane pressure gradient. Diffusion is an efficient transport mechanism for the removal of relatively small solutes, but as solute molecular weight increases, diffusion becomes limited and the relative importance of convection increases.

Continuous hemofiltration utilizes convection as the prevalent mechanism of solute transport (Fig. 7.6.1b and c). Ultrafiltration in excess of the amount required for volume control is produced, and it is partially or totally replaced by replacement fluid. Since replacement fluid is toxin free, the treatment can be used for blood purification and volume control. Continuous hemodialysis utilizes diffusion as the prevalent mechanism of solute transport (Fig. 7.6.1a). Ultrafiltration is obtained exactly in the range of values adequate to maintain patient's fluid control without requirement of fluid reinfusion. Hemofiltration and hemodialysis can be combined and is called continuous hemodiafiltration (Fig. 7.6.1d and e). Dialysate is circulated in countercurrent mode to blood and at the same time ultrafiltration is obtained in excess of the desired fluid loss from the patient. This is totally or partially replaced with replacement fluid. Table 7.6.1 shows the nomenclature of CRRT modes proposed by Acute Dialysis Quality Initiative (ADQI), which is a workgroup seeking to develop consensus and evidence-based statements in the field of AKI [12].

In IRRT, hemodialysis is the most effective to remove small solutes among the three circuit types, but becomes less effective as molecular weights increase (Fig. 7.6.2a). However, in CRRT, because dialysate and ultrafiltrate flow rates are much slower than those in IRRT, there is no difference in small solute clearances among the three circuit types. As the molecular weight increases, the superiority of convection over diffusion becomes obvious (Fig. 7.6.2b). Brunet et al. measured clearances of several solutes during continuous venovenous hemodiafiltration (CVVHDF) at various ultrafiltrate (0–2 l/h) and

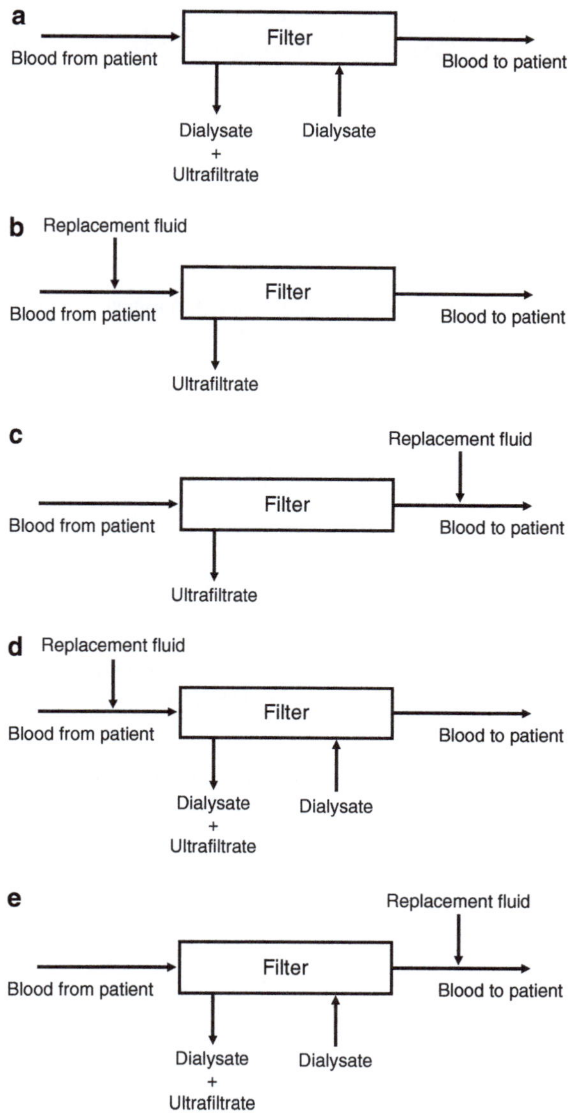

Fig. 7.6.1 Schemes of various circuit types: (**a**) hemodialysis, (**b**) predilution hemofiltration, (**c**) postdilution hemofiltration, (**d**) predilution hemodiafiltration, (**e**) postdilution hemodiafiltration

dialysate (0–2.5 l/h) flow rates [13]. For β2-microglobulin, which has a molecular weight of 11,800 Da, the diffusive clearance rapidly reached a plateau at the dialysate flow rate of 1.5 l/h, with the clearance of 8 ml/min. On the other hand, the convective clearance progressively increased with increasing the ultrafiltrate flow rate, and the clearance of β2-microglobulin was 20 ml/min at 2 l/h. However, the benefit of hemofiltration is offset by its shorter filter life. Proteins also are "dragged" to membrane pores by the high

Table 7.6.1 CRRT nomenclature

Abbreviation	Definition	Description
CAVH	Continuous arteriovenous hemofiltration	Driving force is patient's blood pressure Circuit is arteriovenous Ultrafiltrate produced is replaced with a replacement solution Ultrafiltration in excess of replacement results in patient volume loss Solute removal is through convection
CVVH	Continuous venovenous hemofiltration	Driving force is external pump Circuit is venovenous Other features similar to CAVH
CAVHD	Continuous arteriovenous hemodialysis	Driving force is patient's blood pressure Circuit is arteriovenous Dialysate solution is delivered across membrane countercurrent to blood flow at a rate substantially slower than blood flow rate; typical dialysate flow rates are 1–2 l/h Fluid replacement is not routinely administered Solute removal is by diffusion
CVVHD	Continuous venovenous hemodialysis	Driving force is external pump Circuit is venovenous Other features similar to CAVHD
CAVHDF	Continuous arteriovenous hemodiafiltration	Driving force is patient's blood pressure Circuit is arteriovenous Dialysate solution is delivered across membrane countercurrent to blood flow at a rate substantially slower than blood flow rate; typical dialysate flow rates are 1–2 l/h Ultrafiltration volumes are optimized to exceed desired weight loss and enhance solute clearance from convection Fluid losses are replaced in part or completely with replacement solution Solute removal is both diffusive and convective
CVVHDF	Continuous venovenous hemodiafiltration	Driving force is external pump Circuit is venovenous Other features similar to CAVHDF

transmembrane pressure and block the pores (so-called protein fouling). Ricci et al. compared continuous venovenous hemofiltration (CVVH) and continuous venovenous hemodialysis (CVVHD) in a cross-over study and found that the median filter life was significantly longer during CVVHD (37 h) than CVVH (19 h) [14]. In the BEST Kidney study, CVVH was the most common choice (52.8%), followed by CVVHDF (34.0%) and CVVHD (13.1%) [5].

7.6.3.3 Predilution and Postdilution

Hemofiltration and hemodiafiltration are further classified according to the infusion site of replacement fluid, i.e., predilution and postdilution (Fig. 7.6.1b–e). The infusion site of replacement fluid in the extracorporeal circuit during CRRT has a significant impact on solute removal and therapy requirements. For a given volume of replacement fluid, postdilution CRRT

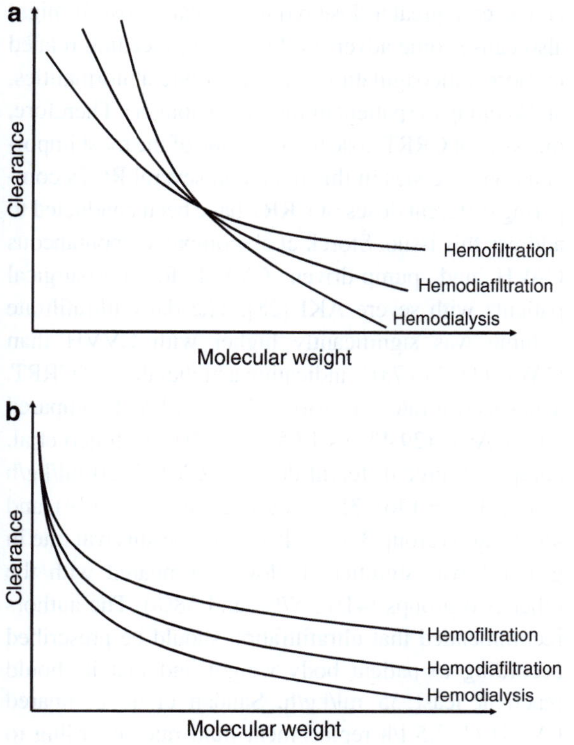

Fig. 7.6.2 Schemes of relationship between molecular weight and solute clearance among different circuit types (hemodialysis, hemofiltration, and hemodiafiltration). (**a**) IRRT, (**b**) CRRT

provides higher solute clearance than does predilution. The relative inefficiency of the latter mode is due to dilution-related reduction in solute concentrations, which decreases the driving force for convective mass transfer. The dilution effect with predilution can be calculated as:

$$\text{Dilution effect} = Qb^* (1-Ht)/(Qb^*(1-Ht)+Qr)$$

Where Qb is the blood flow rate, Qr is the replacement fluid rate, and Ht is hematocrit. Therefore, the relative inefficiency can be partially improved by increasing the blood flow rate. On the other hand, despite its superior efficiency, postdilution is limited inherently by its shorter filter life due to hemoconcentration in the filter. In general, ultrafiltrate flow should not exceed 25% of the blood flow rate.

Therefore, use of predilution reinfusion has an advantage of longer filter patency over postdilution. However, this must be weighed against the predictable dilution-induced reduction in plasma solute concentrations, one of the driving forces for convective solute removal. Whichever dilution method is used, higher blood flow rate can theoretically reduce their shortcomings. In the BEST Kidney study, slightly more than half of patients (58.5%) were treated with predilution [5].

7.6.3.4 Anticoagulation

Anticoagulation is a necessary component of CRRT because blood flow through the extracorporeal circuit causes platelet activation and coagulation cascades, resulting in fibrin deposition on filter membranes. The most common anticoagulant is heparin. In the BEST Kidney study, 42.9% of patients were given heparin for anticoagulation during CRRT [5]. However, the high incidence of bleeding complications secondary to heparin anticoagulation during CRRT have been reported, especially when full heparinization is used (e.g., target activated partial thromboplastin time [APTT] of 1.5–2.0 times normal range) [15]. Low-dose heparin (5–10 IU/kg/h), on the other hand, has been reported to cause fewer bleeding complications, with a shorter filter life [16, 17]. Van de Wetering et al. found that, for every 10-s increase in APTT, the incidence of circuit coagulation was decreased by 25%, while the risk of hemorrhage increased by 50% [18]. Considering the risk of full anticoagulation (bleeding in a critically ill patient) and the possible benefits of low-dose heparinization (reduced cost and workload due to less frequent filter changes), it might be preferable to conduct low-dose heparin anticoagulation during CRRT.

In patients with a high risk of bleeding complications, CRRT without anticoagulation can be used. Indeed, in the BEST Kidney study, no anticoagulation was the second most common anticoagulation method for CRRT (33.1%) [5]. Martin et al. conducted a retrospective study comparing no anticoagulation with low-dose heparinization (100–700 IU/h) and found a similar mean circuit life between the two groups (22.1 vs 24.7 h) [15]. These investigators also found that platelet count was different between the two groups (42 vs 142 $\times 10^3/\mu l$). These findings are consistent with other studies [17]. Platelets are an important factor for clot formation in the circuit [19]. Therefore, CRRT with no anticoagulation appears particularly appropriate in patients with marked thrombocytopenia.

If a patient with a bleeding risk has a very short filter life with no anticoagulation, heparin/protamine regional anticoagulation can be another choice. Uchino et al. observed 31 circuits with regional anticoagulation and found that mean circuit life was 21.2 h with no complication (bleeding or prolonged APTT) [17]. However, there are some concerns about regional anticoagulation with heparin/protamine (e.g., hypotension, meticulous dose adjustment, and risk of bleeding). Therefore, this technique is thought to be a method of rescue anticoagulation in a patient with a high risk of bleeding and a short circuit life in the absence of any anticoagulation.

Several other drugs have been used during CRRT to prolong circuit life: LMWH, citrate, prostacyclin, hirudin, and nafamostat mesilate. Prostacyclin and hirudin have been compared with heparin in randomized controlled trials (RCTs) and did not show a significant increase in circuit life [20, 21]. They also contain their own shortcomings (hypotension for prostacyclin, no antidote available for hirudin). The results of randomized controlled trial (RCTs) comparing LMWH and heparin are controversial [22, 23]. LMWH is renally excreted and could be accumulated in patients with AKI and cause bleeding complications [5]. It is therefore necessary to monitor factor Xa activity to titrate doses of LMWH.

Citrate causes anticoagulation by chelation of ionized calcium. Its effect is reversed by the postcircuit infusion of calcium, so that it does not cause systemic anticoagulation. Citrate has been consistently shown to have a longer filter life than heparin without bleeding complications [24, 25]. However, patients with liver dysfunction cannot metabolize infused citrate at a sufficient rate and may develop severe hypocalcemia [26]. This technique also requires a special dialysate/replacement fluid (containing no calcium or using citrate itself as a buffer).

Nafamostat mesilate is a synthetic serine protease inhibitor, which causes an anticoagulation effect by blocking factors Xa, XIIa, and thrombin. Because of its short half-life (approximately 8 min), it does not affect systemic coagulation [27]. However, nafamostat mesilate is available only in Japan and has not been properly compared with other anticoagulants.

7.6.3.5 Dose

The term "dose" is defined as the amount of CRRT delivered to control uremic toxins. A greater dose of CRRT might improve patient and kidney outcome. However, a greater dose requires greater cost. It might also cause some adverse effects (e.g., bleeding related to more anticoagulation use, electrolyte abnormalities, and keeping the patient immobile for longer). Therefore, the issue of CRRT dose has been one of the most important controversies in this field, and several RCTs comparing different doses of CRRT have been conducted to address this issue. Storck et al. compared spontaneous CAVH and pump-driven CVVH for postsurgical patients with severe AKI [28]. The daily ultrafiltrate volume was significantly higher with CVVH than CAVH (15.7 vs 7.0 l) indicating a higher dose of CRRT. The survival rate was also higher in CVVH compared with CAVH (29.4% vs 12.5%, $p = 0.04$). Ronco et al. compared three different doses of CVVH: 20 ml/kg/h (group 1, $n = 146$), 35 ml/kg/h (group 2, $n = 139$), and 45 ml/kg/h (group 3, $n = 140$) [29]. The survival rate in group 1 was significantly lower compared with the other two groups (41%, 57%, and 58%). The authors recommended that ultrafiltration should be prescribed according to patient body weight and that it should reach at least 35 ml/kg/h. Saudan et al. compared CVVH (1–2.5 l/h replacement fluid rate according to patient's body weight, $n = 102$) and CVVHDF (1–2.5 l/h replacement fluid rate and the addition of 1–1.5 l/h dialysate according to body weight, $n = 104$) [30]. The mean prescribed dose was 25 ml/kg/h in the CVVH group and 42 ml/kg/h in the CVVHDF group. The 28-day survival rate was significantly higher in the CVVHDF group compared with the CVVH group (59% vs 39%, $p = 0.03$).

Therefore, several RCTs published in the last 20 years have shown that increasing dose can improve outcomes in patients with severe AKI requiring CRRT. Although all of these studies were single-center in design, current evidence suggests that the dose of CRRT should be high, e.g., more than 35 ml/kg/h.

7.6.3.6 Other Technical Aspects of CRRT

The evolution of CRRT has been accompanied by a parallel evolution in the related technology. A series of double-lumen catheters has been developed to achieve higher blood flows with lower flow resistance and reduced risk of recirculation [31]. Double-lumen catheters are in some cases substituted by twin separate catheters to maximize blood flow and prevent unwanted recirculation. Several machines have incorporated the heparin pump or other systems for regional heparinization and citrate anticoagulation. In recent years, catheters, blood lines, and filters with heparin bound on the inner surface have been developed. Their use however is still experimental and requires further evaluation. Dialyzers with different membranes have been created making possible to chose among a variety of membrane materials. Membranes with different porosity and ultrafiltration coefficients are available [32]. There is a tendency to increase the filter surface area since the pumped circulation can operate at higher blood flows compared with arteriovenous circuits. A series of online monitoring techniques are today under evaluation including blood volume monitoring and blood temperature monitoring [33, 34]. Finally, a great deal of development has taken place in the operator interface of the CRRT machines. Most of these machines are equipped with large color screens and step-by-step guidelines to prime the circuit and run the treatment smoothly and effectively.

7.6.4 Indications and Timing of Starting CRRT

Whether a patient with severe AKI should receive RRT or can be managed medically is a difficult issue, and very little information is available for it. For example, the most widely used textbook of internal medicine states that the indications of RRT for ARF are "symptoms or signs of the uremic syndrome, management of refractory hypervolemia, hyperkalemia, or acidosis" or a "BUN level of greater than 100 mg/dL" [35]. On the other hand, in the BEST Kidney study, the median blood urea nitrogen (BUN) level was 64.4 mg/dl when CRRT was started, and less than 20% of patients had their CRRT started with BUN higher than 100 mg/dl, suggesting that indications written in textbooks obviously appear outdated. Several reviews for indications of CRRT have been published in the literature [36–38]. Among these, Bellomo et al. proposed criteria for the initiation of RRT in critical ill patients [36]. The criteria consisted of oliguria (less than 200 ml/12 h), azotemia (urea > 30 mmol/l), hyperkalemia (greater than 6.5 mmol/l), acidemia (pH < 7.1), and other uremic symptoms. These criteria are more similar to current practice than those in the textbooks.

However, it is unknown whether earlier start (e.g., before developing severe azotemia) is related to better outcome in patients with AKI or not. If CRRT is started too early, one might treat some patients with CRRT who would actually not require CRRT. On the other hand, if beginning of CRRT is delayed, it also might cause problems, e.g., fluid overload, electrolyte, and acid–base abnormalities, immunosuppression due to uremia, and so on. There have been several studies looking at this issue [39–42]. For example, Gettings et al. retrospectively reviewed 100 adult trauma patients treated with CRRT [39]. Patients were characterized as "early" or "late," based on whether BUN was less than or greater than 60 mg/dl at the beginning of CRRT. Although there was no difference in demographics or laboratory values between the two groups, the "early" group had a significantly higher survival rate than the "late" group (39.0% vs 20%, $p = 0.041$). Kresse et al. compared two periods (period 1: from 1991 to 1993, 128 patients; period 2: from 1994 to 1995, 142 patients) [40]. In period 2, RRT was started earlier compared with period 1 (creatinine 520 vs 250 μmol/l, urine volume 500 vs 900 ml/day). Although there was no significant difference in demographics or etiology of ARF, mortality was lower in period 2 compared with period 1 (59.6% vs 78.9%, $p < 0.001$). However, all of these studies are single-center observational studies, and no randomized controlled trial has been conducted for this issue [39–42].

Therefore, although there is no high-quality evidence (i.e., multicenter RCTs), some epidemiologic studies and physiologic reasoning suggest that early initiation of CRRT might achieve better outcomes for AKI patients, and no evidence exists against such thinking. Early initiation is feasible and physiologically sound, and it should be the approach of choice until one or more RCTs are conducted to provide clinicians with better-quality evidence to guide their practice.

7.6.5 Nonrenal Indications of CRRT

Another issue that needs to be addressed in terms of initiation of CRRT is that of so-called non-renal indications. In patients with multiple organ failure and/or septic shock, CRRT might be able to remove chemical mediators and attenuate the immunologic disequilibrium. Ronco et al. conducted a questionnaire with 345 clinicians who attended in one of two international meetings of critical care nephrology [43]. Fifty-two percent of the respondents reported using CRRT for extended indications even in the absence of AKI and approximately 6% answered "removal of septic mediators" as a reason for initiating CRRT in their ICU. In the BEST Kidney study, 13.6% of patients had CRRT for "immunomodulation" as at least one of the reasons of initiating CRRT [5].

There have been many studies showing that CRRT can remove cytokines and other inflammatory factors from septic patients [44–47]. However, the molecular weights of such substances are too large for them to be removed efficiently by currently available hemofilters. Cole et al. conducted a RCT to evaluate the ability of CVVH (2 l/h) to reduce plasma cytokine concentrations in septic shock patients [48]. These investigators found that CVVH was not associated with an overall reduction in plasma cytokine concentrations. Therefore, CRRT used at current doses with commercially available filters cannot be recommended for patients with sepsis but no AKI.

The negative results have stimulated researchers to the direction of increasing intensity of CRRT to improve the removal capacity of humoral mediators, with increased amount of convection such as high volume hemofiltration or with membranes characterized by increased sieving coefficients. High volume hemofiltration is a pure convective therapy that can be performed with two basic schedules. One is CVVH with a fluid exchange rate of more than 35 ml/kg/h. Technical requirements for this technique consist especially on the increased blood flow rates and the availability of large volumes of replacement fluid. High volume hemofiltration can also be performed for several hours exchanging 6–8 l/h while the patient continues a standard CVVH for the rest of the day. These therapies have been shown to produce a beneficial effect on patient's hemodynamics, with a significant reduction of vasopressor requirement [49].

Large pore size filters also can improve the removal ability of humoral mediators. Morgera et al. used a hemofilter that was designed to increase the in vivo permeability for substances in the molecular weight range of up to 60 kDa [50]. They compared this filter with a conventional filter in patients with sepsis and found significant decline of interleukin-6 and interleukin-1 receptor antagonist plasma levels. They also observed a significant decline in noradrenalin dose over time only in patients treated with the large pore size filter.

Continuous plasma filtration coupled with adsorption is a special technique that consists of two steps: first, blood is circulated through a plasma filter and plasma filtrate is pushed by a pump through a cartridge containing a mixture of hydrophobic resin and uncoated charcoal. Second, the regenerated plasma is returned to the main circuit where blood is reconstituted and eventually dialyzed. Because patient's own plasma is used for reinfusion, there is no need for replacement fluid and unwanted protein losses are avoided. The technique has been effective in reducing the circulating levels of various cytokines and at the same time it has allowed a significant reduction of the pharmacologic requirement to maintain hemodynamic stability [51].

7.6.6 Complications/Problems

Apart from the bleeding complications mentioned above, there are other potential complications of CRRT that physicians need to pay attention to. The most important issue related to conducting CRRT is hemodynamic instability. Although hypotension occurs less frequently during treatment when CRRT is used compared with IRRT, it still needs significant attention. In the BEST Kidney study [5], hypotension related to CRRT occurred in 18.8% of patients, and arrhythmias were observed in 4.3%. Critical arrhythmias (cardiac arrest, ventricular tachycardia, or fibrillation) considered related to CRRT occurred in eight patients, and were fatal in three. When CRRT is started, a patient typically loses the equivalent of a circulating blood volume of approximately 150–200 ml (circuit volume). This acute change in circulating blood volume may induce hypotension in some unstable critically ill patients. Therefore, physicians need to pay the highest level of attention to hemodynamics at the start of CRRT and to consider prophylactic steps (fluid loading before and during initiation, increased vasopressor therapy or both), especially when patients are on a high dose of vasopressors and have a high serum lactate concentration.

Electrolyte abnormalities also need attention. Commercially available replacement/dialysis fluids contain low concentrations of potassium, magnesium, and phosphate because patients with AKI tend to have high blood concentrations of these ions before receiving CRRT. Therefore, after a few days of CRRT, regular monitoring of these electrolytes is required to avoid hypokalemia, hypomagnesemia, and hypophosphatemia.

7.6.7 CRRT Versus IRRT

Choosing CRRT or IRRT has been a matter of debate. CRRT has been reported to offer potential physiologic advantages over IRRT. These potential advantages include greater hemodynamic stability and easier fluid management, better solute control and stable intracranial pressure [2–4, 52, 53].

It is not difficult to understand why CRRT can provide greater hemodynamic stability and easier fluid management. When an anuric patient is given 2 l/day of fluid for nutrition and medication, the same amount of fluid needs to be removed. If second-daily IRRT is used for this patient (4 h for each session), 1 l/h of fluid is taken away from the patient. On the other hand, with CRRT, only 83 ml/h of fluid removal is enough to control the fluid status of the patient. For solute control, one might think that IRRT is better because it uses more dialysate (300–500 ml/min) with a higher blood flow rate (200–300 ml/h) than CRRT. In the BEST Kidney study, the median treatment dose was 2,000 ml/h (=33.3 ml/min) and the blood flow rate was 150 ml/min for CRRT [5]. However, due to the disequilibrium of solutes between the intravascular space and extravascular/intracellular spaces, serum solute concentrations go up soon after IRRT is stopped, which does not happen with CRRT. In a mathematical model, Clark et al. calculated that a patient with a body weight greater than 80 kg could not achieve BUN control of 60 mg/dl even with daily conventional IRRT, while this could be easily achieved with 1.5 l/h of CRRT dose [54]. The disequilibrium could cause relative hypo-osmolarity in the blood, and therefore, intracranial hypertension in patients with brain injury [53].

Whether these physiologic advantages would result in survival benefit remains unknown. Several RCTs have been conducted for this issue [55–59]. None of these studies have shown any benefit of CRRT over IRRT in terms of survival. However, these studies are small and/or contain significant flaws. Nonetheless, even if there was an outcome difference between the two modalities, such differences seem to be relatively small. However, while CRRT has not shown survival benefits over IRRT, it does not necessarily imply that IRRT and CRRT deliver equal outcomes. Renal recovery is another important patient-centered outcome in AKI and might be affected differently by IRRT and CRRT. In theory, due to rapid changes in fluid status and plasma osmolarity, IRRT might often induce a decrease in venous return, blood pressure, and cardiac index. Because of that, there is a possibility that IRRT might cause subclinical renal ischemia and delay renal recovery after AKI. There is some evidence to support this possibility. For example, in an RCT by Mehta et al. [55], CVVHDF was associated with a significantly higher rate of complete renal recovery in surviving patients who received an adequate trial of therapy with no crossover (92.3% vs 59.4%, $p < 0.01$). In a retrospective study, Bell et al. collected data from 2,202 patients treated with RRT for AKI from 32 ICUs in Sweden [60]. Among 944 survivors treated with CRRT, 8.3% never recovered their renal function and became dialysis dependent. On the other hand, the proportion was significantly higher among hemodialysis patients, where 26 patients out of 158 survivors (16.5%) became dialysis dependent.

Nonetheless, the benefit of CRRT over IRRT is unproven and, in such a condition of controversy, there seem to be regional differences in the choice of RRT modes. In a questionnaire study including members of the National Kidney Foundation in the United States, only 3.9% chose CRRT for more than a half of patients with AKI [61]. In a similar questionnaire study done in Canada, it was reported that IRRT was chosen for 71% of patients who required RRT in the ICU [62]. On the other hand, almost all patients with AKI were treated with CRRT in Australia [63]. In Madrid, IRRT and CRRT were chosen in 23% and 72% of cases, respectively [64].

7.6.8 Take Home Pearls

- CRRT may have advantages over intermittent dialysis in terms of hemodynamic stability and easier fluid management, better solute control, and stable intracranial pressure; however, the prospective randomized studies available to date have so far failed to demonstrate that this is associated with improved survival rates.

- The potential advantages of CRRT must be weighed against the fact that this treatment in most cases requires continuous anticoagulation and may thus increase the risk of bleeding complications.

References

1. Uchino S, Kellum JA, Bellomo R, et al. (2005) Beginning and Ending Supportive Therapy for the Kidney (BEST Kidney) Investigators. Acute renal failure in critically ill patients. A multinational, multicenter study. JAMA 294: 813–8.
2. Davenport A, Will EJ, Davidson AM (1993) Improved cardiovascular stability during continuous modes of renal replacement therapy in critically ill patients with acute hepatic and renal failure. Crit Care Med 21: 328–38.
3. Uchino S, Bellomo R, Ronco C (2001) Intermittent versus continuous renal replacement therapy in the ICU: impact on electrolyte and acid-base balance. Intensive Care Med 27: 1037–43.
4. Bellomo R, Farmer M, Bhonagiri S, et al. (1999) Changing acute renal failure treatment from intermittent hemodialysis to continuous hemofiltration: impact on azotemic control. Int J Art Org 22: 145–50.
5. Uchino S, Bellomo R, Morimatsu H, et al. (2007) Continuous renal replacement therapy: a worldwide practice survey. The beginning and ending supportive therapy for the kidney (BEST kidney) investigators. Intensive Care Med 33: 1563–70.
6. Kramer P, Wigger W, Rieger J, et al. (1977) Arteriovenous hemofiltration: a new and simple method for treatment of over hydrated patients resistant to diuretics. Klin Wocherr-Scrift 55: 1121–22.
7. Geronemus R, Schneider N (1984) Continuous arterio-venous hemodialysis: a new modality for treatment of acute renal failure. ASAIO 30: 610–3.
8. Ronco C (1985) Arterio-venous hemodiafiltration (AVHDF): a possible way to increase urea removal during CAVH. Int J Artif Organs 8: 61–62.
9. Oudemans-van Straaten HM, Wester JP, de Pont AC, et al. (2006) Anticoagulation strategies in continuous renal replacement therapy: can the choice be evidence based? Intensive Care Med 32: 188–20.
10. Ronco C, Bellomo R, Acute renal failure in infancy: treatment by continuous renal replacement therapy. In: Ronco C, Bellomo R (eds) Critical Care Nephrology. Kluwer, Dordrecht, pp 1335–50.
11. Ronco C, Ghezzi P, Bellomo R (1999) New perspective in the treatment of acute renal failure. Blood Purif 17: 166–72.
12. Kellum JA, Mehta RL, Angus DC, et al. (2002) The first international consensus conference on continuous renal replacement therapy. Kidney Int 62: 1855–63.
13. Brunet S, Leblanc M, Geadah D, et al. (1999) Diffusive and convective solute clearances during continuous renal replacement therapy at various dialysate and ultrafiltration flow rates. Am J Kidney Dis 34: 486–92.
14. Ricci Z, Ronco C, Bachetoni A, et al. (2006) Solute removal during continuous renal replacement therapy in critically ill patients: convection versus diffusion. Crit Care 10: R67.
15. Martin PY, Chevrolet JC, Suter P, et al. (1994) Anticoagulation in patients treated by continuous venovenous hemofiltration: a retrospective study. Am J Kidney Dis 24: 806–12.
16. Gretz N, Quintel M, Ragaller M, et al. (1995) Low-dose heparinization for anticoagulation in intensive care patients on continuous hemofiltration. Contrib Nephrol 116; 130–5.
17. Uchino S, Fealy N, Baldwin I, et al. (2004) Continuous venovenous hemofiltration without anticoagulation. ASAIO; 50: 76–80.
18. van de Wetering J, Westendorp RG, van der Hoeven JG, et al. (1996) Heparin use in continuous renal replacement procedures: the struggle between circuit coagulation and patient hemorrhage. J Am Soc Nephrol 7; 145–50.
19. Davenport A (1997) The coagulation system in the critically ill patients with acute renal failure and the effect of an extracorporeal circuit. Am J Kidney Dis 30(Suppl. 4): 20–27.
20. Langenecker SA, Felfernig M, Werba A, et al. (1994) Anticoagulation with prostacyclin and heparin during continuous venovenous hemofiltration. Crit Care Med 22: 1774–81.
21. Vargas Hein O, von Heymann C, Lipps M, et al. (2001) Hirudin versus heparin for anticoagulation in continuous renal replacement therapy. Intensive Care Med 27: 673–9.
22. Reeves JH, Cumming AR, Gallagher L, et al. (1999) A controlled trial of low-molecular-weight heparin (dalteparin) versus unfractionated heparin as anticoagulant during continuous venovenous hemodialysis with filtration. Crit Care Med 27; 2224–8.
23. Joannidis M, Kountchev J, Rauchenzauner M, et al. (2007) Enoxaparin vs. unfractionated heparin for anticoagulation during continuous veno-venous hemofiltration: a randomized controlled crossover study. Intensive Care Med 33: 1571–9.
24. Monchi M, Berghmans D, Ledoux D, et al. (2004) Citrate vs. heparin for anticoagulation in continuous venovenous hemofiltration: a prospective randomized study. Intensive Care Med 30: 260–5.
25. Kutsogiannis DJ, Gibney RT, Stollery D, et al. (2005) Regional citrate versus systemic heparin anticoagulation for continuous renal replacement in critically ill patients. Kidney Int 67: 2361–7.
26. Meier-Kriesche HU, Gitomer J, Finkel K, et al. (2001) Increased total to ionized calcium ratio during continuous venovenous hemodialysis with regional citrate anticoagulation. Crit Care Med 29; 748–52.
27. Ohtake Y, Hirasawa H, Sugai T, et al. (1991) Nafamostat mesylate as anticoagulant in continuous hemofiltration and continuous hemodiafiltration. Contrib Nephrol 93; 215–7.
28. Storck M, Hartl WH, Zimmerer E, et al. (1991) Comparison of pump-driven and spontaneous continuous haemofiltration in postoperative acute renal failure. Lancet 337: 452–5.
29. Ronco C, Bellomo R, Homel P, et al. (2000) Effects of different doses in continuous veno-venous haemofiltration on outcomes of acute renal failure: a prospective randomized trial. Lancet 356: 26–30.
30. Saudan P, Niederberger M, De Seigneux S, et al. (2006) Adding a dialysis dose to continuous hemofiltration increases survival in patients with acute renal failure. Kidney Int 70: 1312–7.
31. Jassal V, Pierratos A (1998) Vascular access for continuous renal replacement therapy. In: Ronco C, Bellomo R (eds) Critical Care Nephrology. Kluwer, Dordrecht.

32. Ronco C, Ghezzi PM, Hoenich NA, et al. (2001) Computerized selection of membranes and hemodialysers. Contrib Nephrol 133: 119–30.
33. Ronco C, Brendolan A, Bellomo R (1999) On-Line monitoring in continuous renal replacement therapies. Kidney Int 56(Suppl 72): S8–14.
34. Rahmati S, Ronco F, Spittle M, et al. (2001) Validation of the blood temperature monitor for extracorporeal thermal energy balance during in vitro continuous hemodialysis. Blood Purif 19: 245–50.
35. Brady HR, Brenner BM (1998) Acute renal failure. In: Fauci AS, Braunwald E, Isselbacher KJ, et al. (eds) Harrison's Principles of Internal Medicine, 14th edn. McGraw-Hill, New York, pp 1504–13.
36. Bellomo R, Ronco C (1998) Indications and criteria for initiating renal replacement therapy in the intensive care unit. Kidney Int 66: S106–9.
37. Schetz MR (1998) Classical and alternative indications for continuous renal replacement therapy. Kidney Int 66: S129–32.
38. Palevsky PM (2005) Renal replacement therapy I: indications and timing. Crit Care Clin 21: 347–56.
39. Gettings LG, Reynolds HN, Scalea T (1999) Outcome in post-traumatic acute renal failure when continuous renal replacement therapy is applied early vs. late. Intensive Care Med 25: 805–13.
40. Kresse S, Schlee H, Deuber HJ, et al. (1999) Influence of renal replacement therapy on outcome of patients with acute renal failure. Kidney Int Suppl 72: S75–8.
41. Bent P, Tan HK, Bellomo R, et al. (2001) Early and intensive continuous hemofiltration for severe renal failure after cardiac surgery. Ann Thorac Surg 71: 832–7.
42. Elahi MM, Lim MY, Joseph RN, et al. (2004) Early hemofiltration improves survival in post-cardiotomy patients with acute renal failure. Eur J Cardiothorac Surg 26: 1027–31.
43. Ronco C, Zanella M, Brendolan A, et al. (2001) Management of severe acute renal failure in critically ill patients: an international survey in 345 centers. Nephrol Dial Transplant 16: 230–7.
44. Sander A, Armbruster W, Sander B et al. (1997) Hemofiltration increases IL-6 clearance in early systemic inflammatory response syndrome but does not alter IL-6 and TNFa plasma concentrations. Intensive Care Med 23: 878–84.
45. Kellum JA, Johnson JP, Kramer D, et al. (1998) Diffusive vs. convective therapy: Effects on mediators of inflammation in patients with severe systemic inflammatory response syndrome. Crit Care Med 26: 1995–2000.
46. De Vriese AS, Colardyn FA, Philippe JJ, et al. (1999) Cytokine removal during continuous hemofiltration in septic patients. J Am Soc Nephrol 10: 846–53.
47. Van Bommel EFH, Hesse CJ, Jute NHPM, et al. (1995) Cytokine kinetics (TNFa, IL-1b, IL-6) during continuous hemofiltration: A laboratory and clinical study. Contrib Nephrol 116: 62–75.
48. Cole L, Bellomo R, Hart G, et al. (2002) A Phase II randomized controlled trial of continuous hemofiltration in sepsis. Crit Care Med 30: 100–6.
49. Honore PM, Jamez J, Wauthier M, et al. (2000) Prospective evaluation of short-term, high-volume isovolemic hemofiltration on the hemodynamic course and outcome in patients with intractable circulatory failure resulting from septic shock. Crit Care Med 28: 3581–7.
50. Morgera S, Haase M, Kuss T, et al. (2006) Pilot study on the effects of high cutoff hemofiltration on the need for norepinephrine in septic patients with acute renal failure. Crit Care Med 34: 2099–104.
51. Tetta C, Bellomo R, Brendolan A, et al. (1999) Use of adsorptive mechanisms in continuous renal replacement therapies in the critically ill. Kidney Int 56(Suppl 72): S15–9.
52. Bellomo R, Farmer M, Parkin G, et al. (1995) Severe acute renal failure: a comparison of acute continuous hemodiafiltration and conventional dialytic therapy. Nephron 71: 59–64.
53. Davenport A (1995) The management of renal failure in patients at risk of cerebral edema/hypoxia. New Horizons 3: 717–24.
54. Clark WR, Mueller BA, Kraus MA, et al. (1997) Extracorporeal therapy requirements for patients with acute renal failure. J Am Soc Nephrol 8: 804–12.
55. Mehta RL, McDonald B, Gabbai FB, et al. (2001) Collaborative Group for Treatment of ARF in the ICU. A randomized clinical trial of continuous versus intermittent dialysis for acute renal failure. Kidney Int 60: 1154–63.
56. Vinsonneau C, Camus C, Combes A, et al. (2006) Hemodiafe Study Group. Continuous venovenous haemodiafiltration versus intermittent haemodialysis for acute renal failure in patients with multiple-organ dysfunction syndrome: a multicentre randomised trial. Lancet 368: 379–85.
57. John S, Griesbach D, Baumgartel M, et al. (2001) Effects of continuous haemofiltration vs intermittent haemodialysis on systemic haemodynamics and splanchnic regional perfusion in septic shock patients: a prospective, randomized clinical trial. Nephrol Dial Transplant 16: 320–7.
58. Augustine JJ, Sandy D, Seifert TH, et al. (2004) A randomized controlled trial comparing intermittent with continuous dialysis in patients with ARF. Am J Kidney Dis 44: 1000–7.
59. Uehlinger DE, Jakob SM, Ferrari P, et al. (2005) Comparison of continuous and intermittent renal replacement therapy for acute renal failure. Nephrol Dial Transplant 20:1630–7.
60. Bell M, SWING, Granath F, et al. (2007) Continuous renal replacement therapy is associated with less chronic renal failure than intermittent haemodialysis after acute renal failure. Intensive Care Med 33: 773–80.
61. Mehta RL, Letteri JM (1999) Current status of renal replacement therapy for acute renal failure. A survey of US nephrologists. The National Kidney Foundation Council on Dialysis. Am J Nephrol 19: 377–82.
62. Hyman A, Mendelssohn DC (2002) Current Canadian approaches to dialysis for acute renal failure in the ICU. Am J Nephrol 22: 29–34.
63. Silvester W, Bellomo R, Cole L. (2001) Epidemiology, management, and outcome of severe acute renal failure of critical illness in Australia. Crit Care Med 29: 1910–5.
64. Liaño F, Junco E, Pascual J, et al. (1998) The spectrum of acute renal failure in the intensive care unit compared with that seen in other settings. The Madrid Acute Renal Failure Study Group. Kidney Int Suppl 66: S16–24.

Extended Daily Dialysis

7.7

Danilo Fliser and Jan T. Kielstein

Core Messages

- Key elements defining a renal replacement therapy as extended daily dialysis (EDD) are extended dialysis time (usually 8–18 h) and slow dialysate and blood flow rates.
- Prospective controlled studies in critically ill patients have documented that small solute clearance with EDD is comparable with that of intermittent hemodialysis (IHD) and continuous venovenous hemofiltration (CVVH).
- Patient's cardiovascular stability during EDD is similar to continuous renal replacement therapy (CRRT).
- Nightly EDD treatments have the added benefit of unrestricted access of intensive care unit (ICU) staff to the patient during the day, minimizing interference of renal replacement therapy with other ICU activities.
- EDD combines several advantages of both intermittent and continuous techniques

D. Fliser (✉)
Division of Renal and Hypertensive Disease, Department of Internal Medicine, Saarland University Centre, Kirrberger Strasse, 66421 Homburg/Saar, Germany
e-mail: indfli@uks.eu

7.7.1 Extended Dialy Dialysis: Back to the Roots of Renal Replacement Therapy in Critically Ill Patients

The discussion of extended daily dialysis (EDD) for the treatment of acute kidney injury (AKI) has to begin with the seminal work of Dr W. J. Kolff. Using his dialysis machine made of cellophane tubing (made for sausage casing) wrapped around a cylinder that rotated in a bath of fluid, Kolff started to treat patients in 1943. On 11 September 1945, Maria Schafstaat was the first patient whose life was saved by dialysis [23]. He treated the 67-year-old woman for 690 min (i.e., 11.5 h) with a blood flow rate of 116 ml/min. Therby Dr Kolff defined the key elements of EDD, i.e., prolonged dialysis time with low flow rates. This renal replacement therapy recently has been celebrated as "a new approach" for the treatment for severely ill patients with AKI in the intensive care unit (ICU).

Although both the patient population and the technical equipment have considerably changed, AKI in the ICU is still associated with high in-hospital mortality. This could be explained by the ever-expanding comorbid conditions of ICU patients intensifying the severity of illness [36, 45]. In this patient population, AKI is generally one feature of a multiple organ dysfunction syndrome (MODS). According to results of a large prospective observational study of 29,000 ICU patients in 23 countries, up to 60% of patients with AKI die during their hospital stay [45]. Morever, the development of AKI is thought to be an independent risk factor for in-hospital death [35].

A. Jörres et al. (eds.), *Management of Acute Kidney Problems*,
DOI: 10.1007/978-3-540-69441-0_7.7,

7.7.2 What Led to the Revival of EDD in the ICU?

In light of the unfavorable clinical characteristics of critically ill patients with AKI, physicians caring for these patients have increasingly used continuous renal replacement therapies (CRRTs) such as continuous venovenous hemofiltration (CVVH). These methods seem to offer better cardiovascular stability in the critically ill patient than conventional intermittent hemodialysis (IHD). This opinion has been challenged by observations that if IHD is performed with low blood flow and ultrafiltration rates at the start of the treatment, reduced dialysate temperature along with other measures, procedural morbidity with IHD is comparable with that of CRRT [43]. Furthermore, so far controlled studies [3] and a meta-analysis [46] have not revealed a definitive advantage in terms of patient survival for CRRT as compared with IHD. Hence, the method for renal replacement therapy should be based on the clinical situation, physician proficiency with the available techniques, and logistical capacity of the ICU and dialysis personnel. More important than the choice of renal replacement modality in the ICU may be the delivery of a sufficient treatment dose in critically ill patients [40, 41]. As such, current treatment strategies for patients with AKI in the ICU focus on highly efficacious elimination of uremic toxins and concomitant gentle volume removal. This can be achieved with either daily IHD or high volumes of substitution fluid during CVVH. The procedural costs of these labor-intensive techniques are increasingly prohibitive in their implementation. In addition, both conventional IHD and CRRTs have certain advantages, but also several disadvantages that are summarized in Table 7.7.1.

7.7.3 Clinical Experience with EDD Therapy of Critically Ill Patients with AKI

Several controlled studies and accounts of long-term experience have been published by groups that use EDD to treat ICU patients with AKI [5, 11, 18, 24, 25, 28, 31, 32, 38, 39, 42] (Table 7.7.2). Marshall et al. [30, 31] used a 2008H® machine at a reduced dialysate flow rate of 100 ml/min to treat critically ill patients in whom IHD had repeatedly failed due to intradialytic hypotension, and in patients in whom prescribed solute control goals were not achieved despite daily IHD. Under those circumstances the authors achieved ultrafiltration goals and adequate solute removal in most of their 37 treated patients. The in-hospital mortality rate was not significantly different from expected mortality determined from the APACHE II score. Also, formal training to operate the machines was undertaken by all full-time ICU nurses at the time of the hybrid therapy program inception, consisting of a brief instructional video and a 2-h "hands-on" training session. Inservice was offered on an as needed basis, and has been incorporated into nephrology and ICU nursing orientation

Table 7.7.1 Comparison of continuous renal replacement therapy (CRRT), intermittent haemodialysis (IHD), and extended daily dialysis (EDD)

	CRRT	IHD	EDD
Elimination of uremic toxins	Convective	Diffusive	Diffusive
Membranes	High-flux	Low-flux	Low-flux/high-flux
Dialysate flow	Low	High	Low
Ultrafiltration and solute elimination	Continuous (in theory)	Intermittent (3–5 h)	Intermittent (8–18 h)
Anticoagulation	Continuous	Intermittent (3–5 h)	Intermittent (8–12 h)
Citrate anticoagulation	Yes	Yes	Yes
Nephrology nursing staff	Not required	Required	Required
Required nursing time	High	Absorbes one nurse	Low
Mobilization/diagnostic procedures	Not possible	Possible	Possible
Operating costs	High (mostly for sterile filtration fluid)	Low	Low
Use of standard dialysis machines	No	Yes	Yes
Hemodynamic stability	Excellent	Poor (in some centers)	Excellent
Proven survival benefit compared with other methods	No	No	No

Table 7.7.2 Reports on extended daily dialysis experience

Author (Reference)	Dialysis machines	Blood/dialysate flow rates (ml/min)	Treatment time (h)	Nocturnal treatment
Berbece et al. [5]	Not reported	200/350	8	No
Czock et al. [7]	Genius	150–200/150–200	8	Yes
Fiaccadori et al. [11]	AK200 Ultra	200/100	8–9	No
Kielstein et al. [18]	Genius	200/100	12	Yes
Kielstein et al. [17]	Genius	150–200/150–200	8	Yes
Kumar et al. [24]	2008H[a]	200/300	6–8	No
Lonnemann et al. [28]	Genius	70/70	18	Not reported
Marshall et al. [30]	2008H[a]	200/100	12	Yes
Marshall et al. [31]	2008H[a]	200/100	12	Not reported
Marshall et al. [33]	4008S ArRT-Plus	250–350/200	8	No
Morgera et al. [37]	Genius	180–200/180–200	4–6	No
Naka et al. [38]	Not reported	100/200	6–8	Not reported
Ratanat et al. [39]	Not reported	200–250/67–150	6–12	Not reported
Schlaeper et al. [42]	2008H[a]	100–200/100–200	8–24	Yes
VA/NIH ATN study	Not reported	215/245	8	Yes

[a]Modified for extended daily dialysis treatment

programs and quarterly skills updates. Two months after the introduction of EDD, satisfaction of ICU nurses was formally assessed. When compared with CRRT, all felt that EDD was technically easier and all preferred the hybrid technique to CRRT [14].

Another US center compared EDD with standard CVVH in a prospective study [24]. No differences in mean arterial blood pressure or use of catecholamines were observed between the treatment groups, despite similar median net daily ultrafiltration rates. By contrast, requirement for anticoagulation was significantly less in patients treated with EDD. The authors recently published an account of their long-term experience with EDD [25]. They concluded that this technique is well tolerated and offers many of the benefits of continuous techniques, but is technically much simpler to perform. In this program, the nephrology nursing staff was always in-house with a response time of less than 5 min to the bedside. ICU nursing satisfaction with hybrid therapy was assessed as at least equal to CVVH [25].

We use the Genius® single-pass dialysis system to treat patients with AKI in the ICU. The technical principle underlying this standard IHD machine is based on the very first dialysis systems, the "tank" or "batch" devices as described in detail elsewhere [18]. This simple yet highly efficient treatment modality fulfills all ICU requirements: it offers immediate, highly effective dialysis therapy for acute hyperkalemia, whereas for less urgent indications treatment durations can be extended up to 24 h. In a prospective randomized controlled study in ventilated critically ill patients suffering from oliguric AKI, we could demonstrate that 12-h EDD treatments performed with this machine achieve urea reduction rates comparable to those achieved with 24 h of CVVH, even though a substitution fluid exchange rate of at least 3 l/h was used with the latter [18]. These data are in line with other studies [5] supporting kinetic models which indicate that both CVVH and EDD provide very effective control of azotemia in hypercatabolic AKI patients [27]. Moreover, cardiovascular parameters assessed online via invasive monitoring were not significantly different during CVVH and EDD despite comparable ultrafiltration. In our institution the acute dialysis fellow discusses the required dialysis prescription on his/hers twice-daily rounds on the 12 ICUs. Provision, initiation, and discontinuation of hybrid treatments is always done by the nephrology nurse while hourly monitoring variation of ultrafiltration, troubleshooting, and other responsibilities are shared.

Taken together, a growing body of evidence suggests that EDD, at absolutely equivalent hemodynamic stability, is as efficacious as classical CVVH. The significantly reduced need for heparin with EDD can be a decisive advantage, especially in patients at high risk of bleeding [18, 30]. Another consideration in favor of EDD is the closed system. The forty and more times a CRRT system is opened to connect a bag of replacement fluid and discard the used filtrate (given a substitution rate of 37.5 ml/kg/h in a 100 kg patient) represent considerable risk of bacterial contamination, especially if bicarbonate-based buffers are used. EDD of any kind does not involve this risk. Finally, nocturnal EDD allows unrestricted access of the ICU staff to patients for daytime procedures, thereby minimizing disruption of ICU activities by renal replacement therapy [18, 30]. In general, there are no practical differences with respect to performing daytime and nighttime EDD. After appropriate training, machines are supervised solely by ICU personnel during the overnight shift, but a dialysis nurse is usually available on-call for advice and troubleshooting.

7.7.4 Quantifying the Dose of EDD and Survival with EDD

Solute and fluid removal in EDD are slower than during IHD, but faster compared with conventional CRRT. So far there is no established parameter for the EDD dose. As there is ongoing uncertainty about the utility of small solute clearance as a determinant of dialysis efficacy in EDD, urea reduction rate and/or Kt/V should be reserved for quantifying the dialysis dose in IHD. Support for the hypothesis that urea reduction rate and/or Kt/V are not suited to quantify the dose of EDD comes from a recent study by Eloot et al. [10]. They showed that despite a comparable Kt/V, the total solute removal for creatinine and urea increased with prolonging dialysis time from 4 over 6–8 h, i.e., indicating better solute removel despite identical Kt/V.

Although prospective clinical trials are still ongoing, currently available observational data suggest that the outcome of patients treated with EDD are neither different from that predicted by their illness severity scores nor different from patients treated with continuous renal replacement therapies. The most robust data come from a study by Marshall et al. which is currently only available in abstract form. A sudden and gradual switch from CVVH to EDD in two hospitals did not reveal any change in health-related mortality of patients with AKI in the ICU. The Veterans Affairs/National Institutes of Health (VA/NIH) Acute Renal Failure Trial Network that primarily evaluated the effect of dialysis dose on mortality in all three treatment modalities (IHD, EDD, CRRT) could not detect any association between outcome (survival, dependence from dialysis) and dialysis dose [1]. The primary publication of this study did not report a difference in mortality between different modalities [1]. The Stuivenberg Hospital Acute Renal Failure (SHARF) study is the only ongoing prospective multicenter randomized clinical trial in EDD. A total of 1,600 consecutive adult patients with AKI from ten participating Belgian ICUs are randomized to either EDD or CRRT. An interim report of the first 996 patients, which has been presented in abstract form, shows no difference in outcomes between modalities.

A multidisciplinary stakeholder committee that comprised representatives from the 18 leading international professional societies of critical care and nephrology, recently identified the question *"What is the optimal 'dosage' of RRT to maximize patient and renal survival?"* as one of the five most important topics of clinical research in this area [8]. In this regard, the results of the Hannover Dialysis Outcome (HAN-D-OUT) study are extremely relevant. In this study we compared standard versus intensified EDD in the treatment of patients with AKI in the ICU. Participants were randomly assigned to receive either standard (i.e., currently recommended) dialysis dosed to maintain plasma urea levels between 120–150 mg/dl (20–25 mmol/l) or intensified dialysis dosed to maintain plasma urea levels below 90 mg/dl (<15 mmol/l). Interestingly, no significant differences between intensified and standard treatment were seen for survival at day 14 (74.4% vs 70.0%) or day 28 (56.5% vs 60.0%), or for renal recovery among the survivors at day 28 (60.5% vs 59.5%). This is in line with the data of the ATN Trial in which intensive renal support in critically ill patients with AKI did not decrease mortality, improve recovery of kidney function, or reduce the rate of nonrenal organ failure as compared with less-intensive therapy involving a defined dose of IHD three times per week and continuous renal replacement therapy at 20 ml/kg/h [1]. As a similar finding was also described for continuous venovenous hemodiafiltration (CVVHDF) with prefilter replacement fluid at an effluent rate of either 35 ml/kg/h (high dosage) or 20 ml/kg/h (standard dosage) [44], the dose–survival relationship seems to plateau. Identifying the breakpoint where the steep dose–survival curve plateus might be important for providing the highest beneficial dose without overusing scarce financial and logistic resources. One important point we have to take into consideration is the fact that intensive therapy does not only lead to an increased elimination of uremic toxins, as vividly illustrated by the rate of hypophosphatemia (17.6% of patients in the intensive therapy group as compared with 10.9% undergoing less-intensive therapy) in the ATN study but will also affect the elimination of life-saving drugs such as antibiotics [1]. The failure to adapt the dosing of these and other drugs might explain why septic patients treated with a higher dose of renal replacement therapy in the ATN trial tended to have a lower survival as compared with the lower intensity group, where underdosing of drugs is less likely.

7.7.5 Technical Modifications of the EDD Technique

An important modification of the EDD technique is the use of regional citrate anticoagulation. Morgera et al. [37] have used the Genius® system together with a low-calcium dialysate concentration (1 mmol/l) infusing a 4% sodium citrate solution into the arterial line of the extracorporal circuit, and adjusted the citrate dose according to the postfilter ionized calcium concentration. They observed no significant untoward effects on blood levels of calcium and sodium, and acid–base values remained equilibrated during citrate anticoagulation. Excellent filter patency and cardiovascular stability of patients were maintained. The EDD technique has been also further extended by introduction of sustained low-efficiency daily diafiltration (SLEDD-f), which combines diffusive and convective solute transport to improve clearance of putative middle molecule inflammatory mediators [33].

7.7.6 The Genius Batch Dialysis System

Although the main operational characteristics of EDD, i.e., long dialysis time and low dialysate and blood flow rates, are not different, the Genius® batch dialysis system has some system immanent specifications that in our view offer additional benefits as compared with other dialysis machines. Currently this dialysis system is only available in Europe and South America. The technical principle underlying Genius® is based on the very first dialysis systems, the "tank" or "batch" devices. Briefly (the technical features are described in detail elsewhere [9, 12]), the dialysis machine does not require the usual infrastructure such as multilocal water supply or waste removal. Ultrapure dialysis fluid from a reverse osmosis system is filled in and removed from the individual machine at a central "filling station," where the sterile dialysis fluid is prepared, filled into the machines, and the used dialysate is drained after the treatment. Further advantages are reduced thrombogenicity (tubing is completely fluid-filled, i.e., air-free), simple and reliable control of volumetric ultrafiltration, 100% bicarbonate ultrapure dialysis fluid (with attendant beneficial effects on patient survival [4]), and the option of individualized treatment duration without software or hardware changes. Performing EDD using the Genius® single-pass system causes slight but significant cooling of the patient. Lonnemann et al. [28], using the 75-l tank of a previous model over 18 h, measured a temperature drop in the venous blood line of the extracorporeal circuit from 35.3 ± 0.7°C to 30.2 ± 0.8°C, which is equal to an average temperature loss of 0.28°C/h. When we performed EDD over a period of 12 h in mainly septic patients, at a blood flow rate of 200 ml/min and a dialysate flow rate of 100 ml/min [18], the core temperature (measured by a thermistor in the femoral artery) decreased slightly but significantly from 37.4 ± 0.3°C to 36.7 ± 0.2°C. The decrease in dialysate temperature and consequently the patient's core temperature could actually be advantageous, as it increases peripheral resistance and improves cardiovascular stability (as observed in patients on chronic HD) [47]. Bicarbonate-based buffers are susceptible to bacterial contamination, especially when the system used for CRRT is frequently opened to connect a bag of replacement fluid and discard the used filtrate [15]. This can occur as often as 40 times per day at a substitution rate of 37.5 ml/kg/h in a 100-kg patient. EDD of any kind does not involve this risk. Moreover, the Genius® system need not be opened at all once filled. Its smooth, crack-free, straight glass surfaces, UV radiator, and requirement for ultrapure water make colonization by microorganisms difficult, and facilitate effective cleansing and sterilization. In one analysis, no bacterial growth was found in spent EDD dialysate, even after 18 h [18, 28]. So, the spent EDD dialysate almost meets the threshold of sterility ($<10^{-6}$ colony forming units/ml) [28]. As backfiltration of pyrogens from contaminated dialysate into the blood can induce a drop in blood pressure during high-flux hemodialysis, the high bacteriological quality of the Genius® dialysate might contribute to cardiovascular stability during EDD. The Genius® apparatus also permits easy access to the entire complement of substances removed during a dialysis session. This feature generates exciting opportunities for clinical research in the fields of uremic toxins [16], pharmacokinetics [6, 7, 17, 21], and intoxications [19, 20, 22].

7.7.7 Removal of Drugs and Toxins

One of the main advantages of EDD is the superb efficacy in terms of removal of uremic toxins. Encouraged by this efficient solute elimination, physicians increasingly use EDD to treat intoxications [9, 19, 20, 22]. The advantages of EDD for this indication include less complications (especially in comparison with charcoal perfusion), and use of regular dialysis machines thus minimizing staff work load. Many case reports of standard dialysis followed by EDD to prevent rebound of the offending toxin have been published [20, 22], but the issue merits further study.

Due to the efficient removal of small solutes by EDD, attention must be paid to vital electrolytes such as phosphate [18]. As such, in institutions that perform EDD on a daily basis, phosphate supplementation is part of the treatment protocol [25, 33]. Furthermore, high efficiency renal replacement therapy such as CVVH or EDD has significant effects on pharmacokinetic and pharmacodynamic properties of most vital drugs administered to critically ill patients. In this respect the degree to which EDD eliminates drugs differs considerably from standard IHD or CRRT, and dosing/pharmacokinetic data obtained from patients receiving either IHD or CRRT might not be applicable to patients treated with EDD. Aiming for increased dialysis dose while adhering to outdated drug dosing recommendations based on old data obtained with, from today's view rather ineffective means of renal replacement therapy may lead to under dosing of important drugs such as antibiotics, a clinical catastrophy that in our view might have influenced the outcome of the ATN trial. Indeed, results from clinical studies have confirmed that there are significant differences in rates of drug removal by EDD compared with IHD and CRRT [6, 7, 11, 17]. Thus, dosing recommendations for patients with AKI in the ICU treated with EDD should become standard in the approval process of new drugs. Until then therapeutic drug monitoring should be used whenever possible, and dosing decisions need to be made on an individual basis.

7.7.8 Economic Considerations

Substantial cost reduction can be achieved if the equipment used for EDD is also used for chronic renal replacement therapy in the same hospital. In fact, all centers offering EDD use various standard IHD machines such as the 2008H® or the Genius® single-pass dialysis system without adding or altering software or hardware. In some hospitals, flexible treatment modalities allow the same machine to be used for two IHD sessions and one overnight EDD treatment in a 24-h period. This dual usage has been recognized by major manufacturers of dialysis equipment. Newer machines like the Fresenius 4008 series (4008K in the USA, 4008S ArRT-Plus [Fresenius Medical Care-Asia Pacific Pty, NSW, Australia] and the 4008S elsewhere) have a built-in option for EDD, which is selected from the startup screen without any delay or requirement for further adjustment. Several economic evaluations have shown EDD to be less expensive than CRRT, both within the setting of the US health care reimbursement scheme and within a more widely applicable nationalized health care system [2, 29]. In general, daily costs for EDD are between six and eight times lower than for CRRT [13, 26]. The main sources of cost savings are reduced staff load and reduced need for industrially produced sterile substitution fluid.

7.7.9 EDD: The "Hybrid" Approach in Terms of Techniques and Specialties

While IHD is a domain of the nephrologists, CRRTs have been performed in ICUs mostly without the involvement of nephrologists. Consequently, the choice of renal replacement therapy may also be seen as a statement of who should care for the patients and thereby represents a source of tension between medical specialties. What do we need a nephrologist for? This question reflects the rather hostile environment in which the Latin phrase *Salus aegroti suprema lex* is not more than paying lip service. In this regard it is of interest that the timing of the nephrology consultation may affect the patient's survival in the ICU. A prospective study in four US teaching hospitals revealed that delayed consultation of the nephrology service was associated with a trend toward increased mortality and morbidity, whether or not dialysis was ultimately required [34]. Most ICUs are run by physicians specialized in intensive care medicine, and nephrologists are not always consulted to provide optimal care including best possible extracorporeal renal replacement therapy for critically ill patients.

The effort to develop a cost-effective and easy-to-handle renal replacement therapy for ARF in the ICU has lead to the development of an alternative technique that combines most advantages of both intermittent and continuous renal replacement therapies. This "hybrid" renal replacement therapy utilizes equipment originally designed for treatment of patients with chronic renal failure and therefore does not require expensive industrially produced substitution fluid. The terms "extended daily dialysis" (EDD) or "sustained low-efficiency dialysis" (SLED) are most widely used for this method. The devices used for EDD are modified standard dialysis machines [5, 11, 24, 25, 31, 32, 42]. EDD offers ample opportunity for a collaborative interaction between nephrologists and intensivists as the nephrology staff is responsible for the prescription, provision, and initiation of the treatment, while responsibilities for monitoring, variation of ultrafiltration, troubleshooting, and discontinuation are shared. This cooperative approach may also promote close collaboration between the two distinct specialties, with opportunities for setting joint therapeutic standards and research programs.

7.7.10 Summary and Outlook

EDD is an increasingly popular renal replacement therapy in critically ill patients with AKI. It can also be employed as a prolonged high-volume treatment of severely ill patients, such as highly catabolic patients with sepsis, because normalization of indicators of uremic intoxication is achieved even in a shorter time than with CVVH [18]. Preliminary data indicate that the survival outcome of patients treated with EDD does not differ from that of those treated with state-of-the-art CVVH, but more definitive information will become available from ongoing multicenter prospective randomized trials. An important aspect of EDD is its ease of use for the ICU staff and its high degree of flexibility, especially when technically simple single-pass batch dialysis systems are employed. Increasingly relevant are economic evaluations that proved EDD to be less expensive than CRRT, both within the setting of the US health care reimbursement scheme and within a more widely applicable nationalized health care system [2, 5]. Moreover, the equipment used for EDD can also be used for chronic renal replacement therapy in the same hospital. In fact, all centers offering EDD use various standard IHD machines without substantial changes in software or hardware. Flexible treatment modalities allow the same machine to be used for daytime IHD sessions and overnight EDD treatment. Moreover, EDD has been proven in many centers to be an excellent area of collaboration between nephrologists and intensivists to provide the best possible treatment to critically ill patients. The high level of satisfaction of all those involved proves this to be a prudent approach.

7.7.11 Take Home Pearls

- The hallmark of EDD are long dialysis hours (8–18 h) and slow dialysate and blood flow rates.
- EDD offers a convenient way to control electrolytes and fluid balance in combination with cardiovascular stability.
- Available data suggest that survival with EDD is not different from other modes of renal replacement therapy.
- Dosing and pharmacokinetic data obtained from patients receiving either IHD or CRRT should not be used for patients undergoing EDD.
- Daily costs for EDD are between six and eight times less than for CRRT.

References

1. Intensity of renal support in critically ill patients with acute kidney injury. N Engl J Med 2008;359:7–20.
2. Alam M, Marshall M, Shaver M, Chatoth D: Cost comparison between sustained low efficiency hemodialysis (SLED) and continuous venovenous hemofiltration (CVVH) for ICU patients with ARF. Am J Kidney Dis 2000;35:A9.
3. Augustine JJ, Sandy D, Seifert TH, Paganini EP: A randomized controlled trial comparing intermittent with continuous dialysis in patients with ARF. Am J Kidney Dis 2004;44: 1000–1007.

4. Barenbrock M, Hausberg M, Matzkies F, de la MS, Schaefer RM: Effects of bicarbonate- and lactate-buffered replacement fluids on cardiovascular outcome in CVVH patients. Kidney Int 2000;58:1751–1757.
5. Berbece AN, Richardson RM: Sustained low-efficiency dialysis in the ICU: cost, anticoagulation, and solute removal. Kidney Int 2006;70:963–968.
6. Burkhardt O, Joukhadar C, Traunmuller F, Hadem J, Welte T, Kielstein JT: Elimination of daptomycin in a patient with acute renal failure undergoing extended daily dialysis. J Antimicrob Chemother 2008;61:224–225.
7. Czock D, Husig-Linde C, Langhoff A, Schoepke T, Hafer C, deGroot K, Swoboda S, Kuse E, Haller H, Fliser D, Keller F, Kielstein JT: Pharmacokinetics of moxifloxacin and levofloxacin in intensive care unit patients who have acute renal failure and undergo extended daily dialysis. Clin J Am Soc Nephrol 2006;1:1263–1268.
8. Davenport A, Bouman C, Kirpalani A, Skippen P, Tolwani A, Mehta RL, Palevsky PM: Delivery of renal replacement therapy in acute kidney injury: what are the key issues? Clin J Am Soc Nephrol 2008;3:864–868.
9. Dhondt A, Verstraete A, Vandewoude K, Segers H, Eloot S, Decruyenaere J, Vanholder R: Efficiency of the Genius batch hemodialysis system with low serum solute concentrations: the case of lithium intoxication therapy. Am J Kidney Dis 2005;46:e95–e99.
10. Eloot S, Van Biesen W, Dhondt A, Van de WH, Glorieux G, Verdonck P, Vanholder R: Impact of hemodialysis duration on the removal of uremic retention solutes. Kidney Int 2007.
11. Fiaccadori E, Maggiore U, Rotelli C, Giacosa R, Parenti E, Picetti E, Sagripanti S, Manini P, Andreoli R, Cabassi A: Removal of linezolid by conventional intermittent hemodialysis, sustained low-efficiency dialysis, or continuous venovenous hemofiltration in patients with acute renal failure. Crit Care Med 2004;32:2437–2442.
12. Fliser D, Kielstein JT: A single-pass batch dialysis system: an ideal dialysis method for the patient in intensive care with acute renal failure. Curr Opin Crit Care 2004;10:483–488.
13. Golper TA: Hybrid renal replacement therapies for critically ill patients. Contrib Nephrol 2004;144:278–283.
14. Hall FS, Shaver MJ, Marshall MR: Daily 12-hour sustained low-efficiency hemodialysis (SLED): a nursing perspective. Blood Purif 1999;17:36A.
15. Kanagasundaram NS, Larive AB, Paganini EP: A preliminary survey of bacterial contamination of the dialysate circuit in continuous veno-venous hemodialysis. Clin Nephrol 2003;59:47–55.
16. Kielstein JT, Boger RH, Bode-Boger SM, Martens-Lobenhoffer J, Lonnemann G, Frolich JC, Haller H, Fliser D: Low dialysance of asymmetric dimethylarginine (ADMA) – in vivo and in vitro evidence of significant protein binding. Clin Nephrol 2004;62:295–300.
17. Kielstein JT, Czock D, Schopke T, Hafer C, Bode-Boger SM, Kuse E, Keller F, Fliser D: Pharmacokinetics and total elimination of meropenem and vancomycin in intensive care unit patients undergoing extended daily dialysis. Crit Care Med 2006;34:51–56.
18. Kielstein JT, Kretschmer U, Ernst T, Hafer C, Bahr MJ, Haller H, Fliser D: Efficacy and cardiovascular tolerability of extended dialysis in critically ill patients: a randomized controlled study. Am J Kidney Dis 2004;43:342–349.
19. Kielstein JT, Linnenweber S, Schoepke T, Fliser D: One for all – a multi-use dialysis system for effective treatment of severe thallium intoxication. Kidney Blood Press Res 2004; 27:197–199.
20. Kielstein JT, Schwarz A, Arnavaz A, Sehlberg O, Emrich HM, Fliser D: High-flux hemodialysis – an effective alternative to hemoperfusion in the treatment of carbamazepine intoxication. Clin Nephrol 2002;57:484–486.
21. Kielstein JT, Stadler M, Czock D, Keller F, Hertenstein B, Radermacher J: Dialysate concentration and pharmacokinetics of 2F-Ara-A in a patient with acute renal failure. Eur J Haematol 2005;74:533–534.
22. Kielstein JT, Woywodt A, Schumann G, Haller H, Fliser D: Efficiency of high-flux hemodialysis in the treatment of valproic acid intoxication. J Toxicol Clin Toxicol 2003;41: 873–876.
23. Kolff WJ: Lasker Clinical Medical Research Award. The artificial kidney and its effect on the development of other artificial organs. Nat Med 2002;8:1063–1065.
24. Kumar VA, Craig M, Depner TA, Yeun JY: Extended daily dialysis: A new approach to renal replacement for acute renal failure in the intensive care unit. Am J Kidney Dis 2000;36:294–300.
25. Kumar VA, Yeun JY, Depner TA, Don BR: Extended daily dialysis vs. continuous hemodialysis for ICU patients with acute renal failure: a two-year single center report. Int J Artif Organs 2004;27:371–379.
26. Lameire N, Van Biesen W, Vanholder R: Dialysing the patient with acute renal failure in the ICU: the emperor's clothes? Nephrol Dial Transplant 1999;14:2570–2573.
27. Liao Z, Zhang W, Hardy PA, Poh CK, Huang Z, Kraus MA, Clark WR, Gao D: Kinetic comparison of different acute dialysis therapies. Artif Organs 2003;27:802–807.
28. Lonnemann G, Floege J, Kliem V, Brunkhorst R, Koch KM: Extended daily veno-venous high-flux haemodialysis in patients with acute renal failure and multiple organ dysfunction syndrome using a single path batch dialysis system. Nephrol Dial Transplant 2000;15:1189–1193.
29. Ma, T., Walker, J. A., Eggleton, K., and Marshall, M. Cost comparison between sustained low efficiency daily dialysis/diafiltration (SLEDD) and continuous renal replacement therapy for ICU patients with ARF. Nephrology (Carlton.) 7, A54. 2002. Ref type: Abstract
30. Marshall MR, Golper TA, Shaver MJ, Alam MG, Chatoth DK: Sustained low-efficiency dialysis for critically ill patients requiring renal replacement therapy. Kidney Int 2001;60:777–785.
31. Marshall MR, Golper TA, Shaver MJ, Alam MG, Chatoth DK: Urea kinetics during sustained low-efficiency dialysis in critically ill patients requiring renal replacement therapy. Am J Kidney Dis 2002;39:556–570.
32. Marshall MR, Golper TA, Shaver MJ, Chatoth DK: Hybrid renal replacement modalities for the critically ill. Contrib Nephrol 2001;252–257.
33. Marshall MR, Ma T, Galler D, Rankin AP, Williams AB: Sustained low-efficiency daily diafiltration (SLEDD-f) for critically ill patients requiring renal replacement therapy: towards an adequate therapy. Nephrol Dial Transplant 2004;19:877–884.
34. Mehta RL, McDonald B, Gabbai F, Pahl M, Farkas A, Pascual MT, Zhuang S, Kaplan RM, Chertow GM: Nephrology consultation in acute renal failure: does timing matter? Am J Med 2002;113:456–461.

35. Mehta RL, Pascual MT, Soroko S, Savage BR, Himmelfarb J, Ikizler TA, Paganini EP, Chertow GM: Spectrum of acute renal failure in the intensive care unit: the PICARD experience. Kidney Int 2004;66:1613–1621.
36. Metnitz PG, Krenn CG, Steltzer H, Lang T, Ploder J, Lenz K, Le G, Jr., Druml W: Effect of acute renal failure requiring renal replacement therapy on outcome in critically ill patients. Crit Care Med 2002;30:2051–2058.
37. Morgera S, Scholle C, Melzer C, Slowinski T, Liefeld L, Baumann G, Peters H, Neumayer HH: A simple, safe and effective citrate anticoagulation protocol for the genius dialysis system in acute renal failure. Nephron Clin Pract 2004;98:c35–c40.
38. Naka T, Baldwin I, Bellomo R, Fealy N, Wan L: Prolonged daily intermittent renal replacement therapy in ICU patients by ICU nurses and ICU physicians. Int J Artif Organs 2004;27:380–387.
39. Ratanarat R, Brendolan A, Volker G, Bonello M, Salvatori G, Andrikos E, Yavuz A, Crepaldi C, Ronco C: Phosphate kinetics during different dialysis modalities. Blood Purif 2005;23:83–90.
40. Ronco C, Bellomo R, Homel P, Brendolan A, Dan M, Piccinni P, La Greca G: Effects of different doses in continuous venovenous haemofiltration on outcomes of acute renal failure: a prospective randomised trial. Lancet 2000;356:26–30.
41. Schiffl H, Lang SM, Fischer R: Daily hemodialysis and the outcome of acute renal failure. N Engl J Med 2002;346: 305–310.
42. Schlaeper C, Amerling R, Manns M, Levin NW: High clearance continuous renal replacement therapy with a modified dialysis machine. Kidney Int Suppl 1999;72: S20–S23.
43. Schortgen F, Soubrier N, Delclaux C, Thuong M, Girou E, Brun-Buisson C, Lemaire F, Brochard L: Hemodynamic tolerance of intermittent hemodialysis in critically ill patients: usefulness of practice guidelines. Am J Respir Crit Care Med 2000;162:197–202.
44. Tolwani AJ, Campbell RC, Stofan BS, Lai KR, Oster RA, Wille KM: Standard versus high-dose CVVHDF for ICU-related acute renal failure. J Am Soc Nephrol 2008;19: 1233–1238.
45. Uchino S, Kellum JA, Bellomo R, Doig GS, Morimatsu H, Morgera S, Schetz M, Tan I, Bouman C, Macedo E, Gibney N, Tolwani A, Ronco C: Acute renal failure in critically ill patients: a multinational, multicenter study. JAMA 2005; 294:813–818.
46. Uehlinger DE, Jakob SM, Ferrari P, Eichelberger M, Huynh-Do U, Marti HP, Mohaupt MG, Vogt B, Rothen HU, Regli B, Takala J, Frey FJ: Comparison of continuous and intermittent renal replacement therapy for acute renal failure. Nephrol Dial Transplant 2005;20:1630–1637.
47. van der Sande FM, Kooman JP, Konings CJ, Leunissen KM: Thermal effects and blood pressure response during postdilution hemodiafiltration and hemodialysis: the effect of amount of replacement fluid and dialysate temperature. J Am Soc Nephrol 2001;12:1916–1920.

Quantifying the Dose of Acute Kidney Replacement Therapy

7.8

Zaccaria Ricci and Claudio Ronco

Core Messages

- During acute kidney replacement therapy the amount (dose) of delivered therapy can be described by various terms: efficiency, intensity, efficacy, frequency, and clinical efficacy.
- Efficiency is represented by the concept of clearance (*K*), that is, the volume of blood cleared of a solute over a given time; the clearance does not reflect the overall solute removal rate but rather its value normalized by the serum concentration.
- Intensity can be defined by the product of clearance and time (*Kt*); this is more useful than clearance alone in comparing various therapies; however, it does not take into account the size of the pool from which the solute needs to be cleared.
- Efficacy is the effective solute removal resulting from the administration of a treatment dose to a patient. It can be described as a fractional clearance of a given solute (Kt/V) where *V* is the volume of distribution of the marker molecule in the body.
- Clinical efficiency can only be assessed by adequately powered prospective randomized clinical studies. The evidence available to date supports the use of at least 35 ml/h/kg for CVVH, CVVHD, or CVVHDF, or 1.2 Kt/V daily intermittent hemodialysis in treating patients with acute kidney failure.

Z. Ricci (✉)
Department of Pediatric Cardiosurgery, Bambino Gesù Hospital, Piazza S. Onofrio 4, 00100 Rome, Italy
e-mail: zaccaria.ricci@fastwebnet.it

7.8.1 Introduction

Five to six percent of critically ill patients admitted to intensive care units (ICUs) develop acute kidney injury (AKI), and more than 70% of them require renal replacement therapy (RRT) [1]. The mortality rate for severe AKI has exceeded 50% over the last 3 decades, and it represents an independent risk factor for mortality of critically ill patients [2–5]. Based on the most recent RIFLE classification, AKI can be stratified into three different classes depending on the degree of severity as assessed by the extent of glomerular filtration rate loss [6, 7]. Current management depends on the level of severity and includes optimization of hemodynamics and fluid status, avoidance of further renal insults, optimization of nutrition and, when appropriate, the prescription of RRT.

Indications for RRT are generally clear for some patients with a "failure" level of AKI (e.g., anuria in the setting of septic shock), while they may require careful assessment in less severe situations (e.g., 12 h of oliguria in a 80-year-old patient with previous chronic renal dysfunction the day after surgery). Strategies to improve patient outcome in AKI may include optimization of delivered RRT dose. This chapter will focus on the concept of RRT dose, the meaning of dose calculation, prescription and delivery in the ICU, and on the current evidence addressing this issue.

7.8.2 Meaning and Different Approaches to RRT Dose

As with any other therapy administered in the ICU, any kind of dialysis has its "dosage." The conventional view of RRT dose is that it is a measure of the quantity

A. Jörres et al. (eds.), *Management of Acute Kidney Problems*,
DOI: 10.1007/978-3-540-69441-0_7.8, © Springer-Verlag Berlin Heidelberg 2010

of blood purified of "waste products and toxins" achieved by means of renal replacement. As this broad concept is too difficult to measure and quantify, the operative view of RRT dose is "synthesized" as the measure of the elimination of a representative marker solute. This marker solute should be reasonably representative of all solutes that are otherwise removed from blood by the kidney. This premise has two major flaws: first, the marker solute cannot and does not represent all the solutes that accumulate during AKI because kinetics and volume of distribution are different for each solute. Then, its removal during RRT is not necessarily representative of the removal of other solutes. This is true both for end-stage renal failure and AKI. Nevertheless, despite all of these limitations, a significant body of data [8] suggests that single solute marker assessment of dose of dialysis appears to have a clinically meaningful relationship with patient outcome and, therefore, clinical utility. The concept of RRT dose is useful also for practical purposes: as it happens for antibiotics, vasopressors, antiinflammatory drugs, mechanical ventilation, etc., the administration of an extracorporeal treatment for blood purification requires the operators to know exactly how and how much treatment should be prescribed and delivered. A deep knowledge and critical analysis of RRT dose may impact patients outcome not only on the basis of scientific results, but also because the treatment is optimally tailored to the patient in terms of schedule of administration, prescribed to delivered ratio, and of technical familiarity with complex machines and different membranes. According to a recent survey on practice patterns in different European centers a large number of operators in the field of acute dialysis seem to be uncertain on treatment prescription [9].

The amount (dose) of delivered RRT can be described by various terms: efficiency, intensity, frequency, and clinical efficacy.

Efficiency of RRT is represented by the concept of clearance (K), i.e., the volume of blood cleared of a given solute over a given time (it is generally expressed as volume over time: ml/min, ml/h, l/h, l/24 h, etc.). K does not reflect the overall solute removal rate (mass transfer) but rather its value normalized by the serum concentration: even when K remains stable over time, the removal rate will vary if the blood levels of the reference molecule change. During RRT, K depends on solute molecular size, transport modality (convection or diffusion), and circuit operational characteristics (blood flow rate [Q_b], ultrafiltration rate [Q_f], dialysate flow rate [Q_d], hemodialyzer type and size). Q_b, as a variable in delivering RRT dose, is mainly dependent on vascular access and operational characteristics of utilized machines in the clinical setting. During convective techniques Q_f is strictly linked to Q_b by filtration fraction (the fraction of plasma water that is removed from blood by ultrafiltration) because it is recommended to keep Q_f below $0.5*Q_b$. During diffusive techniques, when Q_d/Q_b ratio exceeds 0.3, it can be estimated that dialysate will not be completely saturated by blood diffusing solutes. In the absence of a specific solute, clearances of urea and creatinine blood levels are used to guide treatment dose. During ultrafiltration, the driving pressure jams solutes such as urea and creatinine against the membrane and into the pores, depending on membrane sieving coefficient (SC) for that molecule. SC expresses a dimensionless value and is estimated by the ratio of the concentration of the solutes in the filtrate divided by that in the plasma water or blood. A SC of 1.0, as is the case for urea and creatinine, demonstrates complete permeability, and a value of 0 reflects complete rejection. Molecular size over approximately 12 kDa and filter porosity are the major determinants of SC. The K during convection is measured by the product of Q_f times the SC. Thus, there is a linear relationship between K and Q_f, the SC being the changing variable for different solutes. During diffusion, an analogue linear relationship depends on diffusibility of a solute across the membrane. As a rough estimate, we showed that during continuous slow efficiency treatments, urea K can be considered as a direct expression of Q_f and Q_d [10]. K can be normally used to compare the treatment dose during each dialysis session, but it cannot be employed as an absolute dose measure to compare treatments with different time schedules. For example, K is typically higher in intermittent hemodialysis (IHD) than continuous renal replacement therapy (CRRT) and sustained low-efficiency daily dialysis (SLEDD). This is not surprising, since K represents only the instantaneous efficiency of the system. However, mass removal may be greater during SLEDD or CRRT. For this reason, the information about the time span during which K is delivered is fundamental to describe the effective dose of dialysis (intensity).

Intensity of RRT can be defined by the product "clearance × time" (Kt: ml/min * 24 h, l/h * 4 h, etc.). Kt is more useful than K in comparing various RRTs.

However, it does not take into account the size of the pool of solute which needs to be cleared. This requires the dimension of efficacy.

Efficacy of RRT is the effective solute removal outcome resulting from the administration of a given treatment dose to a given patient. It can be described as a fractional clearance of a given solute (Kt/V) where V is the volume of distribution of the marker molecule in the body. Kt/V is a dimensionless number (e.g.: 50 ml/min*24 h/45 l = 3 l/h *24 h/45 l = 72 l/ 45 l = 1.6) and it is an established measure of dialysis dose correlating with medium-term (several years) survival in chronic hemodialysis patients [11–14]. Urea is typically used as a marker molecule in end-stage kidney disease to guide treatment dose (the volume of distribution of urea (V_{UREA}) is generally considered as equal to patient total body water which is 60% of patient body weight), and a Kt/V_{UREA} of at least 1.2 is currently recommended for IHD treatments. However, Kt/V_{UREA} application to patients with AKI has not been rigorously validated due to a major uncertainty about V_{UREA} estimation. Some authors have suggested to express dose as K indexed to patient body weight as an operative measure of daily CRRT: it is now suggested to deliver at least 35 ml/h/kg*24 h [15–17]: if the simplification discussed above (K = ml/h = Q_f or Q_d) can be considered acceptable, this CRRT dose might be expressed in a 70 kg patient as about 2,500 ml/h or 60 l/day of continuous venovenous hemofiltration (CVVH: Q_f*kg*24 h) or dialysis (CVVHD: Q_d*kg*24 h). Interestingly, applying Kt/V_{UREA} dose assessment methodology in such a 70 kg patient, the dosage of 35 ml/h/kg *24 h would be equivalent to a Kt/V of 1.4.

Other authors suggested a prescription based on patient body surface area [18] or on metabolic requirements, based on urea generation rate and catabolic state of the single patient [19]. It has been shown, however, that during a continuous therapy a K less than 2 l/h will almost definitely be insufficient in an adult critically ill patient [20].

Some important caveats must be remarked at this point: the major shortcoming of the traditional solute marker-based approach to dialysis dose in AKI lies well beyond the question of which methodologic application of solute kinetics is better to approach. In patients with AKI, the majority of whom are in intensive care, a solute-limited concept of dialysis dose might result as grossly inappropriate. In critically ill patients the parameters that the "dose" of RRT affects are many more than the simple control of small solutes as represented by urea. They include acid–base control, tonicity control, potassium control, magnesium control, calcium and phosphate control, intravascular volume control, extravascular volume control, temperature control, and the avoidance of unwanted adverse effects associated with the delivery of solute control. These aspects of dose are not currently addressed by any attempt of measure, but should be considered when discussing the prescription of RRT: it is likely that patients die more often from incorrect intravascular volume control than hyperazotemia. It has been show, for example, that restoring an adequate water content in small children is the main independent variable for outcome prediction [21, 22]. This concept is much more important in the critically ill smaller patients, where a relatively larger amount of fluid must be administered to deliver an adequate amount of drug infusion, parenteral/enteral nutrition, and blood derivatives. Furthermore, unlike in the field of chronic hemodialysis, it may be that only major changes in the application of dose (e.g., changing from second daily to daily dialysis while prescribing the same Kt/V) can reasonably be believed to truly deliver a "different" dose in the setting of AKI. More subtle adjustments such as prescribing a calculated Kt/V of 1 versus 1.2 can easily be criticized as being within the calculation error around each prescription and not necessarily representing a reliable change in dose delivery.

7.8.3 RRT Dose Adequacy: Does It Exist?

Despite all the uncertainty surrounding its meaning and the gross shortcomings related to its accuracy in patients with AKI, the idea that there might be an optimal dose of solute removal has obviously a great impact on intensivist and operators in this field. This is likely due to practical reasons ("How should I set the machine?") and to the evidence from end-stage renal disease, where a minimum dose (Kt/V 1.2 thrice weekly) is indicated as standard [13]. The optimistic hypothesis that higher doses of dialysis may be beneficial in critically ill patients with AKI must be considered by analogy and investigated. Several reports exist in the literature dealing with this issue.

Brause and coworkers [23] using continuous venovenous hemofiltration (CVVH), found that higher Kt/V values (0.8 vs 0.53) were correlated with improved uremic control and acid–base balance. No clinically important outcome was affected. Investigators from the Cleveland clinic [24, 25] retrospectively evaluated 844 patients with AKI requiring CRRT or IHD over a 7-year period. They found that, when patients were stratified for disease severity, that dialysis dose did not affect outcome in patients with very high or very low scores, but did correlate with survival in patients with intermediate degrees of illness. A mean Kt/V greater than 1.0 was associated with increased survival. This study, of course was retrospective with a clear post hoc selection bias. The validity of these observations remains highly questionable.

Daily IHD compared with alternate-day dialysis also seemed to be associated with improved outcome in a recent trial [26]. Daily hemodialysis resulted in significantly improved survival (72% vs 54%, $p = 0.01$) better control of uremia, fewer hypotensive episodes and more rapid resolution of AKI. However, several limitations affected this study: sicker, hemodynamically unstable patients were excluded and underwent CRRT instead. Furthermore, it appears that patients receiving conventional IHD were underdialyzed. Furthermore, second daily dialysis was associated with significant differences in fluid removal and dialysis-associated hypotension, suggesting that other aspects of "dose" beyond solute control (inadequate and episodic volume control) might have explained the findings. These observations suggest that further studies should be undertaken to assess the effect of dose of IHD on outcome.

In a randomized controlled trial of CRRT dose, CVVH at 35 ml/h/kg or 45 ml/h/kg was associated with improved survival when compared with 20 ml/h/kg in 425 critically ill patients with AKI [15]. Many technical and/or clinical problems, however, can make it difficult, in routine practice, to apply such a strict protocol with pure postdilution hemofiltration. A survey of several units worldwide found that very few units deliver this intensive CRRT regimen: according to Uchino and coworkers, median unadjusted CRRT dose was 2,000 ml/h and the corrected dose was 20.4 ml/h/kg. Only 11.7% of patients were treated with a corrected dose of > 35 ml/kg/h [27]. Finally, in a study conducted by Ronco et al., the technique of CRRT was CVVH with postdilution, whereas current practice includes a variety of techniques in addition to CVVH, such as continuous venovenous hemodialysis (CVVHD) and continuous venovenous hemodiafiltration (CVVHDF). Equally important is the observation that this study was conducted over 6 years in a single center, that uremic control was not reported, that the study was unblinded, that the incidence of sepsis was low compared with that in the typical populations reported to develop AKI in the world [1], and that its final outcome was not the accepted 28-day or 90-day mortality typically used in ICU trials. Thus, the external validity of this study remains untested.

Another prospective randomized trial, conducted by Bouman et al. [28] assigned patients to three intensity groups: early high-volume hemofiltration (72–96 l/24 h), early low-volume hemofiltration (24–36 l/24 h), late low volume hemofiltration (24–36 l/24 h). These investigators found no difference in terms of renal recovery or 28-day mortality. Unfortunately, prescribed doses were not standardized by weight, making the potential variability in RRT dose large. Furthermore, the number of patients was small, making the study insufficiently powered and the incidence of sepsis low compared with that in the typical populations reported to develop AKI in the world.

Recently, Saudan and coworkers [16] enrolled 371 patients with AKI (102 to CVVH and 104 to CVVHDF) and prescribed 25 ml/h/kg ultrafiltration in the CVVH group and 24 ml/h/kg in the CVVHDF group; patients on CVVHDF were prescribed an adjunctive mean dialysis dose of 18 ml/h/kg. The CVVHDF patients had significantly higher mean urea and creatinine reduction ratios 48 h after the initiation of continuous RRT than did the CVVH patients (50% vs 40%, $p < 0.009$, and 46% vs 38%, $p < 0.014$, respectively). Survival rates at 28 days and 90 days were higher with CVVHDF than with CVVH. Like previous trials, this study is underpowered; furthermore, it confounds the effects of dose and technique by adding dialysis to filtration. Nevertheless, pooled results from the last four studies [15, 16, 26, 28] seem to indicate a very large effect on survival in favor of augmented dosing [29]. Although these data may still not be definitive, the best evidence to date supports the use of at least 35 ml/h/kg for CVVH, CVVHDF, or 1.2 Kt/V daily IHD.

Another fundamental aspect of RRT, significantly affecting the meaning itself of dose, is the relation between prescribed and actually delivered therapy in patients with AKI: delivery of prescribed dose can be limited by technical problems such as access recirculation, poor blood flows with temporary venous catheters, membrane clotting, machine malfunction, and long times required for bag and/or circuit substitution. Clinical issues such as hypotension and vasopressor requirements can be responsible for solute disequilibrium within tissues and organs. These aspects are particularly evident during IHD, less so during SLEDD and even less so during CRRT. Treatment interruptions due to patient need for surgery or other diagnostic procedures should also be considered. In this case IHD might result in a more efficient prescribed to delivered ratio.

In a prospective observational trial [30], it has been clearly shown that downtime (amount of hours spent off an active treatment) adversely affects azotemic control: a significant correlation between downtime and creatinine levels was found ($p < 0.0001$). According to these authors, the downtime should be less than 8 h per day to maintain creatinine and urea concentrations with our operative setting (2 l/h of ultrafiltration): for example if one prescribed an ultrafiltration rate of 35 ml/h/kg, only 23 ml/h/kg would be delivered if downtime was 8 h/day. Evanson and coworkers [31] found that a high patient weight, male sex, and low blood flow were limiting factors affecting IHD administration and that about 70% of dialysis delivered a Kt/V of less than 1.2. A retrospective study by Venkatarman et al. [32] also showed that, similarly, patients receive only 67% of prescribed CRRT therapy. Of note, in the CVVH dose trial [15], only patients who achieved more than 85% of the prescribed dose were included: in order to obtain this goal, compensation for interruptions in treatment due to ICU procedures was made by increasing effluent flow rates in the subsequent hours. A recent prospective trial where CRRT prescribed to delivered ratio was monitored, an average 10.7% ($p < 0.05$) reduction of therapy delivery was found, when compared with prescribed dose [10]. This delivery reduction was sometimes due to the estimation error brought about by the use of dose calculator software and, more often, to the short operative treatment time with respect to prescribed.

These observations suggest that RRT prescriptions for AKI patients in the intensive care unit (ICU) should be monitored closely if one wishes to ensure adequate delivery of prescribed dose and, importantly, to avoid underdialysis.

7.8.4 RRT Dose Delivery: Continuous, Intermittent, Hybrid

According recent international surveys on clinical practice patterns, 80% centers administer CRRT, 17% use intermittent RRT (IRRT), and a very small minority apply peritoneal dialysis (PD) [1, 27, 33]. Interestingly, in many centers intermittent techniques are utilized together with continuous ones, thus evidencing the possibility of multiple prescriptions and practices [9]. Nonetheless, after years of debate, the scientific literature is not able to draw conclusions on how RRT delivery modalities may impact clinical outcomes. Many papers have been published on this issue, and they must be analyzed critically.

From the point of view of a pure clearance-based dose, the RRT modality that provides “more dialysis,” seems to favorably impact the outcome. For example PD, apparently providing less urea clearance per week than IHD, has comparable patient outcomes [34]. The reason for this difference may be that urea is less compartmentalized than other solutes, and equivalent amounts of urea removal where one therapy is intermittent rather than continuous do not represent equivalent therapies for a broader range of solutes. Again, if the critical parameter is metabolic control, an acceptable mean blood urea nitrogen level of 60 mg/dl, easily obtainable in a 100-kg patient with a 2 l/h CVVH, in a computer-based simulation, has been shown to be very difficult to reach even by intensive IHD regimens [35]. In addition to the benefits specifically pertaining to the kinetics of solute removal, increased RRT frequency results in decreased ultrafiltration requirements per treatment. The avoidance of volume swings related to rapid ultrafiltration rates may also represent another dimension of dose where comparability is difficult.

Many randomized controlled trials compared intermittent and continuous RRT, providing so far only conflicting and puzzling results. Basing on actual scientific evidence, the Surviving Sepsis Campaign guidelines for management of severe sepsis and septic shock [17] recently concluded that during AKI, CVVH and IHD should be considered equivalent. A large comparative trial randomized 166 critically ill patients with AKI to either CRRT or IHD [36]. The authors found that the CRRT population, despite randomization, had significantly greater severity of illness scores. Furthermore, despite better control of azotemia and a greater likelihood of achieving the desired fluid balance, CRRT had increased mortality. A smaller trial by the Cleveland Clinic group [37] also failed to find a difference in outcome between one therapy and another. A meta-analysis of 13 studies conducted by Kellum and coauthors [38], which concluded that, after stratification of 1,400 patients according to disease severity, when similar patients were compared, CRRT was associated with a significant decrease in the risk of death. The authors confirmed that a large carefully controlled randomized clinical trial should be undertaken. Another meta-analysis [39] found no difference between the two techniques.

Recently, the Program to Improve Care in Acute Renal Disease (PICARD) Group conducted a retrospective trial and compared the outcomes of different RRT modalities in 368 patients (CRRT [$n = 206$] versus IHD [$n = 192$]) [40]. Within the PICARD cohort, CRRT in comparison with IHD was associated with a significantly higher relative risk for mortality. The authors state that these data provide no evidence for a survival benefit afforded by CRRT. However, the authors admit that patients with CRRT were significantly sicker and that the results could reflect residual confounding by severity of illness. Furthermore they claim that a randomized clinical trial should be conducted "excluding patients with severe hypotension and hemodynamic instability, who may be poor candidates for traditional IHD": probably such a trial would not be of clinical relevance among critically ill patients.

Vinsonneau and colleagues [41] recently conducted a large, prospective, randomized multicenter study in 21 ICUs over a 3.5-year period. The primary end point was the 60-day mortality following the randomization of 360 patients with acute renal failure (ARF) to either CVVHDF or IHD in centers that were familiar with both techniques. The eligibility criteria changed after 8 months due to the inclusion rate being too low. No difference in 28-day, 60-day (CVVHDF 33% vs IHD 32%), and 90-day mortality between the two groups was found, and the authors concluded that all patients with ARF as part of multiple organ dysfunction syndrome can be treated with IHD. The study was well conducted and, at the moment, it is the best example of randomized controlled study comparing effectively the two techniques. Nonetheless, the study started more than 7 years ago, during which time the practices in both CVVHDF and IHD have changed considerably. As stated by Vinsonneau and colleagues, this may have lead to changes in investigator practices during the study period, particularly with respect to the delivered dose of renal support. This possibility, however, is hard to ascertain given that the investigators, by protocol, started therapy with "initial standardized settings" and then adapted these settings to meet individual patient requirements to obtain the metabolic control objectives. Interestingly, the mortality decreased in the IHD arm of the study over the time of recruitment, which reflected a change in practice toward an increase in dialysis prescription. Given the lack of control regarding the dosage in both arms of the study, definitive conclusions are hard to make regarding treatment. As remarked in the accompanying editorial [42], the question of which treatment is better is influenced by the nature of the task. CRRT might be better in terms of total water and solute removal over 24 h and hemodynamic tolerance, but IHD can remove much more water and solute per hour, it does not require continuous anticoagulation, nor complete patient immobilization. Furthermore, the advantages of continuous therapies are largely supported when it is administered without prolonged interruptions, that is often not the case: again, unfortunately the study by Vinsonneau do not provided this information. Finally, if it is true that all patients with ARF as part of multiple organ dysfunction syndrome can be treated with IHD, this means that they can also be safely treated by CVVHDF.

Other reports have drawn similar conclusions [43, 44]. One of the common key point of these recent trials can be, however, that IHD has become safer and more efficacious with contemporary dialytic techniques. Furthermore, a liberal and extended use of CRRT might have become less safe and/or efficacious than previously considered or expected. Over the past 2 decades, however, technical advances in the delivery of IHD have dramatically decreased the propensity of IHD to cause intradialytic hypotension. These advances include the introduction of volume-controlled dialysis machines, the routine use of biocompatible synthetic dialysis membranes, the use of bicarbonate-based dialysate, and the delivery of higher doses of dialysis. Schortgen et al. demonstrated that there was a lower rate of hemodynamic instability and better outcomes after implementation of a clinical practice algorithm designed to improve hemodynamic tolerance to IHD [45]. Recommendations included priming the dialysis circuit with isotonic saline, setting dialysate sodium concentration at above 145 mmol/l, discontinuing vasodilator therapy, and setting dialysate temperature to below 37°C. Thus, the original rationale for the widely held assumption that CRRT is a superior therapy may have dissipated over time.

In conclusion, the question of superiority of a modality for renal support might be artificial. In routine clinical practice, as designed by Vinsonneau protocol, a change from an approach to another seems reasonable when clinical status changes (e.g., from CRRT to IHD when hemodynamics improves or the patient is extubated and vice versa), even if this common sense approach has never been scientifically validated. Randomizing patients to receive one therapy or the other regardless of the conditions might yield results that are difficult to generalize to clinical practice. About 10 years ago, a similar passionate debate on ventilation-weaning strategies (pressure support ventilation versus T-piece spontaneous ventilation versus continuous pressure airway pressure versus synchronized intermittent mandatory ventilation) was ongoing: the scientific community finally agreed that it is difficult to select one method over the other and that the *manner* in which the mode of weaning is applied may have a greater effect on the likelihood of weaning than the *mode* itself [46].

Finally, the design of future trials should include as the primary outcome other parameters than mortality. Recently, the Beginning Ending renal Support Therapy study group reported the results of a prospective observational study on a worldwide large cohort of 54 centers over 1,260 patients treated with RRT for ARF: 1,006 (82.6%) were initially treated with CRRT and 212 with IRRT (17.4%) [33]. Patients treated first with CRRT required vasopressor drugs and mechanical ventilation more frequently compared with those receiving IRRT. Unadjusted hospital survival was lower (35.8% vs 51.9%, $p < 0.0001$). However, unadjusted dialysis-independence at hospital discharge was higher after CRRT (85.5% vs 66.2%, $p < 0.0001$). Multivariable logistic regression showed that choice of CRRT was not an independent predictor of hospital survival or dialysis-free hospital survival. However, the choice of CRRT was a predictor of dialysis independence at hospital discharge among survivors (odds ratio [OR] 3.333; 95% confidence interval [95% CI], 1.845–6.024; $p < 0.0001$). The choice of CRRT as initial therapy probably is not a predictor of hospital survival or dialysis-free hospital survival but is an independent predictor of renal recovery among survivors.

Similar results were presented by other authors. In his randomized controlled trial, Mehta et al. reported that initial CRRT was associated with a significantly higher rate of complete renal recovery than IRRT in the subgroup of surviving patients who received an adequate trial of therapy without crossover (CRRT: 92.3% vs IRRT: 59.4%, $p < 0.01$) [36]. Bell and the Swedish Intensive Care Nephrology Group [47] showed that within 1,102 patients surviving 90 days after inclusion in the cohort, 944 (85.7%) were treated with CRRT and 158 (14.3%) were treated with IHD. Seventy-eight patients (8.3%; 95% CI, 6.6–10.2), never recovered their renal function in the CRRT group. The proportion was significantly higher among IHD patients, where 26 subjects or 16.5% (95% CI, 11.0–23.2) developed need for chronic dialysis. Again, analyzing a smaller cohort, Jacka and coworkers reviewed the records of 116 patients undergoing RRT and realized that renal recovery was significantly more frequent among patients initially treated with CRRT (21/24 vs 5/14, $p = 0.0003$) [48].

Hybrid techniques have come during the last few years as a feasible compromise solution to this eternal dispute. They have been given a variety of names such as slow low-efficiency extended daily dialysis (SLEDD) [49], prolonged daily intermittent RRT (PDIRRT) [50], extended daily dialysis (EDD) [51], or simply extended dialysis [52] depending on variations in schedule and type of solute removal (convective or diffusive). Theoretically speaking, the purpose of such therapy would be the optimization of the advantages offered by either CRRT and IHD, including efficient solute removal with minimum solute disequilibrium, reduced ultrafiltration rate with hemodynamic stability, optimized delivered to prescribed ratio, low anticoagulant needs, diminished cost of therapy delivery, efficiency of resource use, and improved patient mobility. These initial case series have shown the feasibility and high clearances potentially associated with such approaches. A single short-term single-center trial comparing hybrid therapies with CRRT has shown satisfying results in terms of dose delivery and hemodynamic stability [52]. Recently, Baldwin and coworkers randomized 16 patients to 3 consecutive days of treatment with either CVVH (8) or extended daily dialysis with filtration (EDDf) (8) and compared small solute, electrolyte, and acid–base control [53]. They did not found significant differences between the two therapies for urea or creatinine levels over 3 days. All electrolyte derangements before treatment were corrected as a result of treatment, except for one patient in the CVVH group who developed hypophosphatemia (0.54 mmol/l) at 72 h. After 3 days of treatment, there was a mild but persistent metabolic acidosis in the EDDf group compared with the CVVH group.

It is now possible to generate ultrapure replacement fluid and administer it in the ICU with a lower cost than CRRT, in greater amounts and for shorter periods of time. Hemofiltration may be combined with diffusion or pure diffusion can be selected at any chosen clearance for a period of time which can encompass the daytime period with the maximum staff availability or the night-shift period. Thus, the choices are now almost limitless: 3 or 4 h of IHD with standard settings or CRRT at 35 ml/kg/h of effluent flow rate can be selected. SLEDD at blood and dialysate flow rates of 150 ml/min for 8 h during the day or SLEDD for 12 h overnight can be considered as an alternative. Another option might be to use a sequential combination of CRRT, performed during the first 2 or 3 days when the patient is in the hyperacute phase, followed by SLEDD when the clinical situation improves.

Going back to the "ventilation approach," the modes of RRT are beginning to resemble the modes of mechanical ventilation with ventilator settings seamlessly being changed to fit into the therapeutic goals and patient needs and phases of illness. Just as the stereotyped approaches to ventilation are anachronistic and inappropriately try to fit the patient into a fixed therapy rather than tailoring the therapy to the patient, so should RRT be adjusted to fulfill the needs of the patients.

7.8.5 Conclusions

There is urgent need for prospective high-quality and suitably powered trials to adequately address the issue of dose and modality: new high levels of evidence are however coming from two very recent trials. A (small) randomized controlled trial in 200 critically ill patients with AKI concluded that patient survival or renal recovery was not different between patients receiving high-dosage (35 ml/kg/h) or standard-dosage (20 ml/kg/h) CVVHDF [54]. In the second study, under the sponsorship of the US Veterans Affairs/National Institutes of Health (VA/NIH) Acute Renal Failure Trial Network, 1,124 critically ill patients with AKI and failure of at least one nonrenal organ or sepsis were randomly assigned to receive intensive or less intensive RRT [55]. The study was a multicenter, prospective, randomized, parallel-group trial conducted between November 2003 and July 2007 at 27 VA and university-affiliated medical centers. In both groups only hemodynamically stable patients underwent IHD, whereas hemodynamically unstable patients underwent CVVHDF or SLEDD. Patients receiving the intensive treatment strategy underwent IHD and SLEDD six times per week and CVVHDF at 35 ml/h/kg of body weight; for patients receiving the less-intensive treatment strategy, the corresponding treatments were provided thrice weekly and at 20 ml/h/kg. Baseline characteristics of the 1,124 patients in the two groups were similar. The rate of death from any cause by day 60 was 53.6% with intensive therapy and 51.5% with less-intensive therapy (OR, 1.09; 95% CI, 0.86-1.40; p = 0.47). There was no significant difference between the two groups in the duration of RRT or in the rate of recovery of kidney function or nonrenal organ failure. This is the first multicenter clinical trial with adequate statistical power on different RRT strategies, so far. The findings of this study contrast with other single-center trials [15, 16] and are similar to smaller studies by Tolwani and Bouman [28, 54]. However, these results add a high level of evidence to the debate on dialysis dose and are going to be discussed for a long time. Nonetheless, many concerns about external validity of the study have risen. First of all, patients were allowed to be transitioned from one dialysis method to another: in this condition, as discussed above, the dialysis dose is impossible to compare and unlikely to be equivalent. Furthermore, there could be confounding factors if the patterns of use of methods differed between the high-intensity and low-intensity groups. Finally it is not known if the study findings can be generalized to different health care systems from those in the United States and to different RRT approaches (e.g., the sole use of CVVH by many European and Australian centers). In any case, it is possible that strategies other than only increasing RRT dose might help AKI patients. As the accompanying editorial correctly points out, current approaches to dialysis are probably adequate to replace critical functions such as regulation of volume and electrolyte and acid–base homeostasis. Still lacking are methods that efficiently down-regulate the inflammatory response, which might play a major role in the pathophysiology of AKI [56].

Finally, during the Acute Renal Failure Trial Network [55], net ultrafiltration of patients undergoing intermittent techniques (less than 2 l/day) was apparently lower than that of patients undergoing CVVHDF (130 ml/h or 2.7 l/day, considering a median daily duration of therapy of 21 h). In particular, a (nonsignificant) difference was present between net ultrafiltration of intense IHD versus less intense IHD (1.7 vs 2.1 l/day), whereas intense CVVHDF had very similar ultrafiltration rates compared with less intense CVVHDF (130 vs 130 ml/h). Since hypotension events were significantly higher in the group treated with a higher RRT intensity, it might be speculated that these were correlated with an excessively rapid fluid (and solute) shifts of intermittent therapies.

As concluded by the Acute Dialysis Quality Initiative (ADQI) workgroup in 2001 [57, 58], delivered clearance should be monitored during all renal supportive therapies. No recommendations can be made for specific dialysis dosing for patient with specific diseases at this time. A minimum dose of RRT, however, needs to be delivered for AKI: the best evidence to date supports the use of at least 35 ml/h/kg for CVVH, CVVHD, or CVVHDF, or 1.2 Kt/V daily IHD. It should also be recommended that the prescription should exceed that calculated to be "adequate" because of the known gap between prescribed and delivered dose. As the spectrum of RRT has expanded from PD and IHD alone approximately 25 years ago, to the full spectrum of therapy from standard IRRT to high-efficacy CRRT, physicians may ultimately choose to take a much more flexible approach to RRT and RRT dose.

7.8.6 Take Home Pearls

- A comparison of delivered "dose" between the different therapy modalities (intermittent vs continuous, convective vs diffusive) is difficult; technically it can be described by the terms: efficiency, intensity, efficacy, and frequency.
- Above all, the most important parameter is the clinical efficiency of kidney replacement therapies; however, this can only be assessed by adequate clinical studies. Based on the evidence available to date, the use of at least 35 ml/h/kg for CVVH, CVVHD, or CVVHDF, or 1.2 Kt/V daily intermittent hemodialysis is recommended for treating patients with acute kidney failure.

References

1. Uchino S, Kellum JA, Bellomo R, Doig GS, Morimatsu H, Morgera S, Schetz M, Tan I, Bouman C, Macedo E, Gibney N, Tolwani A, Ronco C for the Beginning and Ending Supportive Therapy for the Kidney (BEST Kidney) Investigators. Acute Renal Failure in Critically Ill Patients A Multinational, Multicenter Study. JAMA 2005; 294: 813–818.
2. Lameire N, van Biesen W, Van Holder R, Colardijn F. The place of intermittent hemodialysis in the treatment of acute renal failure in the ICU patient. Kidney Int 1998; 53(Suppl 66): S110–S119.
3. Levy EM, Ascoli CM, Horowitz RJ. The effect of acute renal failure on mortality. JAMA 1996; 275: 1489–1494.
4. DuBose T, Warnock DG, Mehta RL, Bonventre JV, Hammerman MR, Molitoire DA et al. Acute renal failure in the 21st century: recommendation for management and outcomes assessment. Am J Kidney Dis 1997; 29: 793–799.
5. Chertow GM, Levy EM, Hammermeister KE, Grover F, Dailey J: Independent association between acute renal failure and mortality following cardiac surgery. Am J Med 1998; 104: 343–348.
6. Bellomo R, Ronco C, Kellum JA, Mehta R, Palevsky P, The ADQI workgroup: Acute renal failure – definition, outcome measures, animal models, fluid therapy and information technology needs: the Second International Consensus Conference of the Acute Dialysis Quality Initiative (ADQI) Group. Crit Care. 2004; 8(4): R204–212.
7. Mehta RL, Kellum JA, Shah SV, Molitoris BA, Ronco C, Warnock DG, Levin A for the Acute Kidney Injury Network. Acute Kidney Injury Network: report of an initiative to improve outcomes in acute kidney injury. Critical Care 2007; 11: R31.
8. Ricci Z, Bellomo R, Ronco C. Dose of dialysis in acute renal failure. Clin J Am Soc Nephrol. 2006; 1: 380–388.
9. Ricci Z, Ronco C, D'amico G, De Felice R, Rossi S, Bolgan I, Bonello M, Zamperetti N, Petras D, Salvatori G, Dan M, Piccinni P. Practice patterns in the management of acute renal failure in the critically ill patient: an international survey. Nephrol Dial Transplant. 2006; 21: 690–696.
10. Ricci Z, Salvatori G, Bonello M, Bolgan I, D'Amico G, Dan M, Piccinni P and Ronco C. In vivo validation of the adequacy calculator for continuous renal replacement therapies. Critical Care 2005; 9: R266–R273.
11. Gotch F, Sargent J. A mechanistic analysis of the National Cooperative Dialysis Study (NCDS). Kidney Int 1985; 28:526–534.
12. Parker T, Hushni L, Huang W, Lew N, Lowrie E. Survival of hemodialysis patients in the United States is improved with a greater quantity of dialysis. Am J Kidney Dis 1994; 23: 670–680.
13. Eknoyan G, Levin N. NKF-K/DOQI clinical practice guidelines: update 2000. Am J Kidney Dis 2001; 38: 917.
14. Eknoyan G, Beck GJ, Cheung AK, Daugirdas JT, Greene T, Kusek JW, Allon M, Bailey J, Delmez JA, Depner TA, Dwyer JT, Levey AS, Levin NW, Milford E, Ornt DB, Rocco MV, Schulman G, Schwab SJ, Teehan BP, Toto R; Hemodialysis (HEMO) Study Group. Effect of dialysis dose and membrane flux in maintenance hemodialysis. N Engl J Med 2002; 347: 2010–2009.
15. Ronco C, Bellomo R, Homel P, et al: Effects of different doses in continuous veno-venous haemofiltration on outcomes of acute renal failure: a prospective randomised trial. Lancet 2000; 356: 26–30.
16. Saudan P, Niederberger M, De Seigneux S, Romand J, Pugin J, Perneger T and Martin PY. Adding a dialysis dose to

continuous hemofiltration increases survival in patients with acute renal failure. Kidney Int 2006; 70: 1312–1317.
17. Dellinger PR, Carlet JM, Masur H, Gerlach H, Calandra T, Cohen J et al. Surviving Sepsis Campaign guidelines for management of severe sepsis and septic shock. Crit Care Med 2004; 32: 858–873.
18. Brophy PD, Bunchman TE. References and overview for hemofiltration in pediatrics and adolescents. www.pcrrt.com. Last access 23/08/2007.
19. Sigler MH, Teehan BP, Daugirdas JT, Ing TS. Slow continuous therapies. In: Daugirdas JT, Blake PG, Todd SI. Handbook of Dialysis, 3rd edition, 2001, Lippincott Williams & Wilkins Philadelphia (PA) USA.
20. Garred L, Leblanc M, Canaud B. Urea kinetic modeling for CRRT. Am J Kidney Dis 1997; 30(Suppl 4): S2–9.
21. Goldstein SL, Currier H, Graf C, Cosio CC, Brewer ED, Sachdeva R (2001). Outcome in children receiving continuous veno-venous hemofiltration. Pediatrics; 107:1309–1312.
22. Foland JA, Fortenberry JD, Warshaw BL, Pettignano R, Merritt RK, Heard ML, Rogers K, Reid C, Tanner AJ, Easley KA (2004). Fluid overload before continuous hemofiltration and survival in critically ill children: a retrospective analysis. Crit Care Med; 32: 1771–1776.
23. Brause M, Nuemann A, Schumacher T et al. Effect of filtration volume of continuous venovenous hemofiltration in the treatment of patients with acute renal failure in intensive care units. Critical Care Med 2003; 31: 841–846.
24. Paganini EP, Tapolyai M, Goormastic M, Halstenberg W, Kozlowski L, Leblanc M, Lee JC, Moreno L, Sakai K. Establishing a dialysis therapy/patient outcome link in intensive care unit acute dialysis for patients with acute renal failure. Am J Kidney Dis 1996; 28(Suppl 3): S81–S89.
25. Paganini EP, Kanagasundaram NS, Larive B, Greene T. Prescription of Adequate Renal Replacement in Critically Ill Patients. Blood Purif 2001; 19: 238–244.
26. Schiffl H, Lang SM, Fischer R. Daily hemodialysis and the outcome of acute renal failure. N Engl J Med 2002; 346: 305–310.
27. Uchino S, Bellomo R, Morimatsu H, Morgera S, Schetz M, Tan I, Bouman C, Macedo E, Gibney N, Tolwani A, Oudemans-van Straaten H, Ronco C, Kellum JA. Continuous renal replacement therapy: A worldwide practice survey : The Beginning and Ending Supportive Therapy for the Kidney (B.E.S.T. Kidney) Investigators. Intensive Care Med. 2007; 27 [Epub ahead of print].
28. Bouman C, Oudemans-van Straaten H, Tijssen J, et al. Effects of early high-volume continuous veno-venous hemofiltration on survival and recovery of renal function in intensive care patients with acute renal failure: a prospective randomized trial. Crit Care Med 2002; 30: 2205–2211.
29. Kellum JA. Renal replacement therapy in critically ill patients with acute renal failure: does a greater dose improve survival? Nat Clin Pract Nephrol. 2007 Mar; 3(3): 128–129.
30. Uchino S, Fealy N, Baldwin I, Morimatsu H, Bellomo R. Continuous is not continuous: the incidence and impact of circuit "down-time" on uraemic control during continuous veno-venous haemofiltration. Intensive Care Med. 2003; 29: 575–578.
31. Evanson JA, Himmelfarb J, Wingard R, et al. Prescribed versus delivered dialysis in acute renal failure patients. Am J Kidney Dis 1998; 32: 731–738.
32. Venkataraman R, Kellum JA, Palevsky P. Dosing patterns for CRRT at a large academic medical center in the United States. J Crit Care 2002; 17: 246–250.
33. Uchino S, Bellomo R, Kellum JA, Morimatsu H, Morgera S, Schetz MR, Tan I, Bouman C, Macedo E, Gibney N, Tolwani A, Oudemans-Van Straaten HM, Ronco C; Beginning and Ending Supportive Therapy for the Kidney (B.E.S.T. Kidney) Investigators Writing Committee. Patient and kidney survival by dialysis modality in critically ill patients with acute kidney injury. Int J Artif Organs. 2007; 30: 281–292.
34. Depner TA. Benefits of more frequent dialysis: lower TAC at the same Kt/V. Nephrol Dial Transplant 1998; 13(Suppl 6): 20–24.
35. Clark WR, Mueller BA, Kraus MA, Macias WL. Renal replacement quantification in acute renal failure. Nephrol Dial Transplant 1998; 13(Suppl 6): 86–90.
36. Mehta RL, McDonald B, Gabbai FB, et al: A randomized clinical trial of continuous versus intermittent dialysis for acute renal failure. Kidney Int 2001; 60: 1154–1163.
37. Augustine J J, Sandy D, Seifert TH, Paganini EP, A randomized controlled trial comparing intermittent with continuous dialysis in patients with AKI. Am J Kidney Dis 2004; 44: 1000–1007.
38. Kellum J, Angus DC, Johnson JP, et al: Continuous versus intermittent renal replacement therapy: A meta-analysis. Intensive Care Med 2002; 28: 29–37.
39. Tonelli M, Manns B, Feller-Kopman D. Acute renal failure in the intensive care unit: A systematic review of the impact of dialytic modality on mortality and renal recovery. Am J Kidney Dis 2002; 40: 875–885.
40. Cho KC, Himmelfarb J, Paganini E, Ikizler TA, Soroko SH, Mehta RL, Chertow GM. Survival by dialysis modality in critically ill patients with acute kidney injury. J Am Soc Nephrol. 2006; 17: 3132–3138.
41. Vinsonneau C, Camus C, Combes A, Costa de Beauregard MA, Klouche K, Boulain T, Pallot JL, Chiche JD, Taupin P, Landais P, Dhainaut JF, Hemodiafe Study Group. Continuous venovenous haemodiafiltration versus intermittent haemodialysis for acute renal failure in patients with multiple-organ dysfunction syndrome: a multicentre randomised trial. Lancet. 2006; 29: 379–385.
42. Kellum J, Palevsky PM. Renal support in acute kidney injury. Lancet 2006; 29: 344–345.
43. Guerin C, Girard R, Selli JM, Ayzac L. Intermittent versus continuous renal replacement therapy for acute renal failure in intensive care units: results from a multicenter prospective epidemiological survey. Intensive Care Med 2002; 28: 1411–1418.
44. Uehlinger DE, Jakob SM, Ferrari P, Eichelberger M, Huynh-Do U, Marti HP, Mohaupt MG, Vogt B, Rothen HU, Regli B, Takala J, Frey FJ. Comparison of continuous and intermittent renal replacement therapy for acute renal failure. Nephrol Dial Transplant. 2005; 20: 1630–1637.
45. Schortgen F, Soubrier N, Delclaux C, Thuong M, Girou E, Brun-Buisson C, Lemaire F, Brochard L. Hemodynamic tolerance of intermittent hemodialysis in critically ill patients: usefulness of practice guidelines. Am J Respir Crit Care Med 2000; 162: 197–202.
46. Butler R, Keenan SP, Inman KJ, Sibbald, WJ, Block G. Is there a preferred technique for weaning the difficult-to-wean patient? A systematic review of the literature. Crit Care Med 1999; 27: 2331–2336.

47. Bell M; SWING, Granath F, Schon S, Ekbom A, Martling CR. Continuous renal replacement therapy is associated with less chronic renal failure than intermittent haemodialysis after acute renal failure. Intensive Care Med 2007; 33: 773–780.
48. Jacka MJ, Ivancinova X, Gibney RT. Continuous renal replacement therapy improves renal recovery from acute renal failure. Can J Anaesth 2005; 52: 327–332.
49. Marshall MR, Golper TA, Shaver MJ, Alam MG, Chatoh DK. Urea kinetics during sustained low efficiency dialysis in critically ill patients requiring renal replacement therapy. Am J Kidney Dis 2002; 39: 556–570.
50. Naka T, Baldwin I, Bellomo R, Fealy N, Wan L. Prolonged daily intermittent renal replacement therapy in ICU patients by ICU nurses and ICU physicians. Int J of Artif Organs 2004; 27: 380–387.
51. Kumar VA, Craig M, Depner T, Yeun JY. Extended daily dialysis: A new approach to renal replacement for acute renal failure in the intensive care unit. Am J Kidney Dis, 2000; 36: 294–300.
52. Kielstein JT, Kretschmer U, Ernst T, Hafer C, Bahr MJ, Haller H, Fliser D. Efficacy and cardiovascular tolerability of extended dialysis in critically ill patients: A randomized controlled study. Am J Kidney Dis 2004; 43: 342–349.
53. Baldwin I, Naka T, Koch B, Fealy N, Bellomo R. A pilot randomised controlled comparison of continuous veno-venous haemofiltration and extended daily dialysis with filtration: effect on small solutes and acid-base balance. Intensive Care Med. 2007; 33: 830–835.
54. Tolwani AJ, Campbell RC, Stofan BS, et al. (2008). Standard versus High-Dose CVVHDF for ICU-Related Acute Renal Failure. J Am Soc Nephrol 19: 1233–1238.
55. The VA/NIH Acute Renal Failure Trial Network (2008). Intensity of renal support in critically ill patients with acute kidney injury. N Engl J Med [epub ahead of print].
56. Bonventre JV (2008). Dialysis in acute kidney injury – More is not better. N Engl J Med [epub ahead of print].
57. Kellum JA, Mehta R, Angus DC, Palevsky P, Ronco C, for the ADQI Workgroup. The First International Consensus Conference on Continuous Renal Replacement Therapy. Kidney Int 2002; 62: 1855–1863.
58. www.adqi.net

Anticoagulation for Acute Dialysis

7.9

Andrew Davenport

Core Messages

- In patients with acute kidney failure in the intensive care unit, coagulation cascades, platelets, complement, and mononuclear leukocytes may all be activated as part of the generalized inflammatory process. Anticoagulation for extracorporeal procedures thus constitutes a particular challenge. Against this, the risk of bleeding associated with systemic anticoagulation must be carefully balanced.
- If anticoagulant-free intermittent hemodialysis is attempted, blood pump speed should be increased and regular predilutional saline boluses performed. For continuous treatment procedures, small surface area dialyzers/hemofilters should be chosen, intradialyzer/filter hemoconcentration be avoided by using predilutional fluid replacement and the circuit carefully printed to remove all air.
- Systemic anticoagulation may be performed using unfractionated heparin, low-molecular-weight heparins, heparinoids, prostaglandins, or direct thrombin inhibitors such as hirudin and argatroban.
- Regional anticoagulation using citrate is growing in popularity particularly in continuous therapies despite the apparent complexity of using it, and the potential array of metabolic disturbances. It may have advantages in patients at risk of bleeding.

A. Davenport
Royal Free Hospital, Pond Street, London NW3 2QG, UK
e-mail: andrew.davenport@royalfree.nhs.uk

7.9.1 Introduction

The coagulation pathway is traditionally divided into the intrinsic or contact pathway, and the extrinsic pathway (Fig. 7.9.1). Activation of these serine protease cascades results in the creation of the tenase and prothrombinase complexes which form on platelet surface membranes, leading to the generation of thrombin (Fig. 7.9.2), and platelet thrombi. There are a series of natural anticoagulants to regulate the coagulation cascade, including antithrombin, heparin cofactor II, proteins S and C, and tissue factor pathway inhibitor (TFPI). Antithrombin III, a serine protease inhibitor, is the major natural anticoagulant, which not only

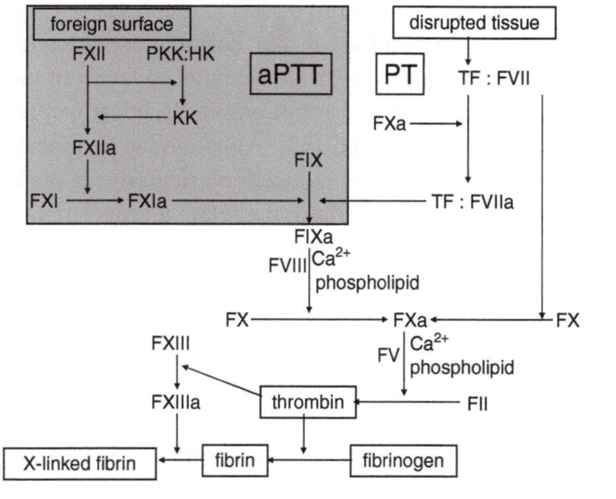

Fig. 7.9.1 The intrinsic coagulation pathway starts with the activation of factor XII, which is accelerated by the conversion of prekallikrein (PK) and high-molecular-weight kallikrein (HK) to kallikrein (KK) leading to increased XIIa generation. Whereas the extrinsic pathway starts with the release of tissue factor (TF) from disrupted endothelium and activated mononuclear phagocytes

A. Jörres et al. (eds.), *Management of Acute Kidney Problems*,
DOI: 10.1007/978-3-540-69441-0_7.9, © Springer-Verlag Berlin Heidelberg 2010

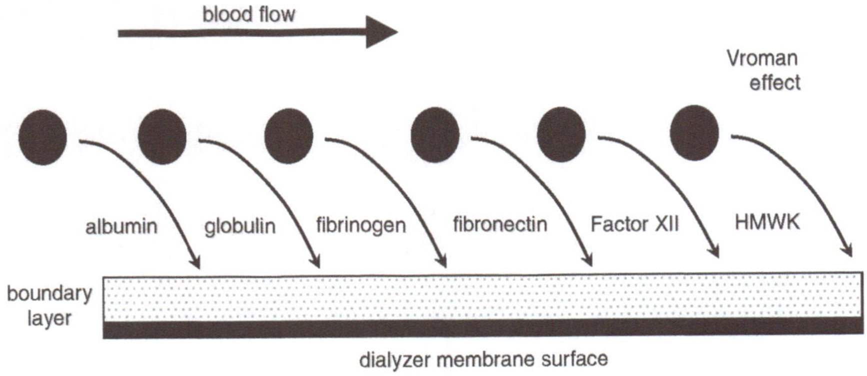

Fig. 7.9.2 Deposition of plasma proteins occurs on the dialyzer membrane, but due to the deposition of their natural inhibitors, contact activation is inhibited

inhibits thrombin, but also factors Xa, IXa, XIa, XIIa, and kallikrein. Heparin cofactor II also inhibits thrombin formation. Protein C, which is carried by complement proteins, regulates the activation of factors V and VIII on endothelial surfaces, in reactions catalyzed by protein S. Similarly, there is a natural inhibitor for the extrinsic system, tissue factor pathway inhibitor (TPFI), which is mainly produced by the endothelium, and its release is stimulated by proteoglycans, including heparins [87].

Many patients with acute kidney injury (AKI), particularly those with multiple organ failure, show activation of both the intrinsic and extrinsic coagulation cascades, with reduced plasma levels of prekallikrein, factors XII, VII, and II, and increased factor XIIa, TF, and thrombin–antithrombin (TAT) complexes [13]. In addition to activation of the coagulation cascades activity, many patients also have reduced levels of the natural anticoagulants: antithrombin III, heparin cofactor II, proteins S and C [77]. Although the peripheral platelet count may be reduced, particularly in those with multiple organ failure, the relative proportion of premature, larger platelets containing RNA is increased, increasing microthrombi formation. In the intensive care unit patient, inflammation with the release of TNF-α tips the balance to coagulation, by both increasing tissue factor and plasminogen activator inhibitor-1 release, whilst reducing endothelial thrombomodulin expression, and protein S by increasing binding to C4b.

Repeated administration of human albumin solutions and other colloid expanders such as dextrans, gelatins, and the high-molecular-weight starches, can potentially increase the risk of bleeding, not only by diluting the plasma concentrations of clotting factors and platelets, but also by reducing von Willebrand factor and platelet adhesiveness [24].

7.9.1.1 Why Do Renal Replacement Therapy Circuits Clot ?

The renal replacement therapy (RRT) circuit has a relatively large surface area, and the simple passage of blood through the extracorporeal circuit could potentially lead to the deposition and subsequent activation of plasma coagulation proteins, on to the dialyzer membrane [40]. In pediatric practice, the relative surface area of the extracorporeal circuit is increased, due to the smaller lumen lines, thus leading to greater surface contact, and circuit clotting is a more common problem than in adult practice.

Although factor XII and high-molecular-weight kallikrein (Fig. 7.9.1) are deposited on to the dialyzer surface membrane due to the Vroman effect (Fig. 7.9.2), studies have failed to demonstrate significant activation of the contact coagulation cascade during RRT [34, 73]. This is probably due to the deposition of their natural inhibitors, so preventing activation of the cascade on the dialyzer membrane.

However, the simple passage of blood through the extracorporeal circuit, and in particular across the dialyzer membrane results in activation of leukocytes, macrophages, lymphocytes, complement proteins, and platelets [65]. Activation starts as blood is sucked into the vascular access catheter, as flow is often nonlaminar, continued by the pressure changes generated by the extracorporeal pump, and then flow through the dialyzer. A series of leukocyte enzymes, called flipase

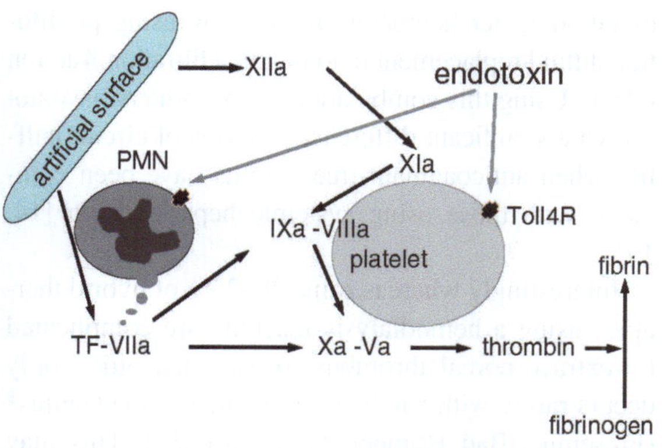

Fig. 7.9.3 Schematic representation of leukocyte activation, in the extracorporeal system leading to tissue factor release which can occur not only by thrombin generation but also by contact activation during passage through the extracorporeal circuit. In the intensive care setting, endotoxin can directly activate leukocytes and platelets via Toll-like receptors

and flopase, regulate the budding, and shedding of cell surface membrane, which becomes a source of tissue factor (Fig. 7.9.3) in the extracorporeal circuit [36]. Activation of both leukocytes and platelets, either as part of the inflammatory process causing AKI, or due to interaction with the RRT circuit, increases the release of cell surface membrane microparticles from leukocytes and monocytes, which are a source of tissue factor, and react with activated platelets to form platelet microthrombi, generating thrombin, and promoting local thrombosis in the extracorporeal circuit.

7.9.1.2 Design of the Extracorporeal Circuit

The key with any extracorporeal circuit design is to minimize the risk of clotting. The greatest pressure drop in the RRT circuit occurs across the vascular access catheter, and so the choice of insertion site, catheter design, composition, and surface coating are important in trying to reduce circuit clotting [14]. When anticoagulant-free or regional anticoagulants are used for continuos renal replacement therapy (CRRT), then the risk of vascular access catheter clotting increases [51]. In pediatric practice, vascular access is even more critical, especially in very small infants when special catheters, with internal lumens of 1.6–2.6 mm are used, and the pressure required to generate flow through these catheters will be proportionately greater. Heparin-coated venous access catheters have been reported to reduce circuit clotting compared with conventional uncoated catheters [17].

After the vascular access catheter, the next major pressure drop occurs as blood flows through the dialyzer membrane. Typically clotting starts first in the outer fibers, as the blood flow is slower compared with the central fiber bundles. The risk of clotting is affected by dialyzer design, including membrane surface area, chemical composition, surface smoothness, geometry, and charge [78]. For example a large surface area will be more likely to result in thrombus deposition, than a smaller surface area, and a reduction in dialyzer surface area has been shown to preserve circuit life, particularly during hybrid therapies [49]. Other studies have shown that membrane biocompatibility impacts on thrombus formation, such that cuprophane membranes generate more PF 1+2, and TATs than polycarbonate-polyether [78], and vitamin E surface coating may also reduce thrombin formation [41]. Membrane charge has also been reported to increase thrombin generation [34], with increased factor XII adsorption, and bradykinin formation [65]. As heparin is negatively charged, by altering membrane surface charge, then heparin can be adsorbed to the dialyzer surface, so potentially allowing anticoagulation-free dialysis [54]. On the other hand, some highly permeable membranes, such as the albufilter (Prometheus®, Fresenius, Bad Homberg, Germany), allow the passage of some clotting factors and natural anticoagulants, so increasing the requirement for heparins.

During hemofiltration, the convective movement of plasma water out through the hemofilter leads to hemoconcentration. If ultrafiltration rates are high then this may additionally result in increased protein deposition or fouling of the hemofilter membrane and the combination with hemoconcentration increase the risk of filter clotting. Thus, administration of the hemofiltration substitution fluid prefilter, minimizes hemoconcentration within the fiber bundles and so reduces membrane clotting compared with postdilutional fluid replacement [12, 19].

Most RRT machines use an occlusive type of roller pump as the blood pump, and the pressure displayed is a time averaged pressure, rather than a dynamic pressure profile [21]. These pressure swings can cause mechanical leukocyte, macrophage, and platelet activation. Some manufacturers have tried to develop alternative pump technology, using a bellows type action Fresenius Accumen® (Fresenius, Walnut Creek, CA, USA), which may reduce extracorporeal clotting [14].

Clotting is often noted in the venous air detector chamber, and thrombus formation is more likely to develop when there is a blood–air interface [47]. To overcome this problem, biomaterials have been developed, that allow gases to escape, but are impermeable to the passage of water. In clinical practice it is important to exclude all air in the RRT circuit prior to starting treatment.

As with all RRT circuits, dialysis lines should be as short as possible, to avoid dependent loops, and inspected regularly to ensure that mechanical kinks do not occur when sedated patients are turned in their beds.

7.9.1.3 Anticoagulant-Free Renal Replacement Therapy

Several centers advocate anticoagulation-free intermittent hemodialysis and CRRT for patients at risk of hemorrhage. The key to success is circuit design and careful priming of the circuit, with special emphasis on removing all air from the dialyzer and lines, and ensuring tight connections to prevent air entry. Most centers utilizing anticoagulant-free CRRT or intermittent dialysis, prime the circuit with heparinized saline, and then flush the circuit with normal saline prior to connecting the patient. The dose of heparin in the priming fluid varies from center to center, from 1,000–20,000 U/l with a priming volume of 1.0–2.0 l [16]. More recently, surface treatment of polyacrylonitrile membranes have allowed more predictable heparin bonding, and successful anticoagulant-free dialysis [54]. Other priming techniques for anticoagulant-free CRRT circuits have included rinsing and priming with human albumin solutions, although the results have been variable [16].

In adult practice, successful anticoagulant-free intermittent hemodialysis is associated with higher blood pump speeds [47], and regular predilutional boluses. Anticoagulant-free CRRT is possible, but requires thought regarding vascular access catheters, preferably large bore, circular diameter with no side holes, placed in the femoral vein, in combination with a biocompatible small surface area dialyzer/hemofilter, and prevention of intradialyzer hemoconcentration by using predilutional fluid replacement to maintain a filtration fraction <25%. Using this combination, many centers have not shown a significant difference in terms of circuit half-life when anticoagulant-free circuits have been compared with those using systemic heparinization [14, 19].

Interestingly whereas some 20–25% of hybrid therapies using a hemodialysis machine are complicated by extracorporeal thrombus formation, clotting only occurs rarely with batch systems, such as the Genius® (Fresenius, Bad Homber, Germany) [33]. This may well be due to the different blood pump technologies used by the two systems, with less leukocyte and platelet activation occurring with the dual chamber pump used by the Genius® system, compared with the standard occlusive roller pump.

7.9.1.3.1 Unfractionated Heparin

Unfractionated heparin (UFH) is a series of glycosaminoglycans (molecular weight range 5–100 kDa), made up of repeating units of sulphated D-glucosamine and D-glucuronic acid. The most active moiety in UFH, a pentasaccharide unit which binds to antithrombin III, causing conformational change, and inactivation of the serine proteases thrombin, factor Xa and factor IXa. Thrombin is most sensitive to this interaction, with heparin binding to both thrombin and antithrombin III. Even if the UFH molecule does not contain the most active pentasaccharide unit, it can still bind to ATIII, electrostatically, if there are more than 18 polysaccharide units. Heparin cofactor II is also catalyzed by heparin, but the anticoagulant effect is only achieved at high concentrations, and is specific for thrombin.

UFH is a systemic anticoagulant, with an action time of 3–5 min. It is not cleared by RRT, but is eliminated in a dose-dependent manner, mainly by hepatic heparinase activity and the vascular endothelium. The half-life (t1/2) is increase in AKI to 40 – 120 min, as normally some 35% is renally excreted.

UFH is a highly negatively charged large molecule, which potentially can be adsorbed to plastics. Thus, when using UFH it is important to use a diluted solution, to both minimize adsorption and also improve thorough mixing with the blood prior to entry into the dialyzer.

Provided there is no increased risk of bleeding, then for intermittent RRT, an appropriate regime would include both a loading dose of 10–20 U/kg, followed by a maintenance dosage of 10–20 U/kg/h, which is terminated 30 min prior to the end of treatment [16]. The dosage schedule for CRRT is similar with a loading dose of heparin (10–20 U/kg) at the start of CRRT, followed by a maintenance infusion of 3–20 U/kg/h [92]. For hybrid therapies using a standard hemodialysis machine, then typically a bolus of 1,000–2,000 IU UFH is followed by a maintenance infusion of 500–1,000 IU/h, aiming for an activated partial thromboplastin time (aPTT) ratio of around 1.5 [56]. Thus heparin requirements using the slow blood pump speeds during extended daily dialysis, tend to be higher than during intermittent hemodialysis.

It is important that UFH is monitored, as individual patients differ in their response, either by bedside testing using the activated coagulation time (ACT), with cuvettes containing an activator of the intrinsic coagulation system, or the laboratory aPTT, aiming for an ACT of 140–180 s, or an aPPT of 100–140 s prior to the arterial port of the dialyzer.

Van der Wetering and colleagues reported a reduced filter patency rate with systemic aPTT times < 35 s [85]. In addition, they also observed that the risk of de novo hemorrhage increased from 2.9 per 1,000 h CRRT when the systemic aPTT was 15–35 s, to 7.4 at an aPTT of 45–55 s [85].

For patients at risk of hemorrhage, the dose of heparin for intermittent RRT should be reduced, to provide minimal heparinization. Most centers give a single loading dose, and then if thrombus forms in the dialyzer or venous air detector, give an additional second small bolus, ~ 50% original load, aiming for a predialyzer whole blood ACT of 120s, and/or aPPT of 80 s. An alternative approach has been to omit the bolus dose, and simply administer an infusion of 15 U/kg/h [66]. Even using low dose heparin (500 U/h) for CRRT in patients at risk of hemorrhage, has not been proven to reduce the risk of bleeding complications [7].

The half-life (t1/2) of UFH is relatively short, and in cases of hemorrhage due to over anticoagulation with heparin, this can be readily reversed with protamine, 1 mg per 1,000 U heparin. Rarely, heparin administration can result in an acute allergic reaction, usually due to pork sensitivity, and also the pseudo-pulmonary embolism syndrome due to heparin-associated antibodies (Table 7.9.1) [20].

Regional Heparinization

Regional heparinization was developed to achieve maximum extracorporeal anticoagulation but with minimum systemic effects, so reducing the risk of hemorrhage. Protamine is a small basic protein with binds to UFH, and the complex is then cleared by the reticuloendothelial system. Protamine is cleaved and then released, which can result in an increase in the protamine half-life with dose and duration of therapy.

As regional heparinization is designed for patients at risk of hemorrhage, then loading doses of UFH are usually conservative (e.g., 5–10 IU/kg), followed by a maintenance dose of 3–12 IU/kg/h [58]. Protamine is then infused postdialyzer starting at a rate calculated on the basis of 1 mg of protamine to neutralize 100 IU of UFH. Monitoring is complex as the aPTT must be

Table 7.9.1 Differences between type I and type II heparin-induced thrombocytopenia (HIT)*

	HIT type I	HIT type II
Frequency	10–20%	2–3%
Timing*	1–4 days	5–10 days
Platelet count	100 × 10^9/l	30–50 × 10^9/l
Antibody-mediated	No	Yes
Thrombosis	No	Yes
Skin necrosis	No	Yes
Repeated circuit clotting	No	Yes
Access thrombosis	No	Yes
Management	Observe, transient	Withdraw all heparins Systemic anticoagulation

HIT type I occurs due to interaction between heparin and platelet factor 4, leading to platelet activation
*HIT type II can occur within 24 h, if previously exposed to heparin

measured both pre and post the UFH infusion and then also post-protamine. Then based on these times the dose of heparin and/or protamine adjusted [45]. Too little protamine and the patient is at risk of hemorrhage, and conversely too much protamine and the RRT circuit may clot or the patient adversely react to protamine.

Comparison of regional heparinization, during spontaneous CRRT, with standard low-dose UFH (500 U/h), was reported to result in a mean 33% increase in filter life and 29% for a pumped CRRT circuit [7]. This data would favor the use of regional heparinization in increasing circuit patency, although in clinical practice, the variability in the amount of protamine required to neutralize 100 IU heparin varies by more than threefold, making it difficult to successfully establish regional heparinization with simple standardized protocols [45].

Protamine has a number of potentially adverse clinical effects, including hypotension, and bronchospasm [45]. When given in large boluses to reverse heparin associated hemorrhage, protamine has been occasionally reported to cause severe anaphylactic reactions [7, 14].

Regional heparinization can not be used with heparin-coated hemofilters/dialyzers, as the protamine binds to the heparin coating, so neutralizing its effect. Protamine has less effect on neutralizing low-molecular-weight heparins (LMWHs), than standard heparin, due to the smaller size of the molecule, and reduced charge. In view of the increased half-life of the LMWHs, regional heparinization with protamine is not recommended.

As patients are given standard heparin, they can still develop the side effects of heparin (see above). Indeed, in some series, there has been no proven reduction in the incidence of hemorrhagic events during regional heparinization compared with standard heparin anticoagulation during CRRT [7].

Recombinant Antithrombin and Unfractionated Heparin

Increased circuit clotting has been reported in patients with reduced antithrombin III activity (<60%) when anticoagulated with UFH [77]. Now that recombinant antithrombin is available, several studies have looked at the effect of administering both antithrombin and unfractionated heparin [26].

For intermittent dialysis, a loading dose of 3,000 IU provides normal antithrombin levels for at least 4 h [53]. In CRRT, a lower loading dose of 1,000 IU, with a continuous infusion of 250–500 IU/h, has been suggested. UFH is then given as a loading dose (5–10 U/kg) at the start of CRRT, followed by a reduced maintenance dose of 3–5 U/kg/h, and adjusted to whole blood clotting time (WBCT) or ACT [16].

Most studies have failed to show that a bolus of antithrombin failed to reduce PF 1+2 or TAT production during dialysis [77]. Although it may prolong CRRT circuit life, in the intensive care unit patient with low antithrombin levels [26, 75]. Until recently most previous studies failed to show any significant duration of extracorporeal circuit life [16]. However, studies using AT-III infusions and maintaining AT-III concentrations > 60% have been effective, although at great expense [26].

Low-Molecular-Weight Heparins

Low-molecular-weight heparins (LMWHs) are glycosaminoglycans with a molecular weight of around 5 kDa. As LMWHs comprise fewer than 18 saccharides, they can not bind to both antithrombin and thrombin simultaneously, thus loosing antithrombin activity compared with standard heparin. As inactivation of factor Xa does not require direct heparin binding, LMWH by activating antithrombin, retains anti-Xa activity.

The currently available LMWHs, ardeparin, certoparin, dalteparin, enoxaparin, nadroparin, reviparin, and tinzaparin differ in size, half–life, and biological activity. The terminal half-life is much greater for the LMWHs than unfractionated heparin, with enoxaparin having the longest at 27.7 h [80]. Compared with standard heparin, LMWHs have been reported to be more effective in reducing fibrin deposition on dialyzer membranes, and extracorporeal clotting, but also less hemorrhagic complications [39]. This appears to be due to both a quicker onset of action that standard heparin, and also less leukocyte and platelet activation [16].

For intermittent dialysis, most adult and pediatric centers use a single loading dose, as this lasts for up to 4 h, or even longer [9, 84]. Tinzaparin has the shortest t1/2 of the LMWHs, and bolus doses of 1,500 IU have been used for dialysis sessions lasting < 4 h and 2,500 for > 4 h. Whereas enoxaparin, with a much longer t1/2 is prescribed according to body weight, 0.7–1.0 mg/kg for patients dialyzing > 4 h, [74]. LMWHs have been successfully used for intermittent dialysis in patients at risk of hemorrhage using reduced doses, for example 0.5 mg/kg enoxaparin.

LMWH by activating antithrombin, retains anti-Xa activity. Thus when monitoring the affect of anticoagulation with LMWH, there is only a modest affect on the aPTT, and special assays are required to determine the inhibition of factor Xa. To titrate the LMWH dose against anticoagulant activity, an anti-Xa assay which omits exogenous antithrombin is required, as otherwise anti-factor Xa activity and the anticoagulant effect of LMWH may not correlate. The recommended anti-factor Xa activity range for standard intermittent hemodialysis is 0.2–0.4 U/mL, and this has been reported to allow successful treatment of patients at risk of hemorrhage [70] (Table 7.9.2). Bedside ACT tests are currently being developed using bovine anti-Xa to help in monitoring of LMWHs.

When LMWHs were first used in CRRT, most centers either used a loading dose followed by a continuous infusion, or gave further bolus doses every 6 h [42, 89]. Although LMWHs are relatively small molecules, they are not significantly cleared during CRRT [77, 87]. More recently LMWHs have been shown to be effective when started as a continuous infusion without a loading dose (e.g., dalteparin 600 IU/h, tinzaparin 400–800 IU/h) achieving a mean anti-factor Xa activity of 0.49 IU/mL, within 1 h of starting CRRT [58, 86]. Recent studies have shown increased circuit survival with LMWHs compared with UFH: for example, enoxaparin given at 0.15 mg/kg bolus followed by a maintenance infusion of 0.05 mg/kg/h, aiming for an anti-Xa activity between 0.25–0.30 IU/L (Table 7.9.2) [43].

If bleeding does occur, then this may be more severe than standard heparin, due to the prolonged half-life.

Table 7.9.2 Dosing schedule for intermittent hemodialysis using LMWH tinzaparin, and subsequent dose alteration according to anti-Xa activity

Duration of dialysis (h)	Tinzaparin bolus dose anti-Xa units
≤ 3	1,500
4	2,500
5	5,000
6–12	2,500 bolus and 2nd bolus after 3 h
Monitor postdialysis anti-Xa activity	
< 0.2 U/ml	↑Bolus dose by 500 anti-Xa units
0.3 – 0.5 U/ml	↓Bolus dose by 500 anti-Xa units
> 0.5 U/ml	↓Bolus dose by 1,000 anti-Xa units

Protamine may only have a moderate effect, and will depend upon the individual LMWH used, and in severe cases fresh frozen plasma, or even activated factor VII may be required [90]. HIT type II may rarely develop with LMWHs [70], and if so then LMWHs must be discontinued.

Heparin-Coated Extracorporeal Circuits

Heparin bonding of cardiopulmonary and extracorporeal oxygenation circuits has been shown to result in a reduction in heparin requirement and risk of hemorrhage. Currently there are heparin-coated venous access catheters and heparin bonded dialyzer membranes (Duraflo®; Baxter, Deerborne, IL, USA), but no completely heparin coated extracorporeal circuit for intermittent hemodialysis and/or CRRT. In addition the surface-treated polyacrylonitrile membrane (Hospal, Lyon, France) readily absorbs heparin, and so can be rinsed with a heparin saline solution (20,000 IU/L), which is then discarded, allowing a 4 h anticoagulant-free dialysis with minimal heparin release to the patient [54].

Heparin-Induced Thrombocytopenia

In the intensive care unit, the usual causes of thrombocytopenia include sepsis and drugs. Fortunately heparin induced-thrombocytopenia (HIT) due to the development of IgG4 antibodies to platelet factor 4–heparin complexes is uncommon, with an estimated incidence of 0–1% [63]. To help in assessing the risk of heparin induced thrombocytopenia, a four T scoring system has been developed (Table 7.9.3) [86]. However, if these antibodies do develop then patients are at risk of not only of vascular access and circuit clotting but also major arterial and venous thrombosis [20]. Once suspected, all heparins, including LMWHs and heparin catheter locks, should be withdrawn until the result of a specific ELISA test is available, and an alternate systemic anticoagulant is required.

Dermatan Sulphate and Danaparoid

Dermatan sulphate is a proteoglycan, which acts as a direct thrombin inhibitor by binding to heparin cofactor II. Trials using either a single bolus dose of 6 mg/kg, or smaller bolus of 4 mg/kg coupled with a continuous

Table 7.9.3 The "4 Ts" scoring system to estimate probability for heparin-induced thrombocytopenia (HIT), prior to laboratory testing for HIT antibodies [86]

Score	2 points	1 point	Zero
Thrombocytopenia x 10^9/l	20–100 or Fall > 50%	10–19 or Fall 30–50%	< 10 or Fall <30%
Timing of onset in fall platelets	5–10 days heparin Rx	> 10 days or timing not evident	< 1 day heparin exposure
Thrombosis or acute systemic symptoms	Proven thrombosis Skin necrosis or acute systemic reaction	Progressive, recurrent, silent thrombosis or erythematous skin lesions	None
Other etiology for thrombocytopenia	None evident	Possible	Probable

Low probability ≥ 3, intermediate probability 4–6, high probability ≤ 6

infusion of 0.65 mg/kg/h, showed that dermatan sulphate was an effective anticoagulant for intermittent hemodialysis, although greater doses were required with polyacrylonitrile membranes [71]. Similar studies have used a bolus of 150 mg followed by 12 mg/h for CRRT.

Subsequently, dermatan sulphate has been superseded by danaparoid, which is a mixture of glycosaminoglycans: 84% heparan sulphate, 12% dermatan sulphate and 4% chondroitin sulphate, derived from porcine intestinal mucosa. Danaparoid exerts its anticoagulant effect predominantly by activating antithrombin, primarily against FXa but also against thrombin. As danaparoid has a minimal effect on platelets, it has been successfully used in the management of patients with heparin induced thrombocytopenia, although there is a potential cross reactivity of < 5% [18]. In the UK and some other European countries, danaparoid is the recommended anticoagulant of choice for cases of HIT [46], whereas in others the direct thrombin inhibitors are preferred. Prior to starting danaparoid in cases of HIT type II, laboratory testing should be undertaken to exclude cross reactivity.

The main disadvantage of danaparoid is the prolonged half-life of around 30 h in renal failure, thus monitoring and adjusting of the loading dose is often based, not on the anti-factor Xa activity at the end of the dialysis session, but on the anti-Xa activity prior to the start of the subsequent dialysis session. In adult practice, an initial loading dose of 3,750 U is recommended (reduced to 2,500 U in patients less than 55 kg), providing there is no additional hemorrhagic risk, and then 2,500 U prior to the subsequent dialysis (2,000 U if under 55 kg), or alternatively start at 35 U/kg. Thereafter the dose is adjusted on the basis of the predialysis anti-Xa activity, and/or the presence of fibrin threads in the dialysis chamber, aiming for intradialytic anti-Xa activity of 0.5–0.8 U/mL [64]. In pediatric practice it has been suggested that a loading dose of 1,000 IU plus 30 IU/kg is used for children under 10 years, and 1,500 IU plus 30 IU/kg for older children. The loading dose then titrated against the subsequent predialysis anti-Xa activity (<0.3 – same bolus, 0.3–0.4 – reduce bolus by 2,500 IU, and if > 0.4 omit bolus dose) [64]. If the same loading dose is continuously used, then the predialysis anti-Xa activity will increase over time due to the prolonged half-life.

For CRRT an initial bolus dose is required, or an alternative approach has been to prime the CRRT circuit with 1,500 IU of danaparoid, followed by an infusion of around 140 IU/h, adjusting the dose according to maintain anti-Xa activity <0.4 [55]. The major problem with danaparoid is the prolonged half-life. If bleeding occurs, there is no simple antidote, and patients may require fresh frozen plasma and/or activated factor VII concentrate [90].

Other proteoglycan based agents have also been used as anticoagulants for hemodialysis, including sulodexide (80% iduroylglycosaminoglycan sulfate and 20% dermatan sulphate).

Heparinoids

Synthetic heparinoids have been developed which just contain the key active pentasaccharide group, which binds antithrombin III. These include fondaparinux and idraparinux. Both of which have prolonged half lives and require anti-Xa monitoring. For example, fondaparinux doses at 2.5 mg alt die has provided sufficient anticoagulation for intermittent hemodialysis [38]. Idraparinux has even a longer half-life and is not recommended as an extracorporeal anticoagulant.

Prostacyclin

Prostacyclin (PGI_2) is a natural anticoagulant produced by endothelial cells, by the breakdown of arachidonic acid. PGI_2, and its analog epoprostenol, are potent antiplatelet agents blocking cAMP, and have been shown to reduce platelet microthrombi during hemodialysis, hybrid therapies and CRRT compared with standard heparin and LMWH [29, 44]. Although both agents are potent arterial vasodilators, most patients do not develop symptomatic hypotension at the doses used (PGI_2 5 ng/kg/min, range 2.5–10 ng/kg/min), as some 40% of the dose is lost during passage through the dialyzer [93]. Hypotension can be avoided by ensuring that patients are not hypovolemic, and by infusing PGI_2 starting at 0.5 ng/kg/min prior to the start of dialysis, and increasing the dose over a few minutes. Fortunately as the half-life is in minutes, any hypotensive episode can readily be reversed by stopping the infusion. As platelet microthrombi are reduced, membrane fouling is less, and dialyzer efficiency increased [52].

Other prostanoids, such as PGE_1 (alprostadil), PGE_2, and PGD also have antiplatelet effects and can be used as extracorporeal anticoagulants. As PGE_1 is metabolized in the lung it has less systemic vasodilatory properties compared with prostacyclin [87]. These prostanoids are not as potent as PGI_2, and hence the dosage of alprostadil recommended is 5–20 ng/kg/min.

PGI_2 does not have any direct effect on the plasma coagulation pathways, so its anticoagulant activity can not be readily assessed, even by thromboelastography [22]. Thrombin generation does occur during dialysis with PGI_2, and therefore some centers have advocated a combination of reduced doses of both heparin and PGI_2 [79, 83], using prostacyclin 2–6.5 ng/kg/min of PGI_2 and/or 2.5–10 ng/kg/min alprostadil with 200–500 U/h of UFH [52, 73].Whereas others have found PGI_2 and prostanoids to be equally effective as heparin in maintaining CRRT circuit life, with better filter patency [23, 28, 44, 72].

When used as the sole extracorporeal anticoagulant, PGI_2 has been shown to significantly reduce the incidence of hemorrhage in patients at risk of bleeding [23, 81], PGI_2 and its analogs are essentially regional rather than systemic anticoagulants. Although PGI_2 has been used in cases of heparin-associated thrombocytopenia, it does not prevent thrombosis and should not be used in cases which require systemic anticoagulation [15].

Direct Thrombin Inhibitors: Hirudin and Argatroban

The direct thrombin inhibitors are typically used in the management of patients with HIT. Hirudin, originally obtained from leeches, is an irreversible thrombin inhibitor, and is now available in recombinant form, lepirudin (6.9 kDa). As hirudin is renally excreted the biological half-life is increased to more than 35 h in renal failure, and has been reported to be even longer in anephric patients. After diluting the lepirudin solution to a concentration of 2 mg/mL, the loading doses used in clinical practice for intermittent hemodialysis have varied from 0.02–0.4 mg/kg (5–30 mg) [18]. The dose of hirudin in the dialysis patient depends upon the dialyzer membrane, as hirudin can pass through plasma filters and also high flux dialyzers (polysulphone > polyacrylonitrile > polyamide), and therefore in these cases a higher loading dose may be required [31]. Whereas cellulosic and polysulphone low flux dialyzers are relatively impermeable. [8]. On the other hand, in approximately a third of patients regularly treated with hirudin develop so-called hirudin antibodies, these reduce hirudin clearance, so potentiating the effect of hirudin, and thus the loading dose needs to be reduced [27].

Whereas a bolus dose of 0.03–0.4 mg/kg (5–30 mg) is usually adequate for intermittent hemodialysis in the acute situation, the dosing for CRRT is more problematical, as hirudin will be cleared during hemofiltration and/or dialysis, and patients are more likely to develop hirudin antibodies, particularly when treated with continuous infusions. Both continuous infusions (0.01–0.02 mg/kg/h), and repetitive boluses (5–10 mg) have been used, aiming for a target aPTT ratio of 1.5–2.0 but <2.5, although bleeding is a potential major problem [35]. To reduce the risk of bleeding one regimen is, a loading dose of 0.4 mg/kg (maximum 30 mg), followed by a further lower bolus dose (0.1 mg/kg) when the aPTTr had fallen to < 1.5, or starting with an infusion of 0.0225 mg/kg/h, then regulating the infusion rate according to aPTTr, so if the aPTTr exceeds 2.5, then stopping the infusion for 2 h and then restarting at 50%, or conversely increasing the rate by 20% if the aPTTr falls below 1.5.

Most centers monitor hirudin using the aPPTr, aiming for a ratio of 1.5–2.5. Unfortunately, the relationship between plasma hirudin concentration and the aPTTr is not linear, and what may appear to be small increases in the aPPTr can correspond to substantial increase in the hirudin concentration, and so increase the risk of hemorrhage [77]. Thus a direct test of thrombin activation – the ecarin clotting time – is advocated (Ecarin activation of prothrombin is independent of cofactors and does not require phospholipid, calcium, or factor Va, and can be performed at the bedside), and other centers measure the plasma hirudin concentration. Bivalirudin, which is used in the cardiological practice is a reversible direct thrombin inhibitor, which has a much shorter half-life compared with hirudin, is a potential alternative, but is not licensed as yet for dialysis.

As hirudin is an irreversible thrombin inhibitor, overdosage, and consequent hemorrhage [48] are serious risks, especially when most centers rely on the aPTT to adjust dosages, and activated factor VII may well be required to stem hemorrhage [91]. Hemodiafiltration can be used to clear plasma hirudin [89], unless the patient has developed antihirudin antibodies, in which case plasma exchange may be helpful.

Occasionally patients have been reported to suffer anaphylactoid reactions to hirudin, and in these cases further hirudin administration is contraindicated.

Argatroban is a synthetic reversible thrombin inhibitor, derived from L-arginine. Unlike hirudin, argatroban is hepatically metabolized, and the recommended starting dose for systemic anticoagulation is 2 μg/kg/min, reduced to 0.5 μg/kg/min in patients with liver disease, aiming for a target aPTTr of 1.5–2.0 [18]. However, argatroban clearance is reduced in renal failure, and in patients treated for more than 24 h, lower infusion rates are often required. Argatroban is not significantly removed by high flux dialyzers and/or hemofilters [69]. In preliminary studies for intermittent hemodialysis the average starting dose was 0.9 μg/kg/min, reducing to a maintenance dose of 0.7 μg/kg/min. The relationship between the plasma argatroban concentration and the aPTTr is relatively steep, so in critically ill patents, even without overt hepatic dysfunction, doses as low as 0.2 μg/kg/min, have been effective in preventing CRRT and/or other extracorporeal devices clotting [5, 62]. Even in patients without over liver disease, small increases in argatroban infusion rate may lead to large increases in the aPTTr, with consequent risk of hemorrhage.

In patients just requiring argatroban for acute intermittent hemodialysis, then providing liver function and baseline clotting studies are normal, an appropriate regime would be a 250-μg/kg bolus followed by a 2-μg/kg/min infusion, stopping the infusion an hour before the end of the dialysis session [62]. However, if patients are already systemically anticoagulated with argatroban, then no adjustment should be required for dialysis [6].

Nafamostat Mesilate

Nafamostat mesilate is a serine protease inhibitor, which essentially acts as a regional anticoagulant, although potentially it inhibits broad enzymatic systems including the coagulation cascades, platelet and complement activation, kinin, and fibrinolysis cascades.

Gabexate mesilate is a short-acting (half-life 80 s) serine protease inhibitor that acts at the same sites as antithrombin, but is not dependent on it for effect [87]. Gabexate has now been superseded by nafamostat mesilate which again has a short half-life of 5–8 min, and some 40% is cleared during passage through the dialyzer [2]. By inhibiting thrombin, factor Xa and XIIa, nafamostat prolongs the WBCT, ACT, and aPTT, thus allowing bedside monitoring. Most experience comes from Japan, where the circuit is usually primed with 20 mg of nafamostat in 1.0 l normal saline, followed by an infusion starting at 40 mg/h during intermittent hemodialysis or CRRT, to maintain a target aPPTr of 1.5–2.0 [57]. Nafamostat contains a cationic portion which binds to negatively charged polyacrylonitrile membranes, and also to some extent to polymethylmethacrylate membranes, if these membranes are used then the nafamostat dose has to be increased, and may not be as effective with PAN 69 dialyzers [3].

Nafamostat has been reported to cause myalgia, arthralgia, eosinophilia, and rarely anaphylactoid reactions and agranulocytosis [16].

7.9.1.3.2 Citrate

Although regional citrate anticoagulation has been used for more than 20 years, it is rarely used for outpatient hemodialysis [68]. Anticoagulation with citrate induces a degree of complexity, as if trisodium citrate is used, then a specialized calcium free, and reduced or bicarbonate free dialysate is required. Calcium is then infused centrally to restore the plasma ionized calcium concentration [39]. Citrate by complexing calcium and reducing calcium concentration, not only prevents activation of the coagulation cascades, but also platelets, during passage through the dialyzer, but does not prevent complement or leukocyte activation [25]. Thus membrane fouling and deposition of fibrin and platelets is much reduced when citrate is used compared with LMWH and standard heparin [39]. The half-life of citrate complex is minutes, and thus citrate is a regional anticoagulant, allowing the successful dialysis of patients at risk of bleeding [25, 68].

Citrate has been used as the anticoagulant for CRRT since the late 1980s, initially for continuous dialysis/hemodiafiltration [59], and more recently for venovenous hemofiltration [67]. As initially there were no commercially available calcium free fluids for dialysate or replacement solutions, a variety of protocols have been developed by different institutions (Table 7.9.4) [50, 59, 67, 82]. In essence all protocols titrate the citrate infusion against the blood flow, typically using calcium free dialysate and/or replacement solutions, and then re-infusion of calcium at central site (Fig. 7.9.4). More recently several investigators have reported that it is possible to use commercial calcium containing solutions when performing continuous hemodiafiltration, although in these cases more citrate is required (Table 7.9.3) [10, 11, 37]. Citrate has been shown to be both a highly effective regional anticoagulant for CRRT, which also reduces the risk of potential hemorrhage [32, 59, 61, 67, 50]. Indeed as citrate is a regional anticoagulant, access problems are a more common cause of circuit clotting, especially if the calcium infusion is returned into the venous dialysis line.

Citrate can also be used to anticoagulate patients treated by hybrid systems, such as the Genius®, and during intermittent hemodialysis and/or hemodiafiltration, using bicarbonate and calcium containing dialysates. Depending upon the concentration of calcium in the dialysate, then additional calcium may or may not be required to maintain normal systemic concentrations [30]. As for CRRT, the citrate infusion is titrated against blood flow, for example with the Genius® system. During dialysis-based treatments, approximately 80% or more of the citrate is removed during passage through the dialyzer, as trisodium citrate is an acidic solution, and when mixed with blood, increases the amount of "free" calcium by changing the binding kinetics between "free" and "bound" calcium, and so increases potential for calcium-citrate clearance [76].

Bedside monitoring is possible by using whole blood activated clotting time (WBACT) (200–250 s); however, most centers adjust the citrate infusion according the post dialyzer calcium concentration (target 0.25–0.35 mmol/L) [50]. The rate of the citrate infusion is dependent upon the blood flow. Thus during hemodialysis and/or hemodiafiltration with blood

Table 7.9.4 Citrate continuos renal replacement therapy (CRRT) anticoagulation protocols, which vary according to dialysis and/or filtration modes and blood flow

Reference	Modality	Blood flow rate ml/min	Citrate infusion mmol/h	Dialysate composition mmol/l	Substitution fluid mmol/l
Mehta [59]	CAVHD[a]	52–125	23.8	Na^+ 117 Cl^- 122.5 Mg^{++} 0.75 Dextrose 2.5%	Na^+ 145 Cl^- 145
Tolwani [82]	CVVHD	125–150	17.5	Na^+ 145 Cl^- 145 Mg^{++} 1.0	None
Bunchman [10]	CVVHD[b]	100	17	Na^+ 140 Cl^- 105 Mg^{++} 0.75 $NaHCO_3^-$ 35	None
Kutsogiannis [50]	CVVHDF	125	25	Na^+ 110 Cl^- 110 Mg^{++} 0.75	Na^+ 110 Cl^- 110 Mg^{++} 0.75 vary $NaHCO_3^-$
Gupta [37]	CVVHDF	150	16.9	Na^+ 132 Mg^{++} 0.75 Lactate 40	Na^+ 154
Cointault [11]	CVVHDF[c]	125	28.3	Na^+ 140 Cl^- 109.5 Ca^{++} 1.75 Mg^{++} 0.50 $NaHCO_3^-$ 32 Lactate 3.0	Na^+ 140 Cl^- 109.5 Ca^{++} 1.75 Mg^{++} 0.50 $NaHCO_3^-$ 32 Lactate 3.0
Palsson [67]	CVVH[d]	180	18.6	None	Na^+ 140 Cl^- 101.5 Mg^{++} 0.75 Citrate 13.3 Dextrose 0.2%

[a]CAVHD - continuous arteriovenous hemodialysis
[b]CVVHD - continuous venovenous hemodialysis
[c]CVVHDF - continuous venovenous hemodiafiltration
[d]CVVH - continuous venovenous hemofiltration

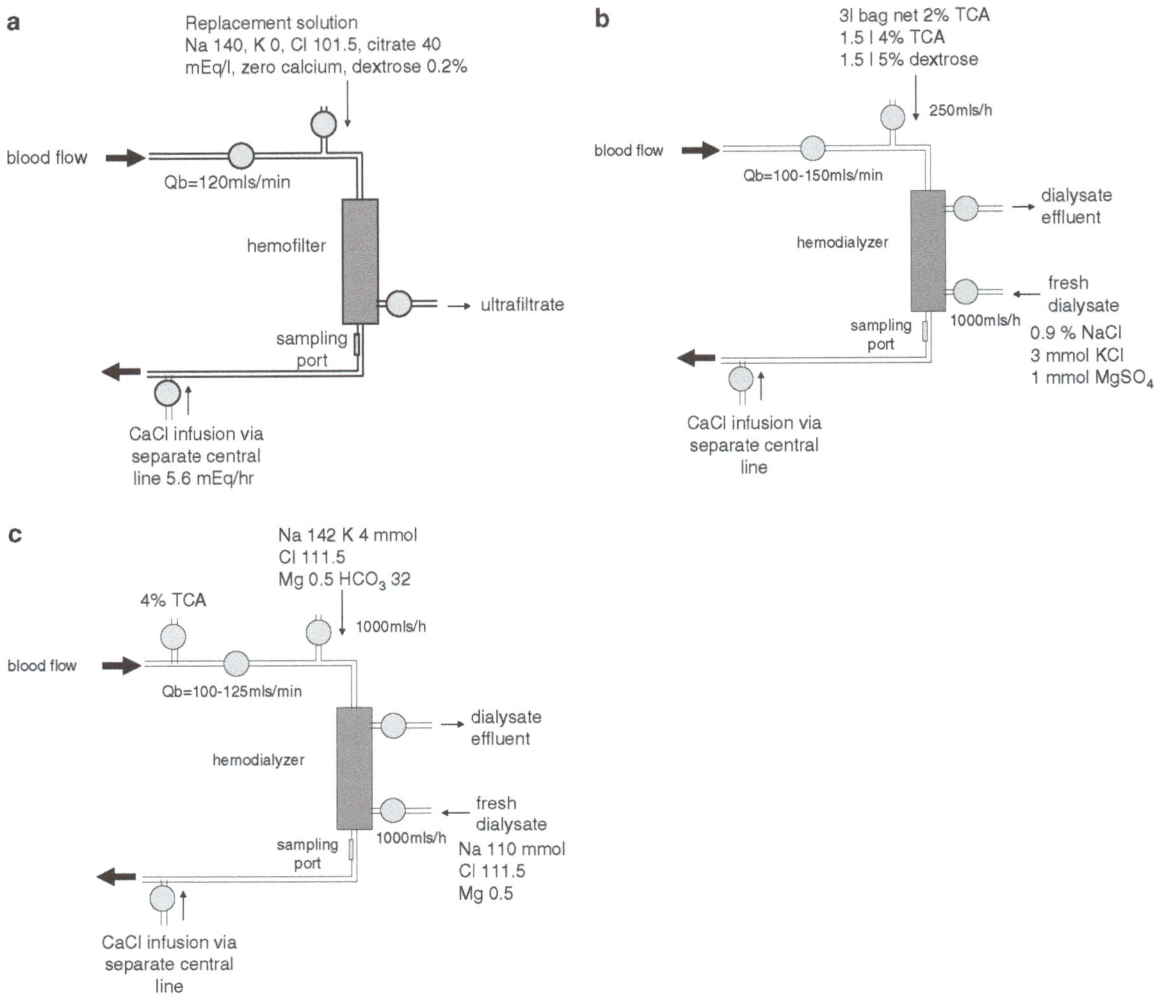

Fig. 7.9.4 Schematic representation of a CRRT circuit for (**a**) predilution continuous venovenous hemofiltration (CVVH), (**b**) continuous venovenous hemodialysis (CVVHD), and (c) predilutional continuous venovenous hemodiafiltration (CVVHDF) using citrate anticoagulation, based on references [50], [82], [67], respectively. Concentrations are expressed in mmol/L unless otherwise specified

flows of 300 mL/min or greater a citrate infusion of 50–60 mmol/h would be appropriate [4]. Whereas during CRRT, with lower blood flow rates, citrate infusion is correspondingly lower (Table 7.9.5). Thereafter, the rate of citrate infusion is adjusted according to the calcium concentration (Table 7.9.5), being reduced if the calcium is less than 0.25 mmol/L, and correspondingly increased when greater than 0.36 mmol/L [50].

Citrate dialysis has been reported to result in citrate intoxication [4], either when citrate is not metabolized rapidly, for example, if there is hepatic failure, or muscle hypoperfusion, and also during isolated ultrafiltration,

Table 7.9.5 Clinical protocol for adjustment of infusion rate of trisodium citrate (TSC) according to ionized calcium concentration, postdialyzer, prior to calcium infusion

Post-dialyzer ionized calcium, mmol/L	Adjustment of TSC infusion rate
> 0.5	↑By 30 mL/h
0.40–0.50	↑By 20 mL/h
0.36–0.39	↑By 10 mL/h
0.25–0.35	No change
< 0.25	↓By 10 mL/h

Table based on reference [50]. Ideal ionized calcium concentration to achieve maximum inhibition of blood clotting is 0.25–0.35 mmol/l [50]

when citrate is not being dialyzed out. Failure to adequately metabolize citrate results in an increased total calcium to ionized calcium ratio (>2.5), due to the accumulation of the calcium–citrate complex, the so-called calcium gap. Not surprisingly this has been most commonly reported in patients with liver failure [60], and should be managed by decreasing the citrate infusion [80]. In addition, citrate has been reported to cause hyperalbuminemia, hyperammonemia, and hypernatremia during sorbent-based dialysis. During CRRT hypernatremia can occur due to the sodium load if trisodium citrate is used, and thus many centers have developed specialized hyponatremic dialysates [59]. Similarly, as each citrate molecule is metabolized through to three bicarbonates, patients are at risk of developing a metabolic alkalosis [12]. To reduce this complication many centers use specialized dialysates and/or replacement solutions with a high chloride load [60]. If bicarbonate dialysate has been used then during intermittent hemodialysis patients can potentially develop profound alkalosis, with paresthesiae, arrhythmia, and even cardiac arrest. There are commercially available zero calcium bicarbonate based dialysates, and in one pediatric study all patients developed a metabolic alkalosis after seven days of CRRT using a bicarbonate based dialysate [10].

To overcome these problems, some have advocated citrate dextrose-A rather than 4% trisodium citrate [32], or reduced the citrate concentration, in combination with a reduced bicarbonate dialysate concentration to 25 mmol/L [10, 12]. Others have reported that when citrate is used for high flux dialysis, additional calcium supplementation is required compared with standard intermittent dialysis, due to increased calcium losses [87]. Hypomagnesemia has also been observed in children treated by CRRT using citrate anticoagulation [81].

Despite the apparent complexity of using citrate, and the potential array of metabolic disturbances, citrate use is growing in popularity for CRRT, as it is a very effective regional anticoagulant, especially in patients at risk of hemorrhage [61].

7.9.1.3.3 Activated Protein C

Protein C is one of the major natural anticoagulants, and normally circulates bound to complement protein 4. When activated it binds to protein S, and inhibits local thrombus formation by inhibiting tissue factor release, blocking the action of coagulation cascade factors VIIIa and Va, so reducing thrombin formation, and also increases fibrinolysis by inactivating plasminogen activator inhibitor-1, and tissue activated fibrinolysis inhibitor and also by blocking thrombin from suppressing thrombolysis. Activated protein C (aPC) is used in the management of patients with critical sepsis, and as it has anticoagulant properties, there have been reports of 3.5–6.8% patients developing serious bleeding [1]. Although, aPC prolongs the aPTT, it may not be sufficient to prevent clotting in extracorporeal circuits, particularly during CRRT. The addition of full dose heparin/LMWHs however, does however significantly increase the risk of bleeding and should be avoided. If possible regional anticoagulants such as citrate, and prostanoids should be considered, or the CRRT circuit carefully designed to be anticoagulant-free.

7.9.2 Summary

Anticoagulation for the patient with acute renal failure in the ICU is more problematical than that for outpatient hemodialysis. As part of the generalized inflammatory process, coagulation cascades, platelets, complement, and mononuclear leukocytes are all activated and will promote thrombus formation in the extracorporeal circuit. Thus more careful thought is required in terms of designing the extracorporeal circuit, particularly for CRRT. In addition the pediatric patient poses greater problems than the adult, due to the relative increase in the extracorporeal surface area, coupled with smaller bore vascular access devices and lower blood pump speeds. The dialyzer/hemofilter should be chosen to minimize bioincompatibility, maximize laminar blood flow and minimize surface area available for contact activation. Similar thought is required for the site and choice of vascular access, and the circuit design for hemofiltration in terms of site of fluid replacement to minimize the filtration fraction.

Although standard unfractionated heparin remains the most commonly used anticoagulant for acute intermittent hemodialysis, hybrid therapies, and CRRT, it does not prevent platelet microthrombi formation and still carries a significant risk of bleeding. LMWHs have an earlier onset of action, and reduce membrane fibrin and platelet deposition compared with standard heparin during intermittent hemodialysis, but have increased half-lives and require specialist monitoring, and as a consequence only have a marginal clinical advantage over standard unfractionated heparin for CRRT. Regional anticoagulants have the combined advantage of reducing the risk of bleeding, and also reducing membrane fouling, so maintaining clearances. Most of these – prostacyclin and other prostanoids and nafamostat – are very expensive and are not for everyday practice. Citrate, although more expensive than heparin, is a very potent alternative. Anticoagulation with citrate does require a degree of complexity, requiring specialized replacement fluids/dialysate, and monitoring to regulate both the rate of citrate and calcium infusions.

In cases of heparin-induced thrombocytopenia type II, which require systemic anticoagulation, the choice lies between danaparoid and the direct thrombin inhibitors, hirudin and argatroban. There is a small risk of cross-reactivity with danaparoid, but the main drawback of danaparoid is the prolonged half-life in renal failure, which can make dosing problematical for CRRT. Hirudin is an irreversible thrombin antagonist, which also has a prolonged half-life. Monitoring can be difficult, as there is no linear relationship between plasma concentration and aPTTr, and hemorrhage is a potential and serious problem. Despite the introduction of hirudin analogs, which are reversible thrombin antagonists, argatroban will probably supersede hirudin for dialysis patients, as it is a reversible thrombin antagonist, which is not affected by renal failure.

7.9.3 Take Home Pearls

- In patients with acute kidney failure in the ICU, anticoagulation for extracorporeal procedures is a particular challenge since coagulation cascades, platelets, complement, and mononuclear leukocytes may all be activated as part of the generalized inflammatory process and may promote thrombus formation in the extracorporeal circuit.
- Systemic anticoagulation may be performed using unfractionated heparin, low-molecular-weight heparins, heparinoids, prostaglandins, or direct thrombin inhibitors.
- Regional anticoagulation may have advantages in patients at risk of bleeding and is mostly performed using citrate.

References

1. Abraham E, Laterre PF, Garg R, et al. (2005) Administration of Drotrecogin alfa (Activated) in Early Stage Severe Sepsis (ADDRESS) Study Group. Drotrecogin alfa (activated) for adults with severe sepsis and a low risk of death. N Engl J Med 353:1332–1341
2. Akizawa T (1990) Beneficial characteristics of protease inhibitor as an anticoagulant for extracorporeal circulation. Rinsho Ketsueki 31: 782–786
3. Akizawa T, Koshikawa S, Ota K et al. (1993). Nafamostat mesilate: a regional anticoagulant for hemodialysis in patients at high risk for bleeding. Nephron 64: 376–381
4. Apsner R, Buchmayer H, Lang T et al. (2001) Simplified citrate anticoagulation for high flux hemodialysis. Am J Kid Dis 38: 979–987
5. Beiderlinden M, Treschan TA, Görlinger K et al. (2007). Argatroban anticoagulation in critically ill patients. Ann Pharmacother.41:749–754
6. Beiderlinden M, Treschan T, Görlinger K et al. (2007). Argatroban in extracorporeal membrane oxygenation. Int J Artif Organs 31:461–465
7. Bellomo R, Teede H, Boyce N (1993) Anticoagulant regimens in acute continuous hemodiafiltration: a comparative study. Intensive Care Med 19: 329–332
8. Benz K, Nauck MA, Böhler J et al. (2007) Hemofiltration of recombinant hirudin by different hemodialyzer membranes: implications for clinical use. Clin J Am Soc Nephrol. v2:470–476
9. Bianchetti MG, Speck S, Muller R et al. (1990) Simple coagulation prophylaxis using low molecular heparin enoxaparin in pediatric hemodialysis. Schweiz Rundsch Med Prax 79: 730–731
10. Bunchman T, Maxvold NJ, Barnett J et al. (2002) Pediatric hemofiltration: normocarb dialysate solution with citrate anticoagulation. Pediatr Nephrol 17: 150–154
11. Cointault O, Kamar N, Bories P et al. (2004).Regional citrate anticoagulation in continuous venovenous haemodiafiltration using commercial solutions. Nephrol Dial Transplant. 19:171–178
12. Davenport A (1996) CRRT in the management of patients with liver disease. Seminars Dial 9: 78–84
13. Davenport A. (1997) The coagulation system in the critically ill patient with acute renal failure and the effect of an extracorporeal circuit. Am J Kid Dis 30(Suppl 4):S20–S27
14. Davenport A (1998) Anticoagulation in patients with acute renal failure treated with continuous renal replacement therapies. Home Hemodial Int 2: 41–60
15. Davenport A (1998) Management of heparin-induced thrombocytopenia during continuous renal replacement therapy. Am J Kid Dis 32: E3
16. Davenport A (1999) Problems with anticoagulation. In Lameire N, Mehta R. Complications of dialysis: recognition and management, Marcel Dekker, Boston
17. Davenport A (2000) Central venous catheters for hemodialysis: How to overcome the problems. Home Hemodial Int 2: 43–45
18. Davenport A (2001) The management of Heparin induced thrombocytopenia during renal replacement therapy. Hemodial Int 3:81–85

19. Davenport A (2003) Pre-dilution or post-dilution fluid replacement for continuous veno-venous hemofiltration: that is the question. Nephron Clin Pract 94:c83–84
20. Davenport A (2006) Sudden collapse during haemodialysis due to immune mediated heparin induced thrombocytopenia. Nephrol Dial Transplant 21: 1721–1724.
21. Davenport A, Will EJ, Davison AM (1990) The effect of the direction of dialysate flow on the efficiency of continuous arteriovenous hemodialysis. Blood Purif 8: 329–336
22. Davenport A, Will EJ, Davison AM (1991) The effect of prostacyclin on intracranial pressure in patients with acute hepatic and renal failure. Clin Nephrol 25: 151–157
23. Davenport A, Will EJ, Davison AM (1994) Comparison of the use of standard heparin and prostacyclin anticoagulation in spontaneous and pump driven extracorporeal circuits in patients with combined acute renal and hepatic failure. Nephron 66: 431–437
24. de Jonge E, Levi M (2001) Effects of different plasma substitutes on blood coagulation. Crit Care Med 29: 1261–1267
25. Dhondt A, Vanholder R, Tielmans C et al. (2000) Effect of regional citrate anticoagulation on leukopenia, complement activation, and expression of leukocyte surface molecules during hemodialysis with unmodified cellulose membranes. Nephron 85: 334–342
26. du Cheyron D, Bouchet B, Bruel C et al. (2006) Antithrombin supplementation for anticoagulation during continuous hemofiltration in critically ill patients with septic shock: a case-control study. Crit Care.10:R45
27. Eichler P, Friesen HJ, Lubenow N et al. (2000) Antihirudin antibodies in patients with heparin Induced thrombocytopenia treated with lepirudin: incidence, effects on aPTT, and clinical relevance. Blood 96: 2373–2378
28. Favre H, Martin Y, Stoermann C (1996) Anticoagulation in continuous extracorporeal renal replacement therapy. Seminars Dial 9: 112–118
29. Fiaccadori E, Maggiore U, Parenti E et al. (2007). Sustained low-efficiency dialysis (SLED) with prostacyclin in critically ill patients with acute renal failure. Nephrol Dial Transplant. 22:529–537
30. Finkel KW, Foringer JR (2005) Safety of regional citrate anticoagulation for continuous sustained low efficiency dialysis (C-SLED) in critically ill patients. Ren Fail 27:541–545
31. Fischer KG, Loo van de A, Bohler J (1999) Recombinant hirudin (lepirudin) as anticoagulant in intensive care patients treated with continuous hemodialysis. Kid Int 72(Suppl): S46–S50
32. Flanigan MJ, Von Brecht J, Freeman RM et al. (1987) Reducing the hemorrhagic complications of hemodialysis: a controlled trial of low dose heparin and citrate anticoagulation. Am J Kid Dis 9:147–153
33. Fliser D, Kielstein JT (2004) A single-pass batch dialysis system: an ideal dialysis method for the patient in intensive care with acute renal failure. Curr Opin Crit Care 10:483–488
34. Frank RD, Weber J, Dresbach H et al. (2001) Role of contact system activation in hemodialyzer induced thrombogenicity. Kid Int 60:1972–1981
35. Gajra A, Vajpayee N, Smith A et al. (2007) Lepirudin for anticoagulation in patients with heparin-induced thrombocytopenia treated with continuous renal replacement therapy. Am J Hematol 82:391–393
36. Gorbet MB, Sefton MV (2001) Leukocyte activation and leukocyte procoagulant activities after blood contact with polystyrene and polyethyleneglycol immobilized polystyrene beads. J Lab Clin Med 137: 345–355
37. Gupta M, Wadhwa NK, Bukovsky R (2004) Regional citrate anticoagulation for continuous venovenous hemodiafiltration using calcium-containing dialysate. Am J Kidney Dis 43:67–73.
38. Haase M, Bellomo R, Rocktaeschel J et al. (2005) Use of fondaparinux (ARIXTRA) in a dialysis patient with symptomatic heparin-induced thrombocytopaenia type II. Nephrol Dial Transplant 20:444–446.
39. Hofbauer R, Moser D, Frass M et al. (1999) Effect of anticoagulation on blood membrane interactions during hemodialysis. Kid Int 56: 1578–1583
40. Holt AW, Bierer P, Berstein AD et al. (1996) Continuous renal replacement therapy in critically ill patients: monitoring circuit function. Anaesth Intensive Care 24:423–424
41. Huraib S, Tanimu D, Shaheen F et al. (2000) Effect of vitamin E modified dialysers on dialyser clotting, erythropoietin and heparin dosage: a comparative crossover study. Am J Nephrol 20:364–368
42. Jeffrey RF, Khan AA, Douglas JT et al. (1993) Anticoagulation with low molecular weight heparin (fragmin) during continuous hemodialysis in the intensive care unit. Int J Artif Organs 17:717–720
43. Joannidis M, Kountchev J, Rauchenzauner M et al. (2007). Enoxaparin vs. unfractionated heparin for anticoagulation during continuous veno-venous hemofiltration: a randomized controlled crossover study. Intensive Care Med 33:1571–1579
44. Journois D, Safran D, Castelain MH et al (1990). Comparison of the antithrombotic effects of heparin, enoxaparin and prostacycline in continuous hemofiltration. Ann Fr Anesth Reanim 9:331–337
45. Kaplan AA. Continuous arteriovenous hemofiltration- and related therapies. In: Jacobs C, Kjellstrand KE,Koch KM, Winchester JF (1996) Replacement of renal function by dialysis. Kluwer, Boston
46. Keeling D, Davidson S, Watson H (2006) Haemostasis and thrombosis task force of the British Committee for standards in haematology. The management of heparin-induced thrombocytopenia. Br J Haematol 133:259–269
47. Keller F, Seeman J, Preuschof L et al. (1990) Risk factors of system clotting in heparin free hemodialysis. Nephrol Dial Transplant 5: 802–807
48. Kern H, Ziemer S, Kox WJ (1999) Bleeding after intermittent or continuous r-hirudin during CVVH. Intensive Care Med 11: 1311–1314
49. Kumar VA, Yeun JY, Depner TA et al. (2004) Extended daily dialysis vs. continuous hemodialysis for ICU patients with acute renal failure: a two-year single center report. Int J Artif Organs 27:371–379.
50. Kutsogiannis DJ, Mayers I, Chi WD et al. (2000) Regional citrate anticoagulation in continuous venovenous hemodiafiltration. Am J Kid Dis 35: 802–811
51. Laliberte-Murphy K, Palsson R, Williams WW et al. (2002) Continuous venovenous hemofiltration as a bridge to liver transplantation. Blood Purif 20: 318–319
52. Langenecker SA, Felfernig M, Werba A et al. (1994) Anticoagulation with prostacyclin and heparin during continuous venovenous hemofiltration. Crit Care Med 22: 1774–1781
53. Langley PG, Keays R, Hughes RD et al. (1991) Antithrombin III supplementation reduces heparin requirement and platelet

loss during hemodialysis of patients with fulminant hepatic failure. Hepatol 14: 251–256
54. Lavaud S, Paris B, Maheut H et al. (2005) Assessment of the heparin-binding AN69 ST hemodialysis membrane: II. Clinical studies without heparin administration. ASAIO J 51:348–351
55. Lindhoff-Last E, Betz C, Bauersachs R (2001) Use of a low-molecular-weight heparinoid (danaparoid sodium) for continuous renal replacement therapy in intensive care patients. Clin Appl Thromb Hemost 7:300–304
56. Marshall MR, Ma T, Galler D et al. (2004) Sustained low-efficiency daily diafiltration (SLEDD-f) for critically ill patients requiring renal replacement therapy: towards an adequate therapy. Nephrol Dial Transplant 19:877–884
57. Matsuo T, Kario K, Nakao K et al. (1993) Anticoagulation with nafamostat mesilate, a synthetic protease inhibitor, in hemodialysis patients with a bleeding risk. Haemostatasis 23: 135–141
58. Mehta RL (1996) Anticoagulation strategies for continuous renal replacement therapies: what works? Am J Kid Dis 28(Suppl 3):S8–S14
59. Mehta RL, McDonald BR, Aguilar MM et al. (1990) Regional citrate anticoagulation for continuous arterio-venous hemodialysis I critically ill patients. Kid Int 38:976–981
60. Meier-Kriesche H-U, Gitomer J, Finkel K et al. (2001) Increased total to ionized calcium ratio during continuous venovenous hemodialysis with regional citrate anticoagulation. Crit Care Med 29:748–752
61. Monchi M, Berghmans D, Ledoux D (2004) Citrate vs. heparin for anticoagulation in continuous venovenous hemofiltration: a prospective randomized study. Intensive Care Med 30:260–265.
62. Murray PT, Reddy BV, Grossman EJ et al. (2004) A prospective comparison of three argatroban treatment regimens during hemodialysis in end-stage renal disease. Kid Int 66:2446–2453.
63. Napolitano L, Warkentin TE, Al-Mahameed A et al. (2006) Heparin induced thrombocytopenia in the critical care setting: diagnosis and management. Crit Care Med 34: 2898–2911
64. Neuhaus TJ, Goetschel P, Schmugge M (2000) Heparin induced thrombocytopenia type II on hemodialysis: switch to danaparoid. Pediatr Nephrol 14:713–716
65. Olbricht C, Lonnemann G, Frei U, et al. (1997) Hemodialysis, hemofiltration, and complications of technique. In Davison AM, Cameron JS, Grunfeld JP, Kerr DNS, Ritz E, Winearls CG. Oxford textbook of clinical nephrology. Oxford University Press, Oxford
66. Ozen S, Saatci U, Bakkaloglu A et al. (1993) Tight heparin regimen for hemodiaysis in children. Int Urol Nephrol 25:499–501
67. Palsson R, Niles JR (1999) Regional citrate anticoagulation in continuous venovenous hemofiltration in critically ill patients with a high risk of bleeding. Kid Int 55:1991–1997
68. Pinnick RV, Wiegmann TB, Diederich DA (1983) Regional citrate anticoagulation for hemodialysis in the patient at high risk for bleeding. N Engl J Med 3:258–261
69. Reddy BV, Grossman EJ, Trevino SA et al. (2005) Argatroban anticoagulation in patients with heparin-induced thrombocytopenia requiring renal replacement therapy. Ann Pharmacother 39: 1601–1605
70. Reeves JH, Cumming AR, Gallagher L et al. (1999) A controlled trial of low molecular weight heparin (dalteparin) versus unfractionated heparin as anticoagulant during continuous venovenous hemodialysis with filtration. Crit Care Med 27: 2224–2228
71. Ryan KE, Lane DA, Flynn A et al. (1992) Antithrombotic properties of dermatan sulphate (MF 701)in hemodialysis for chronic renal failure. Thromb Haemostat 10: 563–569
72. Rylance PB, Gordge MP, Ireland H et al. (1984). Hemodialysis with prostacyclin (epoprostenol) alone. Proc EDTA-ERA 21: 281–286
73. Salmon J, Cardigan R, Mackie I et al. (1997) Singer M. Continuous venovenous hemofiltration using polyacrylonitrile filters does not activate contact system and intrinsic system coagulation pathways. Intensive Care Med 23: 38–43
74. Saltissi D, Morgan C, Westhuyzen J et al. (1999) Comparison of low molecular weight heparin (enoxaparin sodium) and standard fractionated heparin for hemodialysis. Nephrol Dial Transplant 14: 2698–2703
75. Schrader J, Kostering H, Kramer P et al. (1982) Antithrombin III substitution in dialysis dependent renal insufficiency. Dtsch Med Wochenschr 107: 1847–1850
76. Schneider M, Thomas K, Liefeldt L et al. (2007).Efficacy and safety of intermittent hemodialysis using citrate as anticoagulant: a prospective study. Clin Nephrol 68:302–307
77. Shulman RI, Singer M, Rock J (2002) Keeping the circuit open: lessons from the lab. Blood Purif 2002; 20: 275–281
78. Sperschneider H, Deppisch R, Beck W et al. (1997) Impact of membrane choice and blood flow pattern on coagulation and heparin requirement potential consequences on lipid concentrations. Nephrol Dial Transplant 12: 2638–2646
79. Stevens PE, Davies SP, Brown EA et al. (1988) Continuous arteriovenous hemodialysis in critically ill patients. Lancet ii: 150–152
80. Stiekema JC, Van Griensen JM, Van Dinther TG et al. (1993) A cross over comparison of the anti-clotting effects of three low molecular weight heparins and glycosaminoglycuron. Brit J Clin Pharmacol 36: 51–56
81. Swartz RD, Flamenbaum W, Dubrow A et al. (1988) Epoprostenolol during high risk hemodialysis: preventing further bleeding complications. J Clin Pharmacol 28: 818–825
82. Tolwani AJ, Campbell RC, Schenk MB et Simplified citrate anticoagulation for continuous renal replacement therapy. Kid Int 2001; 60: 370–374
83. Turney JH, Fewell MR, Williams LC et al. (1980) Platelet protection and heparin sparing with prostacyclin during regular dialysis therapy. Lancet ii: 219–222
84. Van Biljon I, van Damme-Lombaerts R, Demol A et al. (1996) Low molecular weight heparin for anticoagulation during hemodialysis in children – a preliminary study. Eur J Pediatr 155: 70–73
85. van der Wetering J, Westendorp RGJ, van der Hoeven JG et al. (1996) Heparin use in continuous renal replacement therapies: the struggle between filter coagulation and patient hemorrhage. J Am Soc Nephrol 7: 145–150
86. Voiculescu M, Ismail G, Ionescu C et al. (2002) Anticoagulation efficacy and safety with a low molecular weight heparin – tinzaparin in continuous real replacement therapies. Blood Purif 20: 313p

87. Wartentin TE, Cook DJ (2005) Heparin, low molecular weight heparin, and heparin-induced thrombocytopenia in the ICU. Crit Care Clin 21:513–529.
88. Webb AR, Mythen MG, Jacobson D et al. (1995) Maintaining blood flow in the extracorporeal circuit: hemostasis and anticoagulation. Intensiv Care Med 21: 84–93
89. Willey ML de DS, Spinler SA (2002) Removal of lepirudin, a recombinant hirudin, by hemodialysis, hemofiltration, or plasmapheresis. Pharmacother 2: 492–499
90. Wynckel A, Bernieh B, Toupance O et al. (1991). Guidelines to the use of enoxparin in slow continuous dialysis. Contrib Nephrol 93:221–224
91. Young G, Yonekawa KE, Nakagawa PA et al. (2007) Recombinant activated factor VII effectively reverses the anticoagulant effects of heparin, enoxaparin, fondaparinux, argatroban, and bivalirudin ex vivo as measured using thromboelastography. Blood Coagul Fibrinolysis. 18:547–53
92. Zobel G, Ring E, Rödel S (1995) Prognosis in pediatric patients with multiple organ system failure and continuous extracorporeal renal support. Contrib Nephrol 116: 163–168
93. Zobel G, Ring E, Kuttnig M, Grubbauer HM (1991) Continuous arteriovenous hemofiltration versus continuous venovenous hemofiltration in critically ill pediatric patients. Contrib Nephrol 93: 257–260

Vascular Access for Acute Dialysis

7.10

Bernard Canaud, Leila Chenine, Delphine Henriet, and Hélène Leray-Moragués

Core Message

› Central venous catheters (CVC) are widely used for vascular access in the acute dialysis setting. CVC choice depends on performances (intermittent high flow, continuous low flow), dialysis modality, and acute patient clinical conditions. Catheter insertion has been facilitated and secured by the use of ultrasound devices. Catheter care and handling require complying with strict protocols and best practice guidelines to prevent catheter-related complications (infections, dysfunction). Catheter performances (effective flow, resistance, recirculation) and dialysis efficacy (dialysis dose and adequacy targets) should be regularly evaluated to ensure delivery of adequate dialysis in acute patients. All these aspects are developed in this chapter.

7.10.1 Introduction

Vascular access (VA) is a basic and common tool required to perform acute dialysis or any form of extracorporeal renal replacement therapy [1, 2]. Over the last 2 decades, central venous catheters (CVC) have become the preferred type of vascular access in acute conditions [3]. CVC provides a rapid and easy way for blood access permitting to start immediately dialysis in critically ill renal patient. In most cases, CVC are used temporarily for supporting patient during the failure phase and removed at the time of renal recovery (4–6 weeks later). In some cases, CVC represents a bridging solution to a permanent arteriovenous vascular access when renal function is not recovering and patient turn to chronic renal failure. Despite significant design and material improvements, CVC remains a leading cause of morbidity and mortality in acute renal patients.

Renal replacement therapy in the intensive care unit (ICU) relies on different options that differed essentially by blood flow regime: intermittent dialysis modalities (3–7 sessions a week) require high flow rate to achieve adequate dialysis dose delivery in short duration time; continuous dialysis (24 h/day) or semi continuous modalities (12–18 h/day), are easily satisfied with low flow rate, since long dialysis duration is compensating for low instantaneous clearance. Indication for continuous or intermittent treatment modality relies on hemodynamic stability, patient clinical conditions and physician expert judgment. In theory, CVC design should differ for high and low flow dialysis modalities, but in practice, CVC are very similar and may be used indifferently for both modalities provided they offer low resistance and low recirculation at high flow rate.

In this manuscript, we will address practical questions in order to help physician faced to acute dialysis needs: (1) How to choose CVC for acute dialysis? (2) How to insert, care, and manage CVC in ICU setting? (3) How to evaluate and maintain performances of CVC? (4) How to improve CVC outcomes in ICU?

B. Canaud (✉)
Nephrology, Dialysis & Intensive Care Unit, Renal Research and Training Institute, Lapeyronie University Hospital, CHU Montpellier, 34295 Montpellier, France
e-mail: b-canaud@chu-montpellier.fr

A. Jörres, et al. (eds.), *Management of Acute Kidney Problems*,
DOI: 10.1007/978-3-540-69441-0_7.10, © Springer-Verlag Berlin Heidelberg 2010

7.10.2 How to Choose a CVC for Acute Dialysis?

Catheters are commonly used in intensive care unit to perform acute dialysis. They are easily inserted by physician at bedside under local anesthesia and immediately usable for dialysis. Choosing a CVC for acute dialysis relies however on two basic questions: firstly, what is the design and its impact on the functional characteristics of CVC? secondly, what is the dialysis modality indicated in this acute patient?

7.10.2.1 CVC Material and Design

Several types of hemodialysis CVC are available on the market. Catheters are usually made of polymers (e.g., polyvinyl chloride, polytetrafluoroethylene, polyethylene, polyurethane, silicone elastomer, carbothane) that translate into specific CVC physical and functional characteristics. Catheter design and engineering are important factors contributing to their performances in term of flow, resistance and recirculation [4]. Polymers and surface treatment are crucial factors for CVC hemocompatibility and prevention of complications. Polyurethane and silicone elastomer are now the most widely used material for dialysis CVC.

Catheter stiffness is a physical characteristic that dictates the procedure for percutaneous vein insertion. Catheter rigidity depends mainly on the polymer nature, the plasticizer content and the extrusion mode. Rigid and semi-rigid catheters, usually referred to short-term (acute) catheters, are easily introduced percutaneously using the Seldinger method over a metallic guide wire. However, this stiffness leads to a greater risk of vascular perforation and vascular wall lesion. Now, it must be noted that certain type of catheters made of polyurethane which are semi-rigid at ambient temperature soften up at the body temperature, thereby losing their mechanical aggressiveness. Soft silicone or polyurethane catheters usually referred to long-term (chronic or permanent) catheters. Percutaneous insertion is longer but bears a major advantage that is associated with their subcutaneous tunneling possibility. Several modalities of percutaneous insertion, derived from the Seldinger's method using introducer with sheath dilator (pealable or not) have been developed and substituted to the surgical approach [5]. In addition, long-term CVC beneficiate from a subcutaneous anchoring system (dacron cuff, purse ring suture) that provides a physical barrier against bacterial infection and improves patient's comfort.

Single and double-lumen dialysis CVC are available on the market. Although, two single-lumen catheters (inflow and outflow) inserted in the same central vein are used in some units, catheters featuring a double-lumen design (one arterial port and one venous port) are most popularly used (Fig. 7.10.1). Layout of the lumen and distal ends of catheters may vary considerably from one type to another (Fig. 7.10.2). According to venous and arterial port locations, two main types of catheter may be designed: one with port sites attached in a double-barreled gun fashion (coaxial, double-D, double-O); the other with independent or separated port sites (dual catheter, split catheter) (Fig. 7.10.7 and 7.10.8). From a flow perspective, it has been shown that independent or split catheter lines offered higher and more consistently adequate blood flow than attached ones [6, 7].

New polymer or surface treatment of CVC may reduce substantially the hemoreactivity and the prothrombotic activity of the catheter lines [8, 9]. Introduction of bioactive material with ion bombardment, silver impregnation and anticoagulant or antibiotic/antiseptic are intended to prevent platelet adhesion and subsequent clotting and to prevent bacterial adhesion [10, 11]. Recent studies comparing the incidence of infection using antibiotic or antiseptic impregnated catheters to regular ones have found contrasting results: some confirming the efficacy in reducing streamline infection [12, 13]; others not founding any additive protective effects [14]. However, the true protective effect of this bioactive material is effective on longer period

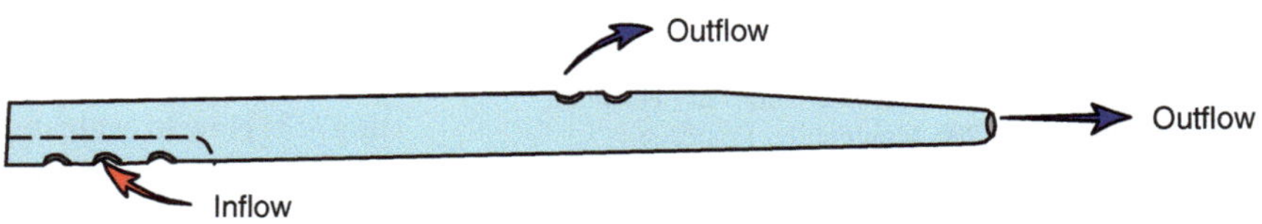

Fig. 7.10.1 Short-term catheter: double-lumen polyurethane catheter

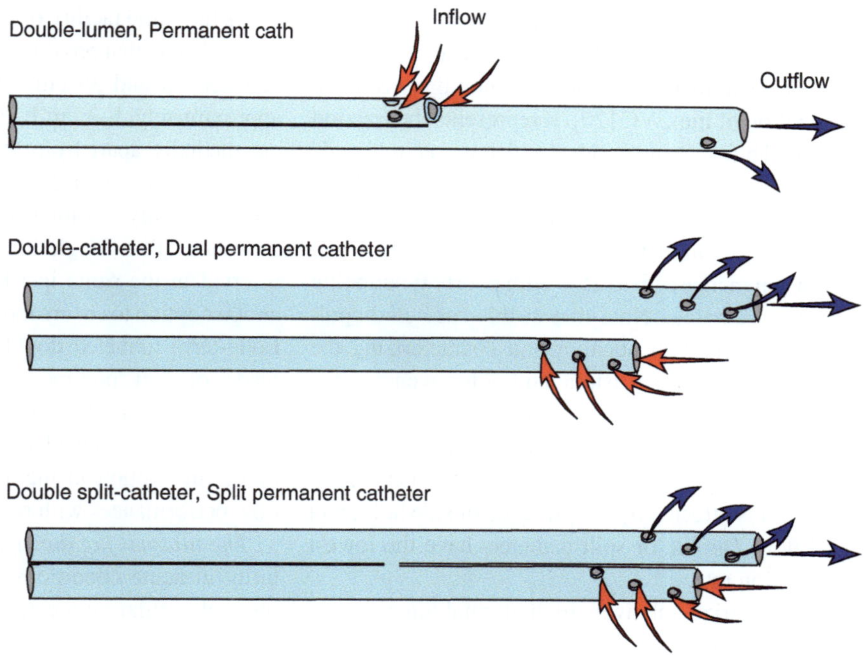

Fig. 7.10.2 Different type of long-term catheters

of time (>6 months) remains to be proved [15]. Catheter locking solution during the interdialytic period, based on antithrombotic/antiseptic mixture, appears more appealing in this context [16, 17]. Locking solutions have been proved highly effective both in reducing significantly catheter-related infection and in preventing bacterial biofilm formation in chronic patients [18]. It remains to be proved that these solutions are applicable to acute setting without risks but this concern deserve further studies [19].

To summarize, one may consider that semi-rigid double-lumen polyurethane catheters are a fairly reasonable choice for a short time use up to 2 weeks, while soft (polyurethane, silicone) double-catheters or double-lumen catheters (long-term or permanent catheters) are a best indication for prolonged renal replacement therapy up to 6 weeks or more.

7.10.2.2 CVC Design and Function

Dialysis adequacy relies on CVC performances, which are dependent on the effective extracorporeal blood flow achieved and the blood recirculation at the tip of catheter.

Catheter geometry and blood viscosity are two main factors conditioning the effective blood flow achieved with CVC. As expressed by the Poiseuille-Hagen law, the resistance (R) opposed to blood flow by CVC is proportional to the pressure generated by the blood pump (ΔP) and inversely proportional to blood flow (Qb) as expressed by the equation $R = \Delta P/\text{Qb}$. Now considering the geometry of the CVC (length, L and radius of the inner lumen r), and the blood viscosity (μ), this equation can rearranged as follows $R = 8\ \mu L/\pi r^4$. From this equation it is clearly shown that flow resistance opposed by a CVC is proportional to the length of the catheter and inversely proportional to the fourth power of its internal lumen radius. In other words, increasing the internal lumen diameter of CVC is much more productive for reducing flow resistance than reducing its length. In addition, it must be acknowledged that CVC resistance is also proportional to blood viscosity, a factor correlated to hematocrit and protein concentration at body temperature.

To prevent clotting and minimize mechanical stress of blood circulating cells it is desirable to maintain laminar fluid profile in CVC. Such a condition is achieved when the forces of friction overcome the dynamic viscosity of the blood, as expressed by the Reynolds number (Re). Re number is directly proportional to the fluid's instantaneous circulatory speed, to the catheter's internal lumen, and inversely proportional to the blood's dynamic viscosity. Thus, Re number translates the blood's dynamic interaction with its CVC contents.

A value less than 2,500 is admitted as being the threshold value to maintain laminar fluid in a catheter.

Blood recirculation is a phenomenon that occurs at the distal tip of the CVC [20]. It represents the fraction of purified blood (venous side), which is "recirculated" on the arterial side and reduces by as much the dialyzer solute clearance. In regular conditions with good CVC functioning, recirculation rate range between 8% and 15%. It can increase up to 25% with poorly functioning or reverse catheters. Note that in this case cardiopulmonary recirculation phenomenon characterizing the arteriovenous access (fistula and arteriovenous bypass) does not exist with venovenous accesses. Recirculation is dependent on the arterial and venous tips positioning and distance apart each other within the vein. It is affected by the presence of side holes and blood flow. Double or split catheters have the lowest recirculation rate.

To summarize, relatively high internal lumen diameter (1.8–2.2 mm) with catheter length (30–40 cm) and low recirculation (<10%) are basic prerequisite for achieving optimal CVC performances.

7.10.2.3 Patient Clinical Condition and Dialysis Modality

Selection of CVC and venous site depend on the clinical condition of the patient and the physician's expertise.

Femoral approach should preferred as first option with critically ill renal patient presenting with respiratory distress (pulmonary edema, respiratory failure), hemodynamic shock or when thoracic access appears risky or because patient's condition dictates prolonged stay in bed (coma, ventilatory assistance, and multiple organ failure). Internal jugular approach is preferable in the absence of thoracic life-threatening conditions. Subclavian access should be reserved for short-term treatment or when no other central vein access options exist.

The femoral approach is the first line for vascular access in emergency [21]. It represents the best choice for renal patient presenting with critical cardiopulmonary condition. Femoral catheterization is also useful in bed-ridden patients with neurologic disorders, ventilatory assistance or multiple organ failure.

Double-lumen polyurethane catheters represent the best option in this case. The right or left femoral vein offers the same facility of insertion. The length of femoral catheters that provide optimal flow performances is between 25 and 35 cm. The insertion site is located approximately 1–2 cm below the crural arcade and 1 cm medially apart from the femoral artery. Although use of such catheters may be extended to several weeks, it is commonly recommended to restrict their use up to 2 weeks. Two single-lumen polyurethane catheters inserted in the same ipsi femoral vein may represent another option to ensure more stable flow performances. Long-term tunneled double-lumen or double-catheter made of soft polymer (polyurethane and silicone) (Fig. 7.10.3) have been used successfully in acute condition [22, 23]. Tunneled CVC offers a new and quite interesting option in the acute setting providing high flow performances with reduced complications [24].

The internal jugular approach has gained in popularity in acute conditions. Irrespective of CVC used, internal jugular vein catheterization entails a reduced

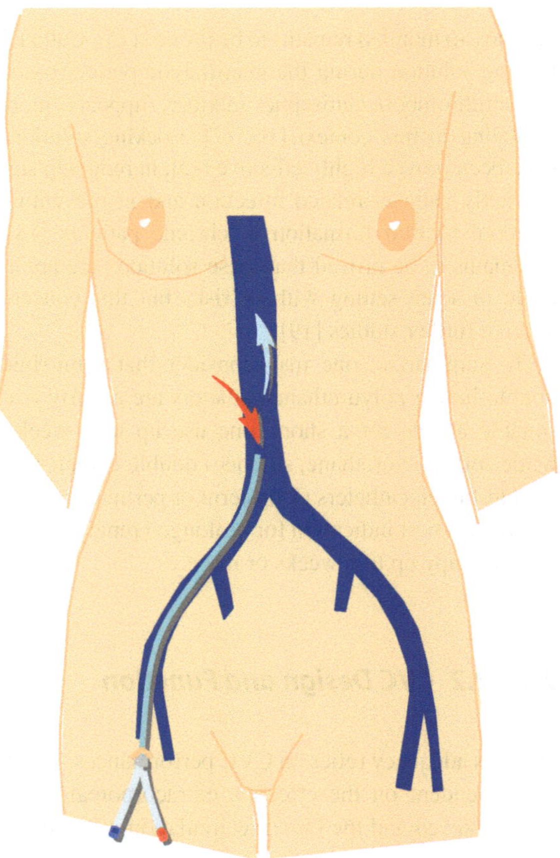

Fig. 7.10.3 Short-term untunneled catheter inserted in the femoral vein with the tip correctly located in the inferior vena cava

incidence of venous thromboses relative to the subclavian access [25, 26]. Due to their location, short-term straight kinked or bent double-lumen jugular CVC bear a higher risk of infection. In addition, short-term jugular CVC does provide neither a comfortable way for patient, nor an easy access for nurses. Short term CVC should be abandoned at the profit of long-term CVC in acute patients. Several studies have proved that long-term tunneled jugular CVC made of polyurethane or silicone catheters may be used in acute patients with excellent results (Figs. 7.10.4 and 7.10.5).

The percutaneous insertion of the catheter into the internal jugular vein is preferably performed in the low position of the Sedillot's triangle. The right internal jugular vein represents the best anatomical option offering a straight and short distance to reach the right atrium. The left internal jugular vein may be indicated as second intent since it is technically more difficult to cannulate and it bears higher risk of vein thrombosis. Subcutaneous tunnel of 10–15 cm on the chest wall below the clavicle with an anchoring system (dacron cuff, purse ring suture) will protect and secure the CVC.

The subclavian approach should be considered as a third line possibility intent in absence of other alternative and for very short-term use. Subclavian cannulation should be restricted to tunneled long-term soft and hemocompatible CVC (Fig. 7.10.6). The right subclavian approach is preferable to reduce malpositioning and dysfunction of CVC. The left subclavian vein is more difficult to cannulate and exposed to a higher risk of left brachiocephalic thrombosis. Shorter cannulae (20–25 cm) are indicated to prevent cardiac trauma on

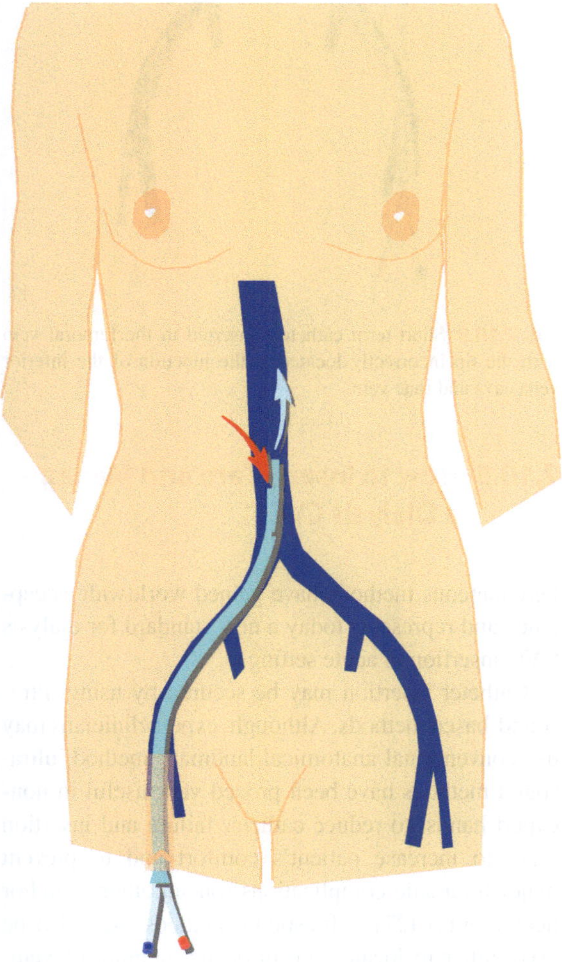

Fig. 7.10.4 Long-term tunneled catheter inserted in the femoral vein with the tip correctly located the inferior cava system

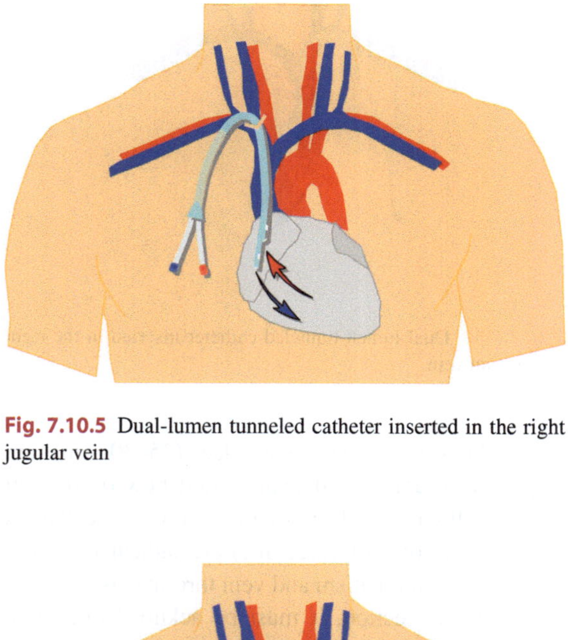

Fig. 7.10.5 Dual-lumen tunneled catheter inserted in the right jugular vein

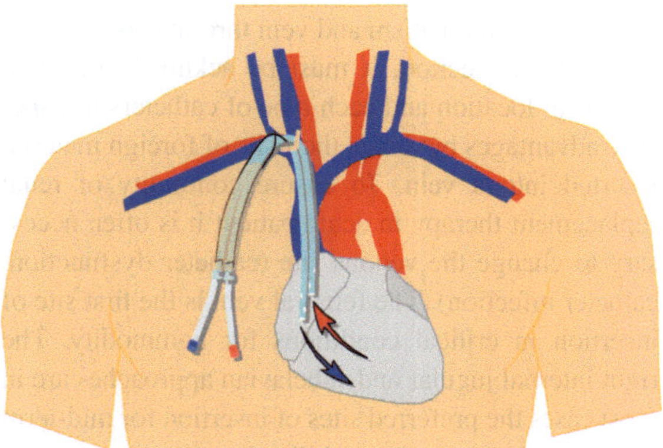

Fig. 7.10.6 Tunneled dual-catheter inserted in the right internal jugular

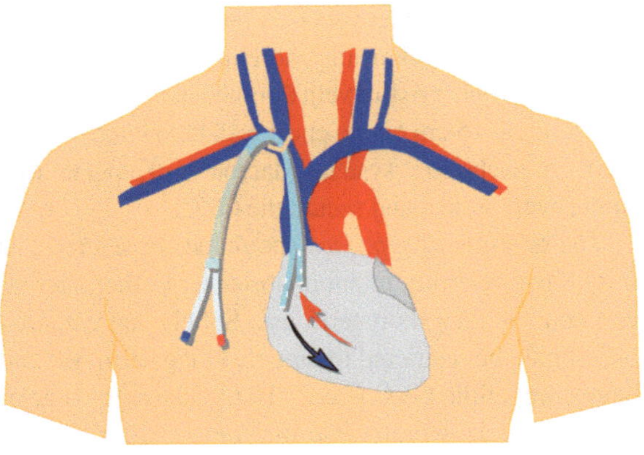

Fig. 7.10.7 Split-catheter inserted in the right internal jugular

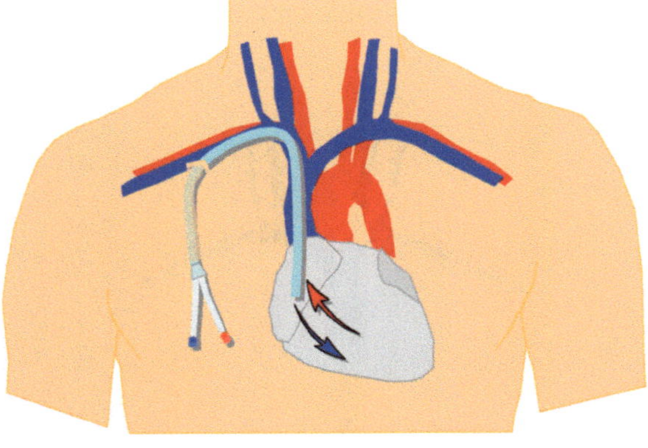

Fig. 7.10.8 Dual-lumen tunneled catheter inserted in the right subclavian vein

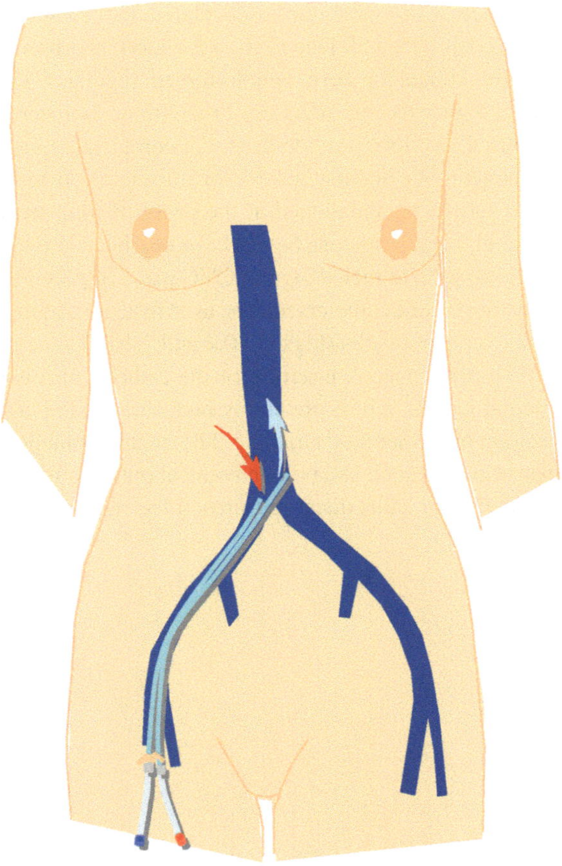

Fig. 7.10.9 Short-term catheters inserted in the femoral vein with the tip incorrectly located at the junction of the inferior vena cava and iliac vein

the right side. Longer cannulae (25–30 cm) are requested to achieve adequate blood flow on the left side. In all cases, soft and hemocompatible catheters (silicone or soft polyrurethane) are indicated to prevent cardiac traumatism and vein thrombosis.

From this section, it must be acknowledged that each vein location and each type of catheters has specific advantages but bears the risks of foreign material inserted into a vein. To ensure continuity of renal replacement therapy in acute patient it is often necessary to change the venous site (catheter dysfunction, catheter infection). The femoral vein is the first site of insertion in critical conditions for commodity. The right internal jugular and subclavian approaches are in most cases the preferred sites of insertion for mid-term use. They facilitate the mobilization of patients (care, physiotherapy, imaging) and should be preferred in conscious or mobile patients.

7.10.3 How to Insert, Care and Manage a Dialysis CVC?

Percutaneous methods have gained worldwide acceptance and represents today a new standard for dialysis CVC insertion in acute setting.

Catheter insertion may be secured by using ultrasound-based methods. Although, expert clinicians may use conventional anatomical landmark method, ultrasound methods have been proved very useful in non-expert hands, to reduce catheter failure and insertion time, to increase patient's comfort and to prevent major traumatic complications (pneumothorax and/or hemothorax) [27]. Ultrasound methods may also be used either to locate vein prior any attempt of venipuncture or to guide directly the vein cannulation at the time of catheter insertion [28].

Basic rules for catheter insertion are well established [29]. Catheter insertion must be performed in a clean room following strict aseptic rules including a meticulous skin preparation and disinfection of the patient, the use of sterile drape, gown, gloves, mask and hat being worn by the operator. Fluoroscopic guidance during the insertion may be used to ensure correct insertion and positioning of the CVC.

Correct positioning of the catheter's tip is essential to prevent CVC dysfunction. Thoracic catheters inserted in the superior vena cava system should have their tips located between the superior vena cava and the right atrium to optimize flow rate (Figs. 7.10.4 and 7.10.5). Chest X-ray checking correct catheter position, tip location and the absence of traumatism must performed prior catheter use (Figs. 7.10.10 and 7.10.11). To ensure safety, semi-rigid catheters should have their tips located in the superior vena cava system (1 or 2 cm above the right atrium) and not in the heart. For a short-term catheter, twenty centimeters is the optimal length when inserted on the right site (internal jugular or subclavian) in an adult. Additional 3–5 cm are required when catheters are inserted on the left side. For a long-term tunneled catheter, 25–30 cm is the optimal length when inserted on the right side (jugular or subclavian) in an adult. Additional 3–5 cm are required when CVC are inserted on the left side.

Femoral catheters accessing the inferior vena cava system should have their tips positioned in the central lumen of the inferior vena cava (Fig. 7.10.3). Thirty to thirty-five centimeters length are needed for short-term femoral catheter to reach the desired location in an adult. For long-term tunneled catheter, 35–40 cm are required to achieve a correct position independently from side. Abdomen X-ray checking correct catheter position of tip is required before use (Fig. 7.10.12).

Catheter care and maintenance are crucial to ensure good functioning and to prevent complications of CVC. In a recent study, it has been shown that accurate placement and appropriate hygienic rules are the best warranty of successful catheter handling [30]. CVC should be ideally used exclusively for renal replacement therapy avoiding their use for blood samples, parenteral feeding and IV injections. Reducing frequency of catheter opening and manipulation reduce the risk of catheter contamination. Nurse training is essential in the prevention of infection and the maintenance of CVC patency. Strict aseptic conditions in catheter handling must be adopted at any time [31, 32]. Interestingly, the use of antiseptic ointment and/or antiseptic protective box on catheter hubs reduces significantly the incidence of bacteriemias [33, 34]. Catheter dressing is highly desirable to protect the emergence of catheters [35]. Indeed, tight occlusive

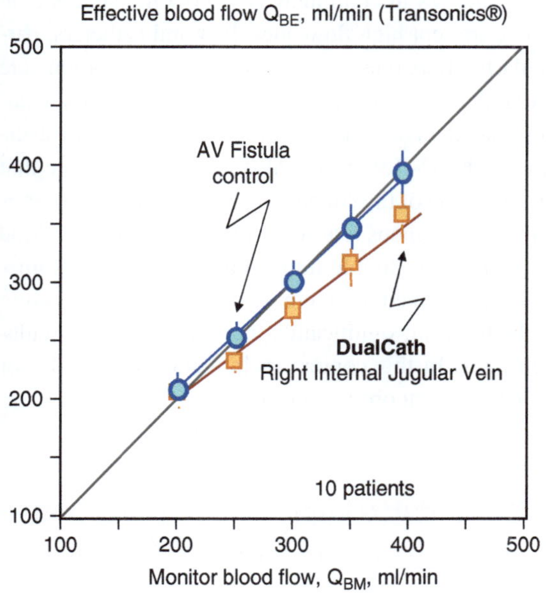

Fig. 7.10.10 Effective blood versus set blood flow on the dialysis monitor. Comparison of DualCath and native AV fistula

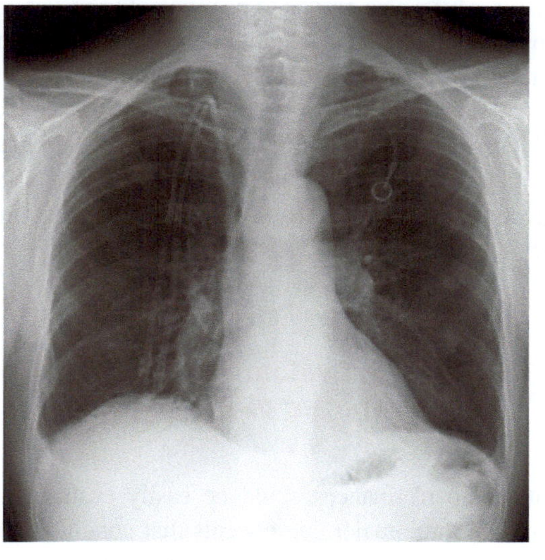

Fig. 7.10.11 Chest X-Ray of a long-term tunneled dual-catheter inserted in the right internal jugular vein with the tip correctly located at the junction of the superior vena cava and the right atrium

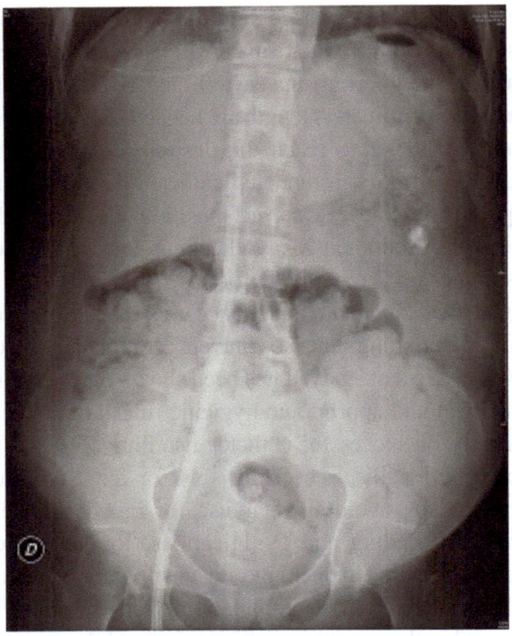

Fig. 7.10.12 Abdomen X-Ray of a long-term tunneled dual-catheter inserted in the femoral vein with the tip correctly located the inferior cava system

polyurethane occlusive dressings promoting moisture and proliferation of cutaneous bacteria are not suitable since they have been associated with an increase risk of catheter infection [36, 37]. Catheter locking solutions based on antithrombotic, antiseptic or antibiotic mixtures have also proved to be efficient in preventing clotting and in reducing endoluminal bacteria contamination [38–41]. Interestingly, it has been found in a recent study that the use of heparin as catheter lock solution may favor the biofilm formation [42]. Catheter decontamination may be achieved in relapsing CVC infection by applying ethanol as adjunctive short time locking solution [43].

7.10.4 How to Evaluate and to Improve Dialysis CVC Performances?

Catheter performances could be easily evaluated in clinic on three major components that conditions the dialysis adequacy: effective blood flow regularly achieved; flow resistance opposed to a preset blood flow; recirculation rate. Effective blood flow may be measured using an external ultrasound monitoring device (Transonics) or calculated by the dialysis machine based on arterial/venous pressure drop [44]. Effective blood is usually 10–20% less than value set on the machine (Fig. 7.10.10).

Flow resistance may be estimated from the pressure measurement recorded by the dialysis machine on the arterial and on the venous side. The negative pressure recorded on the inflow side (arterial line) and the positive pressure recorded on the outflow side (venous line), reflect blood resistance in the extracorporeal circuit. The pressure/blood flow ratio represents an interesting, reliable and simple index that can be used to evaluate resistance and to detect early partial catheter obstruction [45]. In practice, it is convenient to note that the venous pressure is linearly correlated to the blood flow (e.g., for a blood flow rate of 300 mL/min, venous pressure is close to 150 mmHg in a silicone rubber dual catheter device) this relationship could be used to follow the performances of the CVC.

Early catheter mechanical dysfunction is more frequent with double-lumen catheters inserted via the subclavian way than with those inserted in other sites. In these cases, causes of catheter kinking and striction (subclavian pathway or suture) must be ruled out.

Catheter recirculation depends both on catheter type, on insertion site and on blood flow used. Catheter recirculation reduces by as much as the session efficacy. It is worth noting that this phenomenon has fewer consequences in continuous low flow modalities than in intermittent high flow ones. Femoral catheters, particularly short ones, exhibit a high recirculation rate averaging 20% (5–38%). Internal jugular and subclavian catheters have much lower recirculation rate averaging 10% (5–15%). It is also interesting to note that the inversion of the connecting lines (by using the arterial line for venous return and the venous line for blood aspiration) on double-lumen catheters, that is sometimes performed to increase flow when a pressure problem occur, significantly increases blood recirculation rates. In this context recirculation up to 20% or 30% have been observed [46, 47].

7.10.5 How to Improve CVC Outcomes in Intensive Care Unit Setting?

The causes of dialysis CVC dysfunction may be conveniently related to the delay after insertion [48]. Immediate or early dysfunction usually results from mechanical problems, among which are malpositioning of the catheter tip (Fig. 7.10.9) catheter kinking and striction caused by ligatures or aponevrosis [49]. Late dysfunction (more than 2 weeks) are more often caused by thrombotic problems: partial or total obstructive thrombosis of the catheter lumen, thrombosis or stenosis of the cannulated vein, external sheath formation on the catheter distal end (external fibrin sleeve), internal coating of the catheter (endoluminal fibrin sleeve) [50].

Thrombotic complications recognized several causes. Endoluminal thrombosis of the catheter is the most common. This is revealed by intermittent or permanent catheter dysfunction. Catheter may be reopen in these cases by mechanical methods (guide wire brushing) or chemical methods (fibrinolytic). External thrombosis of the catheters caused by fibrin sheath covering the tip of the catheters is relatively frequent but unknown [51]. CVC entrapped in fibrin sleeve requires either a fibrinolysis, an endovascular catheter stripping through femoral vein, or removing or replacement of catheters [52, 53]. Thrombosis of the host-cannulated vein is a more severe situation with potential complication of pulmonary embolism. The incidence may vary from 20% to 70% of reports according to the sites and diagnostic modalities used [54]. Thrombosis of the right atrium is the most serious and potentially lethal complication. Circumstances of discovering CVC thrombotic complications are usually catheter dysfunction, rarely onset of limb edema or unexplained fever. Several factors contribute to the thrombogenicity of the catheter including the catheter (polymer, softness, and surface aspect), the nature and the location of the vein, the duration of cannulation, the clotting and inflammatory state of the patient and the infection of the catheter.

Infections represent a major burden for hemodialysis catheters [55–57]. Non-tunneled polyurethane catheters used as a short-term therapy entail a bacteriemia risk estimated to a median value of 5.9 episodes per 1,000 patient-days in intensive care units [58]. The incidence of bacteriemias varies greatly according units, practice and catheter type [59]. The site of catheter insertion is a major risk factor for CVC infection. Femoral catheter is usually more exposed than subclavian catheter and internal jugular catheter to bacterial contamination [60]. Now, it is worth noting that infectious risk may be significantly reduced in ICU when good nursing practices are applied uniformly [61]. Non-tunneled internal jugular or subclavian CVC bears a higher risk of infections than tunneled and cuffed one [62–64].

Early infection may be related to catheter placement problems or skin and catheter track infection. Placement of a percutaneous catheter disrupts the continuous protecting solution of the skin. Bacterial colonization of the skin is most often incriminated in these catheter infections. The skin acts as a bacterial reservoir and contributes to the subcutaneous penetration of germs along the catheter pathway. Hence, the need to carefully disinfect the skin prior to any catheter insertion, to use full barrier protections and to ensure a particular care in the patients harboring catheters is always suitable [65].

Late infections are associated with endoluminal catheter contamination and the formation of a microbial biofilm. Infectious risk of dialysis CVC does not increase with time spent in ICU [66]. This known risk must minimize through suitable nursing care and handling. Two types of infections are observed with catheters: local infection (skin exit, track infection) and systemic infection (bacteremia, septicemia, infected thrombosis). Skin exit and bacteremia are the most frequent forms of infection [67]. Catheter track infection, septicemia and infected venous thrombosis are most severe form of infections requiring both catheters withdrawal and systemic antibiotic therapy. Endoluminal catheter contamination from hubs may be the source of microbial biofilm. In this case, bacteriae entering into the lumen, adhere onto the catheter surface, growth, produce glycocalyx (slime) and become resistant to antibiotic [68]. Occasionally, bacteria may be released from this biofilm (e.g., higher stress conditions due to blood pump speed) being the source of bacteremia and fever episode. In the event of an unexplained septic condition, it is reasonable to refer first to the role of the catheter as the infection carrier. Several authors have proposed a catheter replacement over a guide wire through the same subcutaneous track [69]. This is an unsafe microbiologically approach that should be abandoned. The insertion of long-term tunneled catheters appears to be more suitable to prevent catheter infection hazards. Now, it must be stressed that strict full barrier protection (gloves, mask, drapes and antiseptic) must be applied for catheter handling and particularly at the time of dialysis connection to prevent contamination of catheter hubs [70].

Stenosis of the host vein is a common risk of catheter [71]. It is more common with than expected with the internal jugular vein and rarely symptomatic [72]. This troublesome complication may compromise future creation of arteriovenous fistula in case of chronic kidney failure.

7.10.6 Conclusion

Central venous catheters are widely used for vascular access in the acute dialysis setting [73]. CVC choice depends on performances (intermittent high flow, continuous low flow), dialysis modality and acute patient clinical conditions. Catheter insertion has been facilitated and secured by the use of ultrasound devices. Catheter care and handling require complying with strict protocols and best practice guidelines to prevent catheter-related complications (infections, dysfunction). Catheter performances (effective flow, resistance, recirculation) and dialysis efficacy (dialysis dose and adequacy targets) should be regularly evaluated to ensure delivery of adequate dialysis in acute patients.

7.10.7 Take Home Pearls

- *Central venous catheters* (CVC) are the preferred type of vascular access for providing renal replacement therapy in acute conditions. CVC remains a leading cause of morbidity and mortality in acute renal patients.
- *Choose a CVC* for acute dialysis relies on cannula design and material that dictates its performances, and on dialysis flow that is indicated (intermittent high flow versus continuous low flow). Semi-rigid double-lumen polyurethane catheters are a fairly reasonable choice for a short time use (less than 15 days). Soft (polyurethane, silicone) tunneled double-catheters or double-lumen catheters are a best indication for prolonged renal replacement therapy (6 weeks or more).
- *Catheter geometry* and blood viscosity are two main factors conditioning the effective blood flow achieved with CVC. To prevent clotting and minimize mechanical stress of blood circulating cells it is desirable to maintain laminar fluid profile in CVC. Blood recirculation is a phenomenon that occurs at the distal tip of the CVC and reduces dialysis dose delivery. Relatively high internal lumen diameter (1.8–2.2 mm) with catheter length (30–40 cm) and low recirculation (<10%) are basic prerequisite for achieving optimal CVC performances.
- The *femoral approach* is the first line for vascular access in emergency. Tunneled CVC offers a new and quite interesting option in the acute setting providing high flow performances with reduced complications. The *internal jugular* approach has gained in popularity in acute conditions. Irrespective of CVC (tunneled or untunneled) used, internal jugular vein catheterization entails a reduced incidence of venous thromboses relative to the subclavian access. The *subclavian approach* should be considered as a third line possibility intent in absence of other alternative and for very short-term use.
- *Percutaneous methods* have gained worldwide acceptance and represents today a new standard for dialysis CVC insertion in acute setting. Catheter insertion may be secured by using ultrasound-based methods. Hygienic rules for catheter insertion are well established and should be followed. Correct positioning of the catheter's tip is essential to prevent CVC dysfunction. Catheter care and maintenance are crucial to ensure good functioning and to prevent complications of CVC.
- *Catheter performances* could be easily evaluated in clinic on three major components that conditions the dialysis adequacy: effective blood flow regularly achieved; flow resistance opposed to a preset blood flow; recirculation rate. Immediate or early dysfunction usually results from mechanical problems, among which are malpositioning of the catheter tip, catheter kinking and striction caused by ligatures or aponevrosis. Late dysfunction (more than 2 weeks) are more often caused by thrombotic problems: partial or total obstructive thrombosis of the catheter lumen, thrombosis or stenosis of the cannulated vein, external sheath formation on the catheter distal end (external fibrin sleeve), internal coating of the catheter (endoluminal fibrin sleeve).
- *Infections* represent a major burden for hemodialysis catheters. The site of catheter insertion is a major risk factor for CVC infection. Infectious risk may be significantly reduced in ICU when good nursing practices are applied regularly. Non-tunneled internal jugular or subclavian CVC bears a higher risk of infections than tunneled and cuffed one. Late infections are

associated with endoluminal catheter contamination and the formation of a microbial biofilm.

References

1. Uldall R. Hemodialysis access – Part A: Temporary. In: Jacobs C, Kjellstrand CM, Koch KM, Winchester JFW (eds) Replacement of renal function by dialysis. Kluwer, Dordrecht, 1996, pp. 277–92.
2. Oliver MJ. Acute dialysis catheters. Semin Dial. 2001; 14(6):432–5.
3. Canaud B, Desmeules S, Klouche K, Leray-Moragués H, Béraud JJ. Vascular access for dialysis in the intensive care unit. Best Pract Res Clin Anaesthesiol. 2004; 18(1):159–74.
4. Curelalu I, Gustavsson B, Hansson AH. Material thrombogenicity in central venous catheterization. II. A comparison between plain silicone elastomer and plain polyethylene, long, antebrachial catheters. Acta Anaesthesiol Scand. 1983; 27:158–64.
5. Canaud B, Leray-Moragues H, Garred LJ, Turc-Baron C, Mion C. Permanent central vein access. Semin Dial. 1996; 9:397–400.
6. Jean G, Charra B, Chazot C, Vanel T, Terrat JC, Hurot JM. Long-term outcome of permanent hemodialysis catheters: a controlled study. Blood Purif. 2001; 19(4):401–7.
7. Trerotola SO, Kraus M, Shah H, Namyslowski J, Johnson MS, Stecker MS, Ahmad I, McLennan G, Patel NH, O'Brien E, Lane KA, Ambrosius WT. Randomized comparison of split tip versus step tip high-flow hemodialysis catheters. Kidney Int. 2002; 62(1):282–9.
8. Baumann M, Witzke O, Dietrich R, Haug U, Deppisch R, Lutz J, Philipp T, Heemann U. Prolonged catheter survival in intermittent hemodialysis using a less thrombogenic micropatterned polymer modification. ASAIO J. 2003; 49 (6):708–12.
9. Eberhart RC, Clagett CP. Catheter coatings, blood flow, and biocompatibility. Semin Hematol. 1991; 28:42–8.
10. Sheng WH, Ko WJ, Wang JT, Chang SC, Hsueh PR, Luh KT. Evaluation of antiseptic-impregnated central venous catheters for prevention of catheter-related infection in intensive care unit patients. Diagn Microbiol Infect Dis. 2000; 38(1): 1–5.
11. Tobin EJ, Bambauer R. Silver coating of dialysis catheters to reduce bacterial colonization and infection. Ther Apher. 2003; 7(6):504–9.
12. Darouiche RO, Raad II, Heard SO, Thornby JI, Wenker OC, Gabrielli A, Berg J, Khardori N, Hanna H, Hachem R, Harris RL, Mayhall G. A comparison of two antimicrobial-impregnated central venous catheters. Catheter Study Group. N Engl J Med. 1999; 340(1):1–8.
13. Chatzinikolaou I, Finkel K, Hanna H, Boktour M, Foringer J, Ho T, Raad I. Antibiotic-coated hemodialysis catheters for the prevention of vascular catheter-related infections: a prospective, randomized study. Am J Med. 2003; 115(5): 352–7.
14. Osma S, Kahveci SF, Kaya FN, Akalin H, Ozakin C, Yilmaz E, Kutlay O. Efficacy of antiseptic-impregnated catheters on catheter colonization and catheter-related bloodstream infections in patients in an intensive care unit. J Hosp Infect. 2006; 62(2):156–62.
15. Bambauer R, Mestres P, Schiel R, Bambauer S, Sioshansi P, Latza R. Long-term catheters for apheresis and dialysis with surface treatment with infection resistance and low thrombogenicity. Therap Apher Dial. 2003 Apr;7(2):225–31.
16. Sodemann K, Polaschegg HD, Feldmer B. Two years' experience with Dialock and CLS (a new antimicrobial lock solution). Blood Purif. 2001; 19(2):251–4.
17. Quarello F, Forneris G. Prevention of hemodialysis catheter-related bloodstream infection using an antimicrobial lock. Blood Purif. 2002; 20(1):87–92.
19. Polaschegg HD, Sodemann K. Risks related to catheter locking solutions containing concentrated citrate. Nephrol Dial Transplant. 2003; 18(12):2688–90.
20. Sherman RA, Matera JJ, Novik L, Cody RP. Recirculation reassessed: The impact of blood flow rate and the low-flow method reevaluated. Am J Kidney Dis. 1994; 23:846–8.
21. Gerasimovska V, Oncevski A, Dejanov P, Polenakovic M. Are ambulatory femoral catheters for hemodialysis a safe vascular access? J Vasc Access. 2002; 3(1):14–20.
22. Montagnac R, Bernard Cl, Guillaumie J, Hanhart P, Clavel P, Yazji J, Martinez LM, Schillinger F. Indwelling silicone femoral catheters: experience of three haemodialysis centres. Nephrol Dial Transplant. 1997; 12:772–5.
24. Klouche K, Amigues L, Deleuze S, Beraud JJ, Canaud B. Complications, effects on dialysis dose, and survival of tunneled femoral dialysis catheters in acute renal failure. Am J Kidney Dis. 2007; 49(1):99–108.
25. Cimochowski GE, Worley E, Rutherford WE, Sartain J, Blondin J, Harter H. Superiority of the internal jugular over the subclavian access for temporary dialysis. Nephron. 1990; 54:154–61.
26. Schillinger F, Schillinger D, Montagnac R, Milcent T. Post-catheterisation vein stenosis in hemodialysis: comparative angiographic study of 50 subclavian and 50 internal jugular access. Nephrol Dial Transplant. 1991; 6:722–4.
27. Defalque RJ, Campbell C. Cardiac tamponade from central venous catheter. Anesthesiology. 1979; 50:249–52.
28. Zollo A, Cavatorta F, Galli S. Ultrasound-guided cannulation of the femoral vein for acute hemodialysis access with silicone catheters. J Vasc Access. 2001; 2(2):56–9.
29. Food and Drug Administration. Precautions necessary with central venous catheters. US Government Printing Office, Washington, DC, 1989, p. 15.
30. Mcgee WT, Ackerman BL, Rouben LR, Prasad VP, Bandi V, Mallory DL. Accurate placement of central venous catheters: a prospective, randomized, multicenter trial. Crit Care Med. 1993; 21:1118–23.
31. Vanherweghem JL, Dhaene M, Goldman M, Stolear JC, Sabot JP, Waterlot Y, Serruys E, Thayse C. Infections associated with subclavian dialysis catheters: The key role of nurse training. Nephron. 1986; 42:116–9.
32. Alonso-Echanove J, Edwards JR, Richards MJ, Brennan P, Venezia RA, Keen J, Ashline V, Kirkland K, Chou E, Hupert M, Veeder AV, Speas J, Kaye J, Sharma K, Martin A, Moroz VD, Gaynes RP. Effect of nurse staffing and antimicrobial-impregnated central venous catheters on the risk for bloodstream infections in intensive care units. Infect Control Hosp Epidemiol. 2003; 24(12):916–25

33. Levin A, Mason AJ, Jindal KK, Fong IW, Goldstein MB. Prevention of hemodialysis subclavian vein catheter infections by topical providone-iodine. Kidney Int. 1991; 40:934–8.
34. Maki DG, Alvarado CJ, Ringer M. A prospective, randomized trial of providone-iodine, alcohol and chlorhexidine for prevention of infection with central venous and arterial catheters. Lancet. 1991; 338:339–44.
35. Le Corre I, Delorme M, Cournoyer S. A prospective, randomized trial comparing a transparent dressing and a dry gauze on the exit site of long term central venous catheters of hemodialysis patients. J Vasc Access. 2003; 4(2):56–61.
36. Conly JM, Grieves K, Peters B. A prospective, randomized study comparing transparent and dry gauze dressings for central venous catheters. J Infect Dis. 1989; 159:310–5.
37. Hoffman KK, Weber DJ, Samsa GP, Rutala WA. Transparent polyurethane film as an intravenous catheter dressing: a meta-analysis of infection rates. JAMA. 1992; 267:2072–6.
38. Bell AL, Gu X, Burczynski FJ, Vercaigne LM. Ethanol/trisodium citrate for hemodialysis catheter lock. Clin Nephrol. 2004; 62(5):369–73.
39. Takla TA, Zelenitsky SA, Vercaigne LM. Effect of ethanol/trisodium citrate lock on microorganisms causing hemodialysis catheter related. J Vasc Access. 2007; 8(4):262–7.
40. Chiou PF, Chang CC, Wen YK, Yang Y. Antibiotic lock technique reduces the incidence of temporary catheter-related infections. Clin Nephrol. 2006; 65(6):419–22.
41. Balaban N, Gov Y, Bitler A, Boelaert JR. Prevention of Staphylococcus aureus biofilm on dialysis catheters and adherence to human cells. Kidney Int. 2003; 63(1):340–5.
42. Diskin CJ, Stokes TJ, Dansby LM, Radcliff L, Carter TB. Is systemic heparin a risk factor for catheter-related sepsis in dialysis patients? An evaluation of various biofilm and traditional risk factors. Nephron Clin Pract. 2007; 107 (4):c128–32.
43. Ackoundou-N'guessan C, Heng AE, Guenu S, Charbonne F, Traore O, Deteix P, Souweine B. Ethanol lock solution as an adjunct treatment for preventing recurrent catheter-related sepsis – first case report in dialysis setting. Nephrol Dial Transplant. 2006; 21(11):3339–40.
44. Canaud B, Leray-Moragues H, Kerkeni N, Bosc JY, Martin K. Effective flow performances and dialysis doses delivered with permanent catheters: a 24-month comparative study of permanent catheters versus arterio-venous vascular accesses. Nephrol Dial Transplant. 2002; 17(7):1286–92.
45. Stroud CC, Meyer SL, Bawkon MC, Smith HG, Klein MD. Vascular access for extracorporeal circulation. Resistance in double lumen cannulas. ASAIO J. 1991; 37:M418–9.
46. Leblanc M, Fedak S, Mokris G, Paganini EP. Blood recirculation in temporary central catheters for acute hemodialysis. Clin Nephrol. 1996; 45:315–9.
47. Level C, Lasseur C, Chauveau P, Bonarek H, Perrault L, Combe C. Performance of twin central venous catheters: influence of the inversion of inlet and outlet on recirculation. Blood Purif. 2002; 20(2):182–8.
48. Leblanc M, Bosc JY, Paganini EP, Canaud B. Central venous dialysis catheter dysfunction. Adv Renal Replace Ther. 1997; 4(4):377–89.
49. Kelber J, Delmez JA, Windus DW. Factors affecting delivery of high-efficiency dialysis using temporary vascular access. Am J Kidney Dis. 1993; 22:24–9.
50. Hoshal VL, Ause RG, Hoskins PA. Fibrin sleeve formation on indwelling subclavian central venous catheters. Arch Surg. 1971; 102:353–8.
51. Oguzkurt L, Tercan F, Torun D, Yildirim T, Zümrütdal A, Kizilkilic O. Impact of short-term hemodialysis catheters on the central veins: a catheter venographic study. Eur J Radiol. 2004; 52(3):293–9.
52. Johnstone RD, Stewart GA, Akoh JA, Fleet M, Akyol M, Moss JG. Percutaneous fibrin sleeve stripping of failing haemodialysis catheters. Nephrol Dial Transplant. 1999; 14(3): 688–91.
53. Alomari AI, Falk A. The natural history of tunneled hemodialysis catheters removed or exchanged: a single-institution experience. J Vasc Interv Radiol. 2007; 18(2):227–35.
54. Trottier SJ, Veremakis C, Oíbrien J, Auer AI. Femoral deep vein thrombosis associated with central venous catheterization: results from a prospective, randomized trial. Crit Care Med. 1995; 23:52–9.
55. Gil RT, Kruse JA, Thill-Baharozian MC, Carlson RW. Triple- vs single-lumen central venous catheters: a prospective study in a critically ill population. Arch Intern Med. 1989; 149: 1139–45.
56. Collignon P, Soni N, Pearson I. Sepsis associated with central vein catheters in critically ill patients. Intensive Care Med. 1988; 14:227–32.
57. Richet H, Hubert B, Nitemberg G. Prospective multicenter study of vascular-catheter-related complications and risk factors for positive central-catheter cultures in intensive care unit patients. J Clin Microbiol. 1990; 28:2520–6.
58. Maki DG. Nosocomial infection in the intensive care unit. In: Parillo JE, Bone RC (eds) Critical care medicine principles of diagnosis and management. Mosby, St. Louis, 1995, pp. 893–954.
59. Eyer S, Brummitt C, Crossley K. Catheter-related sepsis: prospective, randomized study of three methods of long-term catheter maintenance. Crit Care Med. 1990; 18: 1073–8.
60. Oliver MJ, Callery SM, Thorpe KE, Schwab SJ, Churchill DN. Risk of bacteremia from temporary hemodialysis catheters by site of insertion and duration of use: a prospective study. Kidney Int. 2000; 58(6):2543–5.
61. Souweine B, Liotier J, Heng AE, Isnard M, Ackoundou-N'Guessan C, Deteix P, Traoré O. Catheter colonization in acute renal failure patients: comparison of central venous and dialysis catheters. Am J Kidney Dis. 2006; 47(5): 879–87.
62. Pezzarossi HE, Ponce De Léon S, Calva JJ. High incidence of subclavian dialysis catheter-related bacteremias. Infect Control. 1986; 7:596–602.
63. Cheesbrough JS, Finch RG, Burden RP. A prospective study of the mechanisms of infection associated with hemodialysis catheters. J Infect Dis. 1986; 154:579–86.
64. Weijmer MC, Vervloet MG, ter Wee PM. Compared to tunnelled cuffed haemodialysis catheters, temporary untunnelled catheters are associated with more complications already within 2 weeks of use. Nephrol Dial Transplant. 2004; 19(3):670–7.
65. Mermel LA. Prevention of intravascular catheter-related infections. Ann Intern Med. 2000; 132(5):391–402.
66. Souweine B, Traore O, Aublet-Cuvelier B, Badrikian L, Bret L, Sirot J, Gazuy N, Laveran H, Deteix P. Dialysis and central venous catheter infections in critically ill patients: results of a prospective study. Crit Care Med. 1999; 27(11): 2394–8.
67. Safdar N, Maki DG. The pathogenesis of catheter-related bloodstream infection with noncuffed short-term central venous catheters. Intensive Care Med. 2004; 30(1):62–7.

68. Kite P, Eastwood K, Sugden S, Percival SL. Use of in vivo-generated biofilms from hemodialysis catheters to test the efficacy of a novel antimicrobial catheter lock for biofilm eradication in vitro. J Clin Microbiol. 2004 July; 42 (7): 3073–6.
69. Cobb DK, High KP, Sawyer RG. A controlled trial of scheduled replacement of central venous and pulmonary-artery catheters. N Engl J Med. 1992; 327:1062–8.
70. Allon M. Dialysis catheter-related bacteremia: treatment and prophylaxis. Am J Kidney Dis. 2004; 44(5):779–91.
71. Levit RD, Cohen RM, Kwak A, Shlansky-Goldberg RD, Clark TW, Patel AA, Stavropoulos SW, Mondschein JI, Solomon JA, Tuite CM, Trerotola SO. Asymptomatic central venous stenosis in hemodialysis patients. Radiology. 2006; 238(3):1051–6.
72. Wilkin TD, Kraus MA, Lane KA, Trerotola SO. Internal jugular vein thrombosis associated with hemodialysis catheters. Radiology. 2003; 228(3):697–700.
73. Schetz M. Vascular access for HD and CRRT. Contrib Nephrol. 2007; 156:275–86.

Principles and Practice of Acute Peritoneal Dialysis

7.11

Wai-Kei Lo, Sing-Leung Lui, and Terence Pok-Siu Yip

Core Messages

- Peritoneal dialysis (PD) is a well-established renal replacement therapy for patients with acute renal failure (ARF).
- Among its advantages are hemodynamic stability, avoidance of systemic anticoagulation, less labor intensive, and no need for high-tech machines.
- Several clinical studies suggest that outcomes of patients with acute kidney failure treated with peritoneal dialysis are quite comparable to those for hemodialysis.
- Continuous equilibrated peritoneal dialysis is the most commonly adopted form, during which fluid and solute removal can be increased by increasing the cycle frequency and glucose content in dialysate.
- With high-volume peritoneal dialysis, the Kt/V_{urea} achieved can be as high as with standard intermittent hemodialysis.
- The present chapter also discusses prevention and management of complications arising from acute peritoneal dialysis.

7.11.1 Introduction

Peritoneal dialysis (PD) has been established as an effective supportive therapy for patients with acute renal failure (ARF) for fluid control, reduction of uremic status and correction of acid–base and electrolyte disturbances, for more than 30 years. Initially, it was mainly adopted in the form of intermittent peritoneal dialysis (IPD). Subsequently, continuous peritoneal dialysis simulating continuous ambulatory peritoneal dialysis (CAPD) has largely replaced IPD. The development of automated peritoneal dialysis (APD) machines further helps the use of PD for ARF and the development of continuous flow peritoneal dialysis (CFPD) and tidal peritoneal dialysis (TPD). However, despite the lack of studies showing inferior results for PD in ARF in comparison with other forms of renal replacement therapy, there is a global reduction trend in use of PD for ARF. Hyman et al. reported that PD fell from 8% in 1994–1995 to 3% in 1999–2000 in Canada [1]. Even in pediatric patients where PD is still the mainstay of therapy in acute renal failure, the utilization rate fell from 43% to 31% from 1995 to 1999 [2]. This falling trend was largely related to rapid development in the technology and increasing use of continuous veno-venous renal replacement therapy (CRRT) and slow low-efficiency daily hemodialysis (SLEDD) or sustained low-efficiency dialysis (SLED) in the last decade. This is evidenced by the simultaneous fall in utilization of intermittent hemodialysis (HD) during the same period in these reports. A survey involving 54 centers from five continents in 2000–2001 showed that 80% of patients were treated with CRRT, 16.9% with intermittent HD, and only 3.2% with PD [3]. The utilization tends to be higher in developing countries. In Brazil, PD was used in 23% of patients with ARF [4].

Wai-Kei Lo (✉)
Department of Medicine, Tung Wah Hospital, 12 Po Yan Street, Hong Kong
e-mail: wkloc@hkucc.hku.hk

A. Jörres et al. (eds.), *Management of Acute Kidney Problems*,
DOI: 10.1007/978-3-540-69441-0_7.11, © Springer-Verlag Berlin Heidelberg 2010

In the last few years, there has been some growing interest in reestablishing PD as a useful therapy for ARF, particularly in developing countries. In fact, the technology of PD has been advanced quite significantly over the last 2 decades to help reducing the complications of PD and improving the outcome. In addition, there are certain advantages of PD over other forms of renal replacement therapy for ARF, and therefore PD should not be discarded at all.

7.11.2 Advantage of PD for ARF

1. No systemic anticoagulation is required

This is particularly important in ARF following major surgery or when hemorrhage or coagulation disorder is present. The use of anticoagulation with heparin or low-molecular-weight heparin in hemodialysis or CRRT would increase the risk of bleeding. Though heparin-free hemodialysis with saline flushing can be used, the repeated saline flushing would reduce the efficiency of water and sodium removal from the body. Regional citrate anticoagulation is effective, but it is tedious and requires frequent monitoring of the coagulation profile, serum calcium, and bicarbonate level. For PD, no systemic anticoagulation is required and thus it would not increase the bleeding risk. In case intraperitoneal heparin is needed, heparin is not effectively absorbed through peritoneum and therefore there will not be any significant systemic effect on coagulation.

2. Patients on PD are hemodynamically more stable than those on hemodialysis

Many patients with ARF have hypotension and shock, and they tolerate HD or even CRRT poorly. In general, they tolerate PD better than HD or CRRT. Hypotension and arrhythmia are rarely induced by the PD treatment. The reasons include:

(a) No extracorporal circulation causing immediate reduction of blood volume.
(b) Slower fluid removal from the blood volume allowing more time for equilibrium between different fluid compartments.
(c) Slower fall of serum urea level allowing time for equilibrium between intracellular and extracellular urea level. This prevents the acute drop of plasma osmolality as a result of rapid extracellular urea removal that occurs in hemodialysis. Such acute drops of plasma osmolality may cause water shifting from extracellular to intracellular space leading to reduction in plasma volume.
(d) Slower rate of change in electrolyte (potassium and calcium) levels

3. PD may lead to more rapid, and a higher chance of, recovery of renal function

It is well documented that PD preserves residual renal function better than HD in patients with end-stage renal failure. Though the exact mechanism is still unknown, it is generally believed that this is related to the more stable hemodynamics with PD, and possibly also a result of less complement activation and higher middle molecule clearance with PD. The same may apply to PD for acute renal failure. In a retrospective study of 31 patients with ARF from malignant hypertension in the period 1997–2000, 11 out of 20 patients received PD became dialysis free, while none of the 11 patients received HD had recovered their renal function [5]. In another study in 1983, a higher rate of recovery of renal function was noted in patients treated with PD [6]. Randomized controlled studies may better define any beneficial effect of PD in this aspect.

4. Ease of conduction and less labor intensive

Unlike HD or CRRT which requires the availability of high-tech machines, PD can be performed manually without any machines. This is an advantageous feature in developing countries where the economic situation may limit the availability of the expensive dialysis machines. Nursing labor is much less intensive compared with CRRT and is particularly so when automated PD cyclers are used.

In a massive calamity, like an earthquake, involving a lot of victims with ARF, the fixed number of hemodialysis machines limits the treatable number of patients. Water and electric supply to dialysis centers may also be destroyed disrupting hemodialysis service. PD performed manually may be a viable option in such circumstances.

7.11.3 Disadvantages of PD

1. Limited clearance

It is well known that PD provides less small solute clearance compared with hemodialysis. However, it is also well known that chronic PD patient survival is similar to that of chronic hemodialysis patients despite the lower small solute clearance. The exact mechanism is unknown, but it is thought to be related to the more stable homeostasis and possibly higher middle molecule clearance with PD. The minimal weekly solute clearance requirement in terms of Kt/V_{urea} for chronic PD and chronic HD are 1.7 and 3.6, respectively [7–9]. For ARF, there has not been any study on the relationship between solute clearance achieved and patient outcome. The lower clearance achieved with PD always raises a concern on whether PD provides adequate clearance, particularly in patients in a hypercatabolic state.

2. Slower ultrafiltration rate

Fluid removal or ultrafiltration in PD is achieved mainly by the osmotic gradient across the peritoneal membrane contributed by the glucose concentration of the peritoneal dialysate. In chronic PD with four exchanges a day, the amount of ultrafiltration achieved per day is quite variable, and rarely exceeds 2 l a day. The ultrafiltration can be enhanced either by using more high glucose concentration dialysate or by increasing the frequency of exchange. Even with hourly PD cycles, the daily ultrafiltration rarely exceeds 3–4 l a day. In comparison, hemodialysis can easily remove 3–4 l in just 4–5 h, and 1–2 l/h in hemofiltration or CRRT. Therefore in patients with massive fluid overload and/or acute pulmonary edema, PD is not as efficacious as hemodialysis or CRRT in removing the excessive fluid.

3. PD corrects hyperkalemia more slowly than hemodialysis

Many patients with acute renal failure have severe hyperkalemia, particularly the hypercatabolic patients. Compared with HD, PD has a slower potassium removal rate. It is not efficient enough for correction of life-threatening hyperkalemia.

4. PD cannot be used for acute renal failure complicating major abdominal surgery, or in patients with previous major abdominal surgery.
5. In patients with respiratory distress or reduced lung compliance, the instillation of peritoneal fluid may impede diaphragmatic movement causing limitation in lung expansion and worsening hypoxemia.

7.11.4 Outcome of Using PD in Acute Renal Failure

There are very few prospective randomized trials comparing PD with HD in ARF. Most of the published comparison data were based on retrospective analysis. Table 7.11.1 shows some of the published retrospective mortality comparison between PD and HD in acute renal failure according to Ash [10]. There was no major difference in mortality of patients treated with PD or HD. These data were from studies more than 2 decades ago, and the results may therefore not be applicable to the technology today. Furthermore, in these reports, patient condition might have influenced the choice of dialysis modality and produced selection bias for or against PD.

In 2002, there was a published prospective randomized controlled study from Vietnam showing a higher mortality rate of PD compared with hemofiltration for infection-associated ARF [11]. The mortality rate in patients treated with PD was 47%, and with hemofiltration it was 15% ($p = 0.005$). However, this study was heavily criticized, as the PD treatment employed was not quite the standard therapy – using locally produced acetate-based dialysate instead of the standard lactate-based solutions, and rigid uncuffed PD catheters instead of cuffed PD catheters [12–14]. It is well known that rigid catheters are associated with more complications such as leakage and peritonitis,

Table 7.11.1 Mortality comparison in retrospective studies according to Ash [10]

Author	Year	No. of patients	Mortality (%)	
			PD	HD
Orofino	1976	82	52	62
Firmat	1979	1101	50	50
Swartz	1980	45	45	60
Ash	1983	97	38	48
Struijk	1984	45	45	Similar

and acetate-based dialysate may cause hemodynamic instability and is less effective than lactate-based solutions in correcting metabolic acidosis. In fact, only 8 of the 21 patients on PD in comparison with 25 of the 27 patients on hemofiltration achieved normal arterial blood pH at the end of the replacement therapies, and 42% of patients on PD had cloudy effluent but only one was documented to have peritonitis and treated as such. This study used a diagnostic criteria of white blood cell count over 250/mm^3 for peritonitis instead of the commonly used 100/mm^3. This cutoff level is obviously far too high for PD with rapid cycles (30 min cycle in this study), and therefore it was not surprised that many peritonitis cases were not diagnosed and were left untreated, and thus might have resulted in the higher mortality.

In contrast, a recent published randomized controlled study from Brazil showed that the treatment success rate of high-volume PD (2 l/cycle, 18–22 cycles/day for 7 days continuously) using flexible catheters and lactate-based peritoneal dialysate, is similar to daily hemodialysis, with renal recovery 28% and 26%, respectively, and mortality 58% and 53%, respectively [15].

7.11.5 Forms of PD Available

There are several forms of peritoneal dialysis that have been adopted for acute renal failure:

1. Intermittent peritoneal dialysis (IPD)
2. Continuous peritoneal dialysis, or continuous equilibrated peritoneal dialysis (CEPD)
3. Continuous flow peritoneal dialysis (CFPD)
4. Tidal peritoneal dialysis (TPD)

7.11.5.1 Intermittent Peritoneal Dialysis

IPD was the predominant form of PD used in the 1960s and 1970s when uncuffed semirigid catheters were used. It consists of multiple cycles of short dwell for a certain period, usually hourly cycles for 1 to a few days, and then it is stopped and the semirigid catheter is usually removed. It may be restarted later according to the situation of the patient with insertion of another catheter.

7.11.5.2 Continuous Peritoneal Dialysis/ Continuous Equilibrated Peritoneal Dialysis

This is similar to continuous ambulatory peritoneal dialysis (CAPD) but is performed in hospital. With CAPD, usually four to six cycles of PD are delivered per day. For acute renal failure in hospital setting, the number of exchanges per day can easily be increased to eight or even more to increase solute and fluid removal. This is the most commonly adopted form of PD for ARF. When a much higher total volume of PD is used per day, it is often referred as "high-volume peritoneal dialysis" [16].

7.11.5.3 Continuous Flow Peritoneal Dialysis

This is performed with two peritoneal catheters, one for instillation and the other for draining. There is a continuous inflow and outflow of dialysate at 100–300 ml/min to maintain a low concentration of solutes in the dialysate to maximize the diffusion rate of the solute out of the body. It requires implantation of two PD catheters with one catheter tip placed in the pelvic cavity and the other placed toward the diaphragm. Urea removal rate can be two to five times higher than with standard PD [17]. Because of the inconvenience of implanting two catheters, difficulty in controlling the ultrafiltration rate, and the requirement for large amounts of dialysate, it is not widely used.

7.11.5.4 Tidal Peritoneal Dialysis

With a PD cycle, during the late drain phase and early instillation phase, the amount of peritoneal dialysis fluid (PDF) in the peritoneal cavity is small and many areas of the peritoneal cavity are not filled with PDF. The dialysis capacity is quite ineffective in this phase, which may last up to 30 min/cycle (10 min of instillation and 20 min of drainage). It is not so much a problem for CAPD, as the proportion of this ineffective dialysis phase is relatively short compared with the long dwell time. However, in PD with frequent short dwell cycles (e.g., hourly cycles), the proportion of ineffective dialysis increases and the effectiveness of PD is therefore reduced. Tidal PD (TPD) was developed to remove this ineffective dialysis phase by keeping the peritoneal cavity with a certain level of PDF even during the drain phase. Only around 50% of dwell volume PDF (i.e., around 1 l for a 2-l dwell) is drained out, and another 50% will then be instilled. Though this increases the solute removal by reducing the ineffective dialysis phase, the incomplete draining keeps a certain level of urea and uremic toxins in the peritoneal fluid, and thus reducing the concentration gradient achieved. In comparison to conventional continuous ambulatory PD or automated PD, the cost-effectiveness of TPD for treating end-stage renal failure patients is often doubted.

For acute renal failure, the frequency of TPD is usually much higher than that of chronic PD. It can be as frequent as hourly or even shorter cycles. In a crossover study by Chitalia et al. comparing continuous equilibrated PD (2 l, 4 h cycle for 48 h, total 26 l) with TPD (2 l, 20 min cycle with tidal volume 650 ml and tidal drain 750 ml for 12 h, total 26 l) for patients with hypercatabolic acute renal failure, TPD achieved higher urea and creatinine clearance, and ultrafiltration [18]. TPD removed more potassium and phosphate but also significantly more protein and albumin through peritoneum. The cost for TPD was marginally lower at around 10% per session. However, this comparison is only valid if the TPD is performed once every 48 h – but this is not often the case. Solute removal by TPD and continuous equilibrated PD using the same amount of dialysate over the same period of time was also not studied.

7.11.6 Types of Peritoneal Dialysis Catheters for Acute Peritoneal Dialysis

Access to peritoneal cavity is required for peritoneal dialysis. There are mainly two types of peritoneal dialysis catheters for acute peritoneal dialysis:

1. Semirigid straight uncuffed catheters
2. Cuffed flexible silicone catheters

7.11.6.1 Semirigid Straight Uncuffed Catheters

These catheters were in use several decades ago. They can be easily inserted at bed side, with a stiff stylet through a small skin incision over the linea alba in the lower abdomen. Patients are asked to tense up the abdominal wall muscles to allow a clear "give-way" sensation for the operator when the stylet penetrates through the abdominal wall, and/or prior instillation of 1 l of normal saline with an angiocatheter into the peritoneal cavity. The catheter is then advanced forward toward the pelvic cavity and the stylet is then removed. It is then fixed by stitching to the skin at the entrance wound. There is no subcutaneous tunnel. The advantages of these catheters are their easy and quick implantation and removal, but they are prone to leaking, dislodging, wound infection, and peritonitis. The longer these catheters are retained, the higher the chance of peritonitis it will be. Therefore they are seldom used nowadays.

7.11.6.2 Cuffed Flexible Silicone Catheters (Tenckhoff Catheter)

These catheters are basically the same as those used in chronic peritoneal dialysis though single cuffed catheters are often used for easier removal than double cuffed catheters. But in many centers, double-cuffed catheters are routinely used as they can be used continually for long-term PD if patients do not recover from ARF. Tenckhoff catheters are now the standard catheters used even in acute PD. The design of the Tenckhoff catheters, be it straight or swan neck, straight or curled tip, is not very important in either chronic or acute PD [19].

7.11.7 Implantation Technique of Cuffed Silicone PD Catheters

Implantation technique is similar to that of chronic PD: trocar, minilaparotomy, Seldinger technique, laparoscopic, or peritoneoscopic implantation. Implantation with trocar through the linea alba at the lower abdomen can easily be done at bedside, but the risk of leakage is higher compared with other methods. Surgical minilaparotomy is the standard implantation technique in chronic PD. It allows tight closure of the peritoneum around the catheter with a purse string to prevent dialysate leakage even with immediate PD with a 2-l dwell cycle. However, it needs to be performed in the operating theater setting. This may not be possible for critically ill patients, though surgical implantation can also be performed at bedside by experts. Seldinger technique can be used in bedside insertion, and results are as good as surgical minilaparotomy for chronic PD [20]. Laparoscopic-assisted and peritoneoscopic insertion also produces very good results [21, 22], but they also require a proper operating theater setting. However, there are not many comparison reports on these techniques in acute PD, and the results published for end-stage renal failure patients may not apply to ARF patients, as PD is often not started immediately in end-stage renal failure patients. The choice of technique still largely depends on the expertise available. Antibiotic prophylaxis is recommended for implantation of PD catheters as for end-stage renal failure patients [19].

Attention should be paid to patients with gross fluid overload, pulmonary edema, or respiratory distress, because the prolonged supine position during implantation of catheters may worsen hypoxia. In such situations, catheters may be inserted into patients in an inclined position.

7.11.8 The Peritoneal Dialysate

The standard dialysate – lactate-based glucose-containing solutions – for chronic peritoneal dialysis is also used in acute PD. Acetate-based solution is less effective in correcting the metabolic acidosis. In a small-scale study involving 12 pediatric patients with ARF, the use of bicarbonate-based solutions at a level of 38 mmol/l corrected acidosis better by 48 h compared with historical controls with Dianeal® solutions [23]. In a further study on adult patients with shock, using bicarbonate-based solutions corrected metabolic acidosis better and blood pressure was better maintained than with lactate-based solutions [24].

The newer generation of more biocompatible solutions with low glucose degradation products is now commercially available for use in many countries. Some of these have neutral pH or even contain bicarbonate helping correction of acidosis faster. The high biocompatibility may cause less systemic cytokine activation compared with conventional solutions. Whether this would improve the outcome still needs to be studied. Icodextrin solution needs a long dwell time to achieve significant ultrafiltration and is therefore rarely used for ARF.

7.11.9 The Dialysis Prescription

Prescription for peritoneal dialysis basically has to achieve two dimensions of therapy – fluid removal and uremic toxin removal.

7.11.9.1 Achieving Fluid Removal Target

Fluid transport rate, or ultrafiltration rate, across the peritoneum is determined by the net force from hydrostatic pressure gradient + osmotic pressure gradient – oncotic pressure gradient across the membrane. Among these, osmotic gradient is the main adjustable element with PD prescription. The glucose concentrations of the dialysate available are 1.5%, 2.5%, and 4.25% (or 3.89% for dehydrated dextrose). With 1.5% glucose, the dialysate osmolarity is around 347 mOsm/l, higher than the normal serum osmolarity by around 50–60 mOsm/l. Patients with ARF have elevated urea level and sometimes elevated glucose level too, the osmotic gradient will be substantially reduced and ultrafiltration rate may be lower than expected. This may be overcome by using dialysate with higher concentration of glucose. In general, a 1-h cycle of 2 l of 1.5% dialysate may achieve an ultrafiltration rate between 50–100 ml/h. As glucose is gradually absorbed, the osmotic gradient will progressively be reduced with time of dwell, and ultrafiltration rate declines accordingly. Shortening the cycle will help maintaining the osmotic gradient by keeping the dialysate glucose concentration from falling excessively. In patients with gross fluid overload or oliguric patients requiring large amounts of replacement solutions like parenteral nutrition or blood transfusion, hourly cycle dialysis with higher glucose concentration dialysate should be used. However, unlike HD or CRRT where the ultrafiltration rate can be preset and precisely controlled by the machine settings, ultrafiltration rate of PD can only be confirmed after it is started. Therefore frequent monitoring of the ultrafiltration rate and adjustment of the dialysis prescription is needed.

7.11.9.2 Achieving Adequate Uremic Toxin Removal

In chronic PD for patients with end-stage renal failure, adequacy of uremic toxin removal is usually reflected by urea kinetics (Kt/V_{urea}), and creatinine clearance to a lesser extent. The minimal target for Kt/V_{urea} is now generally accepted to be 1.7/week in both anuric and nonanuric patients [8, 9, 25]. However, in acute renal failure, there was no study on the relationship between the levels of peritoneal clearance of these small solutes and patient outcome, and thus no solid recommendation of level of Kt/V_{urea} or creatinine clearance is available. Furthermore, other parameters for adequacy of dialysis in chronic patients recommended, such as clinical well-being, calcium phosphate levels, blood pressure, and ultrafiltration volume, are only applicable in a steady homeostatic status. In theory, because of the acuteness of the condition and existence of hypercatabolic state, higher clearance targets should be achieved.

In chronic PD, Kt/V_{urea} and creatinine clearance are measured when patients are in a steady state, with the formulae using one single plasma urea or creatinine level. In ARF, plasma urea and creatinine levels fluctuate, and mean plasma levels are used for simplicity's sake (see Appendix).

To estimate the amount of dialysate required to achieve a certain level of Kt/V_{urea}, we may use simple calculation based on the total body water (V) and dialysate to plasma ratio of urea in the effluent dialysate. For a 70-kg man with a total body water 42 l, if the equilibration of urea in peritoneal effluent is 80% (for most patients, a urea dialysate to plasma ratio of 0.8 can be achieved with a 3–4 h dwell), to achieve the weekly Kt/V_{urea} 1.75 (i.e., daily Kt/V_{urea} of 0.25), the amount of effluent needed will be 42 l × 0.25/0.8 = 13.2 l. That means he needs at least 2 l × 6 exchanges of dialysate a day, and ultrafiltration volume should be no less than 1.2 l.

To achieve a higher weekly Kt/V_{urea} 2.1 (daily Kt/V 0.3), the amount of daily effluent needed will be 42 l × 0.3/0.8 = 15.8 l. It may be delivered by 2 l cycle for seven to eight exchanges a day, or 2.5 l for six exchanges a day.

Higher clearance can be achieved with more frequent exchanges or with the use of tidal PD or continuous flow PD mentioned above. If hourly cycle is prescribed, 48 l of dialysate will be used over 24 h. As explained earlier, the effective dwell time is only around 30 min. The urea dialysate to plasma ratio is roughly around 0.4, the urea clearance will be 48 l × 0.4 = 19.2 l over 24 h. The Kt/V will be 19.2/42 = 0.46/day, or 3.2/week if the treatment is continued for 7 days. In a study on the use of high volume PD for ARF in a cohort of patients with mean body weight 67 kg [16], prescription with 2 l cycles of 65–80 min/cycle using 36–44 l/day, ultrafiltration achieved were 2 l a day. The Kt/V_{urea} achieved reached 0.55 ± 0.12/day, or 3.8 ± 0.6/week, and solute reduction index (SRI) achieved was 41 ± 9.9.

It has to been kept in mind that adequacy of dialysis based on urea kinetics employed for chronic PD may not be applicable to rapid cycle PD, as short dwell cycles causes greater discrepancy in clearance rate of solutes of different sizes than long cycles.

Stabilization, or even reduction, of plasma urea and creatinine level, and correction of metabolic acidosis, hyperkalemia are also useful tools to assess whether dialysis prescription is adequate or not. In the study by Gabriel et al. described above [16], serum BUN were stabilized after 3 days, and serum bicarbonate and potassium were stabilized after 2 days of high volume PD.

In summary, a standard continuous equilibrated PD prescription for a 70 kg patient should be at least be 2 l every 4 h exchange. In patients with fluid overload, fluid removal can be increased by using more hypertonic solutions or more frequent exchanges. For patients with hypercatabolic state, frequency of exchange can be increased, and/or tidal PD or continuous flow PD may be used to meet the metabolic demand.

7.11.10 Complications of Acute Peritoneal Dialysis

7.11.10.1 Peritonitis

With the use of flexible cuffed PD catheters and automated PD, flush-before-filled connection technique, the risk of peritonitis has been much reduced. However,

Table 7.11.2 Antibiotic dosing recommendation for acute peritoneal dialysis on rapid cycles, based on the modification of "Peritoneal dialysis-related infections recommendation: 2005" of the International Society for Peritoneal Dialysis [19]

	Intravenous loading dose in septic patients	Intraperitoneal loading if a 6-h dwell allows (mg/l)	Intraperitoneal continuous (mg/l), all exchanges
Aminoglycosides			
Amikacin	5 mg/kg	25	12
Netilmicin, tobramycin	1.5 mg/kg	0.6 mg/kg	4
Cephalosporins			
Cefazolin, Cefepime, Ceftazidime	1,000 mg	1 g, or 15 mg/kg	125
Penicillin			
Ampicillin	500 mg	500 mg	125
Vancomycin	1 g	1 g	25
Imipenem/cilastatin	500 mg	500 mg	200

peritonitis is probably still the most important serious complication of peritoneal dialysis. In a study involving 30 patients received 236 sessions of PD, five patients developed peritonitis, and two required catheter removal [16].The cardinal features of peritonitis are cloudy effluent, fever, and abdominal pain. In chronic PD, the diagnosis is confirmed with dialysate white blood cell count greater than 100 cells/mm^3 with >50% neutrophils [26]. However, it is not certain if the same white cell count criteria is applicable to rapid cycle PD, as the rapid exchange may lower the white cell count. But if the count is greater than 100 cells/mm^3, it should be treated as peritonitis. While the effluent is almost always cloudy during peritonitis, fever and abdominal pain may not be present, particularly if the peritonitis is mild, or in case of sedated, ventilated, or critically ill patients.

Apart from the common gram-positive organisms that may be acquired through connection contamination, the critically ill patients are also susceptible to peritonitis from endogenous source, like gram-negative organisms from the gut flora and fungal peritonitis (in particular *candida* peritonitis), as a result of their severely impaired immune system and disturbed gut flora after broad spectrum antibiotics therapy [27, 28]. It may develop as a complication of acute pancreatitis, intestinal obstruction, perforation, or ischemia which are not uncommon in the critically ill patients. The critically ill patients in the intensive care unit are also highly susceptible to hospital acquired infection by organisms like *Pseudomonas* and *Acinetobacter* spp. [29, 30]. In fact, in the recent study of PD in ARF patients by Gabriel et al. [16], pseudomonas and fungus were the major causative organisms.

Once peritonitis is suspected, it should be treated promptly with antibiotics covering both gram-positive and gram-negative organisms. Due to the rapid cycles in acute PD, continuous intraperitoneal administration of antibiotics is recommended. An intravenous loading dose can be given to build up the drug level rapidly. Table 7.11.2 showed some common antibiotics dosage recommendation extracted from the "Peritoneal dialysis-related infections recommendation: 2005 update" of the International Society for Peritoneal Dialysis [19].

7.11.10.2 Catheter-Related Infection

Infection around the exit site of the peritoneal dialysis catheter can occur. Due to the short duration of the dialysis therapy for acute renal failure, incidence of exit site infection for cuffed PD catheters is unknown. Routine mupirocin ointment or gentamicin ointment prophylaxis to the exit site have been shown to be effective in reducing exit site infection and peritonitis in chronic peritoneal dialysis patients [31, 32] and may be considered for acute PD.

7.11.10.3 Complications Related to Catheter Insertion

As with catheter implantation for chronic PD, complications may arise during catheter insertion, including wound bleeding, intraperitoneal bleeding from abdominal wall vessels puncture, omental tear, bowel, and bladder perforation. Serious complication is extremely rare if patients are well prepared for the implantation. Intravenous desmopressin (deamino-D-arginine vasopressin, DDAVP) may be used prophylactically to help reduce uremic bleeding by promoting von Willebrand factor release to shorten bleeding time [33].

Leaking not uncommonly follows insertion of peritoneal dialysis catheter even with cuffed PD catheters, as PD is often needed to start immediately after implantation of catheter. In case of leakage, the dwell volume has to be reduced or peritoneal dialysis be suspended and convert to HD or CRRT. Fibrin glue has been reported to be useful for both treatment and prevention of early peri-catheter leakage and can be considered particularly in children [34, 35]

7.11.10.4 Obstruction of Flow

Catheter blocking may occur with blood clot from intraperitoneal bleeding, fibrin clots, and omental wrapping. Blood and fibrin clot may be prevented by adding intraperitoneal heparin at 500 U/l when the effluent is bloody or contains fibrin. If the catheter is blocked, it may be dissolved by adding 75,000 U of diluted urokinase into the catheter followed by flushing the catheter with peritoneal dialysate [36]. Omental wrapping requires laparoscopic omentectomy or removal and reimplantation. These may not be possible for the critically ill patients. Fortunately, its incidence in acute PD is extremely rare.

7.11.10.5 Increased Intraperitoneal Pressure

The peritoneal fluid may hamper diaphragmatic movement impeding lung expansion. This may be a problem for patients with ventilatory problems. Smaller dwell volume may help in this situation.

Hydrothorax from pleural peritoneal communication through a congenital diaphragmatic defect or weak point has been reported in acute PD in a pediatric patient [37]. It may lead to sudden shortness of breath. Conversion to HD is required.

7.11.10.6 Hyperglycemia

Blood glucose of diabetic patients may be elevated from the absorption of glucose through the peritoneal cavity, especially when higher glucose concentration peritoneal dialysate (e.g., 4.25%) is used. Blood glucose level has to be closely monitored and insulin dosage needs to be adjusted accordingly. Hypoglycemia has to be watched out for when the PD cycle frequency or dialysate glucose concentration is reduced.

7.11.10.7 Hypernatremia

When aggressive ultrafiltration using rapid cycles of high glucose concentration dialysate is achieved, the sodium sieving effect of water being removed in excess of sodium in the first hour of a cycle would lead to water loss in excess of sodium, resulting in hypernatremia. This should be watched out with frequent plasma sodium level monitoring. If serum sodium level is increasing rapidly, part of the ultrafiltration should be replaced in forms of water orally or in dextrose solution intravenously.

7.11.10.8 Hypokalemia

While PD is less effective than HD in correcting hyperkalemia, hypokalemia may develop in patients with preexisting low serum potassium level, poor oral intake, and on diuretic therapy. Potassium 3.5–4 mmol/l may be added into peritoneal dialysis fluid to prevent or correct hypokalemia.

7.11.10.9 Metabolic Acidosis

The conventional peritoneal dialysate uses lactate as the base buffer. Lactate absorbed during peritoneal dialysis is then converted into bicarbonate to correct metabolic acidosis. However, in patients with liver insufficiency or with lactic acidosis, this may worsen lactic acidosis. Bicarbonate-based dialysate has been demonstrated to be more effective in correcting the metabolic acidosis in acute renal failure [23, 24].

7.11.11 Take Home Pearls

- Peritoneal dialysis is still a valuable renal replacement therapy for patients with acute renal failure, particularly in areas with insufficient hemodialysis or CRRT support.
- Even when adequate hemodialysis and CRRT support are available, there are patients who may benefit from peritoneal dialysis more than from other modes of renal replacement therapy.
- Among its advantages are hemodynamic stability, avoidance of systemic anticoagulation, less labor intensive, and no need for high-tech machines.

Appendix

Calculation of daily Kt/V_{urea} and solute reduction index (SRI): In steady state,

$$Kt/V_{urea}\text{ per day} = \frac{\text{total amount of urea in dialyzate in 24 h}}{\text{plasma urea} \times \text{total body water (L)}}$$

$$\text{or} = \frac{\text{D/P urea ratio of effluent} \times \text{total amount of effluent (L)}}{\text{total body water (L)}}$$

In non-steady state,

$$Kt/V_{urea}\text{ per day} = \frac{\text{mean dialyzate urea}}{\text{mean plasma urea}} \times \frac{\text{24 h effluent volume (L)}}{\text{total body water (L)}}$$

Mean dialysate urea = (first bag effluent urea + last bag effluent urea)/2

Mean serum urea = (pre-dialysis urea + post-dialysis urea)/2

$$\text{Solute reduction index} = \frac{\text{total urea in dialysate (g)} \times 100\%}{\text{(pre-dialysis BUN g/L)} \times \text{TBW (L)}},$$

where BUN is blood urea nitrogen and V is total body water which can be estimated from body weight × 0.6 in males, 0.55 in females, or by Watson formula [38]. However, according to Himmelfarb et al. [39], the urea distribution volume in acute renal failure exceeds total body water as calculated by Watson, by 20%, and therefore the final Kt/V_{urea} or SRI should be multiplied by 0.8.

References

1. Hyman A, Medelssohn DC (2002). Current Canadian approaches to dialysis for acute renal failure in the ICU. Am J Nephrol 22:29–34.
2. Warady BA, Bunchman T (2000). Dialysis therapy for children with acute renal failure: survey results. Pediatr Nephrol 15:11–13.
3. Uchino S, Kellum JA, Bellomo R, et al. (2005). Beginning and ending supportive therapy for the kidney (BEST kidney) investigators. Acute renal failure in critically ill patients: a multinational, multicenter study. JAMA 294:813–8.
4. Gabriel DP, Nascimento GVR, Caramori JT, et al.(2006). Peritoneal dialysis in acute renal failure. Ren Fail 2006; 28: 451–6.
5. Katz IJ, Sofianou L, Butler O, et al. (2001). Recovery of renal function in Black South African patients with malignant hypertension: superiority of continuous ambulatory peritoneal dialysis over hemodialysis. Perit Dial Int 21:581–6.
6. Ash SR, Wimberly AL, Mertz SL (1983). Peritoneal dialysis for acute and chronic renal failure: an update. Hosp Pract 18: 179–87.
7. Hemodialysis Adequacy 2006 Work Group (2006). Clinical practice guidelines for hemodialysis adequacy, update 2006. Am J Kidney Dis 48 (Sl)S2–90.
8. Peritoneal Dialysis Adequacy Work Group (2006). Clinical practice guidelines for peritoneal dialysis adequacy. Am J Kidney Dis 48(S1):S99–163.
9. Lo WK, Bargman J, Burkart J, et al. (2006). The International Society for Peritoneal Dialysis (ISPD) guideline on targets for solute and fluid removal in adult patients on chronic peritoneal dialysis. Perit Dial Int 26:520–22.
10. Ash SR 2004. Peritoneal dialysis in acute renal failure of adults: the under-utilized modality. Contrib Nephrol 144: 239–54.
11. Phu NH, Hien TT, Mai NTH, et al. (2002). Hemofiltration and peritoneal dialysis in infection-associated acute renal failure in Vietnam. New Engl J Med 347:895–902.
12. Bazari H (2003). Hemofiltration and peritoneal dialysis in infection-associated acute renal failure. New Engl J Med 348:858–60.
13. Fruchter O (2003). Hemofiltration and peritoneal dialysis in infection-associated acute renal failure. New Engl J Med 348:858–60.
14. Casserly LM (2003). Hemofiltration and peritoneal dialysis in infection-associated acute renal failure. New Engl J Med 348:858–60.
15. Gabriel DP, Caramori JT, Martim LC, et al. (2008). High volume peritoneal dialysis vs daily hemodialysis: a randomized, controlled trial in patients with acute kidney injury. Kidney Int 73:S87–S93.
16. Gabriel DP, do Nascimento GVR, Caramori JT et al. (2007). High volume peritoneal dialysis for acute renal failure. Perit Dial Int 27:277–82.
17. Ronco C, Amerling R (2006). Continuous flow peritoneal dialysis: current state-of-the-art and obstacles to further development. Contrib Nephrol 150:310–20.
18. Chitalia VP, Almeida AF, Rai H, et al. (2002). Is peritoneal dialysis adequate for hypercatabolic acute renal failure in developing countries? Kidney Int 31:747–57.
19. Piraino B, Bailie GR, Bernardini J (2005). ISPD Ad Hoc Advisory Committee. Peritoneal dialysis-related infections recommendations: 2005 update. Perit Dial Int 25:107–31.
20. Ozener C, Bihorac A, Akoglu E (2001). Technical survival of CAPD catheters: comparison between percutaneous and conventional surgical placement techniques. Nephrol Dial Transpl 16:1893–9.

21. Schmidt SC, Pohle C, Langrehr JM, et al. (2007). Laparoscopic-assisted placement of peritoneal dialysis catheters: implantation technique and results. J Laparoendoscopic Adv Surg Tech 17:596–599.
22. Gadallah MF, Pervez A, el-Shahawy MA, et al. (1999). Peritoneoscopic versus surgical placement of peritoneal dialysis catheters: a prospective randomized study on outcome. Am J Kidney Dis 33:118–22.
23. Vande Walle J, Raes A, Castillo D, et al. (1997). Advantages of HCO_3 solution with low sodium concentration over standard lactate solutions for acute peritoneal dialysis. Adv Perit Dial 13:179–82.
24. Thongboonkerd V, Lumlertgul D, Supajatura V (2001). Better correction of metabolic acidosis, blood pressure control, and phagocytosis with bicarbonate compared to lactate solution in acute peritoneal dialysis. Artif Organs 25:99–108.
25. Dombros N, Dratwa M, Feriani M, Gokal R, Heimburger O, Krediet R, Plum J, Rodrigues A, Selgas R, Struijk D, Verger C, EBPG Expert Group on Peritoneal Dialysis (2005). European best practice guidelines for peritoneal dialysis. 7 Adequacy of peritoneal dialysis. Nephrol Dial Transpl 20 (S9):ix24–ix27.
26. Keane WF, Alexander SR, Bailie GR (1996). Peritoneal dialysis-related peritonitis treatment recommendations: 1996 update. Perit Dial Int16:557–73.
27. Troidle L, Kliger AS, Goldie SJ, et al. (1996). Continuous peritoneal dialysis-associated peritonitis of nosocomial origin. Perit Dial Int 16:505–10.
28. Wang AY, Yu AW, Li PK, et al. (2000). Factors predicting outcome of fungal peritonitis in peritoneal dialysis: analysis of a 9-year experience of fungal peritonitis in a single center. Am J Kidney Dis 36:1183–92.
29. Vincent JL, Bihari DJ, Suter PM, et al. (1995). The prevalence of nosocomial infection in intensive care units in Europe. Results of the European Prevalence of Infection in Intensive Care (EPIC) Study. EPIC International Advisory Committee. J Am Med Assoc 274:639–44.
30. National Nosocomial Infections Surveillance (NNIS) report, data summary from October 1986-April 1996, issued May 1996. A report from the National Nosocomial Infections Surveillance (NNIS) System. Am J Infect Control 24:380–8.
31. Tacconelli E, Carmeli Y, Aizer A, et al. (2003). Mupirocin prophylaxis to prevent Staphylococcus aureus infection in patients undergoing dialysis: a meta-analysis. Clin Infect Dis 37:1629–38.
32. Bernardini J, Bender F, Florio T, et al. (2005). Randomized, double-blind trial of antibiotic exit site cream for prevention of exit site infection in peritoneal dialysis patients. J Am Soc Nephrol 16:539–45.
33. Mannuci PM, Remuzzi G, Pusineri F, et al. (1983). Deamino 8-D-arginine vasopressin shortens the bleeding time in uremia. New Engl J Med 308; 8–12.
34. Joffe P (1993). Peritoneal dialysis leakage treated with fibrin glue. Nephrol Dial Transpl 8:474–6.
35. Sojo ET, Grosman MD, Monteverde ML, et al. (2004). Fibrin glue is useful in preventing early dialysate leakage in children on chronic peritoneal dialysis. Perit Dial Int 24:186–190.
36. Strippoli P, Pilolli D, Mingrone G, et al. (1989). A hemostasis study in CAPD patients during fibrinolytic intraperitoneal therapy with urokinase (UK). Adv Perit Dial. 1989; 5:97–9.
37. Cruces R P, Roque E J, Ronco M R, et al. (2006). Massive acute hydrothorax secondary to peritoneal dialysis in a hemolytic uremic syndrome. Report of a case. Revista Medica de Chile 134:91–4.
38. Watson PE, Watson ID, Bam RD (1980). Total body water volumes for adult males and females estimated from simple anthropometric measurements. Am J Clin Nutr 33:27–39.
39. Himmelfarb J, Evanson J, Hakim RM, et al. (2002). Urea volume of distribution exceeds total body water in patients with acute renal failure. Kidney Int 61:317–23.

Choosing a Therapy Modality for Acute Renal Replacement Therapy

7.12

Achim Jörres and Dinah Jörres

Core Messages

- Prospective randomized clinical trials indicate that the initial choice of intermittent versus continuous renal replacement therapy does not influence overall outcomes such as patient survival or recovery of kidney function.
- The decision for a therapy modality should be made based on the individual clinical situation of the patient, in particular taking into account hemodynamic stability, risk for bleeding, and patient mobility.
- The different treatment modalities should be regarded as complementary rather than being in competition, enabling a switch between modalities if the focus of therapy changes.

7.12.1 Introduction

The initial choice for renal replacement therapy (RRT) in patients with acute kidney failure remains controversial. A major conflict zone is the decision between intermittent and continuous RRT, in particular in cases of critically ill patients who develop kidney failure as part of the multiorgan dysfunction syndrome (MODS) [6, 14]. The proponents of continuous renal replacement therapy (CRRT) point out that the continuous removal of excess water leads to better hemodynamic stability, whilst advocates for intermittent RRT bring into the field safety issues (continuous anticoagulation, bleeding risks, and clotting problems) and higher costs related to CRRT regimes. The actual decision between the two modalities will depend mainly on local experiences and availabilities, factors that are often related to the type of intensive care setting (surgical vs medical). At the end of the day, however, the personal choice and preference of the clinician in charge will play a major role, unless local (or even national) treatment standards prevail. Amidst this discussion, recent years have seen an increasing popularity of the hybrid technique of sustained low-efficiency dialysis ([SLED] or slow extended dialysis). Using extended dialysis time (8–18 h) and slow dialysate and blood flow rates, SLED treatment may result in small solute clearance and cardiovascular stability that is comparable to CRRT but at lower cost, thus combining some of the advantages of CRRT and intermittent renal replacement therapy (IRRT) [7, 9]. To further complicate matters, different therapy modalities are available both in the CRRT and the IRRT domain, including hemodialysis, hemofiltration, and hemodiafiltration procedures. The present chapter sets out to review both the available evidence base and clinical experience that may help to choose between the various treatment options, and to point out patient-related factors that may offer guidance if and when a change of the initial strategy should be considered. The dialytic management of pediatric patients and the use of peritoneal dialysis in adult patients will not be discussed here, as these topics are covered in the respective chapters.

A. Jörres (✉)
Department of Nephrology and Medical Intensive Care,
Charite University Hospital Campus Virchow-Klinikum,
Augustenburger Platz 1, 13353 Berlin, Germany
e-mail: achim.joerres@charite.de

A. Jörres et al. (eds.), *Management of Acute Kidney Problems*,
DOI: 10.1007/978-3-540-69441-0_7.12, © Springer-Verlag Berlin Heidelberg 2010

7.12.2 The "Evidence-Base": Clinical Studies Comparing Outcomes of CRRT and IRRT

Several prospective randomized trials have addressed the question of whether the initial choice of CRRT versus IRRT may influence patient survival and/or recovery of kidney function. A comparison of the study outcomes, however, has to take into account their substantial variability in terms of treatment aspects (e.g., CRRT modality and delivered dose) and patient demographics (e.g., medical vs. surgical, presence of SIRS/sepsis).

Mehta and coworkers [10] randomized 166 patients to receive either daily intermittent hemodialysis or continuous hemodiafiltration with dialysate flow rates of 100 ml/min and ultrafiltration rates between 400 and 800 ml/h. Thirty-two of the 84 patients randomized to CRRT received continuous arteriovenous hemodiafiltration (CAVHDF), the remaining patients were treated with continuous venovenous hemodiafiltration (CVVHDF). Continuous therapy was associated with an increase in intensive care unit (ICU) (59.5 vs 41.5%, $p < 0.02$) and in-hospital (65.5 vs 47.6%, $p < 0.02$) mortality as compared with intermittent dialysis. Complete recovery of renal function was observed in 34.9% of patients, with no significant group differences. Despite randomization, however, there were significant differences between the groups in several covariates independently associated with mortality, including sex, hepatic failure, APACHE II and III scores, and the number of failed organ systems, resulting in a bias in favor of intermittent dialysis.

Augustine and colleagues [1] studied 80 critically ill patients with acute kidney failure requiring dialysis who were stratified by severity of illness and randomized to treatment with continuous venovenous hemodialysis (CVVHD) or alternate-day intermittent hemodialysis (IHD) with a target Kt/V of 3.6/week. In-hospital mortality was 67.5% in the CVVHD group compared with 70% in the IHD group. CVVHD did not lead to an improvement in survival, preservation of urine output, or renal recovery compared with IHD.

Uehlinger and coworkers [17] randomized 125 patients to receive either daily IHD or CVVHDF with combined dialysate and filtrate flow rates of 2,000 ml/h. There was no significant difference between the two groups regarding in-hospital mortality (47% with CVVHDF vs 51% with IHD). Likewise, there was no difference regarding hospital length of stay in the survivors or the duration of RRT required.

Vinsonneau and colleagues [18] performed a prospective randomized multicenter study in 21 medical or multidisciplinary ICUs in France, with 360 patients randomized to receive either daily IHD or CVVHDF – the largest prospective randomized cilnical trial (RCT) to date in this area. Their protocol included detailed guidelines for optimum hemodynamic tolerance and solute removal. The observed rate of survival at 28, 60, or 90 days did not differ between the groups (32% in the IHD group vs 33% in the CVVHDF). There was also no difference between the groups regarding hospital or ICU length of stay or the duration of RRT. Apart from a higher incidence of hypothermia in the CVVHDF group, there was no difference regarding adverse events such as hypotension, bleeding episodes, or thrombocytopenia. Interestingly, only six patients had to switch for unplanned reasons from IHD to CVVHDF (because of persisting hemodynamic instability, technical problems, or protocol violation), while 17 patients had to switch from CVVHDF to IHD (because of contraindication to the use of anticoagulants for high risk of bleeding, insufficient metabolic control, technical problems, recurrent filter clotting despite effective anticoagulation, or protocol violations).

Lins and coworkers [8] randomized 316 patients to daily IHD or postdilution continuous venovenous hemofiltration (CVVH) with filtrate rates of 1–2 l/h. Intention-to-treat analysis showed no significant difference in mortality between the two groups (62.5% in IHD compared with 58.1% in CVVH). This result was confirmed in prespecified subgroup analysis (elderly patients, and patients with sepsis, heart failure, or on ventilation) and after exclusion of possible confounders (early mortality and delayed ICU admission). Moreover, they found no difference in duration of ICU or hospital stay. Renal recovery at hospital discharge was comparable between both groups.

Finally, two large retrospective cohort studies [3, 16] focusing on the recovery of kidney function suggested that CRRT was an independent predictor of improved renal recovery among hospital survivors but confirmed the equal outcome regarding survival between IRRT and CRRT.

Overall, the meta-analysis of the available randomized clinical trials suggests that intermittent hemodialysis and CRRT lead to comparable clinical outcomes [2, 12, 13]. It is at least debatable, however, if the type of studies performed to date have asked the right questions. Critically ill patients with acute kidney failure constitute a profoundly heterogeneous cohort in terms of underlying diseases, concomitant medical/surgical therapies, and intermittent/recurrent complications. Intuitively it would seem improbable that one therapeutic strategy chosen at the beginning will remain the optimal choice throughout the course of events and under all circumstances. Rather it would seem prudent to select a certain mode of RRT based on the individual needs of the patient, thereby carefully weighing up the specific strengths and weaknesses of the various RRT techniques in the context of the current clinical circumstances.

7.12.3 The Clinical Choice of Treatment Modalities

The potential advantages and disadvantages of continuous versus intermittent treatment strategies are summarized in Table 7.12.1. Continuous therapies allow a slow and constant filtration of free water. This facilitates the management of oliguric patients with hyperhydration and/or the requirement of large amounts of intravenous fluids (e.g., parenteral nutrition and antibiotics). The continuous removal of excess body water may constitute a particular advantage in patients with hemodynamic instability and/or the requirement of vasopressors. If CRRT is not practical – e.g., in patients with frequent interventions (diagnostic procedures or surgery) – SLED may be the primary alternative to enable optimal hemodynamic tolerance. CRRT also enables the continuous removal of solutes, thereby avoiding rapid shifts in blood composition and osmolality. For this reason, CRRT is the treatment of choice in patients with intracranial hypertension or in patients at risk to develop cerebral edema. Likewise, CRRT or SLED may facilitate the prevention of the dysequilibrium syndrome in patients with excessive azotemia. On the other hand, IHD effectively and rapidly removes small molecules from patients' blood and may thus be the primary choice in clinical situations where a rapid effect on blood composition is desired, e.g., in acute hyperkalemia or severe metabolic acidosis.

Table 7.12.1 Potential advantages (+) and disadvantages (–) of CRRT, SLED, and IHD

	CRRT	SLED	IHD
Hemodynamic tolerance	++	++	–
Control of hyperhydration	++	++	–
Low risk for dysequilibrium or cerebral edema	++	++	–
Emergency correction of hyperkalemia	––	–	++
Anticoagulation required	––	–	+
Platelet loss/activation	––	–	+
Effect on hyperpyrexia	++	+	–
Patient mobility	–	+	++
Time for interventions	–	+	++
Antibiotic dosing	–	–	+
Loss of nutrients, trace elements, electrolytes	–	+	+
Material costs	––	++	++

CRRT continuous renal replacement therapy, *IHD* intermittent hemodialysis, *SLED* sustained low-efficiency dialysis

In terms of dialysis dose, both intermittent and continuous therapies can be modified to reach the desired treatment intensity. However, high-volume CRRT regimes in particular carry the risk of unnoticed loss of nutrients, vitamins, and trace elements. The same holds true for serum potassium and phosphorus which must be closely monitored and substituted if necessary. Another problem during CRRT is the correct dosage of antibiotics, as limited pharmacologic data is available for the various modalities (CVVH, CVVHD, or CVVHDF). In contrast, during intermittent therapies, a supplemental dose administered after the dialysis session may suffice to maintain adequate plasma levels.

Another important aspect is the effect of extracorporeal circulation on blood coagulation and platelets. Intermittent dialysis can often be performed, at least for 3–4 h, without any anticoagulation at all, provided that proper precautions are taken (e.g., high blood flow and saline flushing). In contrast, both continuous therapies and SLED typically require some form of anticoagulation. Unless regional anticoagulation (ideally with citrate) can be performed, CRRT and SLED are thus not the primary choice when coagulation abnormalities are present or in patients at risk of bleeding complications. Moreover, CRRT may be problematic in patients with low platelet counts as it may result in further reduction of platelet number and function [4, 11].

Dialyzers and hemofilters are effective heat exchangers, thus CRRT may lead to hypothermia which in turn can result in energy loss and reduced hemodynamic stability. On the other hand, this cooling effect of CRRT might be desirable in highly febrile patients with hyperdynamic circulation not responding to conservative treatment. Finally, intermittent dialysis is the method of choice in patients with isolated kidney failure and not requiring intensive care therapy, or in ICU patients in whom an expansion of physical therapy and mobilization is desired.

The choice between continuous and intermittent RRT also brings with it budget implications. Material costs are significantly higher (4–5-fold) for CRRT compared with IHD and SLED which is mainly owing to the fact that replacement fluids are quite expensive. One study calculated that the labor costs for CRRT and IHD were similar, however, the direct cost per treatment was nearly double in CRRT (US $543 vs $282 in IHD) [10]. On the other hand, the actual treatment costs may depend on the local organizational structure of the ICU. If CRRT is performed by the ICU nursing staff, while external personnel need to be brought in to run IHD, the cost calculation might be in favor of CRRT.

7.12.4 Diffusive Versus Convective Treatment Strategies

Whilst intermittent RRT and SLED are almost exclusively performed as hemodialysis, the next step in the decision tree for CRRT is the choice between continuous hemodialysis, hemofiltration, or hemodiafiltration, that is, between diffusive and convective treatment (or both). As the principle of convective elimination is the passage of solutes across a membrane carried by water flux, elimination of all solutes for which a membrane is permeable equals water flux. Convection thus results in uniform clearances of small, middle, and large molecules. In contrast, diffusive clearance of middle and large molecules with low-flux hemodialysis is poor. However, diffusive clearance offers an outstanding efficiency in small molecule removal.

If and how this translates into clinical outcomes is unclear at present. It has been suggested that hemofiltration (HF) and hemodiafiltration (HDF) may reduce the frequency and severity of intradialytic and postdialytic adverse symptoms; however, randomized controlled studies in acute patients comparing intermittent hemodialysis (HD) and intermittent HF or HDF are not available. One prospective randomized study compared high-flux and low-flux intermittent dialysis in 159 patients with acute kidney failure and could not find differences in patient survival or renal recovery [5], indicating that in IHD the flux of the membrane per se does not impact overall outcomes. In the field of CRRT one study compared outcomes between CVVH and CVVHDF: Saudan and coworkers [15] performed a prospective clinical trial in 206 critically ill patients with acute kidney failure who were randomized to receive CVVH (1–2.5 l/h replacement fluid) or CVVHDF (1–2.5 l/h replacement fluid; 1–1.5 l/h dialysate). Twenty-eight-day survival was 39% in the CVVH group compared with 59% in the CVVHDF group ($p = 0.03$). The rate of renal recovery among survivors was not different (71 vs 78% in the CVVH and CVVHDF groups, respectively). The authors concluded that increasing the dialysis dose especially for low-molecular-weight solutes confers a better survival in severely ill patients with acute kidney failure, however, a comparison between CVVH and CVVHDF on the basis of equal treatment dose cannot be derived from these data.

Thus, in the absence of compelling clinical trials, the choice between the various modalities will be made on the basis of practical considerations such as efficacy and risk for clotting (Table 7.12.2). The highest efficacy in terms of solute clearances (small and middle molecular) is achieved by postdilution CVVH. However, this modality requires high blood flow to minimize hemoconcentration in the hemofilter. If sufficient blood flows cannot be achieved, predilution may be required at the expense of significantly reduced (up to 30%) clearances. Alternatively, postdilution CVVHDF may be performed to reduce hemoconcentration. This procedure will result in only slightly reduced middle molecule clearance but conserve a high small solute clearance. Particularly in patients with clotting problems, CVVHD or predilution CVVHDF should be considered, as they avoid hemoconcentration and maintain high small solute clearance.

Table 7.12.2 Comparison of different CRRT modalities

	Clearances[a]		Relative clotting risk
	Small solutes	Middle molecules	
CVVHD	+++	+	Very low
Postdilution CVVH	+++	+++	High
Predilution CVVH	+	+	Low
Postdilution CVVHDF	+++	++	Moderate
Predilution CVVHDF	++	+	Very low

CRRT continuous renal replacement therapy, *CVVH* continuous venovenous hemofiltration, *CVVHD* continuous venovenous hemodialysis, *CVVHDF* continuous venovenous hemodiafiltration
[a]Assumes equal treatment volumes

7.12.5 Take Home Pearls

- There is no compelling evidence base to conclude that one RRT modality has general advantages over the other in terms of overall outcomes such as patient survival or renal recovery.
- Among the practical considerations that should be made to decide which therapy is the optimal choice for a specific time and situation are hemodynamic status, risk of bleeding complications, and desired patient mobility. The focus may change in the course of therapy, and different situations may require a modification of RRT or a switch from one treatment strategy to another.
- In critically ill patients with acute kidney failure, a prudent approach might be to use CRRT for the early treatment of hemodynamic instability, followed by daily SLED for as long as MODS persists, and finally to switch to IHD in the phase when intensive care can be stepped down, but kidney function has not yet recovered.
- The various treatment modalities should be regarded as complementary rather than as in competition.

References

1. Augustine JJ, Sandy D, Seifert TH, Paganini EP. A randomized controlled trial comparing intermittent with continuous dialysis in patients with ARF. Am J Kidney Dis 2004; 44(6): 1000–1007.
2. Bagshaw SM, Berthiaume LR, Delaney A, Bellomo R. Continuous versus intermittent renal replacement therapy for critically ill patients with acute kidney injury: a meta-analysis. Crit Care Med 2008; 36(2):610–617.
3. Bell M, Granath F, Schon S, Ekbom A, Martling CR. Continuous renal replacement therapy is associated with less chronic renal failure than intermittent haemodialysis after acute renal failure. Intensive Care Med 2007;33 (5):773–780.
4. Boldt J, Menges T, Wollbruck M, Sonneborn S, Hempelmann G. Continuous hemofiltration and platelet function in critically ill patients. Crit Care Med 1994; 22:1155–1160.
5. Gastaldello K, Melot C, Kahn RJ, Vanherweghem JL, Vincent JL, Tielemans C. Comparison of cellulose diacetate and polysulfone membranes in the outcome of acute renal failure. A prospective randomized study. Nephrol Dial Transplant 2000; 15(2):224–230.
6. Himmelfarb J. Continuous dialysis is not superior to intermittent dialysis in acute kidney injury of the critically ill patient. Nat Clin Pract Nephrol 2007; 3(3):120–121.
7. Kielstein JT, Kretschmer U, Ernst T, Hafer C, Bahr MJ, Haller H, et al Efficacy and cardiovascular tolerability of extended dialysis in critically ill patients: a randomized controlled study. Am J Kidney Dis 2004; 43(2):342–349.
8. Lins RL, Elseviers MM, Van der Niepen P, Hoste E, Malbrain ML, Damas P, Devriendt J; SHARF investigators. Intermittent versus continuous renal replacement therapy for acute kidney injury patients admitted to the intensive care unit: results of a randomized clinical trial. Nephrol Dial Transplant. 2009;24(2):512–518
9. Lonnemann G, Floege J, Kliem V, Brunkhorst R, Koch KM. Extended daily veno-venous high-flux haemodialysis in patients with acute renal failure and multiple organ dysfunction syndrome using a single path batch dialysis system. Nephrol Dial Transplant 2000; 15(8):1189–1193.
10. Mehta RL, McDonald B, Gabbai FB, Pahl M, Pascual MT, Farkas A, et al. A randomized clinical trial of continuous versus intermittent dialysis for acute renal failure. Kidney Int 2001; 60(3):1154–1163.
11. Mulder J, Tan HK, Bellomo R, Silvester W. Platelet loss across the hemofilter during continuous hemofiltration. Int J Artif Organs 2003; 26(10):906–912.
12. Pannu N, Klarenbach S, Wiebe N, Manns B, Tonelli M. Renal replacement therapy in patients with acute renal failure: a systematic review. JAMA 2008; 299(7):793–805.
13. Rabindranath K, Adams J, MacLeod AM, Muirhead N. Intermittent versus continuous renal replacement therapy for acute renal failure in adults. Cochrane Database Syst Rev 2007;(3):CD003773.
14. Ronco C. Continuous dialysis is superior to intermittent dialysis in acute kidney injury of the critically ill patient. Nat Clin Pract Nephrol 2007; 3(3):118–119.
15. Saudan P, Niederberger M, De Seigneux S, Romand J, Pugin J, Perneger T, et al. Adding a dialysis dose to continuous hemofiltration increases survival in patients with acute renal failure. Kidney Int 2006.
16. Uchino S, Bellomo R, Kellum JA, Morimatsu H, Morgera S, Schetz MR, et al. Patient and kidney survival by dialysis modality in critically ill patients with acute kidney injury. Int J Artif Organs 2007; 30(4):281–292.
17. Uehlinger DE, Jakob SM, Ferrari P, Eichelberger M, Huynh-Do U, Marti HP, et al. Comparison of continuous and intermittent renal replacement therapy for acute renal failure. Nephrol Dial Transplant 2005; 20(8):1630–1637.
18. Vinsonneau C, Camus C, Combes A, Costa de Beauregard MA, Klouche K, Boulain T, et al. Continuous venovenous haemodiafiltration versus intermittent haemodialysis for acute renal failure in patients with multiple-organ dysfunction syndrome: a multicentre randomised trial. Lancet 2006; 368(9533):379–385.

Acute Kidney Replacement Therapy in Children

7.13

Jordan M. Symons

Core Messages

- Choice of dialysis modality and prescription in children requires careful multidisciplinary coordination and must be tailored to the individual patient and clinical situation.
- Peritoneal dialysis has the advantages of simplicity and no need for vascular access and systemic anticoagulation. Patients with severe abdominal pathology may, however, be ineligible as a useable abdomen and functioning peritoneal membrane are mandatory. Peritoneal dialysis may be a poor choice if rapid correction of metabolic/electrolyte state is required.
- Extracorporeal hemodialysis and hemofiltration techniques and systems are well established even for the smallest children and have the advantage of high efficiency and permitting quick correction of metabolic and fluid imbalance. Intermittent hemodialysis may be poorly tolerated, however, by the critically ill patient in whom continuous therapies may be preferable.

7.13.1 Introduction

Acute kidney injury in children may necessitate renal replacement therapy. Critically ill children with oligoanuria may benefit from renal support to permit daily fluid input and prevent volume overload. In addition, children with intoxications, either exogenous (medication overdose or poisoning) or endogenous (e.g., hyperammonemia in the setting of inborn errors of metabolism) may require treatment for removal of toxin and restoration of metabolic balance. All modalities of renal replacement therapy – peritoneal dialysis, hemodialysis, and continuous renal replacement therapy (CRRT) – can be considered for pediatric patients [11, 15].

7.13.2 Peritoneal Dialysis

Peritoneal dialysis has long been a preferred method of both acute and chronic dialysis for children. Peritoneal dialysis, often ignored for adults requiring acute dialysis, can be an effective method for children who require renal replacement in the acute setting [12].

7.13.2.1 Advantages

Peritoneal dialysis is technically simpler than hemodialysis. It does not require sophisticated equipment or staff trained for complex, specialized procedures. The materials required to perform peritoneal dialysis are less expensive than those required for hemodialysis. Vascular access is not required. Without extracorporeal perfusion, there is no need for anticoagulation and

J. M. Symons
Division of Nephrology, Children's Hospital and Regional Medical Center, Department of Pediatrics, University of Washington School of Medicine, 4800 Sand Point Way NE, Seattle, WA 98105–0371, USA
e-mail: jordan.symons@seattlechildrens.org

A. Jörres et al. (eds.), *Management of Acute Kidney Problems*,
DOI: 10.1007/978-3-540-69441-0_7.13, © Springer-Verlag Berlin Heidelberg 2010

the associated risks, such as hemorrhage. The relative inefficiency of peritoneal dialysis may be advantageous in the critically ill child, in whom the slow, gentle removal of molecules may be better tolerated. Peritoneal dialysis may be a particularly good choice for infants and children following surgical correction of congenital heart disease [22].

7.13.2.2 Disadvantages

The relatively slow rate of mass transfer from peritoneal dialysis makes it a poor choice in patients where rapid removal of molecules is necessary, such as acute intoxications. The procedure requires a usable abdomen and peritoneal membrane; patients with severe abdominal pathology may be ineligible. There is risk of peritonitis or other infectious complication, especially in the acute setting. Increased intraabdominal pressure from peritoneal dialysate may compromise diaphragmatic excursion, causing potential respiratory complications in the acutely ill patient [7].

7.13.2.3 Indications

Peritoneal dialysis is a reasonable option for any child who requires treatment for acute renal failure or its complications. It would be a poor choice in the clinical setting where rapid metabolic correction is necessary.

7.13.2.4 Technique

Peritoneal access for dialysis can be achieved through placement of a temporary catheter, inserted percutaneously at the bedside [5]. This technique provides quick access but has been associated with a higher number of complications, including dialysate leak, catheter obstruction from omentum, and injury to intraabdominal contents. Surgical placement of a cuffed peritoneal dialysis catheter requires an operative procedure but may be associated with better catheter function [9]. Recommended waiting periods of 2–6 weeks in the chronic dialysis setting are impractical for acute dialysis; risk for leak from the newly placed catheter can be reduced by using smaller fill volumes and keeping the patient supine.

Lower fill volumes can start at 10 ml/kg (~200 ml/m^2) for the first 1–2 weeks. Increased volumes provide better dialysis but raise the chances for peritoneal leak. Target volumes used for long-term chronic peritoneal dialysis of 40–50 ml/kg (1,200 ml/m^2) may not be necessary in the acute setting, especially if dialysis is provided around-the-clock. Dwell times for acute peritoneal dialysis in children usually vary from 15 to 60 min; shorter dwell times are often employed to increase daily ultrafiltration.

Standard dialysate in the United States uses dextrose to generate an osmotic gradient for ultrafiltration. Commercially available concentrates of dextrose are 1.5%, 2.5%, and 4.25%. Slightly different concentrations of dextrose are available in Europe and Asia. Higher concentrations of dextrose increase ultrafiltration with each dwell period but expose the patient to more carbohydrate; this may lead to hyperglycemia. Icodextrin, a synthetic carbohydrate, is used to improve ultrafiltration during the long dwell in chronic dialysis; as such it is infrequently used for acute peritoneal dialysis. Lactate is the standard base in peritoneal dialysate produced in the United States; bicarbonate-based dialsyate is available commercially outside of the United States. It is our practice to use commercially available dialysate for all clinical settings; rare clinical scenarios may require extemporaneously prepared dialysate from the local hospital pharmacy.

Shorter dwell periods permit a larger number of exchanges to be performed each day. Many patients who require acute dialysis can receive their therapy around-the-clock, maximizing dialysis support and ultrafiltration. This can be advantageous when smaller fill volumes are used and mass transfer with each exchange is not optimal.

The majority of children can receive acute peritoneal dialysis using a cycler, an automated device that fills and drains dialysate and monitors fluid flow. Manual dialysis may be required for patients who require very low fill volumes. With either system, careful attention to sterile technique and maintenance of a closed system is essential to prevent infectious complications.

7.13.2.5 Adequacy and Outcome

While recommendations exist for monitoring of peritoneal dialysis adequacy for chronic maintenance therapy, there are no specific guidelines to determine if acute peritoneal dialysis is "adequate." Monitoring of fluid and electrolyte balance, with noted improvement and stability of markers such as blood urea nitrogen, potassium, sodium, and acceptable status of physical exam findings such as blood pressure and volume status, can guide adjustments to the prescription.

7.13.2.6 Complications

Complications of peritoneal dialysis include mechanical and metabolic problems, and infection. Consider peritonitis in any peritoneal dialysis patient who develops fever, abdominal pain, or cloudy peritoneal effluent. Test the effluent for the presence of leukocytes and send the fluid sample for culture; one should have a low threshold to begin empiric antibiotics to cover gram-positive and gram-negative organisms. Specific guidelines exist for the treatment of peritonitis in the chronic peritoneal dialysis patient [29]; these may be adapted to the acute setting. Severe infection may require removal of the peritoneal dialysis catheter.

The peritoneal dialysis catheter may fail to function properly, with limited flow of fluid in or out of the patient's abdomen. This can be due to malposition, kinking, or occlusion of the catheter. Omentum can obstruct the peritoneal catheter; prophylactic omentectomy is frequently performed when placing a permanent peritoneal dialysis catheter. Fibrin can occlude the intraabdominal ostia of the catheter. Radiographs can confirm appropriate position of the peritoneal catheter. If fibrin occlusion is suspected, intralumenal use of tissue plasminogen activator can be considered [25]. Surgical revision of a poorly functioning catheter may be necessary.

Peritoneal catheters can leak due to increased intraabdominal pressure with instilled dialysate. This is more likely to happen with a percutaneously placed catheter, or when a surgically placed catheter is new and the track around the catheter has not yet fully healed. Leak predisposes the patient to peritonitis. Low fill volumes at initiation reduce the chances of leak. If peritoneal leak occurs, fill volume must be reduced. If leak persists, one must consider discontinuation of peritoneal dialysis and evaluate for other methods of renal replacement.

Patients receiving peritoneal dialysis can develop imbalances of electrolytes and of nutrition. Special attention is required to provide appropriate supplementation to balance for losses in the dialysate. Hypernatremia has been reported in small children receiving short-dwell acute peritoneal dialysis, due to rapid movement of water across the peritoneum with slower equilibration of sodium ("sodium sieving"). Adjustment to intravenous fluids and possibly to the dialysate concentration of sodium may be necessary [20, 28].

7.13.3 Intermittent Hemodialysis

Intermittent hemodialysis has been the traditional modality for acute renal replacement therapy. Techniques established in adults have been adapted for pediatric patients. Successful hemodialysis for children requires experience, making use of special protocols and adapted equipment. Of paramount importance is the skilled dialysis nurse who can monitor the patient and provide safe, effective therapy.

7.13.3.1 Advantages

Hemodialysis is highly efficient, rapidly moving molecules out of the patient and permitting quick correction of metabolic and fluid imbalance. The hemodialysis system does not depend on the health of a native dialyzing membrane as is required for peritoneal dialysis. Pediatric techniques, even for the smallest children, are well established [24].

7.13.3.2 Disadvantages

Compared with peritoneal dialysis, hemodialysis is technically complex and considerably more expensive to perform. The procedure requires specialized equipment and highly trained personnel. Not all facilities have the capability or experience to provide hemodialysis to the pediatric patient. Hemodialysis requires vascular access, which can be difficult to achieve in an acutely ill child. The procedure usually requires anticoagulation, which brings with it risks of hemorrhage. Hemodialysis may be poorly tolerated by critically ill patients, and such risks are magnified in children.

7.13.3.3 Indications

Hemodialysis is indicated for renal failure and any of its complications. It can efficiently correct volume overload and maintain volume control in the oligoanuric patient. It is a superior modality for the treatment of acute intoxication, either exogenous or endogenous.

7.13.3.4 Technique

Acute hemodialysis requires vascular access. On rare occasions a chronic hemodialysis patient will present for acute care; in this situation the patient's long-term vascular access (arteriovenous fistula or subcutaneous dialysis graft) may be used for the acute procedure. The majority of the time the patient does not have vascular access and a hemodialysis catheter must be placed. The preferred vascular access site is the internal jugular vein; good blood flow can be achieved, patient comfort can be maintained, and the patient can be more easily mobilized. Convenience often dictates that a hemodialysis catheter is placed in the femoral position; this can be done at the bedside by the Seldinger technique. Femoral catheters are not appropriate for prolonged use. Temporary uncuffed catheters can be used for short-term courses of hemodialysis; for longer courses, one should consider placement of a tunneled cuffed catheter in the internal jugular position. The subclavian position should be avoided; subclavian catheterization is associated with subclavian stenosis, which limits the possibility of placing a permanent vascular access in the patient if they do not recover renal function and require long-term maintenance hemodialysis. Both temporary uncuffed catheters and tunneled cuffed catheters come in a variety of lengths and diameters to accommodate pediatric patients. Surgical assistance may be necessary, especially for smaller children in whom placement of vascular access can be challenging [2].

Several manufacturers produce small dialyzers and tubing sets for pediatric hemodialysis. It is recommended that the extracorporeal volume (dialyzer and tubing) be limited to 10% or less of the patient's blood volume. For small infants this cannot always be achieved and special priming of the extracorporeal circuit may be required to limit excessive dilution of the patient's hematocrit. It is our practice to prime such circuits with a mix of packed red cells and 5% albumin to a hematocrit of approximately 35%. Larger patients can be primed on with saline or, if there is significant volume overload and no problems with hypotension, the patient can "self-prime," disposing of the saline in the extracorporeal circuit prior to initiation of the treatment.

Blood pump speed depends on the size of the vascular access and the clinical status of the patient. Infants may requires blood flow rates as low as 25–30 ml/min; larger children can dialyze at pumps speeds of 200 ml/min or higher. Dialysate flow rate is often device-specific; flow rates of 500 ml/min are often considered standard. The composition of the dialysate can be adjusted by manipulating the concentrate used to generate the dialysate through the online proportioning system. The clinician must choose an appropriate dialysate composition (potassium, calcium, sodium, bicarbonate) for the metabolic status of the patient and goals of the treatment.

Session length depends on clinical goals. One must consider the level of mass transfer desired in the session and the ultrafiltration target; both will have an effect on the duration of the dialysis session. Due to smaller body water volume, effective clearance can be achieved in pediatric patients using shorter sessions. As in adult patients, initial clearance may need to be limited due to risk of disequilibrium syndrome (see Chapter on Adult Hemodialysis).

An acutely ill child with significant volume overload may require a longer session to permit successful removal of the target volume of fluid. Calculation of session length for lower mass transfer may create a conflict with the desire for a longer session to permit slow ultrafiltration. This can be addressed by using a smaller dialyzer or slower blood flow rate to achieve a lower urea reduction in the extended time required for ultrafiltration. Alternatively, ultrafiltration and dialysis may be performed asynchronously; for example, the clinician may order 3 h of ultrafiltration with dialysis performed for only 1 h of this 3-h session. This will permit slower removal of fluid from the patient while limiting urea reduction.

Anticoagulation goals for pediatric patients are similar to those for adults. Heparin induced thrombocytopenia is very uncommon. Infants have increased risk for intracranial hemorrhage; heparin dose may need to be limited.

Intermittent hemodialysis of the acutely ill child requires close monitoring. Due to smaller intravascular volumes children are more likely to have rapid changes in blood pressure during a hemodialysis session. Bedside tools such as pulse oximetry, cardiac monitoring, and online blood volume monitoring can be useful. The most important requirement for safe, successful hemodialysis of the acutely ill child is the highly skilled dialysis nurse at the bedside.

7.13.3.5 Adequacy and Outcome

Adequacy targets for children requiring acute dialysis have not been established. Overall clinical status of the patient with regard to metabolic and volume status guides ongoing therapy.

7.13.3.6 Complications

Complications for children receiving acute hemodialysis are similar to those for adults. Hemorrhage can occur due to extracorporeal perfusion and systemic anticoagulation. Infection risk is high due to the frequent use of indwelling catheters for vascular access. As noted above, risk for hypotension may be greater in children due to their relatively small size; fortunately, most children do not bring the cardiovascular comorbidities as might be seen in an adult patient. Risk for electrolyte abnormalities may be higher for children, again due to relatively small volume compared with adults. Obtaining and maintaining a functional vascular access may be difficult in children due to small vessels and concomitantly small catheters which may be prone to kinking and thrombosis.

7.13.4 Continuous Renal Replacement Therapy

Continuous renal replacement therapy (CRRT) is being used with greater frequency for critically ill children. Modern CRRT machines permit application of the therapy to even the smallest patients [26]. The technique is highly specialized and may not be available in all centers.

7.13.4.1 Advantages

CRRT has the advantage of being a continuous treatment, providing slow, ongoing support that can maintain metabolic stability and may be better tolerated by the critically ill patient. Theoretical advantages in the setting of sepsis have yet to be proven in pediatric clinical trials. Mass transfer capabilities of CRRT, traditionally thought to be less efficient than those of intermittent hemodialysis, may approach those of traditional hemodialysis therapy when applied to a small pediatric patient.

7.13.4.2 Disadvantages

CRRT has the disadvantages of higher cost and the requirement for specialized equipment and personnel. It is technically complex. Like hemodialysis, extracorporeal perfusion requires vascular access, which may be difficult to achieve in a small child. The risks of hemorrhage and infection exist as they do for hemodialysis, potentially magnified by the continuous rather than intermittent use of the therapy. CRRT is usually only available in the critical care setting.

7.13.4.3 Indications

Indications for CRRT in the critically ill child include renal failure, volume overload, electrolyte disturbances, or other complications of kidney dysfunction in which the slow, continuous nature of CRRT may be advantageous. This is most often seen in the critical care setting with a hypotensive patient who may not tolerate intermittent hemodialysis. CRRT can provide ongoing support for the oligoanuric patient to permit delivery of intravenous fluids, blood products, and nutrition without causing further volume overload. Data in critically ill pediatric patients suggest that volume overload is associated with poor outcome [13, 14, 16]; CRRT can assist in regaining control of volume status, maintaining appropriate fluid balance, or preventing fluid overload in the patient who develops acute kidney injury. CRRT can be used to maintain metabolic stability in those patients who have undergone acute hemodialysis for intoxication (see above) and are at risk for "rebound" of toxin from tissue stores or ongoing generation [18, 19].

7.13.4.4 Technique

Venovenous methods have allowed more pediatric patients to receive CRRT, as compared with older arteriovenous methods which were complicated by problems with filter perfusion and hemorrhage. All modalities of CRRT have been used for children, including low-clearance methods (slow continuous ultrafiltration [SCUF]), convective modalities (continuous venovenous hemofiltration [CVVH]), diffusion-based techniques (continuous venovenous hemodialysis [CVVHD]), and combined methods (continuous venovenous hemodiafiltration [CVVHDF]). The choice may depend on local preference and available technology. No modality has been shown to be superior for pediatric patients as there have been no randomized controlled trials for children.

Vascular access for CRRT is as noted above for hemodialysis. Hemofilter and tubing choices may be limited by the equipment available. Hemodynamically unstable patients, anemic patients, or small children with low intravascular volume may require priming of the CRRT circuit with blood as noted above for hemodialysis.

Hemofilters made with the AN-69 membrane have been implicated in a systemic reaction called the bradykinin release syndrome.[3] This causes bronchospasm and profound hypotension at the initiation of CRRT. It is thought to be related to bradykinin activation upon blood contact with the negatively charged hemofilter. The reaction seems to be exacerbated by metabolic acidosis and seems to be most profound in smaller patients who require blood priming of the circuit. Techniques to mitigate the reaction have been described.[3, 17, 21] Avoidance of the negatively charged AN-69 membrane reduces the likelihood of this reaction.

Blood flow should be adjusted for the overall clinical situation, giving consideration to the patient's hemodynamic status and requirements for successful extracorporeal perfusion, as noted above for hemodialysis.

Choice of infused fluids for pediatric CRRT depends on modality, which may further be dictated by available equipment or local preference. SCUF does not call for any infused fluids; CVVHD requires dialysate, CVVH requires replacement fluids, and CVVHDF requires both. Commercially prepared solutions with physiological electrolyte content are convenient and reduce the possibility of errors from extemporaneously prepared solutions [1]. Since blood flow rate usually exceeds the flow rate of infused fluids, mass transfer in CRRT is dependent on effluent rate and, thus, on the prescribed rate of infused fluids. Higher flow rates will, therefore, increase mass transfer.

Unlike adults, there are no randomized trials in pediatric patients that link infused fluid rate to outcome; the best rate for infused fluids is unknown. A common practice, based on experience, has been to target an infused fluid rate scaled to patient body surface area of 2,000 ml/h/1.73 m^2. This provides flow rates at or above the target of 35 ml/kg/h described by Ronco et al. [23] for adult patients and also provides sufficient mass transfer to balance citrate regional anticoagulation using a well-described protocol (see below) [6]. Division of this rate of fluid between dialysate and/or replacement fluid depends on local practice and clinical objectives, emphasizing diffusion, convection, or combined therapies.

Ultrafiltration goals must be coordinated with the clinical needs of the patient. One should develop an ultrafiltration target with knowledge of the daily fluid input, ongoing losses from the patient, and the level of volume overload that must be corrected. Rate for ultrafiltration may be limited by cardiovascular instability; use of vasoactive medications to support blood pressure can make ultrafiltration more successful. Given concerns for volume overload in the critically ill child, every effort should be made to achieve successful ultrafiltration and maintain appropriate fluid balance.

Anticoagulation for pediatric CRRT has traditionally been with heparin. This system is well established but has the disadvantage of systemic anticoagulation, which must be maintained continuously for maintenance of the CRRT circuit. Regional anticoagulation with citrate has been gaining favor with pediatric practitioners; several protocols have been established and shown to be successful [6, 8, 10]. Children may be at increased risk for citrate overload due to relatively higher citrate delivery compared with body size; for this reason, adequate infused fluids for clearance must be prescribed (see above). Neither heparin nor citrate has yet been proven to be clearly superior for pediatric CRRT; a study comparing the two methods showed equal circuit life span for the two methods but fewer bleeding complications for those circuits anticoagulated with citrate [4]. Clearly inferior was CRRT with no anticoagulation, for which circuit life span was much shorter.

7.13.4.5 Adequacy and Outcome

As previously noted, there are no specific data regarding adequacy for pediatric CRRT. Outcomes have improved with experience [27]. Careful, ongoing review of metabolic balance and ultrafiltration targets during therapy is appropriate.

7.13.4.6 Complications

Complications for children receiving CRRT are similar to those for adults. Hemorrhage and infection remain significant concerns in the setting of continuous extracorporeal perfusion. Ultrafiltration in excess of the patient's ability to tolerate can lead to hypotension; use of vasoactive medications to support blood pressure and careful ultrafiltration targeting can limit this complication. Electrolyte imbalance can occur with continuous diffusion or convection of small molecules; frequent monitoring and adjustment to nutritional support is warranted.

7.13.5 Summary/Conclusions

The pediatric patient who requires renal replacement therapy can benefit from any of the available modalities. Successful therapy requires careful consideration of the special issues related to a small patient, coordination of care between all providers, and ongoing reevaluation and adjustment to prescribed therapy.

7.13.6 Take Home Pearls

- Peritoneal dialysis has the advantages of simplicity and no need for systemic anticoagulation. It requires a useable abdomen and may be a poor choice if rapid metabolic correction is required.
- Intermittent hemodialysis has the advantage of high efficiency, but it may be poorly tolerated by the critically ill patient. The technique is complicated and requires highly skilled personnel at the bedside.
- CRRT may be better tolerated in the unstable pediatric patient. It can be used to maintain metabolic and fluid balance and permit delivery of fluids, medications, and nutrition.
- Choice of dialysis modality and prescription must be tailored to the individual patient and clinical situation.
- Successful therapy requires careful multidisciplinary coordination.

References

1. Barletta J F, Barletta G M, Brophy P D, et al. (2006) Medication errors and patient complications with continuous renal replacement therapy. Pediatr Nephrol 21(6):842–845.
2. Beanes S R, Kling K M, Fonkalsrud E W, et al. (2000) Surgical aspects of dialysis in newborns and infants weighing less than ten kilograms. J Pediatr Surg 35(11):1543–1548.
3. Brophy P D, Mottes T A, Kudelka T L, et al. (2001) AN-69 membrane reactions are pH-dependent and preventable. Am J Kidney Dis 38(1):173–178.
4. Brophy P D, Somers M J, Baum M A, et al. (2005) Multicentre evaluation of anticoagulation in patients receiving continuous renal replacement therapy (CRRT). Nephrol Dial Transplant 20(7):1416–1421.
5. Bunchman T E (1996) Acute peritoneal dialysis access in infant renal failure. Perit Dial Int 16 (Suppl 1): S509–511.
6. Bunchman T E, Maxvold N J, Barnett J, et al. (2002) Pediatric hemofiltration: Normocarb dialysate solution with citrate anticoagulation. Pediatr Nephrol 17(3):150–154.
7. Bunchman T E, Meldrum M K, Meliones J E, et al. (1992) Pulmonary function variation in ventilator dependent critically ill infants on peritoneal dialysis. Adv Perit Dial 8:75–78.
8. Chadha V, Garg, U., Warady, B.A., Alon, U.S. (2002) Citrate clearance in children receiving continuous venovenous renal replacement therapy. Pediatr Nephrol 17(10):819–824.

9. Chadha V, Warady B A, Blowey D L, et al. (2000) Tenckhoff catheters prove superior to cook catheters in pediatric acute peritoneal dialysis. Am J Kidney Dis 35(6):1111–1116.
10. Elhanan N, Skippen P, Nuthall G, et al. (2004) Citrate anticoagulation in pediatric continuous venovenous hemofiltration. Pediatr Nephrol 19(2):208–212.
11. Flynn J T (2002) Choice of dialysis modality for management of pediatric acute renal failure. Pediatr Nephrol 17(1):61–69.
12. Flynn J T, Kershaw D B, Smoyer W E, et al. (2001) Peritoneal dialysis for management of pediatric acute renal failure. Perit Dial Int 21(4):390–394.
13. Foland J A, Fortenberry J D, Warshaw B L, et al. (2004) Fluid overload before continuous hemofiltration and survival in critically ill children: a retrospective analysis. Crit Care Med 32(8):1771–1776.
14. Gillespie R S, Seidel K, Symons J M (2004) Effect of fluid overload and dose of replacement fluid on survival in hemofiltration. Pediatr Nephrol 19(12):1394–1399.
15. Goldstein S L (2003) Overview of pediatric renal replacement therapy in acute renal failure. Artif Organs 27(9):781–785.
16. Goldstein S L, Currier H, Graf C, et al. (2001) Outcome in children receiving continuous venovenous hemofiltration. Pediatrics 107(6):1309–1312.
17. Hackbarth R M, Eding D, Gianoli Smith C, et al. (2005) Zero balance ultrafiltration (Z-BUF) in blood-primed CRRT circuits achieves electrolyte and acid-base homeostasis prior to patient connection. Pediatr Nephrol 20(9):1328–1333.
18. McBryde K D, Kershaw D B, Bunchman T E, et al. (2006) Renal replacement therapy in the treatment of confirmed or suspected inborn errors of metabolism. J Pediatr 148(6):770–778.
19. McBryde K D, Kudelka T L, Kershaw D B, et al. (2004) Clearance of amino acids by hemodialysis in argininosuccinate synthetase deficiency. J Pediatr 144(4):536–540.
20. Moritz M L, del Rio M, Crooke G A, et al. (2001) Acute peritoneal dialysis as both cause and treatment of hypernatremia in an infant. Pediatr Nephrol 16(9):697–700.
21. Pasko D A, Mottes T A, Mueller B A (2003) Pre dialysis of blood prime in continuous hemodialysis normalizes pH and electrolytes. Pediatr Nephrol 18(11):1177–1183.
22. Pedersen K R, Hjortdal V E, Christensen S, et al. (2008) Clinical outcome in children with acute renal failure treated with peritoneal dialysis after surgery for congenital heart disease. Kidney Int Suppl(108):S81–86.
23. Ronco C, Bellomo R, Homel P, et al. (2000) Effects of different doses in continuous veno-venous haemofiltration on outcomes of acute renal failure: a prospective randomised trial (see comment). Lancet 356(9223):26–30.
24. Sadowski R H, Harmon W E, Jabs K (1994) Acute hemodialysis of infants weighing less than five kilograms. Kidney Int 45(3):903–906.
25. Shea M, Hmiel S P, Beck A M (2001) Use of tissue plasminogen activator for thrombolysis in occluded peritoneal dialysis catheters in children. Adv Perit Dial 17:249–252.
26. Symons J M, Brophy P D, Gregory M J, et al. (2003) Continuous renal replacement therapy in children up to 10 kg. Am J Kidney Dis 41(5):984–989.
27. Symons J M, Chua A N, Somers M J, et al. (2007) Demographic characteristics of pediatric continuous renal replacement therapy: a report of the prospective pediatric continuous renal replacement therapy registry. Clin J Am Soc Nephrol 2(4):732–738.
28. Vande Walle J G J, Raes A M, De Hoorne J, et al. (2005) Need for low sodium concentration and frequent cycles of 3.86% glucose solution in children treated with acute peritoneal dialysis. Adv Perit Dial 21:204–208.
29. Warady B A, Feneberg R, Verrina E, et al. (2007) Peritonitis in children who receive long-term peritoneal dialysis: a prospective evaluation of therapeutic guidelines. J Am Soc Nephrol 18(7):2172–2179.

Stopping Acute Kidney Replacement Therapy

7.14

Josée Bouchard, Roy Mathew, and Ravindra L. Mehta

Core Messages

- An important aspect of the management of critically ill patients which is still controversial is the timing of initiation and cessation of renal replacement therapy (RRT).
- Whilst in recent publications, timing of initiation of RRT was listed as one of the top priorities in research on acute kidney injury (AKI), the cessation of RRT has received little attention and has not been studied extensively.
- This chapter provides a conceptual framework for the factors influencing treatment cessation, provides suggestions for techniques to evaluate residual kidney function, and discusses various approaches to optimize the stopping of RRT in patients with AKI.

7.14.1 Introduction

Knowing when to start and when to stop renal replacement therapy (RRT) for patients with acute kidney injury (AKI) are among the unanswered questions for physicians. Several randomized studies have tried to delineate the best modality or the optimal dialysis dose to use in this setting, with inconsistent results. In recent publications, timing of initiation of RRT was listed as one of the top priorities in research on AKI [1]; however, has not been included as a factor in any of the large randomized controlled trials (RCTs) in this area. Similarly, cessation of RRT has received little attention and has not been studied extensively. Several factors influence the need to discontinue RRT. A thorough understanding of the underlying concepts and different strategies for stopping RRT is essential to effectively manage these patients. This article outlines the principles for stopping RRT and provides a framework of reference for clinical practice and research in this area.

R. L. Mehta (✉)
Division of Nephrology, Department of Medicine,
University of California, San Diego, CA 92103, USA
e-mail: rmehta@ucsd.edu

7.14.1.1 Stopping RRT: Key Concepts

A decision to start RRT in a patient with AKI is generally influenced by a real or perceived need for additional renal excretory capacity. There is currently a wide variation in indications and timing of RRT. Acute kidney replacement therapy can either be provided for renal replacement or renal support. The former indication is well-known; patients usually present with advanced loss of kidney function and require dialysis for metabolic and/or volume control indications. On the other hand, renal support is considered when a mismatch occurs between demands and capacity. Common indications for renal replacement therapy include hyperkalemia, metabolic acidosis, uremia or progressive azotemia, and volume overload in the setting of oliguria. Indications for renal support include the delivery of adequate nutrition in a hypercatabolic context and the management of relative fluid overload in patients with AKI. Opinions diverge regarding the use of dialysis for these indications. Once RRT is started, unless the patient has end-stage renal disease (ESRD) and is on maintenance dialysis, there will be a need at some point to stop therapy. In essence, one needs to know when it is appropriate to stop and then how to design and implement a

A. Jörres et al. (eds.), *Management of Acute Kidney Problems*,
DOI: 10.1007/978-3-540-69441-0_7.14, © Springer-Verlag Berlin Heidelberg 2010

plan to stop. There are a limited number of reasons for stopping therapy. These include an improvement in renal function adequate to meet demand, an improvement in the disorder that prompted renal support, or futility. It should be evident that each of these events is influenced by the initial indication for starting RRT and is subject to individual variation. The decision to stop thus requires an appropriate assessment of factors conditioning these events. Once a decision to stop is made, a strategy for stopping must be developed. This requires consideration of additional factors and often involves a modality transition as part of the approach. A key feature common to the decision to stop and the strategy for implementation is the level of renal function. Consequently, techniques to measure or estimate underlying renal function are an essential component.

RRT for AKI is analogous to mechanical ventilation for acute lung injury (ALI). Mechanical ventilation is offered for airway protection or to replace decompensated pulmonary function. In either case the decision to stop ventilation is based on an assessment of the underlying pulmonary function and the ability to sustain adequate oxygenation off ventilation. Various weaning strategies are utilized to individualize the discontinuation of therapy and require an ongoing assessment of underlying lung capacity. When the lung is normal and ventilation was offered for airway protection, e.g., for brain injury or sedation, weaning depends on recovery of an adequate neurological status, whereas in ALI, ventilation can be stopped only when the lung functional capacity is enough to maintain adequate oxygenation and acid–base balance. These concepts are similar for RRT. When RRT is offered for renal support, discontinuation will depend on the state of the original organ that contributed to the increased demand, while if it was initiated for a loss of native kidney function, renal recovery will be the key. Concepts utilized for weaning from mechanical ventilation could similarly be applied for discontinuation of RRT. Based on these concepts it is possible to construct various scenarios and recommendations that can be applied to clinical practice. These are discussed in further detail below.

7.14.1.2 RRT Cessation: When to Stop?

As clearly shown in multiple observational studies, the vast majority of patients requiring RRT will recover enough function not to require long-term renal replacement [2–4]. In fact, even in severe AKI, the median duration of RRT will range from 3 to 6 days [2, 5]. Thus indications for RRT in AKI usually resolve quickly, and daily diligence will be required to evaluate the ongoing need for acute kidney replacement therapy. As for mechanical ventilation, RRT cessation can be delayed due to physicians' lack of attention to details indicating improvement in renal status. Daily screening for kidney function recovery is a vital part of medical evaluation, not only because it assesses the need for dialysis, but also to adjust medication dosages.

7.14.1.2.1 Improvement in Underlying Renal Function (Renal Replacement Indications)

The first step to perform is to review the initial indication for dialysis. We will first address the indications for renal replacement therapy and the ability to stop RRT in relation to these indications. Then the indications for RRT for renal support will be discussed.

Hyperkalemia

Indications for dialysis in hyperkalemia have already been discussed in previous chapters. These indications should be followed to determine if dialysis is required for hyperkalemia. In order to know if it is safe to stop dialysis that has been performed mainly to correct hyperkalemia, several considerations need to be addressed. These considerations include the potassium level after dialysis treatment, the possibility of a rebound in potassium levels shortly after dialysis, and the likelihood of further quick increases in potassium levels. As a general guideline, after dialysis, we are trying to reach a potassium level around 4.0–4.5 mmol/l and even lower if anuria or another condition that quickly increases potassium levels is present.

The dialysis modality used will have an influence on potassium levels after treatment. In continuous renal replacement therapy (CRRT), the serum potassium levels reach a plateau 24–48 h after the initiation of CRRT, assuming that the prescription has not been changed [6]. Rebounds should not occur after treatment cessation. In sustained low-efficiency dialysis (SLED), minimal urea rebound postdialysis has been shown in critically ill patients with AKI (4.1%) [7]. Due to its similar diffusive properties, potassium levels should not rebound significantly after SLED. Intermittent hemodialysis (IHD) provides higher clearance over a short period of time compared with the two previous modalities and should be preferred when high potassium levels are associated with changes on electrocardiogram, unless contraindications are present. In intermittent dialysis, however, the levels of potassium right after the treatment session are lowered by the effect of the low potassium concentration in the dialysate used to correct hyperkalemia. Rebound hyperkalemia may occur over the next few hours due to the rapid shifts of potassium between intracellular and extracellular compartments. Studies in the ESRD population have demonstrated that significant rebound hyperkalemia is more closely related to predialysis potassium levels than to total body potassium [8]. No specific studies have been performed on assessing the rapidity or importance of serum potassium rebound following acute RRT. Medical treatments for hyperkalemia, such as inhaled albuterol, periodically lower the serum potassium level by intracellular shift. When intermittent dialysis is performed shortly after these measures, the potassium removal during dialysis will be reduced and greater rises in postdialysis potassium can occur [9]. In summary, potassium levels should always be checked a few hours after the decision to stop dialysis treatment to guide further management, especially when medical measures to treat hyperkalemia are followed by IHD.

A few conditions can cause a significant release of potassium from cells and require careful monitoring before dialysis is definitely interrupted, such as rhabdomyolysis and tumor lysis syndrome. Hyperkalemia in the setting of rhabdomyolysis is typically significant (>5.5 mmol/l) when the plasma creatine kinase (CK) levels are >15,000 UI/l and when AKI is present [10]. Similarly, hyperkalemia may be persistent in severe tumor lysis syndrome [11]. Another condition merits discussion. In the setting of complete anuria, if hyperkalemia has occurred, it is the norm to pursue the dialysis treatments until improvements in kidney function occur.

Metabolic Acidosis

This disorder is a frequent clinical problem in patients with severe AKI requiring CRRT [12, 13]. However, metabolic acidosis associated with AKI can usually be corrected with bicarbonate and should rarely require urgent dialysis if not accompanied by volume overload or uremia [14]. Nonetheless, normalization of the acid–base balance with the use of CRRT in these patients can usually be achieved within 24–48 h [15]. As the pH and bicarbonate values to initiate dialysis for metabolic acidosis are not supported by any evidence-based data, neither is the threshold for stopping dialysis. In these cases, the dialysis treatment is usually stopped with the resolution of the AKI process.

Metabolic acidosis can also occur in scenarios such as sepsis and shock, usually under the form of lactic acidosis. Correction of metabolic acidosis with dialysis in these conditions depends on the underlying disease process. Paradoxically, even if target bicarbonate values are unknown, normalization of acid–base balance is associated with a clearly better overall prognosis [16]. Thus metabolic acidosis is a marker of the overall patients' condition. Patients who failed to correct their metabolic status are sicker and have much lower chances to stop dialysis in the near future than patients who quickly normalize their acid–base balance.

Another important cause of metabolic acidosis is ethylene glycol or methanol poisoning. These conditions are associated with increased anion and osmolar gaps. In these situations, treatment should be continued until blood pH is normalized and ethylene glycol and methanol concentrations are below 10–15 mg/dl or undetectable if possible [17]. Clinical and metabolic status and toxic alcohol levels should be followed closely after dialysis cessation, since rebounds can occur and a second dialysis might be needed. Finally, metformin-associated lactic acidosis can be an indication for dialysis. Experts suggest its use in critically ill patients with a pH below 7.1, who fail to improve with supportive care, or in whom renal insufficiency is present. No precise criteria for dialysis cessation are established, but dialysis is usually stopped when metabolic status is normalized as the benefits for dialysis are related to the correction of metabolic acidosis [18].

Progressive Azotemia

As mentioned, daily assessment of underlying residual kidney function is critical. The evaluation of underlying residual kidney function will allow determining if the metabolic and volume status can be maintained without the assistance of RRT. The assessment of the kidney function will be different depending on the modality used. In intermittent hemodialysis, the residual kidney function can easily be assessed during the interdialytic period. Two readily available and commonly used tools are the change in serum creatinine and/or blood urea nitrogen (BUN) values, and urine creatinine clearance and volume. Using these tools, a trial of weaning or cessation may be considered when (1) the interdialytic rise in serum creatinine or BUN is less than previous changes of similar duration, (2) the urine output is increasing to above oliguric values (>400 ml/24 h) with comparable demand, and (3) the indication for RRT has resolved. It is well known that changes in BUN and creatinine are imprecise to detect an impending recovery and may lag behind recovery [19]. The change in BUN and creatinine levels can also be modified by the volume status and the catabolic rate. In CRRT, serum markers of kidney function are even less reliable. Theoretically, the continuous dialysis clearance of 25–35 ml/min will stabilize serum markers after 48 h. Then further decreases in serum creatinine in the setting of increasing urine output indicate improving kidney function. In such setting, a trial of weaning or cessation may be undertaken.

Timed creatinine clearance is a well-accepted surrogate for glomerular filtration rate (GFR) in chronic kidney disease due to the steady state in creatinine production and elimination. In AKI and critically ill patients, the urinary clearance of creatinine is less reliable. In a trial including critically ill patients without AKI which compared 24-h urinary creatinine clearance, 30-min urinary creatinine clearance, Cockcroft-Gault estimation of creatinine clearance to inulin clearance, the 24-h and 30-min urinary creatinine clearances had poor correlations with inulin GFR [20]. The mean differences in GFR compared with inulin were 21.6 ± 33.0 ml/min and 25.4 ± 28.3 ml/min, respectively. The urinary creatinine clearance significantly overestimated the clearance compared with the gold standard. Interestingly, Cockcroft-Gault estimations of creatinine clearance seemed to have an excellent correlation to measured kidney clearances in one study involving critically ill AKI subjects [21]. However, this equation is not accurate in obesity, large extracapillary fluids, and severe malnutrition.

Very few studies have looked at urine creatinine clearance values as a guide for CRRT withdrawal. One retrospective study examined the impact of different values of 24-h urine creatinine clearances during CRRT treatments on subsequent successful termination of CRRT. Successful termination of CRRT was defined as the absence of CRRT requirement for at least 14 days following cessation [22]. Urine creatinine clearances less than 15 ml/min (median 12 ml/min) were associated with failure to remain off CRRT, whereas urine creatinine clearances greater than 15 ml/min (median 25 ml/min) showed successful terminations of CRRT in six out of seven patients. These preliminary results suggest that in AKI, a 24-h urine creatinine clearance above 15–20 ml/min may be adequate to support metabolic demands without the need for RRT. Further prospective trials will be needed to support these findings.

A third tool to evaluate kidney function is the osmolar and free water clearances. These concepts seem to have been forgotten over the last years. In 1973, Baek et al. described the utilization of osmolar clearance and free water clearance to predict the development and recovery of ARF in patients without CKD [23]. Osmolar clearance is a rough guide of the concentrating ability of the kidney and corresponds to the product of urine flow rate (ml/h) and ratio of urine to plasma osmolarity (mOsm/L).

$$\text{Osmolar clearance} = \text{urine flow rate} \times \text{urine osmolality}/\text{plasma osmolality}$$

The result is the theoretical volume needed to produce iso-osmolar urine with the present solutes. The difference between the urine output and osmolar clearance is the free water clearance.

$$\text{Free water clearance} = \text{urine flow rate} - \text{osmolar clearance}$$

The normal free water clearance is in the range of –25 to –100 ml/h, which represents hyperosmolar urine. In this study, patients who maintained a free water clearance close to zero despite an increase in urine output demonstrated persistent electrolyte, BUN, and creatinine abnormalities. On the other hand, those who were found to have a progressive negative free water clearance showed improved BUN and creatinine parameters along with recovery from AKI [23]. In a subsequent publication, Baek et al. also demonstrated improved renal electrolyte handling with increasingly negative free water clearance [24]. However, this simple tool is rarely used and the influence of RRT on free water clearance is unknown. Nevertheless, during trials of cessation, calculation of free water clearance may provide an additional tool to assess probability of success off RRT.

Detection of AKI and kidney recovery has usually relied on changes in serum creatinine and urea. Over the last years, several novel biomarkers have been discovered for early diagnosis of AKI, namely cystatin C, neutrophil gelatinase-associated lipocalin (NGAL), interleukin-18 (IL-18), and kidney injury molecule-1 [25]. Some of these markers might eventually be used to predict cessation of RRT. Two biomarkers, urine IL-18 and urine NGAL, have been shown to correlate with renal recovery [26]. In this pediatric study involving 71 patients undergoing cardiopulmonary bypass, both urine IL-18 and urine NGAL at 4 h correlated with days until serum creatinine fell below 50% of baseline. No patient required RRT in this study. Further research is needed to identify biomarkers that might predict later renal recovery following AKI requiring RRT.

Volume Overload

Volume overload, with or without reduced urine output, is a common indication for RRT. In a recent epidemiologic survey, it was reported to be the main indication for RRT in 36% of critically ill patients with AKI [27]. Over the course of the dialysis sessions, several clinical parameters help to assess fluid balance and therefore, the need for further RRT. These parameters include central venous pressure (CVP), pulmonary artery wedge pressure (PAWP), mean arterial pressure (MAP), cardiac output (CO), arterial oxygen saturation to fraction of inspired oxygen ratio (paO_2/FiO_2), weight, input and output, and the presence of edema on clinical exam or chest radiography. These parameters need to be globally assessed in order to determine the volume status. No single parameter is a reliable indicator of volume status. We usually evaluate most of these measurements on a daily basis with the aim of reaching prespecified goals of therapy (i.e., goal CVP of 10–12, oxygen saturation ^{3} 90% on minimum oxygen support, etc.). Once these targets are achieved, the balance between obligatory intake and available intrinsic output is assessed to decide if further dialysis is required. Subsequent dialysis will be needed if there is a mismatch between obligatory intake and available output. No data has shown that this precise method is beneficial and some physicians might stop dialysis sessions earlier. The role of diuretics to promote diuresis in this setting will be discussed in a subsequent section.

Poisoning and Drug Toxicity

Lithium intoxication may require urgent dialysis in some conditions. When hemodialysis is initiated, lithium levels need to be checked regularly and dialysis maintained until the plasma lithium level remains at less than 1 mEq/l for 6–8 h after dialysis [28]. In salicylate poisoning, there are clear indications on when to start hemodialysis, but not on the optimal timing for stopping. In acute poisoning, RRT is indicated when concentrations are higher than >100 mg/dl (7.2 mmol/l). Other indications include altered mental status, pulmonary, or cerebral edema, renal impairment that interferes with salicylate excretion, fluid overload that prevents the administration of sodium bicarbonate and clinical deterioration despite aggressive and appropriate supportive care [29]. Ethylene glycol and methanol poisoning have already been discussed in the section on metabolic acidosis. Hemodialysis has also been shown to be valuable in phenobarbital overdose and is recommended when levels exceed 150 mg/l but no criteria for stopping extracorporeal treatment have been determined [30, 31].

7.14.1.2.2 Improvement in Basic Disorder Requiring RRT (Renal Support Indications)

Relative Volume Overload

Relative volume overload is one of the indications for renal support. As mentioned, renal support can be provided when mismatch occurs between demands versus capacity. There is accumulating evidence that relative volume overload is detrimental in ICU patients, especially in the pediatric population treated with CRRT [32–34]. A multicenter pediatric study showed that the percentage of fluid overload was significantly higher for nonsurvivors versus survivors [33]. Thus the timing for stopping RRT might need to be delayed if relative fluid overload is present. Additional studies are needed to assess the benefit to pursue RRT for relative volume overload.

Hypercatabolism

A relative indication for RRT is hypercatabolism. Critically ill patients with AKI typically have hypercatabolic states due to the increased production of stress hormones and cytokines [35]. These mediators increase proteolysis, glycogenolysis, gluconeogenesis, and lipolysis and result in increased muscle catabolism and urea production. Critically ill patients often receive insufficient nutritional replacement to balance these processes. In the setting of AKI, daily or continuous RRT allows better nutritional supplementation [36]. When should we stop dialysis in this context? Decreased catabolism and increasing anabolism may be some of the parameters to assess for cessation of RRT. The protein catabolic rate (PCR), also called the protein equivalent of nitrogen appearance (PNA), is a measure of catabolism frequently utilized in the ESRD population. This measure has also been utilized in the AKI population and has been shown to be markedly elevated especially when associated with critical illness [37, 38]. No study has determined a precise cut-off to delineate the best timing for cessation of RRT. Nevertheless, if appropriate nitrogen balance can be maintained within the capacity of the kidneys to manage the volume of nutritional supplementation, cessation of RRT may be tried if other conditions for stopping RRT are met.

7.14.1.2.3 Futility

Medical futility has been defined as "medical interventions where either the likelihood of benefit to the patient is exceedingly small, and falls well below a threshold considered minimal, or the quality of outcome associated with the intervention is exceedingly poor, and falls well below a threshold considered minimal" [39]. Acute kidney injury portends an increase in mortality and morbidity and subset of patients will not improve despite appropriate therapy. In this situation, withdrawal of acute care might be envisaged if the therapy is regarded as futile, prolonging an evitable death.

The incidence of withdrawal of life-support treatments in critically ill patients with multiorgan failure has increased over the last decade [40]. In general, decisions to withdraw therapy occur in 10% of all patients from general ICU and are responsible for roughly 40% of all deaths [41]. In one study, the frequency of withdrawal of therapy has been related to occurrence of severe acute renal failure. In this study, life-support withdrawal occurred in 72% of deaths. A prolonged stay in the ICU, defined as well beyond 2 weeks, was associated with withdrawal of care [41]. In a single-center retrospective study involving 179 patients with AKI, therapy was withheld or withdrawn in 21.2% [42]. Withholding or withdrawing treatment was independently associated with age and predicted mortality. Interestingly, chronic medical diagnoses did not influence the decision process.

7.14.1.3 RRT Cessation: How to Stop?

Cessation of RRT can occur in at least three different clinical situations. The first one is a *withdrawal of treatment*, as previously defined. In this situation, dialysis is usually stopped by the patient or his/her family in concert with the attending physician. A consensus decision among the caregivers is often required before the patient and/or family is approached to discuss the situation [42]. To make such a decision, several parameters are assessed such as the severity of the acute illness and its potential of reversibility, the patient's wishes and his or her quality of life. We believe that withdrawal of therapy should be undertaken after a consensus is obtained between the patient, his/her legally authorized representative if applicable, and the physicians. The patient's decision should always be prioritized unless its ability to take a decision is impaired. The second situation is a *trial of therapy*. A trial of therapy usually occurs in the setting of a high probability of mortality regardless of what is provided, yet the small chance of survival warrants therapeutic intervention. A trial of therapy implies that the parameters of success of therapy are clearly defined and a definite time frame for achieving these goals is set, for example, 4 or 5 days. At the end of the time period, the patient's condition is reassessed based on the parameters of improvement agreed upon. If conditions are met, a further trial of therapy may be given; if not, then a discussion with the patient and his/her family needs to be held regarding discontinuation of therapy. The third situation is a condition where "*full treatment options*" are provided and the dialysis is stopped when the patient dies or the patient's renal condition improved. In the latter condition, once the indications for renal replacement are no longer present, and it is deemed safe to "stop dialysis," then two options are available: either stop or wean dialysis sessions.

By stopping dialysis sessions, it is assumed that no further need for dialysis will be required in the next days. The process of weaning dialysis sessions refers to a change in the modality, the frequency or the duration of RRT. For example, stopping CRRT for SLED or IHD, decreasing the frequency of IHD from daily to every other day or reducing the duration of continuous renal replacement therapy CRRT from 24 h/day to 12 h/day are different methods of weaning RRT. The concept of weaning therapy is assessed according to the demand versus the capacity. The following parameters need to be evaluated in this situation: indications for dialysis, hemodynamic status and use of vasopressors, fluid balance, catabolic rate, nutritional status, and the need for patient's mobilization.

A change of modality from CRRT to SLED or IHD is frequent when there is no improvement in kidney function and stabilization of the hemodynamic status. CRRT is renowned for better hemodynamic stability [36] and a recent Cochrane meta-analysis confirmed that patients on CRRT had a reduced risk of requiring escalation of vasopressor therapy [43]. CRRT has also been shown to provide both better fluid balance and nutrition compared with IHD [36]. Thus before switching modality, it is important to ensure that the new modality will allow adequate fluid balance and nutritional delivery. As opposed to CRRT, SLED and IHD will enhance patient's mobility and may decrease costs [44–46].

The concepts of reducing the duration or decrease the frequency of dialysis are not supported by evidence-based medicine. In fact, the concept of dialysis dose has been studied as if a fixed dose was required during AKI [47, 48]. No study has assessed the best approach to adjust dialysis dose parameters over the course of AKI. It is therefore impossible to make formal recommendations on this topic. However, we usually reduce the duration or the frequency when the overall condition has improved, implying that catabolism has returned to normal and hemodynamic status has stabilized, and persistent kidney dysfunction is still present. We always ensure that the determined goal for fluid balance will be reached and that nutrition status is adequate.

For many years, diuretics have been used in an attempt to accelerate the weaning process. The role of diuretics to promote diuresis and reduce the frequency or duration of dialysis remains controversial. Recent meta-analyses do not support the use of loop diuretics to improve renal recovery in AKI [49–51]. However, diuretics may shorten the duration of RRT. Three recent meta-analyses have been performed on this subject. In one, the dialysis duration was shortened by 1.4 days on average [49]. Another did not found a reduction in the number of dialysis sessions [50], while the third meta-analysis showed a trend toward reduction for the number of dialyses [51]. Despite a lack of confirmed efficacy, a multinational survey confirmed that diuretics are commonly used in AKI [52]. Most respondents said that their typical target output was 0.5–1 ml/kg/h. In a trial involving post-cardiac surgery patients comparing two diuretics, patients were taken off CRRT when urine output was at least 0.5 ml/kg/h for 6 h. Both furosemide and torsemide were adjusted to maintain a target urine output between 0.8 and 1.5 ml/kg/h. Both diuretics were able to maintain urine output and 25 out of 29 patients maintained dialysis independence. However, there was no control group without diuretic [53]. In summary, diuretic responsiveness may help to shorten the duration of dialysis, guide cessation of RRT and maintain dialysis independence.

7.14.1.4 Monitoring Treatment Cessation

After RRT has been stopped, unless there has been a dramatic improvement in kidney function, both BUN and creatinine levels should increased because the residual kidney function is lower than the sum of residual kidney function and dialysis clearance. BUN and creatinine levels should reach a plateau within the next 24–48 h. During this period, it is important to assess the urine flow rate to determine if it is sufficient to meet the demand. Both creatinine, BUN, potassium, and bicarbonate levels should probably be checked a few hours after dialysis cessation, every 12 h for the first 24 h and then daily for a few days. In certain circumstances, such as the recent correction of severe hyperkalemia, more frequent laboratory checks should be undertaken.

7.14.2 Take Home Pearls

- Little attention has been given in the literature to the most appropriate timing and method for stopping acute kidney therapy; however, several steps are required to ensure a successful cessation:
  - The initial indication for dialysis should have resolved.

- The demands versus the capacity for fluid balance should at least be proportional.
- There should be signs of kidney function recovery.

- Currently, BUN, creatinine, and urine output are the major tools used to assess kidney recovery. In the near future, other biomarkers might be available to predict improvement in kidney function. Then either a cessation or weaning of therapy should be undertaken and patient's status closely followed in the next hours.
- For the patients whose prognosis is exceedingly poor or who do not present any improvement in their global condition after several days on therapy, withdrawal of therapy or a trial of therapy should be considered.

References

1. Liu KD, Himmelfarb J, Paganini E, et al. (2006) Timing of initiation of dialysis in critically ill patients with acute kidney injury. Clin J Am Soc Nephrol 1:915–9.
2. Bagshaw SM, Mortis G, Godinez-Luna T, et al. (2006) Renal recovery after severe acute renal failure. Int J Artif Organs 29:1023–30.
3. Liano F, Pascual J (1996) Epidemiology of acute renal failure: a prospective, multicenter, community-based study. Madrid Acute Renal Failure Study Group. Kidney Int 50:811–8.
4. Nash K, Hafeez A, Hou S (2002) Hospital-acquired renal insufficiency. Am J Kidney Dis 39:930–6.
5. Uchino S, Bellomo R, Kellum JA, et al. (2007) Patient and kidney survival by dialysis modality in critically ill patients with acute kidney injury. Int J Artif Organs 30:281–92.
6. Uchino S, Bellomo R, Ronco C (2001) Intermittent versus continuous renal replacement therapy in the ICU: impact on electrolyte and acid-base balance. Intensive Care Med 27:1037–43.
7. Marshall MR, Golper TA, Shaver MJ, et al. (2002) Urea kinetics during sustained low-efficiency dialysis in critically ill patients requiring renal replacement therapy. Am J Kidney Dis 39:556–70.
8. Blumberg A, Roser HW, Zehnder C, et al. (1997) Plasma potassium in patients with terminal renal failure during and after haemodialysis; relationship with dialytic potassium removal and total body potassium. Nephrol Dial Transplant 12:1629–34.
9. Allon M, Shanklin N (1995) Effect of albuterol treatment on subsequent dialytic potassium removal. Am J Kidney Dis 26:607–13.
10. Veenstra J, Smit WM, Krediet RT, et al. (1994) Relationship between elevated creatine phosphokinase and the clinical spectrum of rhabdomyolysis. Nephrol Dial Transplant 9:637–41.
11. Cairo MS, Bishop M (2004) Tumour lysis syndrome: new therapeutic strategies and classification. Brit J Haematol 127:3–11.
12. Rocktaeschel J, Morimatsu H, Uchino S, et al. (2003) Acid-base status of critically ill patients with acute renal failure: analysis based on Stewart-Figge methodology. Crit Care 7:R60.
13. Rocktaschel J, Morimatsu H, Uchino S, et al. (2003) Impact of continuous veno-venous hemofiltration on acid-base balance. Int J Artif Organs 26:19–25.
14. Gauthier PM, Szerlip HM (2002) Metabolic acidosis in the intensive care unit. Crit Care Clin 18:289–308.
15. Heering P, Ivens K, Thumer O, et al. (1999) Acid-base balance and substitution fluid during continuous hemofiltration. Kidney Int Suppl:S37–40.
16. Thomas AN, Guy JM, Kishen R, et al. (1997) Comparison of lactate and bicarbonate buffered haemofiltration fluids: use in critically ill patients. Nephrol Dial Transplant 12:1212–7.
17. Kraut JA, Kurtz I (2008) Toxic alcohol ingestions: clinical features, diagnosis, and management. Clin J Am Soc Nephrol 3:208–25.
18. Chu J, Stolbach A (2007) Metformin intoxication. In UpToDate, BD Rose (ed.). Waltham: UpToDate.
19. Mehta RL (2001) Indications for dialysis in the ICU: renal replacement vs. renal support. Blood Purif 19:227–32.
20. Robert S, Zarowitz BJ, Peterson EL, et al. (1993) Predictability of creatinine clearance estimates in critically ill patients. Crit Care Med 21:1487–95.
21. Le Bricon T, Leblanc I, Benlakehal M, et al. (2005) Evaluation of renal function in intensive care: plasma cystatin C vs. creatinine and derived glomerular filtration rate estimates. Clin Chem Lab Med 43:953–7.
22. Shealy CB, Campbell RC, Hey JC, et al. (2003) 24-hr creatinine clearance as a guide for CRRT withdrawal: a retrospective study. Blood Purif 21:192.
23. Baek SM, Brown RS, Shoemaker WC (1973) Early prediction of acute renal failure and recovery. I. Sequential measurements of free water clearance. Ann Surg 177:253–8.
24. Baek SM, Makabali GG, Brown RS, et al. (1975) Free-water clearance patterns as predictors and therapeutic guides in acute renal failure. Surgery 77:632–40.
25. Bagshaw SM, Bellomo R (2007) Early diagnosis of acute kidney injury. Curr Opin Crit Care 13:638–44.
26. Parikh CR, Mishra J, Thiessen-Philbrook H, et al. (2006) Urinary IL-18 is an early predictive biomarker of acute kidney injury after cardiac surgery. Kidney Int 70:199–203.
27. Uchino S, Bellomo R, Morimatsu H, et al. (2007) Continuous renal replacement therapy: a worldwide practice survey: the Beginning and Ending Supportive Therapy for the Kidney (B.E.S.T. Kidney) Investigators. Intensive Care Med 33:1563–70.
28. Hansen HE, Amdisen A (1978) Lithium intoxication (Report of 23 cases and review of 100 cases from the literature). Quart J Med 47:123–44.
29. Traub SJ (2007) Aspirin intoxication in adults. In UpToDate, BD Rose (ed.). Waltham: UpToDate.
30. Jacobs F, Brivet FG (2004) Conventional haemodialysis significantly lowers toxic levels of phenobarbital. Nephrol Dial Transplant 19:1663–4.
31. Palmer BF. 2000. Effectiveness of hemodialysis in the extracorporeal therapy of phenobarbital overdose. Am J Kidney Dis 36:640–3.

32. Gillespie RS, Seidel K, Symons JM (2004) Effect of fluid overload and dose of replacement fluid on survival in hemofiltration. Pediatr Nephrol 19:1394–9.
33. Goldstein SL, Somers MJ, Baum MA, et al. (2005) Pediatric patients with multi-organ dysfunction syndrome receiving continuous renal replacement therapy. Kidney Int 67:653–8.
34. Goldstein SL, Currier H, Graf C, et al. (2001) Outcome in children receiving continuous venovenous hemofiltration. Pediatrics 107:1309–12.
35. Wooley JA, Btaiche IF, Good KL (2005) Metabolic and nutritional aspects of acute renal failure in critically ill patients requiring continuous renal replacement therapy. Nutr Clin Pract 20:176–91.
36. Lameire N, Van Biesen W, Vanholder R (2005) Acute renal failure. Lancet 365:417–30.
37. Leblanc M, Garred LJ, Cardinal J, et al. (1998) Catabolism in critical illness: estimation from urea nitrogen appearance and creatinine production during continuous renal replacement therapy. Am J Kidney Dis 32:444–53.
38. Maxvold NJ, Smoyer WE, Custer JR, et al. (2000) Amino acid loss and nitrogen balance in critically ill children with acute renal failure: a prospective comparison between classic hemofiltration and hemofiltration with dialysis. Crit Care Med 28:1161–5.
39. Jecker NS (2007) Medical futility: a paradigm analysis. HEC Forum 19:13–32.
40. Prendergast TJ, Luce JM (1997) Increasing incidence of withholding and withdrawal of life support from the critically ill. Am J Respir Crit Care Med 155:15–20.
41. Swartz R, Perry E, Daley J (2004) The frequency of withdrawal from acute care is impacted by severe acute renal failure. J Palliat Med 7:676–82.
42. Ho KM, Liang J, Hughes T, et al. (2003) Withholding and withdrawal of therapy in patients with acute renal injury: a retrospective cohort study. Anaesthesia Intensive Care 31:509–13.
43. Rabindranath K, Adams J, Macleod AM, et al. (2007) Intermittent versus continuous renal replacement therapy for acute renal failure in adults. Cochrane Database Syst Rev:CD003773.
44. Hoyt DB (1997) CRRT in the area of cost containment: is it justified? Am J Kidney Dis 30:S102–4.
45. Manns B, Doig CJ, Lee H, et al. (2003) Cost of acute renal failure requiring dialysis in the intensive care unit: clinical and resource implications of renal recovery. Crit Care Med 31:449–55.
46. Vitale C, Bagnis C, Marangella M, et al. (2003) Cost analysis of blood purification in intensive care units: continuous versus intermittent hemodiafiltration. J Nephrol 16:572–9.
47. Ronco C, Bellomo R, Homel P, et al. (2000) Effects of different doses in continuous veno-venous haemofiltration on outcomes of acute renal failure: a prospective randomised trial. Lancet 356:26–30.
48. Saudan P, Niederberger M, De Seigneux S, et al. (2006) Adding a dialysis dose to continuous hemofiltration increases survival in patients with acute renal failure. Kidney Int 70:1312–7.
49. Bagshaw SM, Delaney A, Haase M, et al. (2007) Loop diuretics in the management of acute renal failure: a systematic review and meta-analysis. Crit Care Resusc 9:60–8.
50. Ho KM, Sheridan DJ (2006) Meta-analysis of frusemide to prevent or treat acute renal failure. BMJ 333:420.
51. Sampath S, Moran JL, Graham PL, et al. (2007) The efficacy of loop diuretics in acute renal failure: assessment using Bayesian evidence synthesis techniques. Crit Care Med 35:2516–24.
52. Bagshaw SM, Delaney A, Jones D, et al. (2007) Diuretics in the management of acute kidney injury: a multinational survey. Contrib Nephrol 156:236–49.
53. Vargas Hein O, Staegemann M, Wagner D, et al. (2005) Torsemide versus furosemide after continuous renal replacement therapy due to acute renal failure in cardiac surgery patients. Ren Fail 27:385–92.

Part VIII

Extracorporeal Therapies for Nonrenal Indications

8.1 Extracorporeal Therapies and Immunomodulation During Sepsis

Jörg C. Schefold and Achim Jörres

Core Messages

- A hallmark in the pathophysiology of sepsis is the excessive release of endogenous and exogenous inflammatory mediators.
- Various blood purification techniques aiming at the removal of such mediators have been employed as adjunctive therapy in patients with sepsis.
- Renal-dose hemodialysis and hemofiltration with standard protocols and materials have proved ineffective.
- High-volume protocols and/or use of high cut-off membranes may offer better biochemical efficacy; however, their impact on clinical outcomes is unclear.
- Plasma separation, in particular when combined with (unselective or selective) (immuno-) adsorption procedures, are most promising in terms of mediator clearances.
- Until the clinical efficacy of extracorporeal therapies for immunomodulation during sepsis is demonstrated by clinical trials, they cannot be recommended as standard clinical procedures.

8.1.1 Introduction

Despite recent advances in critical care medicine, the treatment of patients with sepsis remains a major challenge. Sepsis has a rising incidence, a persisting high mortality, and remains a leading cause of acute renal failure (ARF), multiple organ dysfunction, and death. Thus, sepsis is considered to account for a major burden on public health care systems. In the pathogenetic course of sepsis, excessive release of endogenous and exogenous inflammatory mediators such as lipopolysaccharides (LPS), tumor necrosis factor-α (TNF-α), Interleukin-6 (IL-6), and interferon gamma (IFN-γ) occurs. In a complex dynamic control system, inflammatory stimuli then yield the release of antiinflammatory mediators, and activate various pathways including the complement and coagulation cascade. This leads to cellular damage, enhanced apoptosis, and end-organ failure. Importantly, counter-regulatory antiinflammation leads to monocytic deactivation and failure of cellular immunity in a large number or patients. To reduce the levels of circulating mediators, various approaches have been investigated including *selective* and *unselective* intermittent and continuous extracorporeal treatment devices. Today, new blood purification techniques such as selective plasmapheresis and adsorption technologies provide new therapeutic avenues to target key mediators in patients with sepsis.

8.1.2 The Immunopathogenesis of Sepsis: A Role for an Extracorporeal Intervention?

The early proinflammatory phase of sepsis is characterized by an excessive release of proinflammatory mediators in response to a microbial infection [1–3]. Multiple

J. C. Schefold (✉)
Department of Nephrology and Medical Intensive Care, Charité-Universitätsmedizin Berlin, Campus Virchow-Klinikum, 13343 Berlin, Germany
email: joerg.schefold@charite.de

A. Jörres et al. (eds.), *Management of Acute Kidney Problems*,
DOI: 10.1007/978-3-540-69441-0_8.1, © Springer-Verlag Berlin Heidelberg 2010

pleiotropic mediators react in complex feedback-regulated dynamic cascades. Clinically, this is associated with hyperdynamic shock, increased shunting and the development of multiple organ failure (MOF) [1–3]. In cases of persisting inflammation, a prompt induction (mostly within 24 h) of antiinflammatory mechanisms occurs. This includes an increased expression of IL-10 and transforming growth factor-beta (TGF-β) and initiates a compensatory antiinflammatory response syndrome (CARS) [3]. At the cellular level this leads to monocytic deactivation in a large number of septic patients. This has been termed "immunoparalysis" and is characterized by reduced monocytic phagocytotic and antigen-processing capabilities, inadequate antigen presentation, and a reduced liberation of cytokines from respective immune cells [4–10]. Importantly, such functional failure of monocytic immunity has been demonstrated to predict reduced survival in sepsis [5–9]. Immunoparalysis may also induce other "downstream" immune phenomena, such as lymphocyte apoptosis and can be assessed via quantitative standardized measurement of the human leukocyte antigen-DR (HLA-DR) expression on monocytes/macrophages [11]. Today, it is well recognized that most patients die from sepsis in this late "hyporesponsive" phase from secondary "infectious hits" in a state of chronic MOF.

Since the 1980s, a large number of prospective randomized clinical sepsis trials aimed to neutralize LPS or to block single short-lived pleiotropic inflammatory mediators using, e.g., antibody mediated approaches (e.g., LPS, IL-1β, or TNF-α). However, these efforts have largely failed [1–3]. Such failure may be attributable to the unidirectional character of these therapeutic efforts and may be a consequence of an inability to prevent the failure of cell-mediated immunity. Nevertheless, these sepsis trials suggested that the modulation of a single mediator or a single immunologic pathway may not lead to significant benefits with regard to the clinical outcome of septic patients. Thereafter, the scientific focus shifted toward nonspecific methods of influencing the inflammatory response. The impact of extracorporeal interventions to restore an "immunologic homeostasis" in sepsis was then studied in clinical trials using measures of convection, diffusion, and adsorption. The third Acute Dialysis Quality Initiative (ADQI) consensus conference stated that there is a biological rationale for extracorporeal blood treatment (EBT) in sepsis [12]. This is based on the understanding that most molecules of interest are water-soluble and fall into the "middle-molecular-weight category" of 5–60 kDa [13–18]. Of special interest with regard to EBT are LPS, cytokines/chemokines (high mobility group box-1 [HMGB-1] and macrophage migration inhibitory factor [MIF]), activated complement factors (C3a and C5a), coagulation factors, eicosanoids, and leukotrienes.

8.1.3 Continuous Renal Replacement Techniques and EBT in Sepsis

Impaired renal function is an almost obligatory element of septic multiple organ dysfunction syndrome. In sepsis, ARF represents an independent risk factor regarding mortality and should be treated early [19, 20]. ARF itself seems to exert negative immunomodulatory properties, apparently caused by both cellular dysfunction in the uremic environment and reduced tubular degradation of certain inflammatory mediators.

Continuous renal replacement therapies (CRRTs) have been shown to remove various inflammatory mediators from the bloodstream [21]. This was initially demonstrated in pigs that were administered intravenous endotoxin. Improved hemodynamics were found in cases receiving additional hemofiltration [22]. Conversely, infusing healthy animals with an ultrafiltrate of endotoxinemic animals resulted in hemodynamic instability [23]. Today, these studies can be considered the birth of EBT in sepsis. Recently, a number of hypotheses were proposed on how CRRT may affect the sepsis-induced disequilibrium.

First, Ronco and colleagues proposed the "peak concentration hypothesis" [15] suggesting an attenuation of the inflammatory response by hemofiltration of excess cytokines/mediators spilling over to the circulation during peak production. The attenuation of peak inflammatory mediator concentrations by CRRT may beneficially influence the course of the disease [15]. However, it is unclear how the attenuation of peak concentrations would impact local and interstitial space mediator production, as well as whether this would modulate cellular function and, importantly, cell-mediated immunity. A successful potent intervention aiming to cut off peak concentrations would require highly efficient removal procedures, which is most likely not met by renal intensive care unit (ICU) dose (30–50 ml/kg/h) hemofiltration. Alternatively, extracorporeal therapies with higher mediator clearance capacities such as high-volume hemofiltration, techniques using high-permeable membranes, or procedures such as selective immunoadsorption or unselective hemoperfusion might be required to achieve the desired impact on mediator removal. The second hypothesis named the "threshold immunomodulation hypothesis" [24] was proposed by P. Honoré, and focuses on the complexity and nonlinear properties of inflammatory networks. The redundancy of pleiotropic proinflammatory mediators might result in cascades still functioning even if one or few components are blocked. Nonselective filtration-based removal of various mediators might interrupt such cascades, and the depletion of a particular mediator would result in its redistribution from the tissue to the circulation, where it can be removed. This process is postulated to continue up to a "threshold point" at which some cascades shut down and end-organ injury may be stopped [24]. However, although a mediator reduction occurs at the tissue and interstitial space level, it seems difficult to determine when such a "threshold point" is reached. Furthermore, the mechanism by which filtration facilitates mediator flow from the interstitium to the blood compartment remains unexplained. Whilst both abovementioned concepts concentrate on the removal of circulating mediators, the "mediator delivery hypothesis" [24] proposed by J. V. DiCarlo and S. R. Alexander suggests that the kinetics of cytokine removal by filtration mostly depend on interstitial cytokine washout. In this model, the infusion of large volumes of replacement fluid drives a dynamic interstitial circulation that delivers mediators and middle molecular weight molecules from the interstitium via the lymphatics to the bloodstream and thus to various points of elimination [25]. Indeed, it has been demonstrated that with extensive fluid infusion (3–5 l/h), lymphatic flow can increase by about a factor of 20–40 [26]. Thus, this theory suggests that hemofiltration may exert an effect at the lymphatic level rather than by direct removal of mediators.

At present, available data do not allow to conclude which of the above concepts best reflects the observed impact of hemofiltration on patients with sepsis. It seems, however, reasonable to conclude that the ideal immunomodulating strategy would be one that restores immunologic stability and efficiently modulates cellular immune function rather than blindly inhibiting or stimulating one or another component of the complex cytokine network. In addition to CRRT, specific EBT adsorption techniques are currently developed for the discontinuous and continuous treatment of septic patients [13–18].

8.1.4 High-Volume Hemofiltration

Comparative trials of convection and diffusion techniques for EBT in sepsis have demonstrated that middle-molecular-weight molecules and large mediators are more effectively reduced using convective measures [27]. Since the in vivo generation rate of inflammatory mediators is high when compared with urea, high-volume hemofiltration (HVHF) should require a membrane of appropriately high permeability, large surface, and a sieving coefficient close to 1 for molecules up to approximately 60 kDa in order to achieve a significant mediator reduction [13–18]. In addition to convective clearance, adsorption of mediators to synthetic membranes appears responsible for the reduction of the respective molecules [28–30]. Hemofiltration rates were increased in order to amplify the convective clearance and HVHF was developed. Later, HVHF was defined as > 35 ml/kg/h [12] and filtration rates of up to 215 ml/kg/h were investigated. In a controlled randomized landmark trial including 425 ICU patients with ARF (approx. 13% septic patients), Ronco et al. demonstrated that increasing the CRRT filtration dose to 35 ml/kg/h improves survival (57% vs 41%, $p = 0.0007$) when compared with the conventional dose (20 ml/kg/h) [31]. An additional dose increase (45 ml/kg/h) did not lead to furthermore improved survival rates at 15 days after termination of hemofiltration (HF) therapy. Nevertheless, in the subgroup of patients with sepsis, the lowest mortality rate was observed in the group receiving the highest dose [31].

Nonrandomized uncontrolled HVHF studies using different doses of HVHF (mostly 40–70 ml/kg/h) in septic patients and in animals (usually doses of about 100 ml/kg/h) observed improvements in hemodynamics and reduced vasopressor need. Some of these studies even reported improved survival rates [32–38]. Interestingly, one randomized trial demonstrates that out-of-hospital cardiac arrest patients may benefit from very high volume HF (200 ml/kg/h) [36]. In addition to the higher dose being delivered using a constantly high exchange rates (> 45 ml/kg/h), higher doses may also be applied via time-limited (usually 6–8 h) "pulses" of HVHF [35]. Nevertheless, mediator removal from the blood compartment via HVHF is considered unsatisfactory [35, 36]. In addition, due to inconsistent and insufficient data, HVHF therapy cannot currently be recommended as an adjunctive therapy for patients with severe sepsis and septic shock without ARF outside of clinical studies.

8.1.5 High Cutoff Dialysis/Hemofiltration and High-Flux Dialysis

An alternative way to improve the clearance of immune mediators by dialysis and hemofiltration is to increase the pore size of respective membranes (to a cutoff of around 45–100 kDa in human blood, pore size about 0.1 μm). A number of different high cutoff (HCO) membranes with varying chemical compositions (polyamide, polysulfone, polyarylethersulfone, and cellulose triacetate) have been tested in ex vivo and in single-center clinical trials [39]. Recent animal and human pilot studies have demonstrated beneficial effects on hemodynamics and on the levels of immune mediators (e.g., IL-6, IL-1 receptor antagonist [IL-1ra], TNF-α, and soluble TNF-α type 1 receptor) [39–41]. However, the interpretation of the respective data from four pilot trials (two uncontrolled trials, one blinded trial) investigating a total of 70 patients with septic ARF at two centers is difficult, as different HCO membranes, different modalities of blood purification (hemofiltration, hemodialysis, and hemodiafiltration), different (blood, filtration, and dialysate) flows, and different membrane sizes in the range of 1.1–2.2 m^2 were tested. Furthermore, most trials did not include an adequate control group, only partly reported data on hemodynamics, and did not investigate cellular immunity. Nevertheless, in these trials, IL-6 clearances were 40 ml/min at maximum (for HCO CVVH), and were 42 ml/min for IL-1ra. When compared with controls, a significant reduction in IL-6 and IL-1ra was achieved under treatment [42]. Two other pilot trials on HCO-CVVH and HCO-CVVHDF did not report data on hemodynamics [41, 43].

Importantly, the use of high cutoff filters leads to relevant loss of proteins and molecules such as albumin (up to 7.7 g per session under intermittent HCO hemodialysis, molecular weight 66 kDa). Only a few data on the loss of other prognostically important molecules such as coagulation factors exist. Although this might imply a negative prognostic impact on sepsis, plasma albumin levels have also been demonstrated rather stable over HCO treatment [43]. Nevertheless, application of HCO membranes seem to provide more effective means with regard to a more efficient (unselective) removal of middle-molecular-weight molecules. However, the optimal cutoff remains unknown, and it is not clear whether HCO treatment is capable of beneficially modulating cellular immunity. As large-scale randomized studies have not been conducted, adjunctive therapy using high flux dialysis can currently not be recommended outside of clinical trials.

8.1.6 Plasmapheresis/Plasma Separation

Plasmapheresis is a nonselective process aimed to replace patient plasma with replacement fluids (donor plasma or albumin). Early human studies investigating plasmapheresis as an adjunctive sepsis therapy demonstrated that it enables an effective reduction of various inflammatory mediators [44]. The largest prospective randomized study of plasmapheresis in sepsis involved 106 patients [45] in whom treatment was performed within 6 h after establishing of the diagnosis and was repeated once whenever patients did not seem to respond. In each session, a volume of 30–40 ml/kg body weight of plasma was exchanged with an equal volume of fresh-frozen plasma, diluted with a 5% human albumin solution. A trend toward a significant reduction in the APACHE III score and in 28-day mortality (53.8% [28/52] versus 33.3% [18/54], $p = 0.05$) was observed. The relative risk for mortality in the treatment group was 0.61, corresponding to an absolute risk reduction of 20.5%, and a number needed to treat of 4.9 was calculated [45].

8.1.7 Adsorption: Hemoperfusion and Plasma Separation/Adsorption

To further increase the clearance of target molecules, adsorption techniques were developed. This approach employs membranes or surface-bound (mostly polyclonal) antibodies to bind target mediators. The binding of respective molecules to the surfaces/antibodies is a result of hydrophobic interactions, electrostatic attraction, hydrogen bonding and van der Waals forces. In general, *whole-blood-based* (hemoperfusion) and *plasma-based* adsorption techniques are distinguished. Whole-blood-based techniques employ the adsorber in the primary extracorporeal circuit. Plasma-based techniques require a plasma separation procedure to feed a secondary circuit in which plasma is brought in contact with adsorber materials. Severe biocompatibility issues, which have limited this approach in the past, have been overcome. The development of new biocompatible matrices and surfaces presents new opportunities and indications are continuously extended [46]. The key advantage of adsorption technology is its ability to selectively intervene in defined cascades while being both highly biocompatible and potent.

8.1.8 Direct Hemoperfusion/Adsorption

The removal of LPS from the circulation of septic patients via extracorporeal blood purification methods has been considered for decades. A large variety of materials have been analyzed in this regard, and various LPS adsorbers have been developed. Polymyxin B, a neurotoxic and nephrotoxic cationic cyclic decapeptide antibiotic, binds endotoxin. Thus, polymyxin-B was immobilized to polystyrene fibers in a device and septic patients received adjunctive treatment via direct hemoperfusion (reviewed in [47]). A number of nonrandomized pilot trials were performed, mostly in Japan. As far back as 30 years ago, improved hemodynamic stability under LPS adsorption was reported under experimental conditions [48] and recent in vivo results might support these findings [49–51]. A current systematic review of 28 studies (9 randomized trials) with mostly limited methodological quality indicates that adjuvant direct hemoperfusion using polymyxin-B based adsorption might beneficial influence hemodynamics and vasopressor need [47]. Although a relative risk of 0.53 (95% confidence interval, 0.43–0.65) was calculated by the authors of the above-mentioned systematic review [47], no large-scale randomized trials exist, and lower mortality has not been sufficiently demonstrated. In a multicenter randomized study, non-polymyxin-B-based LPS adsorption did not affect the primary end point which was a reduction of the APACHE-II score by > 4 points after 4 days of therapy [52]. In this study, patients were treated daily for 4 days with 1.5-fold of the estimated blood volume being processed over 3–4 h. Other authors confirmed these findings in that sole LPS adsorption did not lead to improvements in morbidity and organ dysfunction [53–55].

8.1.9 Coupled Plasma Filtration Adsorption

Coupled plasma filtration adsorption (CPFA) is a hybrid process using both plasma filtration and plasma adsorption. After plasma separation the plasma passes through a synthetic resin cartridge and a second blood filter or dialyzer might be installed for fluid and small molecular weight toxin removal. The complex intervention which involves a plasma filter, a sorbent cartridge and a dialyzer may be performed for 10 h and can be followed by overnight continuous renal replacement therapy. In experimental animal models of endotoxinemia and in early human sepsis trials, CPFA was demonstrated to unselectively reduce various inflammatory mediators. The approach resulted in improved animal survival and might reduce vasopressor requirements in humans [56–59].

8.1.10 Plasma Filtration/Selective Adsorption

Immunological interventions require evidence of immunological efficacy. Thus, an immunological characterization of study cohorts seems crucial. In particular, early EBT studies with a limited number of study patients mostly did not adequately characterize the patients' immunological status. Nowadays this may be regarded a prerequisite to clinical investigations in sepsis. Not to use an immune-guided approach (including an assessment of cellular immunity) in EBT aiming to reduce immunological mediators may clearly be considered not up-to-date and to be doomed to failure [60]. Thus, it is not clear whether the end points chosen in some of the above-mentioned sepsis EBT trials adequately portray the effectiveness of an immunological intervention.

In a prospective controlled pilot trial, it was therefore investigated whether selective simultaneous LPS, IL-6, and complement factor C5a immunoadsorption leads to improved monocytic function and whether this yields improved organ function [61] in septic patients. As assessed by the monocytic HLA-DR expression, LPS, IL-6, and C5a immunoadsorption resulted in significant improvements in monocytic immunity and this procedure was thus found to reverse immunoparalysis.

Table 8.1.1 Extracorporeal techniques for immunomodulation during sepsis

Procedure	Safety	Biochemical efficacy	Clinical efficacy
(Renal-dose) hemodialysis	+++	-	-
(Renal-dose) hemofiltration	+++	-	-
High-volume hemofiltration	++	(+)	?
High cutoff hemofiltration/ hemodialysis	++	++	?
Hemoperfusion/ adsorption	+	+	?
Plasmapheresis	++	+	?
Plasma separation/ (immuno-) adsorption	++	+++	?

Such reversal of monocytic failure was associated with significantly improved hemodynamics and APACHE II scores in the treatment group [61].

Despite encouraging results in initial clinical applications of whole-blood-based and plasma-based interventions, clinical effectiveness has not yet been sufficiently documented (Table 8.1.1). On the other hand, potential adverse effects of these procedures need to be considered. This may include electrolyte abnormalities; hemolysis or loss of platelets, and loss of functional proteins (coagulation factors and immunoglobulins). Thus, based on available data, such therapies cannot be recommended as standard clinical procedures, that is, outside clinical studies.

8.1.11 Conclusions

In sepsis, the homeostasis of the humoral and cellular immune system is profoundly disturbed. EBT strategies provide a promising approach for the interventional treatment of septic patients. Following consensus recommendations [12], a clear biological rationale for the use of such extracorporeal techniques exists. Thus, a biological rationale also applies for extrarenal indications. However, conventional continuous and discontinuous RRT seem to provide insufficient means with regard to a biologically relevant reduction of target mediators. Modified CRRT techniques, high cutoff membranes, and selective and unselective adsorption devices are currently being researched. Some of these approaches have not only been shown to effectively reduce target mediators, but have also been demonstrated to modulate cellular immunity. However, questions regarding the modality, the right dose, and the right timing remain unanswered. Importantly, due to insufficient data, the use of RRT/EBT techniques in septic patients can not currently be recommended in the absence of renal failure. Patients without renal failure should therefore receive EBT treatment only in the context of clinical trials.

8.1.12 Take Home Pearls

- In sepsis, new extracorporeal blood purification techniques may allow a safe and efficient removal of circulating key inflammatory mediators.
- Future efforts in the field should not only target a reduction in single short-lived pleiotropic inflammatory mediators but also aim to beneficially modulate cellular immunity.
- The clinical efficacy of extracorporeal therapies for immunomodulation during sepsis is not sufficiently documented thus far. A potential influence on mortality from sepsis remains unclear. Adjunctive EBT treatment in sepsis should currently only be performed in the context of clinical trials.

References

1. Hotchkiss RS, Karl IE (2003) The pathophysiology and treatment of sepsis. N Engl J Med 348:138–150.
2. Annane D, Bellissant E, Cavaillon JM (2005) Septic shock. Lancet 365:63–78.
3. Cohen J (2002) The immunopathogenesis of sepsis. Nature 420:885–891.
4. Reith W, LeibundGut-Landmann S, Waldburger JM (2005) Regulation of MHC class II gene expression by the class II transactivator. Nat Rev Immunol 5:793–806.
5. Pachot A, Monneret G, Brion A, et al. (2005) Messenger RNA expression of major histocompatibility complex class II genes in whole blood from septic shock patients. Crit Care Med 33:31–38.
6. Tschaikowsky K, Hedwig-Geissing M, Schiele A, et al. (2002) Coincidence of pro- and anti-inflammatory responses in the early phase of severe sepsis: Longitudinal study of mononuclear histocompatibility leukocyte antigen-DR expression, procalcitonin, C-reactive protein, and changes in

T-cell subsets in septic and postoperative patients. Crit Care Med 30: 1015–1023.
7. Monneret G, Lepape A, Voirin N, et al. (2006) Persisting low monocyte human leukocyte antigen-DR expression predicts mortality in septic shock. Intensive Care Med 32: 1175–1183.
8. Lekkou A, Karakantza M, Mouzaki A, et al. (2004) Cytokine production and monocyte HLA-DR expression as predictors of outcome for patients with community-acquired severe infections. Clin Diagn Lab Immunol 11:161–167.
9. Monneret G, Venet F, Pachot A, et al. (2008) Monitoring immune dysfunctions in the septic patient: a new skin for the old ceremony. Mol Med 14: 64–78.
10. Volk HD, Reinke P, Krausch D, et al. (1996) Monocyte deactivation – rationale for a new therapeutic strategy in sepsis. Intensive Care Med 22(Suppl 4):S474–481.
11. Döcke WD, Höflich C, Davis KA, et al. (2005) Monitoring temporary immunodepression by flow cytometric measurement of monocytic HLA-DR expression: a multicenter standardized study. Clin Chem 51:2341–2347.
12. Kellum JA, Bellomo R, Ronco C, et al. (2005) The 3rd International Consensus Conference of the Acute Dialysis Quality Initiative (ADQI). Int J Artif Organs 28:441–444.
13. Bellomo R, Honore PM, Matson J, et al. (2005) Extracorporeal blood treatment (EBT) methods in SIRS/Sepsis. Int J Artif Organs 28:450–458.
14. Ronco C, Inguaggiato P, D'Intini V, et al. (2003) The role of extracorporeal therapies in sepsis. J Nephrol 16(Suppl 7): S34–S41.
15. Ronco C, Bonello M, Bordoni V, et al. (2004) Extracorporeal therapies in non-renal disease: treatment of sepsis and the peak concentration hypothesis. Blood Purif 22:164–174.
16. Venkataraman R, Subramanian S, Kellum JA (2003) Clinical review: extracorporeal blood purification in severe sepsis. Crit Care 7:139–145.
17. Tetta C, D'Intini V, Bellomo R, et al. (2003) Extracorporeal treatments in sepsis: are there new perspectives? Clin Nephrol 60:299–304.
18. Schefold JC, Hasper D, Storm C, et al. (2007) The extracorporeal treatment of septic patients: is there an extrarenal indication? Intensivmedizin und Notfallmedizin 44:57–63.
19. Kellum JA, Angus DC (2002) Patients are dying of acute renal failure. Crit Care Med 30:2156–2157.
20. Druml W (2004): Acute renal failure is not a "cute" renal failure! Intensive Care Med 30: 1886–1890.
21. Gotloib L, Barzilay E, Shustak A, et al. (1986) Hemofiltration in septic ARDS. The artificial kidney as an artificial endocrine lung. Resuscitation 13:123–132.
22. Stein B, Pfenninger E, Grunert A, et al. (1990) Influence of continuous haemofiltration on haemodynamics and central blood volume in experimental endotoxic shock. Intensive Care Med 16:494–499.
23. Grootendorst AF, van Bommel EF, van der Hoven B, et al. (1992) High volume hemofiltration improves right ventricular function in endotoxin-induced shock in the pig. Intensive Care Med 18:235–240.
24. Honore PM, Joannes-Boyau O (2004). High volume hemofiltration (HVHF) in sepsis: a comprehensive review of rationale, clinical applicability, potential indications and recommendations for future research. Int J Artif Organs 27: 1077–1082.
25. Di Carlo JV, Alexander SR (2005) Hemofiltration for cytokine-driven illnesses: the mediator delivery hypothesis. Int J Artif Organs 28:777–786.
26. Olszewski WL (2003) The lymphatic system in body homeostasis: physiological conditions. Lymphat Res Biol 1:11–21.
27. Brunet S, Leblanc M, Geadah D, et al. (1999) Diffusive and convective solute clearances during continuous renal replacement therapy at various dialysate and ultrafiltration flow rates. Am J Kidney Dis 34:486–492.
28. De Vriese AS, Vanholder RC, Pascual M, et al. (1999) Can inflammatory cytokines be removed efficiently by continuous renal replacement therapies? Intensive Care Med 25:903–910.
29. De Vriese AS, Colardyn FA, Philippe JJ, et al. (1999) Cytokine removal during continuous hemofiltration in septic patients. J Am Soc Nephrol 10:846–853.
30. Kellum JA, Dishart MK (2002) Effect of hemofiltration filter adsorption on circulating IL-6 levels in septic rats. Crit Care 6:429–433.
31. Ronco C, Bellomo R, Homel P, et al. (2000) Effects of different doses in continuous veno-venous haemofiltration on outcomes of acute renal failure: a prospective randomised trial. Lancet 356:26–30.
32. Cole L, Bellomo R, Journois D, et al. (2001) High-volume haemofiltration in human septic shock. Intensive Care Med 27:978–986.
33. Honore PM, Jamez J, Wauthier M, et al. (2000) Prospective evaluation of short-term, high-volume isovolemic hemofiltration on the hemodynamic course and outcome in patients with intractable circulatory failure resulting from septic shock. Crit Care Med 28:3581–3587.
34. Oudemans-van Straaten HM, Bosman RJ, van der Spoel JI, et al. (1999): Outcome of critically ill patients treated with intermittent high-volume haemofiltration: a prospective cohort analysis. Intensive Care Med 25:814–821.
35. Honore PM, Joannes-Boyau O, Gressens B (2007): Blood and plasma treatments: High volume hemofiltration- a global view. Contrib Nephrol 156:371–386.
36. Laurent I, Adrie C, Vinsonneau C, et al. (2005) High volume hemofiltration after out-of-hospital cardiac arrest: A randomized study. J Am Coll Cardiol 46:432–437.
37. Yekebas EF, Eisenberger CF, Ohnesorge H, et al. (2001) Attenuation of sepsis-related immunoparalysis by continuous veno-venous hemofiltration in experimental porcine pancreatitis. Crit Care Med 29:1423–1430.
39. Haase M, Bellomo R, Morgera S, et al. (2007) High cut-off point membranes in septic acute renal failure: a systematic review. Int J Artif Organs 30: 1031–1041.
40. Lonnemann G, Bechstein M, Linnenweber S, et al. (1999): Tumor necrosis factor-alpha during continuous high-flux hemodialysis in sepsis with acute renal failure. Kidney Int Suppl S84–S87.
41. Haase M, Bellomo R, Baldwin I, et al. (2007) Hemodialysis membrane with a high-molecular weight cutoff and cytokine levels in sepsis complicated by acute renal failure: A phase 1 randomized trial. Am J Kidney Dis 50:296–304.
42. Morgera S, Haase M, Kuss T, et al. (2006) Pilot study on the effects of high cutoff hemofiltration on the need for norepinephrine in septic patients with acute renal failure. Crit Care Med 34: 2099–2104.
43. Morgera S, Slowinski T, Melzer C, et al. (2004) Renal replacement therapy with high-cutoff hemofilters: Impact of

convection and diffusion on cytokine clearances and protein status. Am J Kidney Dis 43: 444–453.
44. Leese T, Holliday M, Heath D, et al. (1987) Multicentre clinical trial of low volume fresh frozen plasma therapy in acute pancreatitis. Br J Surg 74:907–911.
45. Busund R, Koukline V, Utrobin U, et al. (2002) Plasmapheresis in severe sepsis and septic shock: a prospective, randomised, controlled trial. Intensive Care Med 28:1434–1439.
46. Bosch T (2003) Recent advances in therapeutic apheresis. J Artif Organs 6:1–8.
47. Cruz DN, Perazella MA, Bellomo R, et al. (2007) Effectiveness of polymyxin B-immobilized fiber column in sepsis: a systematic review. Crit Care 1:R47.
48. Palmer JD, Rifkind D (1974) Neutralization of the hemodynamic effects of endotoxin by polymyxin B. Surg Gynecol Obstet 138:755–759.
49. Yonekawa M (2005) Cytokine and endotoxin removal in critically Ill patients. Ther Apher Dial 9:A37.
50. Uriu K, Osajima A, Hiroshige K, et al. (2002) Endotoxin removal by direct hemoperfusion with an adsorbent column using polymyxin B-immobilized fiber ameliorates systemic circulatory disturbance in patients with septic shock. Am J Kidney Dis 39:937–947.
51. Vincent JL, Laterre PF, Cohen J, et al. (2005) A pilot-controlled study of a polymyxin B-immobilized hemoperfusion cartridge in patients with severe sepsis secondary to intra-abdominal infection. Shock 23:400–405.
52. Reinhart K, Meier-Hellmann A, Beale R, et al. (2004) Open randomized phase II trial of an extracorporeal endotoxin adsorber in suspected Gram-negative sepsis. Crit Care Med 32:1662–1668.
53. Bengsch S, Boos KS, Nagel D, et al. (2005) Extracorporeal plasma treatment for the removal of endotoxin in patients with sepsis: clinical results of a pilot study. Shock 23: 494–500.
54. Amoureux MC, Rajapakse N, Hegyi E, et al. (2004) Endotoxin removal from whole blood by a novel adsorption resin: efficiency and hemocompatibility. Int J Artif Organs 27:480–487.
55. Staubach KH, Boehme M, Zimmermann M, et al. (2003) A new endotoxin adsorption device in Gram-negative sepsis: use of immobilized albumin with the MATISSE adsorber. Transfus Apher Sci 29:93–98.
56. Ronco C, Brendolan A, Lonnemann G, et al. (2002) A pilot study of coupled plasma filtration with adsorption in septic shock. Crit Care Med 30:1250–1255.
57. Tetta C, Gianotti L, Cavaillon JM, et al. (2000) Coupled plasma filtration-adsorption in a rabbit model of endotoxic shock. Crit Care Med 28:1526–1533.
58. Tetta C, Cavaillon JM, Schulze M, et al. (1998) Removal of cytokines and activated complement components in an experimental model of continuous plasma filtration coupled with sorbent adsorption. Nephrol Dial Transplant 13: 1458–1464.
59. Bellomo R, Tetta C, Ronco C (2003) Coupled plasma filtration adsorption. Intensive Care Med 29:1222–1228.
60. Schefold JC, Hasper D, Volk HD, et al. (2008) Sepsis: Time has come to focus on the later stages. Med Hypotheses 71: 203–208.
61. Schefold JC, von Haehling S, Corsepius M, et al. (2007) A novel selective extracorporeal intervention in sepsis: immunoadsorption of endotoxin, interleukin 6, and complement-activating product 5a. Shock 28: 418–425.

Extracorporeal Liver Support

8.2

Gesine Pless and Igor Maximilian Sauer

Core Messages

- In patients with liver failure, the accumulation of lipophilic, albumin-bound toxins occurs which cannot be eliminated by standard hemodialysis and hemofiltration techniques. For this purpose (artificial and bioartificial) liver support systems were developed.
- Extracorporeal systems for artificial liver support include:
  - Molecular adsorbents recirculating system (MARS)
  - Single-pass albumin dialysis (SPAD)
  - Fractionated plasma separation and adsorption (Prometheus)
  - Selective plasma exchange therapy (SEPET)
- Extracorporeal systems for bioartificial liver support include:
  - Extracorporeal liver perfusion (ECLP)
  - HepatAssist
  - Extracorporeal liver-assist device (ELAD)
  - Modular extracorporeal liver support system (MELS)
  - Bioartificial liver of the Academisch Medisch Centrum (AMC-BAL)
- The MARS, SPAD, and Prometheus systems are available for clinical use and are mostly employed either for bridging the patient to transplant or else for bridging to recovery of liver function.
- Positive data exist regarding biochemical efficacy and clinical improvement of certain end points such as hepatic encephalopathy, but adequately powered clinical trials evaluating survival rates are at present lacking.

8.2.1 Introduction

Liver transplantation has evolved since 1963 from an experimental procedure, to the standard treatment for the life-threatening syndrome of liver failure. To address the growing disparity between the numbers of suitable donor organs and patients waiting for transplant, efforts have been made to optimize the allocation of organs, find alternatives to cadaveric liver donation, and develop extracorporeal methods to support or replace the failing organ. Liver support devices are used to improve outcome by providing an environment for regeneration of the patient's organ ("bridging to regeneration") or to support the patient until a liver transplant can be carried out ("bridging to transplantation"). Moreover, an extracorporeal liver support device could be of clinical value in the successful management of critical situations after major liver surgery when applied to patients with a small remnant liver volume.

An extracorporeal liver support system has to provide the main functions of the liver: detoxification, synthesis, and regulation. The critical issue of the clinical syndrome in liver failure is understood to be the accumulation of toxins not cleared by the failing liver. Based

I. M. Sauer (✉)
Department of Surgery, Charité Campus Virchow, Augustenburger Platz 1, 13353 Berlin, Germany
e-mail: igor.sauer@charite.de

A. Jörres et al. (eds.), *Management of Acute Kidney Problems*,
DOI: 10.1007/978-3-540-69441-0_8.2,

on this hypothesis, the removal of lipophilic, albumin-bound substances such as bilirubin, bile acids, metabolites of aromatic amino acids, medium-chain fatty acids, and cytokines should be beneficial to the clinical course of a patient in liver failure. This theory led to the development of artificial filtration and adsorption devices (artificial liver support). The complex tasks of regulation and synthesis remain to be addressed by the use of liver cells (bioartificial liver support).

8.2.2 Artificial Liver Support

Conventional continuous venovenous hemodiafiltration (CVVHDF) has been shown to be effective in the removal of water-soluble toxins. To clear the blood of albumin-bound, hydrophobic substances, additional adsorber or acceptor substances are necessary to enhance mass exchange. Albumin is one of the most obvious acceptor substances, since albumin is the predominant carrier of toxins in the patient's blood.

In 1992, Stange, Mitzner, and Ramlow introduced a detoxification system based on albumin dialysis – the molecular adsorbents recirculating system (MARS). Separated from the patient's blood by a high-flux hemodialysis filter, an albumin solution is circulated in a closed circuit. The albumin acts as the acceptor for the toxins and is partly regenerated by passing an anion exchanger and a charcoal adsorber in a closed circuit and is itself dialyzed (Fig. 8.2.1a) [2, 3]. MARS has become the most frequently applied artificial liver

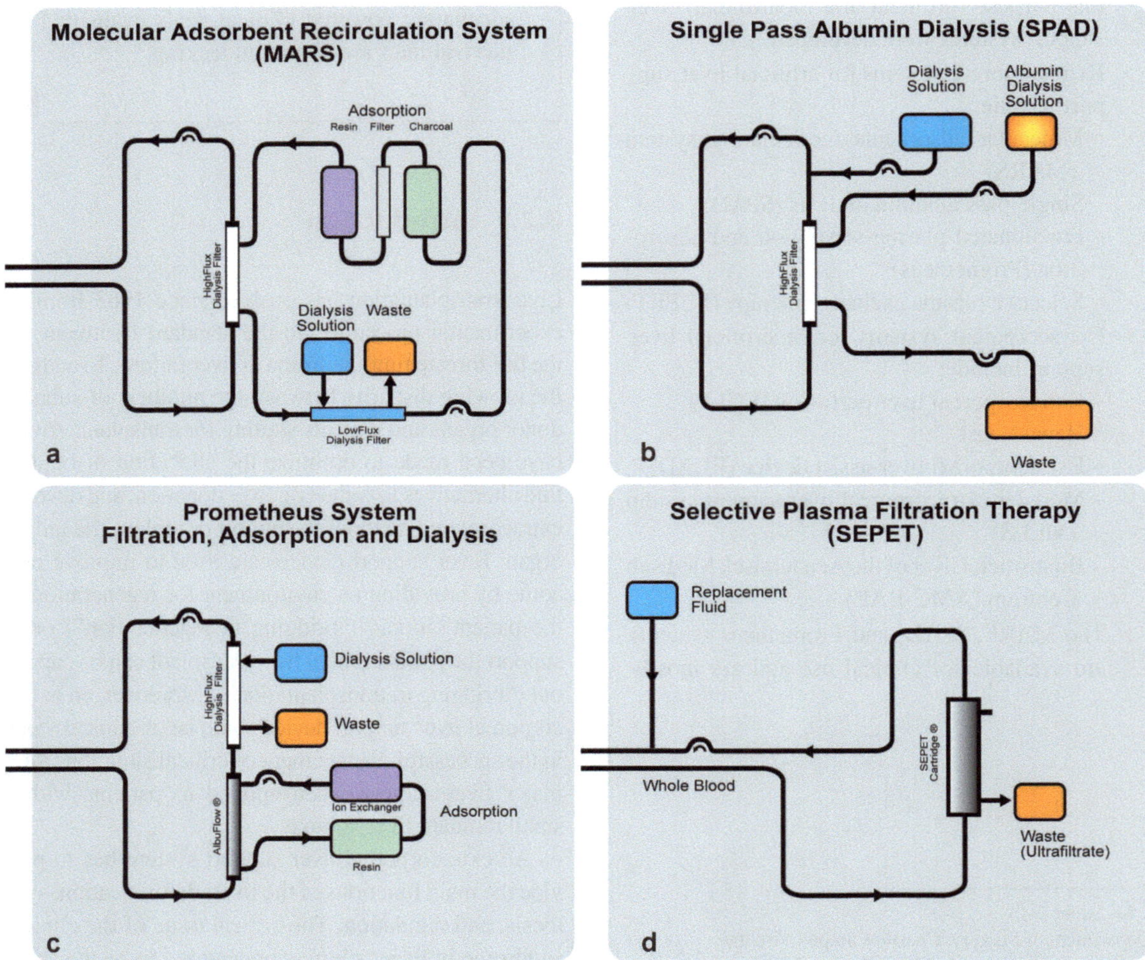

Fig. 8.2.1 Schematic flow diagram for the analysis of different artificial liver support techniques: (**a**) molecular adsorbent recirculating system (MARS), (**b**) single-pass albumin dialysis (SPAD), (**c**) Prometheus, and (**d**) selective plasma exchange therapy (SEPET)

support system. According to the inventors, to date, over 20,000 treatments have been performed in more than 5,000 patients. However, most of the currently published results originate from uncontrolled trials or case report series. The largest randomized controlled trial, performed in Rostock and Essen, Germany, included 24 patients with acute-on-chronic liver failure (ACLF). In this study, MARS treatment was associated with a significant improvement of 30-day survival; however, the 3-month mortality was identical in both groups [2]. A prospective, randomized, controlled, multicenter trial of the efficacy, safety, and tolerability of extracorporeal albumin dialysis using MARS was conducted in 70 patients with advanced cirrhosis. Patients were randomized to MARS treatment and standard medical therapy (SMT) or SMT alone. MARS was provided daily for 6 h for 5 days or until the patient had a 2-grade improvement in hepatic encephalopathy. The improvement proportion of encephalopathy was higher in the MARS group when compared with the SMT group and was reached faster and more frequently than in the SMT group. However, this 5-day study was not designed to examine the impact of MARS on survival [4]. Currently a larger multicenter randomized controlled study with ACLF patients is being conducted in European centers.

Single-pass albumin dialysis (SPAD) is a simple method of albumin dialysis using standard renal replacement therapy machines without an additional perfusion pump system: The patient's blood flows through a circuit with a high-flux dialyzer as used for hemodiafiltration (HDF), similar or identical to that in the MARS system. The other side of this membrane is cleansed with an albumin solution in counter-directional flow to the blood, and is discarded after passing the filter. Continuous venovenous hemodiafiltration (CVVHDF) can be carried out in the first circuit via the same high-flux dialyzer (Fig. 8.2.1b) [1].

SPAD and the MARS were compared in vitro with regard to their detoxification capacity: SPAD showed a significantly greater reduction of ammonia compared with MARS. No significant differences could be observed between SPAD and MARS concerning other water-soluble substances. SPAD enabled a significantly greater bilirubin reduction than MARS. Concerning the reduction of bile acids, no significant differences between SPAD and MARS were seen [5]. The overall performance of MARS and SPAD is limited by the membrane characteristics separating the patient's albumin from the receptor albumin. In addition, MARS has a limited and uncontrolled regeneration capacity of the adsorbers within the circulation circuit. The latter does not apply for SPAD – in this system the receptor albumin is freshly exposed to the membrane and subsequently discarded without regeneration.

The ***Prometheus*** system (Fresenius Medical Care, Bad Homburg, Germany) is a device based on the combination of direct albumin adsorption with high-flux hemodialysis after selective filtration of the albumin fraction through a specific polysulfone filter (AlbuFlow, Fig. 8.2.1c). The Prometheus system is not limited by the albumin-tight membrane like in MARS or SPAD. Falkenhagen et al. introduced the idea of allowing the patient's albumin pass across a size-selective membrane and have this albumin fraction regenerated in a recirculation circuit containing two adsorbers similar to those of MARS. A high-flux dialyzer to remove the water-soluble toxins is in series with the selective filtration. While eliminating some of the membrane resistance, performance is still limited by the albumin regeneration capacity of the adsorbers.

In a first clinical study eleven patients with ACLF and accompanying renal failure were treated with Prometheus on 2 consecutive days for more than 4 h. The treatment significantly improved serum levels of conjugated bilirubin, bile acids, ammonia, cholinesterase, creatinine, urea, and blood pH. Prometheus was proven to be a safe supportive therapy for patients with liver failure [6].

In a randomized crossover study, five patients were treated for ACLF with alternating treatments with MARS and Prometheus. Significantly higher reduction ratios after Prometheus compared with MARS for bilirubin and urea (as marker substances for albumin-bound and water-soluble substances, respectively) were found. Interestingly, reduction of unconjugated bilirubin, a marker for strongly albumin-bound toxins, was exclusively observed in Prometheus-treated patients [7, 8].

In a recent controlled study [9], 24 patients with decompensated cirrhosis were assigned to three groups and either treated with MARS, Prometheus, or received hemodialysis for 6 h. No correlation could be observed between study group and 6-month outcome. A large prospective randomized controlled trial investigating the effect of Prometheus on survival of patients with ACLF (HELIOS study) has been initiated in Europe. First results are expected in 2008 [7].

Selective plasma exchange therapy (SEPET), introduced by Rozga et al. tries to combine the advantages of SPAD with the advantages of Prometheus [10]. Although the fractionated plasma is crossing an albumin-permeable size-selective membrane, similar to Prometheus, there is no regeneration, similar to SPAD. Instead, the albumin fraction containing the toxins from the patients' blood is discarded and replaced by donor plasma (Fig. 8.2.1d). Compared with standard plasma exchange, however, the plasma volume required is significantly reduced. The developers claim that valuable components like hepatic growth factors are retained, while other substances are replaced by the substituted plasma. Selective plasma filtration is a novel approach to blood purification therapy designed to reduce the level of circulating toxins of hepatic and renal failure, mediators of inflammation, and inhibitors of hepatic regeneration.

An open-label uncontrolled phase I study (SEPET Feasibility Trial) has been completed and SEPET has been given the US Food and Drug Administration's Investigational Device Exemption (IDE) status. The clearance enables the company to begin a pivotal clinical phase II/III trial. During the first segment of the trial, five nonrandomized patients will be treated with SEPET to validate the patient selection criteria, clinical protocol, case report forms, and other trial-related documents. During the second segment of the trial, 116 patients will be enrolled in a randomized controlled trial to evaluate the effect on hepatic encephalopathy grade and the 30-day transplant-free survival rate. Pending review and approval by the Data Safety Monitoring Board, the third study segment would permit the size of the trial to be increased by an additional 52 patients.

8.2.3 Bioartificial Liver Support

Bioartificial liver support systems, in contrast to artificial liver support systems, try to address the synthetic and regulatory functions of the liver in addition to the detoxification capacity. Since those functions are numerous, and it is not finally resolved which exact pathways lead to encephalopathy and multiorgan failure, the only way to substitute the liver's synthetic functions is by introducing liver cells into the liver support system. The idea behind this concept is to temporarily support or replace the synthetic functions of the failing liver until either a matching graft is accessible or, in some cases, until the patient's liver is able to regenerate itself. The earliest attempts at something similar to bioartificial liver support systems was **extracorporeal liver perfusion (ECLP)** first applied by Otto et al. in 1958 [11] in preclinical studies with dogs. In 1964, Sen et al. [12] were the first to use extracorporeal liver perfusion in a clinical setting, followed by Eiseman et al. [13]. In EPCL, an explanted liver of xenogeneic or human origin is connected to the patient's circulation via the large graft vessels using surgical techniques. Sen et al. treated five patients with liver failure at the University of Bombay using EPLC with human livers, four of whom died within less than 2 days. One 27-year-old man recovered completely. Eisemann et al. used pig livers for treating eight patients in fulminant liver failure the same year. Within the following decades, about 250 patients were treated with ECLP, mainly with porcine livers. However, the long-term survival rate of these patients did not exceed that of patients receiving standard intensive care treatment [14].

EPLC requires very complicated logistics, since the organ has to be freshly explanted for the treatment session and then connected to the patients' blood circulation. To address these problems, several different liver support bioreactors were developed which enabled cultivation of isolated liver cells in a more suitable mode for integration into clinical perfusion systems and for prolonged cell culture times. Additionally, this approach enables the use cryopreserved cells or proliferating cell lines expanded in a lab. However, one major problem remains: until today, there is no satisfactory cell source to be used in such systems. Several different approaches were made, each of which has different but severe disadvantages.

One possibility is to use xenogeneic cells, most frequently of porcine origin. Those organs and cells are fairly easy to obtain and can be held in supply for the respective patients. However, it is not clear whether interspecies metabolic compatibility is assured in all relevant pathways no longer sufficiently covered by the failing liver. Secondly, there is a substantial risk of xenozoonosis, for example, porcine endogenous retroviruses (PERV) or herpes viruses, although so far, no transmission of PERV could be observed in patients treated with porcine liver cells [15, 16]. Finally, animal protein might lead to allergenic reactions in patients, especially those who are repeatedly treated with xenogenic cells.

Various groups have been using cell lines deriving from human liver tumors. These cells have the advantage of rapid growth and therefore practically unlimited availability. Nevertheless, the cell lines are dedifferentiated and show only some percentage of liver-specific metabolism compared with normal adult liver cells [17, 18]. Since these cells still have tumor characteristics concerning proliferation, the risk of tumor dissemination can not completely be excluded if the cells escape into the patient's circulation, even if several filters are usually included to minimize the hazard.

Primary human liver cells would be the ideal cell type for extracorporeal liver support. The only cell sources for sufficient amounts of primary cells are livers initially explanted for transplantation but subsequently rejected, mainly for steatosis, fibrosis, or trauma. It has to be taken into account that discarded donor organs usually are already histologically impaired and that the cells are additionally stressed by isolation procedures, meaning that their metabolic capacity will be lower than that of cells in the intact liver. Secondly, the logistics of isolating cells from discarded livers and distributing them to the site where they are required is much too complicated to fulfill what is needed here.

To benefit from the advantages of both tumor cell lines and primary liver cells without having to deal with the disadvantages, it would be desirable to establish methods of expanding human liver stem cells, either originating from fetal cell sources or by isolating adult liver stem cells or progenitor cells [19]. However, until today, it is impossible to acquire sufficient amounts of cell material this way.

The only bioartificial liver support system having been evaluated in a prospective randomized controlled clinical study so far is the HepatAssist system by Demetriou et al., in which $5–7\times10^9$ cryopreserved porcine hepatocytes are inoculated into the intercapillary space of a device resembling a modified dialysis cartridge [20, 21]. The patients' plasma ultrafiltrate is fed through the cartridges via an activated charcoal adsorber and an oxygenator.

Smaller series of clinical applications in a phase I trial demonstrated the safety of the system [22–24]. For the controlled trial [25], 171 patients with fulminant or subfulminant liver failure or primary nonfunction of transplanted organ (PNF) were included in the study, 86 of whom received standard intensive care treatment, while the other 85 patients were additionally submitted to HepatAssist treatment. No significant increase in 30-day survival could be demonstrated in the complete patient group. However, a significantly decreased relative risk was observed when excluding the PNF patients, and for the group of liver failure with known etiology (excluding PNF, remaining $n = 85$), a significantly prolonged survival was observed in the HepatAssist group.

The **extracorporeal liver assist device (ELAD)** developed by Sussman et al. uses about 200 g of cells of a cell line originating from human hepatoblastoma (C3A, derived from HepG2) in a similar setting [26, 27]. The cells are inoculated into the extracapillary space, thus being separated from the patients' plasma by hollow-fiber membranes. An integrated charcoal adsorber and a membrane oxygenator support detoxification and maintain the oxygen supply of the cells. ELAD was clinically evaluated in several pilot studies. Between 1991 and 1993, eleven patients were treated, demonstrating the system's safety [28]. In 1996, for a pilot controlled phase I trial [29], 24 patients were assigned to two study groups according to the grade of severity of liver failure. Group I comprised patients with a 50% chance of spontaneous recovery ($n = 17$), while patients in group II fulfilled the criteria for liver transplantation ($n = 7$). The control arm of each group received standard intensive care treatment while the other patients were assigned to the ELAD group. Encephalopathy grade increased in 7 of 12 patients in the control group and in 3 of 12 patients in the ELAD group. The survival rate in the control population of group I exceeded the anticipated 50%, resulting in a survival rate of six of eight patients while seven of nine patients survived in the ELAD group. The clinical course of the first five patients of an open-label, randomized, controlled pilot multicenter study were published in 2002 [30].

The bioreactor introduced by Gerlach et al. in the 1980s and integrated into the **modular extracorporeal liver support system (MELS)** later, displays a more complicated medium/plasma flow. Instead of hollow fibers arranged in parallel in a cylindrical housing similar to a dialysis cartridge, the bioreactor consist of two hydrophilic polyethersulfone membrane bundles and a hydrophobic multilayer hollow-fiber bundle for oxygenation [31–33]. The different bundles each congregate in two opposing ports and are interwoven within the cell compartment to form small repetitive supply subunits. During clinical application, the hydrophilic bundles which serve the supply of cell culture medium to the cell aggregates while in so-called stand-by phase are used for plasma circulation.

The system was charged with freshly isolated primary porcine cells from specific pathogen free (SPF) pigs until 2000 [34]. In a phase I clinical trial, eight patients with acute liver failure (ALF) who all met the criteria for high urgency listing, were treated for 8–46 h until transplant ("bridging to transplantation") [35]. The extracorporeal unit was well tolerated by all patients, who were all transplanted successfully and showed a 5-year survival rate of 100%. Subsequent screening of the patients' plasma for antibodies against PERV was negative in all cases [15].

After the increased discussions about PERV transmission from porcine tissue and with respect to greater biochemical compatibility, cells were thereafter isolated from human donor livers previously accepted for transplant but later discarded due to steatosis, fibrosis, or liver injury. Additionally, the MELS bioreactor was combined with CVVHDF and SPAD for the removal of water-soluble and albumin-bound toxins, respectively [36, 37]. Nine patients with ALF, ACLF, or PNF (each $n = 3$) were treated with MELS containing human cells. The treatment duration ranged from 7 to 91 h. Six patients were successfully bridged to transplant, while two patients died within 10 days of the treatment. One ACLF patient recovered without a transplant and was still alive 2 years after therapy. The treatment showed no adverse effects besides the usual phenomena related with extracorporeal treatment such as decrease in platelets (unpublished results [38, 39]). However, the combination of artificial and bioartificial components makes it hard to discriminate between the effects achieved by either part of the system.

The **bioartificial liver of the Academisch Medisch Centrum (AMC-BAL)** developed by Chamuleau and coworkers in Amsterdam in The Netherlands differs from other clinically applied systems in one major point: instead of separating the patients' plasma from the extracorporally applied liver cells by a membrane, the plasma is in direct contact with the cells. Within a cylindrical housing a nonwoven polyester matrix is spirally wound to provide a scaffold. Arranged between the layers of matrix, hydrophobic hollow fibers streamed with a mix of 95% air and 5% CO_2 serve cell oxygenation. During stand-by, cell culture medium is circulated through the system and a medium reservoir. The matrix offers a large surface enabling the inoculated cells to attach and form aggregates between the fibers [40–42]. The system is charged with about 10×10^9 primary liver cells isolated from pigs.

A preclinical study with the AMC-BAL was performed in anhepatic pigs [42], which were stratified into three groups (each $n = 5$). One group was submitted to intensive care treatment (control I), one was treated for 24 h with bioreactors without cells (control II), and one was treated for 24 h with bioreactors containing autologous cells (AMC-BAL group). Survival time was significantly prolonged in the AMC-BAL group. This group also displayed significantly decreased ammonia blood levels, while bilirubin concentrations were similar in all groups.

Twelve patients with acute liver failure listed for high urgency transplantation were included in a clinical phase I trial [43, 44]. The treatment duration ranged from 4 to 35 h; four patients were treated repeatedly. Eleven patients were successfully bridged to transplant, while one patient's liver function improved during treatment, rendering a transplant unnecessary. No severe adverse events were observed.

8.2.4 Discussion

Over the past 20 years, many liver support concepts have been developed and evaluated. Despite these efforts, none of the devices – neither cell-based nor cell-free – were able to fully meet clinical demands. Twelve trials on liver support systems versus standard medical therapy (483 patients) and two trials comparing different artificial support systems (105 patients) were included in the latest systematic Cochrane Review concerning artificial and bioartificial liver support systems. This analysis indicated that artificial support systems might reduce mortality in acute-on-chronic liver failure. However, the systems did not appear to affect mortality in acute liver failure. Furthermore, no significant benefit in bridging patients to liver transplant was identified. However, an effect on certain clinical parameters and biochemical parameters can be shown for most of the systems and significant improvement concerning encephalopathy was seen [45]. These limited results generate questions: Are the concepts evaluated inadequately? Are the concepts right but their scale too small and performances too low?

Cell-based, bioartificial liver support systems address the complex tasks of regulation and synthesis, but have some biological and physical limitations in common: they use hollow-fiber membranes which limit the mass exchange between the patient's blood and extracorporeal liver cells. Usually, plasma is first separated by a plasma filter and then circulated through the bioreactor, where the cells are again separated from the plasma by a hollow-fiber membrane. The plasma has to pass the barrier twice – firstly to reach the cell compartment and then again to reenter the extracorporeal tubing. This is bound to limit the mass transfer between the cells and the patient's circulation. The blood flow rate of the natural human liver in situ is about 1,500 ml/min, while the perfusion of bioreactors is limited to 100–300 ml/min of plasma. Flow rates are limited by pressure built up in the circulation system due to membranes and tube diameters. Therefore, the maximum clearance rate for any substance in the bioreactor, which involves the plasma volume passing though the bioreactor, must be expected to be much lower than in the human liver [46].

Finally, there is the question of liver cell mass to be discussed. Usually, about 100–200 g of cells are offered in a bioreactor system; Gerlach et al. state up to 600 g cells. In living donation liver transplantation (LD-LTx), a graft size of 40% of the recipient's ideal liver mass is likely to be insufficient for meeting the recipient's metabolic needs, and the recipient is at risk of suffering graft failure [47]. An even larger amount of cells has to be provided when being applied within an extracorporeal circuit – especially because of the physical limitations of bioreactor concepts [46]. However, in clinically applied systems the cell mass was less than 30% of this ideal in all cases, not taking into account that if these cells derive from initially impaired organs, they are most likely to be less metabolically active than healthy liver tissue. The dominating limitation of all cell-based concepts today appears to be the cell source. The use of primary human liver cells is increasingly favored for clinical application, because these cells circumvent several unwanted effects associated with the use of porcine cells (metabolic incompatibility, risk of xenozoonosis) [17, 48, 49] or tumor cell lines (risk of metastases and a lower liver specific metabolic performance) [18]. Discarded donor organs might serve as a source for the isolation of primary human hepatocytes. However, primary human liver cells originating from discarded donor organs – besides their limited availability – have to be regarded as impaired because of histological alteration, preservation, and isolation processes. Until we can establish a reliable, safe, highly metabolically active and easily expandable human cell source, a successful breakthrough in bioartificial liver support systems appears to be unlikely. Thus, most bioartificial devices in use today have an additional detoxification component – either adsorption (e.g., HepatAssist) or albumin dialysis (e.g., MELS) to reduce some of the limitations.

Acceptance of extracorporeal liver support systems by the clinician is currently limited because of the lack of appropriate randomized, controlled, and adequately powered studies. The design of clinical studies concerning liver failure is difficult. In ALF, treatment will be terminated as soon as an organ for transplant is available (usually within 24–48 h after registering as a high urgency candidate). Liver failure – both ALF and ACLF – is a very heterogeneous disease with respect to the capacity of parenchymal regeneration and prognosis. Finally, sensible clinical end points are lacking [50].

The authors of the Cochrane systematic review of clinical trials with liver support systems concluded that randomized trials on liver support systems versus standard medical therapy are warranted. The trend of the data justifies larger trials, preferably involving several clinical sites to increase the external validity.

They ask designers of clinical studies to compare sufficiently the therapeutic potential of one support system to standard medical therapy before such systems are introduced as control interventions to more sophisticated support systems. Such trials should be adequately designed, including centralized randomization (using stratification for important prognostic factors) as well as blinded outcome assessment.

For timely updates on future developments in the field of liver support devices, we recommend the blog of the Working Group Liver Support of the European Society for Artificial Organs (ESAO, www.esao.org).

8.2.5 Take Home Pearls

- A variety of extracorporeal systems for artificial or bioartificial liver support for the removal of lipophilic, albumin-bound toxins in patients with liver failure have been developed.
- The molecular adsorbents recirculating system (MARS), single-pass albumin dialysis (SPAD), and fractionated plasma separation and adsorption (Prometheus) systems have been introduced into clinical practice and were shown to be safe and biochemically effective.
- These systems are mostly used for bridging the patient to transplant or to recovery of liver function; however, few data exist to determine clinical indications, intensity, and duration of therapy with extracorporeal liver support.

References

1. Kreymann B, Seige M, Schweigart U, Kopp KF, Classen M. Albumin dialysis: effective removal of copper in a patient with fulminant Wilson disease and successful bridging to liver transplantation: a new possibility for the elimination of protein-bound toxins. J Hepatol 1999;31:1080–5.
2. Heemann U, Treichel U, Loock J, Philipp T, Gerken G, Malago M, Klammt S, Loehr M, Liebe S, Mitzner S, Schmidt R, Stange J. Albumin dialysis in cirrhosis with superimposed acute liver injury: a prospective, controlled study. Hepatology 2002;36:949–58.
3. Stange J, Hassanein TI, Mehta R, Mitzner SR, Bartlett RH. The molecular adsorbents recycling system as a liver support system based on albumin dialysis: a summary of preclinical investigations, prospective, randomized, controlled clinical trial, and clinical experience from 19 centers. Artif Organs 2002;26:103–10.
4. Hassanein TI, Tofteng F, Brown RS, Jr., McGuire B, Lynch P, Mehta R, Larsen FS, Gornbein J, Stange J, Blei AT. Randomized controlled study of extracorporeal albumin dialysis for hepatic encephalopathy in advanced cirrhosis. Hepatology 2007;46:1853–62.
5. Sauer IM, Goetz M, Steffen I, Walter G, Kehr DC, Schwartlander R, Hwang YJ, Pascher A, Gerlach JC, Neuhaus P. In vitro comparison of the molecular adsorbent recirculation system (MARS) and single-pass albumin dialysis (SPAD). Hepatology 2004;39:1408–14.
6. Rifai K, Ernst T, Kretschmer U, Bahr MJ, Schneider A, Hafer C, Haller H, Manns MP, Fliser D. Prometheus – a new extracorporeal system for the treatment of liver failure. J Hepatol 2003;39:984–90.
7. Krisper P, Stauber RE. Technology insight: artificial extracorporeal liver support – how does Prometheus compare with MARS? Nat Clin Pract Nephrol 2007;3:267–76.
8. Krisper P, Stauber R, Haditsch B, Trauner M, Holzer H, Schneditz D. MARS versus Prometheus: comparison of reduction ratios (RR) as a measure of treatment dose in two different liver detoxification devices. 29th Annual Meeting of The European Association fort he Study of the Liver 2004. Berlin, 2004.
9. Dethloff T, Tofteng F, Frederiksen HJ, Hojskov M, Hansen BA, Larsen FS. Effect of Prometheus liver assist system on systemic hemodynamics in patients with cirrhosis: A randomized controlled study. World J Gastroenterol 2008; 14:2065–71.
10. Rozga J, Umehara Y, Trofimenko A, Sadahiro T, Demetriou AA. A novel plasma filtration therapy for hepatic failure: preclinical studies. Ther Apher Dial 2006;10:138–44.
11. Otto JJ, Pender JC, Cleary JH, Sensenig DM, Welch CS. The use of a donor liver in experimental animals with elevated blood ammonia. Surgery 1958;43:301–9.
12. Sen PK, Bhalerao RA, Parulkar GP, Samsi AB, Shah BK, Kinare SG. Use of isolated perfused cadaveric liver in the management of hepatic failure. Surgery 1966;59:774–81.
13. Eiseman B, Liem DS, Raffucci F. Heterologous liver perfusion in treatment of hepatic failure. Ann Surg 1965; 162:329–45.
14. Pascher A, Sauer IM, Hammer C, Gerlach JC, Neuhaus P. Extracorporeal liver perfusion as hepatic assist in acute liver failure: a review of world experience. Xenotransplantation 2002;9:309–24.
15. Irgang M, Sauer IM, Karlas A, Zeilinger K, Gerlach JC, Kurth R, Neuhaus P, Denner J. Porcine endogenous retroviruses: no infection in patients treated with a bioreactor based on porcine liver cells. J Clin Virol 2003;28:141–54.
16. Di Nicuolo G, van de Kerkhove MP, Hoekstra R, Beld MG, Amoroso P, Battisti S, Starace M, di Florio E, Scuderi V, Scala S, Bracco A, Mancini A, Chamuleau RA, Calise F. No evidence of in vitro and in vivo porcine endogenous retrovirus infection after plasmapheresis through the AMC-bioartificial liver. Xenotransplantation 2005;12:286–92.
17. Morsiani E, Brogli M, Galavotti D, Pazzi P, Puviani AC, Azzena GF. Biologic liver support: optimal cell source and mass. Int J Artif Organs 2002;25:985–93.
18. Stange J, Mitzner S, Strauss M, Fischer U, Lindemann S, Peters E, Holtz M, Drewelow B, Schmidt R. Primary or established liver cells for a hybrid liver? Comparison of metabolic features. Asaio J 1995;41:M310–5.
19. Dan YY, Yeoh GC. Liver stem cells: a scientific and clinical perspective. J Gastroenterol Hepatol 2008;23:687–98.
20. Demetriou AA, Rozga J, Podesta L, Lepage E, Morsiani E, Moscioni AD, Hoffman A, McGrath M, Kong L, Rosen H, et al. Early clinical experience with a hybrid bioartificial liver. Scand J Gastroenterol Suppl 1995;208:111–7.
21. Rozga J, Podesta L, LePage E, Hoffman A, Morsiani E, Sher L, Woolf GM, Makowka L, Demetriou AA. Control of cerebral oedema by total hepatectomy and extracorporeal liver support in fulminant hepatic failure. Lancet 1993; 342:898–9.
22. Hui T, Rozga J, Demetriou AA. Bioartificial liver support. J Hepatobiliary Pancreat Surg 2001;8:1–15.
23. Rozga J, Podesta L, LePage E, Morsiani E, Moscioni AD, Hoffman A, Sher L, Villamil F, Woolf G, McGrath M, et al. A bioartificial liver to treat severe acute liver failure. Ann Surg 1994;219:538–44; discussion 544–6.
24. Mullon C, Pitkin Z. The HepatAssist bioartificial liver support system: clinical study and pig hepatocyte process. Expert Opin Investig Drugs 1999;8:229–35.
25. Demetriou AA, Brown RS, Jr., Busuttil RW, Fair J, McGuire BM, Rosenthal P, Am Esch JS, 2nd, Lerut J, Nyberg SL, Salizzoni M, Fagan EA, de Hemptinne B, Broelsch CE, Muraca M, Salmeron JM, Rabkin JM, Metselaar HJ, Pratt D, De La Mata M, McChesney LP, Everson GT, Lavin PT, Stevens AC, Pitkin Z, Solomon BA. Prospective, randomized, multicenter, controlled trial of a bioartificial liver in treating acute liver failure. Ann Surg 2004;239:660–7; discussion 667–70.
26. Kelly JH, Sussman NL. The hepatix extracorporeal liver assist device in the treatment of fulminant hepatic failure. Asaio J 1994;40:83–5.
27. Wood RP, Katz SM, Ozaki CF, Monsour HP, Gislason GT, Kelly JH, Sussman NL. Extracorporeal liver assist device (ELAD): a preliminary report. Transplant Proc 1993; 25:53–4.
28. Sussman NL, Gislason GT, Conlin CA, Kelly JH. The Hepatix extracorporeal liver assist device: initial clinical experience. Artif Organs 1994;18:390–6.
29. Ellis AJ, Hughes RD, Wendon JA, Dunne J, Langley PG, Kelly JH, Gislason GT, Sussman NL, Williams R. Pilot-controlled trial of the extracorporeal liver assist device in acute liver failure. Hepatology 1996;24:1446–51.

30. Millis JM, Cronin DC, Johnson R, Conjeevaram H, Conlin C, Trevino S, Maguire P. Initial experience with the modified extracorporeal liver-assist device for patients with fulminant hepatic failure: system modifications and clinical impact. Transplantation 2002;74:1735–46.
31. Gerlach J, Schnoy N, Smith MD, Neuhaus P. Hepatocyte culture between woven capillary networks: a microscopy study. Artif Organs 1994;18:226–30.
32. Gerlach JC, Encke J, Hole O, Muller C, Ryan CJ, Neuhaus P. Bioreactor for a larger scale hepatocyte in vitro perfusion. Transplantation 1994;58:984–8.
33. Gerlach JC, Encke J, Hole O, Muller C, Courtney JM, Neuhaus P. Hepatocyte culture between three dimensionally arranged biomatrix-coated independent artificial capillary systems and sinusoidal endothelial cell co-culture compartments. Int J Artif Organs 1994;17:301–6.
34. Gerlach JC, Brombacher J, Kloppel K, Schnoy N, Neuhaus P. Comparison of four methods for mass hepatocyte isolation from pig and human livers. Transplantation 1994; 57:1318–22.
35. Sauer IM, Kardassis D, Zeillinger K, Pascher A, Gruenwald A, Pless G, Irgang M, Kraemer M, Puhl G, Frank J, Muller AR, Steinmuller T, Denner J, Neuhaus P, Gerlach JC. Clinical extracorporeal hybrid liver support – phase I study with primary porcine liver cells. Xenotransplantation 2003; 10:460–9.
36. Sauer IM, Neuhaus P, Gerlach JC. Concept for modular extracorporeal liver support for the treatment of acute hepatic failure. Metab Brain Dis 2002;17:477–84.
37. Sauer IM, Gerlach JC. Modular extracorporeal liver support. Artif Organs 2002;26:703–6.
38. Sauer IM, Zeilinger K, Pless G, Kardassis D, Theruvath T, Pascher A, Goetz M, Neuhaus P, Gerlach JC. Extracorporeal liver support based on primary human liver cells and albumin dialysis – treatment of a patient with primary graft nonfunction. J Hepatol 2003;39:649–53.
39. Sauer IM, Zeilinger K, Obermayer N, Pless G, Grunwald A, Pascher A, Mieder T, Roth S, Goetz M, Kardassis D, Mas A, Neuhaus P, Gerlach JC. Primary human liver cells as source for modular extracorporeal liver support – a preliminary report. Int J Artif Organs 2002;25:1001–5.
40. Flendrig LM, Calise F, Di Florio E, Mancini A, Ceriello A, Santaniello W, Mezza E, Sicoli F, Belleza G, Bracco A, Cozzolino S, Scala D, Mazzone M, Fattore M, Gonzales E, Chamuleau RA. Significantly improved survival time in pigs with complete liver ischemia treated with a novel bioartificial liver. Int J Artif Organs 1999;22:701–9.
41. Flendrig LM, la Soe JW, Jorning GG, Steenbeek A, Karlsen OT, Bovee WM, Ladiges NC, te Velde AA, Chamuleau RA. In vitro evaluation of a novel bioreactor based on an integral oxygenator and a spirally wound nonwoven polyester matrix for hepatocyte culture as small aggregates. J Hepatol 1997; 26:1379–92.
42. Sosef MN, Abrahamse LS, van de Kerkhove MP, Hartman R, Chamuleau RA, van Gulik TM. Assessment of the AMC-bioartificial liver in the anhepatic pig. Transplantation 2002;73:204–9.
43. van de Kerkhove MP, Di Florio E, Scuderi V, Mancini A, Belli A, Bracco A, Dauri M, Tisone G, Di Nicuolo G, Amoroso P, Spadari A, Lombardi G, Hoekstra R, Calise F, Chamuleau RA. Phase I clinical trial with the AMC-bioartificial liver. Int J Artif Organs 2002;25:950–9.
44. van de Kerkhove MP, Di Florio E, Scuderi V, Mancini A, Belli A, Bracco A, Scala D, Scala S, Zeuli L, Di Nicuolo G, Amoroso P, Calise F, Chamuleau RA. Bridging a patient with acute liver failure to liver transplantation by the AMC-bioartificial liver. Cell Transplant 2003;12:563–8.
45. Liu JP, Gluud LL, Als-Nielsen B, Gluud C. Artificial and bioartificial support systems for liver failure. Cochrane Database Syst Rev 2004:CD003628.
46. Iwata H, Ueda Y. Pharmacokinetic considerations in development of a bioartificial liver. Clin Pharmacokinet 2004; 43:211–25.
47. Lo CM, Fan ST, Liu CL, Wei WI, Lo RJ, Lai CL, Chan JK, Ng IO, Fung A, Wong J. Adult-to-adult living donor liver transplantation using extended right lobe grafts. Ann Surg 1997;226:261–9; discussion 269–70.
48. Hammer C. Xenotransplantation for liver therapy or: can porcine hepatocytes generate physiological functions sufficient for a human patient in ALF? Int J Artif Organs 2002;25:1019–28.
49. Alwayn I, Robson S. Understanding and preventing the coagulation disorder associated with xenograft rejection. Graft 2000;4:50–3.
50. O'Grady J. Perspectives and future of artificial and bioartificial devices. In: Artificial Liver Support – Proceedings of the Falk Symposium 145. Dordrecht, The Netherlands: Springer Verlag, 2006.

8.3 Extracorporeal Removal of Drugs and Toxins

James F. Winchester, Nikolas B. Harbord, Pallavi Tyagi, and Herman Rosen

Core Messages

- Indications for extracorporeal removal of drugs and toxins are mostly clinical and include hemodynamic instability; clinical deterioration despite supportive treatment; mental status alteration; and midbrain/brainstem dysfunction resulting in respiratory depression, hypothermia, hypotension, or bradycardia. Further indications are evidence of failure of organ systems; impaired endogenous drug clearance due to cardiac, renal, or hepatic failure; and when a drug or poison can be removed more rapidly compared with endogenous elimination.
- Hemodialysis and hemofiltration techniques are most effective for the elimination of small molecular size, high water soluble compounds with a low degree of protein-binding, a small volume of distribution, and rapid equilibration of drug between plasma and tissues.
- Peritoneal dialysis can also be employed as an acute treatment modality for intoxication with water-soluble, small-molecular-weight solutes but should probably be limited to infants, children, and hemodynamically unstable adults intolerant of a blood circuit or anticoagulation.
- Therapeutic plasma exchange is of clinical utility when blood purification is required for substances with very high molecular weight and/or high degree of protein binding.
- Hemoperfusion is an absorptive modality which effectively can clear substances that are lipid-soluble or as much as 95% protein-bound. It provides superior drug clearance and is the preferred modality for extraction of theophylline, barbiturates, organophosphates, and many hypnotics/sedatives/tranquilizers.

8.3.1 Introduction

The treatment of poisoned or intoxicated patients frequently requires nephrology consultation [1]. In addition to supportive management and treatment of renal failure or electrolyte and acid–base disorders, blood purification may be necessary – active removal of drugs and toxins from the body. Hemodialysis and peritoneal dialysis have been used in the treatment of intoxications since the 1950s [2, 3]; and over time, the indications and technology for extracorporeal therapies have expanded. At present, membranes with large surface areas (high efficiency) and pore-size (high flux), adsorptive perfusion columns, convective modalities, and continuous or extended treatments are widely available.

This chapter will outline the principles of extracorporeal drug removal and the use of particular modalities: hemodialysis, hemofiltration and hemodiafiltration, hemoperfusion, peritoneal dialysis, and therapeutic plasma exchange. The initial approach to the poisoned patient – along with enteric decontamination and enhanced elimination – are beyond the scope of this chapter. Particular consideration will be given to criteria for use of various modalities, available options, and recent advances in extracorporeal therapy. Finally, the

J. F. Winchester (✉)
Division of Nephrology & Hypertension, Department of Medicine, Beth Israel Medical Center, 350 East 17th Street, 18BH20, New York, NY 10003, USA
e-mail: jwinches@bethisraelny.org

A. Jörres et al. (eds.), *Management of Acute Kidney Problems*,
DOI: 10.1007/978-3-540-69441-0_8.3, © Springer-Verlag Berlin Heidelberg 2010

chapter will conclude with a detailed discussion of blood purification with regard to specific poisonings.

8.3.2 Criteria and Considerations for Extracorporeal Therapy

Although discrete indications exist for several intoxications (see Section 8.3.9 Specific Drugs/Poisons), the decision to employ extracorporeal methods is in most cases clinical and first requires assessment of the poisoned patient. Indications include hemodynamic instability; clinical deterioration despite supportive treatment; mental status alteration; and midbrain/brainstem dysfunction resulting in respiratory depression, hypothermia, hypotension, or bradycardia. Further indications are evidence of failure of organ systems; impaired endogenous drug clearance due to cardiac, renal, or hepatic failure; and when a drug or poison can be removed more rapidly compared with endogenous elimination. Finally, dialytic therapies may be indicated to correct concomitant electrolyte and/or acid–base disorders. Intoxicated patients treated with extracorporeal modalities are vulnerable to hypotension – for many clinical reasons and/or the necessary extracorporeal blood volume in the treatment circuit – and may require hemodynamic support. Patients should receive vasopressor infusions distal to any dialyzer or sorbent cartridge with careful monitoring of circulatory status as pressor requirements may change.

Clinicians should be aware of the acute complications possible with extracorporeal therapies. The most frequent complications are intravenous catheter–related and include malfunction (thrombosis or kinking), and rarely hematomas or mechanical problems such as air embolism [4, 5]. Additional risks include hypotension [6], blood loss, arrhythmias [7], and metabolic disequilibria. Although peritoneal dialysis does not involve the risks associated with venipuncture or an extracorporeal blood circuit, peritoneal catheters do predispose to infectious peritonitis [8].

8.3.3 Principles of Extracorporeal Removal of Drugs and Toxins

An understanding of the pharmacologic properties of the offending agent and different principles of drug extraction will allow choice among available modalities. While there is empiric evidence of benefit with extracorporeal therapies in poisoning [9], much of the knowledge regarding solute clearance derives from urea kinetics and the removal of small molecules retained in uremia [10].

Hemodialysis is widely available and the most commonly employed method of extracorporeal drug clearance [1]. Drug removal is governed by both drug-related and dialysis-related factors. Small molecular size (molecular weight < 500 Da), high water solubility, low degree of protein-binding, small volume of distribution (<1l/kg), and rapid equilibration of drug between plasma and tissue are factors that favor drug efflux [11]. On the other hand, clearance is limited with drugs that are largely lipid-soluble or tissue-bound, and exhibit large volumes of distribution and slow plasma equilibration. Factors particular to dialysis include type of blood access, flow rates of blood and dialysate, and the dialysis membrane material, surface area, and pore size/flux. The use of low blood flow rates may prevent hemodynamic instability but necessitate longer or continuous treatments for equivalent clearance. Increasing blood and dialysate flow rates will likely augment drug diffusion (as evident with urea, molecular weight 60 Da) with an eventual plateau at blood flow rates of 300 ml/min and dialysate flow rate of 800 ml/min [12]. Enhanced drug removal can also be accomplished by increasing the surface area (i.e., high efficiency) of the dialyzer.

As the molecular weight of a drug increases, removal is less a function of diffusion than convection – the creation of an ultrafiltrate of plasma through pressure across a membrane [13]. As such, efficient clearance of high-molecular-weight intoxicants is best accomplished with convective modalities such as hemofiltration, and the combined modality hemodiafiltration (also known as high-flux hemodialysis) [14, 15]. However, drugs with molecular weight in excess of 50,000–60,000 Da should not be expected to pass through contemporary high-flux membranes. Similarly, drugs with a high degree of protein binding will not pass into the ultrafiltrate. The convective passage of a molecule across the membrane is described by the sieving coefficient (SC; with values between 0 and 1) [16]; and clearance is equal to the SC multiplied by the ultrafiltration rate. With the convective modalities, clearance of any intoxicant with a SC greater than 0 can be augmented by increasing the ultrafiltration rate.

Continuous treatments are frequently employed in the management of acute kidney injury. However, their utility in the treatment of poisoning is uncertain, and these modalities may not be appropriate for drug removal in acute intoxications [17]. The hemodynamic advantages of low blood flow rates used in continuous renal replacement therapies (CRRTs) in patients with unstable cardiovascular status must be weighed against slower clearances than with conventional hemodialysis. Of course, increased treatment times may result in equivalent total drug clearance. Combined modalities such as sustained low-efficiency dialysis (SLED) with a high-flux membrane – essentially hemodiafiltration with long, discontinuous, treatment time – can provide near equivalent small solute clearance to continuous venovenous hemofiltration (CVVH), although performance diminishes with increasing solute size [18]. Furthermore, SLED appears to more cost-effective and avoids the risks of anticoagulation associated with CRRT [19].

Peritoneal dialysis (PD) can also be used for acute blood purification in the setting of intoxication [20]. Acute PD for this indication requires placement of a catheter (rigid or flexible) through the abdominal wall into the peritoneum, which may not be desirable in select patients. A volume of hypertonic fluid is then instilled into the abdominal cavity, allowed to dwell, and finally drained by gravity and discarded. Solute clearance occurs principally by diffusion down a concentration gradient from the mesenteric arterial vasculature via pores in the peritoneal membrane into the fluid; however, some convective clearance may occur with "solvent drag" [21]. Repeat exchanges allow for cumulative small solute clearance, and total clearance can be determined by factoring the drug level in the fluid by the total drain volume. Unfortunately, peritoneal membrane transport and clearance of small molecules is less efficient than with intermittent hemodialysis. Furthermore, studies using β_2-microglobulin (molecular weight 12,000 Da) suggest that with increased molecular weight, the transport of solutes into the dialysate requires dwells as long as 12 h [22]. The use of automated PD involving continuous and high total volume exchanges has been shown to provide increased small solute removal in patients with acute kidney injury [23]. This benefit may be extrapolated to efficient removal of low-molecular-weight water-soluble toxins. Continuous-flow PD would also theoretically increase clearance of an intoxicant with demonstrable diffusive transport [24]. Finally, sorbent technology may increase the utility of PD in poisoning although extraction may be subject to the limitations of peritoneal solute transport [25]. Interestingly, intraperitoneal nitroprusside and icodextrin appear to augment peritoneal transport [26]. The selection of PD as an acute treatment modality for intoxication should probably be limited to infants, children, and hemodynamically unstable adults intolerant of a blood circuit or anticoagulation. This procedure should also be limited to cases involving intoxication with low-molecular-weight solutes when rapid clearance is required.

Although *hemoperfusion* has been available since the 1940s, it is only occasionally employed for extracorporeal detoxification [1] and has largely been supplanted by advances in dialytic therapies. The procedure involves an extracorporeal blood circuit and passage of anticoagulated blood over a sorbent column containing charcoal or resin. Blood purification is the result of adsorption of solutes of various molecular weights to the perfusion column. Solute properties should determine the choice of column: activated charcoal exhibits higher affinity for water-soluble molecules, while resins have greater affinity for lipid-soluble molecules. The development and approval of engineered sorbent columns employing specific chemical bonds or antigen/antibody binding will advance the treatment of specific poisonings and other conditions such as sepsis and acute kidney injury [27]. Unfortunately, only activated charcoal cartridges are currently available in the United States. Sorbent columns may exhibit saturation with diminished purification in the course of a treatment; and short, intermittent treatments are recommended to improve drug clearance and anticipate "rebound" effect following drug redistribution. Complications specific to hemoperfusion include thrombocytopenia, leukopenia, hypocalcemia, and hypoglycemia.

Therapeutic plasma exchange (TPE), or plasmapheresis, is also occasionally used for extracorporeal treatment of poisoning [28]. The procedure involves passage of blood through a pheresis machine (using either centrifugation or filtration) to separate formed elements from plasma. The cells are then returned to the patient while the plasma containing the poison or offending drug is discarded and replaced with crystalloid, colloid, or fresh frozen plasma (FFP) [29, 30]. Plasma exchange is of clinical utility when blood purification is required for substances with very high molecular weight and/or high degree of protein binding. Drug removal in a single treatment can be calculated by multiplying the volume of plasma removed by the concentration of the drug in plasma. Exchange transfusion, or "whole blood exchange," involves replacement of a patient's blood with donor whole blood. While this procedure is

Table 8.3.1 Drugs and chemicals removed with dialysis

Antimicrobials/anti cancer	Ticarcillin	5-fluorouracil	Lisinopril
Cefaclor	(clindamycin)	(Methotrexate)	Quinapril
Cefadroxil	(erythromycin)		Ramipril
Cefamandole	(azithromycin)	Barbiturates	(Encainide)
Cefazolin	(clarithromycin)		(Flecainide)
Cefixime	Metronidazole	Amobarbital	(Lidocaine)
Cefmenoxime	Nitrofurantoin	Aprobarbital	Metoprolol
Cefmetazole	Ornidazole	Barbital	Methyldopa
(Cefonicid)	Sulfisoxazole	Butabarbital	(Ouabain)
(Cefoperazone)	Sulfonamides	Cyclobarbital	n-Acetylprocainamide
Ceforamide	Tetracycline	Pentobarbital	Nadolol
(Cefotaxime)	(Doxycycline)	Phenobarbital	(Pindolol)
Cefotetan	(Minocycline)	Quinalbital	Practolol
Cefotiam	Tinidazole	(Secobarbital)	Procainamide
Cefoxitin	Trimethoprim		ropranolol
Cefpirome	Aztreonam	Nonbarbiturates	(Quinidine)
Cefroxadine	Cilastatin	Hypnotics, sedatives,	(Timolol)
Cefsulodin	Imipenem	Tranquilizers	Sotatol
Ceftazidime	(Chloramphenicol)	Anticonvulsants	Tocainide
(Ceftriaxone)	(Amphotericin)	Carbamazepine	
Cefuroxime	Ciprofloxacin	Atenolol	Alcohols
Cephacetrile	(Enoxacin)	Betaxolol	Ethanol
Cephalexin	Fluroxacin	(Bretylium)	Ethylene glycol
Cephalothin	(Norfloxacin)	Clonidine	Diethylene glycol
(Cephapirin)	Ofloxacin	(Calcium channel blockers)	Isopropanol
Cephradine	Isoniazid	Captopril	Methanol
Moxalactam	(Vancomycin)	(Diazoxide)	
Amikacin	Capreomycin	Carbromal	Analgesics,
Dibekacin	Pas	Chloral hydrate	Antirheumatics
Fosfomycin	Pyrizinamide	(Chlordiazepoxide)	Acetaminophen
Gentamicin	(Rifampin)	(Diazepam)	Acetophenetidin
Kanamycin	(Cycloserine)	(Diphenylhydantoin)	Acetylsalicylic acid
Neomycin	Ethambutol	(Diphenylhydramine)	Colchicine
Netilmicin	5-Fluorocytosine	Ethinamate	Methylsalicylate
Sisomicin	Acyclovir	Ethchlorvynol	(d-Propoxyphene)
Streptomycin	(amantadine)	Ethosuximide	Salicylic acid
Tobramycin	Didanosine	Gallamine	
Bacitracin	Foscarnet	Glutethimide	Antidepressants
Colistin	Ganciclovir	(Heroin)	(Amitriptyline)
Amoxicillin	(Ribavirin)	Meprobamate	Amphetamines (Imipramine)
Ampicillin	Vidarabine	(Methaqualone)	Isocarboxazid
Azlocillin	Zidovudine	Methsuximide	Mao inhibitors
Carbenicillin	(Pentamidine)	Methyprylon	Moclobemide
Clavulinic acid	(Praziquantel)	Paraldehyde	(Pargyline)
(Cloxacillin)	(Fluconazole)	Primidone	(Phenelzine)
(dicloxacillin)	(Itraconazole)	Valproic acid	Tranylcypromine
(floxacillin)	(Ketoconazole)		(Tricyclics)
Mecillinam	(Miconazole)	Cardiovascular agents	
(mezlocillin)	(Chloroquine)	Acebutolol	Solvents, gases
(methicillin)	(Quinine)	(Amiodarone)	Acetone
(nafcillin)	(Azathioprine)	Amrinone	Camphor
Penicillin	Bredinin	(Digoxin)	Carbon monoxide
Piperacillin	Busulphan	Enalapril	(Carbon tetrachloride)
Temocillin	Cyclophosphamide	Fosinopril	(Eucalyptus oil)

Table 8.3.1 (continued)

Perchloroethylene	Paraquat	Dinitro-o-cresol	Bromide (Copper)*
Thiols	Snake bite	Folic acid	(Iron)*
Toluene	Sodium chlorate	Mannitol	Iodine
Trichloroethylene	Potassium chlorate	Methylprednisolone	(Lead)*
	Miscellaneous	4-Methylpyrazole	Lithium
Plants, animals, herbicides, insecticides	Acipimox	Sodium citrate	(Magnesium)
	Allopurinol	Theophylline	(Mercury)*
Alkyl phosphate	Aminophylline	Thiocyanate	Potassium
Amanitin		Ranitidine	(Potassium dichromate)*
Demeton sulfoxide	Aniline		Phosphate
Dimethoate	Borates	Metals, inorganics (aluminum)*	Sodium
Diquat	Boric acid		Strontium
Glufosinate	(Chlorpropamide)		(Thallium)*
Methylmercury complex	Chromic acid	Arsenic	(Tin)
(Organophosphates)	(Cimetidine)	Barium	(Zinc)

Source: Modified and updated from [129]() implies poor removal
()* removed with chelating age

typically performed in neonatal hyperbilirubinemia, massive drug, or parasite-induced hemolysis, as well as severe sickle cell crisis, exchange transfusion may be considered in some cases of poisoning.

8.3.4 Extracorporeal Modalities – Hemodialysis

Hemodialysis is most frequently employed for blood purification following ingestion of methanol, ethylene glycol, lithium, and salicylates. The use of dialysis for these intoxicants will be discussed in subsequent sections. There are recent case reports of successful dialysis of many substances including other toxic alcohols (glycol mixtures [31] found in brake oil, 2-butoxyethanol [32] found in glass cleaner, diethylene glycol [33] found in paracetamol elixir or Sterno solid fuel, and propylene glycol [34] used as a solvent in intravenous benzodiazepine formulations), perchloroethylene [35], glyphosate-based herbicide (Roundup) [36], star fruit *(Averrhoa carambola)* [37], and metformin (with accompanying type-B lactic acidosis) [38]. Dialysis has been reported to remove iodine [39], silicon [40], and selenium [41]. In many suspected cases of poisoning, early initiation of dialysis is suitable and recommended prior to confirmation of the offending poison or determination of serum concentration. Dialysis also effectively controls ion perturbations that may complicate poisoning, whether iatrogenic, accidental, or intentional: such as hyperkalemia, hyperphosphatemia, or hypermanganesemia following fertilizer ingestion, hypercalcemia following vitamin D intoxication, or hypermagnesemia following excessive cathartic ingestion.

Table 8.3.1 contains a list of drugs and chemicals removed with hemodialysis.

8.3.5 Extracorporeal Modalities – Hemofiltration and Hemodiafiltration

Hemofiltration (HF) and hemodiafiltration (HDF) are not used as frequently for blood purification. Hemodiafiltration is understandably preferred for ingestions accompanied by electrolyte or acid–base perturbations. Although data and clinical experience are limited, these modalities have a particular role in the removal high-molecular-weight intoxicants. For instance, the use of high-flux membranes allow for passage and clearance of large antibiotics such as the aminoglycosides (i.e., gentamicin 477 Da, and tobramycin 1,425 Da) [42] and vancomycin (1,485 Da) [43]. Hemofiltration does not appear to be effective for flecainide overdose [44]. Repeated, extended, or continuous treatments (SLED, CVVHF, or continuous venovenous hemodiafiltration [CVVHDF]) are recommended in ingestions with significant "rebound" potential; such as controlled-release preparations [45], drugs with tight tissue binding or large volumes of distribution or slow equilibration with the plasma (i.e., procainamide [46]). Conversely, clearance of low-molecular-weight drugs with a small volume of distribution and poor protein-binding are more effectively removed with conventional hemodialysis [47]. CVVHDF effectively clears methanol [48] and further appears to be effective in the treatment of lithium [49], salicylate [50], and phenobarbital [51] overdoses. As mentioned previously, continuous treatment modalities may not be preferable to hemodialysis in severe ingestions due to slower intoxicant clearance, although longer treatments can provide equivalent total clearance.

8.3.6 Extracorporeal Modalities – Hemoperfusion

Although rarely employed in blood purification, hemoperfusion provides superior drug clearance and is the preferred modality for extraction of theophylline [52], barbiturates [53], organophosphates [54], and many hypnotics/sedatives/tranquilizers. This absorptive modality effectively can clear substances that are lipid-soluble or as much as 95% protein-bound [55], a distinct advantage over diffusive and convective modalities. Along with plasmapheresis, hemoperfusion is the modality often employed for amanita phalloides mushroom ingestion. The efficacy of charcoal hemoperfusion for treatment of alpha-amanitin toxicity remains uncertain [56], although resin perfusion columns may provide superior clearance without saturation [57]. Charcoal hemoperfusion also does not provide efficient clearance of cardiac glycosides [58], while XAD resin columns [59] and β_2-microglobulin-specific columns [60] appear to be effective. It should also be noted that efficient extraction with hemoperfusion does not confer therapeutic efficacy or survival advantage, as may be the case with paraquat [61]. Hemoperfusion was recently reported to be successful in treating cases of poisoning resulting from the organophosphate dichlorvos [62], the protein-bound chemicals tetramine [63] and fluoroacetamide [64], the antipsychotic clozapine [65], and star fruit (*Averrhoa carambola*) [66]. If clearance is equivalent, dialysis is more cost-effective and preferred to address any concomitant metabolic disorder. Advances in sorbent technology will likely increase the future utility of adsorptive clearance in the treatment of poisoning. Immunoaffinity [67] – using columns of immobilized antibody – and other engineered perfusion columns are some methods which can provide specific adsorptive clearance.

Table 8.3.2 lists some drugs and chemicals removed by hemoperfusion.

8.3.7 Extracorporeal Modalities – Peritoneal Dialysis

Peritoneal dialysis is also infrequently used for extracorporeal removal of toxins. As mentioned, PD should be used for drug removal only in children or when hemodialysis is unavailable or inappropriate. There are reports of successful treatment of poisoning following ingestions of toxic alcohols [68], lithium [69], and salicylates. Bismuth salts [70], chromium [71], and chromic acid [72] have also been treated with PD.

8.3.8 Extracorporeal Modalities – Plasma Exchange and Exchange Transfusion

Some of the toxic conditions that have been effectively treated with plasma exchange include amanita phalloides mushroom ingestion [73, 74] and snake-bite envenomations [75]. Furthermore, replacement of clotting factors with FFP after plasmapheresis has been used for ingestions of Coumadin-like anticoagulants [76]. Successful plasma exchange for acute cisplatin [77] and arsine gas [78] intoxications have also been reported.

Exchange transfusion is effective in cases of methemoglobinemia following exposure to oxidizing agents [79], such as propanil [80], nitrites [81], aniline, and nitrobenzene [82] or dapsone [83]. This modality should be preferred in cases involving severe hemolysis, as with sodium chlorate poisoning [84]. Viper envenomation causing disseminated intravascular coagulation (DIC) [85] has been successfully treated with whole blood exchange. Finally, there are reports of successful use in neonatal caffeine [86] and theophylline toxicity [87], vincristine overdose [88], tricyclic antidepressant, L-thyroxine, verapamil, diltiazem, carbamazepine, mercury, vanadate [89], and cyclosporine [90] toxicity.

Table 8.3.2 Drugs and chemicals removed with hemoperfusion

Barbiturates	Antimicrobials/anticancer	Cardiovascular
Amobarbital	(Adriamycin)	Atenolol
Butabarbital	Ampicillin	Cibenzoline succinate
Hexobarbital	Carmustine	Clonidine
Pentobarbital	Chloramphenicol	Digoxin
Phenobarbital	Chloroquine	(diltiazem)
Quinalbital	Clindamycin	(disopyramide)
Secobarbital	Dapsone	Flecainide
Thiopental	Doxorubicin	Metoprolol
Vinalbital	Gentamicin	n-Acetylprocainamide
	Ifosfamide	Procainamide
	Isoniazid	Quinidine
	(methotrexate)	
	Pentamidine	
	Thiabendazole	
	(5-fluorouracil)	
	Vancomycin	
Nonbarbiturates	Antidepressants /antipsychotics	Miscellaneous
Hypnotics, sedatives and	(amitriptyline)	Aminophylline
Tranquilizers	Clozapine	
	(imipramine)	Cimetidine
	(tricyclics)	(fluoroacetamide)
Carbamazepine		(phencyclidine)
Carbromal		Phenols
Chloral hydrate		(podophyllin)
Chlorpromazine		Theophylline
(diazepam)		
Diphenhydramine		
Ethchlorvynol	Plant and animal toxins,	
Glutethimide	herbicides,	Solvents, gases
Meprobamate	insecticides	Carbon tetrachloride
Methaqualone	Amanitin	Ethylene oxide
Methsuximide	Chlordane	Trichloroethane
Methyprylon	Demeton sulfoxide	Xylene
Phenytoin	Dichlorvos	
	Dimethoate	
Promazine	Diquat	
Promethazine	Endosulfan	
Valproic acid	Fluoroacetamide	
	Glufosinate	
	Methylparathion	
	Nitrostigmine	
	(organophosphates)	Metals
Analgesics,	Phalloidin	(aluminum)*
Antirheumatic	Polychlorinated biphenyls	(iron)*
Acetaminophen	Paraquat	(thallium)
Acetylsalicylic acid	Parathion	
Colchicine	Tetramine	
d-Propoxyphene		
Methylsalicylate		
Phenylbutazone		
Salicylic acid		

() implies poor removal, ()* removed with chelating agent
Source: Modified and updated from [129]

This modality is of uncertain efficacy in carbon monoxide poisoning and appears to be ineffective for quinine intoxication [91].

8.3.9 Specific Drugs/Poisons

8.3.9.1 *Lithium*

Lithium is a cationic alkali metal used as a maintenance treatment for major affective disorders; and is the only mood stabilizer proven to reduce suicide rate in bipolar disorder [92]. This efficacy explains the widespread and continued prescription of lithium despite a narrow therapeutic range and well-described renal [93], neurologic [94], and occasionally, cardiologic toxicity. Lithium is typically available as a carbonate salt and is completely and rapidly absorbed following ingestion, although sustained-release preparations delay absorption and peak concentration by as much as 4 h [95]. The bioavailability of ingested lithium can be reduced by adsorption to orally administered sodium polystyrene sulfonate resin [96]. Lithium exhibits a two-compartment model of distribution with an early rapid phase preceding a slower, wider distribution in total body water (often > 0.5 l/kg body weight); and distribution into the central nervous system (CNS) is further slowed by the blood-brain barrier [97]. This pharmacokinetic profile is responsible for clinical toxicity occurring with chronic overdosage or acute-on-therapeutic ingestions [98]. With blood levels below 1.3 mEq/l, toxicity may be seen in elderly patients. Mild toxicity may be apparent with increasing levels between 1.5 and 2.5 mEq/l followed by moderate toxicity between 2.6 and 3.5 mEq/l, and severe, possibly fatal toxicity with concentrations greater than 3.6 mEq/l.

Extracorporeal blood purification is indicated with any clinically apparent toxicity or levels greater than 2.5 mEq/l [98]; and may be considered if levels plotted on a log-linear scale predict levels exceeding 0.6 mEq/l at 36 h. For lower levels, measures to enhance urinary elimination – isotonic fluid volume expansion and amiloride or triamterene – are generally sufficient. Treatment should continue until levels remain below 1 mEq/l. Hemodialysis and hemofiltration are both effective modalities, and high flux dialyzers should be used if available [99]. Clinicians should be aware of the potential for rebound toxicity following a single hemodialysis treatment, and the need for repeated or prolonged therapy to decrease serum lithium levels.

8.3.9.2 *Salicylates*

Salicylates include acetylsalicylic acid (aspirin), salicylic acid, and methyl salicylate, widely available nonsteroidal antiinflammatory drugs (NSAIDs) used for analgesic, antipyretic, antiplatelet, or antiinflammatory effect. Salicylates are also frequently implicated in accidental and suicidal ingestions and responsible for both acute and chronic toxicity. Acute salicylate intoxication can present with tinnitus or deafness [100], gastrointestinal irritation and ulceration, and both nausea and vomiting. Acid–base disorders are also typical – with early hyperventilation and respiratory alkalosis due to activation of respiratory centers in the medulla. Elevated anion gap metabolic acidosis is common due to retention of salicylate anions and lactic acid production following uncoupled mitochondrial oxidation; which also results in hyperthermia, diaphoresis, and flushing. Further toxicity includes pulmonary edema [101], and cerebral edema with CNS dysfunction presenting as agitation, lethargy, and seizure.

Initial management of intoxication includes gastrointestinal decontamination of recently ingested salicylate, especially enteric-coated preparations, with multiple dose activated charcoal [102]. Urinary alkalinization increases elimination and is also recommended for patients with moderately severe salicylate poisoning who do not meet the criteria for hemodialysis [103]. Hemodialysis is indicated for acutely poisoned patients with evidence of acidosis, CNS dysfunction, pulmonary edema, or levels greater than 80–100 mg/dl. Patients with chronic salicylate intoxication may be symptomatic at lower serum levels, and should be dialyzed for levels > 60 mg/dl. Excellent clearance of salicylate has been reported with both CVVHDF [104] and SLED [105]. Although hemoperfusion is also effective, dialytic methods are preferred to correct any metabolic disturbances.

8.3.9.3 Methanol

Methanol (or methyl alcohol) ingestion typically presents in alcoholic derelicts, after exposure to industrial solvents [106], or in poisoning epidemics involving bootleg or counterfeit liquor [107]. Exposure commonly follows oral ingestion but may result from inhalation or skin absorption. Methanol invasion in an empty stomach occurs with a half-life of only 5 min followed by distribution into a fluid volume greater than 0.7 l/kg of body weight [108]. As with other alcohols, intoxication manifests with inebriation, delirium, and drowsiness, as well as nausea, vomiting, and diarrhea. Only a small percentage of methanol is excreted unchanged; and ingestion and inebriation are followed by a latent period of several hours. Toxicity then results from biotransformation of methanol in the liver and kidneys to formaldehyde and formic acid – the products of the enzymes alcohol dehydrogenase (ADH) and aldehyde dehydrogenase. An osmolal gap may be evident early in presentation (from methanol) followed by closure of the osmolal gap (metabolism of methanol) and generation of an anion gap metabolic acidosis (formate retention). Neurotoxicity is prominent and symptoms include blurred vision, mydriasis (dilated pupils), retinal damage with evident hyperemia, and permanent blindness [109]. Cerebral hemorrhage and necrosis [110] and transtentorial herniation [111] have also been reported. Kussmaul respiration with apnea, coma, and death may result in severe poisoning.

Treatment involves prevention of biotransformation and/or extracorporeal elimination of methanol and any toxic metabolites. Folic or folinic acid administration will promote conversion of formate to water and carbon dioxide [112]. Fomepizole (4-methyl pyrazole or 4-MP) [113] effectively inhibits ADH while ethanol is a favored substrate for ADH metabolism. Although no study has compared their efficacy, fomepizole appears safer – although much more expensive – than ethanol [114]. Low severity methanol poisoning, such as with levels below 20 mg/dl, can likely be treated with bicarbonate and prolonged infusion of fomepizole. However, with fomepizole alone, the formate elimination half-life may be greater than 50–80 h [115]. Most moderate and severe cases of methanol intoxication will be benefit from hemodialysis to rapidly clear methanol and formate (half-life less than 2 h) and correct the accompanying metabolic acidosis [116]. Hemodialysis appears to be superior to CVVHDF for elimination of methanol [117]. Hemodialysis is indicated with any evident acidosis, organ toxicity, or methanol levels greater than 50 mg/dl. Methanol concentration may rebound and treatment should continue until levels remain below 20 mg/dl. It should be noted that fomepizole is dialyzable and infusion should be compensated for elimination during dialysis [114].

8.3.9.4 Ethylene Glycol

Another toxic alcohol is ethylene glycol, widely available as an industrial solvent or automotive "antifreeze." Ingestion is typical in alcoholics, during suicide attempts, or in children and pets attracted to ethylene glycol's sweet taste. Fluorescein dye is frequently added to aid in identification, and may be apparent in the urine postingestion. Enteric invasion is rapid and peak concentration is evident by 1-h postingestion [118]. Inebriation and stupor (with an evident osmolar gap) are likely to be evident postingestion followed by a latent period (typically 12–14 h) preceding organ toxicity and acidosis. Ethylene glycol undergoes rapid biotransformation by alcohol dehydrogenase (ADH) to glycoaldehyde, and subsequently to glycolic acid, glyoxylic acid, and oxalic acid [119, 120]. These organic acid metabolites are toxic to the central nervous system (seizures, cranial nerve paralyses, coma, cerebral edema, and crystal deposition in meningeal blood vessels [121]), and the cardiopulmonary system (congestive heart failure with pulmonary edema and circulatory collapse). Calcium oxalate precipitates in the kidneys causing oliguric acute kidney injury with tubular epithelial vacuolization and interstitial inflammation [122, 123]. Glycolic acid accumulation is responsible for an elevated anion gap metabolic acidosis with severe acidemia [120].

Treatment consists of inhibition of metabolism, correction of metabolic acidosis and, if necessary, extracorporeal elimination of the alcohol and any metabolites. Pyridoxine (vitamin B6) and thiamine (B1) will promote conversion of glyoxylic acid to glycine rather than oxalate [124]. Fomepizole is preferred to ethanol for ADH inhibition and has been demonstrated to prevent metabolite formation, renal injury, and improve acid–base status [125, 126]. Prolonged fomepizole infusion may be necessary, when used without dialysis in patients with preserved renal function, due to the approximate 20 h elimination half-life of ethylene glycol [127]. Acidemia should be corrected with bicarbonate (the same method used during dialysis) as acidosis delays renal clearance and favors tissue penetration of metabolites. Hemodialysis effectively removes ethylene glycol and metabolites and corrects the metabolic acidosis. Although clearance is demonstrable with CVVHDF, this modality is likely to be slower and less efficient than conventional hemodialysis [128]. Extracorporeal elimination is indicated for organ toxicity, acidosis, and when ethylene glycol levels are greater than 50 mg/dl. As with methanol, the potential for rebound may necessitate repeated treatments until levels remain below 20 mg/dl. Fomepizole dosing should be increased during hemodialysis due to elimination.

8.3.10 Take Home Pearls

- The treatment of poisoned or intoxicated patients frequently requires blood purification. Hemodialysis, hemofiltration and hemodiafiltration, hemoperfusion, peritoneal dialysis, and therapeutic plasma exchange are effective methods of extracorporeal drug removal.
- Hemodialysis is widely available and often indicated to correct concomitant electrolyte and/or acid–base disorders. Efficient clearance of high-molecular-weight intoxicants is best accomplished with convective modalities. Low blood flow rates used in continuous renal replacement therapies offer hemodynamic advantages but slower clearance than with conventional hemodialysis. Peritoneal dialysis, hemoperfusion, plasma exchange, and exchange transfusion are also occasionally employed for extracorporeal detoxification.
- The decision to employ these methods is in most cases clinical and requires assessment of the poisoned patient.

References

1. Bronstein AC, Spyker DA, Cantilena LR Jr, et al. 2006 Annual Report of the American Association of Poison Control Centers' National Poison Data System (NPDS). *Clin Toxicol (Phila)*. 2007;45:815–917
2. Linquette M, Goudemande M, Warot P, et al. Acute poisoning by sodium chlorate; anuria; exchange transfusions and peritoneal dialysis. *Echo Med Nord*. 1950;21:269–276
3. Brown IA. The use of hemodialysis in the treatment of barbiturate intoxication. *Minn Med*. 1954;37:650–652
4. Oliver MJ. Acute dialysis catheters. *Semin Dial*. 2001;14: 432–435
5. Schetz M. Vascular access for HD and CRRT. *Contrib Nephrol*. 2007;156:275–286
6. Doshi M, Murray PT. Approach to intradialytic hypotension in intensive care unit patients with acute renal failure. *Artif Organs*. 2003;27:772–780
7. Selby NM, McIntyre CW. The acute cardiac effects of dialysis. *Semin Dial*. 2007;20:220–228
8. Bender FH, Bernardini J, Piraino B. Prevention of infectious complications in peritoneal dialysis: best demonstrated practices. *Kidney Int Suppl*. 2006;103:S44–54
9. Winchester JF. Dialysis and hemoperfusion in poisoning. *Adv Ren Replace Ther*. 2002;9:26–30
10. Clark WR, Winchester JF. Middle molecules and small-molecular-weight proteins in ESRD: properties and strategies for their removal. *Adv Ren Replace Ther*. 2003;10:270–278
11. Maher JF: Principles of dialysis and dialysis of drugs. *Am J Med*. 1977;62:475
12. Ouseph R, Ward RA. Increasing dialysate flow rate increases dialyzer urea mass transfer-area coefficients during clinical use. *Am J Kidney Dis*. 2001;37:316–320
13. Depner T, Garred L. Solute transport mechanisms in dialysis. in *Replacement of Renal Function by Dialysis*, 5th edition, editors Horl W, Koch KM, Lindsay RM, Ronco C, Winchester JF. Kluwer, Dordrecht, 2004:73–93
14. Ledebo I. Principles and practice of hemofiltration and hemodiafiltration. *Artif Organs*. 1998;22:20–25
15. Ronco C, Cruz D. Hemodiafiltration history, technology, and clinical results. *Adv Chronic Kidney Dis*. 2007;14:231–243
16. Clark WR. Quantitative characterization of hemodialyzer solute and water transport. *Semin Dial*. 2001;14:32–36
17. Goodman JW, Goldfarb DS. The role of continuous renal replacement therapy in the treatment of poisoning. *Semin Dial*. 2006;19:402–407
18. Liao Z, Zhang W, Hardy PA, et al. Kinetic comparison of different acute dialysis therapies. *Artif Organs*. 2003;27: 802–807
19. Berbece AN, Richardson RM. Sustained low-efficiency dialysis in the ICU: cost, anticoagulation, and solute removal. *Kidney Int*. 2006;70:963–968
20. Passadakis PS, Oreopoulos DG. Peritoneal dialysis in patients with acute renal failure. *Adv Perit Dial*. 2007;23:7–16
21. Krediet RT. Peritoneal physiology – impact on solute and fluid clearance. *Adv Ren Replace Ther*. 2000;7:271–279
22. Kim DJ, Do JH, Huh W, et al. Dissociation between clearances of small and middle molecules in incremental peritoneal dialysis. *Perit Dial Int*. 2001;21:462–466
23. Gabriel DP, Nascimento GV, Caramori JT, et al. High volume peritoneal dialysis for acute renal failure. *Perit Dial Int*. 2007;27:277–282
24. Ronco C, Amerling R. Continuous flow peritoneal dialysis: current state-of-the-art and obstacles to further development. *Contrib Nephrol*. 2006;150:310–320.
25. Winchester JF, Amerling R, Harbord N, et al. The potential application of sorbents in peritoneal dialysis. *Contrib Nephrol*. 2006;150:336–343

26. Krediet RT, Douma CE, van Olden RW, et al. Augmenting solute clearance in peritoneal dialysis. *Kidney Int.* 1998;54: 2218–2225
27. Winchester JF, Silberzweig J, Ronco C, et al. Sorbents in acute renal failure and end-stage renal disease: middle molecule and cytokine removal. *Blood Purif.* 2004;22:73–77
28. Ibrahim RB, Liu C, Cronin SM, et al. Drug removal by plasmapheresis: an evidence-based review. *Pharmacotherapy.* 2007;27:1529–1549
29. Linenberger ML, Price TH. Use of cellular and plasma apheresis in the critically ill patient: part 1: technical and physiological considerations. *J Intensive Care Med.* 2005;20:18–27
30. Linenberger ML, Price TH. Use of cellular and plasma apheresis in the critically ill patient: Part II: Clinical indications and applications. *J Intensive Care Med.* 2005;20: 88–103
31. Sharma N, Jain S. Toxicity of brake oil. *Emerg Med J.* 2002;19:267–268
32. Gualideri JF, DeBoer L, Harris CR, et al. Repeated ingestion of 2-butoxyethanol: case report and literature review. *J Tox Clin Toxicol.* 2003;41:57–62.
33. Alfred S, Coleman P, Harris D, et al. Delayed neurologic sequelae resulting from epidemic diethylene glycol poisoning. *Clin Toxicol (Phila).* 2005;43:155–159
34. Parker MG, Fraser GL, Watson DM, et al. Removal of propylene glycol and correction of increased osmolar gap by hemodialysis in a patient on high dose lorazepam infusion therapy. *Intensive Care Med.* 2002;28:81–84
35. Choi YH, Kim N, Seo YS, et al. ARF requiring hemodialysis after accidental perchloroethylene ingestion. *Am J Kidney Dis.* 2003;41:E11
36. Sampogna RV, Cunard R. Roundup intoxication and a rationale for treatment. *Clin Nephrol.* 2007;68:190–196
37. Neto MM, da Costa JA, Garcia-Cairasco N, et al. Intoxication by star fruit (Averroes carambola) in 32 uraemic patients: treatment and outcome. *Nephrol Dial Trans.* 2003;18:120–125
38. Guo PY, Storsley LJ, Finkle SN. Severe lactic acidosis treated with prolonged hemodialysis: recovery after massive overdoses of metformin. *Semin Dial.* 2006;19:80–83
39. Kanakiriya S, De Chazal I, Nath KA, et al. Iodine toxicity treated with hemodialysis and continuous venovenous hemodiafiltration. *Am J Kidney Dis.* 2003;41:702–708
40. Fujino Y, Inoue Y, Onodera M, et al. Case of concrete hardener poisoning complicated with acute renal failure treated by hemodialysis. *Chudoku Kenkyu.* 2007;20:263–268
41. Kise Y, Yoshimura S, Akieda K, et al. Acute oral selenium intoxication with ten times the lethal dose resulting in deep gastric ulcer. *J Emerg Med.* 2004;26:183–187
42. Amin NB, Padhi ID, Touchette MA, et al. Characterization of gentamicin pharmacokinetics in patients hemodialyzed with high-flux polysulfone membranes. *Am J Kidney Dis.* 1999;34:222–227
43. Ulinski T, Deschênes G, Bensman A. Large-pore haemodialysis membranes: an efficient tool for rapid removal of vancomycin after accidental overdose. *Nephrol Dial Transplant.* 2005;20:1517–1518
44. Borgeat A, Biollaz J, Freymond B, et al. Hemofiltration clearance of flecainide in a patient with acute renal failure. *Intensive Care Med.* 1988;14:236–237
45. Yildiz TS, Toprak DG, Arisoy ES, et al. Continuous venovenous hemodiafiltration to treat controlled-release carbamazepine overdose in a pediatric patient. *Paediatr Anaesth.* 2006;16:1176–1178
46. Domoto DT, Brown WW, Bruggensmith P. Removal of toxic levels of N-acetylprocainamide with continuous arteriovenous hemofiltration or continuous arteriovenous hemodiafiltration. *Ann Intern Med.* 1987;106:550–552
47. Kay TD, Playford HR, Johnson DW. Hemodialysis versus continuous veno-venous hemodiafiltration in the management of severe valproate overdose. *Clin Nephrol.* 2003;59: 56–58
48. Kan G, Jenkins I, Rangan G, et al. Continuous haemodiafiltration compared with intermittent haemodialysis in the treatment of methanol poisoning. *Nephrol Dial Transplant.* 2003;18:2665–2667
49. Menghini VV, Albright RC Jr. Treatment of lithium intoxication with continuous venovenous hemodiafiltration. *Am J Kidney Dis.* 2000;36:E21
50. Wrathall G, Sinclair R, Moore A, et al. Three case reports of the use of haemodiafiltration in the treatment of salicylate overdose. *Hum Exp Toxicol.* 2001;20:491–495
51. Lal R, Faiz S, Garg RK, et al. Use of continuous venovenous hemodiafiltration in a case of severe phenobarbital poisoning. *Am J Kidney Dis.* 2006;48:e13–15
52. Shannon MW. Comparative efficacy of hemodialysis and hemoperfusion in severe theophylline intoxication. *Acad Emerg Med.* 1997;4:674–678
53. Bouma AW, van Dam B, Meynaar IA, et al. Accelerated elimination using hemoperfusion in a patient with phenobarbital intoxication. *Ned Tijdschr Geneeskd.* 2004;148: 1642–1645
54. Altintop L, Aygun D, Sahin H, et al. In acute organophosphate poisoning, the efficacy of hemoperfusion on clinical status and mortality. *J Intensive Care Med.* 2005;20:346–350
55. Kawasaki CI, Nishi R, Uekihara S, et al. How tightly can a drug be bound to a protein and still be removable by charcoal hemoperfusion in overdose cases? *Clin Toxicol (Phila).* 2005;43:95–99
56. Feinfeld DA, Rosenberg JW, Winchester JF. Three controversial issues in extracorporeal toxin removal. *Semin Dial.* 2006;19:358–362
57. Mydlík M, Derzsiová K, Klán J, et al. Hemoperfusion with alpha-amanitin: an in vitro study. *Int J Artif Organs.* 1997;20: 105–107
58. Clerckx-Braun F, Kadima N, Lesne M, et al. Digoxin acute intoxication: evaluation of the efficiency of charcoal hemoperfusion. *Clin Toxicol.* 1979;15:437–446
59. Mathieu D, Gosselin B, Nolf M, et al. Massive digitoxin intoxication. Treatment of Amberlite XAD 4 resin hemoperfusion. *J Toxicol Clin Toxicol.* 1982;19:931–950
60. Tsuruoka S, Osono E, Nishiki K, et al. Removal of digoxin by column for specific adsorption of beta(2)-microglobulin: a potential use for digoxin intoxication. *Clin Pharmacol Ther.* 2001;69:422–430
61. Castro R, Prata C, Oliveira L, et al. Paraquat intoxication and hemocarboperfusion. *Acta Med Port.* 2005;18:423–431
62. Peng A, Meng FQ, Sun LF, et al. Therapeutic efficacy of charcoal hemoperfusion in patients with acute severe dichlorvos poisoning. *Acta Pharmacol Sin.* 2004;25:15–21
63. Dehua G, Daxi J, Honglang X, et al. Sequential hemoperfusion and continuous venovenous hemofiltration in treatment of severe tetramine poisoning. *Blood Purif.* 2006;24: 524–530

64. Gao Y, Chen YL, Zhong F, et al. Effect of hemoperfusion in treatment of children with acute poisoning. *Zhonghua Er Ke Za Zhi*. 2007;45:665–669
65. He JL, Xiang YT, Li WB, et al. Hemoperfusion in the treatment of acute clozapine intoxication in China. *J Clin Psychopharmacol*. 2007;27:667–671
66. Wu MY, Wu IW, Wu SS, et al. Hemoperfusion as an effective alternative therapy for star fruit intoxication: a report of 2 cases. *Am J Kidney Dis*. 2007;49:e1–5
67. Brizgys MV, Pincus S, Siebert CJ, et al. Removal of digoxin from the circulation using immobilized monoclonal antibodies. *J Pharm Sci*. 1989;78:393–398
68. Vale JA, Prior JG, O'Hare JP, et al. Treatment of ethylene glycol poisoning with peritoneal dialysis. *Br Med J (Clin Res Ed)*. 1982;284:557
69. Hansen HE, Amdisen A. Lithium intoxication. (Report of 23 cases and review of 100 cases from the literature). *Q J Med*. 1978;47:123–144
70. Islek I, Uysal S, Gok F, et al. Reversible nephrotoxicity after overdose of colloidal bismuth subcitrate. *Pediatr Nephrol*. 2001;16:510–514
71. Schiffl H, Weidmann P, Weiss M, et al. Dialysis treatment of acute chromium intoxication and comparative efficacy of peritoneal versus hemodialysis in chromium removal. *Miner Electrolyte Metab*. 1982;7:28–35
72. Kobayashi T, Unishi G, Matsuzaki S, et al. A survival case of acute chromic acid poisoning treated by peritoneal dialysis. *Nippon Jinzo Gakkai Shi*. 1984;26:1259–1261
73. Jander S, Bischoff J. Treatment of Amanita phalloides poisoning: I. Retrospective evaluation of plasmapheresis in 21 patients. *Ther Apher*. 2000;4:303–307
74. Jander S, Bischoff J, Woodcock BG. Plasmapheresis in the treatment of Amanita phalloides poisoning: II. A review and recommendations.*Ther Apher*. 2000;4:308–312
75. Yildirim C, Bayraktaroglu Z, Gunay N, et al. The use of therapeutic plasmapheresis in the treatment of poisoned and snake bite victims: an academic emergency department's experiences. *J Clin Apher*. 2006;21:219–223
76. Gläser V, Seifert R. Successful therapy of phenprocoumon poisoning with plasmapheresis. *Med Klin (Munich)*. 1998;93: 174–176
77. Choi JH, Oh JC, Kim KH, et al: Successful treatment of cisplatin overdose with plasma exchange. *Yonsey Med J*. 2002;43:128–132
78. Song Y, Wang D, Li H, et al. Severe acute arsine poisoning treated by plasma exchange. *Clin Toxicol (Phila)*. 2007;45: 721–727
79. Bradberry SM. Occupational methaemoglobinaemia. Mechanisms of production, features, diagnosis and management including the use of methylene blue. *Toxicol Rev*. 2003; 22:13–27
80. De Silva WA, Bodinayake CK.Propanil poisoning. *Ceylon Med J*. 1997;42:81–84
81. Jansen T, Barnung S, Mortensen CR, et al. Isobutyl-nitrite-induced methemoglobinemia; treatment with an exchange blood transfusion during hyperbaric oxygenation. *Acta Anaesthesiol Scand*. 2003;47:1300–1301
82. Martinez MA, Ballesteros S, Almarza E, et al. Acute nitrobenzene poisoning with severe associated methemoglobinemia: identification in whole blood by GC-FID and GC-MS. *J Anal Toxicol*. 2003;27:221–225
83. Southgate HJ, Masterson R. Lessons to be learned: a case study approach: prolonged methaemoglobinaemia due to inadvertent dapsone poisoning; treatment with methylene blue and exchange transfusion. *J R Soc Health*. 1999;119:52–55
84. Steffen C, Seitz R. Severe chlorate poisoning: report of a case. *Arch Toxicol*. 1981;48:281–288
85. Lifshitz M, Kapelushnik J, Ben-Harosh M, et al. Disseminated intravascular coagulation after cerastes vipera envenomation in a 3-year-old child: a case report. *Toxicon*. 2000;38: 1593–1598
86. Perrin C, Debruyne D, Lacotte J, et al. Treatment of caffeine intoxication by exchange transfusion in a newborn. *Acta Paediatr Scand*. 1987;76:679–681
87. Osborn HH, Henry G, Wax P, et al. Theophylline toxicity in a premature neonate – elimination kinetics of exchange transfusion. *J Toxicol Clin Toxicol*. 1993;31:639–644
88. Kosmidis HV, Bouhoutsou DO, Varvoutsi MC, et al. Vincristine overdose: experience with 3 patients. *Pediatr Hematol Oncol*. 1991;8:171–178
89. Nenov VD, Marinov P, Sabeva J, et al. Current applications of plasmapheresis in clinical toxicology. *Nephrol Dial Transplant*. 2003;18S5:v56–8
90. Kwon SU, Lim SH, Rhee I, et al: Successful whole blood exchange by apheresis in a patient with acute cyclosporine intoxication without long-term sequelae. *J Heart Lung Transplant*. 2006;25:483–485
91. Bateman DN, Blain PG, Woodhouse KW, et al. Pharmacokinetics and clinical toxicity of quinine overdosage: lack of efficacy of techniques intended to enhance elimination. *Q J Med*. 1985;54:125–131
92. Freeman MP, Freeman SA Lithium: clinical considerations in internal medicine. *Am J Med*. 2006;119:478–481
93. Gitlin M. Lithium and the kidney: an updated review. *Drug Saf*. 1999;20:231–243
94. Kores B, Lader MH. Irreversible lithium neurotoxicity: an overview. *Clin Neuropharmacol*. 1997;20:283–299
95. Arancibia A, Corvalan F, Mella F, et al. Absorption and disposition kinetics of lithium carbonate following administration of conventional and controlled release formulations. *Int J Clin Pharmacol Ther Toxicol*. 1986;24:240–245
96. Belanger DR, Tierney MG, Dickinson G. Effect of sodium polystyrene sulfonate on lithium bioavailability. *Ann Emerg Med*. 1992 Nov;21(11):1312–1315
97. Plenge P, Stensgaard A, Jensen HV, et al. 24-hour lithium concentration in human brain studied by Li-7 magnetic resonance spectroscopy. *Biol Psychiatry*. 1994;36:511–516
98. Waring WS. Management of lithium toxicity. *Toxicol Rev*. 2006;25:221–230
99. Peces R, Fernandez EJ, Regidor D, et al. Treatment of acute lithium intoxication with high-flux haemodialysis membranes. *Nefrologia*. 2006;26:372–378
100. Cazals Y. Auditory sensori-neural alterations induced by salicylate. *Prog Neurobiol*. 2000;62:583–631
101. Cohen DL, Post J, Ferroggiaro AA, et al. Chronic salicylism resulting in noncardiogenic pulmonary edema requiring hemodialysis. *Am J Kidney Dis*. 2000;36:E20
102. Chyka PA, Erdman AR, Christianson G, et al. Salicylate poisoning: an evidence-based consensus guideline for out-of-hospital management. *Clin Toxicol (Phila)*. 2007;45:95–131
103. Proudfoot AT, Krenzelok EP, Vale JA. Position paper on urine alkalinization. *J Toxicol Clin Toxicol*. 2004;42:1–26

104. Wrathall G, Sinclair R, Moore A, et al. Three case reports of the use of haemodiafiltration in the treatment of salicylate overdose. *Hum Exp Toxicol*. 2001;20:491–495
105. Lund B, Seifert SA, Mayersohn M. Efficacy of sustained low-efficiency dialysis in the treatment of salicylate toxicity. *Nephrol Dial Transplant*. 2005;20:1483–1484
106. Davis LE, Hudson D, Benson BE, et al. Methanol poisoning exposures in the United States: 1993–1998. *J Toxicol Clin Toxicol*. 2002;40:499–505
107. Paasma R, Hovda KE, Tikkerberi A, et al. Methanol mass poisoning in Estonia: outbreak in 154 patients. *Clin Toxicol (Phila)*. 2007;45:152–157
108. Graw M, Haffner HT, Althaus L, et al. Invasion and distribution of methanol. *Arch Toxicol*. 2000;74:313–321
109. Onder F, Ilker S, Kansu T, et al. Acute blindness and putaminal necrosis in methanol intoxication. *Int Ophthalmol*. 1998–1999;22:81–84
110. Hsu HH, Chen CY, Chen FH, et al. Optic atrophy and cerebral infarcts caused by methanol intoxication: MRI. *Neuroradiology*. 1997;39:192–194
111. Weinberg L, Stewart J, Wyatt JP, et al. Unexplained drowsiness and progressive visual loss: Methanol poisoning diagnosed at autopsy. *Emerg Med (Fremantle)*. 2003;15:97–99
112. Moore DF, Bentley AM, Dawling S, et al. Folinic acid and enhanced renal elimination in formic acid intoxication. *J Toxicol Clin Toxicol*. 1994;32:199–204
113. Brent J, McMartin K, Phillips S, et al. Fomepizole for the treatment of methanol poisoning. *N Engl J Med*. 2001;344:424–429
114. Megarbane B, Borron SW, Faud FJ. Current recommendations for treatment of severe toxic alcohol poisonings. *Intensive Care Med*. 2005;31:189–195
115. Hovda KE, Andersson KS, Urdal P, et al. Methanol and formate kinetics during treatment with fomepizole. *Clin Toxicol (Phila)*. 2005;43:221–227
116. Hantson P, Haufroid V, et al. Formate kinetics in methanol poisoning. *Hum Exp Toxicol*. 2005;24:55–59
117. Kan G, Jenkins I, Rangan G, et al. Continuous haemodiafiltration compared with intermittent haemodialysis in the treatment of methanol poisoning. *Nephrol Dial Transplant*. 2003;18:2665–2667
118. Vasavada N, Williams C, Hellman RN, et al. Ethylene glycol intoxication: case report and pharmacokinetic perspectives. *Pharmacotherapy*. 2003;23:1652–1658
119. Leth PM, Gregersen M. Ethylene glycol poisoning. *Forensic Sci Int*. 2005;155:179–184
120. Jacobsen D, McMartin KE. Methanol and ethylene glycol poisonings. Mechanism of toxicity, clinical course, diagnosis and treatment. *Med Toxicol*. 1986;1:309–334
121. Froberg K, Dorion RP, McMartin KE. The role of calcium oxalate crystal deposition in cerebral vessels during ethylene glycol poisoning. *Clin Toxicol (Phila)*. 2006;44:315–358
122. Stokes MB. Acute oxalate nephropathy due to ethylene glycol ingestion. *Kidney Int*. 2006;69:203
123. Meier M, Nitschke M, Perras B, et al. Ethylene glycol intoxication and xylitol infusion – metabolic steps of oxalate-induced acute renal failure. *Clin Nephrol*. 2005;63:225–258
124. Lheureux P, Penaloza A, Gris, et al. Pyridoxine in clinical toxicology: a review. *Eur J Emerg Med*. 2005;12:78–85
125. Barceloux DG, Krenzelok EP, Olson K, et al. American Academy of Clinical Toxicology Practice Guidelines on the Treatment of Ethylene Glycol Poisoning. Ad Hoc Committee. *J Toxicol Clin Toxicol*. 1999;37:537–560
126. Brent J, McMartin K, Phillips S, et al. Fomepizole for the treatment of ethylene glycol poisoning. Methylpyrazole for Toxic Alcohols Study Group. *N Engl J Med*. 1999; 340:832–838
127. Sivilotti ML, Burns MJ, McMartin KE, et al. Toxicokinetics of ethylene glycol during fomepizole therapy: implications for management. For the Methylpyrazole for Toxic Alcohols Study Group. *Ann Emerg Med*. 2000;36:114–125
128. Christiansson LK, Kaspersson KE, Kulling PE, et al. Treatment of severe ethylene glycol intoxication with continuous arteriovenous hemofiltration dialysis. *J Toxicol Clin Toxicol*. 1995;33:267–270
129. Winchester JF. Active methods for detoxification, in *Clinical Management of Poisoning and Drug Overdose*, 3rd edition, editors Haddad LM, Shannon MW, Winchester JF. WB Saunders, Philadelphia. 1998:175–188

Subject Index

MIX
Papier aus verantwortungsvollen Quellen
Paper from responsible sources
FSC® C105338

If you have any concerns about our products,
you can contact us on
ProductSafety@springernature.com

In case Publisher is established outside the EU,
the EU authorized representative is:
Springer Nature Customer Service Center GmbH
Europaplatz 3, 69115 Heidelberg, Germany

Printed by Libri Plureos GmbH
in Hamburg, Germany